Microbial Disease

Third Edition

Moselio Schaechter, Ph.D.

Distinguished Professor, Emeritus
Tufts University School of Medicine
Boston, Massachusetts
Adjunct Professor
San Diego State University
San Diego, California

N. Cary Engleberg, M.D.

Professor, Departments of Internal Medicine and Microbiology and Immunology
University of Michigan Medical School
Ann Arbor, Michigan

Barry I. Eisenstein, M.D.

Vice President for Research
Beth Israel–Deaconess Medical Center
Professor of Microbiology and Molecular Genetics
Harvard Medical School
Boston, Massachusetts

Gerald Medoff, M.D.

Professor, Department of Microbiology and Immunology and Department of Internal Medicine
Washington University School of Medicine
St. Louis, Missouri

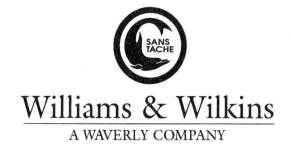

Williams & Wilkins

A WAVERLY COMPANY

BALTIMORE • PHILADELPHIA • LONDON • PARIS • BANGKOK
BUENOS AIRES • HONG KONG • MUNICH • SYDNEY • TOKYO • WROCLAW

Editor: Paul J. Kelly
Managing Editor: Crystal Taylor
Development Editor: Kathleen H. Scogna
Illustrations: Chanksy, Inc.

Printed in the United States of America
First Edition, 1989

Library of Congress Cataloging-in-Publication Data

Mechanisms of microbial disease / [edited by] Moselio Schaechter …
[et al.] — 3rd ed.
   p. cm.
   Includes bibliographical references and index.
   ISBN 0-683-07605-1 (pbk.)
   1. Medical microbiology. 2. Communicable diseases—Pathogenesis.
I. Schaechter, Moselio.
   [DNLM: 1. Communicable Diseases—microbiology. 2. Communicable
Diseases—physiopathology. 3. Bacteria—pathogenicity. 4. Fungi—pathogenicity.
   5. Viruses—pathogenicity. QW 700 M4856 1998]
QR46.M463 1998
616.9—dc21
DNLM/DLC
for Library of Congress
                                98-3835
                                CIP

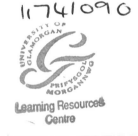

To Edith, Suzy, Joyce, Judy, and the memory of Barbara

Preface

The previous edition of this book has been well received by faculty members and especially by students. Particularly well liked has been our notion of presenting the material in a pathobiological framework and in the context of clinical cases. This format seems to lend itself to an active form of studying and to be easily adaptable to problem-based learning.

This edition reflects many of the rapid changes that have taken place in medical microbiology and infectious diseases. Several new chapters have been added, others have been dropped. Although we have tried to update all the material, we must acknowledge that information in this field is acquired at such dazzling speed that it risks becoming outdated before the ink dries. The format of this edition has also been changed and most of the illustrations are new.

This textbook is intended to be used in courses on medical microbiology and infectious diseases for medical students and other health professionals, graduate students, and advanced undergraduates. In medical schools the topic is often divided between two courses: one on microbiology and another on infectious diseases (frequently embedded within a pathophysiology course). Our intent is to bridge the contents of these two courses by discussing first the major infectious agents as biolog-

ical models (Parts I and II), then presenting ways in which the major systems of the body are affected by infectious diseases (Part III). Since the purpose of this book is to develop a conceptual framework, it highlights certain infectious agents and diseases and does not attempt to present the material in exhaustive fashion.

In many of the chapters on individual infectious agents you will find sections called "Paradigms." Here we discuss certain general principles that are best illustrated with the agents described in that chapter, but which can be applied to others as well.

Following the chapters on each group of infectious agents (bacteria, viruses, fungi, and animal parasites), you will find review charts. Filling in the blank spaces should help you outline the scope of the material, organize your store of information, and prepare yourself for examinations. Only the most common agents of human infectious diseases are listed, with reference to relevant chapters in this book.

Moselio Schaechter
N. Cary Engleberg
Barry Eisenstein
Gerald Medoff

Acknowledgments

Many colleagues and friends have helped us in the past in preparing this book. Their names appear in the previous editions. In this revision, we were helped by Imregard Behlau, Michael Breindl, Latham Claflin, Jenifer Coburn, Wesley Dunnick, Joanne Gilbert, Elizabeth Joyce, Dalia Kalabat, and David Knipe. Our heartfelt thanks go to them for their kind and thoughtful suggestions. We are particularly grateful to our developmental editor, Kathleen Scogna, who, while displaying a keen understanding of what we were trying to say, suggested innumerable apt and original changes. We believe that her efforts greatly contributed to improving this work. Crystal Taylor, our managing editor, orchestrated this project with both patience and imagination. We also thank Matthew Chansky for his imaginative artwork. Our appreciation also goes to Suzy Engleberg, for competently helping us in the demanding job of making the manuscript ready for publication.

Contributors

David W. K. Acheson, M.D.
Assistant Professor, Department of Medicine
Tufts University School of Medicine and Division of
Geographic Medicine and Infectious Diseases
New England Medical Center
Boston, Massachusetts

Elliott J. Androphy, M.D.
Professor, Departmentof Dermatology
Tufts University School of Medicine
Boston, Massachusetts

George M. Baer, D.V.M.
Director, Laboratories Baer
Colonia Condesa, Mexico
Formerly with Department of Health and Human
Services
Centers for Disease Control
Atlanta, Georgia

Neil L. Barg, M.D.
Associate Professor, Division of Infectious Diseases
Department of Internal Medicine
University of Michigan Medical School
Ann Arbor, Michigan

Michael Barza, M.D.
Professor, Department of Medicine
Tufts University School of Medicine and Division of
Geographic Medicine and Infectious Diseases
New England Medical Center
Boston, Massachusetts

Martin J. Blaser, M.D.
Addison B. Scoville Professor and Director, Division
of Infectious Diseases, Department of Medicine
Professor of Microbiology and Immunology Vanderbilt
University School of Medicine and Veterans Affairs
Medical Center
Nashville, Tennessee

Suzanne F. Bradley, M.D.
Associate Professor, Department of Internal Medicine
Faculty Associate, Institute of Gerontology
University of Michigan Medical School
Staff Physician
Veterans Affairs Medical Center
Ann Arbor, Michigan

Daniel K. Braun, M.D. Ph.D.
Clinical Research Physician
Infectious Diseases Therapeutics
Lilly Research Laboratories
Indianapolis, Indiana

John M. Coffin, Ph.D.
Professor, Department of Molecular Biology
and Microbiology
Tufts University School of Medicine
Boston, Massachusetts

Victor J. DiRita, Ph.D.
Associate Professor, Laboratory Animal Medicine Unit
and Department of Microbiology and Immunology
University of Michigan Medical School
Ann Arbor, Michigan

Barry I. Eisenstein, M.D.
Vice President for Research
Beth Israel–Deaconess Medical Center
Professor, Department of Microbiology and Molecular
Genetics
Harvard Medical School
Boston, Massachusetts

N. Cary Engleberg, M.D.
Professor, Departments of Internal Medicine and
Microbiology and Immunology
University of Michigan Medical School
Ann Arbor, Michigan

Roger G. Faix, M. D.
Professor, Department of Pediatrics and
Communicable Diseases
Division of Pediatric Infectious Disease
University of Michigan Medical School
Ann Arbor and Mott Children's Hospital
Ann Arbor, Michigan

Bernard N. Fields, M.D (deceased)
Formerly, Professor
Harvard Medical School
Boston, Massachusetts

Janet R. Gilsdorf, M.D.
Professor, Department of Pediatrics and
Communicable Diseases
Division of Pediatric Infectious Disease
University of Michigan Medical School
Ann Arbor and Mott Children's Hospital
Ann Arbor, Michigan

Sherwood L. Gorbach, M.D.
Professor, Department of Community Medicine
Tufts University School of Medicine
Boston, Massachusetts

Penelope J. Hitchcock, D.V.M
Chief, Sexually Transmitted Diseases Branch
National Institutes of Health
National Institute of Allergy and Infectious Diseases
Bethesda, Maryland

James M. Hughes, M.D.
Director, National Center for Infectious Diseases
Centers for Disease Control and Prevention
Atlanta, Georgia

Adolf W. Karchmer, M.D.
Professor
Harvard Medical School
Chief, Infectious Diseases
New England Deaconess Hospital
Boston, Massachusetts

Gary Ketner, Ph.D.
Professor, Department of Molecular Microbiology and
Immunology
The Johns Hopkins University, School of Public Health
Baltimore, Maryland

Gerald T. Keusch, M.D.
Professor, Department of Medicine
Tufts University School of Medicine Chief, Division of
Geographic Medicine and Infectious Diseases
New England Medical Center
Boston, Massachusetts

George S. Kobayashi, Ph.D.
Professor, Departments of Microbiology and
Immunology and Internal Medicine
Washington University School of Medicine
St. Louis, Missouri

J. Michael Koomey, Ph.D.
Associate Professor, Department of Microbiology and
Immunology
University of Michigan Medical School
Ann Arbor, Michigan

Donald J. Krogstad, M.D.
Henderson Professor and Chair, Department of
Tropical Medicine
School of Public Health and Tropical Medicine
Tulane University
New Orleans, Louisiana

David W. Lazinski, Ph.D.
Assistant Professor, Department of Molecular Biology
and Microbiology Tufts University School of Medicine
Boston, Massachusetts

John M. Leong, M.D., Ph.D.
Assistant Professor, Department of Microbiology
University of Massachusetts Medical School
Worcester, Massachusetts

Zell A. McGee, M.D.
Professor, Departments of Internal Medicine and
Pathology
University of Utah School of Medicine
Salt Lake City, Utah

Gerald Medoff, M.D.
Professor, Departments of Microbiology and
Immunology and Internal Medicine
Washington University School of Medicine
St. Louis, Missouri

Cody H. Meissner, M.D.
Professor, Department of Pediatrics
Chief, Division of Infectious Diseases
New England Medical Center
Associate Professor, Department of Pediatrics
Tufts University School of Medicine
Boston, Massachusetts

Richard M. Peek, Jr.
Assistant Professor, Department of Medicine
Division of Gastroenterology, Department of Medicine
Vanderbilt University School of Medicine
Nashville, Tennessee

Andrew Plaut, M.D.
Professor
Division of Gastroenterology, Department of Medicine
Tufts University School of Medicine
Boston, Massachusetts

William G. Powderly, M.D.
Associate Professor and Co-director
Infectious Diseases Division, Department of Internal Medicine
Washington University School of Medicine
St. Louis, Missouri

Jane E. Raulston, Ph.D.
Research Assistant Professor
Department of Microbiology and Immunology
University of North Carolina School of Medicine
Chapel Hill, North Carolina

Edward N. Robinson, Jr., M.D.
Department of Medicine
University of North Carolina
The Moses H. Cone Memorial Hospital
Greensboro, North Carolina

Moselio Schaechter, Ph.D.
Distinguished Professor, Emeritus
Tufts University School of Medicine
Boston, Massachusetts
Adjunct Professor
San Diego State University
San Diego, California

David Schlessinger, Ph.D.
Professor, Department of Molecular Microbiology
Washington University School of Medicine
St. Louis, Missouri

Arnold L. Smith, M.D.
Professor and Chairman, Department of Molecular Microbiology and Immunology
University of Missouri School of Medicine
Columbia, Missouri

David R. Snydman, M.D.
Professor, Departments of Medicine and Pathology
Tufts University School of Medicine
Director, Clinical Microbiology
New England Medical Center
Boston, Massachusetts

John K. Spitznagel, M.D.
Professor and Former Chairman, Department of Microbiology and Immunology
Emory University School of Medicine
Atlanta, Georgia

Allen C. Steere, M.D.
Professor, Department of Medicine
Tufts University School of Medicine
Chief, Division of Rheumatology
New England Medical Center
Boston, Massachusetts

Gregory A. Storch, M.D.
Professor, Departments of Pediatrics and Medicine
Washington University School of Medicine
St. Louis, Missouri

Stephen E. Straus, M.D.
Chief, Laboratory of Clinical Investigation
National Institutes of Health
National Institute of Allergy and Infectious Diseases
Bethesda, Maryland

Francis P. Tally, M.D
Vice President, Research and Development
Cubist Pharmaceuticals, Inc.
Cambridge, Massachusetts

Donald M. Thea, M.D.
Department of Medicine
Tufts University School of Medicine
Chief, Division of Geographic Medicine and Infectious Diseases
New England Medical Center
Boston, Massachusetts

Debbie S. Toder, M.D.
Assistant Professor, Department of Pediatrics
University of Rochester Medical Center
Rochester, New York

David H. Walker, M.D.
Professor and Chairman, Department of Pathology
University of Texas Medical Branch at Galveston
Galveston, Texas

Ellen Whitnak, M.D.
Professor, Department of Medicine
University of Tennessee College of Medicine
Chief, Infectious Diseases Section
Veterans Affairs Medical Center
Memphis, Tennessee

Marion L. Woods, M.D.
Assistant Professor
Division of Infectious Diseases
University of Utah Medical Center
Salt Lake City, Utah

Priscilla B. Wyrick, Ph.D.
Professor
Department of Microbiology and Immunology
University of North Carolina School of Medicine
Chapel Hill, North Carolina

Victor L. Yu, M.D.
Professor of Medicine
University of Pittsburgh School of Medicine
Chief, Infectious Diseases Service Veterans Affairs
Pittsburgh, Pennsylvania

H. Kirk Ziegler, Ph.D.
Professor, Department of Microbiology and
Immunology
Emory University School of Medicine
Atlanta, Georgia

Contents

SECTION III
Pathophysiology of Infectious Diseases

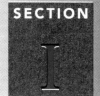

Principles

Establishment of Infectious Diseases

MOSELIO SCHAECHTER

BARRY I. EISENSTEIN

s a student and as a physician you confront a large number of facts about infectious agents and the diseases they cause. How will you manage this large amount of material? Given the magnitude of the task, memorizing bits of information would be difficult and unproductive.

Fortunately, it is possible to develop a conceptual framework on which to hang a multitude of facts. This framework consists of two generalizations that are based on the features that characterize all forms of parasitism:

1. In all infectious diseases, the following events take place :
   Encounter: The agent meets the host.
   Entry: The agent enters the host.
   Spread: The agent spreads from the site of entry.
   Multiplication: The agent multiplies in the host.
   Damage: The agent, the host response, or both cause tissue damage.
   Outcome: The agent or the host wins out, or they learn to coexist.
2. Each of these steps requires the breach of host defenses. The manner in which each parasite combats host defenses distinguishes one parasite from another.

ENCOUNTER

Most of us first encounter microorganisms at birth. Microbiologically speaking, we lead a sterile existence while in our mother's womb. The fetus is well shielded from the microorganisms in the uterine environment by the fetal membranes. Second, the mother is not a likely source of microorganisms for the fetus. The mother's blood carries infectious agents only sporadically and in small numbers. In addition, the placenta is a formidable barrier to the transmission of microorganisms to the fetus. However, such transmission is possible, and some diseases are transmitted to the fetus through the placenta. Examples of these so-called congenital infections are **rubella** (German measles) and **syphilis,** or those caused by **human immunodeficiency virus** (**HIV**) or **cytomegalovirus** (**CMV**).

First Encounters

The first encounter with environmental microorganisms usually takes place at birth. During parturition the newborn comes in contact with microorganisms present in the mother's vaginal canal and on her skin. Thus, the newborn faces the challenge of living in the intimate company with a bewildering number of microorganisms. The mother, however, does not send the newborn into the world totally unprotected. Through her circulation she endows the fetus with a vast repertoire of specific antibodies. Some immunological protection is also provided by the mother's milk (colostrum), which also contains maternal antibodies. However, these acquired defenses soon wane and the child must cope on its own. The microbial challenge is renewed time and again as all of us come in contact with new organisms throughout our lives. Most of these organisms rapidly disappear from the body, whereas others are adroit colonizers and become part of the normal flora. A few will cause disease.

Endogenous vs. Exogenous Encounters

Microbial diseases are contracted in two general ways, exogenously and endogenously.

Exogenously acquired disease

Exogenously acquired diseases are those that result from an encounter with agents in the environment. Thus we "catch" a cold from others, or we get typhoid fever from eating or drinking contaminated food or water. There are various ways in which disease-causing agents can be acquired from the environment: food, water, air, objects, insect bites, or humans or animals with whom we share our environment. Many agents are readily transmitted among humans through the exchange of bodily fluids, for instance by sneezing, touching, or sexual intercourse. The way we encounter a disease agent often suggests a mode of prevention (Table 1.1). Prevention has been successful for many serious epidemics, at least in the developed countries of the world. With the exception of vaccination, most preventive measures involve improvements in sanitation and the standard of living, rather than the employment of medical procedures.

Endogenously acquired diseases

Endogenously acquired diseases are those that are caused by agents present in or on the body. Members of the microbial flora that are normally found on our skin or mucous membranes may cause disease, usually when they penetrate into deeper tissues. Thus, a cut may lead to the production of pus caused by the staphylococci that inhabit the healthy skin. Here, the encounter with the agent took place long before the disease, namely at the time the skin was colonized by the staphylococci. A distinction must be made between **colonization** and **infectious disease.** Colonization denotes the presence of microorganisms in a site of the body, that does not necessarily lead to tissue damage and signs and symptoms of disease. It does suggest, however, that the microorganisms have invaded that site of the body and can multiply there.

The normal flora

The difference between endogenous and exogenous infections is sometimes quite sharp. However, in many other instances the demarcation becomes less clear because it is difficult to define precisely what organisms constitute the **normal flora** (Chapter 2, "Normal Microbial Flora"). For example, some people harbor certain strains of virulent streptococci in their throat for a considerable period of time but only rarely come down with strep throat. Now, before any symptoms arise, we may ask, "Were the streptococci members of the normal flora?" The answer is yes, if by "normal flora" we mean organisms in or on our body that are not in the process of causing disease. The answer is no if we consider that this kind of streptococcus is not found in the throats of approximately 95% of all healthy people. No easy way exists out of this ambiguity, and the terms *exogenous infection* and *endogenous infection* must be used tentatively. Obviously, if we cannot define precisely the composition of normal flora, we cannot always distinguish between endogenous and exogenous infections.

Another reason why the distinction is so vague is that exposure to highly virulent agents does not always lead to disease. For example, even at the height of deadly "black" plague and typhus epidemics, only about half of the population became sick, although most people were likely to have encountered the disease agent.

Thus, the encounter of humans with microbes is quite varied. Each bacterium, virus, fungus, or animal parasite has its quirks and, for that matter, each human being displays an idiosyncratic pattern of responses. Even within one individual, the pattern can change with age, nutritional state, and many other factors.

ENTRY

Most of the tissues we normally think of as being inside of the body are topologically connected with the outside (Fig. 1.1). For instance, the surface of the lumen of the intestine, the alveoli of the lung, the bile canaliculi, and the tubules of the kidney are in direct contact with the exterior environment. In fact, almost all the or-

Table 1.1. Examples of Encounters and Disease Prevention

Type of contact	Example	Type of agent	Source	Strategy for prevention	Preventive aim
Inhalation	Common cold	Virus	Aerosol from infected persons	None	
	Coccidioidomycosis	Fungus	Soil	None	
Ingestion	Typhoid fever	Bacterium	Water, food	Sanitation	Lower infecting dose
Sexual contact	Gonorrhea	Bacterium	Person	Social behavior	Avoid contact
Wound	Surgical infections	Bacteria	Normal flora surroundings	Aseptic techniques	
					Avoid contact
Insect bite	Malaria	Protozoan	Mosquito	Insect control	Eliminate vector

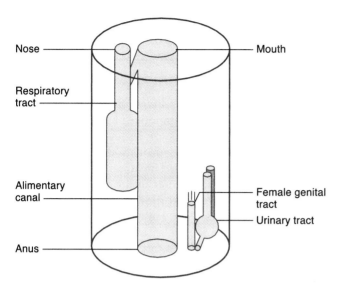

Figure 1.1. A schematic diagram showing the regions of the body in direct contact with the exterior. These include the outer aspect of the digestive, respiratory, and urogenital systems. These systems account for most of the organs of the thorax and abdomen. The main systems that do not have such direct connections are the musculoskeletal, nervous, circulatory, and endocrine. In women, the genital tract is connected to the peritoneal cavity via the fallopian tubes.

gans contained within the thorax and abdomen have this topological characteristic. In principle, an insect could crawl from the mouth to the anus without penetrating any mucous membranes, although it would have to go through several valves and sphincters. In reality, these "external" sites of the body employ powerful mechanisms to keep out invading microorganisms. With the exception of much of the digestive tract and the lower reaches of the genitourinary system, these sites are normally sterile.

The term *entry*, then, can be used in two senses: it means either the **ingress** of microorganisms into body cavities that are contiguous with the outside environment, or the **penetration** of microorganisms into deeper tissue after crossing an epithelial barrier. We discuss both aspects of entry in detail.

Ingress: Entry Without Crossing Epithelial Barriers

Obviously microorganisms enter the intestine by being swallowed and into the lung by being inhaled. External microorganisms can also enter the urinary tract or the genital system. It must also be kept in mind that microorganisms can cause serious diseases without entering deep entry into tissues. Examples of serious infectious diseases that occur without bacterial penetration through epithelial surfaces are **cholera**, **whooping cough**, and infections of the urinary bladder.

Inhalation

To enter the respiratory system, microorganisms face a series of aerodynamic and hydrodynamic obstacles. Microorganisms are inhaled in **aerosol droplets** or **dust particles** contained in the air we breathe. The path that microorganisms must take through the respiratory tract is not a "straight shot"; microorganisms must navigate through complex anatomic structures such as nasal turbinates, the oropharynx, and the larynx. Accordingly, the surgical removal of the larynx (with its nooks and crannies) predisposes an individual to diseases of the lower respiratory tract. Those microorganisms that arrive in the lower reaches of the respiratory tree face the powerful upward sweeping action of the ciliary epithelium. As expected, persons in whom this ciliary elevator is impaired (e.g., heavy smokers) are more likely to get sick with pneumonia. Colonization of these sites requires that the microorganisms be able to stick to the epithelial surface.

Ingestion

When contaminated food or water is ingested, microorganisms face a powerful host defense, the acid in the stomach. The stomach is a chemical disinfection chamber where many microorganisms are destroyed. Its effectiveness in killing microbes, however, is determined by the length of time microorganisms spend in the stomach, which in turn depends on the kind and amount of the food eaten. Even under conditions of greatest destruction, some bacteria and yeasts escape the stomach alive, although their original number may have been reduced one million-fold or more. Although these numbers imply a lot of bacterial killing, some diseases, such as bacillary dysentery, can be acquired from only a few hundred organisms.

Bacteria, fungi, parasites, and viruses that escape this acid barrier enter the duodenum. Here they meet the enzymes of the pancreatic juice, the bile salts, and the strong sweeping force of **peristalsis**. Not unexpectedly, very few microbes gain a foothold at this site or anywhere else in the upper reaches of the small intestine. Toward the ileum, the environment is more favorable to bacterial life, but even here the few organisms that gain a foothold must avoid being washed away. Indeed, bacteria found in this region have special mechanisms that allow them to adhere to the epithelial cells of the intestinal mucosa. As will be discussed in Chapter 2 ("Normal Microbial Flora"), several surface components of these bacteria serve as **adhesins**. The main adhesins are the hairlike pili (fimbriae) and the surface polysaccharides. As mentioned previously, bacteria at this site may cause disease without penetrating the mucosal epithelium. Cholera, and its milder relative, **travelers' diarrhea**, are the manifestations of the local production of powerful toxins in the intestine that affect the epithelial cells. The bacteria that produce these toxins need not enter the host cells to cause disease.

Penetration: Entry into Tissues After Crossing Epithelial Barriers

Penetration into tissues takes many forms. Some microorganisms pass directly through epithelia, especially mucous membranes that consist of a single cell layer. To penetrate the skin, which is tough and multilayered, most infecting agents must be carried across by insect bites or await breaks in the skin surface. On the other hand, certain worms can burrow unaided through the skin and invade the host. An example are hookworms, which may be acquired by walking barefoot on contaminated soil.

To penetrate mucosal epithelial cells, many agents first interact with specific **receptors** on the surface of the host cell. This phenomenon has been studied intensively in viruses, some of which have a complex mechanism for attachment and internalization. For instance, influenza viruses have **surface components** that bind to receptors on the surface of sensitive host cells. Binding is soon followed by the uptake of the virus particles by the cells. These two functions, **attachment** and **internalization**, are also being studied intensively in bacteria. For example, it has been possible to clone bacterial genes that confer the ability to enter cells into strains of bacteria that are normally noninvasive.

Microorganisms may also be actively carried into tissues by white cells or macrophages that lie on the outside of the body. For instance, macrophages that reside in the alveoli of the lungs, known as **dust cells,** can pick up infectious agents by phagocytosis. Most of the time, microorganism-containing macrophages are carried upward on the ciliary epithelium, but occasionally infected macrophages can reenter the body and carry their load of microorganisms into deeper locations. This mechanism of **cell-mediated entry** may function at other mucous membranes as well. It is thought, for example, that HIV, the virus that causes acquired immunodeficiency syndrome (AIDS), may be sexually transmitted by the penetration of virus-laden macrophages from semen.

Insect bites

Insect bites may lead to the penetration of viruses (viral encephalitis or yellow fever), bacteria (plague, typhus), protozoa (malaria, sleeping sickness), or worms (river blindness, elephantiasis). In the case of protozoa and worms, residence in the insect is part of their complex life cycles. The **life stage** of the parasite in the insect is often quite different from that found in the human host. Insects also spread diseases by carrying microorganisms on their surfaces and by contaminating foodstuffs or the skin of a person. A particularly unsavory example of insect transmission is that of the so-called reduviid bugs, which defecate at the same time they bite.

Parasites contained in the insect's feces are then introduced by scratching the bite area. A serious protozoal infection, **Chagas' disease,** is transmitted in this manner.

Cuts and wounds

Penetration from cuts and wounds is a common occurrence that usually goes unnoticed because it does not usually lead to symptoms of disease. For example, brushing one's teeth or vigorously defecating causes minute abrasions of epithelial membranes. A small number of bacteria can then enter in the bloodstream, but they are rapidly removed by the filtering mechanisms of the lymphoreticular system. However, if internal tissues are damaged or the defense mechanisms disrupted, circulating bacteria may gain a foothold and cause serious diseases. An example is **subacute bacterial endocarditis,** a disease which was devastating before the availability of antibiotics. This infection was usually caused by oral streptococci that invaded the heart valves damaged by a previous disease, usually rheumatic fever.

Organ transplants and blood transfusion

Yet another way for organisms to penetrate into deeper tissue is through organ transplants or blood transfusions. For instance, transplants of corneas have been known to result in the infection of recipients with a virus that causes a slow degenerative disease of the central nervous system (**Creutzfeldt-Jakob disease**). Kidney transplants sometimes result in infections by CMV perhaps because the virus resided in the transplanted kidney. However, the transplanted organ is not always the source of infection. Because the immune response of transplant recipients must be suppressed in order to avoid graft rejection, an **endogenous virus** may take advantage of these hosts' weakened defenses and begin to multiply.

Of the infectious agents that may be acquired via blood transfusions, none causes greater concern than HIV. However, many others, such as **hepatitis B virus (HBV)** can also be transmitted in this manner. Screening of blood in blood banks has become imperative.

Inoculum Size

The likelihood that organisms from the flora of the skin or mucous membranes might cause disease depends on many factors. Among them is the size of the **inoculum,** the number of invading organisms. An encounter with a small number of organisms is unlikely to result in an infection; it usually takes many infecting agents to overcome the local defenses. An example that illustrates the importance of inoculum size is infection acquired from contaminated hot tubs. At times the water can become a veritable culture broth with as many as 100 million bacteria (*Pseudomonas*) per milliliter. In such numbers, bacteria that are normally harmless can overcome the normal defenses of the skin and cause skin infection all over the body. Medical professionals are also aware of the importance of inoculum size in infection. For example, before making an incision in the skin, a surgeon prepares the area to reduce the number of bacteria that may invade a surgical wound. Infections are almost inevitable if large numbers of microorganisms are deposited in deeper tissues, either from dirty skin or from contamination by soil or other microbial-rich material. Treatment of patients with open wounds thus requires careful attention to sterile techniques, even in the modern era of powerful antimicrobial drugs.

SPREAD

The term *spread* has two shades of meaning. It suggests direct, **lateral propagation** of organisms from the original site of entry to contiguous tissues, but it can also refer to **dissemination** to distant sites. Either way, microorganisms spread and multiply only if they overcome host defenses. It should be kept in mind that spread can precede or follow microbial multiplication in the body. For instance, the parasite that causes **malaria** enters the body through a mosquito bite and is distributed throughout the bloodstream before it has a chance to reproduce. On the other hand, staphylococci that infect a cut must multiply locally before spreading to distant sites.

The role of **host defenses** in impeding the spread of microorganisms requires a fair understanding of the immune response and of the innate defense mechanisms. Host defenses are discussed in detail in Chapter 6 ("Constitutive Defenses of the Body") and Chapter 7 ("Induced Defenses of the Body") and are a central theme of this book. For now, it is important to keep in mind the dynamic nature of host–parasite interactions: for every defense mechanism in existence, microbes develop strategies to try to overcome it. The host, in turn, adapts to these new challenges, eliciting yet different responses from the agents. This intricate counterpoint is played out, sometimes over extended periods of time, until one of three things happens: (a) the host wins out, (b) the parasite overcomes the host, or (c) host and parasite learn to live with one another in an uneasy truce.

Anatomical Factors

Because the pattern of spread of microorganisms from a given site is often dictated by **anatomical factors,** a knowledge of human anatomy often helps us understand infectious diseases. Consider a localized infection, a bacterial abscess of the lung, as an example. The abscess may burst and allow the organisms to escape into the bronchial tree or, if the abscess is pointed outwards, to the pleural cavity. Spread in one or the other direction has different consequences. In the first case it may lead to a generalized pneumonia; in the second, to pleurisy.

Another example is an infection of the middle ear, a condition more common in children than in adults. This age difference is explained in part by developmental changes that take place in the eustachian tubes with growth. These conduits are nearly horizontal in children and become more steeply inclined with age. For this and other reasons, the eustachian tubes of children do not drain as well as those of adults.

Spread of microorganisms is greatly influenced by **fluid dynamics**. Thus, infected fluids in the interior of the body tend to flow along fascial planes. For example, infection of one site of the meninges will usually result in generalized meningitis, since there are no barriers to impede the spread of the infected cerebrospinal fluid. The same is true for the pleura, the pericardium, and the synovial cavities. Of course, the most extensive liquid system of the body, the blood, is replete with defense mechanisms. All the liquids of the body (blood, lymph, cerebrospinal fluid, synovial fluid, urine, tears, etc.) contain different antimicrobial defense factors that, if overcome, result in disease.

Active Participation by Microorganisms

Infectious agents are not always passive participants in the process of spreading; some actively contribute to it by actively moving. Thus, worms wiggle, ameba crawl, some of the bacteria swim. While some of these movements appear random, others are probably in response to chemotactic signals. Spreading can also be facilitated by chemical rather than mechanical action. For instance, streptococci manufacture a variety of extracellular hydrolases that allow them to break out of the walled defenses erected by the inflammatory response. These organisms make a protease that breaks up fibrin, a hyaluronidase that hydrolyzes hyaluronic acid of connective tissue, and a deoxyribonuclease that reduces the viscosity of pus caused by the release of DNA from lysed white cells. Some bacteria make elastases, collagenases, or other powerful proteases. Such organisms can break through natural surface barriers or can spread through thick viscous pus that would otherwise impede their expansion. At a more superficial site, fungi that cause athlete's foot make keratin-hydrolyzing enzymes that help them spread through the horny layers of the skin. These factors confer clear selective advantages on the microorganisms that produce them.

MULTIPLICATION

Rarely do infectious agents cause disease without first multiplying within the body. As previously stated, the number of microorganisms we inhale or ingest (the size of the inoculum) is usually too small to produce symptoms directly. Infectious agents must reproduce before their presence is felt (Fig. 1.2). One exception to the rule are agents that cause disease through the production of

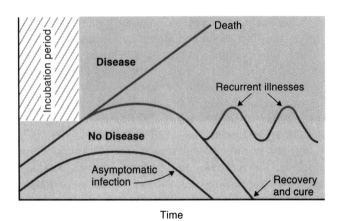

Figure 1.2. Microbial multiplication and clinical manifestations of disease. The number of microorganisms present in a patient must exceed a given threshold to cause disease. If the number is below this threshold, no signs and symptoms of disease will be apparent. In some cases, the numbers oscillate above and below the threshold, resulting in recurrent bouts of disease. Note that this drawing is idealized; in reality, the threshold of overt disease is not fixed but varies with the physiological state of the host.

a toxin, such as *Clostridium botulinum*, which produces botulinum toxin that leads to botulism. This condition is an **intoxication**, not an infection.

In most infections, symptoms manifest some time after the organisms enter the host. This **incubation period** reflects the time needed for the infectious agents to overcome early defenses and to grow to a certain population size. The subject of how hosts defend themselves against microbial multiplication is a lengthy and varied one. Later in this chapter we will discuss how defense mechanisms sometimes go overboard and actually contribute to tissue damage in infections.

The physical environment of the body selects for microorganisms that grow within certain ranges of temperature, osmotic pressure, and pH. Organisms that are almost always found in association with their hosts tend to have a narrow **temperature optimum**. Organisms that are also found in the environment, such as *Pseudomonas*, also grow well at lower temperatures. Some viruses, such as poliovirus, can only replicate just a few degrees over normal human body temperature. Fever, then, may be a defense mechanism that limits the disease. Fungi that cause athlete's foot do not grow well at temperatures above around 30°C and are thus found only on the cooler body surfaces. It follows that in most circumstances these fungi cannot cause internal diseases. As with nutritional requirements, the optimal temperature range for growth is often dictated by the organism's habits.

Subversion of Host Defenses

When a microorganism causes an infection it creates a hostile environment for itself because it impels the host to mobilize defenses that impair the microorganism's growth and threaten its existence. In most cases the host prevails, but the existence of infectious diseases demonstrates that this is not always true and that microorganisms can thwart or evade the host defenses. The microbial countermeasures involved do not contribute directly to tissue damage, yet they can be thought of as virulence factors because they are essential for the microorganism to be pathogenic. Generally speaking, each species of infectious agents develops an individual spectrum of survival strategies. For every successful infection by a microorganism we must ask: **how does it survive in its particular location of the body?** We know some of the answers, but by no means all.

Host defenses do not operate in isolation but are interrelated. The strategies that microorganisms use to subvert them are correspondingly complex. We divide them into those directed against constitutive defenses, **complement and phagocytosis**, and against induced defenses, **humoral and cellular immunity**. Microorganisms invading a host that has not encountered them previously will meet these defenses in this order. Many microbial countermeasures are known from in vitro experimental situations and it is not always possible to determine if they also operate in human disease. This is a subject of intensive research that has clear therapeutic and prophylactic implications.

An example of microbial defensive strategies is to make, or appropriate from the host, a protective covering. This may be an extracellular capsule that blocks recognition and binding by both complement and antibodies, and prevents phagocytosis by leukocytes. This is the strategy of such important mucosal pathogens as the pneumococcus or the meningococcus. Nonetheless, these capsules are themselves immunogenic and antigenic and, therefore, have become the basis of vaccines used to prevent pneumonia and meningitis. Another way that bacteria avoid immune recognition is by altering their surface antigens in a genetically programmed way. Certain pathogens, such as the gonococci or the salmonellae can modify surface structures that are recognized by the immune system.

Many microorganisms survive in the body because they do not cause too much damage to the host (stealth tactics). The best adapted of them cause no disease at all, elicit no inflammatory response, and actually are a help to the host by helping provide nutrients in the GI tract (e.g., vitamin B12), crowding out potential pathogens (on the skin and mucosal surfaces). They may even stimulate the immune system to raise useful cross-protective antibodies (e.g., protection against meningococci may be due to the colonization by related but nonpathogenic commensal species). Among the most successful pathogens are those that cause sexually transmitted diseases. In some people, these bacteria may cause minimal or no disease (e.g., chlamydial infection, gonorrhea), whereas in others, disease comes on slowly or as part of a chronic process (e.g., syphilis). When nonpathogenic strains cause trouble it is a result of their getting into places they don't belong, such as when the mixed flora of the bowel gets into the peritoneal cavity with the rupture of an appendix.

In contrast, the occasional, highly pathogenic invaders with their well-developed set of toxins cause significant acute damage and disease, but may end up killing the host (thus biting the hand that feeds them!). For example, dead end processes like lethal meningitis do not, by themselves, promote bacterial survival.

DAMAGE

There are nearly as many kinds of damage as there are infectious diseases. The type and intensity of the damage depend on the tissues and organs affected, which makes it difficult to make generalizations. An important, if not intuitively obvious point is that damage is not always caused by activities of the invading agent alone, but is often the consequence of a vehement host response. Ask yourself, what causes damage in an infection such as pneumonia due to pneumococci? These organisms make no known toxins and their invasion of the lung alveoli is manifested chiefly by the extensive production of pus in the affected sites. Pus is the result of acute inflammation, the outpouring of white blood cells and liquid from the circulation. Here, as in many other infections, the symptoms of the disease are due mainly to a forceful, if unregulated, host response. In chronic infections, such as tuberculosis, the symptoms of disease can almost invariably be ascribed to the host response, with the microorganism being relatively passive but being able to stimulate the host to respond in a manner that causes the symptoms of the disease.

This is not to say that infective agents are always just innocent bystanders. Some bacteria produce extracellular toxins that are directly responsible for tissue damage. Some of these toxins, such as those of botulism and tetanus, are among the strongest poisons known. Toxins cause damage in various ways: some just help bacteria spread in tissues, others lyse host cells, yet others stop cell growth, and still others exaggerate normal physiological mechanisms. By depressing or augmenting particular functions, toxins may kill a person without directly damaging any cells. No abnormal lesions result—the toxin acts by causing hyperactivity of a normal process.

One of the most dramatic manifestations of infection is cell death. This comes about in a variety of ways: direct action of cytolytic toxins, activation of cell-killing white blood cells, or induction of programmed cell death. The damage caused by the death of tissue cells is most serious when it occurs in essential organs, such as the brain or the heart. It should be noted that in some serious and even life-threatening infectious diseases, cell death is not a distinctive feature even though the agents multiply intracellularly. In the prime example, tuberculosis, the infected cells survive, yet the infection results in far-reaching and pervasive damage. However, cell death is often a prominent feature, especially of acute infections.

With many common bacteria, the so-called Gram-negatives, the host response is elicited by a major component of their surface, a lipopolysaccharide known as **endotoxin.** In small amounts endotoxin elicits fever and mobilizes certain defense mechanisms. In large amounts, it results in shock and intravascular coagulation. Thus, the body response to the presence of these bacteria depends on the **amount** of endotoxin present.

The Immune Response

The immune response is complex and has multiple functions. Due to its complexity, there are many ways in which it may go awry and cause damage. Immune responses are usually classified as "humoral," which leads to the production of circulating antibodies, and "cellular," in which special immune system cells seek out and destroy infected cells. Both responses may cause damage.

Humoral immunity

Infecting agents elicit the formation of specific antibodies. In the circulation and tissues, antibodies combine with the infecting agents or with some of their soluble products. These antigen–antibody complexes evoke an inflammatory response by facilitating the activation of a complex set of serum proteins, the *complement system.* In the presence of antigen–antibody complexes these proteins are activated by a series of proteolytic reactions, the so-called **classical pathway** of activation. Complement can also be activated by the presence of microorganisms alone, resulting in the **alternative pathway.** The products of these proteolytic cleavages are pharmacologically active compounds. Some work on platelets and white cells to produce substances that increase vascular permeability and vasodilation. The result is edema, the outpouring of fluids into tissues. Other complement factors act on white blood cells, some as chemotaxins, others to make bacteria more easily phagocytized. These activities result in both the mobilization of powerful defenses against invading microorganisms, and inflammation.

Antigen–antibody complexes are sometimes deposited on the membrane of the glomeruli of the kidneys, resulting in impairment of kidney function, a condition called **glomerulonephritis.** This condition is seen in the aftermath of certain streptococcal and viral infections. Similar effects also take place in blood vessels, leading to visible skin rashes.

Cellular immunity

A different type of response is expressed via special cells of the immune system and is called **cell-mediated immunity (CMI).** This complex phenomenon leads to the activation and mobilization of macrophages, the powerful phagocytic cells that participate in the later stages of inflammation to clean up debris and remaining microorganisms.

CMI is associated with chronic inflammation, the histological changes that limit the spread of infections but also cause lesions in tissues. These damaging activities are characteristic of chronic infections, often caused by intracellular microorganisms and viruses. An example is chronic tuberculosis, in which the main damage to tissue is due to CMI. The immune response is elicited by the tubercle bacilli, which are able to persist in cells for a long time. Pathological changes associated with CMI lead to the production of **tubercles** or **granulomas,** and eventually to destruction of tissue cells.

It is worth repeating that although the immune responses may cause tissue damage, in most instances the price is well worth it. This point is illustrated in people who have genetic or acquired defects in their immune system. Unfortunately, such people are no longer a medical rarity. The advent and spread of AIDS has placed hundreds of thousands of persons in this category. These patients are ravaged and later killed by microorganisms that cause little or no disease in healthy persons. In the immunocompetent person, for example, active tuberculosis causes much damage but death only occurs after many years. In the immunocompromised patient, the disease can become rampant in a much shorter period.

OUTCOME

No infectious disease, be it mild or life-threatening, is simple. Various properties of the invading agent and the host lead to an intricate and ever-changing interplay. It is not always possible to discern the relative roles of the known properties, let alone those that still await discovery. To complicate matters, humans are beset by a huge number of possible invaders. New ones emerge apparently under our very eyes, to be added to the long list.

The student of medical microbiology therefore faces a demanding challenge. The fascination of the topic may not suffice to overcome the problems inherent in the study of so much detail. The conceptual framework used in this chapter, which is based on the fact that all host–parasite interactions have steps in common, may be useful in mastering many of the details of microbiology. As we indicated at the beginning of this chapter, parasites and host must encounter one another, and the parasite must enter the host, spread, multiply, and eventually cause damage. All these steps require the breaching of host defenses. If these steps are kept in mind, the myriad facts will fall logically into place. You may thereby be able to enjoy one of the liveliest and important subjects in all of biology and medicine!

SUGGESTED READINGS

McNeill WH. Plagues and peoples. Garden City, NY: Anchor Books, 1976.

Mims CA. The pathogenesis of infectious diseases. 4th ed. New York: Academic Press, 1995.

Normal Microbial Flora

BARRY I. EISENSTEIN

MOSELIO SCHAECHTER

The human body normally contains thousands of species of bacteria and a smaller number of viruses, fungi, and protozoa. The great majority are commensal organisms, meaning that they coexist with us without causing harm. The members of the normal flora change with time, but their number at any instant is still formidable. Each of us possesses an individualized spectrum of species and strains. In the words of the Romans, *suum quique*, to each his own.

WHAT IS THE NORMAL FLORA?

Members of the normal flora are defined as those microorganisms that are frequently found on or within the body of healthy persons (Fig. 2.1). Some of these organisms are found in association with the body of humans or animals only; others can also live freely in the environment.

A precise roll-call of the organisms that constitute the normal flora is often possible, a point already discussed in Chapter 1, "Establishment of Infectious Diseases." Consider, for instance, the meningococcus or the pneumococcus, both true pathogens capable of causing meningitis, pneumonia, or septicemia. Both microbes are found in the throats of about 10% of healthy people; thus, they can be counted as members of the normal flora in these individuals but not in 90% of the population. In any one of us they may come and go as sporadic denizens of our throat. Therefore, such organisms should be called **transient** members of the normal flora of some individuals. You are correct if you have already surmised that these pathogens do not usually cause trouble even in colonized individuals. What is not obvious is that disease caused by either of these two organisms does not occur without prior **colonization**. Thus, colo-

nization is necessary, yet insufficient, for meningococcal or pneumococcal disease. But colonization is not a universal prerequisite for all infections, many of which develop soon after entry of the infectious agent into the body without a prolonged period of colonization. Examples are malaria or the common cold.

The problem with many of the definitions in this field is that they are not absolute. The same problems that arise in precisely identifying the normal microbial flora pertain to terms such as **pathogenicity** and **virulence**. As we will see in subsequent chapters, these terms depend not only on properties of the infectious agent, but also on the state of the defenses of the host. Keep in mind, too, that disease is seldom caused by the activities of the agent alone, but often includes the responses of the host. Many of the signs and symptoms of infections are actually due to the host's own inflammatory response to an infection. A good analogy: fire-fighters occasionally augment the property destruction due to fire by producing water damage in their attempts to contain the flames.

The objective of all living organisms, microbes included, is to grow and reproduce. The most successful microbe is the one that can rapidly and efficiently become two microbes. Note that in describing the nature of success among these organisms, "pathogenicity" or "virulence" is not considered. In fact, the most virulent pathogens, those that kill their hosts, may be poorly adapted for survival and represent recent biological associations. After all, why would a guest paying no rent want to set fire to his home? Before exploring the world of pathogens (the "misfits"), it is instructive to first consider our normal guests who behave well. Keep in mind, though, that even the most domesticated among them can cause trouble if given the opportunity.

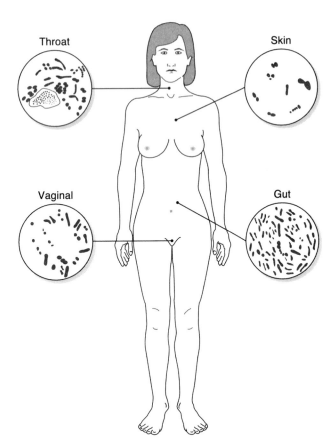

Figure 2.1. The bacterial flora in a healthy person. The typical bacteria seen in the microbe-laden sites of the body are shown in schematic fashion. Gram-positive bacteria are shown in *black*; Gram-negative bacteria are shown in *color*.

WHAT PARTS OF THE BODY ARE INVOLVED?

Let us now consider the parts of the body that are colonized by the normal flora. Those that usually contain large amounts of microorganisms are:

Skin—moist areas especially, e.g., groin, between toes
Respiratory tract—nose and oropharynx
Digestive tract—mouth and large intestine
Urinary tract—anterior parts of the urethra
Genital system—vagina

Bacteria, and to lesser extent, fungi and protozoa, reside and actively proliferate at these sites. Other parts of the body contain small numbers of microorganisms; most of them are in transit and do not usually colonize these sites. Examples include the rest of the respiratory and digestive tracts, the **urinary bladder** and the **uterus**. Finding pathogenic microorganisms at these sites is highly suggestive of disease, but is not proof. At the other extreme are certain tissues and organs that are usually sterile. The presence of microorganisms at these sites is usually diagnostically significant. These sites include **blood, cerebrospinal fluid, synovial fluid,** and **deep tissues** in general.

The number of bacteria in sites that contain thriving microbial communities varies over a wide range. In highly protected areas, bacteria are almost as densely packed as is physically possible. For instance, the gingival pockets around teeth contain wall-to-wall bacteria. Normal feces consist of about one-third bacteria by weight. If the average bacterium is about 1 μm^3 in volume, the densest possible packing would result in a mass of 1×10^{12} per milliliter. Such numbers are actually approached in certain parts of the body. In contrast, sites that are not quite as hospitable, such as the skin, mouth, and vagina, may harbor populations that are of the order of one to ten million bacteria per milliliter of fluid or per gram of scrapings.

HOW DO MICROORGANISMS PERSIST IN THE BODY?

In order to colonize the human body, invading microorganisms must be able to resist host mechanisms that could dislodge or kill them, as well as compete successfully with other microbial species. Picture a bacterial cell entering the mouth and the problems it faces trying to remain at this site. Strong liquid currents will wash it away unless the organism adheres to the surface of the teeth or the mucous membranes. In addition, saliva contains antibacterial compounds, such as enzymes and antibodies; however, these substances are not equally damaging toward all bacterial species. At sites of the mouth that are not exposed to the flushing action of saliva, such as the crevasses of the gums, the organism will find a large resident flora that already occupies likely adherence sites. These resident organisms also produce antimicrobial substances, such as acids derived from their metabolism of sugars, that may be inimical to the invader.

Although certain body sites are normally extensively colonized, only occasionally do these microbes cause trouble at these sites. One example is the dental disease, periodontitis, that results from overgrowth of particular bacterial strains in the gingival crevices and causes gum disease. Another example is the pneumonia that can result when the respiratory defenses are lowered (e.g., from a poor cough reflex due to a stroke or from smoking-induced paralysis of the ciliary clearance mechanisms). Under these conditions, "aspiration pneumonia" is likely to occur. The bacteriologic etiology of such pneumonias is highly dependent on the kinds of organisms that colonize the mouth or throat at the time of the aspiration. If the person is unlucky enough to be colonized with a virulent strain of pneumococcus, only a small amount of material aspirated from the mouth or pharynx into the lungs is sufficient to cause severe pneumonia. In fact, most cases of pneumococcal pneumonia are not associated with obvious aspiration at all, but rather with imperceptible "microaspirations." If the oropharynx is not colonized with virulent bacteria, a significantly larger amount of aspirated material must reach the lungs to cause disease. An example of the factors involved in colonization can be seen by the study of an adhesive protein called **fibronectin**. This protein coats the mucosal surfaces of epithelial cells and has a strong predilection for the so-called Gram-positive organisms (see Chapter 3, "Biology of Infectious Agents"). Fibronectin is probably important in establishing the nature of the bacterial flora in the mouth and pharynx, as suggested by the following findings. The oropharynx of individuals in poor general health, including many hospitalized patients, becomes deficient in fibronectin. With low levels of this protein, Gram-negative organisms tend to displace Gram-positives, in part because the fibronectin-denuded mucosal cells reveal receptors for bacterial surface components called pili or fimbriae, which are adhesive organelles found on Gram-negative, but not on Gram-positive, bacteria. The high incidence of Gram-negative pneumonia in hospitalized patients can be explained in part by these considerations of adherence specificity. In fact, aspiration-related pneumonias, along with catheter-associated infections of the urinary tract and bloodstream (most commonly caused by staphylococci), are the most important causes of hospital-associated (**nosocomial**) infections. These infections exact great cost both in patient lives and the finances of patient care.

The example of the mouth can be extended to the large intestine, the vagina, the perineum, the skin, and other sites that are normally laden with microbes. It follows that colonization by new organisms is an unlikely event and that the successful colonizer must be unusually adept at resisting host and microbial defenses. Colonization of sites that are normally sterile or carry a sparse load of microorganisms, such as deep tissues and the small intestine, is not affected by microbial competition. Not surprisingly, host defenses are typically more intensive at such sites. Few microbes survive the alternating acid and alkaline baths of our upper gastrointestinal tracts or the sea of antibodies, complement, and phagocytic cells that bathes the deep tissues. Obviously, throughout our long history of coexistence and coevolution with the microbial world, our bodies have designated territories that are safe to share and those that are off limits—and to share this space preferentially only with well-behaved guests. Foreign devices, like plastic catheters stuck into arteries and veins, are notorious for upsetting the delicate ecological balance between microbes and host tissues.

The attributes that permit microbes to colonize the body make a long list and, to a large extent, determine what makes each pathogenic organism distinct. Such attributes will be discussed in detail in the chapters on individual organisms. Table 2.1 lists the classes of microbial properties that allow successful colonization.

Table 2.1. Some Issues in Bacterial Colonization

Anti-colonizing property of the host	Examples of how bacteria overcome it
Sweep microbes away by liquid currents	Adhere to epithelial cells (e.g., gonococci stick to the mucous membrane of the urethra)
Kill microbes with the host's phagocytes	Avoid being taken up (e.g., the pneumococcus is surrounded by a slimy capsule that impairs uptake by neutrophils) Kill the phagocyte (e.g., certain streptococci produce a toxin that punches holes in the neutrophil membrane)
Starve microbes for lack of needed nutrients	Derive needed nutrients from host cells (e.g., certain staphylococci lyse red blood cells and use their hemoglobin as a source of iron)

SOME INFECTIOUS AGENTS STRONGLY PREFER CERTAIN SITES IN THE BODY, OTHERS DO NOT

At first glance, it may appear that microorganisms usually cause disease only in specific organs. To some extent, this statement is true: hepatitis viruses affect the liver, encephalitis and rabies virus the brain, the common cold viruses the nasal epithelium. Viruses tend to be more tissue-specific than bacteria, which often show a wide range of **tissue tropism**. Some bacteria, such as the cholera bacillus, have strong predilections (the small intestine, in this case), whereas others (e.g., the staphylococcus) may infect almost any site of the body. In some cases, tissue tropism can be attributed to tissue-specific cellular properties, such as the presence of specific receptors on the surfaces of certain cells (e.g., fibronectin, with its affinity for Gram-positive bacteria). In other instances, physical properties, such as the temperature of the organ, determine the tropism.

The complexities of tissue tropism in bacteria have already been discussed on p. 8 in relation to colonization of the oropharynx. It can also be illustrated with the example of the gonococcus. This bacterium most often causes infection of the urethra, but the throat, rectum, or the eyes may also be affected. Where the lesion occurs in this disease depends on the **site of entry** of the organism. Pharyngeal and rectal gonorrhea are the result of nonvaginal intercourse, whereas ophthalmia (eye infection) is due to the infection of the eyes of a neonate as it passes through the birth canal of the infected mother. Thus, it is clear that the gonococcus has no absolute predilection for the mucous membranes of a given organ. What about other types of tissue? Strains of gonococci that survive in circulation show a marked predilection for certain organs, such as the joints. Thus, gonococcal arthritis is one of the most common complications of gonorrhea. Although the reasons for the site predilection at the joints are known, it is clear that the gonococcus has strong tropism for certain deep tissues, not only for epithelial membranes.

Tissue tropism often relies on the existence of specific receptors on the surfaces of certain cells. This affinity for host cell receptors is seen clearly in viruses and may explain why, in general, these agents show a great degree of tropism. Influenza virus, for example, relies on special glycoproteins found on the surface of respiratory epithelial cells for its attachment. Human immunodeficiency virus (HIV), the virus that causes AIDS, attaches to protein receptors found selectively on certain lymphocytes and macrophages. Other examples include fibronectin in the oropharynx (discussed above), and mucosal cells of the urinary tract in individuals with the P blood-group antigen (99% of the population), which binds *Escherichia coli* carrying P-pilus organelles (see Chapter 3, "Biology of Infectious Agents"). Many research efforts, particularly in novel forms of antiviral therapy, are aimed at discovering ways to neutralize the action of receptors, thereby precluding infection by the agents that recognize them.

The temperature of an organ sometimes determines the location of the infectious agent. Thus, the viruses of the common cold are found in the nasal epithelium and not in internal organs because these agents do not grow at the higher temperature inside the body. Likewise, the spirochete of syphilis is sensitive to higher than normal body temperatures, which induced certain physicians of the pre-antibiotic era to try to cure syphilis by injecting patients with the agent of malaria!

THE ROLE OF THE NORMAL FLORA

The normal flora plays an important role in health and disease, as illustrated by the following examples. The most easily perceptible manifestation of the activities of the normal flora is the production of the various odors associated with epithelial surfaces of the human body. A germ-free human would not need to make use of deodorants.

A Common Source of Infection

The normal flora is the source of many opportunistic infections. When commensal organisms find themselves in unaccustomed sites of the body, they may cause disease. For example, anaerobic bacteria, usually of the genus *Bacteroides*, are carried harmlessly in the intestines of normal persons but produce abscesses if they penetrate into deeper tissues via traumatic or surgical wounds. Staphylococci from the skin and nose, or strep-

tococci and Gram-negative cocci from the throat and mouth, are also responsible for infections of this sort. In fact, *Staphylococcus epidermidis*, the prevalent species on the skin, has a strong predilection for nonspecific attachment to plastic catheters, which occasionally results in severe bloodstream infections in patients with intravenous catheters. Likewise, *E. coli,* a normal inhabitant of the gastrointestinal tract, is by far the most common cause of urinary tract infection. In general, physicians see more patients with disease due to the normal flora than due to agents acquired from outside the body.

These facts point out that the definition of virulence is elusive and that no microorganism is intrinsically benign or pathogenic. Under the right circumstances, any microorganism that can grow in the body can cause disease. However, members of the normal flora do not all have the same pathogenic potential. Some cause disease more readily than others because they are endowed with special virulence properties. For example, peritonitis is caused by the release of intestinal bacteria through a break in the gut wall. The resulting infection is usually caused by a few bacterial species only, a small fraction selected from a large number of species present in the inoculum.

The definition of virulence is not intrinsic to the microorganisms but depends also on the degree of immune competence of the host. Members of the normal flora often invade organs and tissues in immune-compromised patients. Thus, the yeast *Candida*, a harmless commensal in about one-third of normal people, is a common cause of bloodstream infection in patients undergoing vigorous cancer chemotherapy. *Pneumocystis carinii*, a common inhabitant of the lungs of healthy persons, can cause a specific kind of pneumonia and is one of the principal causes of death in patients with AIDS.

Immune Stimulation

Our repertoire of immunoglobulins reflects in part the antigenic stimulation by the normal flora. In general, we do not have high antibody titers to the individual bacteria, viruses, or fungi that inhabit our body. Nonetheless, even in low concentrations these antibodies serve as a defense mechanism. Here, then, is a clear benefit from our normal flora. Among the antibodies produced in response to bacterial stimulation are those of the IgA class, which are secreted through mucous membranes. While the role of these immunoglobulins is not well understood, it seems reasonable that they are an important first line of defense and that they interfere, possibly on a daily basis, with the colonization of deeper tissues by commensal organisms.

Antibodies elicited by the antigenic challenge of the normal flora sometimes cross-react with normal tissue components. A good example are antibodies against ABO blood group antigens. People that belong to the A group have anti-B antibodies and, conversely, B group individuals have anti-A antibodies. People in the O group make both anti-A and anti-B antibodies. You may wonder about the source of antigenic stimulation for these antibodies. On reflection, this source is not obvious. Why should one make antibodies against a blood group different from one's own? Few of us come in contact with red blood cells of a different type, through blood transfusions, with the wrong type blood. The answer to this puzzle is that bacteria from the intestinal flora contain antigens that cross-react with both A and B blood antigens. These constituents are the source of antigenic stimulation. We make antibodies against these foreign blood group antigens but not against those of our own group because we are immunologically tolerant to the "self" antigens but not to the "foreign" ones.

This type of **cross-reactivity** does not usually cause disease. In fact, some evidence demonstrates that cross-reactivity among bacterial antigens can be protective. For example, antibodies raised against various bacteria that normally reside in the bowel have been shown to cross-react with the polysaccharide capsule of meningitis-producing strains of meningococci; the presence of the antibodies is protective against this form of bacterial meningitis. Contrariwise, it is possible for antibodies cross-reactive to microbial antigens to play an insidiously harmful role in health. For instance, the serious disease systemic lupus erythematosus is associated with the production of antibodies against one's own DNA. Some evidence shows the antigens that set off the production of these antibodies are not nucleic acids but may be cross-reacting bacterial lipopolysaccharides.

Keeping Out Invaders

In some sites of the body, the normal flora keeps out pathogens. Commensal bacteria have the physical advantage of **previous occupancy**, especially on epithelial surfaces. Some commensal bacteria produce substances that inhibit newcomers, such as antibiotics or lethal proteins called bacteriocins. It is not surprising, therefore, that colonization by a new species or a new strain is not a frequent event.

This long known fact became relevant once again in the 1970s in connection with experiments performed to assess the safety of new bacterial strains engineered by molecular cloning. The most commonly used organism for this purpose was (and probably still is) a particular strain of *E. coli* called K12. This strain was originally isolated from a person's feces, but has had a long residence in the laboratory. When human volunteers were fed this strain in large numbers, they retained it for only one day. The conventional interpretation is that during its sojourn in the laboratory the strain had lost its colonizing capacity. In other words, this strain can no longer out-compete the resident members of the bacterial flora of the gut.

When the normal flora is nearly wiped out with antibiotics, both exogenous and endogenous microorganisms are given the opportunity to cause disease. For example, the infecting oral dose of a *Salmonella* strain decreases almost a millionfold after mice are given streptomycin. Patients treated with antibiotics that are particularly effective in the gut may suffer from diarrhea, due to the toxins produced from the overgrowth of a particular organism, *Clostridium difficile*. Severe infections with this bacterium result in a serious disease called pseudomembranous colitis (see Chapter 21). This organism is a minor member of the normal flora but can grow to a large population density when its neighbors are suppressed.

A Role in Human Nutrition and Metabolism?

The normal flora of the intestine plays a role in human nutrition and metabolism, but little is known about the extent of this influence. Why has it proved difficult to investigate this role? Obviously, humans cannot be made "germ-free" at will; most of the information comes from work with animals, and its relevance to human nutrition is uncertain. Nonetheless, it is likely that a biomass as huge and metabolically active as that in the large intestine plays a role in the nutritional balance of the host. It is known, for instance, that several intestinal bacteria, like *E. coli* and *Bacteroides* species, synthesize vitamin K, which may be an important source of this vitamin for human beings and animals.

The metabolism of several key compounds involves excretion from the liver into the intestine and their return from there to the liver. This enterohepatic circulatory loop is particularly important for sex steroid hormones and bile salts. These substances are excreted through the bile in conjugated form as glucuronides or sulfates but cannot be reabsorbed in this form. Members of the intestinal bacterial flora make glucuronidases and sulfatases that deconjugate these compounds. The extent to which these activities are physiologically important is not yet known.

A Source of Carcinogens?

The flora of the large intestine may produce **carcinogens**. The compounds we ingest are chemically transformed by the varied metabolic activities of the gut flora. Many potential carcinogens are active only after being modified. Some of the known modifications are carried out by enzymes of intestinal bacteria. An example is the artificial sweetener cyclamate (cyclohexamine sulfate) which is converted to the active bladder carcinogen cyclohexamine by bacterial sulfatases. The importance of the normal flora in production of carcinogens is difficult to assess, but is a subject of considerable scrutiny (Box 2.1).

BOX 2.1. HOW DO WE STUDY THE NORMAL FLORA ?

Much of what we know about the role of the normal flora in nutrition and prevention of disease comes from studying animals reared under sterile conditions, the so-called germ free animals. Rats and mice resemble humans in many physiological properties but differ in important details. Nonetheless, germ-free animal research has produced interesting information.

Small mammals can be reared in the germ-free condition if they are placed in a sterile chamber after a cesarean birth. Chickens can be hatched from eggs whose shell surfaces have been sterilized. The germ-free chamber is provided with gloves and ports to allow manipulation and the exchange of food and other material without breaking the sterile barrier. Many species of animals breed under these conditions and large colonies can be established. It is even possible to obtain germ-free rats and mice from commercial suppliers.

In general, rodents thrive under germ-free conditions as long as their diet is supplemented with vitamins. They even gain weight faster than do conventional animals. As expected, their concentration of immunoglobulins is reduced, especially if the diet is chemically defined and does not contain antigenic compounds. One of the more interesting characteristics of germ-free animals is that the histology of their intestines is quite different from the usual. The most visible difference is in the lamina propria which has only a few lymphocytes, plasma cells, and macrophages. By contrast, in conventional animals, the same tissue is heavily infiltrated with these cells. This finding suggests that the "normal" intestine is in a constant state of chronic inflammation!

THE MEMBERS OF THE NORMAL FLORA

What types of microorganisms constitute the normal flora? The vast majority are bacteria. We also carry viruses, fungi, protozoa, and occasionally worms, but in the healthy person these microorganisms are present in smaller numbers than the bacteria. In the early days of microbiology, it was thought that most bacteria of the body were aerobes or facultative anaerobes. For a long time E. coli was believed to be one of the principal members of the fecal flora. This erroneous conclusion was due to the fact that most of the members of the normal bacteria flora are strict anaerobes and do not grow on media incubated in the ordinary manner in air. Only by using special techniques of anaerobic cultivation has it been realized that in the gingival pocket or in feces, strict anaerobes outnumber the others by 100 to 1 or more. Bacteria do not have to be located far from the air to find themselves under anaerobic conditions, because oxygen has very low solubility in water. Furthermore, the few molecules of oxygen that diffuse into deeper tissue layers are readily used by host cells or by actively metabolizing aerobes and facultative anaerobes. Thus, anaerobic conditions can be found a fraction of a millimeter below the surface.

Table 2.2 shows the distribution and occurrence of the most prominent bacteria in selected parts of the human body. It should be understood that the organisms listed, although the most frequently encountered, represent only a minute fraction of the number of genera and species represented. The total number of taxonomic groups is probably well in the thousands. As an example, in a particularly detailed study, the intestinal flora of a single person alone yielded about 400 distinct species of bacteria.

Newborn babies become colonized very rapidly by a varied microbial flora, especially in their intestine. In animals and probably in humans, different organisms appear according to a specific time sequence. The earliest colonizers are E. coli, streptococci, and some clostridia.

Table 2.2. The Normal Bacterial Flora

| | Examples of frequent types | | | | |
| | Gram-positive | | Gram-negative | | |
	Cocci	Rods	Cocci	Rods	Others
Skin	*Staphylococcus*	*Corynebacterium*, *Propionibacterium acnes*		Enteric bacilli (on some sites)	
Oropharynx	α-Hemolytic streptococci, *Micrococcus*	*Corynebacterium*	*Neisseria*	*Haemophilus*	Spirochetes
Large intestine	*Streptococcus* (enterococci)	*Lactobacillus* *Clostridium*		*Bacteroides* Enteric bacilli	
Vagina	*Streptococcus*	*Lactobacillus*		*Bacteroides*	*Mycoplasma*

Within 24 hours or so, lactobacilli appear and are followed within a few days by the major anaerobes that characterize the normal intestinal flora.

Little is known about why different species vary in their colonizing capacity and in their ability to compete with others. It seems likely that specific properties of bacteria, such as their pili, allow them to attach and survive in different microenvironments within the intestine. Thus, the microbial flora is different at the base of the intestinal crypts, in the mucus that covers the villi, or in the lumen of the gut. Normally, the intestinal flora of one individual is remarkably constant. This stability suggests that each successful colonizer is equipped with powerful devices to withstand the challenge from newly ingested microorganisms

CONCLUSION

Our knowledge about the role of the normal flora in health and disease is derived largely from a few circumstances of uncertain significance: studies with germ-free animals, observation of patients on antibiotics, etc. We are left with the impression that from the immunological and microbiological point of view, the normal flora contributes to the maintenance of health mainly by excluding potential invaders and possibly by long-term immunological stimulation. Nutritionally speaking, the microbial biomass within us plays a role in recycling certain important compounds and probably in supplying vitamin K. However, members of the normal flora are opportunistic pathogens and may cause disease when present in unaccustomed tissues and organs. We do not have the choice of living in a germ-free environment. In a microbe-laden world, it is reasonable to conclude that the normal microbial flora is adapted to do more good than harm.

SELF-ASSESSMENT QUESTIONS

1. Name some infections caused by members of the normal flora and the factors that allow them to cause disease.
2. What is the immunological significance of the normal flora?
3. How does the normal flora ward off colonization by external pathogens?
4. Which portions of the body are usually heavily colonized? Which have a transient microbial flora? Which are usually sterile? What main factors dictate these ecological relationships?
5. Which main groups of bacteria are associated with the heavily colonized parts of the body?
6. What general strategies are available to study the role of the normal flora?

SUGGESTED READINGS

Rosebury T. Life on man. New York: Viking Press, 1969. (A delightful popularization.)

Biology of Infectious Agents

MOSELIO SCHAECHTER

WHAT DO WE WANT TO KNOW ABOUT MICROORGANISMS?

Mainly, we want to know how pathogenic microorganisms harm the host and what we can do about it. This requires more than understanding how they cause disease. For example, features of bacterial anatomy and metabolism have suggested targets for the successful development of powerful antibiotics. Similarly, unraveling details of viral structures and metabolism has led to the production of protective vaccines and to the beginnings of antiviral therapy.

PROKARYOTIC AND EUKARYOTIC PATHOGENS

The world of pathogenic microbiology spans the largest cleft in the living world, that between the prokaryotes and the eukaryotes. Bacteria belong to the prokaryotes, whereas fungi, protozoa, and worms are eukaryotes. Prokaryotes lack nuclei and other internal membrane-bound organelles. They do not carry out endocytosis and are incapable of ingesting particles or liquid droplets. Prokaryotes differ from eukaryotes in important biochemical details, such as the composition of their ribosomes and lipids (Fig. 3.1). Prokaryotes are usually haploid, with a single chromosome and extra-chromosomal plasmids; eukaryotes have a diploid phase and many chromosomes.

Differences in organization between prokaryotes and eukaryotes have important consequences for the way they synthesize certain macromolecules. For instance, the lack of a nuclear membrane allows prokaryotes to simultaneously synthesize proteins and messenger. In other words, translation can be coupled to transcription and begin rapidly on new mRNA chains. In eukaryotes the two processes cannot be directly linked. Transcripts of heterogeneous nuclear RNA must first be processed in the nucleus before they are transported across the nuclear membrane to the ribosomes in the cytoplasm. Only then can eukaryotic protein synthesis take place.

Table 3.1 compares the regulation of gene expression between *Escherichia coli*, a bacterium, and the best known of the unicellular eukaryotes, a yeast. A review of basic biochemistry and molecular biology may be appropriate to understand this material.

PROBLEMS OF UNICELLULARITY

Unicellular organisms, such as bacteria and yeasts, face constant challenges in their environment. The demands made on microorganisms fall into three general categories: **nutrition**, related to the intermittent availability of food; **occupancy**, related to the need to remain in a certain habitat; **resistance** to damaging agents.

A Life of Feast or Famine

Frequently in their existence, microorganisms run out of nutrients. Consider a bacterium that lives in the large intestine of human beings. Every so often, some 20 times a day on average, the ileocecal valve opens and nutrient-rich contents squirt from the small intestine into the cecum. Here, a large bacterial flora rapidly consumes the nutrients, and soon the bacteria are once again deprived of food. Clearly, the different bacteria normally present at this site have adapted to a life of feast and famine. On the one hand, they are able to rapidly utilize nutritional substrates when they become available and to compete efficiently with their microbial neighbors. On the other hand, they have adapted to the lack of nutrients during periods of starvation and also are poised for action whenever nutrients again become plentiful. Two themes emerge in the evolution of such organisms: **efficiency** and **adaptability**. We will see how these two properties are manifested in bacteria.

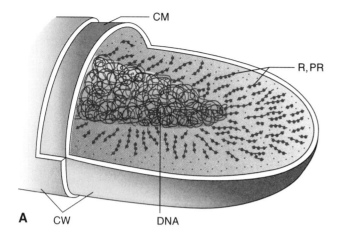

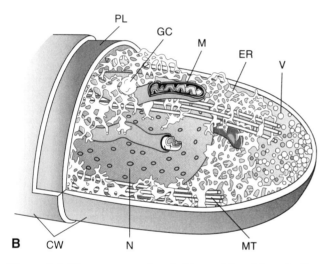

Figure 3.1. Ultrastructure of typical bacterial and fungal cells. **A.** Inside the cell wall (*CW*) and membrane (*CM*), a bacterium is filled with ribosomes (*R*), polyribosomes (*PR*), and proteins. DNA fibrils cluster near the center of the cell in a coiled mass. **B.** The cell wall (*CW*) and plasmalemma (*PL*) of a hyphal tip surround the Golgi complex (*GC*), mitochondria (*M*), vacuoles (*V*), endoplasmic reticulum (*ER*), microtubules (*MT*), and nucleus (*N*) characteristic of the eukaryotic cell.

Colonization and Occupancy

Not all problems in the microbial world are nutritional. In certain environments, such as the intestinal tract, survival depends on being able to remain in a given place and avoid being swept away by liquid currents. Many species of bacteria ensure their occupancy by using mechanisms designed to stick to surfaces. For instance, bacteria attach to the surface of teeth by elaborating adhesive polysaccharides. When polysaccharides build up sufficiently, they form dental plaque. Likewise, in the intestine the abundant microbial flora that adheres to the epithelial wall is different from the one that lives free in the lumen. Note that the "wall" flora faces

different nutritional problems from the "lumen" flora and, consequently, that the selective pressures on these two populations are very different.

Resistance to Damaging Agents

Microorganisms often encounter chemical or physical agents that threaten their existence. Not unexpectedly, they have evolved mechanisms that allow them to cope with these life-threatening challenges. Among the better studied are structural devices and physiological responses that protect microorganisms (up to a point) from such environmental insults as membrane-damaging chemicals, heat, or DNA-damaging radiation. Microorganisms also use genetic strategies to withstand antibiotics and can develop resistance to these substances in a number of ways (see Chapter 5, "Antibacterial Action"). Attempts to rid tissues of pathogenic organisms through the use of antibiotics are counteracted by the mechanisms developed by the organisms to thwart these efforts.

SMALL SIZE PROMOTES METABOLIC EFFICIENCY

The microbial world is composed of small entities, generally below the range of what the unaided human eye can see. Consequently, large numbers can be packed in small volumes. Typical bacteria are of the order of 1 μm in diameter and, if they were shaped like tiny blocks and neatly stacked, 10^{12} would occupy 1 cubic centimeter and weigh about 1 gram. In suspension the turbidity contributed by such small particles is so minimal that a clear fluid like urine becomes visibly cloudy only when bacteria exceed about 1 to 10 million per ml. Each of us currently carries a load of some **10 to 100 trillion** bacteria in our large intestine, greatly surpassing the number of our own eukaryotic cells.

Being small allows microorganisms high metabolic rates because the surface to volume ratio increases as the size of cells decreases. Ultimately, the rate of biochemical reactions is limited by diffusion, and the smaller the cells, the less limiting it is. Consequently, bacteria are in intimate contact with external nutrients and are capable of metabolic rates orders of magnitude higher than those of eukaryotic cells. They can grow extremely fast and some double once every 15 minutes under optimal conditions. One measure of the rapidity of their metabolic flux is that small metabolites (amino acids, sugars and nucleotides—the building blocks of macromolecules) constitute only about 1% of their total dry weight. Some unicellular eukaryotes, such as yeasts and other fungi, have comparable efficiency.

The amazing speed with which these small cells convert nutrients into energy and biosynthetic building blocks requires the coordination of metabolic activities.

Table 3.1. Transcription/Processing of mRNA in Typical Prokaryotes and Eukaryotes

	Escherichia coli (Prokaryote)	Yeast (Eukaryote)
Genomic structure		
Genome organization	Single gene copies	Single gene copies plus repetitive DNA
Chromosomes	One	Many
Ploidy	Haploid	Haploid/diploid cycle
"Cytoplasmic" DNA	Plasmids	Mitochondria, kinetoplasts
Colinearity of gene with mRNA	Precise sequence	Introns within gene
Regulation of gene expression		
Type	Operon-polycistronic mRNA	Single genes
Level	Mostly transcriptional	Often post-transcriptional regulation by protein turnover, etc.
Transcription		
Relation of transcription and translation	Coupled	Uncoupled
mRNA processing	Rare; some cleavages at double-stranded functional domains	Poly(A) at 3'-end, cap at 5'-end; splicing, sites in mRNA
mRNA stability	Unstable	Range of stability; some very stable mRNAs
Translation of mRNA		
First amino acid	Formylated methionine	Methionine
Signal for start	Ribosome binding site preceding AUG	Binding to 5'-end, use of first AUG along mRNA
Initiation factors	Three	>Six
Ribosomes	30S + 50S = 70S "Bacterial" inhibitors	40S + 60S = 80S "Eukaryotic" inhibitors

Features of cell structure and macromolecular synthesis help us to understand how individual species of bacteria maximize their chances for survival and suggest how we may intervene therapeutically against pathogenic organisms and anticipate their defenses.

BACTERIA HAVE COMPLEX ENVELOPES AND APPENDAGES

Going from the outside inwards, bacteria are surrounded by a complex set of surface layers and appendages that differ in composition from species to species. Some of these structures are useful in certain environments only, such as the human body, and may be dispensable under laboratory conditions. These surface components often determine whether an organism can survive in a particular environment and cause disease.

Like all cells, bacteria have an essential structure, the **cytoplasmic membrane**. Most bacteria also possess structures outside the membrane, namely a **cell wall** and some, an **"outer membrane," flagella, pili,** and a **capsule.** These structures can amount to 10 to 20% of the dry weight of the cell (as in other organisms, the wet weight of bacteria is about two-thirds water). The reason for the extra layers outside the cell membrane becomes clear if one considers the stresses that bacteria must face in natural surroundings. For example, intestinal bacteria such as *E. coli* are exposed to bile salts that would dissolve an unprotected cell membrane. Envelope layers and appendages are used by bacteria to adhere to surfaces and also for protection from phagocytes and other threats.

During microbial colonization by microorganisms, the immune system of the host first senses the surface components of the invading microorganisms. Consequently, many of the properties of the surface components are relevant both to the establishment of infection and to the response of the host to the organisms. The strongest antibody response to bacterial antigens is usually directed to surface antigens.

PROTECTION OF THE CYTOPLASMIC MEMBRANE

Bacteria use three principal means to protect their cytoplasmic membrane from environmental stresses, such as low osmotic pressure or the presence of detergents. These solutions are represented by the **Gram-positive, Gram-negative,** and **acid-fast** bacteria. Figure 3.2 illustrates the first two.

The Gram stain (named after an early Danish microbiologist) divides most bacteria into two groups, nearly equal in number and importance. This staining procedure is central in microbiology and, in due course, must

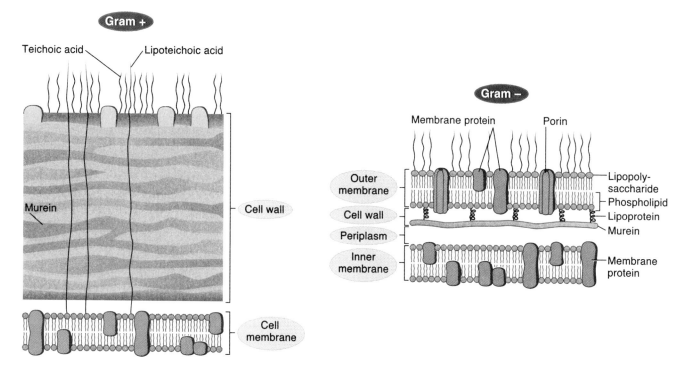

Figure 3.2. The envelope structure of a Gram-positive (*left*) and a Gram-negative (*right*). *OM*, outer membrane; *LP*, lipoprotein; *CM*, cytoplasmic membrane; *PL*, phospholipids. Capsules and appendages are not shown, nor are surface proteins like the M protein of streptococci indicated. Note the 20-fold greater amount of peptidoglycan in the Gram-positive. The outer membrane of the Gram-negative envelopes shows O antigen polysaccharide molecules covering the outer layer. The outer membrane has pores made of trimers of porin, which permit the entry of small hydrophilic molecules.

Table 3.2. Gram Stain and Acid-fast Procedures

Gram stain	Acid–fast stain
1. Stain with crystal violet (purple)	1. Stain with hot carbol–fuchsin (red).
2. Modify with potassium iodide	
3. Decolorize with alcohol; only Gram-positives remain purple	2. Decolorize with acid alcohol; only acid-fast remain red.
4. Counterstain with safranin: Gram-negatives become pink; Gram-positives remain purple	3. Counterstain with methylene blue: acid-fast remain red; others become blue.

---

be learned by every medical student. In brief, Gram staining depends on the ability of certain bacteria (the Gram-positives) to retain a complex of a purple dye and iodine when challenged with a brief alcohol wash (Table 3.2). Gram-negatives do not retain the dye and can later be counterstained with a dye of a different color, usually red. This distinction turns out to be correlated with fundamental differences in the cell envelope of these two classes of bacteria.

The Gram-positive Solution

Gram-positive bacteria protect their cytoplasmic membrane with a thick **cell wall**. The major constituent of the wall is a complex polymer **unique to bacteria**, composed of sugars and amino acids called **murein** or **peptidoglycan** (Fig. 3.3). Murein is the critical component in maintaining the shape and rigidity of both Gram-positives and Gram-negatives, but plays a larger role in protecting the cell membrane of Gram-positives.

How does murein contribute to the defense of cell integrity? Murein is composed of glycan (sugar) chains that are cross-linked to one another via peptides. The overall structure is similar in all cases, but differs somewhat in chemical details (Fig. 3.4). This polymeric fabric is wrapped around the length and width of the bacterium to form a sac of the size and shape of the organism. Depending on the shape of the murein sac, bacteria may be shaped like rods (**bacilli**), spheres (**cocci**), or helices (**spirilla**). The rigid murein corset allows bacteria to survive in media of lesser osmotic pressure than that of their cytoplasm. In the absence of a rigid corsetlike structure to push against, the membrane bursts and the cells lyse. This can be demonstrated experimentally by removing the murein with **lysozyme**, a hydrolytic enzyme present in many human and animal tissues. Treatment with lysozyme causes bacteria to lyse in a low-

N-acetylmuramic acid
N-acetylglucosamine
Cross-linked
peptide

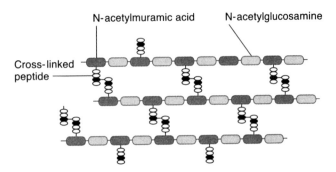

Figure 3.3. Structure of murein. The polysaccharide (glycan) strands consist of alternating units of N-acetyl glucosamine and N-acetyl muramic acid connected to a peptide. Some of the peptides of one strand are cross-linked to those of another. As the result of cross-linking, murein has a two-dimensional structure resembling that of a chain-linked fence. Diaminopimelic acid molecules, shown in *black*, are among the unique chemicals of murein.

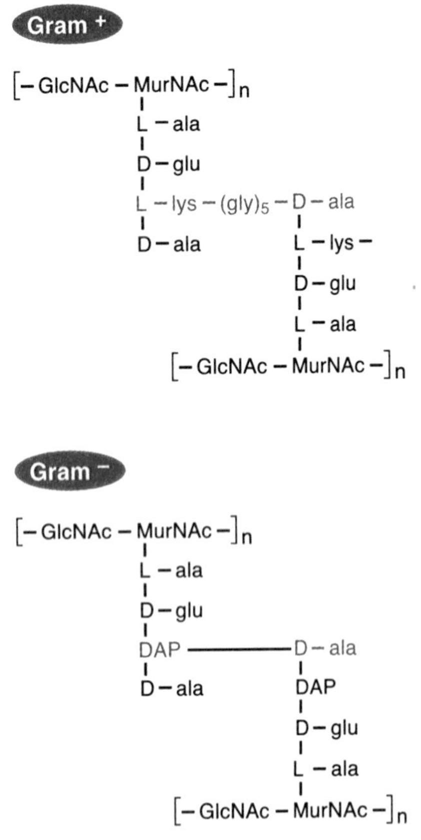

Gram +
[–GlcNAc – MurNAc –]n
L – ala
D – glu
L – lys – (gly)5 – D – ala
D – ala
L – lys –
D – glu
L – ala
[– GlcNAc – MurNAc –]n
Gram −
[– GlcNAc – MurNAc –]n
L – ala
D – glu
DAP
D – ala
D – ala
DAP
D – glu
L – ala
[– GlcNAc – MurNAc –]n

Figure 3.4. Typical composition of murein in Gram-positive and Gram-negative bacteria. In Gram-positives, peptide chains are cross-linked through a peptide (a pentaglycine in *Staphylococcus aureus*) between the free amino group of lysine and the terminal carboxyl group of a D-ala residue. In the Gram-negatives, the cross-link is between diaminopimelic acid and D-ala.

osmotic-pressure environment. If lysozyme-treated bacteria are kept in an isoosmotic medium, they do not lyse but become spherical. Such structures are called **spheroplasts.**

The cell wall of Gram-positives is composed of many layers of the saclike murein, so thick that they impede the passage of hydrophobic compounds. This is because the sugars and charged amino acids of murein make this a highly polar compound. As a result, the cells are surrounded by a dense hydrophilic layer. Thus, many Gram-positives can withstand certain noxious hydrophobic compounds, including the bile salts in the intestine. The feature that makes bacteria Gram-positive—the ability to retain the dye–iodine complex —also seems to depend on the characteristic murein structure of the Gram-positive wall.

Gram-positive walls contain other unique polymers, such as **teichoic acids,** which are chains of ribitol or glycerol linked by phosphodiester bonds (Fig. 3.5). Teichoic acids will be discussed in connection with individual groups of bacteria because at least some of them appear to play a role in pathogenesis.

The Gram-negative Solution

Gram-negatives have adopted a radically different solution to the problem of protection of the cytoplasmic membrane. These bacteria make a completely different structure, an **outer membrane,** which is built up outside the murein cell wall (see Fig. 3.2). The outer membrane is chemically distinct from the usual biological membranes and has built into it the ability to resist damaging chemicals. It is a bilayered structure, but its outer leaflet contains a unique component in addition to phospholipids. This component is a **bacterial lipopolysaccharide or LPS.** LPS is a complex molecule not found elsewhere in nature and one that deserves further attention.

CH2OH
ROC
CH2O
OCH2
ROC
CH2O
Murein
HCO – ala
HCOH
HCO – glu
Murein

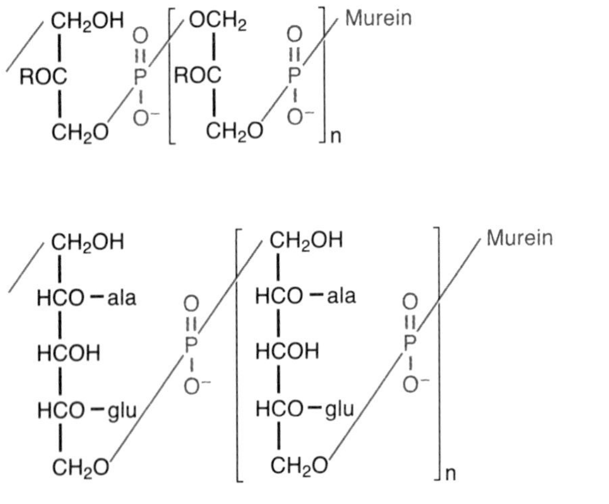

Figure 3.5. Teichoic acid structure. The repeating unit of ribitol and glycerol teichoic acids are shown. The chains in Gram-positive organisms vary in length and amounts.

Bacterial lipopolysaccharide

LPS consist of three components (Fig. 3.6):

- **Lipid A.** This lipid anchors LPS in the outer leaflet of the membrane. Lipid A is an unusual glycolipid composed of disaccharides to which are attached short-chain fatty acids and phosphate groups.
- **The core.** This component consists of a short series of sugars which are nearly the same in most Gram-negative bacteria and includes two characteristic sugars, **keto-deoxyoctanoic acid** (KDO in Fig. 3.6) and a **heptose.**
- **The O antigen.** This is a long carbohydrate chain, up to 40 sugars in length (see Fig. 3.6). The hydrophilic carbohydrate chains of the O antigen cover the bacterial surface and exclude hydrophobic compounds. The importance of the O antigen chains is shown with mutants deficient in their biosynthesis. Mutants that make either no O antigen or merely shortened chains become sensitive to hydrophobic compounds such as bile salts and antibiotics to which the wild type is resistant.

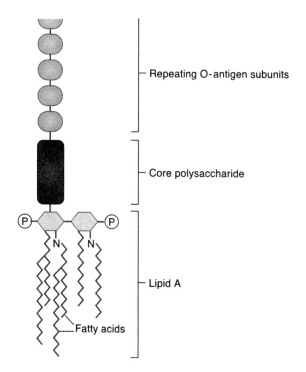

Figure 3.6. The structure of lipopolysaccharide (LPS). LPS consist of three portions: **Lipid A,** a phosphorylated disaccharide to which fatty acids are attached. The fatty acids vary with the organism, but are always responsible for the hydrophobicity of the molecule. In a typical *Salmonella*, region I shows a characteristic series of sugars in the polysaccharide. The **core polysaccharide,** which consists of a variable and an invariant portion. The **O-antigen,** made up of repeating sugar subunits. This portion is highly variable and is the main reason for the different antigenic specificities among Gram-negative bacteria.

Thus, exclusion of hydrophobic compounds in Gram-negative bacteria, as in Gram-positive bacteria, relies on surrounding the cells with hydrophilic polysaccharides, but these polysaccharides differ in structure and organization in the two groups. Because of its lipid nature, the outer membrane could be expected to exclude hydrophilic compounds as well. Seemingly nothing could then cross the outer membrane. Thus, by dealing with the problem of protection of the cytoplasmic membrane, the Gram-negative bacteria appear to have created a new one. How do they transport their nutrients? One solution to this problem would be to use the same active transport devices of the cytoplasmic membrane copied in the outer membrane. However, this solution would not only be wasteful but would probably be incompatible with the protective role assigned to the outer membrane. Once again, bacteria have found an interesting solution: the outer membrane has special **channels** that permit the passive diffusion of hydrophilic compounds like sugars, amino acids, and certain ions. These channels consist of protein molecules with holes, aptly called **porins.** Porin channels are narrow—just the right size to permit the entry of compounds up to 600–700 daltons (Fig. 3.2). The channels are small enough that hydrophobic compounds come in contact with the polar "wall" of the channel and are thereby excluded.

Certain **hydrophilic** compounds that are sometimes necessary for survival are larger than the exclusion limit of porins. These larger molecules include vitamin B_{12}, sugars larger than trisaccharides, and iron in the form of chelates. Such compounds cross the outer membrane by separate, specific permeation mechanisms that utilize proteins especially designed to translocate each of these compounds. Thus the outer membrane allows the passage of small hydrophilic compounds, excludes hydrophobic compounds, large or small, and allows the entry of some larger hydrophilic molecules by especially dedicated mechanisms.

The dual-membrane system of Gram-negative bacteria creates a compartment called the **periplasmic space** or **periplasm** on the outside of the cytoplasmic or inner membrane. This compartment contains the murein layer and a gel-like solution of components that facilitate nutrition. These include degradative enzymes (phosphatases, nucleases, proteases, etc.) that break down large and impermeable molecules to "digestible" size. In addition, the periplasm contains so-called **binding proteins** that help soak up sugars and amino acids from the medium. It also contains enzymes that inactivate antibiotics such as penicillins and cephalosporins, the β-lactamases. The Gram-positive bacteria do not have a defined periplasmic compartment and secrete similar enzymes into the medium.

The outer membrane barrier constitutes both a seeming advantage and a disadvantage to Gram-negative bacteria. For example, some bacteriophages use proteins in the outer membrane as attachment sites for infecting their host bacteria. On the other hand, the outer membrane confers considerable resistance to many antibiotics. Broadly speaking, Gram-negative bacteria are more resistant to many antibiotics, especially penicillin. The peculiarly Gram-negative solution to the problems of protecting the cytoplasmic membrane has unexpected biological consequences. The lipopolysaccharide of the outer membrane is highly reactive in the host. The lipid A component has a large number of biological activities. It elicits fever and activates a series of immunological and biochemical events that lead to the mobilization of host defense mechanisms. In large doses, this compound, also known as **endotoxin**, can cause shock and even death (see Chapter 9, "Damage"). The O antigen portion, as the name denotes, is highly antigenic. O antigens come in many varieties, each defining a species or a subspecies of Gram-negative bacteria.

The Acid-fast Solution

A few bacterial types, notably the tubercle bacillus, have developed yet another solution to the problems of environmental challenge to the cytoplasmic membrane. Their cell walls contain large amounts of **waxes**, which are complex long-chain hydrocarbons with sugars and other modifying groups. Having such a protective cover, these organisms are impervious to many harsh chemicals, including acids. If a dye is introduced into these cells, for instance, by brief heating, it cannot be removed by dilute hydrochloric acid, as would be the case in all other bacteria. These organisms are therefore called acid-fast or acid-resistant (Table 3.2).

The waxy coat is interlaced with murein, polysaccharides and lipids. It enables the organisms to resist the action of many noxious chemicals as well as killing by white blood cells. All this is at a cost; these organisms grow very slowly, possibly because the rate of uptake of nutrients is limited by their waxy covering. Some, like the human tubercle bacillus, divide once every 24 hours.

MUREIN AND ANTIBIOTICS THAT INHIBIT ITS SYNTHESIS

The uniqueness of bacterial murein makes it a natural target for antibiotics. Drugs that block its formation lead to lysis and death of susceptible bacteria. It is not surprising, therefore, that some of the clinically most effective antibiotics, the **penicillins** and the **cephalosporins**, act by inhibiting murein synthesis. They are among the most unequivocally bactericidal antibiotics and among those least toxic to humans. The critical steps in their mode of action is presented in Figure 3.7.

Murein, like many other polysaccharides, is synthesized from nucleotide-bound building blocks. These monomeric units are composed of uridine diphosphate

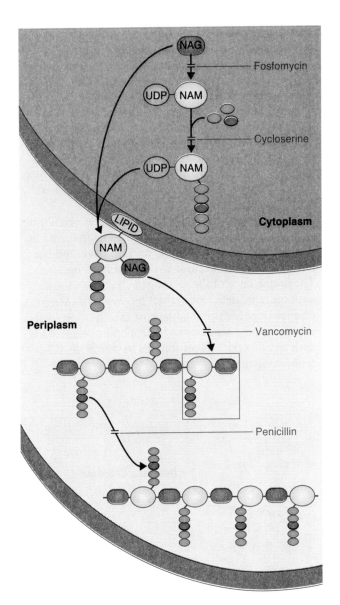

Figure 3.7. Biosynthesis of murein, indicating the site of action of a number of antibiotics. The successive steps occurring in the cytoplasm, at the cytoplasmic membrane, and outside the membrane (in the periplasm of Gram-negatives; in the murein layer of Gram-positives) are indicated, along with the points of attack of cycloserine, bacitracin, vancomycin, and penicillin.

plus either N-acetylglucosamine (GlcNAc) or N-acetyl muramic acid (an unusual sugar, the 3-O-*D* lactic acid derivative of GlcNAc). The latter has a peptide chain attached to it (Fig. 3.3). The monomeric units are made in the cytoplasm and transferred from uridine-diphosphate to a **lipid carrier** in the membrane (Fig. 3.7). Disaccharides are then linked to a growing chain of murein. This step is inhibited by the antibiotic **vancomycin**. Regeneration of the lipid carrier is inhibited by another antibiotic, **bacitracin**.

The final reaction in murein synthesis is transpeptidation. The long chains of disaccharides are cross-linked to make a two dimensional network (Fig. 3.3). The cross-linking reaction consists of forming a peptide bond between D-alanine on one chain and the free N-end of a lysine or a diaminopimelic acid on the other chain. The linkage is formed with the **subterminal** D-alanine, and the **terminal** D-alanine is cleaved away in the process. Thus, the reaction is the exchange of one peptide bond (that between the two D-alanines) with another—a true transpeptidation. **Cycloserine** is an antibiotic that inhibits the ligation of the two D-alanine residues and also inhibits the racemase that forms D-alanine from L-alanine, the common constituent of proteins. The amino acids that make up the peptides vary in different organisms but the D-alanine cross-bridge to either lysine or diaminopimelic acid is universal. This reaction is inhibited by most penicillins and cephalosporins.

The reason why penicillin inhibits transpeptidation may lie in its stereochemical similarity with the D-alanine-D-alanine dimer (Figs. 3.8 and 3.9). In the presence of the drug, the transpeptidase becomes confused: instead of synthesizing an intermediate D-alanine–enzyme complex, it makes a lethal penicilloyl–enzyme complex.

Antibiotics that inhibit murein synthesis almost invariably kill bacteria by lysing them. In contrast with lysozyme, these drugs do not affect murein itself, only its synthesis. How then do they cause lysis? Cells treated with these drugs continue to synthesize their cytoplasmic components and increase in mass. The enlarged cytoplasm is not restrained by a properly cross-linked murein sac, with the result that the cell contents extrude and the cells lyse. Cells that are not growing are not lysed by penicillin—they are not increasing in mass. Consider: would it be advisable to administer an antibiotic that inhibits cell growth at the same time that the patient is receiving penicillin?

Penicillins and cephalosporins have an unusual prop-erty; they bind covalently to certain proteins of the cytoplasmic membrane, the so-called **penicillin binding proteins** (PBPs). These drugs are especially reactive because they have a highly strained β-lactam ring that can be readily hydrolyzed. Individual species of bacteria have a characteristic set of PBPs, each with a different affinity for a given penicillin. These proteins are thought to be involved in the cross-linking of murein. At least three types of PBPs have been distinguished: one seems to be especially involved in the generalized cross-linking that occurs at many points in the periphery of the cell. Another may participate in the special cross-linking at the junction (septum) between separating daughter cells. The third appears to function at points where the nascent murein "turns corners" to determine cell shape. The functional distinction between PBPs has been facilitated by a penicillin called **mecillinam** which binds to only one of these proteins (Fig. 3.9). Mecillinam blocks only part of murein cross-linking, and leads to the release of constraints on the cell shape of *E. coli*. This results in the formation of large, unstable spherical cells that slowly lyse. In mutants resistant to mecillinam, this particular PBP is modified and no longer binds β-lactam antibiotics. These mutants remain susceptible to penicillins that bind to other PBPs.

The simple concept that cells lyse by outgrowing their coats encounters some difficulties. First, in cultures treated with penicillin there is usually a small number of "persisters," bacteria that stop growing but do not lyse. Second, for some types of bacteria, penicillin is bacteriostatic, not bactericidal. These bacteria are called "tolerant." How do we explain "persisters" or "tolerant" bacteria? It appears that tolerant organisms are deficient in

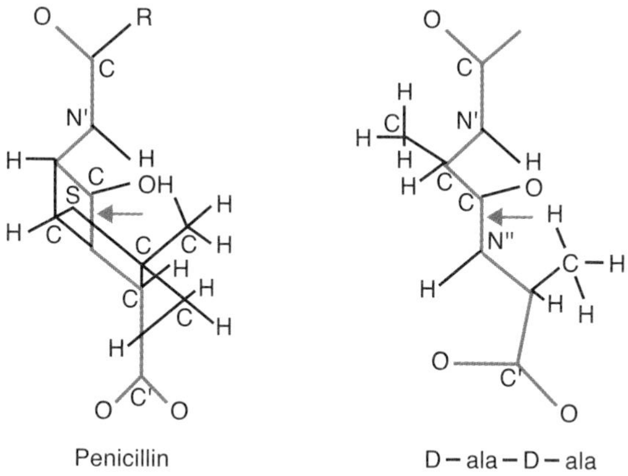

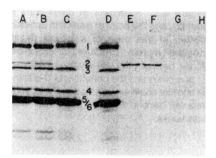

Figure 3.9. Binding of penicillin to membrane proteins (PBPs) of wild-type and mecillinam-resistant *E. coli*. Radioactive penicillin binds to a number of proteins. In the resistant mutant, the only protein to which mecillinam binds is missing. ^{14}C-labeled benzylpenicillin (*A–D*) or mecillinam (*E–H*) were bound to cell envelopes from a wild-type strain and one resistant to mecillinam. The inner membranes were solubilized in detergent and the radioactive proteins separated by gel electrophoresis and detected by autoradiography. Benzylpenicillin binds to 6 PBPs in wild-type cells (*A–B*) and five in the mutant (*C–D*); mecillinam binds only to one protein in the wild type (*E–F*) and not at all in the mutant (*G–H*).

Figure 3.8. The resemblance of part of the penicillin structure to the backbone of D-ala-D-ala is indicated, with the arrows at the bonds broken during covalent attachment to the enzyme involved.

an **autolysin**, a bacterial enzyme that cleaves murein. Bacteria use such an enzyme to break open some bonds of murein at the septum, which permits the separation of daughter cells during cell division. Normally the activity of autolysin is tightly controlled. Treatment with penicillin may arouse it to more unrestrained action. The role of autolysin in penicillin-induced lysis is well illustrated with pneumococci, which are extraordinarily susceptible to lysis. Autolysin-defective mutants are found among penicillin-resistant derivatives; these mutants are not lysed even by strong detergents. Thus, bacteria do not burst easily. Rather than a spontaneous explosion, lysis involves active steps of self-destruction.

There are exceptions to the universal use of murein to maintain bacterial cell integrity. The mycoplasmas are a group of bacteria that have no murein and consequently are not rigid and have almost no defined shape. As expected, they are resistant to penicillin. Some, like an agent of pneumonia, *Mycoplasma pneumoniae,* contain sterols in their membrane, an unusual feature among prokaryotes. It is puzzling how mycoplasmas cope well without a rigid cell wall. Although these organisms are quite delicate in culture, they are common in the human body and in the environment. There are other exceptions to the ubiquity of mureins, especially among a separate of group of bacteria known as the *Archaea.* Thus, there are unorthodox and as yet poorly understood means by which some bacteria safeguard their integrity.

THE CYTOPLASMIC MEMBRANE

The cytoplasmic membrane of bacteria is a busy place. It assumes functions that in eukaryotic cells are divided up among the plasma membrane and intracellular organelles. Most critical is its role in the uptake of substrates from the medium. Bacteria take up mainly small-molecular-weight compounds and only rarely macromolecules and phosphate esters. These compounds are usually hydrolyzed by enzymes in the periplasm or the surrounding medium, and the resulting breakdown products, e.g., peptides, oligosaccharides, nucleosides, phosphate, etc. can then be transported across the cytoplasmic membrane.

The cytoplasmic membrane contains specific carrier proteins called **permeases** that facilitate the entry of most metabolites. In some cases the carrier facilitates the equilibration of a compound inside and outside the cell (Fig. 3.10). However, in most cases carrier-mediated transport requires the expenditure of energy. This permits the internal concentration of certain substances to be as much as 10^5 times higher than that in the medium surrounding the cell.

Transport Across the Cytoplasmic Membrane

The three main versions of transport are illustrated in Fig. 3.10. They are:

A. *Carrier-mediated diffusion,* which takes place when a substance is carried across the membrane down a concentration gradient. An example of a compound that is transported this way is glycerol. This mechanism does not concentrate compounds in the inside of the cells relative to the outside environment. Uptake is driven by intracellular utilization of the compound. For instance, the concentration of free glycerol inside cells is lowered by its phosphorylation to glycerol-3-phosphate. More glycerol is then taken up to equilibrate with the outside concentration.

B. *Phosphorylation-linked transport.* This energy-dependent mechanism is used for the transport of certain sugars. Substances transported in this manner are chemically altered in the process, which is why it is also known as **group translocation**. The example of glucose is shown in Fig. 3.10. The sugar binds to a specific carrier in the membrane (e.g., "enzyme 2"). The glucose-enzyme 2 complex inter-

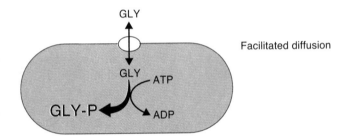

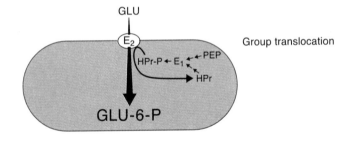

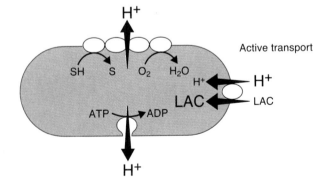

Figure 3.10. Mechanics of transport. Three types of transport in *E. coli* are shown. Facilitated diffusion; group translocation; active transport with the lac permease.

acts with "enzyme 3-phosphate," to yield glucose-6-phosphate which can then be further metabolized (Fig. 3.10).

C. *Active transport,* in which energy is utilized to drive the accumulation of substrate. A substrate, for instance the sugar lactose, is concentrated unchanged inside the cell, which makes the transport of additional molecules energetically unfavorable. In order to drive the transport of lactose, the cells use energy stored in an electrochemical gradient of protons, the **proton motive force.** This gradient is generated by the extrusion of protons from the cell (Fig. 3.10), resulting from the oxidation of metabolic intermediates like NADH or by hydrolysis of ATP. Lactose is accumulated intracellularly by coupling its **energetically unfavorable** transport with the **energetically favorable** reentry of protons into the relatively alkaline cytoplasm of the cell. Thus, transport of this type take place via a **symport,** which requires the simultaneous uptake of molecules, H^+ and sugar.

Each type of transport system involves specific protein molecules. Some of these aid the process by modifying or concentrating substrates in the periplasmic space of Gram-negatives. These **binding proteins** are specific for sugars, nucleotides, etc. The periplasmic space also contains nucleosidases, nucleases, peptidases, proteases, and other hydrolytic enzymes. The actual transport process is carried out by membrane-bound carriers called **permeases,** which are involved in the types of transport mentioned above. We do not have a physical picture of how permeases respond to the proton gradient, but we know that they assume different configurations on the inside and outside of the cytoplasmic membrane. Thus, permeases have a high affinity for substrate on the outside and low affinity on the inside. However they work, they are essential for transport. For example, in the much studied lactose system, cells that lack a functional permease remain impervious to the sugar even when soaked in concentrations approaching syrup!

These various mechanisms of transport are used to different extents by different bacteria. In general, few substrates equilibrate across membranes without the expenditure of energy. Among the energy-requiring mechanisms, "group translocations" are used to a different extent: *E. coli,* for instance, transports a wide variety of sugars in this way, whereas strictly aerobic bacteria use it little. All in all, active transport dominates the repertoire of transport mechanisms in bacteria, especially when nutrients must be concentrated from the medium in order to support cell growth.

The Uptake of Iron

The uptake of iron deserves special mention. Iron is not available in free form in the blood and many tissues because it is bound by proteins like transferrin or ceruloplasmin, yet is essential for the growth of bacteria. Many bacteria that inhabit the human body have developed ingenious mechanisms to obtain the amounts of this element they need for growth. They excrete chelating compounds known as **siderophores** that bind iron with great avidity. Each organism can take up its own particular form of complexed iron; individual complexes are unique enough to be less digestible for other organisms. However, in response to the competition for iron, many bacteria have multiple siderophores and uptake systems, thus trying to gain an edge on the other organisms in the same environment; some can efficiently extract iron from transferrin, an advantage at our own expense.

Other Functions of the Bacterial Membrane

The cytoplasmic membrane of bacteria is also the site where **cytochromes** are located and **oxidative metabolism** is carried out. It thus performs the role of the mitochondria of eukaryotic cells. Another function of the bacterial membrane is to act like a **primitive mitotic apparatus.** It is thought that bacterial DNA is attached to the cell membrane, with each newly replicated molecule adhering to the two sides of the septum made during cell division. When the bacterium divides, each half receives one of the daughter chromosomes.

The membrane is also the location of nascent proteins destined either for secretion or for incorporation in the membrane itself. Some bacteria secrete as much as 10% of all the proteins they make, including toxins and other virulence factors. The nascent peptide chains, containing the hydrophobic "signal sequences" at the N-termini, are translocated from ribosomes across the cytoplasmic membrane by an energy-requiring mechanism. Proteins that are to be secreted are released into the environment while those that become part of the membrane structure are retained within it. Note that in the Gram-negative bacteria there is an added problem, that of transporting proteins to the outer membrane. It is not known exactly how this takes place.

Some bacteria have also an exceptional ability to take up enormously long DNA molecules. The phenomenon was first demonstrated by genetic transformation of pneumococci and occurs among other bacterial species. Some, such as *E. coli,* must be coaxed to take up DNA by the addition of calcium ions. Very little is known about the mechanism of uptake of DNA by bacteria but it appears that, like active transport, it depends on the proton motive force.

In spite of its versatility and range of activities, the cytoplasmic membrane of bacteria is rarely the site of action of useful antibiotics (see Chapter 5, "Biological Basis for Antibacterial Action"). May this be due to its overall similarity in structure to the membranes of eukaryotic cells?

DNA AND CHROMOSOME MECHANICS

The genome of bacteria consists of a **single circular chromosome** of double-stranded DNA. For all its importance, it accounts for only some 2% of the cellular dry weight. The chromosome of *E. coli* has a molecular weight of about 3×10^9 daltons, or about **5 million base pairs**. This codes for about 2–3000 genes, over half of which have been identified. The total description of several bacteria is at hand and that of many more will be forthcoming.

Bacteria must solve a demanding topological problem in organizing their DNA, since it is a long and thin molecule. If stretched out it would be about 1000 times the length of the cell. If a bacterium were to be magnified to the size of a human being, its DNA would be about a mile long. The DNA is coiled in a central irregular structure called the **nucleoid**. Its physical state is unknown and somewhat mysterious, because in the test tube a solution 100 times more dilute is a gel! About all that is known about the physical state of the DNA is that it is twisted into **supercoils** (analogous to twisted telephone coils) and that this condition is indispensable for its organization, its replication, and the transcription of a number of genes. Supercoiling is thought to be achieved by the balance of the action of two topoisomerases. One of these, **DNA gyrase**, introduces supercoils into circular DNA, an action counteracted by a second enzyme, **topoisomerase I**, which relaxes the supercoils by making single-strand nicks.

Like all macromolecular synthesis, DNA replication has three stages: initiation, elongation, and termination. Replication takes place bidirectionally, that is, DNA synthesis starts at a precise place on the chromosome, the **replicative origin**, and proceeds away from it in both directions. The two moving polymerase complexes meet halfway around the chromosome. In order to replicate, the DNA helix in *E. coli* must unwind and rotate at some 6000 rpm. One wonders how this can take place without entanglement of the tightly coiled nucleoid.

The **timing of chromosome replication** is a highly regulated process and is coupled to growth and cell division. At a given temperature the **rate of DNA polymerase movement is nearly independent of the growth rate** of the cells. In *E. coli*, DNA replication takes 40 minutes, whether the cells are growing slowly or fast. In slowly growing cells, e.g., those dividing once every 100 minutes, one round of synthesis occurs in each division cycle, and no DNA is synthesized during the remaining 60 minutes. In very fast growing cells (dividing, for example, every 20 minutes), initiation of rounds of replication is adapted to produce new chromosomes as often as the cell divides (Fig. 3.11). Since each chromosome requires 40 min to be synthesized, replication will initiate again on a strand, long before its own replication has completed. Thus chromosome replication in bacteria is

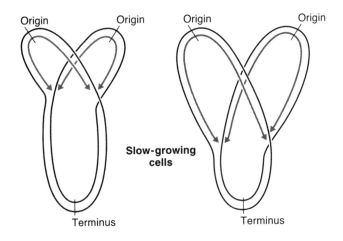

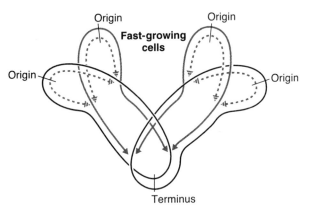

Figure 3.11. Replication of DNA in slow and fast-growing *E. coli*. Replication begins at a specific site, the **origin**, and proceeds in both directions toward a **terminus**. The process takes about 40 minutes at 37°C. In a culture doubling every 20 minutes, this requires that the process initiate every 20 minutes, that is, before the previous round of replication has terminated. In such cultures the DNA is undergoing **multifork replication**.

regulated by how often the process gets started, i.e., by the frequency of initiation of DNA synthesis.

How Do Antibiotics Inhibit DNA Metabolism?

Most inhibitors of DNA replication bind to DNA and are too toxic for clinical use. An interesting exception is **metronidazole**, a drug which is itself inert, but which can be selectively modified to an active form by some bacteria. This compound contains a nitro group that must be **partially** reduced to render the molecule active. Full reduction to the amino state makes the molecule inactive again. Partial reduction is achieved by anaerobic bacteria but only rarely by the cells of the human body or by aerobic bacteria.

Partially reduced metronidazole is incorporated into the DNA of the bacteria. This is an example of **lethal synthesis** since the metronidazole-containing DNA molecules are unstable. It follows that metronidazole and related drugs are particularly useful against anaerobic bacteria and against amoebas, which also grow anaerobically. These drugs, however, are not ideal. To a small extent, the partial reduction to active agents occurs in normal tissue, leading to possible mutagenesis and perhaps carcinogenesis as well.

Other DNA inhibitors act selectively by binding to specific enzymes. **Nalidixic acid,** for example, inhibits DNA gyrase and is bactericidal. Whether it binds to the counterpart human enzyme in vivo is not known, but it is relatively nontoxic. A class of antibacterial compounds, called the **quinolones,** interfere with DNA gyrase.

GENE EXPRESSION: UNIQUENESS OF PROKARYOTIC RNA POLYMERASE AND RIBOSOMES

The bacterial cytoplasm is composed largely of proteins (about 40% of the dry weight, with about one million molecules per cell) and RNA (up to 35% of the dry weight in rapidly growing cells). Bacterial **ribosomes** have smaller subunits (30S and 50S vs. 40S and 60S) and smaller RNA molecules than do their eukaryotic counterparts. Bacterial ribosomal RNAs, combined with 21 and 35 different proteins, respectively, make up the ribosomal subunits. These join together in the complete ribosomes which move along messenger RNA molecules to synthesize proteins.

The large requirement for proteins makes **protein synthesis** the **principal biosynthetic activity** of rapidly growing bacteria. A large proportion of a bacterium's energy and metabolic building blocks is devoted to the assembly of the protein synthesizing machinery, including ribosomes and RNA polymerase. Over a considerable range of growth rates, **RNA is made at a rate proportional to the number of RNA polymerase molecules** engaged in the process of transcription. Likewise, the rate of protein synthesis is proportional to the cellular concentration of ribosomes. This suggests that the rate of polymerization of single chains of RNA or protein remains constant whether cells are growing rapidly or slowly. Remember that this is also true for DNA replication (see above). Thus, the synthesis of the principal macromolecules of bacteria is **regulated mainly by the frequency with which each chain is initiated** and **not** so much by altering their rate of manufacture of each molecule (the speed of **chain elongation**).

Cells growing rapidly increase the frequency of initiation of RNA or protein synthesis by an analogous mechanism to that used to generate chromosomes more often than once every 40 minutes. As one RNA polymerase molecule moves away from the start site on the DNA, another can become engaged, so that a single gene can be concurrently transcribed into many RNA molecules. Likewise, a single mRNA can be translated by many ribosomes simultaneously, creating a structure called a polyribosome or polysome.

Antibiotics That Inhibit Transcription and Translation

Antibiotics may act selectively at **initiation** or **elongation** of macromolecular synthesis. For example, **rifampin,** a powerful inhibitor of bacterial transcription, acts at the initiation step. How does it recognize this step? This drug binds strongly to molecules of RNA polymerase that are floating freely in the cytoplasm, but much less well to polymerase molecules that are bound to DNA. As a result, a polymerase that is bound to DNA and has initiated RNA synthesis will not be inactivated by rifampin until it completes its round of RNA synthesis and is released from the DNA. Rifampin is clinically useful, particularly in the treatment of tuberculosis and leprosy, in part because it is relatively nontoxic. The reason is that mammalian RNA polymerases do not bind rifampin.

The largest class of **clinically useful antibiotics,** apart from the β-lactams, consists of those that **inhibit protein synthesis.** Some of them work by binding to ribosomes, either to the large or the small subunit (Table 3.3). The reason that bacteria are selectively targeted is that the ribosome of prokaryotes is different from that of eukaryotes. Among these ribosomally active antibiotics are **chloramphenicol, lincomycin,** and **erythromycin,** which **block the formation of peptide bonds** by binding at or near the aminoacyl tRNA binding site on the large ribosomal subunit. After some time, the previously synthesized peptidyl tRNA is released and hydrolyzed. The ribosomal subunits are then released from the mRNA and are free to rejoin other mRNA molecules to start another abortive cycle. This leads to a truncated version of the ribosome cycle (Fig. 3.12). As a result, when these antibiotics are withdrawn, many free ribosomes are present and ready to resume normal protein synthesis. This explains why the **action of these drugs is reversible** and why these antibiotics are **bacteriostatic** and not **bactericidal.** It should be pointed out that this does not necessarily diminish their usefulness. When bacteria are kept in check by bacteriostatic drugs, they are usually cleared from tissues by the body defense mechanisms.

One important group of protein synthesis inhibitors, the **aminoglycosides,** is **bactericidal.** How they kill bacteria has not yet been satisfactorily explained, but we have some hints. Aminoglycosides, like **streptomycin, kanamycin** and **neomycin,** are taken up by bacteria and bind to the smaller 30S ribosomal subunit. This is their critical site of action, as demonstrated by the finding that a single amino acid change in a mutated 30S ribosomal protein leads to resistance to these drugs. Binding of aminoglycosides has many effects on ribosome function; for instance, the interaction of the 30S and 50S

Table 3.3. Antibiotics—Mechanisms of Action of Commonly Used Antimicrobial Agents	
β-lactams—Murein synthesis inhibitors	
Penicillins and cephalosporins	Interfere with cell wall biosynthesis through interaction with penicillin-binding proteins; autolysis
Polyenes—Inhibitors of membrane function	
Amphotericin B	Bind to sterols in eukaryotic cell membranes, leading to membrane leakiness and, at high levels, lysis
Sulfonamides—Folate antagonists	
Sulfanilamide	Competitive inhibitor of dehydropteroate synthesis; blocks synthesis of tetrahydrofolate, and cell-linked metabolic pathways
Aminoglycosides—Protein synthesis inhibitors	
Streptomycin Kanamycin Neomycin Gentamicin Amikacin Tobramycin	Bind to 30S subunit of bacterial ribosome. Cause translational misreading and inhibit elongation of protein chain; kill by blocking initiation of protein synthesis
Other protein-synthesis inhibitors	
Chloramphenicol Erythromycin Lincomycin	Bind to ribosome 50S subunit; inhibit protein synthesis at chain elongation step
Fusidic acid	Blocks protein synthesis by interaction with soluble elongation factor G (the translocation factor)
RNA synthesis inhibitors	
Rifampin	Binds to bacterial RNA polymerase and blocks transcription (synthesis of RNA) at initiation step
DNA synthesis inhibitors	
Nitrofurans Metronidazole	Partially reduced nitro groups give addition products on DNA that lead to cidal strand breakage
Nalidixic acid Novobiocin Ciprofloxacin and other quinolones	Interfere with DNA replication by inhibiting the action of DNA gyrase
Mercury salts, organomercurials	Inhibit protein function by interaction with sulfhydryl groups

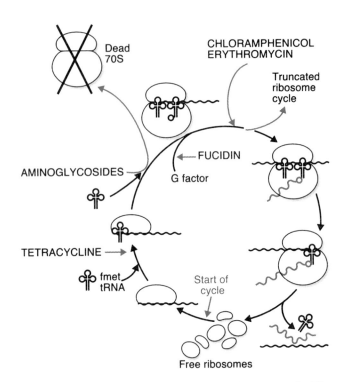

Figure 3.12. Antibiotic blockage of the ribosome cycle. The normal cycle of 30S and 50S subunits in and out of polysomes is recalled, with the assembly of a 70S initiation complex, elongation of the polypeptide chain as the ribosome moves across the mRNA, and release of all components on completion of the polypeptide. Points of blockage by antibiotics are shown. Tetracycline inhibits aminoacyl tRNA binding; cidal aminoglycosides provoke formation of "dead" aberrant initiation complexes; fucidin blocks translocation by elongation factor G; and others block elongation, leading to premature dissociation of the active complex.

subunits becomes tighter, and the elongation of peptide chains is inhibited. Typical of the action of this group of antibiotics is the accumulation of free ribosomes as aberrant 70S particles and not as 30S and 50S subunits. This coincides with cell death. Accumulating 70S ribosomes result from abortive attempts to initiate protein synthesis and do not function appreciably in protein synthesis. However, they bind to mRNA and thus block the function of ribosomes that are still unaffected by the drug. The inhibition of protein synthesis by aminoglycosides is apparently irreversible because once the drug is taken up it cannot be removed from the cell. Thus, cells treated with these drugs cannot recover, which is one reason why the aminoglycosides are bactericidal.

CAPSULES, FLAGELLA, AND PILI: HOW BACTERIA COPE IN DIFFERENT ENVIRONMENTS

The morphological variety of bacteria is not limited to walls and membranes. Some bacteria, but by no means all, have other exterior structures such as **capsules, flagella,** and **pili.** These components are dispensable, that is, they are important for survival under certain circumstances but not others. The **capsule** is a slimy outer coating made by certain bacteria. Under laboratory conditions the capsule is not needed and the organisms may grow well without it. Capsules usually consist of high-molecular-weight polysaccharides that make the bacteria very slippery and difficult for white blood cells to phagocytize. As you will see, pneumococci, meningococci, and other bacteria that are likely to encounter phagocytes during their infective cycle are indeed encapsulated. In the laboratory, colonies of encapsulated bacteria on agar plates are viscous and shiny. Colonies of nonencapsulated organisms are usually smaller and appear dull.

Protruding through the surface layers of many bacteria are two kinds of filaments, **flagella** and **pili** (also called **fimbriae**) (Fig. 3.13). Flagella are long, helical filaments that endow bacteria with motility. Many successful pathogens are motile, which probably aids their spread in the environment and possibly in the body of the host. Depending on the species, a single bacterial cell may have one flagellum or many flagella (Fig. 3.14). In some, the flagella are located at the ends of the cells (polar) and in others at random points around the periphery (peritrichous, or "hairy all over"). This distinction is useful in taxonomy and in diagnostic microbiology. Pili are involved in the attachment of bacteria to cells and other surfaces (see below)

Bacterial Chemotaxis

The movement caused by flagella is used by bacteria for **chemotaxis,** i.e., movement toward substances that attract and away from those that repel. Considerable research has shown that bacterial chemotaxis is based on the following sophisticated mechanism: flagella spin around from their point of attachment at the cell surface. Each flagellum has a **counterclockwise helical pitch** and when there are several on one bacterium, they array themselves into coherent **bundles** as long as they all rotate counterclockwise. When the flagella are arranged in these bundles, they beat in the same sense and the bacteria **swim in a straight line** (Fig. 3.15). However, when flagella rotate clockwise they get in each other's way and cannot form bundles. As a result, the bacteria **tumble** in random fashion. The two types of motion, swimming and tumbling, account for bacterial chemotaxis. In the absence of **attractants** or **repellants,** bacteria alternate indifferently between swimming and tumbling. When an attractant is sensed, swimming lasts longer than tumbling, whereas swimming stops more quickly when a repellant is present. The net result is movement toward attractants and away from repellants. Little is known about the role of chemotaxis in pathogenesis, but it would be surprising if it were not important in some instances in guiding bacteria toward cellular targets or possibly away from white blood cells.

Bacterial Adhesion and Pili (Fimbriae)

Whether by active chemotaxis or by more passive mechanisms, microorganisms are attracted to specific tissues. Sometimes this **tissue tropism** results from the selective survival of the organism in a particular environment; for example, the fungi that cause athletes' foot cannot grow at 37°C, which explains why they are found only on the skin and not in the interior of the body. In other cases, tropism involves **attachment** of surface components of the organisms to **specific receptors** present on the cells of certain tissues. The bacterial structures most often involved in attachment are the **pili.** These are filaments shorter than flagella and distributed,

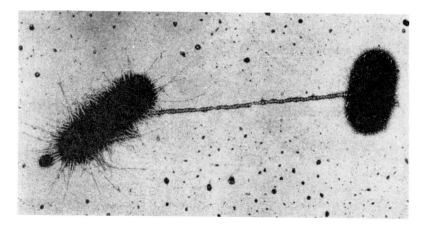

Figure 3.13. *Escherichia coli mating.* The cell covered with numerous appendages (pili or fimbriae) is a genetic donor connected to a recipient cell (without appendages) by the so-called F pilus. The F pilus is a specialized structure (sex pilus) itself controlled by genes on the fertility, or F plasmid.

The F pilus has been labeled by special virus particles that infect donor cells via the F pilus. The other pili surrounding the cell have no role in conjugation but are required by *E. coli* for colonization and pathogenicity in the intestinal and urinary tracts of humans and animals.

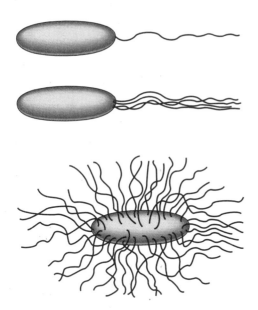

Figure 3.14. Arrangement of flagella in some types of bacteria.

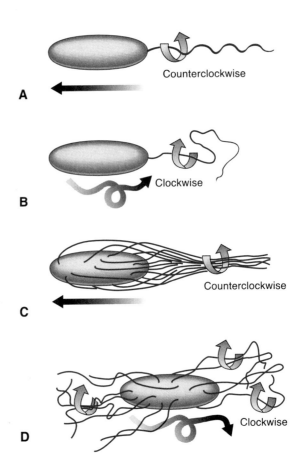

Figure 3.15. Flagellar arrangement and motility. A. A bacterium moving smoothly right to left when its single polar flagellum rotates *counterclockwise*; this is the same direction as the thread of the helix formed by the flagellin molecules in the flagellum. **B.** The same bacterium tumbles generally left to right when the flagellum rotates *clockwise*. **C and D.** With a peritrichous bacterium, *counterclockwise* rotation (**C**) produces a coherent bundle of flagella and smooth movement; the tumbling produced by *clockwise* rotation is extreme (**D**).

often in large numbers, over the surface of some bacteria. Bacteria that can conjugate have, in addition, specialized **sex pili.** These are rather different structures from the "common pili." They are much longer and link the donor (male) and recipient (female) cells during transfer of DNA by conjugation. Sex pili are usually coded for by genes carried on "fertility" plasmids (Chapter 4, "Genetics").

How Bacteria Change Their Surface Components

Pili allow bacteria to adhere to the surface of host cells, or, in the case of sex pili, to other bacteria. Virtually all Gram-negative bacteria possess "common pili," which help them adhere to mucosal surfaces throughout the gastrointestinal tract. Individuals under high physical stress, such as those ill enough to be in the hospital, tend to lose an adhesive protein found in the mucosa of the oropharynx, **fibronectin,** which preferentially binds to Gram-positive bacteria. Under these circumstances of fibronectin depletion, the common pili help the Gram-negative bacteria colonize the mouth and throat much more avidly than normal. Specialized strains of *E. coli* that cause traveller's diarrhea possess an additional type of pilus that allows adherence to cells of the small intestine where the bacteria secrete a toxin that causes the symptoms of the disease. Other strains of *E. coli* that cause urinary tract infection have been found to possess yet another form of pilus ("P-pili") that specialize in adherence to the urinary tract. Likewise, pili are essential for gonococci to infect the epithelial cells of the genitourinary tract, again by facilitating bacterial adherence and colonization.

Pili have other roles in disease. Like capsules, they can be antiphagocytic. They are also highly changeable and permit some organisms to put on a succession of disguises which enables them to outflank the immune system. This has been studied in detail in the gonococcus. Gonococci have a large number of genes that code for variants of the protein, **pilin,** that polymerizes to form pili. Each version of pilin is antigenically distinct and elicits the formation of different antibodies. In the presence of antibodies to one type of pilin, there is rapid selection for variants of gonococci that have switched to the synthesis of another antigenic type of pilin. Thus they keep one step ahead in this quick-change scenario. Only one (or a few) of the large repertoire of pilin genes is active at any time. The molecular basis for the shift from one pilin to another is that pilin genes contain two types of sequences: one codes for a constant portion of the pilin protein that is not very antigenic, the second codes for a variable region that is highly antigenic. At intervals, a constant region will recombine with a variable region to form a gene that codes for a complete pilin protein. The result is that many varieties of pilin genes can arise and be expressed, allowing the organisms to survive for long times in the face of the host immune response. It is easy to see why attempts to immunize against gonococci using a particular pilin vaccine have failed so far.

Such specific rearrangements of portions of genes are not unique. A comparable shuffling of constant and variable portions of genes gives rise to the magnificent variety of antibodies made by the body. In microorganisms, analogous mechanisms have been found in yeast, in the bacteria that cause relapsing fever (*Borrelia*), and in the protozoa that cause sleeping sickness (trypanosomes). By a related mechanism organisms that cause food poisoning and other illnesses, the *Salmonella*, undergo rapid changes between expression and nonexpression of genes that code for the protein of flagella. This change in flagellar synthesis is called **phase variation** and is based on the control of a gene for flagellar protein. The gene can be inverted on the chromosome and can only be read in one of the two orientations.

NUTRITION AND ENERGY METABOLISM

Bacteria survive and grow in a large variety of habitats. Whatever the habitat, all bacteria must synthesize cellular constituents in a coordinated manner in order to grow. The required building blocks must either be provided at suitable levels in the medium or be synthesized in proper amounts by the organisms themselves. With regard to their nutritional requirements, bacteria can be divided into two large groups: In one are the **photosynthetic** or **chemosynthetic** bacteria that subsist on CO_2 and minerals, using either light or chemical energy. The other includes all the **organisms that need preformed organic compounds**. All pathogenic microorganisms fall in the second group, but within it they have many gradations of nutritional needs. Some, like *E. coli*, are satisfied with glucose and some inorganic material (Table 3.4). Other pathogenic bacteria, like their human host, are unable to make one or more essential metabolites—vitamins, amino acids, purines, pyrimidines, etc.—which must be supplied as growth factors.

Bacteria also have a wide range of responses to oxygen. At the extremes are the **strict aerobes,** which must have oxygen to grow. An example is the tubercle bacillus, which thrives in the portions of the body that are better oxygenated, such as the lungs. At the other extreme are the **strict** or **obligate anaerobes,** bacteria that cannot grow in the presence of oxygen, such as the organisms that cause botulism and tetanus. The largest number of bacteria that are medically important can grow whether or not oxygen is present. They are called

Table 3.4. Glucose Minimal Medium

	Per liter	Main source of
Na_2HPO_4	6.0 g	P, buffering power, osmotic strength
KH_2PO_4	3.0 g	P, buffering power, osmotic strength
NH_4Cl	1.0 g	N
$MgSO_4$	0.012 g	Mg, S
$CaCl_2$	0.011 g	Ca
Glucose	2.0 g	Energy, carbon building blocks

pH adjusted to 7.0.

facultative anaerobes, and include *E. coli* and other intestinal bacteria.

These differences in the response to oxygen mirror the way bacteria oxidize substrates to obtain energy. Strict aerobes carry out **respiration** only, the process in which the **final electron acceptor** in a series of coupled oxidation-reductions is **molecular oxygen**. Strict anaerobes carry out **fermentation**, where the final electron acceptor is an **organic molecule**. Examples of organic electron acceptors are pyruvate, which is reduced to lactate in the lactic acid fermentation, or acetyl-CoA, which is reduced to alcohol in ethanol fermentation. Facultative anaerobes are capable of either form of metabolism, depending on whether oxygen is present or absent. Thus, they will respire in its presence and ferment in its absence.

Per molecule of substrate oxidized, respiration yields more energy than fermentation. Therefore, fermentative organisms must turn over more substrate to obtain the same amount of energy. The industrial microbiologist takes advantage of this for the purpose of maximizing either the yield of cell mass or the amount of metabolic products formed. Under what conditions of oxygenation would you grow yeast in a fermentation tank if the intended product were a) yeast cake, or b) alcohol?

We have mentioned that *E. coli* can use glucose as its sole organic source. It can also utilize other compounds, like lactose, fructose, or one of several amino acids. The list includes some 30 known substances, but this is not particularly impressive compared to species of *Pseudomonas*, which can grow on any of several hundred organic compounds. No wonder such nearly omnivorous *Pseudomonas* have been used by genetic engineers to construct strains for use in the degradation of environmental pollutants. And no wonder *Pseudomonas* species are omnipresent in the water supply and the soil where they can take advantage of a great variety of substrates.

Although these bacteria can manage on meager solutions of glucose and a few salts, they do not disdain richer fare. When *E. coli* is given a mixture of amino acids, sugars, vitamins, etc., it will use the compounds provided rather than making them endogenously. The result is sparing of energy and biosynthetic potential, and faster growth. In the laboratory it is possible to culture bacteria in media that are truly spartan, the so-called **minimal media**, which are water solutions of glucose, ammonia, phosphate, sulfate, and other minerals (Table 3.4). Conversely, they can be grown in a rich medium, a **nutrient broth** that contains meat extract and soluble partial hydrolysates of complex proteins. Add **agar** to these solutions and you have the corresponding **solid media**.

Some bacteria can grow only in complex media and have nutritional requirements that rival or exceed those of humans. The organisms are said to be **nutritionally fastidious**. This is characteristic of highly parasitic species that are found in close association with the rich environment of the human body. Examples of these organisms are the staphylococci or the streptococci which can grow only if provided with a long list of compounds. As expected, bacteria that can get by with only a few nutrients, *E. coli* or *Pseudomonas*, are found also in less enriched habitats, like bodies of water. The ecology of an organism usually gives good hints of its nutritional requirements.

Certain bacteria cannot grow in artificial media at all and only replicate inside host cells. These bacteria, like *Chlamydia*, are known as **obligate intracellular parasites**. Other bacteria, such as *Treponema pallidum* (the causative agent of syphilis) or *Mycobacterium leprae* (leprosy) should be able to grow on laboratory media because they grow extracellularly in the host. However, microbiologists have not been able to figure out how to get them to do it.

GROWING AND RESTING STATES

When bacteria find themselves in a suitable environment they grow and eventually divide. The time it takes for a bacterium to become two is called the **generation time** or **doubling time**. For example, *E. coli* requires about 20 minutes to double in rich nutrient broth and 1 to 2 hours in minimal medium at 37°C. Growth will go on until the population reaches a certain cell density when the nutrients in the environment become exhausted or toxic metabolites accumulate. Until this occurs, the bacteria grow in an unhindered manner and are physiologically all alike. This condition is called **balanced growth**, since all cell constituents will increase proportionally over the same period of time. Such a steady state does not exist for long in nature since the environment usually undergoes rapid changes.

The Measurement of Bacterial Growth and a Few Definitions

How is bacterial growth measured? The most direct way is to take samples at different times and count the number of bacteria under a microscope using a hemocytometer chamber. This tedious procedure has been superseded by electronic particle analyzers which detect bacteria as tiny semiconductors in an electric field. Either of these procedures measures the number of bacteria as physical particles. In other words, they give the body count, with no discrimination between living and dead bacteria. This is known as the **total count**. The total count can also be conveniently estimated by measuring a property proportional to the number of bacteria present, for instance, the turbidity of a liquid culture.

Often it is important to determine the number of **living** or **viable** bacteria. This number is determined by a **colony count**, which is carried out by placing an appropriate dilution on solid growth medium. Since colonies arise from living bacteria, the number of colonies multiplied by the dilution factor is the number of **colony-forming units** or **CFUs** originally present. Note that if bacteria grow in clumps, like staphylococci, or chains, like streptococci, the number of CFUs is an underestimate of the total number of living bacteria present.

The Law of Growth

Balanced growth can be described mathematically as follows. Let N be the number of bacteria and t the time, then

$$dN/dt = Nk$$

where k is the **growth rate constant**. By integration we obtain the **growth law**:

$$N_t = N_{0_0}e^{kt}$$

where N_t is the number of bacteria at time t and N_0 is the initial number of bacteria at time $= 0$. This describes a **geometric progression**, which holds for many natural phenomena. In situations that lead to cell death (for instance, sterilizing heat or antiseptic chemicals) the decrease in viable bacteria is often described by the same equation, but with a negative constant. The same equation also describes the decay with time of a radioactive isotope or the kinetics of degradation of unstable messenger RNA molecules in cells.

Growth in the Real World

If balanced growth went unchecked, a single bacterium dividing twice an hour would produce a mass as large as that of the earth in just 2 days. Instead, when bacteria grow to a certain density, they either exhaust required nutrients or they accumulate toxic levels of metabolites (Fig. 3.16). They may run out of the carbon source, a required inorganic compound, or essential amino acids or vitamins. For aerobic bacteria, crowding leads to the exhaustion of oxygen since it is poorly soluble in water. Toxic metabolites may be hydrogen peroxide for some anaerobes that lack catalase, or acids formed by fermentation, which results in a pH too low

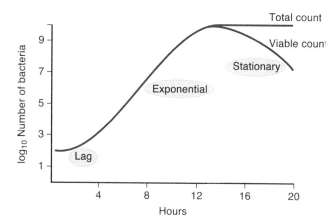

Figure 3.16. The growth of a bacterial culture. Bacteria in the inoculum sometime resume growth slowly (**lag phase**, hours 0–5). They then enter the **exponential phase** of growth (hours 5–10). When foodstuff is exhausted or toxic material accumulates, they enter the **stationary phase** (hours 10 onward). During the stationary phase bacterial cultures sometimes lose their viability, as reflected in the **viable count**, often without losing cell integrity (maintaining a constant **total count**).

to be compatible with growth. Which of these factors actually slows down growth first depends on the strain of bacteria and on the composition of the culture medium. For example, in a well-buffered medium *E. coli* may exhaust nutrients before the pH drops, while the converse may be true in poorly buffered media. The stage of the culture where growth stops is known as the **stationary phase.**

The explosiveness of exponential growth means that even a small number of bacteria may rapidly initiate an infection. An example of unhampered growth that leads to dangerous illness is acute bacterial meningitis in a child. Bacteria that cause this disease, like the meningococcus, grow so rapidly in the patient that the physician may have to intervene with great speed to avoid a fatal outcome. On the other hand, not all pathogens grow fast. For example, tubercle bacilli divide every 24 hours or so even under optimal conditions. The disease they cause is chronic and takes considerable time to be manifested.

In the tissues of the body, bacteria are often **stressed** by nutritional limitations or by the damaging action of the defense mechanisms. Consequently, bacterial populations in the body are rarely fully viable. To permit them to adapt to such conditions, bacteria do not cease all metabolic activities when they stop growing. Instead, they may cease net growth but continue some synthetic activities that permit them to make specific constituents needed for adaptation. To use a laboratory example, when *E. coli* cultures exhaust glucose they continue to carry out a low level of protein synthesis, sufficient to adapt to the utilization of other nutrients, such as other sugars that may be present. Energy and building blocks

are supplied by turnover of cell material that is not needed in the stationary phase. A major source of amino acids are ribosomes and preexisting proteins that are present in excess under these conditions. Their breakdown products can also be oxidized to supply energy. This process of feeding on itself allows adaptability and postpones death, which might otherwise occur by random degradative events in the absence of synthetic activities.

Bacteria are exposed to countless kinds of **injury** and have developed special adaptive mechanisms to cope with many of them. For example, damage to the DNA of *E. coli* by ultraviolet light activates a set of genes that code for proteins capable of repairing this damage. This is known as the **SOS response.** Other protective responses are turned on when bacteria are starved for the source of carbon, nitrogen, or phosphorus, when the temperature is raised abruptly, or when anaerobic cultures are suddenly exposed to oxygen. In each case, the rapidity of adaptation is a tribute to the powers of bacterial adaptation.

Even when they are **not growing**, bacteria can still **cause damage** to their host. In the first place, nongrowing bacteria are still immunogenic and can elicit immune responses with both beneficial and detrimental results. In the second place, production of toxins often starts or accelerates when bacteria enter the stationary phase. In some cases, we can fathom the reason for this timing because toxin production provides certain bacteria with nutrients. For example, some streptococci make enzymes that lyse red blood cells and proteases that degrade hemoglobin. The organisms are thus supplied with amino acids plus a source of iron. Why do these organisms make their hemolysins mainly in the stationary phase? Clearly, as long as they are growing they must already be supplied with enough iron and needed amino acids. Why should they then expend energy to make hemolysins?

Cessation of growth of some bacteria initiates **sporulation.** This results in the production of metabolically inert spores that are extraordinarily resistant to chemical and physical insults. During sporulation the "mother cell" is eventually lysed. The cytoplasmic contents that are released sometimes contain large amounts of toxins. This happens in tetanus, gas gangrene, and other diseases caused by sporulating bacteria.

The relationship between microbial growth and pathogenesis is far from simple but should be kept in mind when attempting to understand the etiology and course of infections.

MECHANISMS OF ADAPTATION

Both over short periods and throughout evolutionary times, bacteria are selected for their efficient and economical ways of coping with the environment. **Ineffi-**

cient strains are rapidly lost in competition with others that use their resources more effectively. Metabolic efficiency is characterized by metabolic **parsimony**, that is, bacteria tend not to make compounds they cannot use at the time. There are important exceptions to this statement, but, by and large, it illustrates the economy and efficiency of the bacterial way of life.

We know a great deal about the mechanisms bacteria use to adapt to changing environmental conditions. As more information is gathered, it becomes evident that there is a large number of mechanisms operating specifically under given circumstances. To use a specific example, take a culture of *Escherichia coli* growing in a minimal medium and add to it an excess of the amino acid leucine. Within seconds, the endogenous synthesis of leucine will be stopped and the cells will utilize the exogenously supplied leucine exclusively. From the point of view of the economy of the bacteria, this is desirable, as it saves the metabolic energy expended for biosynthesis of leucine. The same phenomenon occurs if other amino acids, purines, pyrimidines, or other metabolites were added.

Regulation of Enzyme Activity

How did the bacteria switch off the synthesis of leucine? When the enzymes of the metabolic pathway dedicated to the synthesis of leucine were studied, it was found that the first enzyme in the pathway is inhibited by leucine, and will not function in its presence. This inhibition is due to **allosteric** properties of the enzyme, that is, its ability to change conformation by the binding of an effector, in this case leucine. Why was the first enzyme and not the others in the pathway affected? The reason is economic, because by stopping the flow of substrates at the very beginning of the pathway there is no waste of unusable metabolites. This effect is known as **feedback** or **end-product inhibition**.

Regulation of Enzyme Synthesis

Feedback inhibition suffices to stop the synthesis of leucine in the leucine-fed culture. If this were all, the organisms would still synthesize the biosynthetic enzymes for leucine, at a cost of considerable energy. This is wasteful and would place the organisms at a selective disadvantage vis-à-vis more efficient ones. To avoid such an unnecessary expenditure, the cell rapidly turn off the synthesis of the enzymes of the leucine biosynthetic pathway. How is this done? It is a characteristic of prokaryotic cells that the enzymes involved in a metabolic pathway are often strung together in a multigenic segment of DNA called an **operon**. **Transcription** of all the genes of an operon into mRNA can be turned on or

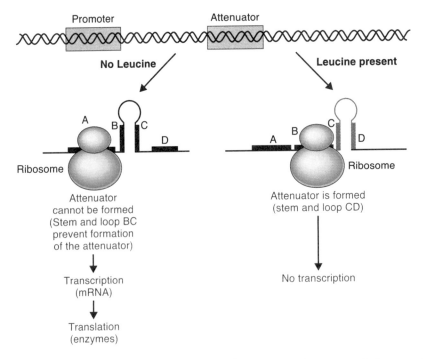

Figure 3.17. Regulation of enzyme synthesis by attenuation. Transcription stops when a **termination stem and loop structure** involving sequences C and D is formed. The left side of the drawing shows how the absence of leucine causes ribosomes to stop at sequence A and to prevent the formation of the CD stem and loop structure. This allows RNA polymerase (not shown) to continue transcription past this region. On the right side, when leucine is present, ribosomes continue to sequence B, allowing the formation of the CD termination stem and loop structure. In this case, RNA polymerase cannot proceed and transcription stops.

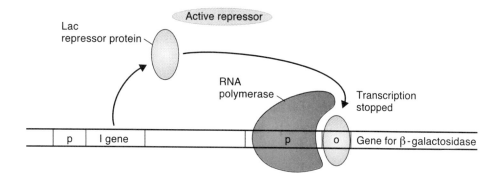

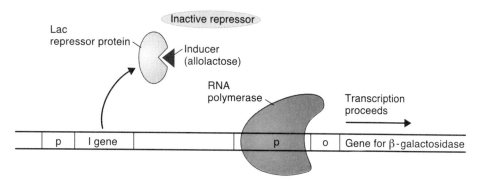

Figure 3.18. The Operon model: regulation of β-galactosidase synthesis by repression. The repressor protein for the genes encoding enzymes for lactose utilization exists in two states, active, when the sugar inducer is absent, and inactive, when the inducer is present. The top of the figure shows that when the inducer (a derivative of lactose, allolactose) is absent, the repressor is in the active form and binds to the operator, thus preventing transcription from taking place. In the bottom of the figure, the repressor is inactivated by the inducer and cannot bind to the operator. Transcription can now proceed and the enzyme β-galactosidase is formed.

off together by throwing a single regulatory switch. At one end of the operon where transcription starts, there is a series of regulatory sequences that do not code for amino acids but are recognized by the regulatory mechanisms. One of these sequences is the **promoter** site, where RNA polymerase binds to initiate the synthesis of mRNA. We will discuss two such mechanisms of **regulation of gene expression** used to switch operons on and off.

The operons involved in the biosynthesis of amino acids, such as leucine, are sometimes regulated by a mechanism called **attenuation**. This is how it works, still taking leucine as an example. A small stretch of mRNA is synthesized from the beginning of the coding sequence of the leucine operon, regardless of the presence or absence of leucine. The RNA polymerase now encounters a region called the **attenuator**, where, in the presence of leucine, **transcription is terminated**. This achieves the desired effect of not making the unneeded biosynthetic enzymes. In the absence of leucine, when the biosynthetic enzymes become essential, the secondary structure of the nascent mRNA at the attenuator region is altered

in such a way that transcription, and therefore translation, can proceed. Details of how this works are shown in Fig. 3.17.

Another mechanism for turning on or off the synthesis of enzymes is found in the case of many enzymes involved in the utilization of sugars. Taking the utilization of lactose as an example, if this sugar were the sole carbon source, the bacteria must make the enzyme β-galactosidase, which is necessary to convert lactose into glucose and galactose. In the absence of lactose, as in the case of a culture growing solely on glucose, the synthesis of β-galactosidase is unnecessary and wasteful. This is how the synthesis of the enzyme is regulated (Fig. 3.18). At the beginning of the operon, just past the promoter, there is a regulatory sequence known as the **operator**, where a protein called the **repressor** binds. When the repressor binds to the operator, transcription cannot begin. In the presence of lactose, the repressor undergoes a conformational change to render it incapable of binding to the operator. Note that the lactose repressor is an allosteric protein, capable of undergoing conformational changes under the influence of an effector. The result is that when lactose is added to a culture, the repressor becomes inactive and cannot bind to the operator, thus allowing the synthesis of β-galactosidase to proceed. β-galactosidase is an example of an **inducible enzyme**, one made on demand, as contrasted with a **constitutive enzyme**, one that must be made at all times, such as RNA polymerase. In the case of β-galactosidase, lactose (or, more precisely, one of its metabolites) is known as the **inducer**.

An Overview of Regulation

Regulation of gene expression by attenuation, repression, or other mechanisms results in the relatively rapid switching of gene expression on and off. The reason is that, in bacteria, mRNA molecules are relatively short-lived and undergo rapid turnover. Thus, after the synthesis of an enzyme is stopped, the amount of residual enzyme produced will be very small. In addition, what enzyme is left may be subject to feedback inhibition and little of its product will be made. Note that all forms of regulation come at energy cost. Thus, feedback inhibition requires that the protein be more complex than just what is needed for catalytic activity. Regulation of enzyme synthesis by attenuation depends on the synthesis of a stretch of mRNA that will not be used if the enzymes of the operon are not made. Using a repressor to regulate an operon likewise requires the constitutive synthesis of protein repressor molecules. The energy cost of making regulatory devices is weighted against the greater disadvantage that cells would have in not being able to switch on and off major biosynthetic pathways. Thus, free living cells such as bacteria must balance their powers of efficiency and adaptability

The theme of efficiency and adaptability to environmental changes recurs throughout this book, especially when considering how microorganisms cope with the changes they encounter when entering the body and certain of its tissues and organs.

SELF-ASSESSMENT QUESTIONS

1. What distinguishes prokaryotes from eukaryotes? Compare a typical bacterium and a typical eukaryotic cell.
2. Discuss the physiological and structural consequences of bacteria being small.
3. What are the structural features of a "typical" bacterium? What distinguished Gram-positives from Gram-negatives?
4. Describe the outer membrane of Gram-negatives and discuss its role in bacterial ecology and virulence.
5. How does penicillin work?
6. What are the principal mechanisms used by bacteria to take up substrates?
7. Discuss DNA replication in *Escherichia coli.*
8. Is it clear to you why some protein-synthesis-inhibiting antibiotics are bacteriostatic? Discuss why some others are bactericidal.
9. Discuss the role of bacterial flagella and pili in growth and pathogenesis.
10. What are the main ways in which bacteria derive their energy? What is the relation between this and how they cope with oxygen?
11. Discuss the law of bacterial growth and some of its consequences in the real world.
12. Discuss the difference between regulation by feedback inhibition and by control of gene expression.
13. Give two examples of regulation of enzyme synthesis in bacteria.
14. What happens when bacteria are exposed to potentially lethal challenges, such as high temperature?

SUGGESTED READINGS

Neidhardt FC, Ingraham JL, Schaechter M. Physiology of the bacterial cell. Sunderland, MA: Sinauer Assoc, 1990.

Neidhardt FC, et al. *Escherichia coli* and *Salmonella typhimurium.* 2nd ed. Washington, DC: American Society for Microbiology, 2 vols, 1996. This is an encyclopedic treatise on the structure, function, and heredity of these organisms.

Genetics of Bacterial Pathogenesis

MOSELIO SCHAECHTER

BARRY I. EISENSTEIN

N. CARY ENGLEBERG

In this chapter, we discuss concepts of bacterial genetics that are relevant to the study of pathogenic mechanisms. We assume that the reader has a general background in molecular biology and microbial genetics and is familiar with basic aspects of this subject.

INTRODUCTION

The traits that render certain bacteria pathogenic are known as **virulence factors**. In a narrow sense, this term refers to substances produced by a microorganism that can harm the host. The classic examples of virulence factors are bacterial toxins, discussed in Chapter 9, "Damage by Microbial Agents." More recently, the term has come to mean any component of the microbe that is required for or that potentiates its ability to cause disease. According to this expanded definition, even a substance that, when purified, is nontoxic to host tissue could be considered a virulence factor if its absence would make the microbe significantly less capable of causing disease (less virulent). Excluded from the definition are any genes (and gene products) essential for normal growth of the microbe. Thus, a factor required by a bacterium for growth in a laboratory medium is not considered a virulence factor, whereas a factor that enhances the ability of the bacterium to invade the human bloodstream is.

Virulence factors are now commonly studied via a genetic approach. The hallmark of such investigations is the comparison of the behavior of **isogenic** strains in an appropriate model of infection. Isogenic strains consist of a wild type parent and a mutant that is **genetically identical to its wild-type parent except for a single mutation**. Models of infection range from the use of experimental animals to tissue or cell cultures employed in studies of bacterial adherence, invasion, or propagation. However, the genetic approach is not the only one used to study virulence factors. Researchers have traditionally studied the toxins biochemically; detailed structure–activity relationships allow researchers to determine precisely the "active site" of the toxin molecule and how it works. Another nongenetic approach is epidemiological and involves the correlation of the virulence of naturally isolated strains with their clinical properties. In fact, most toxins have been discovered using these correlations.

Virulence is always multifactorial, since the infection process is invariably complex. In order for a pathogenic microorganism to cause disease, different virulence factors have to come into play at each stage of the process. For a given pathogen, the major research goals are to determine:

- What virulence factors are involved in the infection.
- How these factors are involved in the establishment of the disease.
- If virulence genes turned regulated. In particular, do special environmental signals induce the microbe to turn the expression of virulence genes on or off? How are such signals discerned and transduced by the microorganisms?

Each infectious agent has its own repertoire of virulence-related functions. Nevertheless, it has now been recognized that many microbes share similar approaches to similar biological problems. In the chapters that follow, these motifs are presented in sections called **paradigms**.

A GENETIC APPROACH TO STUDYING VIRULENCE FACTORS

Let us now assume that we wish to study a certain virulence factor, for instance one involved in the attachment of a pathogenic bacterial species to the surface of host cells. A common approach is to **clone** candidate genes that encode this trait and insert these genes into bacterial species that are normally incapable of attachment. The mutated bacterium—-the bacterium that has incorporated the new genes into its genome—must then be **isolated** from all others. Isolation is usually accomplished by **selecting** the bacteria that have the desired trait. Further studies on their virulence can then be performed.

The steps of the process are as follows:

1. The first step in cloning the gene or genes is to purify the DNA of the pathogenic donor organism and to cut the DNA into a large number of fragments, one of which encodes the attachment factor.
2. Fragments are individually **spliced** into **plasmids** that are used as genetic carriers or vectors.
3. The collection of spliced plasmids are introduced by **genetic transformation** or other manipulation into a recipient strain that is incapable of attaching to host cells.
4. Among the transformed bacteria carrying spliced plasmids, clones that are able to attach to host cells are **selected**.
5. To definitively establish that the gene actually encodes for the attachment mechanism, the gene is **mutated** to an inactive form and then exchanged for the native gene in bacteria of the donor virulent strain. The resulting strain should have the mutant phenotype, i.e., the bacteria should be unable to attach to host cells.
6. If the protein product of the gene can be purified, its amino acid sequence can be compared to that inferred from the DNA sequence. Sequence information is often used to study the structure and biochemical activity of a protein, in this case, its ability to bind directly to animal cells.

We will now discuss these approaches to microbial genetics and their underlying concepts in detail. We will occasionally digress from the central theme when it becomes necessary to make other points of interest.

The first step in gene cloning is to cut purified donor DNA in a test tube using **restriction enzymes**. These nucleases are "molecular scissors" that cut both strands of the DNA at specific sequences, producing pieces of different length called **restriction fragments**. The length of a fragment depends on the distance between two neighboring recognition sequences.

Several hundred restriction enzymes with different specificities, nearly all the product of different bacteria, are currently commercially available. The sequence on the DNA recognized by a given restriction enzyme may be four, five, or more bases long. The number of cuts made in a piece of DNA depends on the frequency of occurrence of such sequences; thus, enzymes that recognize shorter sequences make more cuts than those that recognize longer sequences. For example, an enzyme that recognizes a four-base sequence will, in principle, cut on the average once every 256 nucleotides ($1/4^4$), whereas one that recognizes a six-base sequence cuts on the average once every 4096 nucleotides ($1/4^6$). In reality, the DNA sequence of organisms is not a random array; thus, these numbers are only approximations. Many restriction enzymes make staggered cuts on each of the DNA strands, thus leaving single-stranded overlapping ends at the site of the cut, whereas others cut precisely across the double strand, resulting in blunt ends (Fig. 4.1).

Restriction enzymes are not merely laboratory tools but also have important biological functions. They serve to protect the organisms from foreign DNA. How do restriction enzymes distinguish foreign DNA molecules from the bacterium's own DNA? In addition to making a specific restriction enzyme, each species is also capable of modifying the corresponding DNA sequence by **methylation**. The bacterium's methylated DNA is resistant to the restriction enzyme whereas the foreign, unmethylated DNA will be cleaved. Such systems protect cells, for example, from killing by certain viruses.

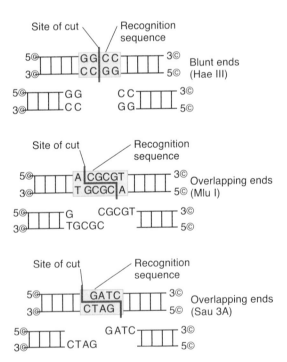

Figure 4.1. Restriction enzymes. The recognition sequence and site of cuts of three restriction enzymes are shown. Restriction enzymes are known by a three-letter abbreviation of their bacterial species of origin (Hae, *Haemophilus aegypticus*; Mlu, *Micrococcus luteus*; Sau, *Staphylococcus aureus*.)

Molecular Cloning

The general strategy for cloning a gene involves introducing a mixture of restriction fragments, one of which contains the desired sequence, into a suitable recipient organism. The mixture contains thousands of DNA fragments; only a few of the recipient cells will contain the gene of interest. Therefore, the suitable recipients must be isolated by taking advantage of some property that allows them to be selected. Thus, a key aspect of this strategy and, indeed, one of the most powerful aspects of microbial genetics, is the ability to select rare events. To use a simple example, one can spread 100 million or more sensitive bacteria on the surface of an agar plate containing an antibiotic and have a few colonies (clones) of drug-resistant mutants grow out after incubation. Thus, one can study with ease events that happen with a frequency of 1×10^{-8} or even less. This figure is of the same order of magnitude as the ratio of the size of a needle to that of a medium-sized haystack!

A second problem arises. Most restriction fragments are not capable of replicating inside bacteria. In order to preserve and amplify the desired fragment, it must be incorporated into DNA molecules capable of self-replication. This incorporation is achieved by "splicing" the fragments to be cloned into a DNA carrier molecule or **cloning vector.** If the chosen restriction enzyme makes staggered cuts, it will produce fragments with overlapping ends (see Fig. 4.1). When such restriction fragments are placed in the proper conditions of ionic strength and temperature, the overlapping ends will join (**anneal**) by forming hydrogen bonds between their complementary purine and pyrimidine bases (see Fig. 4.1). Often the cloning vector is a plasmid.

What Are Plasmids?

Plasmids are autonomously replicating (extrachromosomal) double-stranded DNA molecules. Most are covalently linked DNA circles. Plasmids are a dispensable addition to the genetic material of most bacteria, but often encode properties that are required for survival in specific environments, such as those in the human body. Plasmid-less strains of many species can usually grow in laboratory media but are not normally found in nature.

The most medically relevant plasmid-encoded properties are antibiotic resistance and virulence factors. Plasmids exist in many varieties, differing in size, genetic composition, and ability to be transferred between bacteria. They range in size from those that carry some 100 genes to those that have only about 5 genes. Like the bacterial chromosome, plasmids regulate their own replication. Thus, each plasmid constitutes an independent replicating entity known as a **replicon**, which possesses its own **origin of replication** and **regulatory proteins.**

The number of plasmids per cell depends on how closely their replication is linked to that of the chromosome. In some cases, the connection is close and the number of plasmids (**copy number**) is small, sometimes just one or two per cell. This type of control is characteristic of large plasmids. Small plasmids tend to be present in high numbers, sometimes as many as 50–100 copies per cell. Such plasmids are useful in genetic engineering work, which requires that the product of a particular gene be expressed in large amounts.

Some plasmids mediate their own transfer between bacteria of the same or different species. These plasmids are known as **conjugative plasmids.** The F factor involved in *E. coli* conjugation is one of the best studied examples. Such plasmids carry genes encoding products, such as the sex pilus, that are involved in cell-to-cell contact. Many antibiotic-resistance plasmids are also conjugative. Some plasmids are promiscuous in their ability to replicate in different hosts, and these plasmids are most likely to spread drug resistance between unrelated bacterial species. Such plasmids have contributed to the dramatic increase in antimicrobial resistance in natural populations.

Using Plasmids in Genetic Engineering

An example of how restriction fragments can be spliced into a plasmid is shown in Figure 4.2. The loosely joined donor and recipient DNA molecules are covalently linked using the enzyme DNA ligase. Note that a large number of different molecules will result from this annealing and ligation, most of them irrelevant to the study. From this complex mixture, how does one find the molecules that contain the gene in question? Notice that if the chromosome of the donor is cut into more than 1000 fragments, the chances of finding the desired clone are less than 1 in 10^3.

Plasmids are useful in cloning technology because they contain their own replication origin. If the donor DNA is to cause a stable change in a recipient bacterium, it must be replicated. A donor DNA molecule that cannot replicate is lost from the population, without further genetic consequences (see Fig. 4.3). Intracellular DNA replication requires that the DNA molecule possess a replicative origin, a sequence recognized by specific protein initiation factors that allow the replication process to start. Bacterial chromosomes have a single replicative origin (unlike eukaryotic cell chromosomes, which have several origins each). When a bacterial chromosome is cut into fragments, most of them will not contain the origin and therefore will not be able to carry out independent replication. One way to ensure that DNA fragments will replicate is, therefore, to **splice** them into DNA molecules that possess a replicative origin, such as a plasmid.

The plasmid DNA containing spliced donor DNA is now introduced into recipient bacteria by a process called **genetic transformation.**

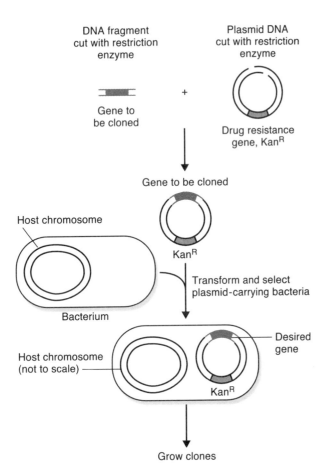

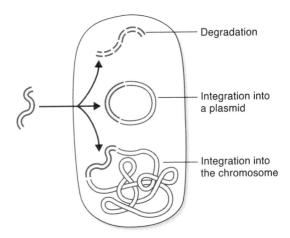

Figure 4.3. Possible fate of DNA introduced into bacteria. *Linear* DNA is degraded unless it is integrated into a stable replicon, such as a plasmid or the chromosome of the recipient bacterium. If the DNA is in *circular* form and is capable of replication, it can propagate and become a plasmid. Neither linear nor circular DNA will survive the restriction enzymes of the cell unless they are properly methylated.

Figure 4.2. Engineering a plasmid for molecular cloning. The DNA containing a desired gene and that of a plasmid vector are cut with a restriction enzyme that produces overlapping ends. When the two kinds of DNA are mixed, some of the cloned DNA will hybridize to the plasmid DNA at the complementary sequences of their protruding ends. The molecules can now be covalently linked (using DNA ligase) to yield a new plasmid that contains the desired gene. The plasmid containing the desired gene can now be used to transform suitable bacteria. These are grown to yield a clone of bacteria carrying the desired gene.

Genetic Transformation

Transformation consists of the exchange of genetic material between bacteria by way of DNA. Some bacteria take up DNA spontaneously from the medium and incorporate it into their genomes. Such strains are said to be **competent.** Bacteria are not necessarily competent at all times and competence may be an inducible property. Pneumococci, for instance, become competent when their culture reaches the stationary phase of growth. At that time some of them secrete a protein called **competence factor** which induces other cells in the culture to become competent. Competence factors induce competence by exposing DNA-binding proteins on the bacterial cell surface.

Other species do not have an innate mechanism for

DNA uptake but may be coaxed to incorporate DNA if their surface properties change. In *E. coli*, altering membrane permeability by adding calcium ions allows this normally recalcitrant species to take up DNA. This **artificially induced competence** is used extensively in genetic engineering experiments.

How do competent bacteria ensure that DNA from other species are not taken up randomly, which could threaten their genetic stability? Bacteria employ several mechanisms to recognize "self" from "nonself," other than the restriction enzyme systems already mentioned. Certain bacterial species, such as *Haemophilus influenzae*, are quite discriminating and take up DNA from the same or related species only. How does this organism recognize that the DNA is homologous? On its membrane, *Haemophilus* carries a protein that binds specifically to an 11–base pair sequence. This protein is frequently found in *Haemophilus* DNA, but it is rare in other species. Note that a given 11–base pair sequence occurs at random once in 4^{11} (or about 5 million bases), and that a typical bacterial chromosome is 3–5 million base pairs in length. Thus, this "password" is unique to *Haemophilus* and serves to distinguish "self" DNA from "nonself" DNA. In *Haemophilus*, as in many other Gram-negatives, DNA is taken up as a double strand, but only one strand participates in recombination with the host genome.

Other bacterial species, such as the pneumococcus, are indiscriminate in their uptake of DNA. One strand of the foreign DNA is degraded on the bacterial surface, and the other is incorporated into the cell. Recognition of foreign now takes place intracellularly. The strand that is taken up will undergo recombination with the genome of the recipient only if it has nearly the same sequence of bases, that is, if it is homologous. Heterologous DNA, on the other hand, is rapidly degraded with no genetic consequence.

In *E. coli*, transformation is a relatively rare event and only a small proportion of the cells in the population (at most, 1 in 1000) can be expected to contain any DNA from the donor bacteria. Because so few of the cells are successfully transformed, at most one in a million bacteria in a culture will contain the gene of interest. Thus, it becomes important to first discard the 999/1000 or so bacteria that failed to take up any DNA and keep the bacteria that did. Such **transformants** can be selected by a simple strategy. A cloning vector that encodes an easily selectable property, e.g., resistance to an antibiotic, in this case ampicillin, can be chosen and added to the culture. Only the bacteria that take up the plasmid will grow in an ampicillin-containing agar medium and make individual colonies, whereas the bacteria that do not take up the plasmid do not grow on this medium. Ampicillin resistance is a **selectable marker** that allows investigators to isolate the few bacteria that take up donor DNA from the majority that do not. Note that each ampicillin-resistant clone is likely to contain a different restriction fragment of the donor bacteria. The collection of such clones is collectively known as a **genomic library** of the donor organism (Fig. 4.4). Only a few of these clones will have been transformed for the desired gene. How these bacteria are isolated will be discussed under "Selection and Characterizion of the Desired Clone."

Transformation is not the only way to introduce foreign genes into bacteria (see Fig. 4.5). DNA can be introduced using a **bacteriophage** or **phage**. This procedure is known as **transduction**. The third major way that foreign DNA is taken up by a host is by **conjugation**, which involves cell-to-cell contact. The choice of technique used to introduce DNA depends on the recipient bacterial species and on details of the experimental strategy.

Bacteriophages

Bacteriophages or phages are viruses that infect bacteria (Fig. 4.6). They have been intensively studied and play an important role in genetic experimentation. Like all viruses, phages are composed of either DNA or RNA (never both) surrounded by a protein shell called a **capsid**. Some bacteriophages have a **tail** structure and tail fibers that are involved in attachment to the host bacteria. The nucleic acid may be double-stranded or single-stranded. In some phages, the capsid is surrounded by a lipid-containing layer that probably plays a role in the attachment of the phage to host cell membranes. Other phages contain proteins and other non-nucleic acid constituents within their capsids. In size and shape, phages

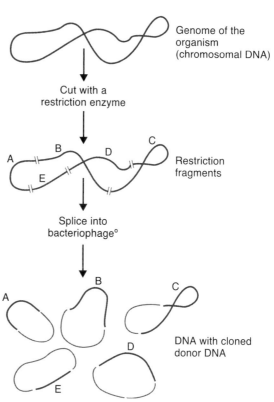

Creating a genomic library

Figure 4.4. Creating a genomic library. The DNA of an organism is cut into restriction fragments (here shown as *A* through *E*) which are annealed to the DNA of a phage. After ligation, these molecules are packaged in vitro into a mature phage that can be used to infect recipient bacteria.

range from the very small (containing about 6 genes) to the large and complex (with more than 100 genes). Details of the biology of viruses are described in Chapter 31, "Biology of Viruses."

Phages are of two general types, virulent and temperate (Fig. 4.7). In each type, the life cycle begins when the phage attaches to the host bacteria via proteins that recognize specific receptors on the host membrane. Like all viruses, phages lose their structural integrity during their replication. Their capsid and nucleic acid separate, usually soon after attachment to the host bacteria. In typical cases, the nucleic acid is injected into the host cells and the capsid remains on the outside. In the case of **virulent phages**, viral nucleic acid replicates rapidly after it enters the host bacterium and yields tens, hundreds, or even thousands of copies. Independently, the capsid proteins are synthesized and, together with the viral nucleic acid and other constituents, assemble to make the complete virus particle, called a **virion**. Phage virions are released by lysis of the host cell or extrusion though the membrane. This sequence of events is known as the **lytic cycle**, because the host bacterium is eventually destroyed.

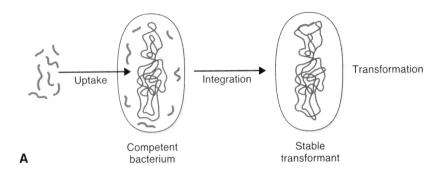

A

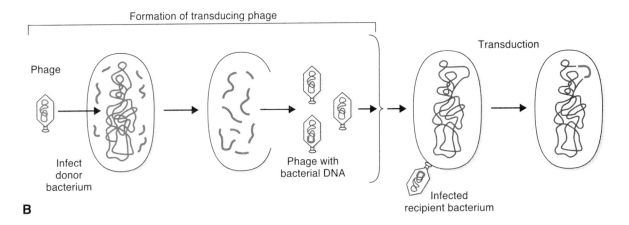

B

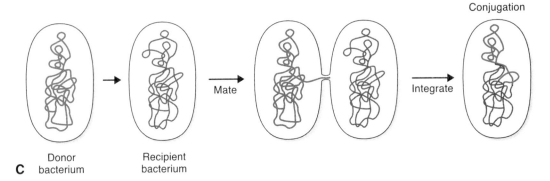

C

Figure 4.5. Methods to introduce DNA into bacteria. **A.** Transformation, using naked DNA. **B.** Transduction, using phages. **C.** Conjugation, using cell-to-cell contact.

Depending on environmental conditions, **temperate phages** may go through a lytic cycle, as described for virulent phages, or an alternative cycle called a **lysogenic cycle.** In the lysogenic cycle, phage genes are repressed. Instead of replicating inside the host cell, the viral nucleic acid integrated into the host genome. Such phages always contain double-stranded DNA, not RNA. Integration is a special type of genetic recombination, which results in an extension of the host genome by the amount of viral genome incorporated. The integrated phage genome is known as the **prophage.** Host cells that carry a prophage are called **lysogens,** and the process in which a prophage is integrated into a host genome is known as

lysogeny. With some *E. coli* phages, such as **Mu,** the prophage integrates at many sites on the chromosome. With other phages, such as **lambd** (λ), integration takes place primarily at a single specific site on the *E. coli* chromosome.

In some cases, the lysogenic phage carries one or more genes that profoundly affect the virulence of the host bacterium. A classic example is that of phage β, which infects *Corynebacterium diphtheriae*, the causative agent of diphtheria. Diphtheria toxin (see Chapter 9, "Damage by Microbial Agents") is encoded by the phage genome; only lysogenic bacteria, therefore, are capable of producing the disease diphtheria.

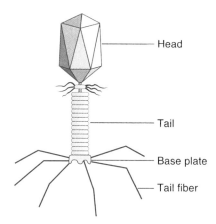

Figure 4.6. Structure of phage T4. T4 is a phage that infects *E. coli* and is representative of a family of large and complex viruses.

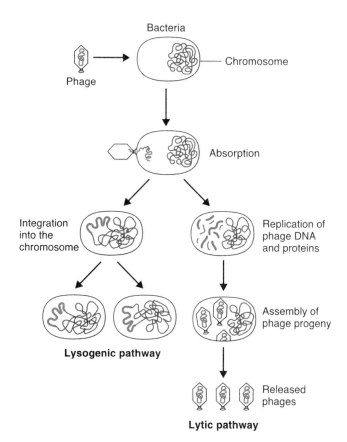

Figure 4.7. Lysogenic and lytic pathways of phage development. After adsorption of the phage attaches to the host bacterium and penetration of the phage DNA enters the host, one of two events are possible, depending on environmental conditions. The lysogenic pathway leads to the stable integration of the phage genome into that of the host. The lytic pathway leads to phage multiplication and the eventual release of new phage particles.

How do we know that a bacterium is lysogenic, that is, that it contains a prophage? Such cultures grow normally and do not readily reveal the presence of their viral passenger. It is often possible to reverse the lysogenic state, that is, to have the prophage become **derepressed** and enter a lytic cycle. This event happens spontaneously, albeit rarely, or can be induced by physical or chemical agents such as ultraviolet light or nitrosoguanidine.

When the prophage DNA enters the lytic cycle, it is cut ("excised") from the chromosome; it may not do so precisely, but may include a few of the bacterial genes adjacent to its site of integration in the chromosome. Such viruses are capable of transporting these genes from their cells of origin to other cells, that is, they can **transduce** the recipient cells. How does this take place?

A Transduction: Phage-Mediated Mechanism To Exchange DNA Between Bacteria

Transduction is the introduction of genetic material into bacteria by the use of the phage infection apparatus. Phages capable of transduction may be temperate phages which, when excised from the chromosome, vary. As noted in the previous section, during excision of the prophage from the bacterial chromosome, the prophage may pick up some of the adjacent bacterial genes. Such imperfect cutting may result in phage DNA particles that cannot replicate because too much of their own genome is replaced by host DNA. These **defective phages** can infect new hosts only once. However, during infection, the phage introduces the bacterial genes into the new host. Although, this infection is a "dead end," it does result in a change in the genetic make-up of the recipient cell. This process is known as **specialized transduction** because transduction is limited to the genes that are adjacent to the prophage on the chromosome. Certain phages, such as lambda (λ), integrate only at specific sites on the host DNA; transduction is limited to the genes to the right and the left of this site. The Mu-type phages, which integrate at many sites, pick up any physically contiguous genes and thus can transduce a large number of genes from donors to recipients.

During the assembly process of some phages (whether temperate or virulent), the capsid may not be filled with viral DNA, but may pick up any DNA in its surrounding. Fragments of chromosomal DNA from the host that are generated during lytic infections can thus be packaged into capsids, making phage particles that are incapable of reproduction. However, they can still attach to new host cells and inject their DNA. The particles produced from this process are called **pseudovirions**. Because any gene from the donor can be involved, this type of transfer is called **generalized transduction**. Pseudovirions can also be created artificially by carrying out the viral assembly process in vitro using the components of the capsid and any DNA molecules, including those that are produced by cloning techniques. Pseudovirions can be created using capsids of a wide variety of viruses and can be useful DNA delivery systems, not just to bacteria but also to eukaryotic cells.

Conjugation Another Way to Exchange Genes Among Bacteria

Bacterial genetic material can also be exchanged by a more conventional mechanism, **sexual conjugation**. In bacteria, sexual conjugation is the one-way transfer of genetic material from a donor cell to a recipient cell in a mating pair (Figs. 3.13 and 4.8). The process requires cell-to-cell contact. Most bacteria are not genetically endowed to carry out conjugation; to be able to conjugate, they must contain **conjugative plasmids** that possess the necessary genes. For instance, the F plasmid of *E. coli* codes for several conjugative functions, including a **sex pilus**, a specialized structure that differs from the other, so-called common pili (or fimbriae) in that it functions as a conjugal bridge between donor and recipient bacteria. The transfer of the DNA is a complex process and conjugation requires the products of some 20 plasmid genes. Transfer takes place by a special form of replication of the F plasmid in the donor cell, as shown in Figure 4.8. The process begins at a special site on the plasmid DNA called the **transfer origin**.

In general, conjugative plasmids bring about the transfer of their own DNA only and not that of the chromosome. However, if a conjugative plasmid becomes integrated into the chromosome, it will transfer not just itself but also the chromosomal genes that are covalently attached to it. In principle, the entire chromosome could be transferred to a recipient cell during conjugation. However, transfer of the DNA is relatively slow, requiring about two hours for the passage of the entire chromosome. The bridge between the two cells is fragile and seldom persists that long. Thus, in many instances, the only portion of the donor DNA to transfer is that proximal to the origin of transfer. The closer a gene is to the transfer origin, the sooner it will be transferred. The timing of transfer is therefore related to the position of the gene on the chromosome, a fact that has been used to map the *E. coli* genome by a series of timed coitus interruptus.

Selection and Characterization of the Desired Clone

Let us now assume that suitable recipient bacteria have received a desired gene from a donor strain by one of the three major mechanisms of genetic exchange, transformation, transduction, or conjugation. How can one isolate the bacteria that contain the desired gene from the great majority that do not? Obviously, testing each of the recipient bacteria, a brute-force approach, would be extraordinarily demanding due to the thousands of colonies that have to be tested individually. Note that selection of drug resistant clones (as described on pp. 15 and 16) reduces the choice to cells that take up DNA from the medium, a 1000-fold saving in effort. However, the plasmid DNA used for cloning is not composed of identical molecules because, in the process of splicing, only very few of them result in the desired new combination. Thus, even though cells that received plasmid DNA can be readily selected, most will not contain the new gene. In order to obtain these cells, further selection steps are necessary.

Finding a desired gene among a collection of clones depends on selecting for the phenotype of the desired gene. In the example we have used, the cloning of a gene for bacterial adherence, it is possible to select for adhering organisms by exposing the bacterial mixture to cultured animal cells and washing away the nonadherent bacteria. Such procedures are seldom completely effective because some "negatives" may also attach, albeit with lesser efficiency. For this reason, such a procedure constitutes an **enrichment**, rather than a perfect selection. Repetition of the procedure may improve the enrichment.

Often, a desired gene does not impart a selectable property on the bacterium (usually *E. coli*) into which it is cloned. For example, a toxin or enzyme that is critical to virulence in a pathogen offers no selectable phenotype when its gene is cloned into *E. coli*. In such cases, it may be possible to **screen** for the presence of the gene. One approach to screening is to test for the function of the gene product. For example, many pathogenic bacteria produce cellular toxins that lyse red blood cell, i.e., **hemolysins**. It might be possible to select clones containing the gene or genes encoding an hemolysin by plating them on agar containing red blood cells and looking for colonies with a clear zone around them. Alternatively, if

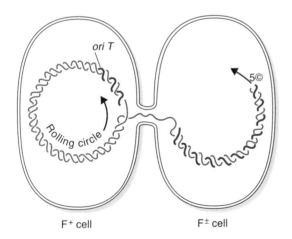

Figure 4.8. Transfer of F plasmid from an F⁺ to an F⁻ cell. A single DNA strand generated by replication is transferred from the donor to the recipient cell. The complementary strand is then synthesized in the recipient to reconstitute the complete F plasmid.

a functional assay is not available, the desired clone can be detected with antibodies made against the purified product from its original source.

Assuming that we have successfully obtained bacterial clones that carry a desired trait, such as adherence to animal cells, what have we found out so far? We can conclude that the gene imparts the ability to adhere to the recipient strain. However, the gene came from a different species or strain; thus, the result does not strictly prove that this gene is responsible for the invasiveness of the original organism. Although this point may seem pedantic, it needs to be investigated for the following reason. The two species involved differ considerably in their genetic make-up (i.e., they are not isogenic) and it is possible that in one of them the adhesion gene that was cloned acts together with some other gene product to facilitate invasion.

To establish whether the cloned gene acts alone, the gene must be mutated, then reintroduced into the original donor bacteria and exchanged for the resident wild type gene. Cells containing the mutated gene would then be impaired in adhesion. What kinds of mutants should be used in such experiments? Let us consider the choice of mutants available to bacterial geneticists.

Mutants and Mutations

Mutants are organisms that differ genetically from the **wild type**, the kind found most abundantly in nature. For a mutant to be useful for experimental study, it must differ not only in its **genotype** (its DNA sequence), but also in a demonstrable property, its **phenotype**. Mutants arise by **mutation**, defined as changes in the coding sequence of genes. **Spontaneous mutations** are rare, generally occurring for a given gene once in 10^6 to 10^9 cell divisions. This frequency can be increased many fold by **mutagenesis,** the process of making mutations.

It is easy to see how mutations in dispensable functions may be obtained and studied. How can we study mutations in functions that are essential for growth, since, by definition, they will be lethal? For this purpose, geneticists use **conditional mutants.** These mutants have a mutation that is expressed under one condition but not another. For example, a mutation in RNA polymerase may be expressed at high temperature, e.g., 40°C, but not at 30°C. A culture of such a **temperature-sensitive mutant** can be maintained and grown at the lower (**permissive**) temperature, but its defect will manifest at the higher (**nonpermissive**) temperature.

Mutations arise by a variety of alterations in the DNA (Fig. 4.9). Some of these changes are relatively small, such as single base substitutions. Others involve a greater amount of DNA, either by deletion, insertion, or inversion of more than one base pair of DNA. Mutations are often the result of errors during DNA replication. Most such errors are corrected by the replication machinery, but a few escape.

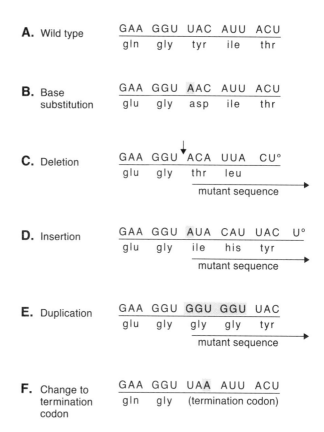

Figure 4.9. Different kinds of mutations. A short stretch of DNA and the corresponding amino acids are shown. **A. *Wild type.* B. *Base substitution.*** A uracil (*U*) is substituted with an adenine (*A*), changing the codon from one encoding for tyrosine (*tyr*) to asparagine (*asp*). Such a mutation may or may not affect the activity of the protein product. **C. *Deletion.*** One of the uracils (*U*) is deleted, changing the sequence of the amino acids encoded further downstream. **D. *Insertion.*** An adenine (*A*) is inserted, changing the sequence of the amino acids encoded downstream. **E. *Duplication.*** The codon GGU is duplicated twice. **F. *Change to termination codon.*** Changing the cytosine (*C*) in the codon UAC alters it into termination codon UAA. Peptide synthesis stops at this site.

Deletions, insertions, and changes to termination codons may or may not affect the activity of the protein product, depending on how far along the coding sequence they are. If close to the sequence coding for the amino terminus of the protein, the effect may not be as great as if located near the carboxy terminus.

The rate of mutagenesis can be increased one-thousand to one-million fold by the addition of mutagenic agents. Many chemical and physical agents are mutagenic; many of these agents are normally present in the environment. Some are chemical analogs of the DNA bases that lead to the replacement of one base by another (e.g., guanine for adenine). Base substitutions may not affect the encoded protein because the genetic code is redundant (i.e., 64 possible codons encode only 20 amino acids plus 3 "stop" codons). Thus, many muta-

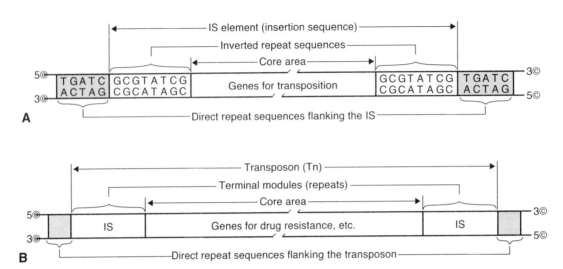

Figure 4.10. Insertion sequences and transposons. A. Insertion sequence (IS element). B. Transposon (*Tn*).

tions will not be expressed and therefore will appear to be **silent.**

In a **missense mutation,** one amino acid in a protein is substituted for another. Such a change does not always affect the function of the encoded protein, but when it does, the defect in the protein will result in a **mutant phenotype.** If the mutation is a change from an amino acid–specifying codon to a **stop codon** (e.g., UAA) in protein synthesis, this **nonsense mutation** will result in a **truncated protein.** Ionizing radiation and certain alkylating agents lead to the deletions of one or more bases. A single base deletion results in a **frameshift mutation,** in which the triplet code is read in a different frame, producing a totally different sequence of amino acids in a peptide. Larger deletions may also result in a frame shift (if they involve bases in numbers other than 3 or its multiples), but in every case lead to the formation of incomplete, often inactive proteins. An alternative class of large-scale changes is the **insertion** of genetic material. Such insertions are usually obtained by the introduction of **transposable elements,** an important addition to the strategic tools employed in modern genetics. Insertions usually inactivate a protein because they introduce a string of irrelevant amino acids into its amino acid sequence. Both deletions and insertions can be detected by biochemical means, such as using restriction enzymes.

Transposable Elements—"Hopping Genes"

Transposable elements ("hopping genes") are DNA segments that can be inserted into a DNA molecule. These elements can also be excised from a DNA molecule. Thus, these elements can "hop" from one chromosomal location to another, from a chromosome to a plasmid, or vice versa. The two steps, **integration** and **excision,** are carried out by different mechanisms. In addition, there are two varieties of transposable elements: **insertion sequences** have the minimal genetic in-

formation for transposition; **transposons** carry extra genes in addition to those required for transposition.

The integration of a transposon or an insertion sequence within a gene disrupts the gene and constitutes an insertion mutation.

Insertion sequences (IS elements) are relatively small DNA sequences, about 1–2 kilobases long, with two characteristic properties. First, they contain specific sequences located at their ends that are **inverted repeats** of one another (Fig. 4.10). These sequences are required for the integration process. Second, these sequences are recognized by enzymes encoded within the IS elements that carry out integration into a target site.

Transposons (Tn) are more complex DNA sequences capable of insertion into a genome. For this reason, transposons are commonly used by scientists to locate genes of interest. That is, a transposon may be introduced into a pathogen, and the progeny may then be screened for loss of a specific virulence trait. The interrupted gene is likely to play a critical role in the expression of that trait, and it can be easily located or cloned since it now contains an antibiotic resistance gene (from the transposon). Transposons integrate by several distinct mechanisms, one of which resembled the mechanism used by IS elements. Transposons are useful in genetic engineering because they carry extraneous genes which may be of clinical interest, such as those for antibiotic resistance (Fig. 4.10).

Certain plasmids, e.g., the widely distributed R plasmids, carry one or more drug-resistance transposons. The ability of these determinants to hop from one plasmid to another provides bacteria with the ability to adapt to a hostile environment, such as a hospital, which is usually inundated with antibiotics. In these types of environments, bacteria may become resistant to antibiotics by acquiring resistance genes. Because of selective pressure, R plasmids may acquire many transposons with new drug resistance genes. Since many of these R plasmids are conjugative, **multiple drug resistance** can spread among different types of bacteria with the use of a single antibiotic in the environment. Under such conditions, although only one resistance gene is being selected, the other genes are carried from one bacterial strain to another as fellow travelers.

Recombination

Most organisms have the natural capacity to incorporate added DNA into their genome. For single-cell organisms such as bacteria, this process is essential if they are to exploit their version of "sex" to generate genetic diversity. When bacteria conjugate, some of the genes from the donor may be incorporated into the chromosome of the recipient by the process of **recombination**. As with sex in higher organisms, recombination in bacteria allows for more mixing of genes, more diversity among individuals, and an enhanced likelihood of producing organisms that will compete successfully in the evolutionary contest. Interestingly, the proteins that mediate recombination are some of the same molecules that repair DNA when it becomes damaged by chemicals or radiation.

To understand how scientists can exploit this phenomenon for their own purposes, we need to examine briefly the process of recombination. Recombination occurs by two kinds of site recognition, called homologous and site-specific.

Homologous recombination takes place when the donor DNA is substantially similar to sequences on the host chromosome. Sequence homology must be sufficient to allow the first step in recombination, namely the pairing of the two regions. The paired molecules then undergo a reaction known as a **crossover**. If two crossovers take place along the same chromosome, the entering donor DNA replaces the resident sequences (Fig. 4.11). As we have observed, this process requires that the donor and recipient DNA be somewhat similar. After all, the recipient bacterium needs to incorporate "better" versions of the genes it already has. It has no use for completely unrelated foreign DNA.

Site-specific recombination does not require extensive sequence homology between the recombining DNA molecules. Instead, this process depends on the activity of specific **integrases**, enzymes that recognize a specific short DNA sequence as a site for recombination. This method of recombination is used by temperate phages or transposable elements to integrate into the chromosome.

Geneticists make abundant use of homologous recombination to introduce mutated genes into microorganisms. When a mutated copy of a gene is introduced into cells by transformation, conjugation, or transduction, only rarely will a cell undergo two crossovers, replacing the resident gene with the mutated one. Since recombination is such a rare event, how can one be sure to

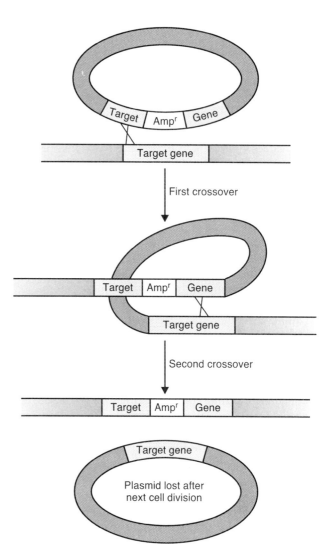

Figure 4.11. Replacing a wild type gene in the chromosome with a mutated gene. A donor strain is transformed with a plasmid that has two characteristics: (1) it is incapable of replication in the new host, and (2) it carries the target gene that has been inactivated by insertion of the gene for ampicillin resistance (amp^R). Transformants can be selected by virtue of their ampicillin resistance. Such strains arise by two crossovers between the chromosome and the plasmid within the gene under study. These strains will have a mutant phenotype because the mutant gene substituted for the wild type.

select organisms in which the exchange has occurred? One way is to insert a selectable gene (e.g., an antibiotic resistance gene) within the mutated gene. In addition, the mutated gene is typically cloned on a genetic element that cannot be maintained after it is introduced into the pathogen, e.g., on a plasmid that cannot replicate within the recipient organism. After introduction into the pathogenic strain, the organisms are grown in media containing the selecting antibiotic. During growth, organisms that lose the mutated gene will not survive. And since the mutated gene cannot be maintained on its plasmid, surviving organisms will be those in which the mutated (selectable) gene has been introduced onto the chromosome. This is most likely to occur by recombination in a region of DNA homology. A single crossover event will result in the entire plasmid integrating into the chromosome at the recombination site. A second recombination can result in the excision of the resident gene with the plasmid. The "exchange" of the mutated and resident genes occurs after both recombinational events, i.e., **double homologous recombination** (Fig. 4.10).

The Arrangement of Genes on the Chromosome

A distinguishing characteristic of a gene is its location on the chromosome. Until recently, the location of genes was established chiefly by their **linkage** or proximity to genes whose location has been previously determined. The degree of linkage is determined by the frequency of recombination that takes place between two genes: The closer they are, the less the chance that a recombination event will occur between them (Fig. 4.12). This method is being rapidly superseded by examination of **genomic sequences**. Bacterial genomes are being sequenced at an increasing rate and soon we will have the entire sequences of representatives of the major classes of bacterial pathogens. Many genes involved in microbial virulence tend to be similar in different species, thus, candidate virulence genes will increasingly be found by scanning a genome and looking for similarities to known virulence factor genes in model organisms.

A major discovery emerging from genetic studies of pathogenic bacteria is that virulence-related genes are often situated within continuous segments ("islands") of

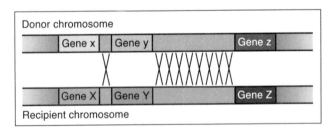

Donor chromosome

As a result of this recombination, strains like this:

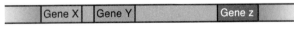

are 8 times more common than strains like this:

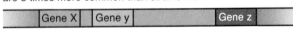

Therefore, genes X and Y are more closely linked than genes X and Z

Figure 4.12. The distance between genes on the chromosome defines their degree of linkage. The smaller the distance separating two genes, the fewer crossovers that will take place, and the greater the linkage.

the chromosome. These **pathogenicity islands** are long stretches of DNA that may have been acquired by transduction via phages or by conjugation with other organisms. Pathogenicity islands are located at specific locations on the bacterial chromosome. Like transposons, these DNA segments have terminal repeats, which suggests that pathogenicity islands may have been integrated into the chromosome by recombination at specific sites. Pathogenicity islands encode a number of genes required for infection, such as those required for the formation of pili (adhesins required for some bacteria to bind to host cells) or secretion of toxins. This finding is epidemiologically important because it suggests that a harmless bacterium may become pathogenic in a single step. This contrasts sharply with the idea that pathogenicity evolved by stepwise mutations or the acquisition of virulence genes one at a time. Pathogenicity islands have been found in a number of bacteria, including certain diarrhea-producing strains of *E. coli*, *Salmonella*, *Shigella*, the cholera bacillus, and the plague bacilli.

Characterizing the Product of a Gene

How does one characterize the protein encoded by a gene? Often it is easy to recognize that a protein is present in a wild type strain but absent in a mutant. For example, because certain bacterial adhesion proteins are located in the cell membrane, it has been relatively straightforward to establish their absence in preparations from mutant strains. In other cases, the presence or absence of a protein can be determined by analyzing the majority of a cell's protein by two-dimensional electrophoresis. In such experiments, thousands of individual proteins appear as spots at characteristic locations; thus, the presence or absence of a given protein can be determined. In addition, truncated or otherwise inactive proteins can be identified after precipitation with specific antibodies made against the wild type protein. Thus, a number of techniques permit identification of the protein that is likely to correspond to the gene under study. But can one determine with certainty that a given protein is encoded by a given gene?

The most direct way to identify the gene that encodes a specific protein is to juxtapose the sequences of the DNA and the protein. To conclude that a gene encodes a particular protein, the amino acid sequence of the protein must be shown to match the sequence of the corresponding triplet codons on a stretch of DNA according to the rules of the genetic code. In reality, demonstrating the correspondence between the two sequences can be a demanding task. The usual strategy is to carry out this work in steps. The first step is to estimate the length of the protein and of the gene. If a protein can be identified as a specific band in polyacrylamide gel electrophoresis, it is easy to determine its approximate molecular weight. When the sequence of the region of the DNA becomes known, the presence of a gene can be established by inspection. A gene can be defined as a DNA sequence spanning a **start codon** (the one coding for the first amino acid of the protein) and a **termination codon**, as long as both are in the same translational reading frame (that is, they are separated by trios of bases only). The stretch of DNA defined by the start and stop codons is known as an **open reading frame (ORF)**.

Determining the Number of Genes That Code for a Certain Trait

Let us assume that DNA sequencing and protein experiments strongly suggest that a gene encodes a certain protein. How can one tell if this gene is the only gene involved in the phenomenon under study? Could other genes be necessary for the expression of the particular trait? In order to determine whether a gene acts alone, a **complementation test** can be performed. This test consists of obtaining a number of independent mutations and introducing them two at a time into the same bacterium. As the test is usually performed, one of the mutations is carried on the chromosome, the other on a plasmid. Under these circumstances, if the trait were carried by two genes encoding for two individual proteins, say A and B, a mutant in A would make normal B product and vice versa. In this case, a complete set of A and B proteins would be made, the two mutations would **complement** each other, and the bacterium would have a positive phenotype. On the other hand, if the trait were

determined by one gene only, complementation could not occur.

CONCLUSION

The experiments discussed in this chapter demonstrate how the combined use of genetics, biochemistry, and cell biology help us to better understand the mechanisms of microbial pathogenesis. In situations in which the prime virulence factor is a toxin (as will be discussed in subsequent chapters), the biochemical approach is often the most direct means to determine the mechanism of pathogenesis. However, when dealing with more complex microbial–host interactions, the genetic approach provides the first means to dissect the many factors involved so that they can be meaningfully analyzed.

SUGGESTED READINGS

Dorman CJ. Genetics of bacterial virulence. Boston: Blackwell, 1994.

Groisman EA, Ochman H. Pathogenicity islands: bacterial evolution in quantum leaps. Cell 1996;87:791–794.

Lewin B. Genes V. Oxford: Oxford University Press, 1994.

Maloy SR, Cronan JER Jr, Freifelder D. Microbial genetics. 2nd ed. Boston: Jones & Bartlett, 1994.

Salyers AA, Whitt DD. Bacterial pathogenesis: a molecular approach. Washington: ASM Press, 1994.

Snyder L, Champness W. Molecular genetics of bacteria. Washington: ASM Press, 1997.

Biological Basis for Antibacterial Action

DAVID SCHLESSINGER

BARRY I. EISENSTEIN

Killing microorganisms is relatively simple as long as it is not selective. Microorganisms can be killed by heat, radiation, strong acids, etc. Targeting specific microbes while sparing host cells and tissues is much more difficult. According to Paul Ehrlich (the forerunner of modern chemotherapy), what we want is a "specific chemotherapy." We are indebted to the microorganisms themselves for producing many chemotherapeutic agents, the antibacterial antibiotics.

We discuss how antibiotics act in Chapter 3, "Biology of Infectious Agents." In this chapter we discuss the biological basis for the actions of these drugs, including how bacteria defend themselves against them. This chapter focuses on antibacterial drugs. Antiviral drugs are discussed in Chapter 43, "Strategies to Combat Viral Infections"; antifungal drugs in Chapter 45, "Introduction to the Fungi and the Mycoses"; antiprotozoal drugs in Chapter 50, "Blood and Tissue Protozoa" and Chapter 51, "Intestinal and Vaginal Protozoa"; anthelminthic drugs in Chapter 52, "Intestinal Helminths" and Chapter 53, "Tissue and Blood Helminths."

HOW AND WHEN WERE ANTIBIOTICS DISCOVERED?

One way organisms in the environment—soil, water, or areas of the human body—attempt to gain an advantage over other organisms is by secreting specific chemicals. Some secrete antibiotics, while others employ more subtle methods of competition. In Chapter 3, "Biology of Infectious Agents," we mentioned that microorganisms secrete iron-chelating compounds and are capable of reabsorbing their own iron-bearing products. In this manner, these microbes reduce the iron concentration to

levels that do not permit the growth of other organisms that cannot scavenge iron. Thus, in complex environments, competition for nutrients combines with the action of antibiotic substances to produce a balanced microbial ecology.

In the last 30 years, we have taken advantage of this natural warfare for our own purposes: we borrow antibiotics from one organism to combat others. The result has been a medical revolution of immense proportions. Figure 5.1 shows the increase in human longevity since the introduction of antibiotic therapy. But because we now take for granted the use of antibiotics, it is difficult to recapture the early impact of modern chemotherapy. Ask older family members how they feared the loss of a loved one from pneumonia or postoperative infection, or talk to older physicians about how powerless they were when treating children with meningococcal meningitis or subacute bacterial endocarditis.

However, there is a price to pay for our therapeutic progress. The selective pressure exerted by antibiotics on bacteria is so great that within one human generation they have responded by becoming resistant, often to several antibiotics.

The first important antimicrobial agents were not true antibiotics but synthetic **antimetabolites**. Ehrlich's seminal work derived from his findings that dyes used in histochemistry became bound to cell-specific receptors. "Why then," he asked, "should not such dyes be made toxic for specific organisms?" Ehrlich's intuition was validated by workers in the mammoth German chemical industry, who systematically synthesized thousands of compounds and tested them for biological effects. In 1934, Domagk found that one of these compounds, Prontosil, cured a fatal streptococcal infection in mice. It was then shown that Prontosil was inactive in pure cultures of

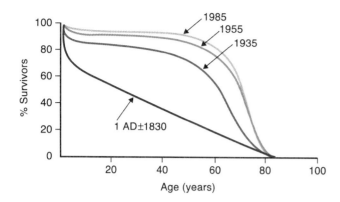

Figure 5.1. Survival of human populations as a function of age. Average life expectancy (50% level) remained at 25 until 1830. Between 1830 and 1935, the impact of sanitation, public health, and immunization extended the life expectancy. Antibiotics (along with better nutrition and health education) added an average of another 8 years. Note that more recent medical breakthroughs have not extended average life expectancy very much.

bacteria in vitro but was hydrolyzed in vivo to the active drug, **sulfanilamide**. Cures with this first sulfa drug, or **sulfonamide**, were soon reported. These findings gave impetus to the efforts to purify penicillin, a true antibiotic first detected by Fleming as the product of a mold in 1928. A new era had arrived; the search for new antimetabolites and antibiotics has continued ever since.

WHAT IS THE BASIS FOR SELECTIVE ANTIMICROBIAL ACTION?: THE EXAMPLE OF SULFONAMIDES

Early on researchers discovered that extracts from yeast contain a substance that antagonizes the action of sulfonamides. When purified, this substance was found to be *p*-aminobenzoic acid (PAB; Fig. 5.2), a component of folic acid. The similarity in the structure of the PAB and sulfanilamide is obvious. Following this lead, hundreds of thousands of antimetabolites have been tested for possible therapeutic value. In the sulfa class alone, thousands of derivatives with small and large modifications have been studied; about 25 of them are still in use.

The competition between sulfonamide and PAB in bacteria is illustrated in Figure 5.3; when more sulfonamide is added, proportionally more PAB is required to counteract its action. This type of antagonism is called **competitive inhibition**. The mechanism of action of sulfanilamide was clarified when the function of PAB became better known. Because PAB is a constituent of folic acid (see Fig. 5.2), it was inferred that sulfa drugs inhibit the synthesis of this vitamin and thus the coenzymes that contain it. The main coenzyme is tetrahydroformyl folic acid, which functions in reactions that add a carbon unit to synthesize nucleosides and certain amino acids (see

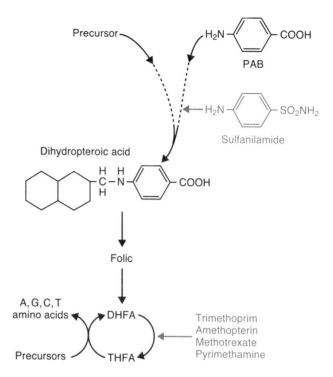

Figure 5.2. Inhibition of folic acid synthesis (by sulfa) and function (by other antibacterial drugs). The addition of sulfanilamide instead of *p*-aminobenzoic acid to dihydroxypteroic acid inhibits the synthesis of folic acid. In addition, the resulting analog functions as a "lethal product."

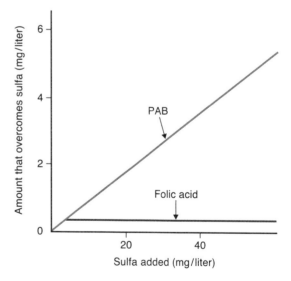

Figure 5.3. PAB overcomes sulfa addition competitively; folic acid, noncompetitively.

Fig. 5.2). Therefore, researchers reasoned that folic acid should suppress the action of sulfa drugs, and further, that if bacteria were given enough folic acid to satisfy their growth requirements, no amount of a folic acid inhibitor synthesis could suppress their growth. Unlike the case of PAB, antagonism of sulfas by folic acid is **non-**

competitive. This expectation was subsequently confirmed (see Fig. 5.3).

The effectiveness of sulfa drugs against bacteria depends on the different ways body cells and bacteria synthesize and use folic acid. Body cells require *preformed* folic acid, which explains why they are unaffected by sulfonamides. Sulfonamides inhibit the *synthesis* of this compound, not its *utilization*. On the other hand, the folic acid we require must be present in the circulation and tissues. Why then can't bacteria use and escape sulfonamide action? The reason seems to be that many bacteria that make folic acid lack a system for the uptake of preformed folic acid and cannot benefit from its presence in the environment. These bacteria must synthesize their own folic acid, which makes them susceptible to sulfa drugs. Folic acid everywhere, and not a molecule to save them!

WHAT LIMITS THE EFFICACY OF ANTIMICROBIAL DRUGS?

The mechanism of action of a drug is only one of the properties that determines its potential usefulness. You will learn of many others, e.g., pharmacodynamics, cost, and the likelihood of patient compliance. Here we consider briefly three kinds of limitations on the efficacy of antimicrobial drugs that are related directly to their modes of action: the speed with which the drugs work, the sensitivity of the microbial target, and the side effects on the host.

Speed of Action

The practical efficacy of drugs sometimes depends on how fast they stop bacteria in their tracks. The case of sulfanilamide is instructive: when the drug is added to a culture of susceptible bacteria, they continue to grow for about two to four generations before their growth is inhibited (Fig. 5.4). The reason for this delay is that each bacterium contains enough preformed folic acid to meet the demands of up to 16 daughter cells. Only after 16 cells are formed does the drug become effective. Inhibition by sulfonamides, then, is dependent on the continued growth of the bacteria.

Other things being equal, a **bactericidal** agent, one that kills microorganisms rapidly, is preferable to a **bacteriostatic** one that inhibits growth reversibly. Organisms that remain alive in the presence of a drug may still harm the host, either by continuing to produce toxins or by becoming resistant to the drug and eventually resuming growth. Bactericidal drugs have been clearly shown to work better when the body's defenses are insufficient to clear the invading agents. Important examples are bacterial endocarditis, bacterial meningitis, and infections in patients with low numbers of circulating neutrophils (agranulocytopenia). Nevertheless, the preference for bactericidal agents depends on the circumstances.

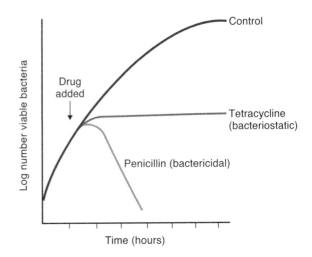

Figure 5.4. The effect of bacteriostatic and bactericidal drugs on the growth of bacteria. Note that certain bacteriostatic drugs may not inhibit growth for some time. In the case of sulfa drugs, this lag is due to the time required to use up preformed folic acid in the bacteria.

For example, an inhibitor of protein synthesis, such as erythromycin, is bacteriostatic but stops the synthesis of protein toxins abruptly. In contrast, penicillin kills bacteria but not immediately: during the lag before the drug exerts its lytic effect, the organisms continue to produce toxins. In experimental infections of mice with an agent of gas gangrene, *Clostridium perfringens*, a static drug protected the animals better than a cidal one. In practical terms, static antibiotics are also generally effective. Ultimately, inhibition of bacterial growth gives the defense mechanisms of the body an opportunity to get rid of the organisms.

The distinction of *static vs. cidal* should not be taken as absolute. First, the action of a drug may differ in different organisms. For example, the modified aminoglycoside spectinomycin is static for *Escherichia coli* and cidal for gonococci. Second, some drugs show odd kinetics of action that make them difficult to classify. For example, rifampin rapidly kills 99% of *E. coli* cells in vitro, but is static for the remaining 1%, perhaps because these bacteria are particularly resistant during a phase of their cell cycle. In other cases, a combination of two static drugs may achieve a cidal action. Despite these ambiguities, the criterion of static vs. cidal is generally useful in considering the outcome of drug therapy. In the future, drugs may be developed that work in other ways, such as the ability to inhibit virulence factors (e.g., toxins or adhesins). Notice that such drugs would not affect the growth of microorganisms in vitro, thus their action would only be manifested in vivo.

Sensitivity of the Target

The efficacy of antimicrobial drugs depends on the degree of sensitivity of the intended target organisms. Every agent is effective against a defined range or **spec-**

trum of organisms. Broad-spectrum antibiotics, which are effective against a wide range of bacteria might be thought to be preferable to drugs with narrow spectra. However, several practical considerations, such as cost, argue against the widespread use of broad-spectrum antibiotics. These drugs should be reserved for appropriate situations, as in cases when the etiological agent cannot be determined before therapy begins, or for immunocompromised patients who may be subject to simultaneous infection by several agents.

The spectrum of microbial susceptibility depends not only on the organisms but also on the conditions of the infection. For example, aminoglycosides are taken up poorly by bacteria under anaerobic conditions. Thus, these drugs are ineffective against anaerobes. Also, the level of a drug achievable at the site of infection limits its usefulness. For example, nitrofurantoin is concentrated in the urine and is effective in many cases of urinary tract infections. However, the rapid excretion of this drug prevents it from reaching effective levels in tissues or blood.

Side Effects

An important limitation is that antimicrobial drugs may have side effects on the host. In antimicrobial chemotherapy, the object is to optimize the **therapeutic index**, the ratio between the effective and the toxic dose. It is important to keep in mind that the degree of selectivity chosen depends on the plight of the patient. Certain inhibitors of folic acid metabolism, e.g., methotrexate, are very toxic in humans and are used as anticancer agents. For some patients, there is no choice.

Infectious agents that do not penetrate into deep tissues are special cases in therapy. Topical applications for skin infections are less likely to produce side effects. This lack of side effects permits extensive use of agents, such as the antibacterial drug polymixin and the antifungal antibiotic nystatin, that can harm host cell membranes. Drugs against intestinal worms, which are topologically located outside body tissues, are also less likely to cause side effects.

Often, astute clinical observation can turn side effects to advantage, sometimes outside the field of antimicrobial pharmacology. Some derivatives of sulfonamides have a diuretic effect and cause blood acidosis and alkaline urine. Although these effects are weak, they led to the synthesis of an important group of modern diuretics. Similarly, some sulfa drugs produce hypoglycemia, which led to the development of new drugs for the treatment of diabetes.

HOW ARE ANTIBIOTICS SELECTIVE?

In the case of sulfa drugs, selectivity is based on the fact that bacteria, but not humans, must synthesize their own folic acid. Any step in metabolism, unique to

microorganisms or not, is a potential target for antimicrobial action. All that is needed is selective toxicity. In the same pathway as that affected by sulfonamides, the drug **trimethoprim** blocks the function rather than the synthesis of folic acid (Fig. 5.2). Trimethoprim inhibits the enzyme dihydrofolate reductase which catalyzes the reduction of dihydrofolate to tetrahydrofolate. This enzyme is necessary for human cells as well as for bacteria, but the amount needed to cause 50% enzyme inhibition is 0.005 mM for bacteria, 0.07 mM for protozoa, and 250 mM for mammals. Thus the drug can be used against bacteria and protozoa without harming humans.

This example of efficacy is based on the relative insensitivity of the host compared to bacterial targets. In another instance, e.g., tetracycline, both host cells and bacteria are sensitive to the drug. However, bacteria, unlike mammalian cells, concentrate the antibiotic. As a result, tetracycline is effective against even intracellular organisms (e.g., chlamydiae).

The armamentarium of antimicrobials includes drugs that affect the synthesis or function of every class of microbial macromolecules. Extreme selectivity is achieved when the biochemical target is absent in the host cells. The best examples are the penicillins, which affect the biosynthesis of the murein layer of the bacterial cell wall (Chapter 3, "Biology of Infectious Agents"). No comparable structure exists in mammalian cells, which are totally insensitive to the action of these antibiotics. Nonetheless, even penicillins can have two undesirable side effects. Some individuals cannot take them because they have a strong allergic reaction. Also, administration of ampicillin, one of the most widely used penicillins, may lead to the destruction of the normal bacterial flora, particularly of the gut. This effect can lead to colitis, overgrowth by fungi, and other complications. Even a nearly perfect antibiotic comes with a price tag.

HOW DO PATHOGENS CIRCUMVENT THE ACTION OF ANTIBIOTICS?

The destructive power of antibiotics is so pervasive that within years of their introduction resistant organisms may supplant susceptible ones. At what point in the action of antibiotics does resistance come into play? The activity of antimicrobial drugs can be broken into a sequence of three steps: First, the drugs must associate with the bacteria and penetrate their envelope. Second, they must be transported to an intracellular site of action. Third, they must bind to their specific biochemical target. Resistance to drugs may occur at each of these steps. Pathogenic microorganisms, like sophisticated biochemists, have developed a multitude of ways to become resistant. The clinically relevant mechanisms of resistance include:

- Synthesis of enzymes that inactivate the drug
- Prevention of access to the target site by inhibiting uptake or increasing excretion of the drug
- Inactivation of the drug
- Modifying the target site

All these mechanisms have been recognized in clinical pathogens, but the most common is the last one. Some of the examples introduced in Chapter 3 are treated more fully below. A more extensive list of mechanisms of antibacterial resistance is shown in Table 5.1.

The β-Lactams and Enzymes That Inactivate Them

In Chapter 3, we summarized the effects of penicillins and cephalosporins on cell wall formation and their consequences for bacterial survival. This group of drugs is large, and for various reasons, their efficacy varies greatly.

These antibiotics contain a β-lactam ring (Fig. 5.5). Particular side chains located on the β-lactam ring permit the drugs to penetrate the outer membrane of Gram-negative bacteria, thus extending the list of susceptible organisms. In effect, these drugs become "broad-spectrum antibiotics" by virtue of their β-lactam rings. Other chemicals allow these drugs to be more easily absorbed or more resistant to stomach acid, thus making them effective oral chemotherapeutic agents.

An example of drug development is the transformation of cephalosporin. The original drug is more resistant to inactivating enzymes than penicillin but is less potent. The addition of new side chains created a so-called second generation of cephalosporins with greater potency, especially against Gram-negatives. A third generation with a somewhat different spectrum has been synthesized by replacing the sulfur in the ring nucleus with an oxygen (see Fig. 5.5). Cephalosporins in this class have two important advantages. First, they extend the spectrum of activity to organisms that were resistant to most of the previous cephalosporins such as *Pseudomonas* and *Haemophilus influenzae*. Second, unlike the previous cephalosporins, they penetrate well into the central nervous system. This ability has made them especially useful in the treatment of Gram-negative meningitis.

The bactericidal action of the β-lactam antibiotics requires the following steps:

1. Association with the bacteria;
2. In Gram-negatives, penetration through the outer membrane and the periplasmic space;
3. Interaction with penicillin-binding proteins on the cytoplasmic membrane;
4. Activation of an autolysin that degrades the cell wall murein.

The principal mechanism of resistance to the β-lactams is the elaboration of inactivating enzymes, the **β-lactamases**. So far, more than 100 β-lactamases have been identified, a small number of which account for most of the clinically encountered resistance. They can be divided into two categories, the penicillinases and the cephalosporinases. A fair degree of crossing over occurs

Table 5.1. Most Common Mechanisms of Resistance to Antibacterial Agents

Agent	Plasmid-borne	Resistance mechanism
Penicillins & cephalosporins	Yes	Hydrolysis of β-lactam ring by β-lactamase
Chloramphenicol	Yes	Acetylation of hydroxyl groups of chloramphenicol transacetylase; interference with transport into cell
Tetracyclines	Yes	Exit pump pushes drug out of cell
Aminoglycosides (Streptomycin, kanamycin, gentamicin, tobramycin, amikacin, etc.)	Yes	Enzymatic modification of drug by R plasmid encoded enzyme; drug has reduced affinity for ribosome, and transport into cell is reduced
Sulfanilamides	Yes	Sulfanilamide-resistant dihydropteroate synthase
Trimethoprim	Yes	Trimethoprim-resistant dihydrofolate reductase
Erythromycin	Yes	Enzymatic modification (methylation of 23S ribosomal RNA)
Lincomycin	Yes	RNA of susceptible cells converts ribosome to drug resistance (unable to bind inhibitor)
Mercury (merthiolate)	Yes	Enzymatic reduction of mercury salts to metallic state and vaporization
Nalidixic acid, rifampin nitrofurans, ciprofloxacin, etc.	No	Spontaneous mutation of gyrase, other target enzymes
Methicillin	No	Change in penicillin-binding protein (not in β-lactamase)
Vancomycin	Yes	Change in binding site in the peptidoglycan target

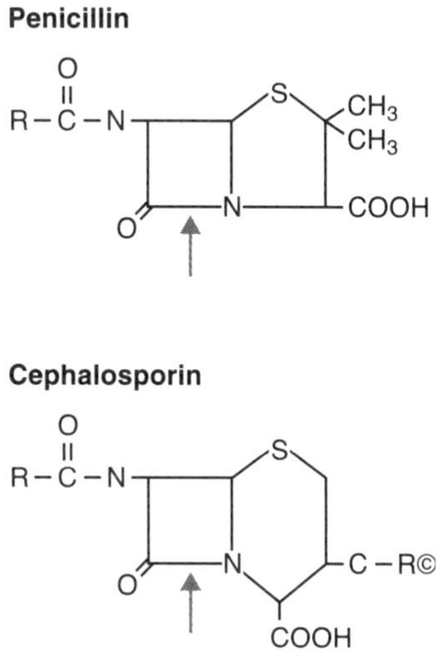

Penicillin

Cephalosporin

Figure 5.5. Core structure of penicillins and cephalosporins. The R groups specify the particular antibiotic; *arrow* indicates the bond broken during function and during inactivation by β-lactamases.

within these categories, i.e., a cephalosporinase may also inactivate a penicillin and vice versa, but with different efficiency.

In general, Gram-positive bacteria such as the staphylococci produce extracellular β-lactamases. Secreted into the medium, these enzymes destroy the antibiotic before it comes in contact with the bacterial surface. Gram-positive β-lactamases are often made in large amounts after induction by the corresponding antibiotic. Adding more drug only induces the formation of greater amounts of enzyme, and as a result, resistance usually cannot be overcome even with massive doses. In the Gram-negatives, β-lactamases are found in the periplasm or bound to the inner membrane. They are often constitutive; that is, they are produced at a constant rate that does not increase with the addition of greater amounts of the drugs. Therefore, resistance in these organisms can sometimes be overcome with higher doses of antibiotic.

β-lactamase-dependent resistance to penicillins and cephalosporins is widespread among pathogenic bacteria. It has become so common in staphylococci, both those acquired in hospitals and in the community, that infecting strains of these organisms must be considered penicillin-resistant unless proven otherwise by antibiotic susceptibility tests.

The development of β-lactam resistance among the Gram-negatives differs from that of the Gram-positives. With few exceptions, like the gonococcus, these organisms are resistant to the first drug of this group, the original penicillin G. However, when challenged with the newer drugs to which they are susceptible, the Gram-negatives have been more slow to develop resistance. For

example, prior to 1974, *H. influenzae*, an important pathogen in meningitis and pulmonary infections, was universally susceptible to the penicillin derivative ampicillin. This antibiotic was considered the drug of choice in treatment of *H. influenzae* infections. However, in 1975, it became apparent that 10–20% of the isolates of *H. influenzae* elaborate an ampicillin-degrading β-lactamase. This enzyme is encoded in a highly promiscuous plasmid, which probably accounts for the rapid spread of ampicillin resistance in this organism.

A similar reversal has occurred with the gonococcus. This organism used to be universally susceptible to penicillin, although higher levels of the drug have been gradually required over the last 30 years. In 1976, highly penicillin-resistant strains were isolated in two widely separated areas of the world. The gene coding for this resistance is carried on a transposon, which hops to other strains of gonococci and to other aerobic Gram-negatives. Thus, we can no longer rely on penicillin as the universal agent for the treatment of gonorrhea.

These examples illustrate the role of transferable genetic elements in the spread of β-lactamase resistance. The role of plasmids and transposons in the transfer of resistance has increased in importance since the early days of the antibiotic era. The first strains that became antibiotic-resistant harbored chromosomal genes, and only later were they replaced by strains with plasmid-borne resistance. The result is an increase in the spread of resistance to previously susceptible organisms. Thus, not only has resistance increased in *H. influenzae* and gonococci, but resistance in other previously highly susceptible organisms, such as the pneumococci, has been reported. If this pattern spreads further to include other important β-lactam susceptible pathogens, such as the meningococci and certain streptococci, it would be a serious blow to our ability to treat some important infectious diseases.

Other mechanisms of resistance to β-lactams have been reported. In a few instances, bacterial resistance has been attributed to poor penetration of the drugs or to mutations in the penicillin-binding proteins. This type of resistance sometimes takes on global proportions in the staphylococci. Some strains of *Staphylococcus aureus* become resistant to most of the known penicillins and cephalosporins, including a rather different one called methicillin. For this reason, these strains have the blanket designation of *m*ethicillin *r*esistant *S*taphylococcus *a*ureus, or **MRSA**. They are responsible for some of the worst outbreaks of hospital-acquired infection in recent history. These strains can only be treated successfully with another inhibitor of cell wall synthesis, vancomycin, a cyclic glycopeptide antibiotic. However, resistance to vancomycin has also been reported (see below).

Finally, certain strains of pneumococci and staphylococci are inhibited rather than killed by certain levels of β-lactams. This form of partial resistance is called **toler-ance**. In the case of tolerant pneumococci, the drugs are bacteriostatic and not bactericidal because these strains lack sufficient levels of the suicidal autolysin. Bacterial tolerance may possibly explain some of the relapses that occur following treatment of staphylococcal and strep-tococcal infections. However, compared to drug inacti-vation by β-lactamases, tolerance accounts only for a small percentage of clinically important resistance.

Antiribosomal Antibiotics

The effectiveness of the second largest class of anti-bacterial agents, the antiribosomal antibiotics, is based on structural differences between the ribosomes of bac-teria and those of eukaryotic cells. In eukaryotic cells, ri-bosomes have larger RNA molecules and more protein components. Typical drugs of this group, such as strep-tomycin or erythromycin, bind to bacterial but not to mammalian ribosomes. The difference is not always ab-solute and does not completely explain the selective tox-icity of all the drugs of this class. First, some antibiotics like tetracycline target mammalian and bacterial ribo-somes in vitro. Second, mammalian cells have bacterial-like ribosomes in their mitochondria, and these are sen-sitive to many of the drugs of this class. Researchers believe that these drugs are not toxic because they can-not pass through the plasma membrane. However, some patients experience damage to their bone marrow after treatment with chloramphenicol. This damage may re-sult from the selective uptake of the drug into the mito-chondria of highly oxidative bone marrow stem cells.

Other toxic side effects of these antibiotics cannot be anticipated from their mechanisms of action. Examples are chelation of magnesium by tetracyclines with atten-dant bone and tooth malformation in children, or toxic-ity of various aminoglycosides for the eighth cranial nerve. Another significant complication is the inhibition of the normal bacterial flora, as seen in the diarrhea that results from treatment with some of these drugs.

Tetracycline—Resistance by Drug Excretion

Resistance to antiribosomal antibiotics can take many forms because these drugs must go through many steps to reach their targets. Tetracycline, for example, must:

1. Bind to the cytoplasmic membrane, which, in the case of Gram-negatives, requires passage through the outer membrane and the periplasmic space; and
2. Be transported across the cytoplasmic membrane by an active transport mechanism. This transport mechanism involves two components, an initial rapid uptake and a second phase of slower uptake.

Resistant strains do not accumulate tetracycline within the cell. The reason is not, as might be expected, failure to take up the drug. Rather, the intracellular con-centration is kept low by an exit mechanism that actively excretes the drug. Tetracycline resistance has been found in almost all bacteria, including gram-positives and gram-negatives, aerobes, and anaerobes.

Chloramphenicol—Resistance by Drug Inactivation

Many kinds of bacteria have become resistant to chloramphenicol since its introduction. Recent examples of resistance to this drug have been seen in outbreaks of bacillary dysentery and typhoid that occurred in Central America and Mexico in the late 1960s and the early 1970s. Since chloramphenicol was considered the drug of choice for these diseases, it was widely administered. Patients did not respond to the treatment, and many died.

Bacterial resistance to chloramphenicol is mediated by two mechanisms. First, a bacterial enzyme **acetylates** it to an acetyl or diacetyl ester. The acetylated deriva-tives are biologically inert because they cannot bind to the ribosomes. **Acetyl transferase** is the enzyme respon-sible for the widespread resistance to chloramphenicol in aerobic bacteria, both Gram-positives and Gram-neg-atives. The genes coding for this enzyme are plasmid-borne. The second mechanism for chloramphenicol in-activation has been demonstrated in anaerobic bacteria, which reduce a *p*-nitro group on the molecule.

Vancomycin—Resistance by Modifying the Target (Cell Wall)

Vancomycin, a glycopeptide antibiotic in constant clinical use since the 1950s, has been a mainstay of ther-apy for Gram-positive infections, particularly strains of staphylococci and a type of streptococci, the enterococ-cci. Since this antibiotic is given intravenously, it is typ-ically reserved for hospitalized patients, many with nosocomial (hospital-acquired) infections. Vancomycin has been particularly valuable against MRSA strains for which it is typically the only useful drug available.

Since the late 1980s, however, many strains of ente-rococci have acquired resistance to vancomycin via a set of plasmid-borne genes. These genes act in consortium to produce an altered cell wall peptidoglycan precursor. Instead of the usual D-alanine-D-alanine terminus, these modified precursors have D-alanyl-lactate. The normal D-alanine-D-alanine is the target for vancomycin, where-as the modified terminus is not. Bacteria with the modi-fied terminus are resistant to vancomycin.

Many patients infected with vancomycin-resistant strains of enterococci are essentially untreatable, since these strains are also resistant to other antibiotics. A great concern is that plasmid-borne genes encoding van-comycin resistance may be transferred to staphylococci, raising the possibility that MRSAs, which are more per-vasive and virulent pathogens, will become untreatable. If these strains take hold and become more prevalent, we would revert to a situation equivalent to that of the pre-antibiotics era.

The Macrolides—Resistance by Modifying the Target (Ribosomes)

The macrolide antibiotics, another important group, are represented in clinical medicine by erythromycin, lincomycin, and clindamycin. The target of these drugs can be modified in a particularly interesting way, by methylation of the 23S ribosomal RNA of susceptible Gram-positive bacteria. This modification renders the 50S ribosomal subunits resistant to the drugs. The **methylase** involved is usually made from a plasmid gene under highly regulated conditions: little enzyme is formed during normal bacterial growth, but it is rapidly synthesized in the presence of a macrolide.

The Aminoglycosides—Resistance by Transport or Drug Inactivation

Perhaps the most complex mechanism of action of all antiribosomal antibiotics is that of the aminoglycosides. They go through the following steps:

1. Penetration of the outer membrane of Gram-negatives.
2. Association with a two-stage active transport system. This system is one-way and irreversible, unlike that of tetracycline or most metabolites.
3. Binding to the 30S ribosome subunit to inhibit protein synthesis, primarily at or near the initiation step, and to increase "miscoding" by the ribosomes that still manage to function. Miscoding results in "nonsense proteins."

Two major mechanisms of resistance to aminoglycosides have been recognized in Gram-negative bacteria. The first is the **inactivation of their transport;** this mechanism of resistance occurs in anaerobic bacteria. The second, which involves **inactivating enzymes,** is the most common mechanism in clinical isolates. Many distinct enzymes that inactivate these drugs have been identified in coliforms, pseudomonads, and staphylococci. Each one can inactivate more than one aminoglycoside, but usually not all of them. Thus, a given strain can become resistant to, say, streptomycin, kanamycin, and tobramycin, but remain fully susceptible to amikacin. Usually, the aminoglycoside-inactivating enzymes are encoded by genes carried on plasmids or transposons, and more than one enzyme may be carried by one plasmid.

SELECTIVITY AND LIMITATIONS OF ANTIFUNGAL AGENTS

As we move up the phylogenetic tree and consider eukaryotic pathogens, the differences between host and parasite begin to narrow. For example, most of the antibiotics that inhibit fungal ribosomes are active against human ribosomes and are therefore useless. Therapeutic agents against fungi, viruses, and animal parasites are often quite toxic. Nevertheless, antifungal agents with selective toxicity do exist.

Especially interesting examples are the polyenes (Chapter 45, "Introduction to the Fungi and the Mycoses"), which bind more avidly to the ergosterol in the membranes of fungi than to cholesterol in the membranes of higher eukaryotes. The margin of safety is often considerable. For example, yeasts are about 200-fold more sensitive to the polyene antibiotic amphotericin B than are cultured human cells. Amphotericin B is one of the few antifungal compounds that is sufficiently nontoxic to be used systemically. However, its efficacy is limited: at higher effective doses, it also damages membranes of kidney cells.

The imidazoles are another group of antifungal agents that have greater specificity for the fungal than for the animal cytochrome P450 demethylase involved in sterol synthesis. These antifungal agents can be used topically to treat local infections or systemically to treat invasive disease (see Chapters 45–47 on the mycoses).

Griseofulvin, a potent antifungal agent (Chapter 48, "Subcutaneous, Cutaneous, and Superficial Mycoses"), binds tightly to newly formed keratin and is effective against many superficial skin and nail infections. The required levels are sufficiently nontoxic to allow oral use for extended periods, although at higher levels cytotoxicity and carcinogenesis have been demonstrated in animal studies.

IF ONE ANTIBIOTIC IS GOOD, ARE TWO BETTER?

A potent argument for counteracting drug resistance in microorganisms can be made for the administration of several antibiotics at once. Drug-resistant mutants occur with frequencies of 10^{-6} to 10^{-9} per generation. Thus, outgrowth of resistant bacteria can easily take place and become a significant clinical risk. But two antibiotics given simultaneously can theoretically reduce the chance that a bacterium will completely evade antibiotic destruction. For example, assume that resistance to drug A has a frequency of 10^{-6} per generation. If drug B has a similar frequency of resistant mutants and is given simultaneously, the chance of a single bacterium becoming resistant to both antibiotics is 10^{-6} times 10^{-6}, or 10^{-12}, which is vanishingly small.

An excellent example of this concept currently in practice is combined therapy with sulfamethoxazole and trimethoprim. Although both drugs act on one-carbon metabolism, their sites of action are different and resistance to one does not influence resistance to the other.

Another example is antifungal therapy by the joint administration of amphotericin B and 5-fluorocytosine. The two act synergistically because 5-fluorocytosine is highly toxic in high doses, but can be used effectively at

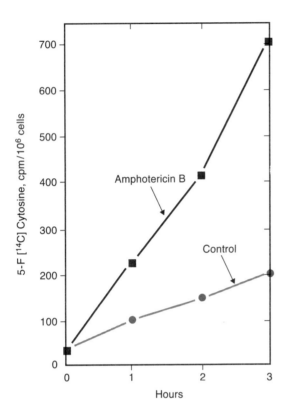

Figure 5.6. The synergistic activity of amphotericin B and 5-fluorocytosine. The uptake of labeled 5-fluorocytosine into growing *Candida albicans* is shown in the presence and absence of 0.2 μg/ml amphotericin B.

lower blood levels if the fungal membrane is selectively perturbed to become more permeable (Fig. 5.6).

The use of drugs in combination is not without problems. In fact, three outcomes are possible:

1. **Synergism.** For example, when penicillin is given along with streptomycin, the penetration of streptomycin is often enhanced.
2. **Antagonism** by one of the two drugs. Thus, when chloramphenicol is given with penicillin, it blocks protein synthesis, preventing the cell growth that is required for penicillin to cause lysis. The result is dominance by the weaker, bacteriostatic drug.
3. **Indifference.** Each drug works no better and no worse alone or in combination with the other.

Further cautions are warranted with multiple drug administration. Thus, drugs may show **synergism in toxicity,** as well as in antimicrobial action (an example is the heightened damage to the kidney by the joint administration of vancomycin and an aminoglycoside). Finally, in a hospital setting, the main sources of drug resistance are the members of the resident bacterial flora. Therefore, the decision to administer multiple drugs and which ones to choose should be governed by the spectrum of multiple drug resistance of the dominant organisms in that hospital.

ARE SUPERGERMS A THREAT?

Some of the genes that lead to antibiotic resistance are chromosomal and thus are part of the patrimony of the bacterial species. Many of these genes are plasmid-borne and are probably acquired from other bacteria (see Table 5.1).

Resistance genes, both chromosomal and on plasmids, predate the use of antibiotics. Such genes have been found in strains stored before the introduction of the drugs or in isolates from areas where antibiotics have never been deliberately introduced. The selective pressure of the widespread use of antibiotics has resulted in an increasing frequency of resistant bacteria. In broad terms, the spread of resistance genes increases with the usage of drugs in a particular geographic area or medical center. Multiple resistance genes may accumulate in a given strain by the effective mechanism of gene transposition (see Chapter 4, "Genetics of Bacterial Pathogenesis"). This process could lead to the emergence of "supergerms," microorganisms resistant to a large number of antimicrobial agents. Near-supergerm status has been achieved by occasional isolates that are resistant to 15 or more antibiotics! Particular examples are strains of enterococci (see p. 11) that are resistant to all available antibiotics and carry a high mortality rate when associated with bacteria.

Not all species have the potential to become supergerms. Some species have probably not developed an effective system of DNA transfer. Others have a transfer system that is limited in its ability to spread multiple drug resistance. For example, staphylococcal plasmids usually do not bear multiple drug resistance genes. They are usually transferred by phage transduction, and this mode of transmission may restrict the size of the DNA that can be transferred. Meningococci, group A streptococci, and the spirochete of syphilis by and large remain as susceptible to penicillin today as they were when the drug was first used.

The threat of accumulating resistance factors is nevertheless quite real. During the six years following the introduction of penicillin, resistant hospital isolates of *S. aureus* climbed from a very low level to more than 80% of the total. As mentioned above, drug-resistant strains of gonococci, *H. influenzae,* and pneumococci have recently been discovered. With the successive accumulation of resistance to many penicillinase-resistant penicillins, other agents of greater toxicity, such as vancomycin, have been reluctantly restored to clinical use.

CONCLUSION

The countermeasures taken against resistant organisms include the continued development of more effective antibiotics (such as the cephalosporins). Certainly the war between therapy and resistance mechanisms is unlikely to abate, but the battles must continue to be won. The alternative would be to give up what many physicians and historians of science regard as the difference between modern medicine and the Dark Ages.

SELF-ASSESSMENT QUESTIONS

1. Prepare yourself to give a short talk to lay persons about the history and importance of antibiotics in medicine. What points would you emphasize?

2. Describe the mode of action of sulfonamides. What is meant by competitive and noncompetitive inhibition? What is the basis of their selective toxicity?

3. Distinguish between bactericidal and bacteriostatic drugs. Under what conditions is one type preferable to the other?

4. What are the general mechanisms for bacterial resistance to antibiotics? Give examples of each class.

5. Discuss the steps required for β-lactam antibiotics activity. Which steps are commonly modified in resistant mutants?

6. Describe the mode of action of the following protein-synthesis inhibiting antibiotics: tetracycline, chloramphenicol, macrolides, and aminoglycosides. What steps become modified in resistant mutants?

7. Discuss the general mode of action of antifungal drugs.

8. Discuss two reasons for the use of multiple antibiotics to treat a patient. Why is it sometimes undesirable?

SUGGESTED READINGS

Bennett PM, Chopra I. Molecular basis for β-lactamase induction: bacteria. Antimicrob Agents Chemother 1993;37:153–158.

Gold HS, Moellering RC Jr. Antimicrobial resistance. N Engl J Med 1996;335:1445–1453.

Hunter PA, Darby GK, Russel NJ, eds. Fifty years of antimicrobials: past, perspectives and future. Cambridge: Cambridge University Press, 1995.

Levy S. The antibiotic resistance paradox. New York: Plenum, 1992.

Levy S. Active efflux mechanisms for antimicrobial resistance. Antimicrob Agents Chemother 1992;36:695–703.

Shaw KJ, Rather BN, Hare RS, Miller GH. Molecular genetics of aminoglycoside resistance genes and familial relationships of the aminoglycoside-modifying enzymes. Microb Rev 1993;57:138–163.

Speer S, Shoemaker N, Saylers A. Resistance to tetracycline: mechanisms and transmission. Clin Microb Rev 1992; S:387–399.

Constitutive Defenses of the Body

JOHN K. SPITZNAGEL

DEFENSES AGAINST MICROORGANISMS

We humans have a unique ability to shape our environment. In good part, our sanitary lifestyle determines the extent to which we encounter exogenous microorganisms, including potential pathogens. Our health is influenced by such external factors as cleanliness and nutrition. Thus, defenses against infectious diseases begin with the way we affect our environment and one another. For example, poor children who live in crowded, inadequately ventilated housing and eat a diet lacking in proteins, are much more likely to contract infectious diseases such as tuberculosis. The reason is twofold: poor nutrition diminishes the effectiveness of body defenses, and crowding makes the encounter with tubercle bacilli more frequent. The adults in such families may already have tuberculosis and, in close quarters, become a ready source of contagion. Defenses against such events are clear: they include good nutrition, adequate housing, and treatment of the ill. While these favorable conditions occur readily in an affluent society, they have to be fostered with care and sacrifice in the developing countries of the world.

Physicians share with others their concern for defense against infectious diseases. Good food in sufficient quantity, uncontaminated water, and freedom from insects and rodents—all these are the primary business of the sanitary engineer and the social scientist. Other activities are mainly medical, such as immunization, and treatment of human carriers or patients likely to contribute to the spread of disease.

We will leave this subject to Chapter 56, "Epidemiology". For now we will continue with the body's own defense mechanisms.

PHYSICAL AND CHEMICAL BARRIERS TO ENTRY

Throughout life, the body surfaces tolerate a rich and complex flora that is usually harmless but can cause op-portunistic infections. In contrast, domains of the body just a few micrometers beneath the epidermis or the mucous membranes are usually free of microorganisms. Host defenses intensify as microorganisms encounter the skin and the mucous membranes. In this and the next chapter we will explore how the body maintains this microbial gradient, from microorganism-associated surfaces to aseptic inner- and intracellular tissue domains. The question is important because a breakdown of this gradient is usually what infection is about.

The Skin

Before microorganisms can enter the normally aseptic regions of the body they must pass through the barriers of the skin, the conjunctivae of the eye, or the mucous membranes of the respiratory, alimentary, or urogenital tracts. Each barrier has its own protective mechanisms (Table 6.1). For example, the low pH of the stomach effectively kills many bacteria and viruses. The skin is bathed with oils and secretions from the sebaceous and sweat glands. These secretions contain fatty acids that are inhibitory to bacterial growth. The skin further rids itself of adherent microorganisms by desquamation, as the keratinized squamous cells are steadily sloughed off and replaced with new layers. This formidable barrier is seldom breached except by injuries such as burns, cuts, or wounds. Once they have traversed the skin, microorganisms encounter powerful defenses in the underlying soft tissues. However, these defenses do not work at full capacity under all conditions. For instance, abrasions or lacerations impair the local vascular and lymphatic circulation and interfere with soluble and cellular defense mechanisms, thus rendering the underlying connective tissue vulnerable. When this occurs, substantially fewer microorganisms are required to cause infection. This effect is seen in chronically debilitated patients who suffer

---

Table 6.1. Constitutive Defenses: Barriers to Infection

Physical		
System or Organ	Cell Type	Clearing Mechanism
Skin	Squamous	Desquamation
Mucous membranes	Columnar nonciliated (e.g., gastrointestinal tract)	Peristalsis
	Columnar ciliated (trachea)	Mucociliary movement
	Cuboidal ciliated (e.g., nasopharynx)	Tears, saliva, mucous, sweat
	Secretory (various)	Antimicrobial compounds, flow of liquids

Chemical		
System or Organ	Source	Substance
Skin	Sweat, sebaceous glands	Organic acids due to skin bacteria
Mucous membranes	Parietal cells of stomach	Hydrochloric acid, low pH
	Secretions	Antimicrobial compounds
	Neutrophils	Lysozyme, peroxidase, lactoferrin
Lung	A cells	Pulmonary surfactant
Upper alimentary	Salivary glands	Thiocyanate
	Neutrophils	Myeloperoxidase
		Cationic proteins
		Lactoferrin
		Lysozyme
Small bowel and below	Liver via biliary tree	Bile acids
	Gut flora	Low-molecular-weight fatty acids

---

from decubitus ulcers (bed sores) that become contaminated and are constantly infected with normally harmless organisms on the skin. When an injury introduces foreign bodies, such as splinters or particles of soil, the impairment of the defensive mechanisms is even more profound.

The Mucous Membranes

The mucous membranes of the mouth, pharynx, esophagus, and lower urinary tract are composed of several layers of epithelial cells, whereas those of the lower respiratory, gastrointestinal, and upper urinary tracts are delicate single layers of epithelial cells, often endowed with specialized functions. Membranes of the alveoli and the intestine are thin because they serve as exchangers of gases, fluids, and solutes. They are easily traumatized, especially when subjected to high pressure or abrasions. In fact, trauma occurs daily in the colon during defecation and in the mouth during vigorous tooth brushing.

Many mucous membranes are covered by a protective layer of **mucus**, which provides a mechanical and chemical barrier, yet permits proper function. Mucus is a giant cross-linked gel-like structure made up of glycoprotein subunits. It entraps particles and prevents them from reaching the mucous membrane. Mucus is hydrophilic and allows diffusion of many substances produced by the body, including antimicrobial enzymes such as lysozyme and peroxidase. Its rheological properties enable it to bear substantial weight and yet be readily moved by the motion of the cilia of the underlying cells.

Asepsis of deep tissues depends heavily on complex antimicrobial mechanisms, some of which are constitutive, others inducible. The constitutive systems are known collectively as the **inflammatory response** and the inducible systems as the **immune response**.

INTERNAL CONSTITUTIVE DEFENSES—INTRODUCTION

When a microorganism crosses the protective epidermis of the skin or the epithelia of mucous membranes it encounters constitutive defense mechanisms. These mechanisms are called constitutive because they do not require previous contact with the invading microorganisms (see Table 6.1). **Inflammation**, or the **inflammatory response**, the most powerful of these defenses, is not manifested in all tissues at all times but must be called up. Inflammation is elicited by a complex set of alert signals and pharmacological mediators, some of which are part of an intricate collection of interacting serum proteins called the **complement system**. This system is never completely inactive, and is normally in an idling state. Its activity is greatly increased, usually locally, by the presence of microorganisms in tissues. An important consequence of these activities is the recruitment of **phagocytes,** white blood cells that ingest and often kill invading bacteria and other microorganisms.

Early investigators believed that constitutive mechanisms lacked the potency of the **inducible** immune response (Chapter 7, "Inducible Defenses"). Researchers gradually learned that the two responses are interrelated: the inducible response cannot be expressed in the absence of constitutive mediators. It is now clear that these mediators sound the alarm for the inducible response. In the meantime they hold the invading microorganisms at bay. The two systems act synergistically to provide a magnificently enhanced defense system. The body then becomes: "A Fortress built by Nature for herself against Infection . . . ," to appropriate what Shakespeare said (in a different context).

INFLAMMATION

Inflammation is defined as the process that occurs in tissues as the reaction to injury. Early signs of inflammation are confined locally and include pain, swelling, or both, and a sense of heat and throbbing of the injured part. The inflamed site appears red, shiny, and hot and painful to the touch as the result of alterations in local blood vessels and lymphatics. These rapid changes, which are called **acute inflammation,** are dynamic and undergo predictable and continued evolution. The tissues may return to normal or become scarred. The outcome depends on the extent of damage done by trauma, by the infecting microorganisms, or by the inflammatory response itself. If acute inflammation does not cure the problem, it may change character and become a **chronic inflammation.** Although both processes are essential for defense, they can damage the structure and function of tissues.

What are the underlying changes in acute inflammation? Briefly, the blood supply to the affected part increases due to vasodilatation. How does this take place? Endothelial cells synthesize a series of special proteins (selectins, immunoglobulin-like molecules, and cytokines, see below) that allow capillaries to become more permeable to fluid and large molecules such as antibodies and complement components. Inflammation thus allows these components to enter the tissues. White blood cells, first neutrophils and later monocytes, accumulate on the increasingly sticky endothelium of inflamed capillaries. More and more white blood cells cross between the capillary endothelial cells by **diapedesis,** migrate into surrounding tissue, and move by chemotaxis toward the injured site. Thus, redness and increased heat are due to greatly increased blood flow in the area. Swelling is caused by the outpouring of fluid and white blood cells. In mild inflammation, the fluid

has a low protein content, as in the contents of a blister, which is called the **serous exudate.** In severe inflammation, the fluid is known as **fibrinous exudate** because it is rich in fibrinogen and other proteins, and eventually clots due to fibrin formation. Pain is caused by the release of chemical mediators (see below) and by the mechanical compression of nerves.

An important consequence of inflammation is that in inflamed tissues the pH is decreased owing to the production of lactic acid by the inflammatory cells that enter the area. Low pH itself is antimicrobial. Moreover, the antimicrobial action of small-molecular-weight organic acids is enhanced at low pH. In addition, low pH may alter microbial sensitivity to antibiotics and antimicrobial tissue peptides, making them either more resistant or more sensitive. The oxygen tension in inflamed tissue also changes, first increasing when circulation is increased by vasodilation, then decreasing when circulation is impaired by edema, necrosis, or vascular spasm.

Molecular Mediators of Inflammation and the Acute Phase Response

How does the body respond to microorganisms in the inflammatory response? During inflammation, a series of complex events takes place that eventually result in the production of **chemical mediators,** substances that are responsible for the signs of inflammation, vascular permeability, vasodilation, and pain. The earliest events that result in the formation of these mediators are the activation of complement or the blood clotting cascade, which, in turn, are activated by the presence of microorganisms.

The list of mediators is formidable, and we will mention only a few of the main players. Among the best known chemical mediators is **histamine,** which dilates blood vessels and increases their permeability. Histamine is made by mast cells and its release is induced by three small peptides called **anaphylatoxins C3a, C4a,** and **C5a** that are produced by activation of the complement system.

Other inflammatory mediators include the so-called **kinins** (Table 6.2), small basic peptides that alter vascular tone, increase permeability, and initiate or potentiate the release of yet other mediators from leukocytes. The best known is **bradykinin,** whose potency in increasing vascular permeability rivals that of histamine. Kinins are produced by cleavage of precursor proteins, called **kininogens,** by activation of the clotting cascade, or by release from granulocytes. A key compound in these complex interactions is the **Hageman factor,** which induces the production of kinins after it is activated during inflammation. One of the compounds that elicits the activation of Hageman factor is the **endotoxin** (lipopolysaccharide) of Gram-negative bacteria, which explains in part how the presence of these microorganisms can elicit an inflammatory response.

Table 6.2. Some Constitutive Defenses

Ions and Small Molecules	Source	Function
Reduced oxygen species, OH·/, H_2O_2 O_2^-, OH· H_2O_2	Phagocytes, occasionally bacteria	O_2 tension in tissues influences microbial growth; reduced oxygen molecules are antimicrobial
Chloride ion	Body fluids	Cl^- combines with myeloperoxidase and H_2O_2 to form a potent antimicrobial system
Hydrogen ion	Phagocytes (and other cells)	Antimicrobial in high concentrations
Fatty acids	Metabolites (of phagocytes and other cells)	Most antibacterial at low pH
Platelet-activating factor (an alkylacetyl glycerophosphocholine)	Leukocytes and many other cells	Multiple effects: platelet aggregation and degranulation; activates monocytes but inhibits T lymphocyte proliferation

Single Protein Systems	Source	Function
Lactoferrin	Neutrophils, other granulocytes	Binds iron, limits bacterial growth
Transferrin	Liver	Binds iron, limits bacterial growth
Interferons	Virus-infected cells	Limit virus multiplication
Cytokines (various interleukins, tumor necrosis factor)	Various cells of the immune system	Affect function and proliferation of cells of the immune system
Lysozyme	Neutrophils, macrophages, tears, saliva, urine	Antimicrobial for many bacteria (degrades murein)
Fibronectin	Macrophages, fibroblasts	Opsonin for staphylococci

Complex Protein Systems	Source	Function
Complement cascade	Macrophages, liver cells	Products increase vascular hepatic permeability, cause smooth parenchymal cells muscle contractions; chemotactic; opsonize bacteria; bactericidal
Coagulation system Kinins	Produced by the action of specific proteases (the kallikreins) on certain liver glycoproteins called kininogens)	Permeability, vasodilation, increase vascular permeability, pain
Fibrinopeptides	Fibrinogen	Chemotactic
Hageman factor	Clotting cascade	Triggers several inflammatory events in the coagulation system

Other mediators, the **leukotrienes** and the **prostaglandins,** act on the motility and metabolism of white blood cells. Prostaglandins formed in the hypothalamus also act on the thermoregulatory centers of the brain and cause fever. Aspirin and indomethacin prevent the effects of prostaglandins by inhibiting their synthesis. Note that in preventing the synthesis of these compounds, these drugs remove an important warning sign that infection may be present.

During inflammation, certain proteins that participate in various aspects of inflammation are released (chiefly) from the liver. Collectively, their rise in concentration in serum is known as the **acute phase response.** The length of the list of mediators readily illustrates how complex inflammation really is. However, there is even

more. Once the white blood cells are mobilized and participate in the inflammatory response, they make a family of mediators known as **cytokines** which have been implicated in several important aspects of the inflammatory and the immune response.

Cytokines

A microorganism in host tissues triggers alarm systems that, in Shakespeare's words, "Cry havoc and let slip the dogs of war." If inflammation and collateral tissue damage are the havoc that ensues, the phagocytes and lymphocytes summoned are the dogs of war. Commanding these impressive host responses are the cytokines, proteins secreted by the macrophages and lymphocytes. Cytokines (literally, "cell movers") are

Table 6.3. Components of the Complement System[a]

Component	Role in the Complement Cascade
Classical pathway	
C1q	Binds to Fc region of Ig in Ab–Ag complexes; this binding leads to the activation of C1r
C1r	C1r is cleaved on activation to generate $\overline{C1r}$, a smaller fragment of C1r, which is a serine protease that cleaves C1s
C1s	C1s is cleaved to produce a fragment $\overline{C1s}$, a serine protease; this, in turn, cleaves C4 and C2
C4	Is split by $\overline{C1s}$ into the anaphylatoxin C4a, and the protein C4b which binds to the surface membrane and becomes part of the C3 convertase
C2	Binds to C4b and is cleaved by $\overline{C1s}$ into C2b, which is a serine protease component of the C3/C5 convertase, and C2a that diffuses away
C3 (also part of the alternative pathway)	Cleaved by C2b into the anaphylatoxin C3a, and the protein C3b which is an opsonin and is also part of the C3/C5 convertases
Alternative pathway	
Factor B (Bf)	Analogous to C2 in the classical pathway
Factor D (D)	A serine protease that activates factor B by cleaving it
Membrane attack complex (MAC)	
C5	Cleaved by the convertase complex; C5a is an anaphylatoxin, C5b is the anchoring protein for C6
C6	Binds to C5b and this complex becomes the anchor for C7
C7	Binds to the C5b, C6 complex and then C5b, C6, C7 inserts into the membrane and becomes an anchor for C8
C8	Attaches to C5b, C6, C7 and produces a stable membrane-associated complex that can bind C9
C9	Polymerizes at the site of the C5–C8 complex; this completes formation of the fully lytic MAC
Complement receptors	
Complement receptor type 1 (CR1)	Accelerates dissociation of the C3 convertases, enhances phagocytosis of C3b- or C4b-coated microorganisms
Complement receptor type 2 (CR2)	Clearance of complement-containing immune complexes, cell surface receptor for Epstein-Barr virus (EBV)
Complement receptor type 3 (CR3)	Adhesion protein (integrin family), important in phagocytosis of iC3b-coated microorganisms
Complement receptor type 4 (CR4)	Member of the integrin family of proteins, important in phagocytosis of iC3b-coated microorganisms

[a] The proteins that regulate complement activity are listed separately in Table 6.5.

induced by and interact with many systems in distant cells, adjacent cells, and the cells that produce them. The number of cytokines is impressive; at least twelve called **interleukins** (abbreviated IL plus a number) have been described, and several similar proteins known by other names have also been recognized. Cytokines play important roles in the induction of the immune response as well as in inflammation, and so they are described in greater detail in Chapter 7, "Induced Defenses" (see Table 7.3).

Several cytokines are so important to inflammation that they should be mentioned here (see Table 6.2). IL-l is involved in many inflammatory events, including production of fever, induction of adherence proteins on en-

dothelial cells, enhancement of vascular permeability and coagulation, and induction of the respiratory burst in neutrophils and monocytes. In the hypothalamus, IL-1 acts by stimulating its target cells to express prostaglandins that in turn act on other cells. Another cytokine, **tumor necrosis factor (TNF)** has many activities including the capacity to kill tumor cells, cause cachexia (wasting) in infection and in cancer, and induce fever. IL-6 has multiple effects, but one of its most interesting actions is to induce the synthesis of acute phase proteins by the liver. IL-8 released by mononuclear phagocytes and endothelial cells in response to IL-l and TNF is a powerful chemotaxin and activator of oxygen radical production by neutrophils and macrophages. It contributes to accumulation of pus in inflammation. **IL-12** is the most powerful stimulant of natural killer (NK) cells and causes them to secrete increased amounts of a protein called γ-interferon which enhances the ability of macrophages to kill intracellular organisms, a key step in cell-mediated immunity (see Chapter 7, "Induced Defenses").

From the microorganism's point of view, the actions of cytokines are beneficial to the host and detrimental to the infecting agent. However, powerful substances like cytokines can and do contribute to local and general tissue damage. Nevertheless, the overall effect of the cytokines is to orchestrate the protective mechanisms of the host. In fact, patients who cannot mount inflammatory responses rapidly succumb to infections.

COMPLEMENT

Activation of the Classical and Alternative Pathways

The complement system is extraordinarily complex. It has many components that are known by unfamiliar names (see Table 6.3), it mediates a large number of biological effects, and it interacts with other complex systems, such as blood clotting and specific immune responses. Because the complement system plays an essential role in health and disease, some familiarity with it is needed.

The complement system derives its name from the original belief that it "complements" or "completes" the action of antibodies. Only later did researchers realize that it plays a crucial role in body defenses even in the absence of specific antibodies. The complement system is constitutive and, in the immunological sense, nonspecific. The complement system is normally barely "on," and must be **activated** in order to become a significant part of the defense mechanisms (Fig. 6.1). Once activated, it functions to enhance the antimicrobial defenses in several ways:

- It makes invading microorganisms susceptible to phagocytosis.
- It lyses some microorganisms directly.
- It activates antimicrobial systems of phagocytes.
- It produces substances that are chemotactic for white blood cells.
- It promotes the inflammatory response, as we have already seen.

The complement system can be activated in one of two ways. The two activation pathways are known as **classical** and **alternative** (Fig. 6.1). Each pathway starts out separately but the two eventually converge to make the same end products. The classical pathway is usually set in motion by the presence of antigen–antibody complexes. It is the most prominent of the two and was described first, hence its name. The alternative pathway is

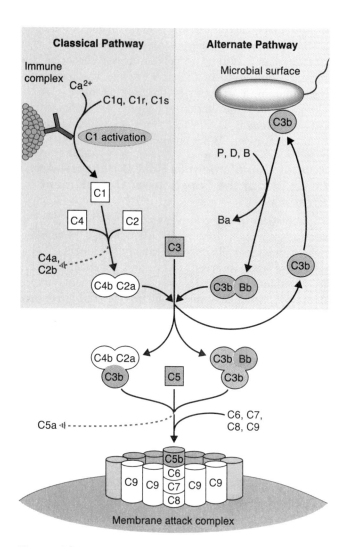

Figure 6.1. Activation of complement through the classical and alternative pathways.

elicited independently of antibodies (Fig. 6.1), often by bacterial surface components, such as lipopolysaccharides. In either case, activation results from **proteolytic cleavage** of inert larger proteins. Some important steps in activation by either pathway depend on the function of **protein complexes** made by binding several of the cleaved fragments.

Nomenclature

The complement system comprises as many as 30 proteins, most of which are present in serum and a few that are part of cell membranes. The nomenclature of complement components is complicated by their sheer numbers and by the chronology of their discovery. The major components of the classical pathway are designated by the letter C followed by a number, for example, C3 (see Table 6.3). When the component is cleaved in the process of activation, its fragments receive an additional letter, **a** or **b**. Thus, **C3a** and **C3b** are the products of proteolytic cleavage of C3. The "a" usually designates a small soluble peptide, whereas "b" denotes a larger peptide that may bind to cell surfaces. When cleavage products bind to form an active enzyme, the complex is indicated by a superscript bar, for example C4b2b. Components of the alternative pathway are designated by letters, such as **B, D, P**, except for **C3b**, which is formed by both pathways. What an alphabet soup this is!

Role of Complement in Host Defenses—An Overview of the Functions of Complement Proteins

Activation of the complement system is involved in several important aspects of host defenses. Hereditary defects in almost all the complement components (Table 6.4) have been observed. Individuals genetically unable to manufacture some of the crucial complement components are particularly susceptible to bacterial infections. Although many of these individuals live healthy lives, some develop life-threatening conditions. These individuals are also subject to unusual noninfectious disease, such as systemic lupus erythematosus.

Two activities of complement are specifically directed toward enhancing phagocytosis, which is probably the most effective of the constitutive defenses against microorganisms. These activities are the recruitment of white cells by **chemotactic proteins**, such as C5a (Fig. 6.2), and the facilitation of phagocytosis by proteins called **opsonins** (Fig. 6.3).

Other components of complement make the so-called **membrane attack complex**, which is responsible for the lysis of bacteria, some viruses, and foreign cells. They may even lyse infected tissue cells that appear alien because they display viral or other foreign proteins in their cell membrane. This activity is particularly important in killing bacteria that resist phagocytosis, such as meningococci and gonococci. Indeed, genetic deficiencies of the proteins involved in the formation of the membrane attack complex result in increased susceptibility to infections by these particular organisms (see Table 6.4).

Complement activation induces the inflammatory response via the formation of Il-1, TNF, and anaphylatoxins. These activities can be considered beneficial, insofar as the inflammatory response helps fight invading microorganisms. However, they also have negative effects which can be quite severe. In persons with hypersensitivity disorders, the inflammatory response damages sensitive tissues, especially by causing leukocytes to secrete their lysosomal enzymes in inappropriate ways. These diseases include rheumatoid arthritis, serum sickness, and infective endocarditis.

The Crucial Step in Complement Activation: Cleavage of C3

The two pathways of complement activation converge at a key biochemical step, the **cleavage of component C3** (see Fig. 6.1). From this point on, the remaining steps of both pathways are the same. The enzymes responsible for this activity, **C3 convertases**, yield fragments **C3a** and **C3b**. Both of these components are pharmacologically active. C3a is an anaphylatoxin, and C3b has several functions: it is an opsonin, and it also binds to platelets to induce the release mediators of inflammation. In addition, C3b becomes part of the C3 convertase of the alternative pathway to stimulate its own synthesis and participates in the subsequent steps of complement activation.

The action of either C3 convertase is potentially dan-

Table 6.4. Hereditary Complement Deficiencies and Their Role in Microbial Pathogenesis

Affected Component	Defective Function	Infectious Disease Associations
Classical Pathway		
C1q, C1r, or C1s	Activation of the classical pathway	Susceptibility to pyogenic infections
C4	Activation of the classical pathway	Susceptibility to pyogenic infections
C2	Activation of the classical pathway	Susceptibility to pyogenic infections
C3	Activation of the classical and alternative pathways	Pyogenic infections; these may be frequent and can be fatal
	Opsonization	
	Phagocytosis	This deficiency points out the central importance of C3 in handling these microorganisms
Alternative Pathway (Note: no known defect in factor B)		
D	Activation of the alternative pathway	Susceptibility to pyogenic infections
P	Activation of the alternative pathway	Frequent pyogenic infections; fulminant meningococcemia
Attack complex		
C5, C6, C7, C8, C9	MAC formation and cell lysis	Enhanced susceptibility to disseminated *Neisseria* infections

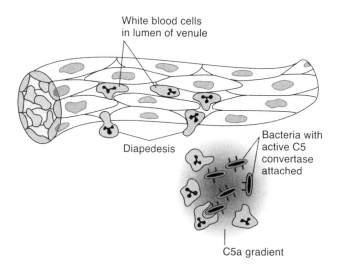

Figure 6.2. Chemotactic action of C5a diffusing from bacteria toward a postcapillary venule.

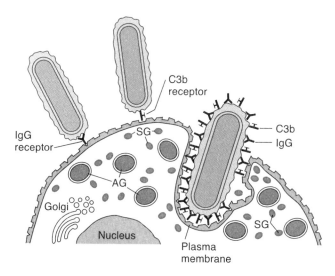

Figure 6.3. Opsonization enhances phagocytosis. This schematic representation shows how *Escherichia coli* is opsonized with immunoglobulin (*IgG*) and complement component *C3b*. The Fc and C3b ligands on the bacteria attach to the phagocyte through specific receptors. The mechanism of this interaction probably resembles that of a zipper or, perhaps, the fabric Velcro. Thus, sequential binding leads to the ingestion of the bacteria by the phagocytic membrane, until the vesicle formed is pinched off as a new organelle inside the phagocyte. Meanwhile, degranulation, the fusion of granules with the phagocytic vesicle, forms a chamber in which bacteria are destroyed. The secondary granules (*SG*) and the azurophil granules (*AG*), also known as primary granules, fuse their membranes with that of the nascent phagosome, thus making a phagolysosome. As phagocytes tend to be "sloppy" eaters, there is some "drooling" and the enzymes and surfactant proteins enter the surrounding fluid, contributing to the tissue changes of inflammation.

gerous, since it produces mediators of inflammation that would damage tissues if produced in large amounts. It is not surprising, therefore, that the body contains powerful **convertase inhibitors**. These inhibitors are discussed below (see "The Regulation of Complement Activation").

C3 Convertase of the Alternative Pathway

How is the alternative pathway activated? C3 is constantly cleaved even without complement activation. Such cleavage generates C3b in plasma, but normally specific inhibitors inactivate most of these fragments. In the presence of microorganisms, some C3b fragments survive by binding covalently to their surface. Such **surface-bound C3b** is protected from inactivation and can participate in subsequent complement reactions. Thus, the alternative pathway is elicited by the stabilization of C3b, which may be caused by the presence of microorganisms.

C3 Convertase of the Classical Pathway

Activation of complement by the classical pathway usually occurs in the presence of antigen–antibody complexes and thus is set off as the result of an induced immunological response. It may, however, be elicited in the absence of antibodies. The classical pathway involves a protein complex called **C1** and two proteins, **C2** and **C4**. C1 is unusual in structure and function: it is composed of three proteins, **C1q**, **C1r**, and **C1s**. C1q is made up of six subunits, each shaped like a tulip (Fig. 6.4).

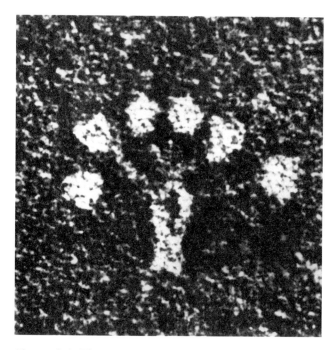

Figure 6.4. Electron micrograph of complement component C1q ×500,000. In this lateral view, six terminal subunits are connected to a central subunit by fibrillar strands.

Complement activation by this pathway proceeds as follows: The globular "head" of C1q binds to the Fc portion of antibodies in antigen–antibody complexes and other compounds that elicit the activation by the classical pathway. This binding of C1q converts C1r to a protease that carries out the next step in the pathway, the cleavage of C1s. The activated enzyme C1s in turn cleaves **C2** and **C4** into fragments $\overline{C4b2b}$ which become the **C3 convertase** of the classical pathway. This process resembles the formation of the alternative pathway C3 convertase in that $\overline{C4b2b}$, like C3b, binds covalently to nearby membranes and escapes inactivation. This process is also subject to positive feedback, and the production of this convertase may also be amplified as ever more C3 molecules are converted to C3b peptides.

Late Steps in Complement Activation: The Membrane Attack Complex (MAC)

Once C3b is formed by either pathway, the downstream steps in complement activation can take place (see Fig. 6.1). Eventually, **C5** is cleaved to produce two important fragments, C5a and C5b. **C5a**, like C3a, is an anaphylatoxin, as well as a powerful chemoattractant for phagocytes. The other fragment, **C5b**, is involved in making the final product of the complement cascade, the **membrane attack complex**. This armor-piercing weapon can punch holes in bacteria and, in some cases, in tissue cells (Fig. 6.5). The MAC damages cells and bacteria by the insertion of donut-shaped multimers of C9 (which are assembled with the help of components C5b, C6, C7, and C8) into their membranes. The resulting hole makes cells permeable to ions and metabolites. Water enters the cells and raises their pressure, which eventually causes the cells to lyse.

Regulation of Complement Activation

The complement system is programmed to destroy. It must, therefore, be strictly regulated. Fortunately, its spontaneous activation in the blood is closely controlled by several mechanisms. Both fluid-phase and membrane-bound proteins inhibit components of both the classical and alternative pathways (Table 6.5). For example, the formation of the C3 convertase of both pathways is inhibited by **decay accelerating factor** (DAF). DAF is a membrane glycoprotein, found on many cell types, that inhibits the formation of the C3b convertase (see Fig. 6.1). Complement activities are regulated at many other stages as well (Table 6.5) and this careful control underscores the damage that complement components, if unchecked, are capable of inflicting on normal cells and tissues.

The importance of these inhibitory proteins is also seen in persons who lack them because of genetic defects. For example, deficiency of H or I protein, is associated with **recurrent pyogenic infections**. Such conditions arise from faulty complement regulation, which leads to the imbalance in the concentration of certain complement components. The genetic deficiency of C1 esterase inhibitor permits activation of the classical pathway with the uncontrolled production of anaphylatoxins. The result may be **hereditary angioedema**, a potentially fatal condition that causes laryngeal edema and airway obstruction. Another serious hereditary disease, **paroxysmal nocturnal hemoglobinuria**, manifests as bouts of intravascular hemolysis due in part to complement lysis. This condition results from defective function of inhibitory proteins on the surface of red blood cells. Each red blood cell binds as many as 1000 molecules of C3b per day. The reason these cells are not normally lysed is that they have inhibitory proteins on their surface. In patients with this disease, these inhibitors do not function because they are not properly inserted in the red blood cell membrane.

Microbial View of Complement and Other Defenses in Plasma

Complement killing by insertion of the MAC affects not only bacteria but also **enveloped viruses**. Not sur-

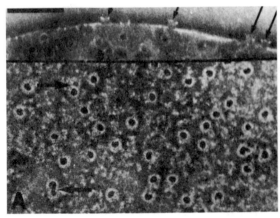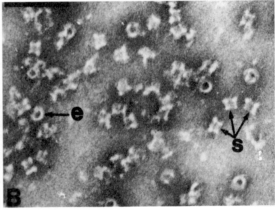

Figure 6.5. Membrane attack complex (MAC) seen under the electron microscope. **A.** MACs inserted into complement-lysed red blood cell membranes. On top portion, MACs are shown in their lateral projections. **B.** Isolated MACs in a detergent solution. *e*, a MAC on end. *s*, MACS on their side.

Table 6.5. Proteins That Regulate Complement Activity[a]

Component	Function
Soluble serum proteins	
C1 inhibitor (C1 INH)	Inhibits C1̄r and C1̄s and prevents their participation in the classical pathway
C4 binding	Binds to C4b and enhances the decay of the protein (C4bp) classical pathway C3 convertase
Factor H (H)	Binds to C3b and enhances the decay of the alternative pathway C3 convertase
Factor I (I)	Proteolytically inactivates C4b and C3b
Properdin (P)	Binds to the C3–C5 convertase and stabilizes it
Anaphylatoxin (ANA-IN) inactivator	Proteolytically inactivates the anaphylatoxins, C3a, C4a, and C5a
S-protein (S) (vitronectin)	Inhibits insertion of the MAC into the lipid bilayer by binding to the C5b-7 complex
Integral membrane proteins	
Complement receptor type 1 (CR1)	Accelerates dissociation of both C3 convertases
Membrane cofactor protein (MCP)	Cofactor for factor 1–mediated cleavage of C3b
Decay accelerating factor (DAF)	Accelerates dissociation of both C3 counvertases
Membrane inhibitor of reactive lysis (MIRL, CD59)	Prevents MAC formation
Homologous restriction factor (HRF)	Blocks MAC insertion into the surface of cells

prisingly, sensitive microorganisms have evolved countermeasures, some of which are discussed in Chapter 8 ("The Parasite's Way of Life"). An interesting example of microbial defenses against complement is provided by herpes simplex virus (HSV). One of the glycoproteins of HSV, glycoprotein C, contains a region that has an amino acid sequence similar to that of part of complement receptor Type 1 (CR1). This amino acid sequence allows glycoprotein C to bind complement component C3b, thereby interfering with the rest of the complement cascade and with complement-mediated killing of the virus.

Complement is not the only component of blood capable of killing bacteria. The enzyme **lysozyme** also plays an important role, although it affects certain kinds of bacteria only. Lysozyme is found in most body secretions and is present in blood in large amounts (4 μg/ml). It specifically cleaves bacterial cell murein at its sugar backbone. Lysozyme is the only enzyme with this activity present in vertebrates. It may well represent an adaptive mechanism that keeps animals from becoming deposits of murein and chitin. This is fortunate because these two compounds activate complement and are therefore highly inflammatory.

Lysozyme acts mainly on **Gram-positive bacteria**, although many bacterial species have evolved resistant modifications of their cell wall chemistry. Gram-negative bacteria, however, are resistant because their murein substrate is shielded by their outer membranes. In this case, lysozyme may work synergistically with complement. If the outer membrane of Gram-negatives is disrupted by the MAC of complement, murein is then available for degradation by lysozyme. Despite the im-

pressive effects of complement and lysozyme, it should be emphasized that many bacteria are resistant to them. This does not diminish the importance of the so-called **serum bactericidal activity** in destroying invading bacteria. However, inherited lysozyme deficiency in humans has not been described, thus it is difficult to assess the real contribution of this enzyme.

Leukocyte Chemotaxins—Sounding the Alarm

We have already seen that a product of complement activation, C5a, is an attractant for neutrophils and monocytes. It is not the only one; chemically distinct **chemotaxins** are also made by bacteria and by nucleated blood cells. Prominent among the latter are the leukotrienes, which are lipid products of cell membrane metabolism, and IL-8, a product of monocytes and macrophages.

The chemotaxins made by bacteria have an interesting origin. Many bacterial proteins "mature" after their synthesis, when a peptide is clipped off from their N-terminus. The first amino acid in these peptides is N-formyl-methionine, the initiator amino acid in procaryotic protein synthesis. Eukaryotic cells do not use this device. These cleaved peptides are recognized by the host as strong chemoattractants for phagocytes. They differ in activity depending on their amino acid sequence, some being remarkably potent. N-formylmethionyl-leucyl-phenylalanine, for example, is active at concentrations of 10^{-11} molar! In this way, living bacteria loudly advertise their presence as they synthesize their proteins.

Chemotaxins enhance and direct the motility of phagocytic cells. As these compounds diffuse from their source, a concentration gradient is formed in the surrounding tissues. If the tissues are inflamed, neutrophils are already poised for action on the vascular endothelia. When neutrophils sense the chemotaxins, they travel along the gradient, cross the endothelial cells, and move in tissues toward the microorganisms. This chemical homing mechanism guides the neutrophils precisely and efficiently to their targets.

Opsonization and Opsonins

Normally, phagocytic cells are not equipped for highly efficient uptake of particles. Unless stimulated by substances called **opsonins**, neutrophils, for example, will phagocytize only a relatively small proportion of bacteria present. The term *opsonin* is related to the Latin word *opsonium*, which means "relish," an apt term for making bacteria more appetizing to phagocytes.

Several substances normally serve as opsonins, among them the **C3b** component of complement and antibodies. C3b binds covalently to the surface of bacteria and forms a ligand that is recognized by receptors on neutrophils, monocytes, and macrophages. Microorganisms coated with C3b become anchored to the surface of phagocytes, which facilitates their uptake. Four receptors for C3b and its various cleavage products are located on white blood cells. These receptors are called **CR1, CR2, CR3,** and **CR4,** for "complement receptor" (see Table 6.3).

In a following section we discuss how antibodies also function as opsonins, and how these alter the metabolism of phagocytes to make them more effective in taking up and killing microorganisms.

PHAGOCYTES: THE MAIN LINE OF CONSTITUTIVE DEFENSE

Of all the constitutive antimicrobial defenses of the body, the most potent is the cellular response. It consists of the influx of neutrophils, eosinophils, and monocytes into infected tissues. You should be versed in the properties of these cell types (Table 6.6).

Neutrophils

Neutrophils are actively motile phagocytic cells produced in the bone marrow (Table 6.6). They differentiate from stem cells over a period of about 2 weeks. During this time they produce two kinds of microscopically visible granules, first the azurophil, and later the specific granules (Table 6.7). When they mature, in numbers of about 10^{10} per day, about 5% of them enter the peripheral blood and circulate for an average of 6.5 hours. Half of these neutrophils enter the capillary bed where they "**marginate**," that is, they adhere to the endothelium of venules. In response to distress signals from the tissues (complement components, cytokines such as IL-1), the endothelium in the involved region expresses a set of adhesion molecules that bind more firmly to the neutrophils. When summoned by chemotaxins, the neutrophils cross the endothelium by diapedesis through the cell junctions, traverse the basement membrane, and enter the extravascular tissue spaces (see Fig. 6.2).

As we have seen, neutrophils and monocytes can be enticed into foci of infection by gradients of chemoattractant molecular fragments generated by the complement system of the host and the formylated byproducts of microbial protein synthesis. But what ensures that these phagocytes will arrive precisely where they are needed?

The answer to the question is that neutrophils and monocytes, as well as the endothelial cells to which they must adhere, become **sticky** (see Fig 6.2). The molecular explanation is simple; it is due to sugars on glycosylated

---

Table 6.6. The White Blood Cells

Phagocyte	Source	Function
Neutrophil	Bone marrow via stem cells to peripheral blood	Adherence, chemotaxis, diapedesis Phagocytosis Degranulation Antimicrobial action, oxidative and nonoxidative
Eosinophil	Similar to neutrophil	Antiparasitic action, nonoxidative and oxidative
Monocyte	Bone marrow via stem cells Promonocyte to peripheral blood	Adherence, chemotaxis Diapedesis Phagocytosis Antimicrobial actions, secretion of cytokines
Macrophage	Monocytes of the peripheral blood	See monocytes Synthesis of important molecules, including complement components Lysozyme, II-1, II-8, tumor necrosis factor and other cytokines, plasminogen activator, other proteases, undefined mediators and important cell membrane components including MHC class I and II product (see Table 6.7). Immunologic functions include but are not limited to antigen processing, antigen presentation, etc.

Table 6.7. Substances Associated with the Azurophil and Specific Granules of Neutrophils

	Antimicrobials		
Granule Type	O_2-Independent	O_2-Dependent	Other
Azurophil	CAP57[a] CAP37 BPI[b] Elastase Cathepsin G Defensins[c] Lysozyme	Myeloperoxidase[d]	
Specific	Lactoferrin Lysozyme	NADPH oxidase[e] cofactors	Bacterial chemotaxin receptors C5a receptors Collagenase Gelatinase Vitamin B_{12}-binding protein

[a] CAP signifies cationic antimicrobial proteins.

[b] Bacterial permeability–inducing protein.

[c] Low-molecular-weight cationic antimicrobial proteins.

[d] Myeloperoxidase together with C1 and hydrogen peroxide form a potent antimicrobial system.

[e] This enzyme complex forms with fusion of specific granule membranes with the cytoplasmic membrane. The specific granules are believed to contribute the cytochrome component of the complex and the flavoprotein, while the neutrophil cytoplasmic membrane contributes an NADPH oxidase to the complex.

surface proteins. The **glycoproteins** involved include several **receptor molecules** on the endothelial cells and on the phagocytes. However, stickiness introduces a problem: blood cells that originate in the marrow must enter the bloodstream and be able to circulate there without sticking too firmly. For their part, the endothelial cells lining the blood vessels must avoid becoming too sticky, thus permitting the circulation of the blood cells. At the proper time, however, both leukocytes and endothelial cells must be able to stick to each other. The transition from loosely adherent to tightly adherent is critical for the leukocytes to leave the circulation and move through the tissues. Clearly leukocytes and endothelial cells are subject to regulatory mechanisms that induce stickiness of these cells at the proper time. Complement fragments such as C5a and cytokines such as IL-l, TNF, and IL-8 play such directive and regulatory roles, attracting leukocytes and stimulating endothelial cells, upregulating their stickiness and causing them to produce additional cytokines and prostaglandins.

The importance of glycoprotein receptors for endothelial cells that are present on neutrophils is illustrated in people with congential defects in these proteins. Neutrophils of these patients are unable to pass through the vascular endothelium, and, in addition, fail to orient, bind, and ingest particles. Such defective neutrophils are unable to form pus. Patients with this condition are said to have congenital **leukocyte adhesion deficiency (LAD)** and suffer recurrent, often fatal infections. The reason that neutrophils of LAD patients do not pass through

endothelia is that their receptors fail to bind to the endothelial cells. The reason for failure to bind to and ingest bacteria is that one of the receptors (called Mac-1), which normally binds the complement opsonin C3b, is defective. These molecules are of great interest to the pharmaceutical industry, where efforts are being directed toward the discovery of drugs to control leukocyte adhesion functions.

In a healthy person, sticking of leukocytes to endothelial surfaces is most intense in the submucosa of the alimentary tract. The large intestine has an enormous microbial population just one cell layer away from the host's aseptic tissues. This abundant flora generates large amounts of chemotaxins that recruit the bulk of the normally available neutrophils. Thus, the submucosa of the gut is in a constant state of inflammation, which keeps the microbial flora of the lumen in check. Failure of the bone marrow to make neutrophils due to toxic chemicals, or radiation, or other reasons, results in infections that emanate from the gut.

Monocytes and Macrophages

Slower to arrive at the sites of microbial invasion are the **monocytes**. These circulating members of the mononuclear family eventually settle in tissues and become known as resident **tissue macrophages**. Although monocytes and macrophages share a common progenitor with neutrophils, their kinetics of maturation and appearance are substantially different. Unlike the neutrophils, monocytes continue to differentiate after they leave the bone marrow. Most importantly, monocytes and macrophages represent both constitutive and inducible defense mechanisms, a point that will be elaborated further (see Chapter 7, "Induced Defenses"). From now on, it is important to know that these mononuclear cells become involved in cooperative interactions with the cells of the immune system and play a crucial role in **cell-mediated immunity**.

In general, monocytes and macrophages come into play slowly, often hours after neutrophils have been actively combating invading microorganisms. Neutrophils play a role in recruiting mononuclear cells because they release a granule protein (CAP 37) that is a potent attractant specific for monocytes. The delay in monocyte activity is seen in patients who become neutropenic from chemicals or radiation. If the neutropenia develops slowly, there is time for monocytes to replace the disappearing neutrophils. The risk of infection is much smaller in these patients than in those with an abrupt onset of neutropenia.

Tissue or resident macrophages exist throughout the body and have different names and functions, depending on the tissue. Thus, they are called Kupffer cells in the liver, alveolar macrophages in the lungs, osteoclasts in the bone, and microglia in the brain, etc. All these tissue macrophages phagocytize invading microorganisms. Tissue macrophages contribute greatly to the inflammatory response by releasing IL-1, which enhances sticking of neutrophils to the capillary endothelia, and TNF, which activates newly arrived neutrophils. In addition, tissue macrophages release an activator of the acute phase reaction (Il-6) and an attractant for neutrophils (Il-8). These macrophages are replenished by the arrival and differentiation of monocytes from the bone marrow. The most active macrophages arise from monocytes delivered to sites of inflammation.

Eosinophils

The eosinophils parallel the neutrophils in lifestyle and function. However, their target is animal parasites more than bacteria. Indeed, the increase of these cells in the circulation, **eosinophilia**, is the hallmark of multicellular parasitic diseases such as schistosomiasis or trichinosis. The reason for this specificity is not known. It has been shown that the cytoplasmic granules of the eosinophils carry large amounts of an enzyme known as **eosinophil peroxidase**, as well as specific cationic proteins. These compounds have the power to kill certain parasites. Thus, eosinophils have an anti-infectious armamentarium similar to that of neutrophils, but specifically targeted to certain protozoa and worms.

How Do Neutrophils Kill Microorganisms?

Once near their microbial target, neutrophils must do several things to carry out their antimicrobial action. To destroy microorganisms, they must attach and ingest the organisms, either spontaneously or with the aid of opsonins, and then kill them (see Figs. 6.3, 6.6, and 6.7).

The membrane of neutrophils contains the receptors for chemotaxins and opsonins. After chemotaxins bind to them, the receptor molecules are internalized and replaced with new ones. What makes chemotaxis so effective is that neutrophils are unusually motile. Neutrophils move by rearranging together their cytoplasmic microfilaments and their microtubules. Actin and myosin in microfilaments are affected by a protein, gelsolin (which invites the comparison of neutrophils with muscle cells), which results in a morphological alteration of the cell shape. During chemotaxis, the portion of the cell that faces upstream in the chemotactic gradient forms a structure called a **lamellopodium**, where the cytoplasm is densely packed with microfilaments. The portion of the cell that faces downstream in the gradient forms a knoblike structure, the **uropod**.

Enfolding of bacteria or other particles of suitable size takes place by formation of a pouchlike structure, the **phagosome**, which invaginates, displacing the nucleus and the granules toward the uropod (see Figs. 6.6, 6.7, and 7.5). The cytoplasmic granules soon discharge their contents into the phagosome by fusion of their membranes, forming a new structure known as the

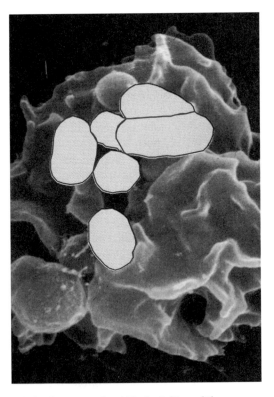

Figure 6.6. Phagocytosis of *Escherichia coli* by a neutrophil. Neutrophils were incubated with *E. coli*. After 60 seconds, one bacterium is partially engulfed into a phagosome, a cluster of bacteria are attached to the neutrophil surface. Scanning electron micrograph, ×19,000. The bacteria are highlighted in false color.

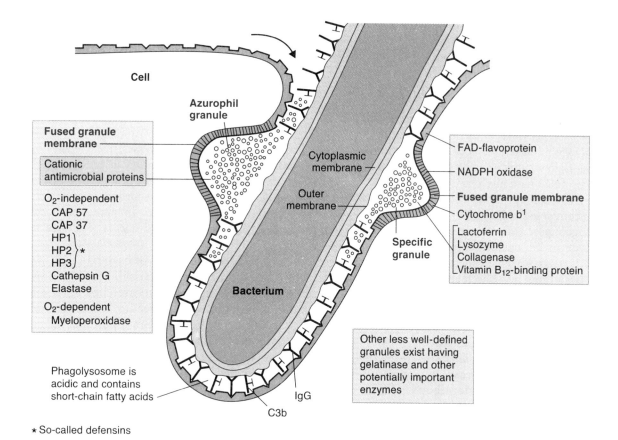

Cell

Azurophil
granule

**Fused granule
membrane**

Cationic
antimicrobial proteins

O$_2$-independent
CAP 57
CAP 37
HP1
HP2 ⟩ ∗
HP3
Cathepsin G
Elastase

O$_2$-dependent
Myeloperoxidase

Cytoplasmic
membrane

Outer
membrane

Bacterium

FAD-flavoprotein

NADPH oxidase

Fused granule membrane

Cytochrome b^1

Lactoferrin
Lysozyme
Collagenase
Vitamin B$_{12}$-binding protein

Specific
granule

Phagolysosome is
acidic and contains
short-chain fatty acids

IgG

C3b

Other less well-defined
granules exist having
gelatinase and other
potentially important
enzymes

∗ So-called defensins

Figure 6.7. Fusion of the phagosome and the granules. Fusion between the membranes of the specific granules and the cytoplasmic membrane, together with proteins from the cytosol completes the enzyme complex that generates reduced oxygen species, including the H$_2$O$_2$ that forms antimicrobial compound, with chloride and myeloperoxidase. Fusion of the specific and azurophil granules with the phagosome activates the oxygen-independent antimicrobial mechanisms.

Specific granules appear to fuse first. They deliver several proteins to the phagolysosomes; lysozyme will attack the murein

of many bacteria and lactoferrin binds iron tenaciously, denying bacteria this essential metal. Lactoferrin bound to iron also has direct antimicrobial action. The azurophil granules release highly complex mixtures including cationic antimicrobial proteins BPI/CAP57, CAP37/azurocidin, and the defensins. Two proteolytic enzymes, cathepsin G and elastase, as well as lysozyme, are also delivered by azurophil granules. Finally, oxygen-independent antimicrobial action is also mediated by hydrogen ions and short-chain fatty acids produced by the glycolytic metabolism of the neutrophil.

phagolysosome. The phagolysosome quickly pinches off from the plasma membrane and becomes a separate cytoplasmic organelle. By the time the pinching off is completed, the fusion of the granules is well under way and bacteria are already coated with antibacterial proteins. Thus, like poisonous snakes that disable their prey before swallowing it, neutrophils kill bacteria before they completely ingest them.

Bacteria become enfolded into the plasma membrane of the neutrophils by a zipper-like action, with the receptors on the phagocyte surface progressively attaching to the ligands on the bacterial surface (see Figs. 6.3 and 6.7). This binding stimulates two mechanisms that lead to killing of bacteria. One mechanism is set in motion by a vigorous burst of oxidative metabolism that leads to the production of hydrogen peroxide and other compounds lethal to microorganisms (Fig. 6.7). This is the

oxygen-dependent killing. The second mechanism also results in the discharge of toxic compounds from the granules into the phagosome. This is known as **oxygen-independent killing.** The granules of these cells may be considered to be enlarged lysosomes, packed with large amounts of powerful hydrolytic enzymes and other active substances. They are contained within unit membranes (see Fig. 6.7). **Azurophil,** or **primary granules,** contain a variety of enzymes and several cationic proteins that are also powerfully antibacterial (see Table 6.7). **Specific,** or **secondary,** granules contain a cytochrome, the iron-binding protein lactoferrin, that binds vitamin B$_{12}$, as well as a collagenase.

Oxygen-dependent killing

How does the oxidative process kill microorganisms? This mechanism is complex and involves several different radicals and chemical species. A highly active, multi-component **NADPH oxidase** rapidly reduces molecular oxygen to superoxide, O_2^-, that in turn becomes H_2O_2 in the following reaction:

$$2O_2^- + H_2O \rightarrow H_2O_2 + O_2$$

The components of the NADPH oxidase include at least four proteins. Two of them, **Phox 91** (phox stands for phagocyte oxidase), a cytochrome, and **Phox 22** are inserted into the cytosolic membrane by fusion of the specific granules with the phagosome. There, they are joined by cytosolic proteins **Phox 47** and **Phox 67** to form the completed oxidase.

Hydrogen peroxide, while bactericidal, does not work alone in killing microorganisms within phagocytes. Rather, an enzyme called **myeloperoxidase** converts chloride ions into the highly toxic **hypochlorous ions**, the same chemical found in common bleach (see Fig. 6.7 and Table 6.7). Myeloperoxidase is delivered to the phagolysosome by fusion of the azurophil granules.

The importance of these oxidative processes in neutrophil microbicidal action is illustrated in children with **chronic granulomatous disease,** a congenital defect caused by mutations involving the NADPH oxidase Phox proteins, most often Phox 91. Such defects render the phagocytes incapable of producing the reduced oxygen products. The cells can phagocytize and degranulate, but they fail to kill the ingested bacteria. Interestingly, microorganisms that lack catalase, such as the streptococci, obligingly release H_2O_2 into the phagocytic vacuole when phagocytized, thereby committing suicide. Thus pneumococci (a species of streptococci) do not cause disease any more frequently in such patients than they do in normal persons. The incidence of chronic granulomatous disease is about 4 per million. Mutations involving Phox 91 comprise 50–60% of the cases of chronic granulomatous disease and are X chromosome-linked. These patients develop subcutaneous abscesses, lung abscesses, hepatic abscesses, lymphadenitis, pneumonias, and osteomyelitis.

Oxygen-independent killing

Oxygen-independent killing mechanisms are also triggered by the binding of opsonized bacteria to the plasma membrane of neutrophils (see Fig. 6.7, Table 6.7). Specific granules seem to fuse to phagosomes first and deliver several bactericidal proteins, including lysozyme, the enzyme that disrupts the cell wall of many bacteria and lactoferrin, an iron-binding protein that effectively reduces the amount of iron available to the microorganisms. The azurophil granules discharge **antimicrobial cationic proteins** into phagosomes. Some of these proteins are "amphipathic" (partly hydrophilic and partly hydrophobic), and thus resemble other surface-active agents. Apparently, these proteins disrupt the outer membrane of Gram-negative bacteria and kill them by causing leakage of vital components. Each of these substances has a unique antimicrobial spectrum, but they tend to affect Gram-negative bacteria more than Gram-positives. The activity of these proteins may account for the survival of some children with chronic granulomatous disease.

The oxygen-independent mechanism also accounts for bacterial killing under the highly anaerobic conditions found in deep abscesses. Deficiencies in cationic proteins have been described in patients with chronic skin infections and abscesses. A genetic disease known as the **Chediak-Higashi syndrome** is caused by the formation of large granules in neutrophils, which are poorly functional and substantially reduce the killing power of these cells.

How do various kinds of bacteria differ in their sensitivity to the two bactericidal mechanisms of neutrophils? In general, organisms found in the gut, such as Gram-negative rods, are readily killed by the oxygen-independent mechanism. Gram-positive bacteria of the kind found on the skin and in the upper respiratory epithelia tend to be resistant to oxygen-independent killing and are killed chiefly by the oxygen-dependent pathway. Does this reflect the abundance of oxygen in the skin and its absence in the gut?

Killing by monocytes and macrophages

Together, monocytes and macrophages serve to mop up what is left at the scene of the battle between microorganisms and neutrophils. They phagocytize the microorganisms and the debris left by neutrophils. Their mechanisms of chemotaxis, phagocytosis, and microbial killing resemble those of the neutrophils. **Nitric oxide** (NO), a simple chemical made by macrophages in some animal species as the result of activation by γ-interferon and TNF, has been shown to play an important role in the killing of microorganisms by macrophages in mice. However, persistent efforts have failed to show that human macrophages make this chemical in significant amount. In humans, fibroblasts, some neurons, and cells of the vasculature make small amounts of NO. Thus, it is conceivable that this chemical may perform other important functions in humans.

An important point is that these cells, unlike the neutrophils, continue to differentiate after they leave the bone marrow and become activated when properly stimulated. In addition, these versatile cells synthesize several complement components and cytokines. Activated macrophages phagocytize more vigorously, take up more oxygen, and secrete a large quantity of hydrolytic enzymes. In general, they are better prepared to kill microorganisms and, appropriately, have been called the "angry" macrophages. Macrophage activation is elicited by substances made in response to the presence of microorganisms, like complement fragment C3b or γ-interferon. They are also activated by a variety of other compounds, such as endotoxin of Gram-negatives. Some bacteria, fungi, and protozoa can grow within unstimulated macrophages, but in general they are killed when these cells become activated.

Perhaps the most important property of macrophages is their participation in the induction of specific immune responses. In this role of living garbage collectors they help rid the body not only of invading microorganisms but also of tumor and other foreign cells by stimulating the development of the lymphocytes involved in the immune response. In turn, they respond to signals from some of these lymphocytes which stimulate their differentiation and activation. In this way, macrophages and the cells of the induced immune system communicate with each other. In fact, they carry out an animated conversation that results in a strong interaction between the constitutive and induced systems of defense.

SUGGESTED READINGS

Abbas AK, Lichtman AH, Pober JS. Cellular and molecular immunology. 3rd ed. Philadelphia: WB. Saunders, 1997.

Bachner RL. Chronic granulomatous disease of childhood: clinical, pathological, biochemical, molecular, and genetic aspects. Pediatr Pathol 1990;10:143–153.

Cotran RS, Kumar V, Robbins SL. Pathologic basis of disease. 5th ed. Philadelphia: WB. Saunders, 1994.

Densen P, Clark RA, Neuseef WM. Granulocytic phagocytes. In: Mandell GL. Principles and practice of infectious diseases. 4th ed. N.Y.: Churchill Livingstone, 1995.

Mims CA, Dimmock NJ, Nash A, Stephen J. Mims' pathogenesis of infectious diseases. 4th ed. San Diego: Academic Press, 1995.

Roitt IM, Brostoff J, Male DK. Immunology. 4th ed. London: Gower Medical Publishing, 1996.

Spitznagel JK. Antibiotic proteins of human neutrophils. J Clin Invest 1990;86:1381–1386.

Induced Defenses of the Body

H. KIRK ZIEGLER

CONSTITUTIVE VS. ACQUIRED IMMUNITY

As discussed in the previous chapter, constitutive immune responses are those that do not depend on prior exposure to the invading agent. These mechanisms are relatively nonspecific and constitute the initial lines of defense against invading pathogens. In contrast to constitutive immunity, specific acquired defense reactions are highly selective for nonself entities such as invading microorganisms, and are qualitatively and quantitatively altered by antigenic exposure. The two salient hallmarks of these reactions are **specificity** and **memory**.

HUMORAL AND CELLULAR IMMUNITY

Immunity can be broadly classified as either **humoral** or **cellular**. This distinction is based on the ability to transfer resistance to normal animals or humans using either the serum (humors) or the cells of the immune donor. Specific humoral immunity results from the action of proteins in serum, the **antibodies**, whereas cellular immunity (**cell-mediated immunity**, or **CMI**) is mediated by **T lymphocytes**.

The relative importance of humoral and cellular immunity varies with the type of pathogen and the site of infection. For example, resistance to a toxin may be predominantly humoral, as antibodies bind to and neutralize the injurious activity of the toxin. Also, antibody binds to antigen, which makes it easier for phagocytic cells to ingest it and to activate the complement systems (Chapter 6, "Constitutive Defenses"). In contrast, pathogens that can multiply within host cells are not accessible to antibody. Immunity to such microbes requires the cooperative efforts of T lymphocytes and macrophages. This reaction is mediated by the secretion of soluble factors called cytokines, which are released by T cells and macrophages (Chapter 6, "Constitutive Defenses"). Certain cytokines called macrophage-activat-

ing factors enhance the cell-killing functions of macrophages, allowing them to kill intracellular microbes. Also, cell-mediated immunity can be expressed by the direct action of a subset of T cells termed cytotoxic T lymphocytes. These cells recognize foreign or nonself antigens on the surface of infected cells. For example, cytotoxic T lymphocytes can lyse virus-infected cells early in the virus infection cycle, that is, before mass production of virus progeny occurs. Thus, specific acquired immunity is expressed either by direct cell–cell interaction or secretion of antibodies and cytokines.

SPECIFICITY: SELF–NONSELF DISCRIMINATION

Immunological defenses are based on the ability to recognize **self** from **nonself**. This recognition maintains the individuality and integrity of the organism. Self may be defined as the tissues, cells, and molecules that are an integral part of the organism, encoded by the genome. Nonself is everything else. In general, the immune system recognizes entities in the nonself world, antigens, and responds in a way that eliminates the antigens from the self environment. In humans, if the nonself entity is a pathogenic microorganism, the process is directed toward the successful resolution of an infection.

The maintenance of individuality or integrity of an organism is fundamental to its survival. Immunological defenses are normal biological phenomena common to all living organisms, including microorganisms. For example, bacteria use nucleases to fight invading DNA that could contaminate their genome and elaborate toxic substances to conquer their immediate environment. Some parasites use camouflage by coating themselves with host antigens. Viruses ensure their survival by "hiding" in host DNA. When the survival needs and defenses of microbes conflict with ours, the result is the pathology of infectious disease. Or, as Lewis Thomas said, "Disease usually results from inconclusive negotiations for symbiosis, an overstepping of the line by one side or the other, a biological misinterpretation of the boundaries." From a microbial point of view, there is little to be gained by causing disease. Pathogenicity is the side effect of the border dispute. In fact, many of the symptoms of infection are caused not by the presence of the microbe, but rather by the immune defense mechanisms invoked. Our arsenal for fighting a microbe is so powerful we are possibly in more danger from ourselves than from the microbe. We live in a war zone in the midst of exploding devices: we are mined.

What is the cost of maintaining individuality via defense reactions? Perhaps we "pay the price" by getting old and dying: One explanation of aging is that tissue degeneration is caused by the protracted battle of self and nonself with the resulting accumulation of damage. The immune system makes occasional mistakes in discriminating self from nonself (autoimmune reactions). Effector molecules activated during border disputes with microbes can damage host cells and tissues. And sacrificing a few cells for the good of the organism, as occurs with the "micro-amputations" that take place in the destruction of virus-infected cells, is a sound but ultimately damaging strategy. Thus, the challenge of the immune system is to provide an efficient and powerful means for recognizing the millions of different components of the nonself world and to respond with minimal damage to our own tissues. To meet this challenge, nature has provided higher animals with highly specific immune defenses which are evoked only when needed. This is called specific acquired immunity.

Immunological Memory

The immune system is able to remember prior exposure to an antigen and to respond more rapidly and strongly on a repeat exposure. Immunization exploits this feature of the immune system. To illustrate the concept of immunization, consider mice infected with a microbial pathogen (Fig. 7.1). Groups of immunologically naive (normal) mice are injected with different numbers of organisms, and their survival is noted after an appropriate period of time. With 10^4 bacteria, one-half of the animals die, thus defining a so-called lethal dose 50% ($LD_{50} = 10^4$). If the same experiment is performed with the animals that have recovered from the first infection (e.g., those animals receiving, for instance, 10^3 organisms), it now takes 10^7 microbes to kill half the animals. These animals have acquired enhanced resistance or immunity to the pathogen by prior antigenic exposure, i.e., they remember their previous history. The specificity of this acquired immunity is illustrated by the observation that such animals are no more resistant to an antigenically unrelated pathogen than are normal controls. Thus, the immune system has remembered the specific prior insult and has successfully adapted to maintain the

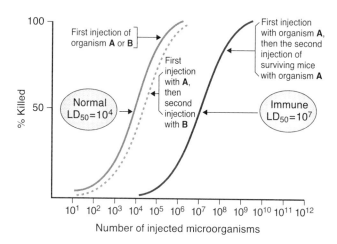

Figure 7.1. Specific acquired immunity. In this experiment groups of animals were injected as indicated with antigenically unrelated pathogenic microorganisms designated *A* and *B*. The percentage of animals killed by the infection is plotted as a function of the number of microorganisms injected into each animal. Note that animals that receive a first injection with microbe A are resistant or immune to secondary challenge with microbe A.

health of the organism. This capacity is termed **immunological memory.**

The reaction evoked the first time an antigen is encountered is called the **primary immune response,** that caused by subsequent encounters with the same antigen, the **secondary responses** (Fig. 7.2). If the **amounts of antibody** generated in a primary and a secondary response are measured, marked differences are noted (Fig. 7.3). The secondary response occurs after a **shorter lag period;** it is of greater intensity and it has a longer duration. In addition, different kinds of immunoglobulins are produced in the secondary response.

The faster and stronger secondary response (also called the **anamnestic** or **memory response**) results from clonal selection and differentiation that occur during the primary response. The clonal proliferation of lymphocytes is followed by a dual pathway of differentiation of both B- and T-cell lineages. By yet unknown mechanisms, some of the progeny become effector cells—cells capable of causing an immediate effect, whereas others become memory cells. In general, effector cells are active for a finite and usually short period of time. For example, plasma cells are the effector cells of the B-cell lineage; cytotoxic cells are one type of effector cells of the T-cell lineage. Immunological memory is due to the fact that the **memory lymphocytes** are long lived and can persist for years. They are capable of rapid differentiation into effector cells when stimulated with antigen. B-cell lineage cells are poised to rapidly secrete large amounts of antibody when appropriately activated by secondary contact with antigen.

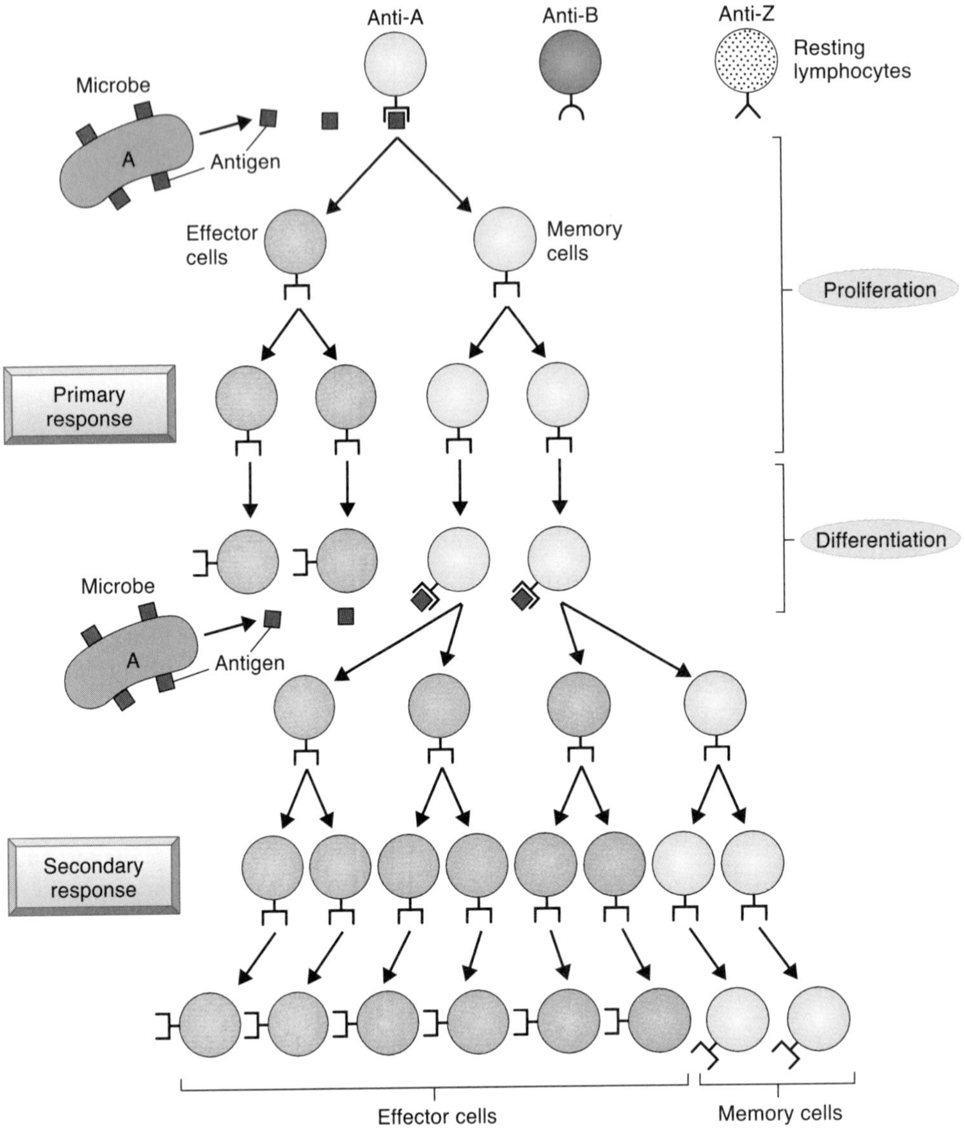

Figure 7.2. Clonal selection. When an antigen (designated by the *squares*) is introduced into the immune system, the antigen binds to clones of lymphocytes with receptors for that antigen. This binding initiates the proliferation and differentiation of the lymphocytes indicated. (Lymphocyte clones reactive with other antigens [e.g., circles and triangles, not shown] are not stimulated.) As such, antigen is said to **select** certain clones for proliferation. Note that upon secondary contact with the same antigen, a relatively large number of clones (memory cells) can interact with the antigen. Memory cells account for specific immunological memory. This process occurs with both B and T lymphocytes. For simplicity, the function of antigen-presenting cells and other molecular interactions are not shown.

Clonal Selection—The Central Paradigm of Immunology

The specificity and memory of acquired immunity is mediated by lymphocytes and their receptors through a process of **clonal selection** (Fig. 7.2). The clonal selection hypothesis suggests that there are millions of different lymphocytes, each with receptors specific for a particular antigen. These lymphocyte surface receptors consist of an immunoglobulin on B lymphocytes and a related protein on T lymphocytes called the T-cell receptor.

When an antigen binds to its specific receptor on a lymphocyte, that particular lymphocyte proliferates and differentiates. The result is the clonal expansion of the lymphocytes of that specificity. Thus, specific immunological memory is due to the predominance of clones of lymphocytes of a particular specificity. In the example described above (Fig. 7.1), the specifically immune mice can handle a larger number of microbes because they now have many more lymphocytes with receptors specific for the microbial antigens.

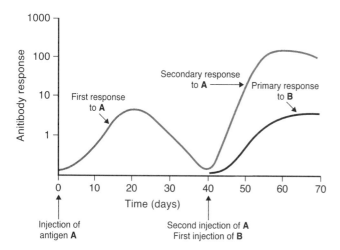

Figure 7.3. Primary and secondary immune responses. The antibody responses to antigens *A* and *B* are shown as a function of time after primary and secondary stimulation with antigens as indicated. Note the faster and stronger secondary response to antigen A.

IMMUNOLOGICAL TOLERANCE

A major question in immunology is: How does the immune system distinguish self from nonself? There are two possible explanations. One is that the genes coding for the antigen receptors specific for self molecules are simply not present in the genome. The other (and correct one) is that the immune system is intrinsically capable of responding to both self and nonself entities but that mechanisms exist to prevent potentially disastrous reactions to self. The existence of autoimmune diseases (immune responses to self components that result in pathology) indicates that at least some self-recognition can occur.

Several experimental observations indicate that the immune system "learns" not to respond to self components early in development. For example, if an antigen is injected into a mouse at birth, when the immune system is still immature, it will not respond to that antigen when becoming an adult. A similar phenomenon occurs in genetically different twins that have shared a common circulation before birth. They do not react to the tissue antigens of their partner. Thus, their immune systems learn to tolerate a normally foreign antigen as if it were a self component. The state of antigen-specific immunological unresponsiveness is called **acquired immunological tolerance**. Immunological tolerance may be thought of as "negative immunological memory"; prior exposure to antigen results in a decreased response (rather than a heightened one) to the antigen. Like immunological memory, immunological tolerance is an active response that requires antigenic exposure and is mediated by lymphocytes.

Under special circumstances, immunological toler-

ance can be demonstrated in immunologically mature animals. Tolerance can be induced by intravenous injection of soluble protein antigen in either very large or in repeated small amounts. Also, the use of immunosuppressive treatments, such as x-rays or certain immunosuppressive drugs, can promote the induction of tolerance. Both T cells and B cells can be "tolerized" experimentally.

If tolerance to self breaks down, autoimmune disease may result. For example, in systemic lupus erythematosus (SLE), patients produce antibodies to their own nucleic acids and, in myasthenia gravis, to acetylcholine receptors. Both result in severe chronic illnesses. Multiple sclerosis, a disease characterized by chronic demyelination of the central nervous system (CNS), is thought to result from T-cell reactivity to CNS-associated self proteins. The onset of certain autoimmune disorders is often associated with microbial infections, which suggests that microbial products may somehow alter self components or modulate the processes that normally maintain tolerance to self components.

The precise mechanisms of immunological tolerance are not known. There are three major possibilities for which experimental evidence exists. 1) Clones of lymphocytes potentially reactive to a particular antigen may be eliminated. For the T-cell lineage, this **clonal deletion** is thought to occur in the thymus during T-cell maturation. In fact, many newly made T cells do not leave the thymus because they are the "forbidden" self-reactive clones. Clonal deletion has also been observed to occur with B cells, but this process may be less frequent than in T cells. 2) Specific clones may be present but may have received negative signals through their receptor systems and thus may be less responsive to antigen. Immature B lymphocytes behave in this manner. This functional inactivation has been termed **clonal anergy**. Functional inactivation of T cells has also been observed when antigen is provided in the absence of a second costimulatory signal from antigen-presenting cells. 3) The response of lymphocyte clones may be actively inhibited by the action of **suppressor T cells**. However, the precise role of suppressor cells remains controversial.

The issue of tolerance induction is of obvious importance in **organ transplantation**, since the immune response represents a major barrier to graft survival. Also, intelligent intervention in the control of disease caused by too much immune reactivity (autoimmunity and hypersensitivity), or too little (immunodeficiencies and infections), will require a thorough understanding of these regulatory pathways.

In many ways the immune system is analogous to the nervous system. Both are comprised of very large numbers of phenotypically distinct cells. These cells interact in positive and negative ways, and this cellular network is dispersed throughout the body to patrol and guard its identity. Both systems are involved in pattern recognition. With a keen sense of touch, the immune system has the precise capacity for discrimination. It can distinguish proteins that differ in only one amino acid and can perceive differences between isomers of simple chemicals. Collectively, the cells of the immune system have intelligence and morality in telling the good (self) from the bad (nonself), with a memory that lasts a lifetime. Both systems rely on effective intracellular communication via synaptic transmission of chemical signals. However, unlike the hard wiring of the nervous system, the immune system employs transient mobile interconnections among cells with a dynamic and renewable capacity.

THE CELLULAR BASIS OF IMMUNE RESPONSES

Lymphocyte Function

To supply strong and appropriate immune defenses, nature has imposed a division of labor among lymphocytes. **B lymphocytes**, when stimulated by antigens and the appropriate products of other lymphocytes and macrophages, proliferate and differentiate into plasma cells whose sole purpose is to synthesize and secrete **antibody** molecules. Each of these antibody "factories" can secrete thousands of molecules per second. Plasma cells are so committed to synthesis and secretion that they are incapable of further growth, and die after several days. In general, the specificity of the secreted antibody is identical to the blueprint present on their cell surfaces as the antigen receptor. Thus, B lymphocytes with a given receptor specificity expand clonally to increase their numbers, which then undergo differentiation to plasma cells. Each of these groups of cells is capable of secreting a large number of similar yet functionally specialized antibodies—what a well-designed system for acquiring heightened reactivity to the nonself world!

In contrast to B cells, antigen activation of **T lymphocytes** does not lead to the production of secreted forms of antigen-receptor molecules. Rather, differentiated T cells express their functions through direct cell–cell interaction and via the secretion of **cytokines**. There are several functionally distinct subsets of T cells. **Helper T cells** help other cells perform optimally; they help B cells make antibody, T cells become cytotoxic, and macrophages kill microbes. **Cytotoxic T cells** recognize and destroy cells infected with microbial pathogens such as viruses. **Suppressor T** cells downregulate the activity of B cells and other T cells. Thus, the functional diversity of T lymphocytes is expressed by separate subsets of cells.

Lymphocytes are all morphologically similar, but can be identified by **surface markers** (Table 7.1). These markers are also known as **differentiation antigens** because they appear at certain stages of lymphocyte differentia-

Table 7.1. Human T-lymphocyte Markers

| Surface marker | | |
T designation	Cluster designation	Cellular distribution
T_3	CD3	Mature T cells
T_4	CD4	Helper/inducer T cells
T_8	CD8	Cytotoxic/supressor cells

tion. Mature human T cells express characteristic proteins called CD3. Helper T cells bear the CD4 protein. Cytotoxic T lymphocytes (CTL) and suppressor T cells express the CD8 marker. In peripheral blood, about 45% of the lymphocytes are CD4 positive and 30% are CD8 positive. (The rest are null cells [more later] and B cells). These markers can be used for diagnostic purposes. Patients with AIDS, for example, have low numbers of CD4+ cells, which indicates an immunodeficiency.

Lymphocyte Development

Lymphocytes are found in the blood, lymphoid tissues, the lymph, and in smaller numbers in tissues throughout the body, especially at sites of inflammation. The total number of lymphocytes in humans is large (about 2×10^{12}), and the total mass of the immune system is comparable to that of the liver or the brain. Like other blood cells, lymphocytes are derived from the pluripotent hemopoietic **stems cells** in the fetal liver and the bone marrow of adults. Lymphocyte development occurs by two major pathways corresponding to the two major subsets, B and T lymphocytes (Fig. 7.4).

In the T-lymphocyte pathway, the progeny of stem cells migrate from the bone marrow and enter the thymus. In this central or primary lymphoid organ, the development of **thymus-derived (T) lymphocytes** takes place. Here they "learn" to express receptors for antigens and to select appropriate specificities. Researchers are beginning to better understand this "thymic education" process. Molecules produced by thymic epithelial cells and macrophages play important roles in both positive and negative selection of thymocytes that bear appropriate receptors. During development in the thymus, there is an ordered expression of surface markers. As T cells leave the thymus they express CD3 and either CD4 or CD8. At this point, these T cells are functionally mature. Upon exiting the thymus, the lymphocytes travel to the secondary or peripheral lymphoid organs, where responses to foreign antigen occur and mature lymphocyte function is expressed. The peripheral lymphoid organs include the spleen, lymph nodes, and gut-associated lymphoid tissue (Peyer's patches, appendix, tonsils, and adenoids).

The other major lymphocyte population, the **B cells**, are so named because in birds their development is dependent on maturation in a central lymphoid organ called the bursa (B) of Fabricius. Mammals have no bursa of Fabricius; B-cell development probably occurs in the hemopoietic tissue and in secondary lymphoid organs.

While lymphocyte development is dynamic and continues throughout the life of mammals, the importance of primary lymphoid organs is easily demonstrated in young animals. For example, removal of the thymus at birth prevents the development of T cells and results in severely impaired immune responses in the adult. However, if the thymus is removed from adult animals, little if any deficit in immune responsiveness occurs. This is because lymphocytes are relatively long lived, and possibly because other sites of lymphocyte development take over in adults.

The separate developmental pathways of B and T lymphocytes in humans was first illustrated in genetic immunodeficiencies. For example, the DiGeorge syndrome results in a selective decrease of T lymphocytes, while patients with X-linked agammaglobulinemia (Bruton's disease) have normal T-cell function but cannot make antibodies.

Lymphocyte Circulation

Lymphocytes patrol the body from their home bases in the lymphoid organs. The majority of T cells, and some B cells, continuously recirculate between the blood and lymph. They leave the bloodstream by traversing specialized endothelial cells in venules and enter the tissues. Molecules known as **homing receptors** are present on the lymphocyte surface. These receptors recognize other molecules known as **vascular addressins** on endothelial venules, and this interaction facilitates lymphocyte homing to particular tissues. Other molecules of the **integrin family** are involved in nonorgan-specific binding to endothelial venules. After passing through the tissues and patrolling for antigens, these lymphocytes travel via the fluid flow and accumulate in lymphatic vessels that connect to a series of downstream lymph nodes. From there they enter progressively larger lymphatic vessels and eventually complete their round trip by passing back into the blood via the thoracic duct. This recirculation promotes the contact of lymphocytes with antigens and ensures that information about a localized antigenic insult is dispersed throughout the body. Thus, systemic immunity is produced.

The pattern of lymphatic circulation and the structure of the lymph nodes both play important roles in immune responsiveness. Consider a microbe that has penetrated the defenses of the skin and is present in the extracellular fluid in the tissues. Through the inflammatory response, the microbe will be swept by the fluid flow into the blind-end afferent lymphatics present in almost all

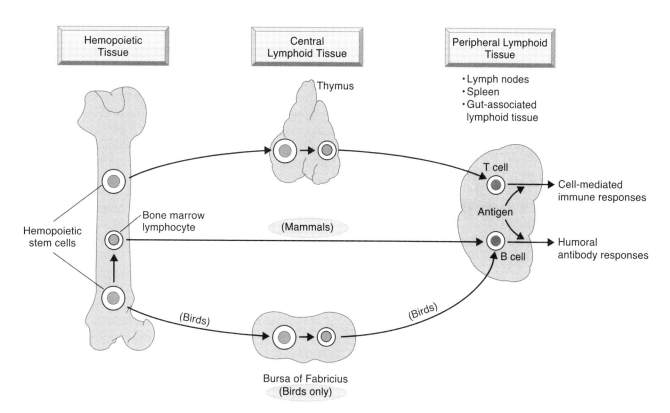

Figure 7.4. Lymphocyte development. The development of functional T and B lymphocytes occurs in primary lymphoid organs and the response to antigen takes place in peripheral lymphoid tissue. B and T lymphocytes have different pathways of development.

tissues (notable exceptions include the central nervous system and the placenta). The lymph is deposited into a meshwork of lymphoid cells which are able to bind and ingest the microbe. These cells are collectively referred to as the **lymphoreticular system** and include macrophages and comparable cells with different names, depending on their characteristics and anatomical locations. These sticky cells are arranged in a filterlike array interspersed with lymphocytes and are the site where the antigen is trapped. The immune system has the invading microbe right where it wants it, bound by cells capable of "processing" and "presenting" the antigen and surrounded by the lymphocytes poised to engage it with specific receptors. ("Go ahead, make my day.") As a consequence of the filtering action of the lymph node, the lymph exiting the node via the efferent lymphatic vessel and ultimately emptying into the blood is microbe-free, or in other words, sterile. The antigen trapped in the lymph node then initiates the immune response.

Cellular Cooperation and Lymphocyte Activation

Most immune responses require intimate cellular cooperation among the lymphocytes, macrophages, and other accessory cells. These cells communicate with each other by direct cell–cell interactions and by secreting cytokines, as illustrated in Figure 7.5. Electron micrographs of lymphocyte–macrophage interactions are shown in Figure 7.6.

In order to differentiate into antibody-secreting cells, B lymphocytes must interact with T lymphocytes and be stimulated by their cytokines. The probable steps involved are:

1. **Binding** of antigens to B cells via their immunoglobulin receptors.
2. Processing and "**presentation**" of the antigen to T cells. This involves the proteolysis of protein antigens in lysosomes and/or endocytic vesicles, and the transfer of resulting antigen fragments to the B-cell surface, where they can be recognized by receptors on T cells (Fig. 7.5).
3. Direct delivery of T-cell derived cytokines to B cells by cell-to-cell contact. This combination of signals drives the proliferation of B cells and their differentiation into plasma cells. Thus, by presenting antigens on their surface, B cells get efficient help from T cells.

Macrophages and dentritic cells also contribute to lymphocyte activation by elaborating several **cytokines** (e.g., **interleukin 1** [IL-1] and **interleukin 2** [IL-2]) and by processing and presenting antigens to T cells. The resulting activated T lymphocytes communicate with B cells and macrophages via the release of a variety of cytokines. These include growth- and differentiation-promoting factors such as IL-2 and IL-4.

All of this activity in the secondary lymphoid organs alters the lymphocyte traffic patterns and structure of the lymph node. After an antigen is trapped, there is an initial period (about 24 hours) of decreased flow of lymphocytes from the node followed by an increased flow. Vessels dilate, blood flow increases, and lymphocytes proliferate. These events cause the nodes to enlarge, hence the classic "swollen glands" that often accompany infection. Lymphocytes specific for the antigen in question appear to localize at the site of the immune response, the nodes where the antigen is trapped.

ANTIGENS

Any organic macromolecule can potentially act as an antigen. In descending order of antigenicity, proteins, polysaccharides, lipids, and nucleic acids can be antigenic under the correct circumstances. The portions of an antigen that combine with the antigen-binding site of lymphocyte receptors are called **antigenic determinants** or **epitopes**. The size of an antigenic determinant may be as small as several amino acids or sugar molecules. Since most antigens are large molecules, they can have many epitopes and thus can stimulate many different lymphocyte clones. Such a response is called **polyclonal**. When one is dealing with the response of a single clone of cells—a situation achievable only under special circumstances—the response is called **monoclonal**. Antigens are classified according to the relative thymus dependency of the antibody response. While all B-cell responses are enhanced by the action of helper T cells, certain antigens can elicit antibody production without T cells. Such antigens, called **T-cell-independent antigens**, have many repeats of an epitope and/or have the ability to cause B cells to proliferate. Many of these antigens are associated with bacterial cell envelopes; lipopolysaccharide from Gram-negative bacteria and pneumococcal capsular polysaccharide are two examples. This direct elicitation of antibody may play an important role in the rapid immune response to bacterial invasion.

Antigenicity is the ability of a molecule to interact with an immune recognition molecule such as an antibody. **Immunogenicity** is the ability of a molecule to elicit an immune response. This definition is operational and depends on many factors. In general, large molecules with multiple antigenic determinants are more antigenic than small molecular weight substances. Very small compounds, called **haptens**, can elicit an immune response but only when coupled to a larger molecule called a **carrier**. Examples of haptens are simple sugars, certain drugs (e.g, penicillin) and chemical side chains, such as dinitrophenyl groups, which are used experimentally. Also relevant are the dose of antigen, the route of immunization, and the presence of **adjuvants,** agents that enhance the immune response. From a microbiological view, live microorganisms are gener-

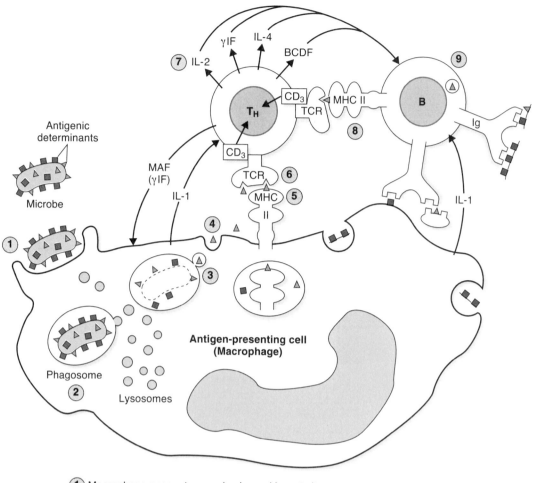

1. Macrophage encounters a microbe and ingests it
2. Microbe engulfed in phagosome
3. Microbe antigen is processed
4. Antigen is "sent" to macrophage surface
5. Antigen binds with MHC II
6. T_H binds to antigen/MHC II complex
7. T_H releases cytokines
8. B-cell binds to antigen/MHC II complex on T_H
9. B-cell binding and cytokines stimulate proliferation of B-cells into plasma cells

Figure 7.5. Complex cellular cross-talk. Both macrophages and B cells express class II MHC gene products and can present antigen to helper T cells. Helper T cells are activated via the T-cell receptor and produce a shower of cytokines that have powerful and diverse effects on the cells of the immune system. Cells of the Th1 phenotype produce cytokines which lead to activation of macrophages; cells of the Th2 phenotype produce cytokines that stimulate B cells and antibody production, while simultaneously inhibiting the Th1 effects.

ally better antigens and make better vaccines than dead ones. Most relevant to immunogenicity is the degree of difference between the antigen molecule and any analogous structure present as self. In general, the greater degree of phylogenetic difference between self and nonself, the greater the immune response.

THE HUMORAL IMMUNE RESPONSE; FOCUS ON IMMUNOGLOBULINS

Structure and Function

The term *antibody* is usually used for **immunoglobulins** that have specific antigen-binding capacity. Im-

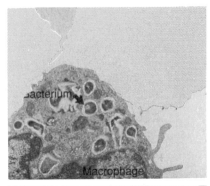

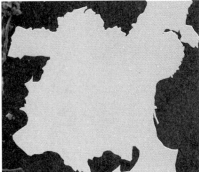

Figure 7.6. Electron micrographs of T cell–macrophage interactions. In these photographs, T cells are recognizing bacterial antigens on the surface of macrophages. Transmission electron microscopy is used in Figure 7a and scanning electron microscopy is used in Figure 7b. Note the bacteria present in the phagosomes of macrophages (7a) and the extensive membrane–membrane interaction between T cells and macrophages. This interaction is antigen-specific (i.e., mediated by the T-cell receptor) and requires the expression of class II MHC gene products by the macrophage. See Figure 7.5 for schematic view of molecular interactions.

munoglobulins play two roles and exist in two structurally different forms: as **membrane receptors** on resting B lymphocytes and as major **secretory products** of fully differentiated plasma cells. Antibody can bind antigen and then mediate several other activities or functions in the interaction with other cells and molecules of the immune system.

Antibody molecules fall into several different yet related classes. Consider the secreted immunoglobulin of the G class (IgG) as the prototypical structure (see Fig. 7.7). This immunoglobulin is a Y-shaped protein with identical antigen-binding sites at the tip of each arm. With these two binding sites it is called **bivalent**. The proteolytic enzyme papain cuts the antibody molecule into functionally distinct Fc and Fab fragments. The **Fab fragments** are the cleaved arms of the Y and have **antigen-binding** ability. The tail of the Y is called the **Fc fragment** because it is easily crystallizable. The Fc portion directs important functions of antibody other than antigen binding. These effector functions include complement

activation and interaction with specific Fc receptors (Chapter 6, "Constitutive Defenses"). Different classes of antibody molecules may have identical antigen-binding sites but different Fc parts, therefore supplying different functions.

The multiple binding sites of an antibody molecule enable it to cross-link soluble antigen molecules into a large lattice, provided the antigen has three or more antigenic determinants. When this complex of antigens and antibodies reaches a certain size, it comes out of solution. This process is called **immunoprecipitation**. Antigen-binding and cross-linking reactions are aided by the flexibility of the parts of the molecule where the arms meet the tail, the so-called **hinge region**. Within the lattice of bound antigens and antibodies, many Fc parts are displayed. The Fc fragments can then work cooperatively in a multivalent fashion that enhances their binding avidity to cells with Fc receptors and to the C1 component of complement. Immunoglobulin G (IgG) consists of four polypeptide chains, two identical **light (L) chains** (each about 220 amino acids) and two identical **heavy (H) chains** (each about 440 amino acids). The chains are held together both by covalent interchain disulfide bonds and noncovalent interactions. Each antigen-binding site is formed by a portion of both a heavy chain and a light chain. The Fc part is composed of the carboxy-terminal halves of the two heavy chains.

Both heavy and light chains are composed of repeating segments or **domains** that fold independently to form compact functional units. Each domain, about 110 amino acids long, has one intrachain disulfide bond and a characteristic three-dimensional structure called the **immunoglobulin fold**. Each domain is a sandwich of 3 and 4 antiparallel polypeptide strands in a β-sheet configuration.

Immunoglobulin Classes

In mammals, there are five major **immunoglobulin classes** or **isotypes**. The classes of antibody differ in structure and function, as summarized in Table 7.2. Classes are based on differences in the heavy chains. The isotypes are called IgM, IgD, IgG, IgE, and IgA with their respective heavy chains designated by the Greek letters, μ, δ, γ, ϵ, and α. There are two different types of light chains, λ and κ. The heavy chains determine the unique biological activity of the different isotypes. A single antibody molecule has only one type of heavy chain; it can have either two κ or two λ light chains, but never one of each. This distribution ensures that both antigen-binding sites are identical.

IgG

IgG is the major class of immunoglobulins present in the blood. It is produced in greater amounts in the secondary response than in the primary response. IgG can activate complement, bind to phagocytes via its Fc part,

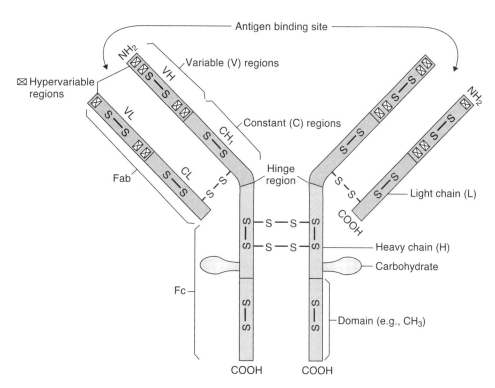

Figure 7.7. Structure of IgG. Immunoglobulin of the IgG class is composed of two heavy and two light chains. Note that portions of the amino terminal regions of both heavy and light chains form the antigen-combining sites. The Fc part is formed by the heavy chains alone.

Table 7.2. Human Immunoglobulins

Isotype	Structure	Concentration in serum mg/m;	No. of heavy chain domains	Distinguishing feature of functions
IgM	B cell	1.5	5	First in development and response
IgD	B cell	0.03	5	B-cell receptor
IgG		12.5	4	Opsonin, ADCC
IgE	Mast cell or basophil	0.00005	5	Allergic response
IgA	Secretory component	0.05 3.5	4	In secretions (GALT)

participate in antibody-dependent cell-mediated cyto-toxicity (ADCC) with killer (K) cells (see null cells below), and cross the placenta to supply some protection to neonates. In humans, there are four major subclasses of IgG: IgG1, IgG2, IgG3, and IgG4. These subclasses differ in their ability to activate complement (IgG4 doesn't) and to bind to macrophage Fc receptors (IgG1 and IgG3 do).

IgM

IgM is the major product in the primary immune response and is the predominant antibody produced in response to thymus-independent antigens. Secretory IgM consists of five copies of the basic four-chain unit (2 light + 2 heavy chains) and therefore has 10 antigen-binding sites. This multivalency promotes its ability to cross-link, while its multiple Fc parts make it a very efficient activator of complement. IgM also contains an extra protein called the J (joining) chain which aids in the polymerization process within plasma cells. The large size of IgM (about 970,000 daltons) confines it to the blood, and it is not found in substantial quantities in tissues.

Membrane IgM is an important antigen receptor on B cells. It is an integral membrane protein, anchored by a hydrophobic carboxy terminus. Unlike secreted IgM, but resembling IgG, membrane IgM is a four-chain structure with two antigen-binding sites. Its heavy chain is the first to be produced during B-cell development. It may be important as a receptor of signals that lead to clonal anergy and immunological tolerance. Membrane IgM may be constitutively expressed on both resting and memory B cells. Plasma cells do not express a membrane form of immunoglobulin.

IgD

IgD is another membrane immunoglobulin predominantly found on resting B cells. Human IgD is also a four-chain molecule like IgG, but it has a very long hinge region. Its very low concentration in the blood may be explained by its sensitivity to proteolysis at the hinge region and the rarity of IgD-secreting plasma cells. Its only function may be as a membrane receptor for antigen. During B-cell ontogeny, IgD is expressed after IgM. The appearance of IgD renders the B cell functionally mature.

IgA

IgA is present in seromucous secretions such as milk, tears, saliva, perspiration, and secretions of the lung and gut. Small amounts are also found in the blood. In secretions, IgA molecules consist of two copies of IgG-like molecules covalently attached via disulfide bonds with an intervening J chain. They are also associated with another protein called the **secretory component,** which is synthesized by epithelial cells. The secretory component is a portion of an integral membrane protein called the poly Ig receptor, which plays a key role in the transport of IgA across the epithelial cells into the lumen. Secretory component, which is attached to secreted IgA, also acts as a stabilizer and provides protection against proteolytic activity present in secretions. IgA is synthesized at a very high rate in the lymphoid tissue of the gut, especially the Peyer's patches. The body produces amounts of IgA equal or greater to those of any other immunoglobulin class. IgA can neither activate complement nor bind well to Fc receptors, but it may play an important role in preventing the attachment and subsequent invasion of pathogenic microbes, a kind of strategic defense initiative at the external surface.

IgE

IgE is the antibody class that occurs in serum at the lowest concentration. IgE is responsible for the clinical manifestations of allergies such as hay fever, asthma, and hives. Its Fc region specifically binds to very high-affinity receptors present on the surfaces of mast cells and basophils. Cell-bound IgE then serves as a receptor for antigen. The cross-linking of these receptors by antigen causes the release of a variety of biologically active agents. One such agent, histamine, causes smooth muscle contraction and increases in vascular permeability. These effects may have some protective function by enhancing the influx of cells, antibodies, and complement into the site of inflammation. IgE may also be important in the response to parasitic infection (principally by worms) as it is often greatly elevated in the serum of patients with these diseases. IgE participates in antibody-dependent cell-mediated killing of parasites by macrophages and eosinophils, cells that possess low-affinity Fc receptors specific for IgE. Is the price for allergy worth paying because IgE defends us against parasites?

Membrane and Secreted Immunoglobulins

With the possible exception of IgD, all immunoglobulins exist in two versions: a membrane form and a secreted form. The membrane form has an extra carboxy terminal portion on the heavy chain that anchors it to the membrane and perhaps plays a role in signal transduction. For example, memory B cells that are "ready" to secrete IgG contain a membrane form of IgG. Upon activation by antigen, the switch from the membrane form to the secreted form occurs via an alteration of mRNA mediated by differential RNA processing.

Structural Basis of Antigen-binding Specificity

Each class of antibodies includes millions of different molecules, each with unique antigen-binding specificity and amino acid sequence. This diversity provides the variety of functions of each isotype and the multitude of specific antigen-binding sites required for a sophisticated mobile defense system. However, diversity presents formidable genetic problems. Their solution involves some very special mechanisms of gene expression. For example, immunoglobulins turned out to be the first known exception to the "one gene, one polypeptide" rule.

Each light chain and heavy chain consists of two major regions: **variable** and **constant** regions. These were originally identified by comparing the amino acid sequences of different immunoglobulin molecules. As the names imply, the sequences in the constant regions are similar, whereas the variable region sequences differ considerably from antibody to antibody.

In light chains, the carboxy-terminal halves of chains of the same type (κ or λ) have the same sequence, while the amino-terminal part are different. In heavy chains, a variable region of similar size (about 110 amino acids) is present at the amino terminus, while the rest of the molecule is rather constant. Within the variable regions, differences are clustered into three regions of the light chains and four heavy chains. These regions, each about 4–12 amino acids long, are known as **hypervariable regions**. From x-ray diffraction studies, it is now clear that the variable regions of the light and heavy chains are so folded that the hypervariable regions form an antigen-binding pocket that can accommodate an antigenic determinant the size of several sugars or amino acids. Thus, the amino-terminal variable parts of the light and heavy chains form the antigen-binding site. Their amino acid differences provide the structural basis for the diversity of antigen-binding function.

The interaction of antigen with antibody is a reversible **bimolecular reaction**. Unlike enzyme–substrate reactions, neither of the reactants is permanently altered. The binding of antigen to the antigen-combining site is mediated by the sum of many noncovalent forces such as hydrophobic and hydrogen bonds, van der Waals forces, and ionic interactions. Since these forces are effective at short distances, a tight fit takes place when the surfaces are complementary, that is, if the size and shape of the antigen fits to the combining site on the antibody. The "goodness of the fit" or binding strength is referred to as **affinity**. Affinity can be determined experimentally by quantitating the affinity constant of the antigen–antibody interaction. **Avidity** of the antigen–antibody interaction is the total binding strength of all the sites together; the multivalency of IgM, for example, increases the avidity.

Antibody Specificity and Quantitation

Specificity is defined as the ability of antibodies produced in response to an antigen to react with that antigen and not with others. Antibodies can be incredibly specific. They can discriminate atomic differences between simple chemicals and single amino acid substitutions in proteins. Antibodies may bind to more than one

antigen molecule; these events are called **cross-reactions**. For example, antibody raised to antigen X may cross-react with antigen Y, which is due to the presence of a similar molecular configuration on the two antigens.

Specificity can be improved and cross-reactions minimized by the use of **monoclonal antibodies**. By a procedure illustrated in Figure 7.8, cells can be generated that secrete homogeneous antibody molecules with a single kind of binding site. An antibody-forming B cell is fused with a myeloma cell resulting in a hybrid cell (called a **hybridoma**) with the combined properties of both fusion partners: the ability to secrete specific antibody and the ability for rapid and sustained growth. The use of special culture media that permit the growth of only the hy-

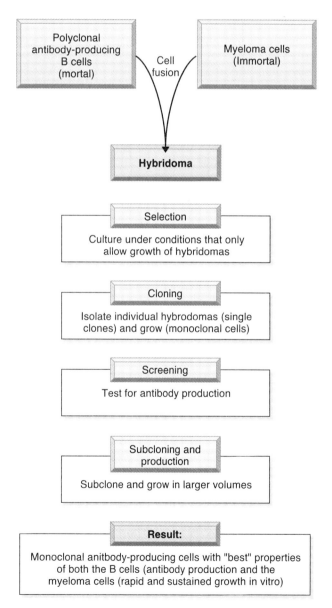

Figure 7.8. Production of monoclonal antibodies. Sequential steps in the procedure used to generate monoclonal antibodies are illustrated.

brid cells, coupled with methods for isolation of the progeny of individual hybridomas, results in the propagation of monoclonal antibody-producing cells. This procedure has revolutionized biology and medicine by making unlimited quantities of homogeneous antibodies available for a variety of applications.

There are numerous methods for detecting both antibodies and antigens. Some methods rely on the ability of antibodies to precipitate antigen which can be visualized or quantitated: these include quantitative immunoprecipitation, immuno-double diffusion (Ouchterlony test), single radial immunodiffusion (SRID or Mancini test), immunoelectrophoresis (IEP), etc. Other tests rely on antigen–antibody interactions that are detected by coupling antibody or antigen with a radioactive tracer (radioimmunoassay [RIA]), an enzyme (enzyme-linked immunosorbent assay [ELISA]), or a fluorescent compound (immunofluorescence or fluorescence immunoassays [FIA]). These tests are described in Chapter 55, "Diagnostic Principles." Still other assays utilize the ability of antibody to cross-link and agglutinate antigen-bearing cells (e.g, antibodies to red cells can be detected by hemagglutination) or activate complement when bound to antigen (complement fixation test).

Evolution of the Immunoglobulin Supergene Family

As previously discussed, the heavy and light chains are composed of homologous domains, and each domain has a characteristic three-dimensional structure called the immunoglobulin fold. The homology among the domains suggests that the immunoglobulin chains arose in evolution by a series of **gene duplications** of the basic 110-amino acid unit. It is now clear that the immunoglobulin fold is a fundamental structural unit that defines a whole family of homologous proteins, called the **immunoglobulin supergene family** (Fig. 7.9). Members of the family include immunoglobulin, the T-cell receptor, molecules of the major histocompatibility complex (MHC), and other lymphocyte surface proteins such as CD4, and CD8. Recent counts show that there are 1397 protein domains of the family expressed by cells of the immune system, the nervous system, and others. New members of the family will undoubtedly continue to be detected.

It is possible that the supergene family evolved to supply a common function to the family members. It is clear that the functions of the domains of immunoglobulin heavy and light chains are to interact, to stabilize the immunoglobulin molecule, and to form the antigen-binding site. Similarly, the family may have evolved to mediate cell–cell interactions via significant binding affinity between family members, as discussed below.

Generation of Diversity (G.O.D.)

One major challenge to the immune system is to provide millions, perhaps billions, of antibodies specific for almost any antigenic determinant. The remarkable aspect of antibody diversity is how this is achieved without requiring an unreasonably large amount of genetic material.

Immunoglobulins are produced from **three groups** of similar genes on separate chromosomes, corresponding to the κ light, λ light, and heavy chains, respectively. Each gene pool contains many variable region genes (and subdivisions of variable gene segments), located at a distance upstream from the constant region genes. During B-cell development, variable genes are **translocated** to a position closer to a particular constant gene. In this way, the chains (composed of variable and constant regions) are transcribed and translated. The first translocation that occurs in B-cell development brings a particular variable region gene segment close to the μ-constant gene and thus leads to the expression of heavy chains for IgM. Other translocations occur during this differentiation, so that a particular variable gene is connected more closely to other heavy-chain constant genes, allowing the expression of other isotypes of antibody (Fig. 7.10). This phenomenon is called **class switching**. These events occur by a process known as **site-specific recombination**, which depends on specific recombination sequences flanking each gene segment. These translocations also account for the fact that different classes of antibody may have the same antigen-binding specificity.

It is in the recombination of variable region genes that the conservation of genetic information is most prominently displayed. Variable-region genes are actually composed of two or three separate variable gene segments. A **segment** is defined as a contiguous stretch of DNA that is ultimately translated into a portion of the mature polypeptide. Two segments code for the variable region of each light chain: they are called V for variable and J for joining segments. Three segments are involved for heavy chains: V, D (diversity), and J segments (see Figs. 7.10 and 7.11). During assembly of a complete variable region gene, these segments are brought into proximity to permit transcription. These different V, J, and D segments allow many unique combinations to be created by somatic recombination, thereby increasing antibody diversity. For example, variable-heavy-chain genes may be made up of about 200 V segments, 10 D segments, and 4 J segments. Random combination could produce 8000 ($200 \times 10 \times 4 = 8000$) unique variable heavy chains. Similarly, if the 200 or so variable light-chain κ gene segments were to recombine with the 4 J segments, about 800 unique variable genes would be generated. Also, since the antigen-binding site is generated by both heavy and light chains, the random association of H and L chains could yield about 6.4 million ($8000 \times 800 = 6,400,000$) different antibody molecules. (This process is like creating a large number of different meals in a Chinese restaurant by choosing one

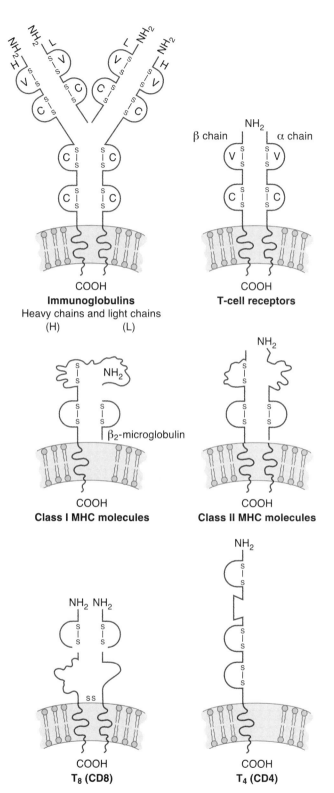

Figure 7.9. The immunoglobulin supergene family. Schematic diagrams of some of the members of the immunoglobulin supergene family are shown. Immunoglobulin, β_2 microglobulin, and class I MHC have been studied by x-ray diffraction and the three-dimensional structure is known. Other structures are predicted from the amino acid sequence inferred from the nucleotide sequences of cloned genes. Homology units (or domains) are depicted by intrachain disulfide-bonded loops. These loops represent globular domains each of which has a polypeptide chain folded into a β-pleated sheet configuration. Irregular loops represent imperfect folding into such a configuration.

from column A, one from column B, and so on. See Figure 7.11. The number of gene segments differs in various species, but the mechanisms are the same.)

Additional diversity can be created by the mistakes made during the cutting and joining of the V, D, and J segments, known as junctional diversity. **Nucleotide ad-**dition during the joining process also increases diversity in heavy chains. Also, **point mutations** in and around the V region genes can occur. This is called **somatic mutation**. These mechanisms probably increase antibody diversity by a factor of 10 to 100. Somatic mutation may play an important role in antibody production during

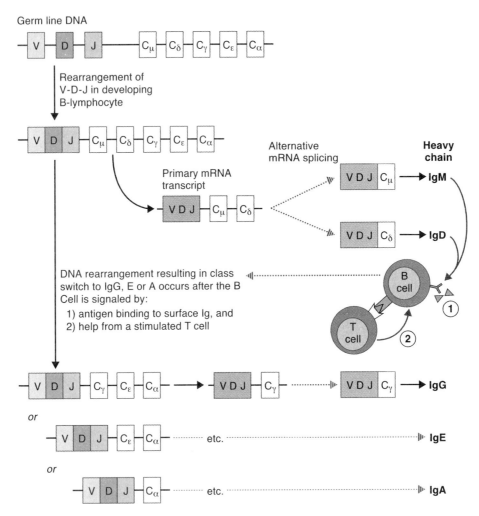

Figure 7.10. Organization and expression of immunoglobulin heavy-chain genes. The gene rearrangements that occur during B-cell development and the response to antigen are depicted. DNA segments that encode for individual portions of the mature protein are carried separately in the *germ line DNA*. These gene segments must rearrange as indicated in order for expression to occur. The joining of a given variable gene to different constant region genes permits the production of different isotypes (classes) of antibody with identical antigen-binding characteristics. The genes are not drawn to scale, and many details are omitted for simplicity.

secondary responses to antigen. Such mutations "fine tune" the affinity of a particular antibody. Additionally, somatic mutations may reflect the immune system's attempt to "anticipate" changes in antigens. For example, the genes of an invading microorganism are subject to mutations that can potentially change antigens to a form unrecognizable by a particular antibody and thus evade the immune response. Antibody genes may also "gamble" that somatic mutations in variable genes produce changes in the binding site that complement changes in the antigen, thus permitting successful recognition and destruction of the invader.

Thus, somatic recombination of segments, junctional diversity, somatic mutation, and combinatorial joining of light and heavy chains all act to increase antibody diversity for possibly 10^8 different antibody molecules.

This huge repertoire is apparently sufficient to deal with the antigenic universe. But, antibody diversity is only half of the story. The other arm of immune defense, the T lymphocytes, can likely generate, by similar mechanisms, a repertoire of millions or billions of antigen-binding molecules (the T-cell receptor, TCR).

T LYMPHOCYTES AND CELL-MEDIATED IMMUNITY

Cell-mediated immune reactions are those mediated by the thymus-derived T lymphocytes. Like B lymphocytes and the antibody responses, T lymphocytes can specifically recognize and react to highly diverse structures. Both types of lymphocytes respond to antigen and mediate memory responses by clonal selection. However, T-cell antigen recognition and function differ from B cells in several important aspects:

- There are several **functionally distinct categories** of T cells: cytotoxic cells, inducer or helper cells, and suppressor cells.
- T cells recognize antigen when it is associated with proteins of the **major histocompatibility complex** (MHC). More will be said about MHC encoded proteins later in this chapter. In general, cytotoxic T cells recognize antigen only when it is associated with "class I MHC" molecules, whereas helper T cells recognize a molecular configuration formed by the physical association of processed antigen with "class II MHC" molecules.

- The **developmental pathways** are different: T cells depend on the thymus for important differentiation and selection events.
- A number of lymphocyte **accessory molecules**, important for T-cell activation, are not expressed by B cells.
- The **receptor for antigen** used by T cells is related to immunoglobulin, but is structurally and genetically distinct. In general, the T-cell receptor is not designed to be a secretory product like antibody.

T-Cell Receptor Complex

T cells recognize and respond to antigen by using integral membrane glycoproteins called the **T-cell recep-**

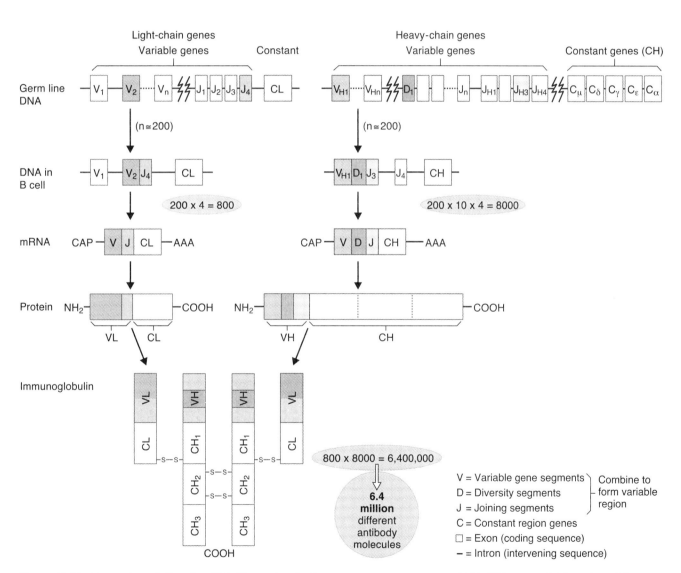

Figure 7.11. Generation of diversity. This illustration depicts the mechanism by which a large number of unique immunoglobulin molecules are created. The number of unique variable regions and antigen-combining sites created at each step is calculated. For example, with heavy chains the 200 *V* segments can combine with any of the 10 *D* segments and 4 *J* segments to create 8000 different variable regions. The number of *V*, *D*, and *J* segments present are, in some cases, minimal estimates and the actual numbers of segments vary among different species. A similar mechanism occurs for the generation of diversity in T-cell receptors (not shown).

tors (TCR). There are two types of TCR. The most completely characterized receptor is a disulfide-linked heterodimer of two polypeptide chains, designated α and β, each having a molecular weight of about 40–50 kilodaltons. The other receptor has two similar chains designated γ and δ. Each chain contains N-terminal variable regions unique to particular clones of T cells and carboxy-terminal constant regions shared among T cells. This basic structure has been identified on both helper T cells and cytotoxic T cells. The receptor(s) for antigen on suppressor T cells has not been identified.

The T-cell receptor has a domain structure homologous to immunoglobulin, which places it in the Ig supergene family. Like immunoglobulin, T-cell receptors are constructed by somatic recombination of genes carried separately in the genome. For example, α-chain genes include a single constant region which contains about 50 J segments and about 75 V segments. Upstream of the genes for the β constant region, there are about 12 J segments, 2 D segments, and about 25 V segments. In both chains, junctional diversity and nucleotide addition increase the repertoire, but somatic mutation does not appear to play a role in increasing diversity. Like diversity created with the construction of an immunoglobulin gene, many different unique α, β, γ, and δ chains can be constructed by the random combinations of V, J, and D segments. By combinatorial associations of different chains a very large repertoire of T-cell receptors can be potentially generated. Interestingly, there appears to be much greater junctional diversity in TCR genes than in Ig genes and the repertoire of TCRs may be even greater than for antibodies. This diversity is certainly comparable to that of antibody diversity and large enough to deal with the antigenic universe.

How does the triggering of these receptors translate into the expression of function? We know that other membrane proteins of T cells are involved in as yet poorly understood but well established accessory roles. One of these is designated the **CD3 complex**. The CD3 complex is a group of five major proteins noncovalently linked to the T-cell receptor. Although the CD3 complex must be present for proper T-cell function it does not bind directly to antigen. It appears to be involved in transmitting signals to the cell interior that result in cell activation.

Functional T-Cell Subpopulations

T lymphocytes are divided into three main functional groups: cytotoxic T cells, helper or inducer T cells, and suppressor T cells. They may also be subdivided on the basis of differential T-cell receptor expression and cytokine production.

Cytotoxic T cells

Cytotoxic T lymphocytes can specifically recognize and destroy cells that carry foreign antigens on their surface, the so-called **antigen-presenting cells**. They defend us against certain viral diseases (and probably bacterial diseases caused by intracellular pathogens) by reacting with antigens expressed on the surface of infected cells. Prevention of viral replication results from their ability to recognize very low levels of antigen and to kill infected cells before production of virus progeny. Intimate effector cell–target cell interaction is required for killing. This cellular adhesion is aided in an undefined way by lymphocyte-function-associated molecules such as LFA-1, CD8, CD28, and others. Following binding to the target cell, the CD8 molecule and the CD3 complex are involved in expression of lytic function.

The mechanism of killing is not certain, but the most attractive hypothesis is termed the granule exocytosis model. Evidence exists that the T cell secretes a protein called **perforin** from intracellular granules onto the target cell membrane. This protein then assembles into amphipathic channel-forming structures—analogous to the membrane attack complex of complement—that cause permeability changes in the target cell and eventual osmotic lysis. Cytotoxic T lymphocytes may also induce a nuclease activity in the target cell that destroys both cellular and viral DNA. It is clear that the effector T cell is not damaged in this process and can kill multiple target cells.

Helper T cells

Helper or inducer T lymphocytes are essential for optimal proliferation and differentiation of B cells and cytotoxic T-cell precursors. They are also important for increasing the ability of macrophages to ingest and destroy microbial pathogens and to kill tumor cells. They display characteristic surface markers including CD3 and CD4. CD3 is involved in signal transduction and CD4 stabilizes cellular interactions by binding to portions of the class II MHC molecules present on B cells and macrophages.

When activated, T-helper cells release a variety of **cytokines**. These include several interleukins such as IL-2 and IL-4 which stimulate lymphocytes, and macrophage-activating factors such as γ-interferon. The properties of some cytokines are summarized in Table 7.3. There are too many cytokines to list completely here. For example, at the last count there are 15 interleukins.

Because of their secretory function, many, if not all, of the activities of helper T cells can be duplicated by the appropriate mix of active cytokines. However, the most efficient delivery of helper T-cell-derived cytokines to B cells and macrophages is accomplished by the direct physical interaction between the cells. This occurs when antigen is presented by B cells so that helper T cells interact with it on the B cell's surface. Likewise, macrophage activation via helper T-cell-derived γ-interferon is aided by macrophage-mediated antigen presentation. Thus T cells form synaptic-like junctions with in-

Table 7.3. Cytokines

Name	Major cellular source	Major activities
Interleukin-1 (IL-1)	Macrophages, others	Costimulates various cells (e.g., T cells), induces fever
Interleukin-2 (IL-2)	T cells (Th1)	Induces proliferation of activated T and B cells
Interleukin-3 (IL-3)	T cells (Th1 and Th2)	Induces growth of bone marrow stem cells
Granulocyte–macrophage–colony stimulating factor (GM-CSF)	T cells (Th1, $\pm$ Th2)	Induces growth of granulocytes and macrophages
Interferon-gamma (γ-IFN)	T cells (Th1)	Activates macrophages, NK cells; promotes MHC expression; induces B-cell differentiation and IgG2a synthesis
Tumor necrosis factor (TNF-α)	T cells (Th1, $\pm$ Th2), macrophages	Activates monocytes, macrophages and PMNs; induces fever
Interleukin-4 (IL-4)	T cells (Th2)	Activates B cells; promotes IgG1 and IgE response; inhibits macrophages activation
Interleukin-5 (IL-5)	T cells (Th2)	Induces proliferation of eosinophils
Interleukin-6 (IL-6)	Macrophages, T cells (Th2)	Activates B cells; induces acute-phase protein release
Interleukin-10 (IL-10)	T cells (Th2)	Inhibits Th1, inhibits macrophage cytokines
Interleukin-12 (IL-12)	Macrophages, B cells	Enhances Th1 development and activity

teracting cells and the directional release of cytokines may be more analogous to neurotransmitters than hormones.

Suppressor T cells

Suppressor T cells downregulate the response of B cells or other T cells to antigens. They remain the most enigmatic regulatory T cell. One thing that is clear is that they regulate responses in an antigen-specific manner. Suppression can be mediated by soluble factors from suppressor T cells. The current confusion about suppressor T cells will only be mitigated when their antigen receptors are characterized and the mechanisms involved in their postulated roles in cellular interactions elucidated.

Other T-Cell Subsets

T cells can be classified according to the type of T-cell receptor expressed. T cells that express the α/β TCR are found in blood and peripheral lymphoid tissue. Current dogma about T cells is derived exclusively from the study of α/β T cells. T cells that express the γ/δ TCR are found in epithelial tissue in significant numbers and in very high proportion as compared with α/β T cells. Because of their epithelial localization, it is thought that γ/δ T cells play important roles in initial defense at external boundaries. Although it is clear that γ/δ T cells do play an important role in early defense against microbial pathogens, little is known about their mechanism of antigen recognition. It is known that γ/δ T cells elaborate γ-interferon in response to cytokine signals and can kill infected cells in a selective manner.

Another classification of T-cell subsets is based on cytokine production. One type of helper T cell, termed Th1, secretes cytokines such as IL-4 and promotes B-cell development and antibody production. Another T cell, the Th2 cell, elaborates IL-2 and γ-interferon. Th1 cells participate in cell-mediated and immunity and delayed-type hypersensitivity reactions. Th1 cells help B cells, whereas Th2 cells help macrophages (and other T cells). The preponderance of Th1 or Th2 cells can profoundly influence the outcome of infectious disease. For example, Th1 cell are required for immunity to intracellular pathogens. Because Th1 and Th2 development is mutually antagonistic, a Th2 response can be made to the detriment of host defense to certain pathogens. Th1 and Th2 cells communicate via the action of the cytokines.

Null cells or "third population cells"

In addition to B and T lymphocytes, other functionally important cells exist that do not display the classical surface markers and functions of T cells, B cells, and macrophages. As the name "null" implies, these cells lack the readily detectable markers and functions of macrophages, B cells, and T lymphocytes. While their lineage remains unclear, they are generally considered to be lymphocyte-like. This group includes cells of two functions: **natural killer (NK)** cells and **killer (K)** cells, which are responsible for **antibody-dependent cell-mediated cytotoxicity (ADCC)**.

NK cells can efficiently kill certain types of tumor- and virus-infected cells, but without the precise specificity displayed by cytotoxic T lymphocytes. NK cells do not require the thymus for development. NK cells have prominent cytoplasmic granules and therefore have been called **large granular lymphocytes** (LGL). These granules contain perforin and other lytic agents. Granule exocytosis, as described for the cytotoxic T cell, is the likely mechanism of killing by NK and K cells.

K cells express high-affinity Fc receptors which are employed to recognize and destroy antibody-coated cells. IgG is the predominant class responsible for directing the specificity of cytotoxic activity of K cells. These cells can kill certain bacteria and mammalian cells.

K cells and NK cells are either the same population of cells or part of largely overlapping subsets. The activity of both NK and K cells is increased in response to cytokines such as γ-interferon, and they can proliferate in response to IL-2. NK cells themselves can also produce cytokines such as γ-interferon IL-2 and IL-12.

MACROPHAGES

Macrophages play an important role in cell-mediated immunity. Macrophages develop from **myeloid stem cells** in the bone marrow. There, as **promonocytes**, they undergo intense proliferation (driven by colony stimulating factor). These cells then enter the blood, where they are called **monocytes**. After several days in the blood, they seed various tissues as **mature macrophages**. Macrophages are called several names and have specialized functions depending on their anatomical location. For example, in the lung they are called alveolar macrophages; in the brain, microglial cells; in the liver, Kupffer cells; and in the skin, Langerhans cells.

In general, mature macrophages have a limited ability for proliferation. Thus, the increase in number of monocytes in the blood (monocytosis) or at inflammatory sites is not due to local proliferation but rather to greater influx from the bone marrow. Macrophages are readily distinguished from lymphocytes by function, morphology, and surface markers. Unlike lymphocytes, macrophages have horseshoe-shaped nuclei, prominent cytoplasmic granules, and the ability to ingest particles and to adhere to surfaces. While macrophages play crucial roles in constitutive defense reactions, as described in Chapter 6 ("Constitutive Defenses"), their most important roles may be related to their symbiotic relationship with lymphocytes. Macrophages activate lymphocytes by processing and presenting antigen and by elaborating molecules such IL-1 and IL-12. Conversely, lymphocytes activate macrophages through the elaboration of cytokines.

One such group of cytokines is known as **macrophage-activating factors** (MAF), the most well-defined of which is γ-interferon. This cytokine augments a variety of macrophage functions, such as antigen presentation, phagocytic functions involving complement component C3b and antibody fragment Fc, and destruction of intracellular microbial pathogens and extracellular tumor cells.

Macrophages probably have several mechanisms for expression of cytocidal function. In addition to those discussed in Chapter 6 ("Constitutive Defenses"), activated macrophages secrete **tumor necrosis factor** (TNF). TNF has several biological activities, including tumor-killing and antiviral effects. Macrophages also release other antiviral substances, α- and β-interferons. The expression of macrophage-mediated cytotoxicity is dramatically affected by a number of bacterial products such as lipopolysaccharide (LPS) from Gram-negative bacteria (Chapter 3, "Biology of Infectious Agents" and Chapter 9, "Damage"). LPS dramatically increases macrophage cytolytic activity and other defensive activities.

The growth and differentiation of macrophages from bone marrow–derived stem cells is mediated by the colony stimulating factors, working in synergy with cytokines. Other T-cell-derived cytokines are thought to be important for the accumulation of macrophages at certain inflammatory sites; macrophages are attracted to sites where macrophage chemotactic factor(s) are present and are prevented from leaving by migration inhibitory factor(s).

ANTIGEN-PRESENTING AND DENDRITIC CELLS

Any cell with the ability to present antigens to lymphocytes is functionally classified as an antigen-presenting cells. Such cells include macrophages, B cells, and dendritic cells, all of which appear to have several required functions:

- Antigen binding
- Antigen processing
- Expression of class II MHC gene products (see below)
- Elaboration of IL-1

Dendritic cells get their name from their long slender processes and irregularly shaped nuclei. They are effective antigen-presenting cells and are thought to be important in cooperative interactions with lymphocytes, especially during primary immune responses. They are found in small numbers in lymphoid tissue, and their lineage is unclear. They have little or no phagocytic activity and carry neither B- nor T-cell receptors. They do have Fc receptors, C3 receptors, and express class II MHC proteins. There are several kinds of these cells, each with somewhat different locations and functional properties: lymphoid, follicular, interdigitating dentritic cells, and Langerhans cells.

The various cells involved in immune responses are shown in Table 7.4. In summary, the relationships among lymphocytes and their products are so intricate

Table 7.4. Cells of the Immune System

Cell	Surface components	Function
T lymphocytes	T$_3$	Involved in cell-mediated immunity
Helper T cells (T$_H$)	T$_4$	Recognizes antigen with class II MHC; promotes differentiation of B cells and cytotoxic T cells; activates macrophages
	T-cell receptor complex: α, β dimer associated with T$_3$	
Cytotoxic T cells (CTL)	T$_8$	Recognizes antigen with class I MHC; kills antigen-expressing cells
γ/δ T cells	Probably all T$_4$ and T$_8$ negative	Respond to commonly encountered microbial antigens perhaps at epithelial boundaries; MHC restriction and function unknown
B lymphocytes	Surface immunoglobulin, Fc receptors, class II MHC	Recognizes antigen directly; differentiates into antibody-producing plasma cells, antigen presentation
Large granular lymphocytes (LGL) K cells	Fc receptor	Kills antibody-coated cells (ADCC)
NK cells	Receptor for target "antigen" unknown	Kills cells with some selectivity
Macrophages	Fc receptor, C3 receptor; some have class II MHC; can bind to wide variety of substance via surface "receptors"	Antigen presentation; phagocytotic killing of microbes and tumor cells; secretion of IL-1
Dendritic cells	Fc receptor, C3 receptor, class II MHC	Antigen presentation
Mast cells (tissues) and basophils (blood)	High-affinity receptors for IgE	Allergic responses; histamine release
Neurophils	Fc receptor, C3 receptor, C5 receptor and FMLP receptor	Phagocytosis and killing of bacteria, yeast, and fungi
Eosinophils		Phagocytosis and elimination of parasites

and interdependent that it is difficult to speak of an individual cell without reference to other members of the partnership. Like the nervous system, it is difficult to appreciate the function of an individual neuron without understanding the collective activities of networks of functioning cells and molecules. Thus, a major challenge for the future is to define the rate-limiting steps of the various cellular and molecular interactions and to understand the regulation of immune physiology.

MAJOR HISTOCOMPATIBILITY COMPLEX (MHC)

The MHC consists of proteins originally discovered as being responsible for the rejection of tissue or organ grafts. Only later did it become clear that the MHC performs a far more crucial role, that of helping T cells recognize foreign antigens. The MHC has played several tricks on immunologists. One trick was that they made us focus first on issues concerning graft rejection and tissue

transplantation between members of a species. While such strong transplantation antigens are indeed encoded by the MHC (hence the name), the importance of hindering organ transplantation makes no immediate sense for survival value and for the normal protective immune responses against pathogenic microbes. In addition, susceptibility to certain diseases is associated with certain alleles of MHC genes. For example, it remains a mystery why people with a particular MHC allele (HLA B27) are at a 300-fold greater risk of developing the degenerative disease ankylosing spondylitis. There are ideas, of course! One of the most popular is that a surface antigen of the microbe associated with ankylosing spondylitis, *Klebsiella*, mimics the host HLA-B27 molecule, and therefore the host is unresponsive to the microbe. Other mysteries of the MHC include the control of mating behavior by the MHC. Mating is disfavored among mice with similar MHC genes, which may serve to increase genetic polymorphism. Interestingly, mice can smell minor differences in the MHC expressed by other mice. Strange but true.

Straight Dope On MHC

Unless we are being tricked again (doubtful), we now believe that the main role of the MHC is in mediating cell–cell communication. MHC-encoded cell-surface proteins "hold" foreign antigens in the "proper" configuration for recognition by T cells and serve to "guide" the appropriate subpopulation of T cells to the appropriate antigen-expressing surface. Thus, T cells recognize foreign antigens in association with self-MHC molecules.

Chemistry and Cellular Location of MHC

Two structurally and functionally different classes of MHC molecules exist, conveniently termed class I and class II. As summarized in Table 7.5, these classes differ in genetic loci, chain structure, cell distribution, and function with different T-cell subsets. In general, class I molecules direct the activity of CD8+ cytotoxic T lymphocytes. Class II guide the function of CD4+ helper T cells

Mature class I molecules are composed of **two subunits**, a single 345 amino acid polypeptide encoded by the MHC and a smaller protein called **β-2-microglobulin**. The class I chains are **integral membrane proteins**. The three-dimensional structure of a human class I MHC molecule has been determined. MHC molecules are members of the immunoglobulin supergene family as they share structure in the membrane proximal domains. β-2-microglobulin is also homologous to immunoglobulin constant regions. Class II molecules (also called Ia molecules or DR antigens) are structured from two noncovalently linked glycoproteins, an α-chain (MW about 33,000 Da) and a β-chain (MW about 28,000 Da). Each chain is a **transmembrane protein** with two external domains. For both class I and class II proteins, the two membrane distal domains form a characteristic structure with two alpha helical regions bordering the floor of a β-pleated sheet. This region binds antigenic peptides for presentation to T cells.

Class I gene products are expressed on almost all nucleated somatic cells. In contrast, class II molecules normally have a more restricted cell distribution. All B cells and some macrophages, dendritic cells, thymus epithelial cells, and activated T cells express class II molecules. Many cell types (including epithelial, endodermal, and parenchymal cells) express class II under certain abnormal clinical situations, such as graft rejection and autoimmune diseases.

The cellular distribution of class I and class II molecules is thought to reflect differences in their function. Cytotoxic T cells patrol the tissues "looking for" abnormal cells such as potentially dangerous cancer cells or virus-infected cells. The advantage of recognizing both class I and foreign antigen is that the cytotoxic T cell can focus its function on the source of the potential trouble. Cytotoxic T cells can destroy infected cells before pathogenic progeny are formed. This cellular surveillance by cytotoxic T cells requires the global expression of class I molecules. In contrast, the more restricted expression of class II molecules directs the function of helper T cells to the cells requiring the help: B cells and macrophages. Thus, during evolution, T-helper cells "learned" to recognize antigens associated with B cells and macrophages, while cytotoxic T cells "learn" to pay attention to all somatic cells expressing suspicious structures—alterations of self.

MHC Genetics

Both class I and class II MHC proteins are encoded by several genes called HLA (genes for class I molecules are called HLA-A, HLA-B, and HLA-C; genes for class II molecules, HLA-DP, HLA-DQ, and HLA-DR). The HLA genes are the most polymorphic group of genes known in higher vertebrates. There is a very large number of different alleles (alternate forms of the same gene) within a species. For example, hundreds of different class I glycoproteins can be expressed by all the individuals of species. However, the diversity of MHC proteins differs from that of antibody molecules. Thus, MHC genes do not undergo somatic rearrangements like immunoglobulin and T-cell receptor genes. Each of us can make millions of different antibody molecules, but we inherit only a single MHC allele at each locus from each parent. Thus, MHC polymorphism must be involved in survival of the species, not of the individual.

Table 7.5. Properties of Class I and Class II MHC Proteins

	Class I	Class II
Genetic loci	HLA-A, HLA-B, HLA-C	HLA-D (DP, DQ, DR)
Chain structure	45,000 mol wt glycoprotein + β_2-microglobulin	α-chain (33,000 mol wt) β-chain (28,000 mol wt)
Cell distribution	Almost all nucleated somatic cells	B cells, some macrophages dendritic cells, thymus epithelial cells, and activated T cells
Functions in presenting antigen to	Cytotoxic T cells (CD8+ cells)	Help T cells (CD4+ cells)

Immune response genes (Ir genes) are the class II MHC genes that control responses of helper T cells (similar control of cytotoxic T lymphocytes by class I MHC genes also occurs). Certain MHC alleles are associated with low responsiveness, while others determine high responsiveness to a particular antigenic determinant. Because these effects are antigen-specific, a given individual or group of inbred animals can be a low responder to antigen X but a high responder to antigen Y. Although high responsiveness is dominant, under certain circumstances a cross between two allelically dissimilar low responders can yield a high responder. This results from the creation of a unique class II molecule by combinatorial association of an α chain from one parent with a β chain from the other (or vice versa).

What Do MHC Molecules Do?

MHC molecules **physically interact** with antigen. This binding is required for effective immune responses and probably serves as the basis for immune response gene control. Class II molecules from high responders can bind processed antigen, but low responder class II molecules cannot bind the antigenic determinant in question.

Exogenous protein antigens are **endocytosed** by antigen-presenting cells such as macrophages and then degraded by **proteolysis** in acidic lysosomal/endosomal compartments. Processing occurs by means of a cytoplasmic proteosome (a proteolytic macromolecule), and a peptide transporter permits access to the **endoplasmic reticulum**. Peptide epitopes derived from this degradation are then bound to nascent class II MHC molecules and transported via the Golgi apparatus to the cell surface. When the protein antigen is foreign to the antigen-presenting cell (such as a viral protein), MHC class I molecules bind the antigenic peptides derived from processing of the antigen. The interaction between foreign peptide and MHC class I probably occurs in the endoplasmic reticulum. The peptide–MHC complex is then transported to the cell surface.

Some bacterial antigens, such as the staphylococcal enterotoxins, bind outside the peptide binding groove of the MHC class II molecules and are recognized by large numbers of T cells. Since the frequency of enterotoxin-sensitive T cells is much higher than that of regular antigens, these enterotoxins have been called **superantigens** (Chapter 9, "Damage"). Because of the large number of activated T cells after exposure to enterotoxins, there are complications such as shock and fever that can lead eventually to death.

The interaction among the T-cell receptor, the MHC molecules, and the foreign processed antigen may be thought of as a triple complex in which each component of the complex interacts with the other two (see Fig. 7.12). Accessory molecules such as CD4 and CD8 contribute to cell–cell interaction through associations with class II and class I MHC molecules.

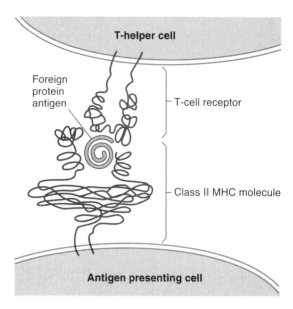

Figure 7.12. The interaction of the TCR, processed peptide antigen, and class II MHC molecule. MHC molecules bind antigenic peptides in a selective manner. The MHC molecule has a peptide-binding groove composed of polymorphic residues in two helices over a floor of conserved residues in a β-pleated sheet. The processed antigenic peptide of between 8–20 amino acids in length fits into the groove like a "hot dog in a bun." Residues of TCR interact with the antigenic peptide and with the MHC molecule.

The basis for strong T-cell reactions to foreign MHC molecules, as in those reactions leading to transplantation rejection, is not yet clear. One possibility is that foreign MHC molecules present on the grafted tissue collectively resemble the complex between self MHC and foreign peptides. In this model, T cells reactive with self MHC plus foreign peptides would cross-react with nonself MHC on the graft. Through fighting infectious disease, the immune system generates a large group of specificities for peptide–MHC complexes and some of these react well with nonself MHC.

Since the MHC controls immune responsiveness, does MHC polymorphism have survival value? Consider an epidemic within a species caused by a highly pathogenic microorganism that is weakly immunogenic. This hypothetical microbe may have antigenic determinants that bind poorly to most kinds of MHC molecules. In this "Andromeda Strain" scenario, MHC polymorphism may increase the likelihood that at least certain members of the species would have the "right" MHC molecules (high responders) and make a protective response to the pathogen. At least some members of this species would survive.

In summary, the MHC is crucial to the understanding of T-cell specificity and function. We know that these molecules bind antigenic determinants and guide the activities of T-cell subsets. MHC molecules can transport antigenic determinants from the inside of the antigen-presenting cell, where processing occurs, to the cell surface, where recognition can occur (see Fig. 7.5). MHC molecules may also protect portions of antigens from complete degradation. Additional roles for the MHC may be as unambiguous markers for self that maintain the critical process of tolerance to self tissue. The MHC may even constitute a "leftover" recognition system from the days when we were swimming about in primordial ooze trying to reject the dissimilar and bind to the similar. Their possible role as cell interaction molecules in developmental processes has also not been overlooked. Clearly, all the answers about these crucial molecules are not in. Are we being tricked again? Let's hope not.

REGULATION OF THE IMMUNE RESPONSE (IMMUNOREGULATION)

The immune response to foreign antigen must be regulated. Otherwise, once it were initiated, our bodies would fill up with lymphocytes and antibody. There are five major ways by which the immune response is downregulated. These involve: the limited life span of effector cells; antigen removal; antibody feedback; suppressor cells; and the idiotypic network.

1. The first regulation system is the simplest. The immune response is self-limiting because the functional life span of effector cells is short. For example, plasma cells can live only a few days.
2. Since continuous production of effector cells requires antigen, another way to downregulate the response is to remove the antigen. This is, in fact, the primary goal of the protective immune responses. The elicited antibody combines with antigen and the resulting immune complexes are more rapidly removed by the garbage collectors of the body, the cells of the lymphoreticular system. For example, proteins are rendered nonantigenic by complete digestion to amino acids in the lysosomes of macrophages. Such antigen degradation is more efficiently performed by activated macrophages.
3. Another fundamental mechanism is **feedback regulation** by antibody. Soluble antibody can mask antigenic determinants and prevent binding to B-cell receptors. Also, the Fc parts of the antigen-bound antibody can cross-link Fc receptors on the B cell and thereby "switch off" for B-cell proliferation and differentiation.
4. **Suppressor cells** regulate immune responses via complex regulatory cell circuits. Suppressor T cells are generated in response to increased numbers of helper T cells. Thus, helper T cells activate suppressor T cells that in turn downregulate the helper T cells. This feedback pathway allows the activity of both cells to be self-regulating. The action of sup-

pressor cells may be mediated by soluble suppressor factors which are molecularly heterogeneous. However, the exact nature of these cells and molecules has not been established and remains controversial.

5. The fifth and most intriguing way by which the immune response is regulated involves the so called **idiotypic network** as proposed by Niels Jerne. He proposed that the antigen-combining sites of the lymphocyte's antigen receptors are themselves antigenic. He called the antigens associated with the combining sites **idiotypic determinants** (also called **idiotopes**). Because an individual idiotope is present in very small concentrations in the body, immunological tolerance to self idiotopes is not established. Thus, immune responses can be generated to self idiotypic determinants. Antibodies raised against these determinants can prevent the binding of antigen to the antibody. Consequently, antigen can block the interaction of the anti-idiotypic antibody with idiotypic determinants on the target antibody. These facts suggested to Jerne the network theory (see Fig. 7.13).

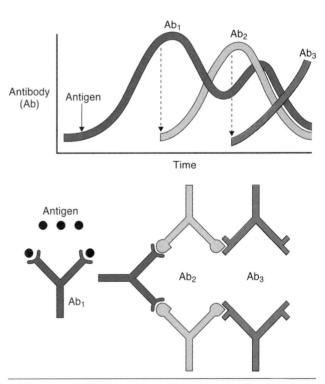

Ab₁ directed against antigenic determinant (epitope)
Ab₂ directed against idiotypic determinant (idiotope) of Ab₁
Ab₃ directed against idiotope of Ab₂

Figure 7.13. The idiotypic network. The amount of antibody produced is plotted as a function of time after injection of foreign antigen. When antibody-1 (directed against the epitope of the antigen) reaches a high concentration, it is sensed by the immune system and antibody-2 is made against the idiotope (or variable region) of antibody-1. A similar reaction then occurs with antibody-3 and so forth.

The network theory is based on two functions of the antibody molecules: its traditional role in binding antigen and a nontraditional role as an antigen. When animals are immunized with antigen X, the concentration of anti-X antibody is greatly increased. This increase in anti-X antibody is then perceived by the immune system, and antibody reactive to the idiotypic determinants of anti-X antibody is generated. The anti-idiotypic antibody can then elicit the production of another wave of antibody. Thus, antigen X stimulates anti-X antibody (Ab_1) that stimulates anti-(anti-X antibody) antibody (Ab_2) that stimulates anti-[anti-(anti-X antibody) antibody] antibody (Ab_3), and so on. Each response wave, however, is dampened by regulatory mechanisms.

The network theory allows the immune system to regulate itself using only itself. Idiotypic determinants may be thought of as the "internal images" of the external antigens. In other words, antibody against an antigen-binding site "looks like" the antigen. Because some antibodies are made even in the absence of foreign antigen, a vast number of immune responses are always going on. These internal reflections, a web of opposing immune responses, are in a dynamic equilibrium (a kind of immunological "muscle tone"). According to the network theory, what we perceive as an immune response when foreign antigen is introduced is simply the perturbation of the preexisting network and the establishment of a new position of equilibrium.

Anti-idiotypic antibody can regulate immune responses in both positive and negative ways. Anti-idiotypic antibody can be used instead of antigen to immunize animals; their potential utility as vaccines has been well demonstrated in mice and rats. Inhibition, rather than activation, occurs when the anti-idiotypic antibody is of a class that can bind complement and Fc receptors. In this case, it is likely that the anti-idiotypic antibody suppresses responses by eliminating the clones of lymphocytes that express the idiotypic determinant.

It's all a matter of molecular complementarity. "Nature (the idiotypic network), she shows us only surfaces, but she's a million fathoms (receptors) deep," said Ralph Waldo Emerson.

IMMUNOPATHOLOGY

Immunopathology refers to disease caused by inappropriate immune responses. Immune responses that fail to distinguish self from nonself may result in **autoimmune diseases**. Exaggerated or inappropriate immune responses are called **hypersensitivity reactions**. And defects in defense reactions, which cause recurring infections, are known as **immunodeficiency diseases**. Thus, immune responses that are misdirected, too strong, or too weak can result in pathology.

Autoimmune Diseases

Autoimmune reactions are those directed against the body's own tissues, cells, or molecules. These reactions occur when the regulatory events involved in immunological tolerance are subverted or otherwise malfunction. Self antigens, or **autoantigens**, are the targets of autoimmune reactions. Autoantigens may be intracellular components, receptors, cell membrane components, extracellular components, plasma proteins, or hormones. Depending on the autoantigen, the disease may be organ-specific (e.g., Graves' disease with the primary site in the thyroid gland) or nonorgan-specific (e.g., systemic lupus erythematosus with symptoms affecting many systems). Both antibody and T-cell responses to self antigens may cause disease.

Tissue damage by the immune response may be caused by the sharing of antigenic determinants between host and parasite. Given the biological relationships of hosts and parasites, it is not surprising that microorganisms and vertebrates sometimes share antigenic determinants. However, it is not known how host determinants elicit an immune response, since they should be recognized by the body as "self" and tolerance to such antigens should be established.

Autoimmune reactions have been implicated in two puzzling disorders that follow infections by certain streptococci (Chapter 12, "Streptococci"). Rheumatic fever and glomerulonephritis are uncommon but severe sequels of otherwise mundane "strep throats." We know that antigens in the cell walls of the infecting streptococci cross-react with components of heart muscle or kidney glomeruli, and that antibodies reactive with self tissues are present in such patients. However, the precise role of autoimmune reactions in these diseases is still unclear.

Since immunological tolerance to self components hidden from the immune system cannot be established, immune responses to self antigens occur when these sequestered antigens are released or abnormally expressed. Tissue and cellular damage may result in the release of antigenic intracellular molecules. The resulting immune reactions may cause continued cellular trauma, the further release of sequestered antigens, and perpetuation of the inflammatory process. Self components present in organs that lack conventional lymphatics and thus frequent contact with lymphocytes, such as the central nervous system, may elicit strong immune responses in an unusual context. For example, in experimental animals, injection of self CNS tissue mixed with an adjuvant may cause a demyelinating encephalitis that resembles the human disease multiple sclerosis. It is also thought that the abnormal expression of class II MHC gene products on cells other than antigen-presenting B cells and macrophages may initiate and perpetuate local immune reactions to self antigens on these cells.

Autoimmune disease may also result from alterations of self components by environmental agents. For example, one class of autoimmune hemolytic anemias is known to be drug-induced. The drug may bind to red cells and permit immune responses to the drug-associated self components. Conceivably, alterations of self components by interactions with microbial products may also contribute to autoimmune reactions. Additionally, many microbial agents are able to polyclonally activate lymphocytes and thus possibly bypass the normal regulatory pathways that maintain tolerance to self.

Finally, it is important to note that self-reactivity may occur in the absence of pathology. The idiotypic network, for example, initiates a web of responses to self idiotopes. Also, the association of a particular disease with autoimmune reactions does not necessarily imply a direct cause-and-effect relationship. An autoreaction may be secondary to the pathological changes caused by another mechanism.

Hypersensitivity Reactions

The term **hypersensitivity** is used for immune responses that occur in an exaggerated or inappropriate manner. None of the many clinical manifestations of hypersensitivity is pleasant. As the name implies, hypersensitivity reactions occur in individuals who have been previously sensitized to the antigen; in other words, they are secondary responses. They have been classified by Gell and Coombs into four major types according to the speed of the reaction and the nature of the immunological reactions involved. Despite these separate groupings, hypersensitivity reactions rarely, if ever, occur in complete isolation from each other. Nonetheless, these groups are useful conceptual frameworks for review of immune reactions (Fig. 7.14). Types I, II, and III are antibody-mediated while type IV is cell-mediated.

Type I or immediate hypersensitivity

Type I hypersensitivity reactions are also called **allergic reactions,** and the antigens involved are called **allergens.** These occur within minutes of exposure to antigen. The cross-linking of mast cell–bound IgE by the allergen triggers the release of vasoactive amines that produce inflammation. It is not known why some antigens elicit IgE production and cause such responses. While it is not entirely clear why only certain individuals suffer from these reactions, genetic control by class II MHC genes plays a significant role. Examples include allergic asthma, hay fever, urticaria, and anaphylactic reactions to insect venom.

Type II or cytotoxic hypersensitivity

Antibody binding to cell surface antigens is followed by **antibody-dependent cell-mediated cytotoxicity (ADCC)** by K cells or complement-mediated lysis. Examples of type II diseases include transfusion reactions, hemolytic disease of newborns, and certain drug allergies resulting in hemolytic anemia. Tissues can also be damaged by cytotoxic T lymphocytes but these diseases are discussed below as a form of cell-mediated hypersensitivity.

Type III or immune complex–mediated hypersensitivity

This kind of immunopathological damage is caused by the activation of complement by immune complexes (via the classical pathway) and the mobilization of white blood cells, especially neutrophils. Antigens may be soluble or associated with small particles like viruses. The antigen–antibody complex activates the complement pathway, and the resulting complement fragments (C3a, C5a, see Chapter 6) cause an inflammatory response. The vascular permeability changes and influx of neutrophils (and later macrophages) elicits symptoms like fever, skin rash, and arthritis. Thus, the deposition of antigen–antibody complexes in certain tissues can elicit inflammatory reactions that result in damage and disruption of normal organ function. The site of deposition of immune complexes dictates the type of pathology. Why complexes show affinity for particular tissues (kidney, joints, etc.) is not clear, but certain hemodynamic factors as well as the size of the immune complexes are thought to be critical. A relatively high or persistent antigen load characterizes these conditions. Hypersensitivity reactions may result from persistent infection with certain bacteria (streptococcal infections), viruses (hepatitis B), parasites (the *Plasmodium* agents of malaria), or worms (filariae, the agents of elephantiasis). Examples of type III reactions include glomerulonephritis, alveolitis, and certain autoimmune diseases.

Type IV cell-mediated reaction or delayed type hypersensitivity (DTH)

This is so named because symptoms appear at least 24–48 hours after antigen exposure. These reactions are caused by the activation of T cells, the release of cytokines, and the subsequent influx of macrophages to the site. Allergic contact dermatitis (e.g., poison ivy) and the skin test for exposure to tubercle bacilli, called the tuberculin test, are examples of DTH reactions.

Cell-mediated hypersensitivity is often characteristic of infections by intracellular slow growing pathogens, typified by the tubercle bacilli or by *Histoplasma capsulatum*, the agent of histoplasmosis. Circulating antibodies here play a minor role because the organisms are shielded in their intracellular location. Chronic inflammations are usually manifestations of cell-mediated immune reactions. These reactions may result in a lesion called the **granuloma**, a densely packed collection of macrophages which fuse to produce characteristic giant cells, surrounded by epithelioid cells and lymphocytes. Granulomas are usually slow progressing but active lesions. As the host attempts to contain the infection, the microorganisms continue to grow intracellularly at slow rates. Whether the lesion progresses or resolves depends on many factors, principally the rate of release of antigens from the organism.

A prototype of this kind of hypersensitivity reaction

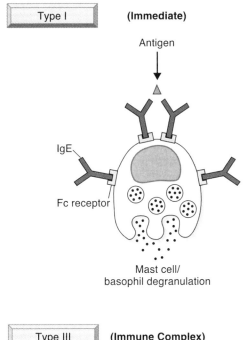

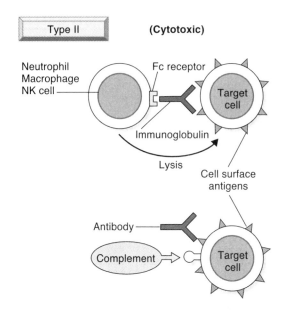

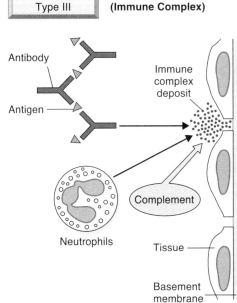

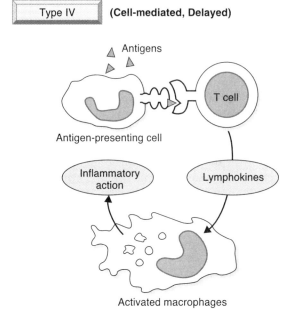

Figure 7.14. Hypersensitivity reactions. Hypersensitivity reactions are secondary responses to antigen that occur in an exaggerated or inappropriate form. These reactions have been classified by Gell and Coombs into four major types. Type I, II, and III are antibody-mediated while type IV is cell-mediated. Serious pathology can result from these reactions.

is the disease leprosy. It is caused by an organism called *Mycobacterium leprae*, a relative of the tubercles bacillus. These organisms survive inside monocytes, probably because they possess a thick layer of wax (see Chapter 3, "Biology of Infectious Agents," and Chapter 23, "Mycobacteria"). In one form of the disease, lepromatous leprosy, the organisms elicit the production of granulomas that damage sensory nerves, which results in anesthesia of fingers or whole limbs. Because the patient has little feeling in the affected areas, they are subject to re-

peated trauma and secondary infection by bacteria. This cycle of injury and repair leads to some of the deformities characteristic of untreated cases of the disease.

While CD4-expressing T cells are most noted for their release of cytokines and elicitation of DTH reactions, CD8-bearing T cells can also release cytokines and participate in cell-mediated immunity. In experimental animals, CD8$^+$ cells have been shown to play a protective role in cutaneous leishmaniasis (*Leishmania* are protozoan parasites) and in immunity to certain intracellular bacteria. Whether these effects are due to cytokine elaboration and/or the direct cytotoxic effector function of such cells is unclear.

The tissue-damaging effect of cytotoxic T lymphocytes has been noted in the immunopathology of persistent viral infection. Infection of mice with lymphocytic choriomeningitis virus (LCMV) is a good example. LCM is relatively noncytopathic. When injected into neonatal mice a persistent infection is produced. The mice, even as adults, remain healthy. In contrast, the injection of adult mice with the virus causes rapid death from meningochoroidoencephalitis. However, death is prevented in adult mice by immunosuppression with x-irradiation, thymectomy, or pharmacological means. Thus, it is the immune response to the virus (cytotoxic T lymphocytes) rather than the virus itself that causes death. Neonatal mice are not killed by the virus because they are immunoincompetent and presumably develop tolerance to viral antigens as in the process of developing tolerance to self antigens. Similar mechanisms may be involved in the chronic infection of humans with measles virus which can cause a severe degenerative disease and death due to subacute sclerosing panencephalitis (SSPE). It is believed that the immunopathology associated with a variety of persistent virus infections may be due at least in part to the action of cytotoxic T lymphocytes and other immunological mechanisms (see Chapter 34, "Paramyxoviruses").

Immunodeficiencies

Perhaps the most serious forms of pathology involving the immune system results from the loss of immune function. Immunodeficiency diseases may be acquired or congenital. Congenital immunodeficiencies are tragic "experiments of nature" that have proven to be important tools for defining the differentiation pathways of lymphocytes described above. Of the acquired immunodeficiencies, the most worrisome example is, of course, the acquired immunodeficiency syndrome or AIDS. In AIDS, the virus binds to the CD4 protein of helper T cells and destroys them. The reduction in the number of CD4$^+$ helper cells produces a profound immunosuppression that leads to severe infections with commensal and normally avirulent microorganisms. *Pneumocystis carinii* pneumonia, herpes simplex infections, candidiasis, and disseminated Kaposi's sarcoma are some of the more common manifestation of AIDS. (See Chapter 38, "Retroviruses," for further discussion of AIDS and its opportunistic diseases.) Thus, the AIDS virus has developed an ingenious and nefarious strategy for survival: infection and destruction of the very cells that could help the host fight back. AIDS patients succumb not to HIV infection itself, but rather to overwhelming opportunistic infections. A better understanding of the immune system and of HIV offers hope for the future.

THE INTEGRATION OF DEFENSE MECHANISMS

As previously discussed (in Chapter 6, "Constitutive Defenses" and this one), higher animals have a multitude of means to discriminate self from nonself and to maintain the integrity and health of the individual. Nature has provided a system with many layers of defensive fail-safe mechanisms. The advantages of this layering should be obvious: failure at any one level can often be compensated by success at another. These different defense reactions differ in terms of speed, specificity, and strength, but they are interactive and cooperative.

More primitive defense reactions, such as the toxins and enzymes of procaryotic organisms or the phagocytic cells of invertebrates, were not discarded during the development of the more sophisticated specific acquired immune responses of mammals. Instead, the new mechanisms of defense were layered on top of the older ones. And, most importantly, the specific induced defenses evolved to interact with the primitive innate or constitutive defense reactions, so that both types of reactions work best in concert. To prevent infectious disease, humans may avoid contact with microbes, prevent their entry (keep them on the epithelial side), or destroy them if they breach the defensive barriers. Here, we review briefly the defense reactions against a microbe once it has gained entry. Multiple defense reactions will be emphasized.

Gauntlet of the Body's Defenses

Consider a microbe running the gauntlet of immune defenses in a human being. There are three phases in these defenses. In the first stage, the immune system senses the microbe as foreign and constitutive defense reactions are expressed. In the second stage, the foreign entity is processed by cells and the specific immune response is initiated. In the third phase, the constitutive defense reactions interact with the induced defense reactions, resulting in the efficient elimination of the invading microbe. The importance of each of these stages in host defense varies with the invading organisms and their principal pathogenic mechanisms.

Stage 1. Constitutive (Innate) Defenses: Detection of Foreign Invaders

Important reactions in the first or detection stage involve complement, interleukins, interferons, phagocytes, killer cells, and other elements of the inflammatory response. Through random collisions and ill-defined attachment mechanisms, phagocytes have the intrinsic ability to ingest and destroy microbes. Phagocytic activity is amplified by activation of complement and by white blood cell chemotaxis. Important events include the recruitment of phagocytes, especially the faster neutrophils, in response to microbial products such as the bacterial chemotaxin formyl-met-leu-phe (Chapter 6, "Constitutive Defenses"). If the alternative pathway of complement is activated, the movement of phagocytes toward the microbe is aided by C5a. Complement activation may also generate the opsonin C3b, which promotes phagocytosis of the microbe as well as the membrane attack complex, which can lyse certain bacteria and viruses.

The concerted action of these cells and molecules may result in death and digestion of microbes. If a microbe fails to negotiate this first level of the gauntlet, no further action is required by the immune system. In fact, specific lymphocyte responses are not even elicited. However, if destruction is incomplete, the short-lived neutrophils begin to disintegrate, and the later-arriving macrophages come into play. Macrophages play important roles as garbage collectors and domestic engineers, as they arrive to digest debris and remaining microbes. Macrophages also play perhaps an even more important role as a liaison between phagocytes and lymphocytes in initiating the next stage of immune defense.

Stage 2. Specific Immune Responses

The second stage of immune defense is the generation of specific immune responses. This stage is also called the afferent immune response. Macrophages process microbial antigens and express them on their cell surface in association with class II MHC gene products. In this form, antigens are recognized by helper T lymphocytes (CD4+). Virus-infected cells that have escaped constitutive defenses express viral antigens on their surface in association with class I MHC gene products. These antigen–MHC complexes are recognizable by the precursors of cytotoxic T lymphocytes (CD8+). Still other microbial antigens may remain relatively intact and thus interact directly with the receptors on B lymphocytes.

The engagement of antigen-specific receptors and the subsequent cellular and molecular interactions lead to proliferation and differentiation of lymphocytes. This process of clonal selection and memory cell production accounts for specific acquired immunity. Effector cells (e.g., plasma cells and cytotoxic T cells) are also generated in this process. Such cells and/or their products may then mediate several important functions in the third and final stage of immune defenses, the specific, amplified, efferent phase.

Stage 3. Specific and Amplified Efferent Phase

The third stage involves the concerted action and cooperation of both constitutive and specific acquired immune responses. In this stage, the host uses every means available to eliminate the invader. Thus, this stage is not just a simple addition or layering of the specific induced defenses over the constitutive defenses, but also the synergistic effect of both. For example, antibody helps activate complement more efficiently via the classical pathway. In turn, complement activation makes for more

efficient killing of microbes and accelerates chemotaxis and opsonization by phagocytes. Antibodies neutralize toxins that impair the function of leukocytes and prevent the invasion of new microbes. Antibodies also enhance and direct the function of the large granular lymphocytes (NK cells and the K cells) to perform antibody-dependent cell-mediated cytotoxicity (ADCC).

In this stage, functions and products of T lymphocytes also play key roles in amplifying constitutive defense reactions. Notably, macrophage-activating factors elaborated by T cells dramatically improve the phagocytic killing mechanisms. For example, cytokines increase the expression of macrophage Fc receptors, which in turn promotes the function of antibody as an opsonin. Macrophage activation by T lymphocyte cytokines is especially important in the elimination of intracellular pathogens that have managed to escape initial destruction and live inside macrophages. Cytokines released by T cells (e.g., γ-interferon) also increase the expression of MHC molecules on macrophages and other cells and thus augment antigen presentation.

These are just a few of the examples by which products of induced defenses interact with constitutive defense mechanisms during the elimination of invading microbes. If this array of cooperative defenses were not impressive enough, there is an even more intelligent strategy for defense. Even after the successful resolution of the infection, the immune system quietly waits, anticipating the next encounter with the microbe. Immunological memory ensures that the next response to the microbe will be even stronger and faster and more interactive with constitutive defense reactions.

CONCLUSION

Our immune system faces three major challenges in maintaining our health: (1) How to distinguish an apparently infinite array of foreign antigens and ensure that a specific response is made even when antigen is present in small concentrations; (2) How to ensure that the response is appropriate to the foreign agent so that the foreign agent is eliminated; and (3) How to avoid responding to self antigens and damaging self. The immune system meets these challenges with specific acquired immune responses. Such responses have been described as a "microcosm of evolution operating on somatic cells."

SUGGESTED READINGS

Abbas AK, Lichtman AH, Pober JS. Cellular and molecular immunology. 3rd ed. Philadelphia: WB Saunders, 1997.

Janeway C Jr, Travers P. Immunobiology. The immune system in health and disease. 2nd ed. Current Biology/NY: Garland Publishing, 1996.

Kuby J. Immunology. 3rd ed. New York: WH Freeman, 1997.

Roitt IM, Brostoff J, Male DK. Immunology. 4th ed. London: Gower Medical Publishing, 1996.

The Parasite's Way of Life

MOSELIO SCHAECHTER

BARRY I. EISENSTEIN

N. CARY ENGLEBERG

In view of our long acquaintance with infectious diseases, it is not surprising that we tend to take an anthropomorphic view of our relationship with our microbial neighbors. Often, we use analogies to war, e.g., microbial "attack" or "invasion" is repelled by host "defense systems." In reality, the most important driving force for microbes is not aggression, but survival and reproduction. To succeed in this mission, many have evolved the ability to persist in the body, only incidentally causing disease. These microbes act much less like invaders and more like unwanted house guests. Whether as aggressive pathogens or harmless commensals, microbial agents face many problems in their association with the host. In order to survive, microbes must:

- Avoid being washed away (surface colonization)
- Find a nutritionally compatible niche
- Survive the constitutive and induced defenses
- Transfer to a new host

Every successful commensal or pathogen has evolved a specific repertoire of strategies to face these challenges. These strategies are discussed in detail in the chapters on individual agents. Here, we present an overview of the mechanisms involved.

SURFACE COLONIZATION

Picture a microbe entering the mouth and imagine the obstacles it faces trying to remain at this site. Strong liquid currents would wash it away unless the organism can adhere to the surface of the teeth or mucous membranes. At places not exposed to the flushing action of saliva, such as the crevices of the gums, the organism would encounter a large **resident flora** that already occupies potential adherence sites. Occupancy here is indeed a good part of the law!

Colonization of microorganisms to host surfaces involves both microbial and host factors. Microorganisms elaborate substances or organelles that are involved in the adherence and are known as **adhesins** (Table 8.1). In most cases, adhesins bind to special **receptors** on host surfaces. Both adhesins and receptors are usually highly specific for the species of microorganisms and the host.

We present here a few examples of bacterial adhesins. Some Gram-negative bacteria position their adhesive molecules on the tips of long, slender structures (fimbriae pili) as if "reaching out" for the host cell surface. Fimbrial adhesins interact with structural constituents of host epithelial cells, often glycolipids. In other Gram-negative bacteria, adhesins are found directly on the cell surface and not on protrusions. An example of such an adhesin, **invasin**, is a protein that recognizes normal cellular receptors on host cells called **integrins**. Integrins are receptors primarily involved in other processes, such as the adherence of white blood cells to endothelial surfaces, but here they are usurped by bacteria for their own use. Binding of bacteria via integrins results in an intimate association between the bacterium and the host cell membrane. Such an appropriation of normal host functions by microorganisms is a recurrent theme in pathogenic microbiology. In Gram-positive bacteria, the interplay between adhesins and host cell receptors is different. A receptor for certain Gram-positive bacteria is the protein **fibronectin,** which normally coats the mucosal surfaces of epithelial cells. Fibronectin plays an important role in selecting the kind of the bacterial flora in the mouth and pharynx, as suggested by the finding that the oropharynx of individuals in poor general health, including many hospitalized patients, is deficient in fibronectin. With low levels of this protein, Gram-negative organisms tend to displace Gram-positive bacteria, in part because the fibronectin-denuded mucosal cells

Table 8.1. Bacterial Adhesins	
Gram-negative bacteria	Gram-positive bacteria
Pili (fimbriae)	Surface proteins
Surface proteins (nonpilar)	Capsules
Capsules	

reveal the receptors for Gram-negative fimbrial adhesins. The greater incidence of pneumonia caused by Gram-negative bacteria in hospitalized patients can be explained in part by such adherence specificity.

The mouth, large intestine, vagina, perineum, skin, and other sites are normally laden with bacteria. Since these bacterial populations are fairly stable, it follows that colonization by new organisms is an unlikely event. The successful colonizer must be unusually adept at outmaneuvering the resident microorganisms. On the other hand, microbial competition is not usually an important factor in colonization of sites that are normally sterile or carry a sparse load of microorganisms, such as all the deep tissues or the small intestine.

Obviously, in our long history of coexistence and coevolution with the microbial world, our bodies have learned what territory is safe to share and what is off limits. And, we've managed to share this space preferentially with well-behaved guests. Foreign devices, like plastic catheters inserted into arteries and veins, may upset the delicate ecological balance between microbes and host tissues, in part because they allow bacteria and fungi to bypass the normal defenses, and in part because they potentiate growth by those organisms with special ability to stick well to plastics (e.g., strains of *Staphylococcus epidermidis*, which are otherwise harmless skin residents. See Chapter 11, "*Staphylococcus*").

FINDING A NUTRITIONALLY COMPATIBLE NICHE

To microbes, the human body would seem to be a rich nutritional environment. Body fluids such as plasma contain sugars, vitamins, minerals, and other substances that can be used for growth by bacteria, fungi, and animal parasites. Still, bacteria grow sparsely on fresh plasma in a test tube. The major reason is the presence of antimicrobial substances, such as lysozyme, constituents of the complement system, and antibodies, and the scarcity of available iron. In addition, some nutrients are in short supply in body fluids. Plasma and most other body fluids, for example, contain very little **free iron**. This metal is highly insoluble and must be combined with avid iron-binding proteins for transport. The lack of free iron significantly limits the growth of bacteria in the body, as bacteria need iron for the synthesis of their cytochromes and other enzymes. The body may

even further sequester iron in response to microbial invasion. When a sufficient number of organisms enters the body, iron-binding proteins are poured into plasma and tissue fluids, and the normally low amount of available iron is further reduced. Many bacteria respond to this challenge by excreting highly iron-avid compounds (chelators). After capturing an iron molecule, these compounds may contact another bacterium and deliver the iron to specific bacterial receptors (Chapter 3, "Biology of Infectious Agents"). Other bacteria possess surface molecules that can "steal" iron from the host's iron-binding proteins. Certain bacteria (e.g., some streptococci) scavenge intracellular iron by making toxins that destroy host cells, such as red blood cells.

Some microorganisms use specific nutrients found only in certain sites of the body. Thus, mouth strains of streptococci are adept at using dietary sucrose, which gives them a growth (and colonization) advantage over bacteria that cannot. Even more startling is the example of brucellosis in cattle. Brucellosis is a systemic disease in humans and other animals. In addition, brucellosis causes abortion in cattle and a few other animal species. The reason for this species-specific abortion is that cattle and some other animals, but not humans, contain in their placenta a 4-carbon sugar, erythritol, for which the organisms have a special affinity.

The spectrum of nutritional requirements of microorganisms that live in the body reflects their ecological habits. For instance, many of the bacteria that are found mainly in the human body, such as staphylococci or certain streptococci, have complex nutritional requirements and need several amino acids and vitamins for growth. Organisms that are found both in the body and in soil or water are usually much less picky and can fulfill their organic requirements with simple carbon compounds. Examples are *Escherichia coli* and many *Pseudomonas* that can grow in laboratory "minimal media." Another connection between physiology and ecology is illustrated by a bacterium's oxygen requirements. Many of our most heavily colonized sites, e.g., the periodontal spaces and the colon, are anaerobic. Not surprisingly the bacteria found in those sites are overwhelmingly anaerobic, with very few strict aerobes present.

SURVIVING THE CONSTITUTIVE AND INDUCED DEFENSES

Many of the bacteria that enter the body do not survive owing to the physical barriers and inhospitable microenvironments that they encounter. These factors are the first lines of host defense against infection. However, over millennia of coevolution with their bacterial neighbors, mammals have also developed second lines of defenses to deal with those microbes that manage to evade the first-line defenses. How do microbial agents overcome these powerful defense mechanisms? How do they avoid the action of complement and phagocytosis or evade antigenic recognition by the host immune system?

Defending Against Complement

The most effective way to protect against the antimicrobial action of complement is to prevent its activation. Bacteria prevent complement activation several ways (Table 8.2). One is by **masking** surface components that activate the alternative pathway. Lipopolysaccharides of Gram-negative bacteria, teichoic acids of Gram-positive bacteria, and other microbial structural components are potential complement activators. Meningococci and pneumococci are examples of bacteria that prevent complement activation by secreting a capsule that covers these activators (Fig. 8.1).

Table 8.2. Some Microbial Anticomplement Strategies

1. Mask activating substances
   a. Coating with capsule (e.g., staphylococci)
   b. Coating with IgA antibodies (e.g., meningococci)

2. Appropriate inhibitor of activation to their surface
   Binding factor H by *E. coli*, group B streptococci
   Binding decay accelerating factors by schistosome
   Mimicking component C4bp by vaccinia virus

3. Cover up target of membrane attack complex (e.g., *E. coli*, salmonellae)

4. Inactivate complement chemotaxin C5a (e.g., group A streptococcus, *Pseudomonas aeruginosa*)

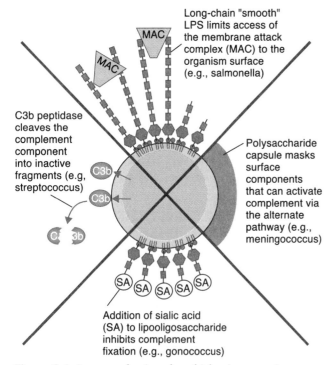

Long-chain "smooth" LPS limits access of the membrane attack complex (MAC) to the organism surface (e.g., salmonella)

C3b peptidase cleaves the complement component into inactive fragments (e.g, streptococcus)

Polysaccharide capsule masks surface components that can activate complement via the alternate pathway (e.g., meningococcus)

Addition of sialic acid (SA) to lipooligosaccharide inhibits complement fixation (e.g., gonococcus)

Figure 8.1. Some mechanisms by which microorganisms may prevent harmful effects of complement.

Some organisms take advantage of the host's own mechanism for avoiding complement activation. Most host cells incorporate sialic acid, a sugar that inhibits complement activation into their surface molecules. Many bacteria achieve the same protection by incorporating sialic acid into their capsular polysaccharides. When they grow in tissues, gonococci add sialic acid to the terminal sugar of their lipopolysaccharide, which makes them resistant to complement lysis. Meningococci employ a different strategy to avoid complement activation. These bacteria become coated with **circulating IgA antibodies,** a class of immunoglobulins that do not activate the complement cascade (a "wolf in sheep's clothing" strategy). This coating prevents other kinds of antibodies capable of setting off complement activation by the classical pathway from reaching the surface of the organisms.

Certain viruses have also evolved mechanisms to prevent complement activation. For example, herpes simplex virus has an **envelope glycoprotein** that binds **complement component C3b,** thus inhibiting activation by the alternative pathway (Chapter 41, "Herpesvirus"). Vaccinia virus infected cells secrete a virally encoded protein that shares amino acid homology with a complement control protein (C4bp). C4bp binds to the C4b fragment. By mimicking the action of the host C4bp, the virus limits complement activation by the classical pathway and causes the accelerated decay of C3 convertase. Mutants of vaccinia virus that lack the protein produce smaller, more rapidly healing skin lesions in experimental animals.

Some Gram-negative bacteria, such as *Salmonella* or *E. coli*, do not prevent formation of the complement membrane attack complex, but rather, hinder its access to its target, the bacterial outer membrane. "Smooth" strains, which have a long O antigen polysaccharide chain, do not allow access of the membrane attack complex to their outer membrane, while "rough" mutants, which have little or no O antigen, are readily killed by it. The presence or absence of the O antigen correlates well with pathogenicity. Smooth strains tend to be virulent, while rough strains are not. However, capsules and other protective surface structures come with a price: most of them are highly antigenic and in time elicit the production of anticapsular antibodies that enable the activation of complement by the classical pathway. Notice that these organisms defend themselves better against the more immediate host defense, activation of complement by the alternative pathway, than against later events, the formation of antibodies.

Subverting Phagocytosis

Microorganisms employ a number of strategies to avoid being killed by phagocytes. The host attempts to overcome these microbial countermeasures, and, in turn, these efforts are answered by yet other microbial tactics. A point must be made at the outset: being phagocytized by a cell is not necessarily a bad thing from the microbe's point of view. Some microorganisms are able

Table 8.3. Microbial Strategies to Evade Phagocyte Function

Antiphagocyte activity	Mechanism	Examples
Avoiding being phagocytized		
Diversion (to nonproductive use)	Activate complement C5a Leucoaggregation Pulmonary sequestration	Streptococci Gram-negative enterics
"Playing hard to get"	Slimy capsule on organisms	Pneumococci, meningococci, *Haemophilus influenzae*, *Bacteroides fragilis*, many others
	M protein	Group A streptococci
	Pili	Gonococci
Humiliation	Release of adenylate cyclase leading to high cAMP levels; all phagocyte functions depressed	*Bordetella pertussis* (toxin)
Paralysis	Make cells unresponsive to chemotactic factors	*Capnocytophaga* Tubercle bacilli
	Induce inhibitors of migration	Leprosy bacilli
	Inactivate chemotaxins (C5a)	*Pseudomonas* (elastase)
After being phagocytized		
Murder	Membrane lysis	Streptococci (streptolysin O) *Pseudomonas* (exotoxin A) *Staphylococcus aureus* (α-toxin)
Indifference (resist lysosomal enzymes)		*Salmonella enterica* var. *typhimurium mycobacteria* spp. *Leishmania* spp.
Disablement (inhibit phagosome–lysosome fusion)	? ?	Tubercle bacilli *Legionella pneumophila* *Toxoplasma gondii*
Disablement (inhibit oxidative killing)	Inhibit respiratory burst Catalase breaks down H_2O_2	Virulent salmonellae *Legionella pneumophila* *Listeria monocytogenes* *Staphylococcus aureus*
Escape (from phagosome into cytoplasm)	Pore-forming hemolysins? Phospholipase?	*Listeria monocytogenes* *Shigella* Rickettsiae Influenza viruses

to grow within host cells, where they are shielded from antibodies and certain antimicrobial drugs.

We present here a few examples of strategies used by microorganisms to withstand the killing power of phagocytic cells. Various aspects of phagocytosis are affected, from the arrival of the phagocytes at the scene to the killing powers of phagocytic cells (Table 8.3).

Inhibiting phagocyte recruitment and function

We have already seen that some microorganisms prevent the activation of complement. In doing so, they prevent the secondary release of neutrophil chemotaxins and opsonins, thus reducing the risk of encountering these cells as well as their function. Other organisms (e.g., *Bordetella pertussis*, Chapter 19) directly inhibit neutrophil motility and chemotaxis by producing a toxin that increases cyclic AMP to inhibitory levels. Group A streptococci produce a **C5a peptidase** which specifically inactivates this chemotactic product of the complement cascade.

Microbial killing of phagocytes

Some pathogenic bacteria produce exotoxins called **leukocidins** that kill neutrophils and macrophages. These soluble products work at a distance and thus may protect bacteria before the phagocytes come near them. In many cases, however, microbes kill after they are ingested. In this strategy, the phagocyte commits suicide by carrying out phagocytosis (see Chapter 9, "Damage by Microbial Agents"). Typical leukocidin producers are highly invasive bacteria, such as *Pseudomonas*, staphylococci, group A streptococci, and the clostridia that cause gas gangrene. The yersiniae produce proteins that are injected directly into host cells and interfere with cellular activation (see paradigm, Chapter 17, "Invasive and Tissue-damaging Enteric Bacteria").

Escaping ingestion

A notable microbial counterdefense to phagocytosis is the capsule. One of the more captivating visual experiences in microbiology is to watch a preparation of live neutrophils and encapsulated pneumococci under the microscope: each time a neutrophil attempts to embrace a pneumococcus, the slimy bacterium squeezes away with what looks like total indifference, and repeated attempts are no more successful. The picture changes when a small amount of capsule-specific antiserum is added: now the neutrophils have no trouble engulfing the now opsonized pneumococci. Anticapsular antibodies thus provide protective immunity against infection by encapsulated bacteria. However, bacteria have evolved measures to counter opsonization either by complement components or by specific antibodies. Any mechanism that inhibits activation of complement (see above) or synthesis or activity of antibodies (see below) will reduce the probability of opsonization.

Staphylococci, streptococci, and probably other bacteria have evolved a mechanism to reduce opsonization even when antibodies are present: they make a surface component, **protein A**, that binds to IgG molecules by the "wrong" end, the Fc portion (see Chapter 11, "Staphylococcus"). These antibodies cannot act as opsonins because they cannot bind to the Fc receptors on phagocytic cells, not to mention that their Fab region is "waving in the breeze." It is not known to what extent this antiphagocytic mechanism plays a role in actual infections.

How microorganisms survive inside phagocytes

Microorganisms have many ways to survive once they are taken up by host cells:

- Inhibition of lysosome fusion with phagosomes. When lysosomes fuse with phagosomes, they release powerful microbicidal substances (see Chapter 6, "Constitutive Defenses"). Inhibiting this fusion clearly benefits intraphagosomal microorganisms, such as the agents of tuberculosis, psittacosis, or Legionnaires' disease. How this inhibition is accomplished is not well understood, but it is thought that compounds secreted or present on the surface of the microorganisms modify the phagosome membrane in some way.
- Escape into the cytoplasm. The shigellae, *Listeria monocytogenes*, and the rickettsiae cross the membrane of the phagocytic vesicle, the phagosome, and enter the cytoplasm. Since lysosomes do not release their contents in the cytoplasm, the microorganisms are protected from lysosomal enzymes in this site. This escape is accomplished by destroying the phagosomal membrane. *L. monocytogenes* secretes a pore-forming toxin, **listeriolysin**, which is required for the phagosomal escape. A surface-bound phospholipase may also be responsible for weakening the phagosomal membrane.

- Resistance to lysosomal enzymes. Some microorganisms are innately resistant to the lysosomal enzymes and survive in the phago-lysosome, the vesicle formed by fusion of the lysosomes with the phagosomes. Examples are protozoa called *Leishmania*, which cause several severe tropical diseases. Resistance of leishmaniae to lysosomal enzymes may be due to resistant cell surfaces and, in addition, to the excretion of enzyme inhibitors. Note that the pH of the phago-lysosome may be as low as 4, which means that leishmania can thrive in an extreme environment.
- Inhibition of the phagocytes' oxidative pathway. Some microorganisms, such as *Legionella*, inhibit the hexose-monophosphate shunt and oxygen consumption in neutrophils, thus reducing the respiratory burst used by these cells for killing engulfed microorganisms. Others, e.g., some staphylococci, produce a powerful catalase which breaks down the hydrogen peroxide necessary for oxidative killing.

Intracellular life

Many bacteria, protozoa, and fungi have adapted to intracellular existence within the host. This lifestyle is obviously obligatory for viruses, but not so for organisms capable of free existence. The advantages of such existence are clear: while inside host cells, the organisms are protected from antibodies and some antimicrobial drugs. However, intracellular residence is not without peril and requires ingenious forms of adaptation. An intense subject of current research, intracellular existence requires the expression of specific microbial genes and the usurpation of normal cell functions. Here are some of the issues associated with intracellular existence.

- Penetration. Penetration of the host cell is not a problem for "professional phagocytes," such as neutrophils and macrophages, but it is not a normal activity for other types of cells. Here, penetration is often induced by microbial activities, including binding to specific receptors and sending signals to the interior of the cell that stimulate uptake by rearrangements of the cellular cytoskeleton.
- Surviving host cell defenses. As mentioned already, microorganisms have developed a wide repertoire of strategies to avoid or resist antimicrobial factors such as the lysosomal contents. So successful are some parasites that they grow within dedicated antimicrobial cells, such as macrophages. Members of the *Ehrlichia* thrive even within the most powerfully antimicrobial of cells—the neutrophils!
- Transmission to other cells. When the growth of microorganisms results in the lysis of the host cell, transmission via the blood or body fluids can take place directly. Other organisms do not impair the

cell's integrity, but instead can spread from cell to cell directly, without exposing themselves to the extracellular environment. Several viruses spread by causing infected cells to fuse with uninfected, neighboring cells. The histopathology associated with these viral infections (e.g., herpes simplex virus, varicella zoster virus, respiratory syncytial virus) are notable for the formation of **syncytia** and **multinucleated giant cells**. More recently, it has been learned that certain bacteria are also able to spread directly from one cell to another. This type of spread is accomplished by making intricate use of the host cytoskeleton. For example, *L. monocytogenes* (Fig. 8.2) are able to induce polymerization of actin at one of their ends, which results in the formation of a cytoskeletal scaffold at one end of the bacterium. In the electron microscope, this scaffold can be visualized as a "cometlike" trail behind the bacterium, with actin polymerizing at the "head" and depolymerizing throughout the "tail." As more and more actin polymers are formed at the bacterial surface, the organisms are actually pushed ahead and can be observed microscopically to be moving through the host cell cytoplasm. If the bacteria reach the cell membrane, they literally push out fingerlike projections, each containing one bacterium. These projections are driven into adjacent cells, where they are eventually engulfed and snipped off. The organisms must now cross two sets of membranes, one from the original cell, the second from the neighboring cell. When they have crossed these membranes, the bacteria are now in the cytoplasm of a new host cell.

Subverting the Immune Responses
Immunosuppression

Some infectious agents protect themselves by inducing a general suppression of the host immune responses. The outcome is that the host now becomes susceptible to all kinds of agents and the threat to survival is heightened. Such patients may suffer from several concurrent infections, which expands considerably the complexities of their clinical problem. The ability of infectious agents to cause immunodeficiency has reached its known limit with acquired immune deficiency syndrome (AIDS). Immunodeficiency in this disease is especially profound because human immunodeficiency virus (HIV), the AIDS virus, infects the CD4+ (inducer-helper) subset of lymphocytes (see Chapter 6, "Constitutive Defenses"), leading to the collapse of the immune system, (see Chapter 38, "The Human Retroviruses").

The regulatory interactions of the immunocompetent cells may go awry even when lesser changes are introduced into the network. Long before AIDS, it has been known that infection with measles virus is immunosuppressive. It had been noticed, for example, that tuberculosis is more common in a community after widespread measles outbreaks. Immunosuppression has been found to follow other viral infections as well, e.g., hepatitis B and influenza. These viruses function more subtly than HIV, impairing the function of lymphoid or myeloid cells without causing major structural changes.

In some cases, immune suppression results from inhibition of the synthesis or of the function of selected cytokines, which stimulate the proliferation and differentiation of lymphocytes. Cytokines, themselves the secreted

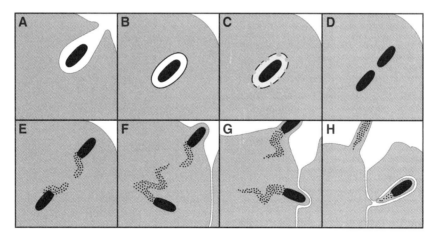

Figure 8.2. Actin-dependent intracellular motility and itercellular spread. (A) The bacterium is ingested by conventional phagocytosis and resides briefly in a mebrane-bound pagosome. (B), (C) The ingested bacterium lyses the pagosomal membrane surrounding it. (D) After escaping into the cytoplasm, the organism may divide. (E) Actin polymerizes at one pole of each bacterium. (F) Continued actin polymerization forms scaffolding that propels the bacteria through the cytoplasm in random directions. (G) Both bacteria encounter the cell membrane and continue to move outward; one is pushing toward a second cell, the other into an extracellular space. (H) The second cell has ingested one of the bacteria, its actin tail, and some of the cell membrane and cytoplasm from its neighbor. Eventually, this bacterium will be released into the cytoplasm of the second host cell.

products of inflammatory and immuno-directed cells, act to amplify the inflammatory response (see Chapter 6, "Constitutive Defenses"). Mycobacteria, certain viruses, and some multicellular parasites have been shown to affect different steps in the cytokine cascade, perhaps thereby enhancing the pathogen's persistence in the host.

Diversion of lymphocyte function—the superantigens

Certain bacteria and viruses have evolved a particularly insidious strategy to subvert the immune response. Instead of suppressing immune functions, they actually stimulate them, but in a manner that squanders these important defensive tools in a nonproductive way. An example are toxins made by certain streptococci, called **superantigens**, which stimulate a **nonspecific T-cell response**. A large subpopulation of T cells are stimulated by superantigens, but these cells have specificities that are mostly unrelated to streptococcal antigens. This misdirection of the immune response not only keeps the host from mounting a proper response, but also unleashes a toxic cascade of cytokines.

Understanding how superantigens work requires you to revisit the mechanism of antibody formation (see Chapter 7, "Induced Defenses"). Normally, antigen-presenting cells display on their surface peptides derived from antigens they engulfed. Such peptides are "presented," i.e., reach the cell surface, in association with MHC II molecules (see Fig. 7.12). These complexes are recognized by T cells, setting in motion the processes of cell-mediated immunity or specific helper functions to enhance antibody production. Superantigens take a shortcut; they bind directly to both the MHC molecule (but not at the antigen binding groove) and the T-cell receptor (but not at the antigen-recognition sites (see Fig. 8.3) Because it is not dependent on specific antigen recognition, superantigen binding occurs on the surface of many more antigen-presenting cells than is usual and thus leads to the diversion of these cells to nonproductive uses. To give an idea why these compounds are known as superantigens, consider that normally 1 in 10,000 antigen-presenting cells is stimulated by processed antigens, whereas the figure for superantigens is as high as 1 in 5.

Masquerading by changing antigenic coats

Certain bacteria, viruses, and protozoa are unusually adept at frustrating immune recognition by changing their surface antigens. The classical cases are trypanosomes, gonococci, the agents of relapsing fever, and influenza viruses. (See the paradigm, Chapter 14, "Neisseriae.")

- **The case of the trypanosomes.** One of the best studied examples of antigenic variation is seen with the protozoan that causes sleeping sickness, *Trypanosoma brucei*. The organism affects humans and domestic animals and infects the blood and interstitial fluids. Thus, the organisms are exposed to circulating antibodies. Trypanosomes are covered with a thick protein coat called **variable surface glycoprotein**, which undergoes periodic antigenic changes during the infection. These parasites have several hundred genes that encode for different antigens, but they express only one at time (see Chapter 50, "Blood and Tissue Protozoa"). When antibodies against one type are made, the number of parasites in the blood of an infected host drops, but they are soon replaced by a new antigenic type. There can be many successive waves of antigenically different parasites in a single host. Thus, protective immunity does not function in the long term against this master of disguise.

- **Antigenic variation in bacteria.** Like the trypanosomes, some bacteria can also switch their surface antigens. One example is the gonococcus, which undergoes periodic changes in **pilin**, the protein that makes up its pili, the apparent means of attachment of host cells (see Chapter 3, "Biology of Infectious Agents" and Chapter 14, "Neisseriae"). The borreliae also undergo antigenic variation of their major surface antigen in a manner that is analogous to the

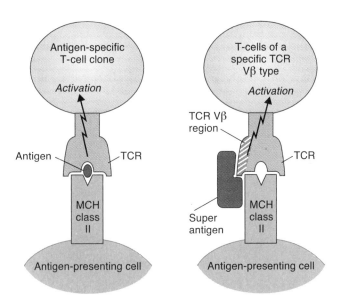

Figure 8.3. A comparison of antigen-mediated and superantigen-mediated T-cell activation. Both antigens and superantigens bring antigen-presenting cells and T cells together. Antigens (in conjunction with MHC II) interact with the specific antigen-binding domain of the T-cell receptor (TCR). In contrast, superantigens form a bridge between the two molecules that does not involve the antigen binding groove. Instead, they bind to a portion of the TCR, the Vb domain. Every T-cell has a TCR with one of numerous Vb types. Each superantigen binds preferentially to one Vb type and can activate any T-cell carrying that type, regardless of the specificity of the TCR for antigen.

trypanosomes (see Fig. 8.4). Thus, the surface of these organisms displays a highly variable antigenic profile to the host immune system.

■ **Influenza viruses.** The tendency of influenza to reappear in a population on a regular basis is due in part to the great ability of influenza viruses to change its antigenic composition. This is also the major obstacle to the development of a truly effective vaccine against this disease. Unlike the processes of antigenic variation described above with trypanosomes and gonococci, antigenic changes in these viruses do not emerge repeatedly within individual hosts. Instead, the novel antigenic types develop gradually in a population of viruses over the course of an epidemic season. Minor changes are called **antigenic drift** and occur every 2 or 3 years. Major antigenic changes, called **antigenic shifts,** take place every 10 years or so. These changes involve two surface proteins, a **hemagglutinin** that serves to bind to cell surface receptors, and a **neuraminidase** that changes these re-

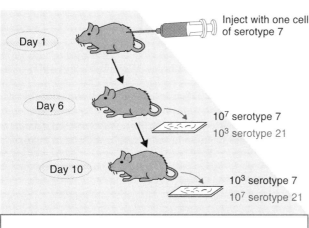

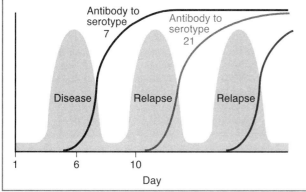

Figure 8.4. An experimental infection in which the development of type-specific antibodies against *Borrelia* **sp. is associated with the emergence of new antigenic types.** The emergence of each new type is associated with a relapse of disease; hence the common name for these borrelia infections—"relapsing fever." The rapid emergence of the new antigenic types is mediated by successive DNA rearrangement (see the paradigm in Chapter 14, "Neisseria" for more details).

ceptors. How these proteins are involved in attachment and penetration of the virus is discussed in Chapter 36, "Influenza Virus."

Proteolysis of Antibodies

A number of bacteria—gonococci, meningococci, *Haemophilus influenzae*—and some dental pathogenic streptococci make extracellular proteases that specifically inactivate antibodies of the secretory IgA class. They cleave IgA molecules at the hinge region to yield complete but relatively ineffective fragments. The proteases are present in active form in tissues and fluids infected by the bacteria that produce them. Nonpathogenic relatives of these organisms are protease-negative. The absence of proteases in nonpathogenic bacteria suggests, although it does not prove, a role for IgA proteases in pathogenesis.

In some instances, it is known that when an organism cleaves IgA, the Fab fragment remains attached. The attached Fab fragment makes the antigens unavailable for binding by intact antibody molecules. This phenomenon has been called **fabulation** (after "Fab") and may serve to protect organisms from antibodies. Fabulation may be more widely used by pathogens than is currently known.

Viral latency

The more chronic an infection, the more lasting must be the mechanisms for microbial evasion of host defenses. This tenet is well-illustrated in herpes infection. To limit access from circulating defenses, herpes viruses do not usually enter the extracellular fluid but pass from cell to cell via cytoplasmic bridges. Also, even intracellular herpes viruses have a major mechanism for evading attack, **latency**, whereby they reside within nerve cells but do not proliferate (see Chapter 41, "Herpes Virus"). In these circumstances, viruses are not affected by antibodies, cell-mediated immunity, or interferon. They can then survive for long periods of time in the presence of well-developed host defense mechanisms. Later—often when the host defenses have subsided—the viruses may reactivate to cause disease and perhaps even cancer.

TRANSMISSION TO A NEW HOST

Infectious agents are carried into a new host via food, drinks, aerosols, bites, sexual contact, or by introduction into a wound from the skin or soil. Although these modes of transmission may seem passive, many infectious agents actually contribute actively to their transmission to new hosts. They do this in at least two ways:

■ Many microorganisms differentiate into a "**transit form,**" a stage in their life cycle that helps them survive in the environment and in reservoirs, or, if vector-borne, in insects. Among the animal parasites, transit forms usually differ greatly in structure and function from those that cause disease in the host, as in the case of the protozoa that cause malaria, or the worms. Note that living reservoirs and vectors shield infectious agents from deleterious environmental factors and obviate the need for the transit form to be highly resistant.

- In certain bacteria, such as the chlamydiae, the transit form (here called the elementary body) becomes encased in a tough envelope composed of highly cross-linked proteins (see Chapter 27, "Chlamydiae"). The chlamydiae elemental body is thus reminiscent of the environmentally tough form *par excellence*, the bacterial spore. In other bacteria, e.g., the enterics, the changes are more subtle and are revealed at the level of selective expression of certain genes, such as those involved in entering the stationary phase of growth. An emerging subject of study is how infectious agents "know where they are," that is, how they express different sets of genes outside and inside the body. The problems of transit are minimized when contact between hosts is direct and does not involve prolonged exposure of the agents to the environment. It may not be a coincidence that many of the agents of sexually transmitted diseases do not appear to have developed tough transit forms. For example, the gonococci, the treponemes of syphilis, and HIV are particularly sensitive to drying and chemicals (chlamydiae may be an exception).
- Microorganisms can actively potentiate their spread from one host to another, thus providing themselves with new feeding grounds. Examples are organisms that cause diarrhea (e.g., *Vibrio cholerae*, pathogenic strains of *E. coli* or *Shigella*), which is an effective way of spreading large amounts of bacteria-laden intestinal contents in the environment. Agents that induce coughing (e.g., *M. tuberculosis*) lead to their dispersal via aerosols, and those that produce exudative lesions on the skin (e.g., *Streptococcus pyogenes*) are transmitted through the contamination of objects or skin.

- Some of the mechanisms developed by microorganisms for actively enhancing their transmission seem fiendishly clever. For example, the agent of plague, *Yersinia pestis*, is transmitted from an infected human to another by the bite of fleas. These bacteria increase the efficiency of this transmission greatly by making the flea feel hungry. How do the bacteria enhance the fleas' appetite? The plague bacilli reproduce within the digestive tract of infected fleas, eventually causing blockage. To ward off starvation, such "blocked fleas" feed repeatedly and, in each feeding attempt, regurgitate some of the contaminated material, thus increasing the chances of infecting a new host. The mechanism of blockage is not wholly understood but may involve either the coagulation of the ingested blood or the accumulation of the bacteria themselves. Not all pathogens that are transmitted by insects use such a mechanism, but it would not be surprising that many microorganisms alter an arthropod vector's behavior to enhance their survival and transmissibility.

SUGGESTED READINGS

Bliska JB, Galan JE, Falkow S. Signal transduction in the mammalian cell during bacterial attachment and entry. Cell 1993;73:903–920.

Cotter PA, Miller JF. Triggering bacterial virulence. Science 1996;1183:273.

Fearon DT, Locklsey RM. The instructive role of innate immunity in the acquired immune response. Science 1996;272: 50–54.

Finlay BB. Bacterial virulence factors. Scientific American Science and Medicine 1995;16(May/June).

Finlay BB, Falow S. Common themes in microbial pathogenicity revisited. Microb Molec Biol Rev 1977;61:136–169.

Marrack P, Kappler J. Subversion of the immune system by pathogens. Cell 1994;76:323–332.

Roth JA, Bolin CA, Brogden KA, Minion FC, Wannemuehler MJ. Virulence mechanisms of bacterial pathogens. 2nd ed. Washington, DC: ASM News, 1995.

Salyers AA, Whitt DD. Bacterial pathogenesis: a molecular approach. Washington, DC: ASM Press, 1994.

Damage by Microbial Agents

MOSELIO SCHAECHTER

Infectious diseases inflict as many kinds of damage to host tissues and organs as there are such diseases. It is no wonder that this topic constitutes a large and varied section of any pathology textbook. Because the types and intensity of damage depend on the biology of the agent, the sites affected, and immunological and other factors, it is difficult to make generalizations. Nevertheless, damage in infectious processes may be loosely categorized as due to direct actions of the agents or to responses of the host to their presence. However, these actions are interrelated, and both categories of actions are usually present during any one disease. We start this chapter with a brief overview of the types of damage. This discussion is followed by a more intensive presentation on bacterial toxins.

AN OVERVIEW OF THE MECHANISMS THAT CAUSE DAMAGE IN INFECTIONS

Cell Death

The most dramatic effect of an infection, if not always the most evident one, is the death of cells in host tissues. The effect of cell death depends on (1) the cells involved, (2) the number of cells infected, and (3) the speed with which the infection proceeds. If the cells belong to an essential organ, such as the heart or the brain, the outcome is likely to be serious and could even be fatal. For example, myocarditis, the infection of the heart muscle, is sometimes a fulminating disease when it is caused by an agent called coxsackievirus. Coxsackievirus is also thought to kill the insulin-producing cells of the islets of the pancreas and may be one of the causes of infantile diabetes. Two mechanisms lead to cell death: cell lysis and programmed cell death.

Lysis of host cells

Lysis of host cells occurs in several ways:

- The invading organisms produce toxins that affect the integrity of the cell membranes. For example, in patients with **gas gangrene**, red blood cells are lysed by membrane-destroying toxins made by the organisms. These mechanisms are discussed in detail below.
- The agents multiply intracellularly, leading to cell lysis. This mechanism is seen in **Rocky Mountain spotted fever,** which derives its name from the skin rash produced when endothelial cells of small vessels are killed by the intracellular growth of the infecting rickettsiae.
- The infected cells are killed by killer lymphocytes as the result of **cell-mediated immunity.** This mechanism is often seen when agents such as viruses or the tubercle bacilli grow intracellularly without directly causing lysis.

Programmed cell death (apoptosis) of infected cells

Programmed cell death is a normal part of the mammalian cell cycle that ensures the maintenance of healthy cells. Some microorganisms, such as the agents of dysentery (the *Shigella*), usurp this process when they invade cells. This mechanism may explain why the agents survive after being taken up by phagocytes. Some viruses, such as herpes viruses or HIV, also stimulate cells to undergo premature apoptosis. In contrast, other viruses, such as the Epstein-Barr virus, can block apoptosis and thereby immortalize the host cell.

Pharmacological Alterations of Metabolism

Certain infectious diseases do not involve the direct killing of cells. Among these are some of the most severe diseases, such as **tetanus, botulism,** or **cholera.** They are caused by bacterial toxins that alter important aspects of metabolism in ways that resemble the action of hormones or other pharmacological effectors. In all these diseases, the affected cells remain intact. The mechanism of action of these toxins is discussed in detail below.

Mechanical Causes

If infectious agents are large enough and present in sufficient numbers, they may obstruct vital passages. Such mechanical obstructions occur, although rarely, in children with an overload of worms in their intestines. A heavy infestation with the large roundworm *Ascaris* (15–35 cm long and about 0.5 cm thick) may result in the occlusion of the intestinal lumen. A single worm may also migrate into the common bile duct and obstruct the passage of bile.

More often, mechanical obstruction results not from the infectious agents alone but from the inflammatory response of the host elicited by their presence. An example is the disease **elephantiasis**, an enormous swelling of limbs or scrotum caused when small worms, the filariae, become lodged in lymphatics. Their presence sets off a tissue reaction that occludes the vessels, causing swelling and tissue hypertrophy.

Almost any duct or tubelike organ, thick or thin, may be obstructed by infections, sometimes with life-threatening consequences. Examples include inflammation of the epiglottis, which may impede the passage of air; infection of the meninges, which can result in hydrocephalus (a dilatation of the cerebral ventricles due to obstruction of the flow of cerebrospinal fluid); infection of the prostate, which may obstruct the flow of urine from the bladder; and an inflammatory reaction to the eggs of the liver fluke, which may result in severe disturbances of the portal circulation

Damage Due to Host Responses

Counterintuitive as it may seem, the symptoms of infectious diseases are seldom produced by the microorganisms alone but result in part from the host's response to their presence. The host response is rarely so finely tuned that it does only what is necessary to combat infection. An example is gonorrhea, which has as its main symptom the production of copious pus in the ureter. The gonococcol organisms set off the host response, but it is the inflammation itself, with its accompanying copious pus production and swelling, that accounts for the symptoms. Likewise, in many chronic infections, such as tuberculosis, the damage to tissues is caused by the effects of chronic inflammation.

Although the overemphatic expression of the host response contributes greatly to the immediate signs and symptoms, it helps the host survive in the long run. This point is well illustrated by tuberculosis, a disease that is usually chronic and whose patients survive for many years. However, if the host response is defective, as in AIDS, tuberculosis can cause a rapidly progressing lethal infection. The principal manifestations of the host response to infection are damage due to **inflammation** and the **immune response**. The importance of these mechanisms cannot be overemphasized. They operate both in acute and chronic diseases and may manifest either locally or systemically. The mechanisms involved in inflammation are discussed in detail in Chapter 6, "Constitutive Defenses of the Body," and those involved in immunopathology in Chapter 7, "Induced Defenses of the Body." These aspects of damage will be further emphasized in chapters on individual diseases, where you will find that they occupy center stage. To pique your curiosity, consider that the inflammatory response places patients with a brain abscess at risk of dying, an overwhelming activation of the **complement** system kills patients suffering from septicemia, an autoimmune response causes rheumatic fever, and cell-mediated immunity is responsible for most of the manifestations of chronic tuberculosis. In certain circumstances, it makes sense to intervene by attenuating the inflammatory response.

BACTERIAL TOXINS

Definitions

Bacterial **toxins** are substances that alter the normal metabolism of host cells with deleterious effects on the host. They are the salient feature of some bacterial diseases and are responsible for their main signs and symptoms. Knowing how they work helps us understand the pathophysiology of many infectious diseases and, in some instances, reveals important facts about normal processes. The role of a few toxins in causing disease has been studied in detail, but most toxins await further study. Individual toxins are treated in detail in the chapters on specific bacterial pathogens. Here, we discuss the basic concept of how bacterial toxins cause damage in the host. Traditionally, toxins are associated with bacterial diseases. However, it seems quite possible that toxins play important roles in diseases caused by fungi, protozoa, and worms.

Two types of toxins exist: **exotoxins** and **endotoxins**. Exotoxins are proteins produced by bacteria that are usually secreted into the surrounding medium, but are sometimes bound to the bacterial surface and released upon lysis. In contrast, endotoxins are the lipopolysaccharides of the outer membrane of Gram-negative bacteria and act as toxins only under special circumstances.

Bacterial exotoxins vary in their specificity; some act on certain cell types only, whereas others affect a wide range of cells and tissues. Some bacteria make a single toxin, while others are known to produce 10 or more (Table 9.1). Some bacteria, like the pneumococci, make no known toxins and probably cause disease by mechanisms that do not involve them.

For each toxin-producing pathogen, it would be ideal to know whether the toxin is important in the process of infection. To find out, we may ask:

- Does the toxin alone, in purified form, produce damage (in experimental animals or cells in culture, of course)?

Table 9.1. Major Toxinogenic Organisms

Toxin	Effects	Mechanism
Bacillus anthracis		
Protective antigen	Required for other toxins	"B" components
Edema factor	Edema	Internal adenylate cyclase; calmodulin-dependent
Lethal factor	Pulmonary edema	Kills certain cells (All three factors together give vascular, permeability, neurotoxicity)
Bordetella pertussis		
Adenylate cyclase	Inhibits, kills white cells	Adenylate cyclase; can be calmodulin-independent
Pertussis toxin	Many hormonal effects	ADP-ribosylation of G-binding protein
Tracheal cytotoxin (others)	Kills cilia-bearing cells	?
Campylobacter jejuni		
Enterotoxin	Diarrhea	Cholera-like
Clostridium botulinum		
Botulinum toxin	Neurotoxin	Blocks neuromuscular junctions; presynaptical flaccid paralysis
Clostridium difficile		
Enterotoxin	Hemorrhagic diarrhea	Acts at membranes
Cytotoxin	Cytoplasmic; cells lose filaments	
Clostridia		
α-toxin	Necrosis in gas gangrene; cytolytic, lethal	Phospholipase C
β-toxin	Necrotic enteritis	?
Enterotoxin (others)	Food poisoning; diarrhea	Cytoxin; damages membranes
Clostridium tetani		
Tetanus toxin	Spastic paralysis	Inhibits GABA and glycine release from nerve terminals at inhibitor synapsis
Corynebacterium diphtheriae		
Diphtheria toxin	Kills cells	ADP-ribosylates elongation factor 2
Escherichia coli (and often other enterics)		
Heat-labile enterotoxins	Diarrhea	Identical to cholera toxin
Cytotoxin	Hemorrhagic colitis	Like *Shigella* toxin
Legionella pneumophila		
Cytotoxin	Lyses cells	?
Listeria monocytogenes		
Listeriolysin	Membrane damage	Like streptolysin O
Pseudomonas aeruginosa		
Exotoxin A (others)	Kills cells	Like diphtheria toxin
Shigella dysenteriae		
Shigella toxin	Kills cells	Inactivates 60S ribosomes
Staphylococcus aureus		
α-toxin	Hemolytic, leukocytic, paralysis of smooth muscle	Lytic pores in membranes
β-toxin	Cytolytic	Sphingomyelinase
δ-lysin	Cytolytic	Detergent-like action
Enterotoxins	Food poisoning (emesis, diarrhea)	Superantigens
Toxic shock syndrome toxin(s)	Fever, headache, arthralgia, neutropenia, rash	Mediated through IL-1 induction
Exfoliating (others)	Sloughing of skin ("scalded skin syndrome")	?
Streptococcus pneumoniae		
Pneumolysin	Cytolysin	Similar to streptolysin O
Streptococcus pyogenes		
Streptolysin O	Cytolysin	Cholesterol target
Erythrogenic toxin (others)	Fever, neutropenia, rash of scarlet fever	Mediated through IL-1
Vibrio cholerae		
Cholera toxin (others)	Diarrhea	Hormone-independent activation of adenyl cyclase
Yersinia enterocolitica		
Heat-stable enterotoxin	Diarrhea	Like *E. coli*

- Is virulence quantitatively correlated with toxin production?
- Can a specific antibody (antitoxin) prevent or alleviate the manifestations of the disease?
- If toxin production is impaired by a mutation in the pathogen, is the disease process affected?

In cases in which a toxin is important, we may want to know:

- What is its mechanism of action?
- Why is it specific for certain cells or tissues?
- Does the pathogen make other toxins? Do they interact with one another?

The answers come easiest when the action of a single toxin accounts for the symptoms of the disease, which is the case in cholera, diphtheria, tetanus, and botulism. In contrast, many pathogenic bacteria, such as staphylococci and streptococci, make several toxins. In such multifactorial situations, the importance of individual toxins is difficult to assess.

Production of Toxins

Toxins share with antibiotics an ambivalent position in the life of the organisms that produce them. On one hand they are dispensable: they are not necessarily required for growth. On the other hand, they may be essential for the survival and spread of the bacteria under certain conditions.

Reflecting the dispensability of toxins, the genes that encode them are frequently carried by DNA elements that are themselves dispensable: **plasmids** and **temperate bacteriophages**. The location of these genes on mobile DNA molecules ensures that the ability to produce toxin may rapidly spread to nontoxigenic bacteria. Conversely, the property may also be lost from the bacteria by "curing" the cells of plasmids or prophages.

Some toxins are produced continuously by growing bacteria; others are synthesized when the cells enter the **stationary phase**. The latter is often also true for antibiotics and other "secondary metabolites," which are produced as growth stops or slows down. In some instances, producing toxin only when growth slows makes teleological sense. For example, certain toxins help bacteria obtain nutrients that have become scarce. Thus, high levels of diphtheria toxin are produced only when the diphtheria bacilli run out of iron. Since very little free iron exists in normal tissues, it is believed that the organisms obtain free iron by lysis of the cells killed by the toxin.

Sporulating bacteria sometimes release toxins during **spore formation**. In this process the bacterial cells in which the spores are formed eventually lyse, leading to the liberation of cytoplasmic proteins—including toxins—that may have accumulated. Examples are toxins made by the organisms that cause botulism, gas gangrene, or tetanus, which are all members of the genus *Clostridium*. In a heterogeneous environment, such as a contaminated wound, some organisms are growing while others are sporulating. In this type of environment, toxins will be produced continuously during the course of the infection.

A particularly interesting attribute of certain pathogenic bacteria is their ability to secrete toxins and other virulence factors by a mechanism that senses the presence of host cells. This so-called **contact-dependent** or **type III** secretion is turned on when the bacteria come in contact with host cells. The stimuli provided by the host cells are not well characterized, but include temperature, oxygen tension, and salt concentration. Contrast this type of protein secretion with those that do not require contact with host cells (these are called types I and II). The requirement of bacteria–host cell contact for this type of secretion allows a more intimate delivery of virulence factors to the target cells. Virulence factors are thus delivered more efficiently and are not as likely to elicit an immune response that might neutralize them. Bacteria that use this mechanism include *Salmonella*, *Shigella*, cholera bacilli, and plague bacilli. (For more details, see Paradigm in Chapter 17.)

Mechanism of Exotoxin Action

Bacterial toxins work at extraordinarily low levels of concentration and include the **strongest poisons** known. One gram of tetanus, botulinum, or shigella toxin can kill about 10 million people; thus, one pound would just about do in all of mankind. One hundred-fold more is required for the action of diphtheria toxin, and one thousand-fold more for others (for example, *Pseudomonas* A toxin).

A particularly interesting aspect of the action of certain toxins is that they are able to subvert the normal antibody response. Acting as so-called **superantigens**, some toxins cause the production of large amounts of nonspecific antibodies, not just those directed against themselves. Such antibody production is wasteful and inefficient in combating infection. This intriguing aspect of how microbes can "twist" a normal body response is described in Chapter 8, "The Parasite's Way of Life."

Toxins that help bacteria spread in tissues

Certain toxins contribute to disease without affecting any particular type of host cells. These toxins include degradative enzymes that function as **spreading factors** by facilitating the dispersal of infecting organisms. For example, some streptococci secrete a **hyaluronidase** that breaks down hyaluronic acid, the ground substance of connective tissue. They also secrete a **DNase**, which thins pus made viscous by the DNA released from dead white blood cells. A streptococcal protein, **streptokinase**, apparently works by binding to and activating plasminogen. Plasminogen is then converted to plasmin, the serum protease that in turn attacks fibrin clots. In this way, streptokinase eliminates fibrin barriers that may be in the way of invading streptococci.

Similar roles have been suggested for the **collagenases** and **elastases** produced by other organisms. Such "meat tenderizers" are unregulated forms of enzymes that also exist in the uninfected host, but whose activity is normally under control.

Toxins that lyse cells

A large and common class of toxins kill host cells by destroying their membranes. They act either as **lipases** or by inserting themselves in the membrane to form pores.

1. An example of a lipase toxin is a **lecithinase** formed by the clostridia of gas gangrene. This enzyme lyses cells indiscriminately because its main substrate, phosphatidylcholine (lecithin), is ubiquitous in mammalian membranes. Several toxins of this sort are known as **hemolysins** because they are usually detected by their ability to lyse red blood cells. However, they affect other cells as well, including white blood cells. Organisms that elaborate lipase toxins thus eliminate potential host defenses and at the same time create a necrotic, nutritionally rich anaerobic milieu in which they thrive.
2. The other class of membrane-damaging toxins are those that insert themselves in membranes to make **protein pores**. These channels make the membranes more permeable. Water pours into the cytoplasm and the cells begin to swell. When this process continues beyond a certain point, the cells burst. Even at toxin concentrations too low to cause lysis, cellular functions may be severely damaged by slight perturbations of permeability that may cause leakage of potassium ions needed for protein synthesis and cell viability. Thus, low levels of this kind of toxin effectively inhibit the function of the phagocytes, the first line of host defense.

The pattern of ion leakage and of subsequent damage is similar for many of these toxins. Working nonenzymatically, they employ a mechanism similar to that of the membrane attack complex of complement (see Chapter 6, "Constitutive Defenses of the Body"). The pores formed by the complement complex as well as by the pore-forming bacterial toxins consist of fortified protein structures that are unusually resistant to proteases and detergents. This general resistance very likely contributes to the stability of the toxin at the cell surface.

An example of a toxin that works in this manner is the α-toxin of *Staphylococcus aureus*. This toxin is a **homogeneous pore former**; i.e., each pore has the same number of protein molecules (see Fig. 6.5 for similar-looking channels produced by the membrane attack complex of complement). The **heterogeneous pore formers** constitute another class of membrane-damaging toxins.

These toxins make pores that vary in size and in the numbers of monomer molecules involved. The prototype of this class is **streptolysin O**, one of the toxins produced by certain streptococci. Streptolysin O ("O" for "oxygen labile") binds to cholesterol in the cell membrane. The free toxin is inactivated by cholesterol, but once it is incorporated in the membrane, it becomes impervious to it. For unknown reasons, streptolysin O lyses red blood cells but not neutrophils or macrophages. Nevertheless, low levels of this toxin contribute indirectly to the death of these white blood cells because the toxin acts preferentially on the membranes of lysosomes, releasing their hydrolytic enzymes. The result is damage to the cytoplasmic contents, leading to a suicidal type of cell death. In addition, the lysosomal enzymes released from killed neutrophils damage the surrounding tissue. The heterogeneous pore formers demonstrate that pores made by toxins need not be large or well-defined to cause widespread damage.

Toxins that block protein synthesis

In contrast to the toxins that act on the surface of cells, which are highly variable in structure and mode of action, those that act inside cells have a number of similarities (Fig. 9.1):

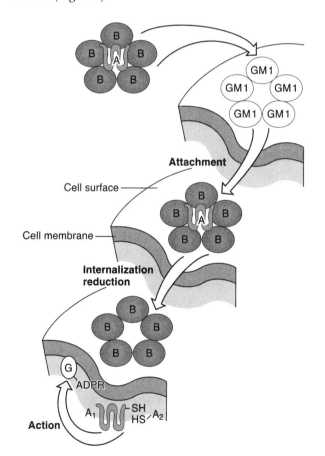

Figure 9.1. Cholera toxin becomes active. The *B* ("binding") component probably incorporates into the membrane by binding to a ganglioside receptor (*GM1*), and the *A* ("active") component enters the cell.

- Most of these toxins have two portions, one involved in binding to the cell membrane, the other responsible for the toxic activity. In some toxins, these two activities are carried out by a single polypeptide chain, in others by two different chains. These chains are called **A** for "active" and **B** for "binding," and these toxins are known as **A-B toxins.**
- Binding to the membrane is usually followed by **receptor-mediated endocytosis** and internalization of the toxin, or, alternatively, by direct passage through a pore.
- Once inside the host cell, the A moiety is often still inert. For example, diphtheria, cholera, tetanus, and shigella toxins are all synthesized as inactive precursors that must be activated to become toxic. Activation usually takes place by proteolytic cleavage and reduction of disulfide bridges.
- Many of these toxins have a common mode of action: they catalyze the transfer of the adenosine diphosphate group from the coenzyme NAD to target proteins. These **ADP-ribosyltransferases** are exemplified by diphtheria toxin, cholera toxin, and exotoxin A of *Pseudomonas aeruginosa.*

A well-studied example of protein synthesis–blocking toxins is **diphtheria toxin**, which consists of a single polypeptide chain with A and B portions. When the toxin binds to a cell membrane receptor, the molecule is cleaved at a protease-sensitive site between the A and B portions, which remain covalently associated by disulfide linkage. The entire receptor–toxin complex then enters the cell by receptor-mediated endocytosis, just like hormones and certain viruses. Once inside the endosomal vesicle, reduction of the disulfide bond separates the toxin into its A and B portions. The acidic conditions within the vesicle promote insertion of the B chain into the endosomal membrane, which facilitates the passage of fragment A into the cytosol. Thus, both endocytosis (passage across the cell membrane) and membrane translocation (out of the vesicles and into the cytoplasm) are required for fragment A to reach the cytoplasm and begin its toxic action.

The A fragment resists denaturation and thus remains active for a long time inside cells. Its ability to remain active accounts in part for its potency: a single molecule can kill a cell. Killing takes place by a specific mechanism of protein modification, **ADP-ribosylation.** Many toxins are capable of this reaction, but diphtheria and *Pseudomonas* A exotoxins target a specific protein, **elongation factor 2 (EF-2)**, a factor in eukaryotic protein synthesis that catalyzes the hydrolysis of GTP required for the movement of ribosomes on mRNA. The reaction is:

$$\text{EF-2} + \text{NAD}^+ \rightarrow \text{ADPR—EF-2} + \text{H}^+$$

EF-2 protein is the only known substrate for diphtheria and *Pseudomonas* exotoxin A toxins. The reason for this specificity is that EF-2 contains a rare modification in one of its histidine residues, and it is this site that these toxins target for ADP-ribosylation. Mutant cells in which this histidine is not modified are resistant to the toxins. The addition of ADP-ribose inactivates EF-2 and kills cells by an irreversibly blocking protein synthesis.

Pharmacological toxins

Another kind of toxin elevates or depresses normal cell functions but does not kill target cells. Some toxins of this type act by elevating the intracellular level of **cAMP,** to which many physiological functions are sensitive. Pathogens employ several mechanisms to elevate cAMP inside cells. Some pathogens make a toxin that alters the activity of the adenylate cyclase of host cells, others secrete an adenylate cyclase to make more cAMP from ATP, and still others pour out cAMP directly.

One of the best studied of the toxins that modify the host's adenylate cyclase is **cholera toxin.** The target tissue for this toxin is the epithelium of the small intestine. The toxin has separate A and B subunits: the B component has specific affinity for the intestinal epithelial mucosa (see Fig. 9.1). As with diphtheria toxin, the A subunit ADP-ribosylates a target protein, a GTPase that functions in the production of cAMP. When the GTPase is modified by the toxin, cAMP synthesis becomes unregulated, and cAMP is made in large amounts. By an incompletely understood process, this overproduction of cAMP provokes loss of fluids and the copious diarrhea characteristic of cholera.

To understand how cholera toxin elevates the cAMP level, let us examine how the synthesis of this compound is regulated normally, an intricate business. The adenylate cyclase complex is membrane-bound in the intestinal cells and includes two proteins known as **G protein,** the **cyclase** itself (Fig. 9.2). G protein has two conformational states: when it binds GTP, it stimulates adenylate cyclase to make cAMP; when it binds GDP, it is inactive. This stimulatory effect is normally of short duration, because G protein is also a GTPase that cleaves GTP to GDP. The activity of adenyl cyclase is thus determined by the balance of binding and hydrolysis of GTP by G protein. How does cholera toxin act to increase the level of cAMP? Cholera toxin promotes the "active" state of G protein by the ADP-ribosylation of one of its arginine residues. G protein is now locked in the conformation that stimulates adenylate cyclase. The interminable synthesis of cAMP provokes the movement of massive quantities of fluid across the intestinal membrane and into the lumen of the gut.

Activation of adenylate cyclase by ADP-ribosylation is a strategy adopted by a number of other diarrhea-producing enterotoxins, such as the labile toxin or LT enterotoxin of *Escherichia coli.* Other toxins, such as that produced by *Bordetella pertussis,* the agent of whooping cough, raise cAMP in leukocytes. Phagocytic cells are of-

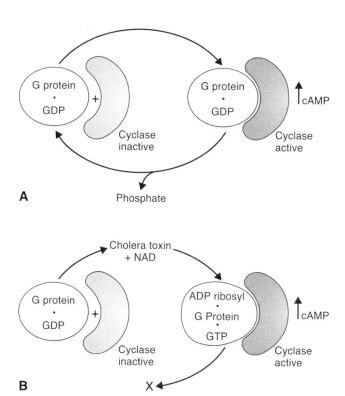

A

Phosphate

B

X

Figure 9.2. The action of cholera toxin. Gs, R, and cyclase all interact with the membrane. **A.** Gs protein binds *GTP*, stimulated by the complex of R protein and its cognate hormone. With GTP bound, Gs protein activates adenyl cyclase. **B.** *Cholera toxin* riboslylates Gs protein which now cannot hydrolyze GTP and remains in the stimulatory GTP-bound form. The result is continued synthesis of *cAMP* from adenyl cyclase.

ten an important target of these toxins because excess cAMP impairs their motility and ability to migrate toward invading bacteria (chemotaxis).

The different effects of cholera toxin and pertussis toxin on the host also illustrate the importance of the site of bacterial colonization. Both toxins have similar biochemical activities, but their distinct effects reflect the different location of the organisms in the body.

Toxins that block nerve function

Among the most lethal toxins known are those of tetanus and botulism, which are produced by members of the anaerobic spore-forming genus *Clostridium*. Both toxins act on the nervous system: **tetanus toxin** produces irreversible muscle contraction, while **botulinum toxin** blocks muscle contraction.

Tetanus and botulinum toxins, like diphtheria toxin, consist of single polypeptide chains (molecular weight about 150,000 daltons) which contain putative A and B regions. Both are metalloproteases and work by clipping proteins involved in neurotransmission. They bind to **ganglioside receptors** which, in this case, are specific to nervous tissue. These toxins are also activated by prote-

olysis and disulfide reduction, and they function intracellularly. Tetanus and botulism toxins are similar proteins, sharing considerable amino acid homology and biochemical activity. Both are peptidases that act on **synaptobrevins**, proteins found in the neurons' synaptic vesicles and responsible for the release of neurotransmitters and inhibitory mediators.

Tetanus bacilli rarely move from their location in wounds, and their toxin acts at a distance on the central nervous system. Tetanus is one of the best examples of a disease that results from the action of a single toxin at a distant target. Once bound to cell membranes, tetanus toxin is internalized, probably by receptor-mediated endocytosis, and flows via retrograde transport through axonal processes to the spinal cord. There the toxin degrades synaprobrevins, thus inhibiting the release of **inhibitory neurotransmitters** such as γ-aminobutyric acid from inhibitory interneurons. The excitatory and inhibitory effects of motor neurons become increasingly unbalanced, which leads to rigid muscle contraction. In some cases, this may lead to spasms of the respiratory muscles and death due to decreased ventilation.

Unlike tetanus toxin, botulinum toxin is seldom produced in wounds but is made in contaminated food kept under anaerobic conditions, e.g., improperly sterilized canned beans or sausages. The disease is therefore a true intoxication: it does not require the presence of the organisms to cause signs and symptoms. Botulinum toxin is not destroyed by proteases of the digestive tract, apparently because it protects itself by complexing with other proteins. In fact, intestinal proteases activate the toxin, which is a single polypeptide chain with A and B portions.

In contrast to tetanus toxin, botulinum toxin affects peripheral nerve endings. Once across the gut lining, it is carried in the blood to neuromuscular junctions. There it binds to gangliosides at motor nerve endplates, where it is taken up. Subsequent events are biochemically similar to those of tetanus toxin, but here they result in a presynaptic block of the release of acetylcholine. The interruption of nerve stimulation causes an irreversible relaxation of muscles, leading to respiratory arrest. It is not entirely understood how botulinum and tetanus toxins lead to such different physiological effects, given their biochemical similarity. Perhaps the reason lies in differences in the specificity of the binding domains of the two toxins. Botulinum toxins bind preferentially to peripheral neurons, tetanus toxin to central nervous system neurons. However, this alone does not explain how the two toxins affect different neuroactive compounds.

Immune Protection Against Exotoxins

Because toxins are foreign proteins and are antigenic, **immune protection** of the host is an optimistic possibility. For some diseases, such as tetanus, the clinical disease itself does not confer immunity to subsequent infections, probably because the toxin is produced in amounts too small to be an effective immunogen. On the other hand, vaccination and treatment with **antitoxins** have been used successfully against tetanus and other diseases. Of course, active immunization cannot be carried out by injecting the toxins themselves. Fortunately, some toxins can be modified chemically to retain their immunogenicity while losing their toxicity. Such **toxoids** are commonly used for the prevention of *d*iphtheria and *t*etanus (as part of the widely used *DPT* shots). Initial doses in the first months of an infant's life are effective, and boosters every 10 years are sufficient to maintain immunity. As may be anticipated, infection by the organisms can still occur in individuals immune only to the toxin, but serious disease does not ensue.

In a nonimmune individual, antitoxin must be administered rapidly to be effective. Once toxins are bound to the cells, antitoxins do not usually work because the toxins are rapidly internalized and become unavailable to the antibody molecules. Another serious drawback of this "passive immunization" is that the antitoxin is usually produced in horses or other animals. As a result, antitoxin administration can lead to **serum sickness**, an immune reaction against foreign proteins.

Recombinant DNA technology may refine some of the vaccination procedures, and it may soon be possible to immunize using tailor-made fragments of the toxin. The B fragments of A-B toxins seem to be particularly promising candidates, because antibodies which prevent binding of a toxin block the initial steps of toxin action. In the absence of the A fragment, the B fragments are innocuous and could be administered with little risk.

Not all toxin-mediated diseases respond to vaccination. In particular, vaccines against cholera administered systemically have limited value. Protection here requires the intestinal secretion of IgA antibodies against the toxin (to prevent its action) and against the bacterial adhesins (to prevent colonization of the bacteria). Vaccines administered by injection give poor or short-lived protection, in part because they do not induce the formation of effective amounts of IgA antibodies.

Bacterial toxins are also being used in attempts to make them useful delivery systems for drugs, such as coupling a specific antibody to an A subunit of a toxin. The antibody would then seek out the specific cell, and the toxin fragment would kill it. The results of these attempts have thus far been equivocal and have often been accompanied by side effects. Nonetheless, the idea of turning toxins to advantage remains appealing.

Endotoxin: Sometimes a "Toxin," Usually an Immunostimulant

Endotoxin is the **lipopolysaccharide** (LPS) of the outer membrane of Gram-negative bacteria (see Fig. 3.2) and plays an important role in the diseases caused by these organisms. At low concentrations, endotoxin elicits a series of **alarm reactions**: fever, activation of complement by the alternative pathway, activation of macrophages, and stimulation of B lymphocytes. At high concentrations, it produces **shock** and even death. The term endotoxin is misleading on two counts—it is not "endo" (internal), and it exerts its toxic effects only at high concentrations.

Endotoxin and exotoxins differ in important ways. Unlike exotoxins, endotoxin is not a protein but rather a complex molecule with some exotic chemical constituents not found elsewhere in nature. Most exotoxins have a single mode of action. Endotoxin, on the other hand, induces many different pharmacological and immunological changes at low and at high concentrations. Our knowledge of endotoxin is still fragmentary, and at times, its study stirs up considerable controversy. As you will see, endotoxin is full of surprises.

Chemistry of endotoxin

The complex chemistry of endotoxin does not, as yet, shed light on how it works. As discussed in Chapter 3, "Biology of Infectious Agents," bacterial lipopolysaccharide is composed of **three parts**: a glycophospholipid, called **lipid A**; a **core** of sugars, ethanolamine and phosphate; and the **O antigen**, a long side chain of species-specific, often unusual sugars (see Fig. 3.6). Of these parts of the molecule, only lipid A is active; the others serve as carriers. Lipid A alone is water-insoluble and inert, but its activity is restored when complexed even with large-molecular-weight carriers, such as proteins. The structure of lipid A is unusual: it contains uniquely short fatty acids (12, 14, and 16 carbons in length), some with hydroxyl groups.

Major effects of endotoxin

Endotoxin has seemingly different effects at high and low concentrations (Fig. 9.3): At the low range of concentrations it sets off a series of alarm reactions, at high range it induces **shock**. The extent to which these complex events overlap depends not only on the amount of endotoxin, but also on the route of injection and the previous exposure of the host to this substance.

The primary targets for endotoxin are four kinds of cells: the mononuclear phagocytes (peripheral blood monocytes, macrophages of the spleen, bone marrow, lung alveoli, peritoneal cavity, and Kupffer cells), **neutrophils, platelets**, and B lymphocytes. These cells probably possess specific endotoxin receptors, although at present the existence of these receptors is still in question.

The alarm reactions to endotoxin

Fever. In the words of Lewis Thomas, endotoxin acts like propaganda: it tells the body that bacteria

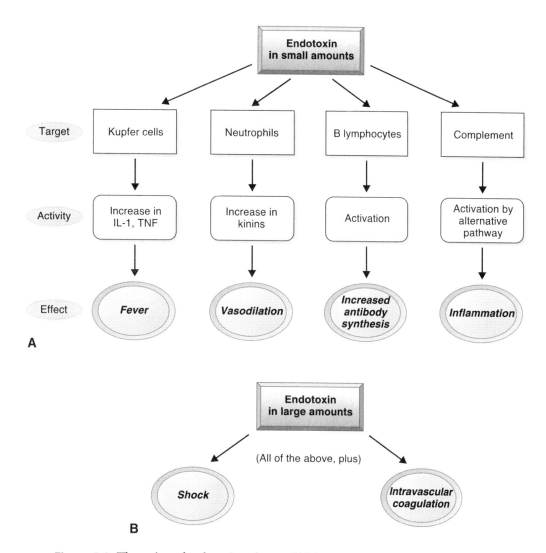

Figure 9.3. The action of endotoxin at low and high concentrations. See text for details.

are present. Extremely small amounts of endotoxin are **pyrogenic**, that is, it elicits **fever**, a common sign of infection. About 100 nanograms (0.1 microgram) of endotoxin injected intravenously in an adult human volunteer produce a measurable pyrogenic response. Note that this amount comes from about ten million enteric bacteria, which is not a particularly large amount of microbial mass; the normal intestinal flora contains perhaps one million times more bacteria. If all the endotoxin in the bowel were to enter the bloodstream and if fever followed an absurdly linear response, body temperature would rise to about one million degrees! Obviously, the amount of endotoxin that spills over from the gut into the portal circulation is probably quite small. Nonetheless, this amount of endotoxin serves in healthy people as a constant low-level stimulation of the immune response without pathological manifestations. Low titers of antibodies to endotoxin are found in most healthy persons.

Fever produced by endotoxin induces the release of proteins known as **endogenous pyrogens** from mononuclear phagocytes. The best known of these proteins are **interleukin-1** and **tumor necrosis factor**, which set off a complex series of events known as the **acute phase response** (Chapter 6, "Constitutive Defenses of the Body"). Gram-positive bacteria also induce fever but, lacking endotoxin, they elicit it through their cell wall components, which also causes the release of interleukin-1 and tumor necrosis factor.

Activation of complement. Endotoxin activates complement by the alternative pathway (see Chapter 6, "Constitutive Defenses of the Body"). At low endotoxin concentrations, the events most likely to be of consequence to the bacteria are the production of the **membrane attack complex**, plus phagocyte chemotaxis and opsonization. Neutrophils are called up and, because of the opsonizing effect of C3b, become available for phagocytosis. Complement activation also leads to the production of **anaphylatoxins**

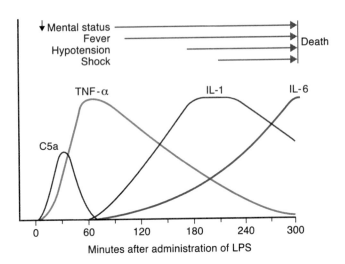

Figure 9.4. Release of mediators of sepsis following the experimental injection of LPS. TNF-α triggers the release of IL-1. These cytokines act synergistically to induce the damaging effects of sepsis. Other cytokines, such as IL-6, are released as a consequence of this synergy. IL-6 does not produce shock, but the level of IL-6 release is highly correlated with death from septic shock.

(C3a, C5a), which lead to increased capillary permeability and release of lysosomal enzymes from neutrophils (degranulation). Thus, endotoxin elicits an inflammatory response.

Activation of macrophages. Endotoxin activates **macrophages**; that is, it stimulates them to increase their production of lysosomal enzymes, to speed up the rate of phagocytosis, and to secrete some of their hydrolases into the medium. Once activated, macrophages become superb scavengers and are able to handle larger numbers of invading microorganisms. Their exuberance even extends to killing certain cancer cells, partly by direct attachment and partly by releasing proteins such as tumor necrosis factor. The ability of endotoxin—via macrophages—to limit the growth of certain tumors has been recognized for some time and is the subject of continued investigation. Endotoxin derivatives belongs to a class of potential anticancer agents known as **biological response modifiers,** which are currently being evaluated for use in clinical work.

Stimulation of B lymphocytes. By inducing the release of interleukin-1, endotoxin induces B lymphocytes (but not T lymphocytes) to divide. B lymphocytes mature into antibody-producing cells, thus adding to resistance to infection by increasing the level of antibodies. In this capacity endotoxin is an **immunological adjuvant.**

Effects of high amounts of endotoxin—shock

The full panoply of the activities of endotoxin is more emphatically displayed when it is administered in large amounts (Fig. 9.4). The full scope of endotoxin activity is seen fortunately rarely, in a condition known as **bacterial sepsis.** In sepsis, the body is overwhelmed by bacteria, often Gram-negative bacteria such as *E. coli*, *P. aeruginosa*, or meningococci (see Chapters 14, "Neisseriae: Gonococcus and Meningococcus," 19, "*Bordetella pertussis* and Whooping Cough," and 64, "Intravascular Infection"). The result is a frequently lethal condition known as **endotoxic shock,** which manifests as a serious drop in blood pressure, **hypotension,** and **disseminated intravascular coagulation.**

Hypotension is caused by a complex series of reactions elicited by endotoxin. It has recently been proposed that the key mediators in endotoxin-induced hypotension are, once again, tumor necrosis factor and interleukin-1. The extent of hypotension is considerably reduced by the administration of antisera against tumor necrosis factor or interleukin-1 prior to the injection of endotoxin. An earlier view is that decreased resistance of peripheral vessels results from a buildup of vasoactive amines (histamine and kinins). Considerable work is being carried out to clarify the situation and to understand the molecular basis for endotoxin shock.

Disseminated intravascular coagulation (DIC) is the deposition of thrombi in small vessels, with consequent damage to the areas deprived of blood supply. The effect is most severe in the kidneys, where it leads to cortical necrosis. Other organs affected include the brain, lungs, and adrenals. In some cases of meningococcal infection, adrenal insufficiency due to infarction leads to rapid death, a condition known as the **Waterhouse-Friderichsen** syndrome. Endotoxin contributes to coagulation of blood in three ways: (1) it activates clotting factor XII (the so-called Hageman factor), to set off the intrinsic clotting cascade; (2) it causes platelets to release the contents of their granules, which are involved in clotting; and (3) it prompts neutrophils to release proteins known to stabilize fibrin clots.

In conclusion, endotoxin is the visiting card of Gram-negative bacteria. When it is noticed, the body sets off a series of alarm reactions that rapidly help it fend off the invaders. These include the mobilization of neutrophils, the activation of macrophages, and the stimulation of B lymphocytes. In large amounts, endotoxin becomes deserving of its name and induces shock and widespread coagulation. This suggests that we have evolved successful defense mechanisms against Gram-negative bacteria but have not developed ways of regulating them in every instance.

SELF-ASSESSMENT QUESTIONS

1. Discuss how certain toxins lyse host cells.
2. Describe how A-B toxins attach to and enter cells.

3. Which group of toxins has no obvious B portion?

4. What is the basis for believing that diphtheria toxin causes the main clinical features of this disease?

5. How does cholera toxin act?

6. Compare and contrast the mode of action of tetanus and botulinum toxins.

7. What are the ideal properties of a toxoid to be used for vaccination?

8. What are the main differences between exotoxins and endotoxins?

9. Contrast the local and systemic activities of low concentrations of endotoxin.

10. Discuss the effects of high concentrations of endotoxin.

SUGGESTED READINGS

Alouf JE, Freer J, eds. Sourcebook of bacterial toxins. San Diego: Academic Press, 1991.

Bhakdi S, Tranum-Jensen J. Alpha-toxin of *Staphylococcus aureus*. Microb Rev 1991;55:733–751.

Johnson HM, Russell JK, Ponzer C. Superantigens in human disease. Sci Amer 1992(Apr);266:92–101.

Moss J, Iglewski B, Vaughan M, Tu AT. Handbook of natural toxins. Vol 8. Bacterial toxins. New York: Marcel Dekker, 1995.

Schiavo G, Benfenati F, Poulain B, Rossetto O, Polverino de Lauretto P, DasGupta BR, Montecucco C. Tetanus and botulinum-B neurotoxins block neurotransmitter release by proteolytic cleavage of synaptobrevin. Nature 1992;359: 832–835.

Infectious Agents

Bacteria
Viruses
Fungi
Animal Parasites

Bacteria

Introduction to the Pathogenic Bacteria

MOSELIO SCHAECHTER

Thousands of species of bacteria, both harmless and pathogenic, are found in association with the human body. Although you need to know only the principal bacteria, even these comprise a long list. But knowing the taxonomy of bacteria may help you make important diagnostic and treatment decisions. For example, it is helpful to know that staphylococci and streptococci both belong to a group called the Gram-positive cocci, that *Escherichia coli* is classified among the Gram-negative enteric bacteria, that the tubercle bacillus belongs to the acid-fast bacteria, and so forth.

In this chapter, we will use a simplified, practical scheme to divide the main pathogenic bacteria rather than the organizational scheme used in the science of bacterial taxonomy (Fig. 10.1). In broad terms, medically interesting bacteria belong to one of two large categories:

- The "typical" bacteria, rods and cocci (spheres) that lack unusual morphological features. These "garden variety" bacteria can be subdivided into the Gram-positive and Gram-negative bacteria, and each of these categories can be further divided into rods and cocci.
- Those that do not fall in this group.

Like all other forms of life, bacteria are named by their genus, as in *Escherichia*, and species, as in *coli*. Conventionally, after its first use in a text, the genus name is shortened to the first letter, e.g., *E. coli*. Many bacteria also have common names, usually related to the main disease they cause, e.g., the "cholera bacillus," the "tubercle bacillus." Sometimes, the origin of the genus and species names is interesting and useful to know. Many bacterial names honor famous microbiologists (e.g., *Escherichia* is named after Dr. Escherich;

Salmonella after Dr. Salmon, not the fish), but some names are descriptive. For instance, *pyogenes* (as in *Streptococcus pyogenes*) indicates that the bacteria leads to pus production, and *nana* (dwarf) signifies that *Hymenolepis nana* is the "dwarf" tapeworm.

A confusing aspect of bacterial taxonomy is that considerable variety usually exists within a species. Thus, a *Staphylococcus aureus* isolated from another patient may be distinctly virulent, whereas another strain of the same bacterium may not be. These isolates are called **strains.** This point is well illustrated by the many strains of *E. coli*: this designation includes the strain commonly used in molecular biology research, known as K12, as well as less benevolent strains that cause infection of the intestine, the urinary bladder, or the meninges. All are *E. coli*, but each is a different strain.

THE "TYPICAL" BACTERIA

The **Gram stain** property reflects fundamental differences among bacteria; these differences lie mainly in their permeability properties and surface components. The chief differences that the Grain stain illustrates are the presence of an outer membrane in the Gram-negative bacteria and of a thick **murein** layer in the Gram-positive bacteria (Chapter 2, "Normal Microbial Flora"). These organisms can also be divided into rods and cocci, yielding four categories in which to classify them (Fig. 10.2).

Because the Gram stain reflects such fundamental differences among bacteria, Gram-positive bacteria differ more from Gram-negative bacteria than cocci differ from rods. For instance, the Gram-positive streptococci are closely related to the lactobacilli, which are Gram-positive rods; however, the streptococci are quite distant from Gram-negative cocci such as the gonococci. Gram-

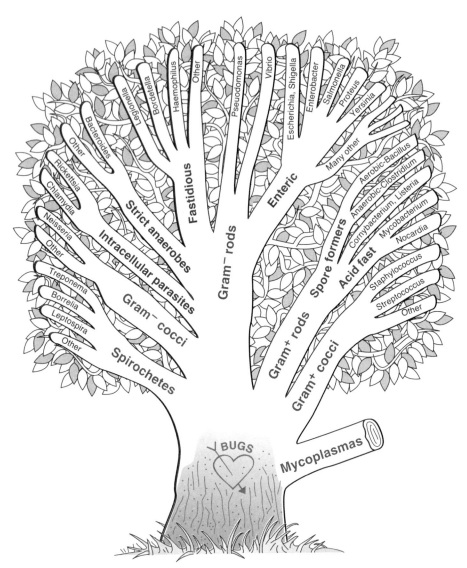

Figure 10.1. The major groups of medically important bacteria. This illustration is a practical representation of the principal groups of pathogenic bacteria. It is meant to be a study aid, not a taxonomic or phylogenetic tree.

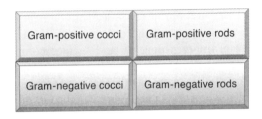

Figure 10.2. The "Big Four" typical bacteria.

positive bacteria accept the Gram stain and appear dark violet, whereas Gram-negative bacteria do not accept the stain and appear red. (See Chapter 3, "Biology of Infectious Agents" and Table 3.2 for details).

The four categories presented in Fig. 10.2 are fairly evenly represented in the normal flora of the mouth, the pharynx, and the large intestine; major pathogens, however, are represented in fewer numbers. The Gram-positive cocci and the Gram-negative rods are the most common agents of infection, followed by the Gram-negative cocci and the Gram-positive rods.

The Gram-positive Cocci

The streptococci

Streptococci grow in chains of spherical cells—like strings of pearls—and constitute a large and diverse group. Streptococci are subdivided according to the changes they produce when grown on agar-containing blood. Thus, β-**hemolytic** streptococci (or "beta strep"), which cause most streptococcal infections, lyse red blood cells signified by a clear area around the colonies. The α-**hemolytic** streptococci produce a different change and cause the hemoglobin within the red blood cell to turn green. Other streptococci do not change the blood at all. Many streptococci strains are nonpathogenic and are found in the environment as well as in the normal human intestine. Some strains are associated with dairy products and contribute to the manufacture of cheese.

Streptococci do not carry out respiration, only fermentation. Fermentation is characteristic of anaerobic bacteria, and indeed some streptococci are strict anaerobes. However, most of the pathogenic species of streptococci grow in air, and they are thus described as **oxygen-tolerant anaerobes**. Streptococci usually grow in small colonies on agar. Streptococci produce many extracellular proteins, some of which are virulence factors that assist the organisms in spreading throughout tissues and damaging host cells.

The main pathogens in this genus are the β-hemolytic strains. These strains are further subclassified into groups by the presence of different cell wall polysaccharides. Of all the groups (A through T), the most important strains in human disease are those of group A. The full taxonomic name of these organisms is *Streptococcus pyogenes*, but they are often referred to as "group A strep." They cause "strep throat," infections of soft tissues and other serious infections. These infections may cause serious complications, such as rheumatic fever or glomerulonephritis. α-hemolytic streptococci include one main pathogen, the pneumococcus, or the main agent of bacterial pneumonia, and other, mainly opportunistic species.

The staphylococci

The three main species of staphylococci are *S. aureus*, *S. epidermidis*, and *S. saprophyticus*; however, few others exist. Thus, this group is not as diverse as the streptococci. Under the microscope, staphylococci look like arrays of buckshot or bunches of grapes (*staphylo* comes from the Greek word for grapes). They are more robust than streptococci and are able to withstand many chemical and physical agents; these qualities make it difficult to eradicate them from the human environment. Their colonies on agar are larger than those of the streptococci and they are aerobes.

Staphylococci are found in many sites of the body, especially on the skin. They are the most likely organisms to cause pus in wounds and may produce serious infections in deep tissues, such as osteomyelitis (infection of the bone marrow) or endocarditis (infection of the heart valves). Like the streptococci, they also secrete a large number of extracellular enzymes and toxins. One enzyme, **coagulase**, clots plasma and is useful in classification as only the most pathogenic species of the genus, *S. aureus*, produces this enzyme.

Gram-negative Cocci

Gram-negative cocci include several genera of medical importance, the most important of which is the *Neis-*

seria. This genus includes many organisms found in the healthy mouth and pharynx and two important pathogens, the **gonococcus** and the **meningococcus**. Like all Gram-negative bacteria, they possess an outer membrane that contains endotoxin (lipopolysaccharide). The gonococcus obviously causes gonorrhea, and the meningococcus causes meningitis and a severe septicemia.

Gram-positive Rods

Abundant in the environment, this group includes bacteria that only infrequently cause diseases, at least in the developed regions of the world. One, diphtheria, was a deadly disease in children until vaccination nearly eradicated it. The agent of diphtheria is called *Corynebacterium diphtheriae* and has many relatives called the **diphtheroids**. The diphtheroids are common inhabitants of the skin and mucous membranes and can cause opportunistic infections. (Note that *diphtheria* has two h's.)

In the human environment, the most common organisms in this group are the **spore-forming rods**. They are the largest of the typical bacteria, comprising 5 to 10 times the volume of an average *E. coli*, and measure about 1 μm^3 in length. They are divided into two genera: the **aerobic** *Bacillus*, which contains only one important pathogenic species, *B. anthracis*, which causes anthrax; and the **strict anaerobes**, which are members of the genus *Clostridium*. Clostridia are medically important because they include species *C. botulinum*, which cause botulism; *C. tetani*, the agent of tetanus; and several other species that produce gas gangrene (most commonly *C. perfringens*). Symptoms of these diseases are caused by powerful exotoxins. Among the most commonly encountered clostridial diseases is pseudomembranous colitis, caused by *C. difficile*.

Another important pathogen among the Gram-positive rods is *Listeria monocytogenes*, which occasionally causes serious infections in infants and in adults who are immune-compromised.

Gram-negative Rods

The enteric bacteria

The Gram-negative rods are a large group of bacteria and include many important pathogens. The **enteric bacteria** are among the most clinically important of the Grain-negative rods. Their paradigm is *Escherichia coli*, the typical bacterium *par excellence*. The enteric bacteria (or family *Enterobacteriaceae*) comprise many genera, including the *Salmonella* of typhoid fever and food poisoning and the *Shigella* of bacillary dysentery. All enteric bacteria grow readily on laboratory media, make middle-sized colonies (usually less than one millimeter across) on agar and do not form spores or have special cell arrangements. Many, but not all, are motile. They are divided into two main groups: those that ferment lactose (*E. coli* and others) and those that do not (*Salmonella, Shigella*). Although many pathogens are non-lactose fermenters, this rule is not absolute, and many exceptions exist. Relatives of the enteric bacteria include the organisms that cause plague and certain intestinal infections (*Yersinia*).

Among their more distant relatives are Gram-negative rods that differ in metabolism and somewhat in morphology. These include the genus *Pseudomonas* and the cholera bacillus, *Vibrio cholerae*. A close relative of *Vibrio* is *Campylobacter jejuni*, a common agent of infectious diarrhea, and an organism implicated in gastritis and gastric ulcers, *Helicobacter pylori*. Pseudomonads, as the members of the *Pseudomonas* are sometimes called, are often found in aqueous environments, such as rivers, lakes, swimming pools, and tap water; these environments are thus frequent sources of human infection.

The "fastidious small gram-negative rods"

Besides the organisms mentioned above, the Gram-negative rods include an important and heterogeneous group of genera. They can be lumped, somewhat arbitrarily, into a group that may be awkwardly described as the "fastidious, small, Gram-negative rods" because they have complex nutritional requirements and tend to be smaller than, for example, *E. coli*. Included in this group are the following genera: *Haemophilus* which cause pneumonia and meningitis, *Bordetella* (whooping cough), *Brucella* (brucellosis), *Francisella* (tularemia), *Bartonella* (cat-scratch fever), and others. *Pneumophila*, the agent of Legionnaires' disease, is also a small Gram-negative rod but varies considerably from the others in its habitat (soil, water) and chemical composition.

The strictly anaerobic gram-negative rods

Lastly, an important group of Gram-negative rods is distinguished by its strictly anaerobic way of life. Clinically, the most noteworthy of these organisms belongs to the genus *Bacteroides*. These bacteria are common in the human body and are often the most frequent members of the intestinal flora. They are also found in the gingival pockets that surround the teeth. Although the bacteria are usually harmless, members of this genus may cause serious disease when deposited in deep tissues; for example, if they are associated with peritonitis, the abdominal infection that results from the outpouring of intestinal contents into the peritoneum. These organisms usually do not cause disease alone but are found in association with other bacteria, thereby causing mixed or polymicrobial infections. They will not reproduce if incubated aerobically and require special anaerobic techniques for their growth and detection.

THE "NOT SO TYPICAL" BACTERIA

This taxonomic hodgepodge includes organisms that have special shapes, sizes, or staining properties. They do not have many features in common, other than their medical importance. Each group, then, stands alone.

The Acid-Fast Bacteria

This group is almost synonymous with the genus *Mycobacterium*, which includes the **tubercle bacillus**, *M. tuberculosis*, and the **leprosy bacillus**, *M. leprae*. Acid fastness refers to the ability of these organisms to withstand many chemicals; as such, they must be stained by a special procedure (Chapter 3, "Biology of Infectious Agents"). They are surrounded by a waxy envelope that can only be penetrated by dyes if the bacteria are heated or treated with detergents. The Gram stain is irrelevant for these bacteria because they do not take up regular dyes.

The special staining procedure used for acid-fast bacteria is called the **Ziehl-Neelsen** technique (Table 3.2). Its most frequently used modification consists of treating smears with a solution of a red dye (fuchsin) that contains detergents. After washing, the smear is treated with a solution of 3% hydrochloric acid that removes the dye from all bacteria except the acid-fast organisms. The preparation is then exposed to a blue dye that counterstains all other bacteria, white blood cells, etc. Tubercle or leprosy bacilli, the "red bugs," are clearly visible against the blue background.

Several species of mycobacteria found free living in the environment may cause opportunistic infections, especially in immune-compromised patients. These environmental species used to be called **atypical acid-fast bacilli**. Among the most commonly encountered of these bacteria are members of a complex known as *Mycobacterium avium-intracellulare*. All mycobacteria grow slowly and are quite resistant to chemical agents, but not to heat.

Because these organisms sometimes form branches that vaguely suggest the fungi, the name of this genus contains the root word for fungus (*myco-*). Even more akin to fungi in morphology are relatives of the mycobacteria called the *Actinomycetes*. These organisms take up the Gram stain and are Gram-positive. Some are also weakly acid-fast. They form true branches and long filaments with complex structures, a feature that places them among the most highly differentiated of the procaryotes. There are two pathogenic genera, *Nocardia*, which are aerobic, and *Actinomyces*, which are strict anaerobes. Bacteria of these genera cause certain forms of pneumonia and soft tissue infections. A generally nonpathogenic genus, *Streptomyces*, includes organisms that make important antibiotics (streptomycin, tetracycline, etc.)

The Spirochetes

These bacteria are helical and are shaped like a spring (not a screw). They include the agent of syphilis, *Treponema pallidum*, the species name ("pale") of which refers to the fact that these organisms are so thin that they do not take up enough dye to be readily seen under the microscope. Unstained, they can be seen with a phase contrast or a darkfield microscope. The spirochetes of syphilis are not readily cultivated in the laboratory.

Other spirochetes include the genus *Leptospira*, which cause a disease called icterohemorrhagic fever, and *Borrelia recurrentis*, the agent of relapsing fever. Lyme disease (named after the town in Connecticut) is also caused by a spirochete, *Borrelia burgdorferi*, and is one of the most important spirochetoses in the Eastern and Western United States.

The Chlamydiae

The chlamydiae are small, strictly intracellular bacteria that cannot be grown in artificial media. They are among the smallest cellular forms of life but have a fairly complex life cycle. Their morphological form when they are growing inside cells differs from their form when they are in transit between cells. *Ehlamydia trachomatis* is the most common cause of sexually transmitted disease (chlamydial urethritis) and other more unusual infections. *C. pneumoniae* is an agent of pneumonia in young adults. These organisms set up housekeeping within phagocytic vesicles of their host cells and obtain their energy from them.

The Rickettsiae

Like the chlamydiae, the rickettsiae are also small, intracellular bacteria. These bacteria cause epidemic typhus, Rocky Mountain spotted fever, and other diseases. Included in this group is the genus *Ehrlichia*, which infect white blood cells in humans and animals. Each species is transmitted by the bite of different arthropod species (lice, fleas, ticks, etc.), with the exception of *Coxiella burnetii*, the agent of Q fever, which may also be acquired by inhalation. Rickettsiae are small, rod-shaped bacteria that lack distinctive growth cycle stages.

The Mycoplasmas

Perhaps most evolutionarily distant from all other bacteria, these organisms lack a rigid cell wall. They are almost plastic in structure, grow slowly on laboratory media, and have special nutritional requirements. The most unique of these requirements is the need for sterols, which are not required by any other group of bacteria. Mycoplasmas lack murein and, consequently, are resistant to penicillin and other cell wall antibiotics. The oldest known human pathogenic mycoplasma is *Mycoplasma pneumoniae*, which causes a form of pneumonia. Others, such as *Ureaplasma ureae*, have been implicated in different diseases.

Mycoplasmas resemble wall-less forms of regular bacteria that are produced in the laboratory, the so called L-forms. Regular bacteria take on the same amorphous appearance as the mycoplasma when their cell walls are removed with lysozyme or when murein synthesis is inhibited with penicillin. Cell lysis usually occurs, but if the L forms are placed in a hypertonic medium they can be grown in colonies that resemble those of the mycoplasmas. However, the similarity is only superficial. L-forms usually revert to the regular bacterial form when they are removed from lysozyme or penicillin. Mycoplasmas, on the other hand, do not. Mycoplasmas also differ in terms of their degree of relatedness to all other bacteria as measured by DNA hybridization.

CURRENT CONCEPTS REGARDING THE MICROBIAL FLORA

Many microorganisms can be seen under the microscope but cannot be cultured. Some are suspected of causing important diseases, but the point has been difficult to establish without pure cultures. New technologies have allowed scientists to make some progress in this area. For example, an organism that is visible but not culturable has been detected in tissues of patients with a disease called cat-scratch fever; this organism is suspected of being the causative agent. The DNA of the suspected organism has been isolated from tissues and amplified by a technique called the polymerase chain reaction (PCR; see Chapter 55, "Diagnostic Principles"). Hybridization studies with this DNA have revealed that the organism may be related to the rickettsiae. In time, information obtained by these and other methods may help establish the etiologic role of the organism.

Cloning techniques have been useful in studies of well-known but noncultivatable bacteria, such as the treponeme of syphilis or the mycobacterium of leprosy. The genes of these agents have been introduced into surrogate organisms, such as *E. coli*, and many of the protein gene products have been studied, especially with regard to their immunological properties.

More and more possible agents of disease are being recognized and studied because of the ecological disturbance introduced by the human immunodeficiency virus (HIV) and other agents of immunosuppression. Bacteria, viruses, fungi, protozoa, and worms that were previously unknown or known to be present only in animals or the environment have now joined the list of potential or known human pathogens (Chapter 54, "Addressing Emerging Infectious Diseases"). The combination of new technologies and the changes in the human immune condition will undoubtedly lead to the discovery of many more agents of infectious diseases. At the same time, with progress in sanitation and vaccination, many of the classic infectious pathogens are waning in importance. The list of important pathogens is constantly changing.

Despite these changes, many things remain the same. Over the hundred years or so that microorganisms have been studied in the laboratory, they have exhibited remarkable genetic constancy. For instance, the staphylococci or streptococci of today fit their original descriptions from the end of the last century. Likewise, a microbiologist from Koch's laboratory would have no problem correctly identifying a modern strain of *Escherichia coli* or tubercle bacilli. On the other hand, important changes have occurred practically before our eyes. Virtually all the pathogenic bacteria have become significantly more resistant to every new antibiotic that has been introduced in the last five decades. For example, pathogenic staphylococci are now almost universally resistant to penicillin, although in the 1950s, when the drug came into general use, their ancestors were sensitive to it.

In many of the following chapters on individual infectious agents you will find sections called paradigms. These sections highlight points of general relevance to the understanding of microbial pathogenesis.

Staphylococci: Abscesses and Other Diseases

FRANCIS P. TALLY

Key Concepts

Staphylococci:

- Are pyogenic ("pus-forming") bacteria.
- Cause different diseases, including abscesses, food poisoning, and toxin-related diseases (toxic shock and scalded skin syndromes). If the organisms enter the bloodstream, they may cause osteomyelitis and endocarditis.
- Include *Staphylococcus aureus, Staphylococcus epidermis, Staphylococcus saprophyticus* (which almost exclusively causes urinary tract infections), and others.
- Possess a variety of virulence factors; *S. aureus* possesses cell-wall factors (peptidoglycan, teichoic acid, and protein A), catalase, coagulase, and toxins. Some strains produce β-lactamase (an enzyme that breaks down penicillin).
- Infections are treated with antibiotics, although antibiotic resistance to penicillin and other antibiotics is a problem.

Staphylococci (Gram-positive cocci) are among the most common of the **pyogenic** or pus-producing bacteria. They can produce local abscesses in almost any place in the body, from the skin (furuncles or "boils") to the bone (*osteomyelitis*). Occasionally, they cause more specific diseases such as *endocarditis*.

Staphylococci produce a number of toxins and enzymes. These products act locally mainly to help them withstand **phagocytosis** by **neutrophils**. They are among the most adaptable of the pathogenic bacteria and are difficult to eliminate from the human environment. Thus, they are responsible for many hospital-acquired infections. Some staphylococcal strains also produce special toxins that cause diseases, such as food poisoning, toxic shock syndrome, and a disease of children called "scalded skin syndrome."

■ CASE

Mr. S., a 45-year-old pastry chef, cut his left forearm with a knife while working. Over the next week, he noticed swelling, redness, and warmth at the site. He thought his symptoms were a reaction to the cut, but after 4 more days he developed fever with shaking chills and came to the emergency room with severe low back pain. Physical examination revealed a fever of 39.4°C and a swollen left forearm with an area of central softness, indicating an abscess. He had tenderness to pressure over his lower spine.

The laboratory reported that he had a high white blood cell count. A Gram stain of pus aspirated from the forearm showed Gram-positive cocci in clusters (Fig. 11.1). *Staphylococcus aureus* was cultured from the pus. Blood cultures were positive for the same organism. A nuclear bone scan showed increased uptake of the third lumbar vertebra, suggesting osteomyelitis (Fig. 11.2). The organism was resis-

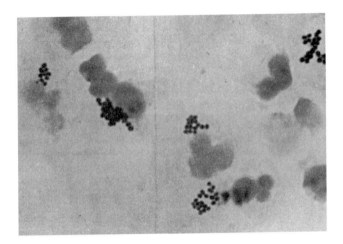

Figure 11.1. Gram stain of *S. aureus* in pus.

tant to penicillin but sensitive to oxacillin, which was used to treat Mr. S. with good results.

The day after Mr. S. was admitted to the hospital, the local public health department was notified that eight restaurant customers had developed severe vomiting and diarrhea 4 to 6 hours after eating there. Health department investigators learned that six of the eight persons who had diarrhea had eaten cream pie, whereas only 1 of 15 patrons who were well ate pie. Cultures of remaining cream pies in the restaurant refrigerator were positive for *S. aureus*. A preformed staphylococcal toxin called enterotoxin A was detected in the cream pies. The organisms from the contaminated food belonged to the same phage type (see below) as those isolated from the patient's abscess and blood, and were therefore likely to be the same.

A number of questions arise:

1. What was the source of the organisms that infected Mr. S.?
2. What contributed to the development of the abscess in the skin?
3. How did *S. aureus* invade his bloodstream?
4. How did *S. aureus* cause infection in the bone?
5. What caused the food poisoning in the patrons of Mr. S.'s restaurant?
6. What are the properties of *S. aureus* that allow it to cause such different types of disease?

The case of Mr. S. illustrates several features typical of staphylococcal infections. The initial lesion, a "boil," was mild and localized. Boils are the most common manifestation of staphylococcal disease. Boils are usually self-terminating, although in Mr. S.'s case the infection moved to the bloodstream, a complication that can be life-threatening. The only apparent metastatic focus of Mr. S.'s infection was a vertebral bone infection (osteomyelitis), a slowly progressive, localized form of *S. aureus* infection. Had he developed metastatic infection

of the heart valve (endocarditis) or a brain abscess, he would have been at immediate and serious risk.

S. aureus causes more frequent and more varied diseases than perhaps any other human pathogen (Table 11.1). Some of these diseases are caused by a variety of bacterial factors that act together to facilitate the growth of the organism and promote localized tissue damage

Table 11.1. Diseases Caused By Staphylococci

Skin and soft tissue infections
  Furuncles, carbuncles
  Wound infections (traumatic, surgical)
  Cellulitis
  Impetigo (also caused by streptococci)
Bacteremia (frequently with metastatic abscesses)
Endocarditis
Central nervous system infections
  Brain abscess
  Meningitis—rare
  Epidural abscess
Pulmonary infections
  Embolic
  Aspiration
Musculoskeletal infections
  Osteomyelitis
  Arthritis
Genitourinary tract infections
  Renal carbuncle
  Lower urinary tract infection
Toxin-related diseases
  Toxic shock syndrome
  Scalded skin syndrome
  Food poisoning (gastroenteritis)

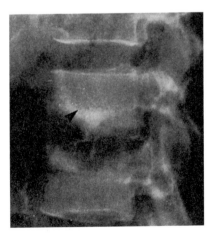

Figure 11.2. X-ray of vertebrae showing infection of the intervertebral disk space. Compare the sharp edge of the normal vertebral plates (above and below) with the ragged eroded edges of the involved vertebral plates (*arrow*).

(such as in Mr. S.'s case of wound infection and osteomyelitis). Other diseases (such as staphylococcal food poisoning) are attributable to specific toxins produced by certain staphylococcal strains. Among the more specialized, toxin-related staphylococcal diseases are the **toxic shock syndrome (TSS)** and **staphylococcal scalded skin syndrome (SSSS)**. TSS is caused by a specific toxin from localized areas of staphylococcal growth (such as wound infections). SSSS, a serious condition that predominantly affects children, also results from trivial staphylococcal infections caused by strains elaborating a different toxin.

STAPHYLOCOCCUS

Staphylococcus aureus is a large, Gram-positive coccus that grows in clusters. It is one of the hardiest of the non-spore-forming bacteria and can survive for long periods on dry inanimate objects. It is also relatively heat-resistant. These properties permit *S. aureus* to survive in almost any environment in which humans coexist.

The genus *Staphylococcus* includes several species (Table 11.2). The most ubiquitous *Staphylococcus* species is *Staphylococcus epidermidis*, which is found on the skin of most people and only infrequently causes disease. *S. aureus* is less common but generally more pathogenic. The species name *aureus* means "golden," and refers to bronze pigmentation of *S. aureus* colonies (other species colonies are white). A third species, *Staphylococcus saprophyticus*, is unique in that it apparently causes only urinary tract infections. The genus *Staphylococcus* contains other species that occasionally cause disease; these species are described in standard microbiological texts. The three species mentioned suffice for our purposes.

It is relatively easy to identify staphylococci in the laboratory. All members make large, creamy colonies on nutrient agar, and in a Gram stain they look like clusters of grapes (*staphylo* is derived from the Greek word for grape clusters) *S. aureus* is best distinguished from other species of the genus by using the **coagulase test**. Coagulase, an enzyme that clots plasma, is made by *S. aureus* but not by the other staphylococci.

Within a species of staphylococci, individual strains can be identified by differences in their resistance to a panel of antibiotics, or more commonly, by a procedure called **phage typing**. This procedure involves determining the sensitivity of a strain to a variety of standard bacteriophages. Its usefulness in epidemiology can be seen in our case report: finding the same pattern of phage sensitivity in the isolates from Mr. S.'s abscess and from the contaminated cream pies served to establish their epidemiological link. Newer molecular techniques for typing staphylococci based on the DNA sequence of the bacterial chromosome provide greater discrimination than phage typing between outbreak-related and non-outbreak-related strains.

Encounter

Staphylococci share their environment with that of human beings. They live on people and survive on inanimate objects or surfaces (fomites), such as bedding, clothing, door knobs, etc. Humans are the major reservoir for *S. aureus*. The organisms frequently colonize the external nares and are found in approximately 30% of normal individuals. However, studies of individuals over time have found that up to 90% of people will be colonized in the nares with *S. aureus* at some point. The organisms can also be found transiently on the skin and oropharynx and in feces. Staphylococci are well-equipped to colonize the skin because they grow at high salt and lipid concentrations.

The ability of *S. aureus* to colonize the skin and mucosal surfaces has been associated with a bacterial cell surface protein that binds to **fibronectin**, an extracellular matrix protein. A fibronectin-binding protein (FNBP) has been identified on the surface of *S. aureus*. FNBP allows *S. aureus* to attach to exposed fibronectin in wounds and thus it is an important virulence factor for the invasion of deeper tissues. *S. aureus* also has receptors for **collagen IV** and **sialoprotein**, important components of connective tissue, bones, and joints. Receptors are also present for **laminin**, a protein which is present in basement membranes of epithelial and endothelial linings.

Staphylococci spread from person to person, usually

Table 11.2. Properties of Various Species of Staphylococci

Species	Frequency of disease	Coagulase	Color of colonies	Mannitol fermentation	Novobiocin resistance
S. aureus	Common	+	Bronze	+	−
S. epidermidis	Common	−	White	−	−
S. saprophyticus	Occasional	−	White	−	+
Others—Different responses by individual species					

via hand contact. They can also spread by aerosols produced by patients with pneumonia. Infants are colonized with staphylococci shortly after birth, acquiring the organism from people in their immediate surroundings. Some people will become carriers for prolonged periods of time, while others will harbor the organisms only intermittently. For unknown reasons, people in certain occupations, including physicians, nurses, and other hospital workers, are more prone to colonization. Also, certain patient groups, including diabetics, patients on hemodialysis, and chronic intravenous drug abusers have a higher carriage rate than the general population.

ENTRY

Staphylococci and most other bacteria do not usually penetrate into deep tissue unless the skin or the mucous membranes are damaged or actually cut. Skin damage may be caused by burns, accidental wounds, lacerations, insect bites, surgical intervention, or associated skin diseases. In Mr. S.'s case, the organisms penetrated via a cut. If present in very large numbers, some bacteria are able to enter spontaneously and cause disease. This scenario occurs in cases of poor hygiene or prolonged moisture of the skin, which permit the growth of large numbers of staphylococci. It is not known if these infections are due to spontaneous penetration or if the organisms enter through inapparent cuts and abrasions.

SPREAD AND MULTIPLICATION

Once they have entered tissues, survival of staphylococci depends on several factors: the number of entering organisms, the site involved, the speed with which the body mounts an inflammatory response, and the immunological history of the person. When the inoculum is small and the host is immunologically competent, infections by these and other organisms are usually stopped. Nonetheless, staphylococci possess a particularly complex but effective pathogenic strategy, and even healthy persons may be unable to combat *S. aureus*. Luckily, the area of inflammation most often remains localized, and the organisms are contained.

DAMAGE

Local staphylococcal infections lead to the formation of a collection of pus called an **abscess**. Abscesses in the skin are called boils, or, in medical parlance, furuncles. Multiple interconnected abscesses are called carbuncles. Alternatively, staphylococci may spread in the subcutaneous or submucosal tissue and cause a diffuse inflammation called **cellulitis**. In most cases, these skin infections are caused by *S. aureus* and not by the other staphylococcal species.

The development of an abscess is a complex process that involves both bacterial and host factors (Fig. 11.3). The early events are characteristic of an **acute inflammatory reaction**, with the rapid and extensive participation of neutrophils. Chemotactic factors, derived both from bacteria and complement, are made in large amounts. However, some staphylococci not only survive this onslaught but are even capable of killing and lysing many of the neutrophils that have ingested them. The lysed neutrophils pour out large amounts of lysosomal enzymes, which damage surrounding tissue.

The host responds to this focal inflammation by surrounding the area with a thick-walled fibrin capsule. The center of the abscess is usually necrotic and consists of the debris of dead neutrophils, dead and live bacteria, and edema fluid. An abscess, then, is a well-defined area in tissue that contains pus. From the point of view of the host, it represents a containment of invading organisms in one site. However, the cost of this containment is that serious symptoms may develop if the abscess is located in vital parts of the body.

Staphylococcal infection involves a titanic struggle between the white blood cells and the invading organisms (see Fig. 11.3). Despite an impressive array of virulence factors, *S. aureus* do not always win the struggle; neutrophils usually gain the upper hand. The importance of neutrophils in containing staphylococcal infections is evident in children with a hereditary defect in phagocyte function called **chronic granulomatous disease** (Chapter 66, "Sexually Transmitted Diseases"). This fatal disease is characterized by frequent and serious infections with *S. aureus*. Neutrophils of these patients are unable to make sufficient hydrogen peroxide to set off the oxidative killing pathway. In these children, the balance between staphylococci and phagocytes is clearly shifted toward the microorganisms.

S. aureus produce an unusually large number of virulence factors which either prevent the bacteria from being phagocytized or help them to survive in phagocytes after they are ingested. These factors include soluble enzymes, toxins, and cell-envelope constituents. This formidable list invites speculation: why are so many virulence factors needed? Perhaps these factors do not individually impart virulence, but act in concert to permit the pathogen to cause disease. Or perhaps different factors are important in different sites of infection. More detailed genetic study of these molecules is needed to answer this puzzling question.

What are the main factors that allow staphylococci to defend themselves against neutrophils? First, the cell surface of staphylococci plays an important defensive role. *S. aureus* are sometimes surrounded by a **capsule** that may inhibit phagocytosis, but its role in virulence is far less significant than the capsules of meningococcus or pneumococcus. **Peptidoglycan** in the cell wall of *S. aureus* activates complement by the alternate pathway, thus contributing to the inflammatory response. Note

PARADIGM ■ ■ ■

The Multifactorial Nature of Pathogenesis

Staphylococci are classic representatives of a group of bacteria referred to as *pyogenic*, or pus-producing. How do the pyogenic bacteria cause disease? Despite significant progress in the understanding of bacterial pathogenesis at the cellular and molecular level, a complete answer to this question has not yet been found. The main reason is that the pathogenesis of pyogenic infections is clearly complex and multifactorial.

Like many other pyogenic bacteria, staphylococci elicit inflammation by secreting leukocyte **chemotaxins** plus a large number of **toxins** and **enzymes** that enhance the response. Some of these proteins, such as leukocidin, kill neutrophils; others, such as catalase, inhibit their antibacterial activities. Other factors, e.g., coagulase, are involved in extracellular changes that favor abscess formation. Although many of these bacterial products have been purified and their activities characterized, the precise role that each plays in the actual infectious process has been difficult to assess. An approach is needed that integrates the whole infectious process while at the same time focusing attention on the activity of a single factor. The best way to carry out the approach would be to construct a **mutation** in a gene that encodes a factor of interest, then compare the mutant carrying this mutant with its **isogenic** parent in some appropriate experimental model of disease. This comparison should allow the determination of what effect the loss of the particular factor plays in the disease. The process could then be repeated for each of the potential virulence factors.

How does one choose the virulence factor to focus on? In toxin-related diseases, such as TSS or SSSS, one can readily generate the following experimental observations confirming the central importance of the respective toxins: (a) purified toxin reproduces the disease in animals or humans, (b) specific antibody against toxin prevents the disease, (c) mutation of the toxin gene results in a strain that does not cause the disease, and (d) transfer of the toxin gene to a non-disease-causing strain enables the recipient's strain to cause the disease. This evidence clearly demonstrates that the toxin gene and the toxin it encodes are central to the disease.

For many years, investigators have tried to identify a single staphylococcal toxin that is central to the pathogenesis of wound infections. However, no single toxin or exoprotein has been found that can cause all the features of a wound infection in animals or humans. It may be that multiple factors are required to produce this particular disease. As a first step in the process of making

sense of multifactorial pathogenesis, the investigator often seeks an **epidemiologic correlation** between a large number of bacterial strains associated with a particular infection and a bacterial trait. In the case of *Staphylococcus*, it has long been known that strains isolated from severe lesions tend to belong to *S. aureus*, which can be distinguished from other staphylococcal species by virtue of secreting **coagulase**, an enzyme that clots plasma. The fact that **coagulase-positive** staphylococci are, epidemiologically speaking, more virulent suggests that coagulase is an important factor in the pathogenesis of staphylococcal infections, but it does not prove it. At this stage of the investigation, there is **correlation** without direct evidence of **causation**. Moreover, questions would still remain about the role of other possible virulence factors of *S. aureus*.

Researches addressing these issues have constructed isogenic strains of *S. aureus* that contained mutations in various putative virulence genes (i.e., genes for traits that were epidemiologically correlated with virulence). These strains were tested in a mouse mastitis model, in which the organisms were injected into the mammary glands. The resulting histopathologic changes were reproducible and could be readily recorded. Researches found that coagulase-negative mutants were less virulent than the wild type. It was shown, moreover, that mutants defective in either α-**toxin** or β-**toxin** were even more attenuated in virulence. It is important to note that infection and tissue damage still occurred; it was simply less pronounced than with the wild type strain. Furthermore, double mutants, defective in both factors, had markedly lower virulence than either single mutant, suggesting that both factors are needed and that they do not cause disease in the same manner (i.e., their effects are additive or even synergistic). Other factors, e.g., **protein A** on the surface of the organisms, did not appear to be important in causing the short-term mastitis. This is not the end of the story, though. Recently, some doubt has been raised about the role of coagulase because, in contrast to these studies with animal models of infection, a newer study has recently shown that coagulase-negative mutants are no less virulent than the wild type! Obviously, one or both of these studies may be flawed. Each may be valid in its respective model system, but neither may be highly relevant to human disease. After all, an animal model does not replicate human disease precisely. It appears that wound infections are highly complex events that require a multiplicity of virulence factors acting in concert.   EDITORS

---

that in this regard staphylococcal peptidoglycan resembles the endotoxin of Gram-negative bacteria. Another important cell wall constituent is **teichoic acid,** a polymer of ribitol and glycerophosphates (see Chapter 3, "Biology of Infectious Agents"), which also appears to

be involved in complement activation and possibly in the adherence of these organisms to mucosal cells.

A fourth wall component, **protein A,** has an unexpected property: it binds to the Fc terminus of immunoglobulin G (see Fig. 11.3). This binding incapaci-

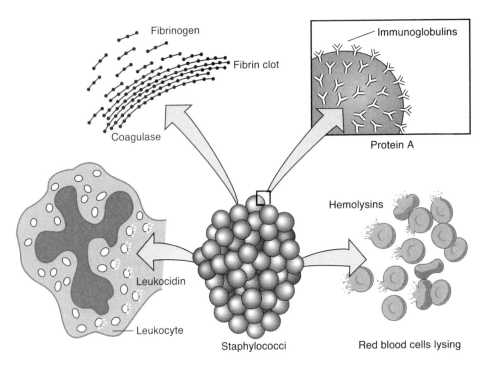

Figure 11.3. Virulence properties of *S. aureus* in pus and abscess formation.

tates antibody function of these molecules since their business end, the Fab portion, is now dangling away from the surface of the organisms. As a result, the amount of Fc residues available for attachment to phagocytes is reduced, thereby reducing opsonization. Protein A is also released into the environment surrounding bacterial growth, where it may bind free antibodies in the same manner.

In addition to these components, *S. aureus* secretes several enzymes and toxins that are almost certainly directed toward the struggle with phagocytes (see Fig. 11.3). **Catalase** converts hydrogen peroxide to water and may help counteract the neutrophils' ability to kill bacteria by the production of oxygen free radicals. **Coagulase** converts fibrinogen to fibrin and may help prevent the organisms from being phagocytized, since white cells penetrate fibrin clots poorly.

Several **pore-forming toxins** are perhaps the most important virulence factors of *S. aureus*. The molecules damage not only phagocytic cells, but also other cells (e.g., vascular endothelium, renal endothelium, neurons, myocardial cells). All of these toxins exert their effect by creating channels in cell membrane which significantly disturb cellular homeostasis. One group of these toxins (α-, β-, γ-, and δ-toxins) have been traditionally referred to as **hemolysins** because they lyse red blood cells contained in blood agar plates. However, this effect does not appear to play a role in human infection. γ-toxin and a related toxin called **leukocidin** are particularly effective in damaging neutrophils. As in many other bacteria, these virulence factors are controlled by a two-

component regulatory system, called **Agr**, or **accessory gene regulator** (see paradigm, Chapter 19, "*Bordetella pertussis*").

Several other proteins made by *S. aureus* probably enhance its virulence by damaging tissues. Many strains make a **hyaluronidase** which hydrolyzes the matrix of connective tissue and perhaps facilitates bacterial spread along tissue planes. Most strains also make lipases, proteases, DNAases, and others which may also act as **virulence enhancers**.

In addition to the tissue-damaging factors of staphylococci, they also produce substances that make them more difficult to treat with antibiotics. The most clinically significant example of these substances is β-**lactamase**, a powerful enzyme that hydrolyzes the classical penicillins. It is found in about 90% of *S. aureus* strains and is responsible for their infamous penicillin resistance, which was identified in the late 1940s and spread rapidly around the world.

In Mr. S.'s case, the organisms escaped from the abscess in the skin and entered way into the bloodstream. This outcome is unusual, since most local staphylococcal diseases are self-limiting by spontaneously draining through the skin; they do not typically result in metastatic infections. In healthy individuals, organisms that escape from a local abscess are usually destroyed by the clearance mechanisms of the blood and the lymph. Mr. S. did not appear to have impaired defenses, although impairment could have been temporary. On the other hand, the "shower" of organisms from the skin lesion could have been so great that it overwhelmed the capacity of the body to destroy them. When staphylococci become implanted in deep tissues, they tend to colonize tissues that have been previously traumatized by physical trauma, disease, or surgical intervention. Otherwise, the site of metastatic infection seems random and is probably dictated by the clearing capacity of the organ and the amount of blood flowing through it. The main sites of metastatic abscesses are the highly vascularized organs: bones, joints, lungs, and kidneys. Immunocompromised patients frequently have multiple staphylococcal metastases, which can lead to serious and often fatal diseases.

Once implanted in deep tissue and able to survive, staphylococci elicit an inflammatory reaction similar to that of skin abscess. In the words of Pasteur, osteomyelitis is a "boil of the bone. . ." (Chapter 61, "Skin and Soft Tissue"). The consequences of abscess formation in deep sites depend on their location. Nowhere is it more devastating than in the heart or the brain. However, if the function of the organ is not directly compromised, staphylococcal abscesses can persist for a considerable period of time and cause relatively mild symptoms. These symptoms tax the diagnostic acumen of the physician.

Other Species of Staphylococci

S. epidermidis, the common inhabitant of the normal skin, rarely causes disease. However, infections with *S. epidermidis* and other coagulase-negative staphylococci are found with increasing frequency in patients with implanted artificial devices, such as prosthetic joints or intravenous catheters. When defense mechanisms are impaired, *S. epidermis* can cause serious infections, like septicemia and endocarditis. A potential virulence factor of these organisms is an exopolysaccharide **slime layer** that has been found in over 80% of disease-causing isolates. It is thought that this slime layer allows the organisms to stick to the surface of plastics used in various devices.

S. saprophyticus may be the most highly specialized staphylococcus in terms of pathogenicity because it is almost entirely associated with urinary tract infections, particularly cystitis in young women. The reason for this specialization is not yet known, but it seems likely that this organism has unique properties that allow it to bind the epithelium of the urethra or the bladder.

STAPHYLOCOCCAL TOXIN DISEASES

In contrast to these classical complicated infections, staphylococci also cause three toxin-related diseases. The symptoms of each of these diseases are caused by a different toxin. The first is called **scalded skin syndrome** (SSS), a life-threatening disease which mainly affects children. SSS causes extensive sloughing of the skin. A toxin known as **exfoliatin** causes these symptoms in laboratory animals. Its role has been clearly established because the administration of specific antitoxin prevents the skin lesions in humans or mice.

A second disease caused by a toxin, called **toxic shock syndrome** (TSS), is characterized by fever, skin rash, hypotension, and the dysfunction of several essential systems. The disease was originally associated with the use of highly absorbent tampons, which apparently foster the growth of the organisms. Nowadays, TSS more commonly follows staphylococcal infection of traumatic or surgical wounds, and it occurs in men as well as women. The toxin involved cannot be studied as readily as exfoliatin because it does not cause all the symptoms of the disease in laboratory animals. It does cause fever by the same mechanism as the endotoxin of enteric bacteria, namely by stimulating the formation of interleukin-1, the endogenous pyrogen. It can be clearly implicated in staphylococcal toxic shock because it has been found in all strains isolated from patients with this disease and only rarely in other isolates.

Finally, a group of staphylococcal **enterotoxins** are a major cause of **food poisoning**, as in our case report. These toxins can cause disease even in the absence of the organism. They cause intensive intestinal peristalsis, apparently by working directly on the vomiting control center of the brain. They are heat-stable and are not necessarily destroyed by cooking. These toxins cause signs and symptoms that mimic the disease when administered to laboratory animals. Note that the same strain of *S. aureus* can cause several of the diseases mentioned. In the case described here, a single strain was responsible for Mr. S.'s bone and soft tissue infection, as well as for food poisoning in the people who ate the pastries prepared by him.

All of these toxins belong to a large family of related Gram-positive exoproteins that act as **superantigens**. If these proteins enter the bloodstream, they may nonspecifically activate large subsets of T-cells and induce cytokine production that may produce the signs of septic shock.

DIAGNOSIS

Recognizing staphylococcal infections is not usually a difficult diagnostic problem, and they are among the most frequent infections seen both in the community and in the hospital. A localized abscess in a seriously ill patient should be aspirated and the contents examined by Gram stain and culture. Clusters of large, Gram-positive cocci point to staphylococcal infection. The patient's blood should also be cultured to determine if the organisms have invaded the bloodstream. A common problem of blood cultures is the difficulty in distinguishing between *S. aureus* and coagulase-negative staphylococci, since the latter is a common contaminant and is considered pathogenic only under special circumstances. The coagulase test serves to distinguish these two species.

TREATMENT

A staphylococcal abscess, such as those seen in Mr. S., should be drained and an appropriate antibiotic should be administered. The bacteria will probably be resistant to penicillin. Semisynthetic penicillins and cephalosporins that are resistant to staphylococcal β-lactamase may be useful. Methicillin was the first of many semisynthetic penicillins with this property. However, a race between the synthetic chemists and the organisms has now appeared, because no sooner are new drugs introduced than reports of staphylococcal resistance begin to appear. During the 1970s and 1980s, a disturbing increase in numbers of *S. aureus* and coagulase-negative staphylococci resistant to these β-lactamases occurred. Infections with either of these organisms require treatment with vancomycin which, in such cases, is becoming the drug of last choice.

Methicillin resistance (and resistance to all other semisynthetic penicillins and cephalosporins) is mediated by the production of a novel penicillin binding protein (PBP2a) in *S. aureus*. PBP2a is able to maintain cell wall integrity during growth and cell division when the usual enzymes are inhibited by β-lactam antibiotics. The protein is encoded by a chromosomal gene called *mecA* that has also been found in coagulase-negative staphylococci. Researchers believe that *S. aureus* may have been acquired by the gene from their nonpathogenic relatives. In 1992, 32% of U.S. nosocomial *S. aureus* isolates and 75% of *S. epidermidis* isolates were methicillin-resistant. In many hospitals, the frequency of resistance may be even higher. Methicillin resistance has spread to all hospitals, including small community hospitals. It is a serious clinical and economic problem, since treatment of these infections often requires the use of vancomycin, an antibiotic that is more difficult to administer and more expensive than the penicillins. Quinolone antimicrobial agents had been used to treat methicillin-resistant staphylococcal infections. Unfortunately, resistance to these antibiotics has also developed rapidly. Sixty to 70% of methicillin-resistant *S. aureus* isolates are also quinolone-resistant.

Other classes of antibiotics (e.g., aminoglycosides, macrolides) may be useful second-line agents in the treatment of certain kinds of staphylococcal infections (particularly in penicillin allergic patients), although some strains are resistant to them as well. The choice of drugs should be based on the antibiotic sensitivity of the infecting strain and the special characteristics of the patient.

Today, the great concern is that the staphylococci will acquire the genes that encode vancomycin resistance in the enterococci (see Chapter 20, "Clostridia"). The transfer of this resistance has been accomplished under laboratory conditions, but fortunately, such strains have not yet appeared in the natural world. If they should emerge, we may one day face the daunting problem of common and potential dangerous staphylococcal infections with no effective antibiotics at our disposal.

Over the years, vaccines have been developed for the treatment of recurrent, recalcitrant staphylococcal infec-tions and to prevent the carrier state. Success has been limited, probably because circulating antibodies play a relatively minor role in these infections.

CONCLUSION

Staphylococci are potent pathogens, widely found in the human environment, and may cause a variety of infections. They are hardy organisms that can survive under adverse conditions. They possess a large number of virulence factors that allow them to cause serious diseases by different mechanisms. The most common diseases caused by these versatile pathogens are pyogenic infections, sometimes leading to the formation of abscesses in deep tissues. They can also cause distinct disease entities by making specific toxins. Staphylococci have acquired antimicrobial resistance promptly after the introduction of new antibiotics. Currently, many strains are resistant to all but one or two available antibiotics, and the prospect of the emergence of a strain resistant to all available antibiotics is a serious concern.

SELF-ASSESSMENT QUESTIONS

1. What general types of diseases are caused by staphylococci? Which are the most frequent and serious?
2. What are the structural, physiologic, and ecologic characteristics of the staphylococci? Which are the main types?
3. For each of the different staphylococcal diseases, describe how the organisms are encountered?
4. How do staphylococci enter deep tissues? How do they set up residence? How do they cause disease? Why are these questions particularly difficult to answer for some staphylococcal infections but not for others?
5. How does the body respond to different staphylococcal infections?
6. What are the therapeutic problems encountered in different staphylococcal infections? How has this changed through recent history?

SUGGESTED READINGS

Gemmell CG. Staphylococcal scalded skin syndrome. J Med Microbiol. 1995; 43:318–327.

Foster TJ, McDevitt, D. Surface-associated proteins of *Staphylococcus aureus:* Their possible role in virulence. FEMS Microbiol. Letters 1994;118:199.

Radetsky P. The rise and (maybe not the) fall of toxic shock syndrome. Science 1985;85:72.

Sheagren JN. *Staphylococcus aureus:* the persistent pathogen. N Engl J Med 1984;310:1386 (Part l), 1437 (Part 2).

Todd JK. Staphylococcal toxin syndromes. Annu Rev Med. 1985;36:337–347.

Tranter HS. Foodborne staphylococcal illness. Lancet 1990; 336:1044–1046.

CHAPTER

12

Streptococci

ELLEN WHITNACK

NEIL L. BARG

Key Concepts

The streptococci:

- Can be classified according to hemolysis pattern, Lancefield group, or species. This chapter discusses all the streptococci excluding the pneumococcus, which is covered in Chapter 13, "Pneumococcus."
- Include Group A streptococci (*Streptococcus pyogenes*), which causes "strep throat," scarlet fever, and impetigo. Rheumatic fever and glomerulonephritis are nonsuppurative sequels of strep infection.
- Include Group B streptococci (*Streptococcus agalactiae*), the leading cause of neonatal sepsis and meningitis; Groups C and G streptococci, which cause infections similar to Group A infections; minute-colony streptococci, which cause abscesses; Group D streptococci, which include the enterococci and nonenterococci; and viridans streptococci, which cause subacute bacterial endocarditis and dental caries.

The streptococci are a heterogeneous group of bacteria comprising species that colonize and infect humans and animals. In humans, they cause many diseases, including strep throat, neonatal meningitis, brain abscess, endocarditis, and gangrene. Members of this diverse group of organisms share several features. They exhibit Gram-positive staining and grow in chains resembling short strings of beads. They also undergo fermentative (anaerobic) metabolism, although most streptococci are oxygen-tolerant and grow readily in air. (Strictly anaerobic streptococci are in a different genus—*Peptostreptococcus*—and are discussed in Chapter 15, "*Bacteroides*").

Streptococci are classified in three different ways, each of which has some clinical significance.

- Hemolysis pattern: When grown (as is customary) on blood agar, which is red and nearly opaque, streptococcal colonies may be surrounded by a zone of partial hemolysis with a greenish discoloration of the hemoglobin (α-hemolysis) or a clear zone of complete hemolysis (β-hemolysis). No zone surrounds nonhemolytic (γ-hemolytic) streptococci. The toxins that cause the hemolysis are neutralized in body fluids and do not cause hemolysis in vivo.
- **Lancefield group:** Streptococci may be grouped serologically according to their major cell-wall carbohydrate antigens. Groups are lettered A through T; however, some streptococci cannot be assigned to any of these groups.
- **Species:** Like other bacteria, streptococci are grouped into species according to their metabolic reactions in various culture media. Several dozen species exist.

These classifications are independent of one another, in that a given species may encompass more than one group or hemolysis pattern and vice versa. The result is a fearful muddle, but fortunately the classification can be simplified for clinical purposes. We will use a scheme shown in Figure 12.1, which is a slightly condensed ver-

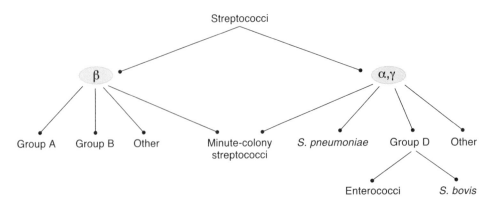

Figure 12.1. A classification of streptococci. β-hemolytic streptococci are sometimes called simply "hemolytic streptococci." α- and γ-hemolytic streptococci are lumped because most species or groups on this side of the diagram include strains of both hemolytic patterns. Often such organisms are called "viridans" (greening) streptococci after the greenish color seen in α hemolysis.

sion of one actually used in many hospital laboratories. The pneumococcus (*Streptococcus pneumoniae*) is so important that it is covered in a separate chapter (Chapter 13, "The Pneumococcus"). In this chapter, we discuss the remaining groups. Pride of place is given to the group A streptococcus, because it has caused the greatest variety of diseases, killed the most people, and stimulated the most research.

GROUP A STREPTOCOCCI

■ CASE 1

J., a 6-year-old boy, came home from school tired and cranky. By suppertime he was hot and flushed and complained of a sore throat. He refused to eat and vomited once. His mother took him to an evening clinic, where his temperature was noted to be 39.4°C. The physician found that J. had a red throat with grayish-white exudate on both tonsils and his cervical lymph nodes were enlarged and tender. A throat swab was taken for a rapid enzyme immunoassay to detect streptococcal group A antigen; it was positive. The physician said that if J. could take medicine three times a day for 10 days without fail, he could avoid a shot. J. nodded vigorously to this suggestion; his mother looked dubious. J. got a shot of a long-acting penicillin preparation. Two days later, he had recovered.

■ CASE 2

The year was 1846, the place, the Allgemeines Krankenhaus in Vienna. Frau M., a 31-year-old woman, had been delivered of her fourth child on the previous day after 36 hours of labor. She had lost quite a bit of blood and had been pale, weak, and restless all afternoon. Early in the evening she suddenly had a shaking chill, then a high fever. The lochia (postpartum uterine discharge) became thin and

malodorous. By midnight, Frau M. was delirious, with a weak, thready pulse; by morning, she was dead. Hers was the sixth such case of childbed fever on Division A that week.

The following questions arise:

1. Is "strep throat" a trivial disease? Why is treatment important?
2. Why did J.'s physician insist on 10 days of treatment and use long-acting instead of regular penicillin?
3. Were J.'s sore throat and Frau M.'s death caused by the same kind of streptococci?
4. How do people "catch" streptococci? Are they part of the normal bacterial flora?
5. J.'s throat showed purulent inflammation. Is pus typical of streptococcal diseases? Do streptococci cause pus by the same mechanisms as, say, the staphylococci?

Most group A streptococci are β-hemolytic and belong to the species *Streptococcus pyogenes*; for practical purposes, "group A strep" and "*S. pyogenes*" are synonyms. This organism has caused human disease since antiquity but seems to have reached the peak of its virulence in the 19th century, when it was a dangerous scourge. Indeed, until the middle of the present century, serious streptococcal diseases were common and much feared. **Strep throat** and **scarlet fever** (strep throat with a red skin rash) were dreaded for their frequent complications which include peritonsillar abscess ("quinsy"), otitis, mastoiditis, bacteremia, sepsis, and meningitis. As recently as the 1930s, group A streptococci were the most common cause of **sepsis**, accounting for perhaps two-thirds of the cases. Streptococcal pharyngitis (J.'s problem) was not infrequently followed by **acute**

rheumatic fever, an inflammatory disease affecting the heart and joints that could permanently damage the heart valve and lead to lifelong disability and early death from embolic stroke, bacterial endocarditis, or heart failure. Entire wards—indeed, entire hospitals—were once devoted to the care of children with acute rheumatic fever. Group A streptococcal **pneumonia** was noted for its aggressiveness and its tendency to produce large empyemas (collections of purulent fluid in the pleural cavity). **Impetigo**, itself a trivial streptococcal skin infection, could be followed by **acute glomerulonephritis**; this problem could also occur following strep throat.

Streptococcal infections of the soft tissues were often fatal; **erysipelas**, an infection of the skin and subcutaneous tissues, swept through Civil War encampments "like a scythe," as historian James McPherson describes. Streptococcal **necrotizing fasciitis** and myositis could complicate any wound with lethal results unless the infected tissue was excised or amputated. Combat surgeons dreaded "hospital gangrene," as streptococcal necrotizing fasciitis was called, and to this day, battle-casualties are routinely treated with prophylactic penicillin.

Finally, the group A streptococcus was the most common cause of Frau M.'s affliction, **puerperal or childbed fever** (postpartum endomyometritis and sepsis). It was this organism that Ignaz Semmelweis was unknowingly combating when, suspecting contagion via material carried on the hands of physicians who had performed autopsies, he required doctors attending parturient women at the Allgemeines Krankenhaus to disinfect their hands with chloride of lime. The death rate fell from 9.92% in 1847 to 1.27% two years later, earning Semmelweis a permanent place in the medical pantheon, although not in his lifetime.

Simple strep throat and impetigo are still common infections, but the incidence of serious streptococcal infections, as well as rheumatic fever, has been decreasing throughout this century and particularly since World War II, at least in developed countries. The nature of the organism seems to have changed. Perhaps improved living standards (better hygiene, less crowding), along with the widespread use of penicillin, have interfered with the rapid person-to-person transmission of the organism necessary for maximal expression of its virulence factors. As of the mid-1980s, serious streptococcal disease seems to be nearly extinct.

However, in 1985, an outbreak of rheumatic fever occurred in Salt Lake City. Although the outbreak was nothing like the old days, it was dramatic nonetheless: 18.1 cases per 100,000 children per year, which represented an eightfold increase over the previous 15-year average. Subsequently, outbreaks occurred in several other locations, particularly in the Ohio valley, and an increased incidence of acute rheumatic fever over baseline levels was reported nationwide. At the same time, case reports of invasive streptococcal infections began to accumulate. For instance, streptococcal pneumonia killed Jim Henson, creator of the Muppets. An even more dramatic—if not melodramatic—illness to gain attention in recent years is **streptococcal toxic shock syndrome (strep TSS)**. This sepsis-like condition with shock and multiorgan failure kills up to a third of its victims, including healthy young people, despite antibiotic treatment. In contrast to staphylococcal TSS (Chapter 11, "*Staphylococcus*"), strep TSS often coexists with bacteremia, necrotizing fasciitis, or both. The fasciitis may begin at a site of trivial trauma, or it may be blood-borne. This feature of the illness has earned the infecting strains the sobriquet "flesh-eating bacteria" from the tabloid press. The resurgence of invasive infections such as these has stimulated a renewed interest in the group A streptococcus, together with apprehension at the return of an old enemy.

ENCOUNTER

Group A streptococci live on human skin and mucous membranes; pharyngeal carriage rates among school-aged children in the winter months can be as high as 20%. The organism spreads from person to person, asymptomatically for the most part, probably by infected droplets and perhaps by hand-to-hand-to-mouth contact. Food-borne outbreaks of streptococcal pharyngitis occur occasionally when food handled by a carrier is allowed to stand at room temperature. In the case of skin and wound infections, additional modes of transmission by fomites such as towels, shed skin scales, and direct skin-to-skin contact seem likely.

ENTRY

The first step in the establishment of a streptococcal infection, as for all epithelial infections, is adherence of the bacteria to epithelial cells. Adherence allows the organisms to multiply without being swept away by fluid secretions. The first streptococcal **adhesin** to be described was **lipoteichoic acid (LTA)**. Teichoic acid and LTA are constituents of the cell envelope of many Gram-positive bacteria (Chapter 3, "Biology of Infectious Agents"). The LTA of group A streptococci is a polymer of about 25 glycerolphosphate subunits with a lipid (palmitate) attached at one end. Streptococci with abundant LTA on their surfaces are generally sticky, but they also interact specifically with **fibronectin**, a host protein that coats the epithelial cells of the oropharynx. This interaction is mediated by the lipid moiety. It is unusual for a hydrophobic structure of any size to protrude from a cell surface, and it is thought that the LTA may be

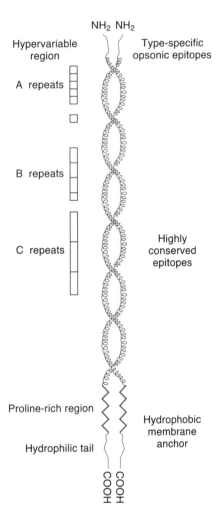

Figure 12.2. Group A streptococcal M protein. M protein molecules are typically about 500 residues long. They are anchored in the cell membrane by a hydrophobic sequence near the carboxy terminus; they then traverse the cell wall via a sequence rich in glycine and proline, and finally emerge to project from the cell wall as fibrils. The fibrils are mostly α-helical, and contain two or three blocks of repeating amino acid sequences. There is a seven-residue periodicity in the placement of hydrophobic amino acids that favors a coiled-coil conformation, so that each fibril actually consists of two α-helical M molecules wound about each other. The proximal portion of the molecule binds the complement control protein factor H. The amino-terminal halves, despite their structural heterogeneity, retain the ability to bind fibrinogen, which protects the organism from nonspecific opsonization by the alternative pathway of complement.

forced into this inside-out orientation due to the binding of its polyglycerol phosphate backbone to surface proteins. In recent years, several more adhesins have been discovered, including F protein, a fibronectin-binding protein found in many streptococcal strains. These adhesins may be critically important for adherence of the strains that possess them.

SPREAD

The spread of group A streptococci in tissues seems to depend on how the infection is acquired. Infections of the skin or mucous membranes usually remain well localized. Impetigo, at worst, becomes an inflamed ulcer called ecthyma. Pharyngeal infections may be locally very severe, with necrosis and abscess formation in and around the tonsils and, occasionally, with seeding of the bloodstream; however, spread to adjacent tissues is uncommon. When spread does occur, the result is usually facial erysipelas. Streptococci can infect other epithelia of the upper respiratory tract, such as the sinuses and the middle ear, where again they may be locally invasive, as in mastoiditis. Only a few cases of TSS with strep throat have been reported.

In contrast, streptococci infecting deeper tissues (as in a wound) may spread rapidly. The reason for this rapid spread may be that streptococci secrete digestive enzymes including proteases, hyaluronidase, DNase, and streptokinase. **Streptokinase** binds to host plasminogen to form complexes that catalyze the conversion of plasminogen to plasmin, which, in turn, degrades fibrin and a number of other proteins. (A similar enzyme secreted by group C streptococci has been used as a "clot-buster" to open the coronary arteries of patients with heart attacks.) Together, these enzymes allow the streptococcus to break down almost any large molecule in its path, permitting rapid spread through tissues. Indeed, pus from streptococcal infections is characteristically thin and runny because the large molecules responsible for the viscosity of pus—principally DNA and fibrin—have been degraded. It is not surprising, therefore, that *Clostridium perfringens*, the agent of classical gas gangrene, elaborates many of the same kinds of enzymes (see Chapter 20, "Clostridia").

MULTIPLICATION

To multiply in tissues, streptococci must avoid phagocytosis. Resistance to phagocytosis is the best understood virulence mechanism of the group A streptococcus. At least two surface molecules are responsible for this resistance: **M protein**, a rod-shaped molecule that projects from the surface of the bacterial cell as a layer of fuzz, and **hyaluronic acid**, which forms a mucoid capsule. A C5a peptidase, which inactivates a potent phagocyte chemotaxin made during complement activation (Chapter 6, "Constitutive Defenses"), may be an additional resistance factor.

M Protein

M protein (Fig. 12.2) is the most important antiphagocytic factor of *S. pyogenes* and is the central player in *streptococcal pathogenesis*. This protein is required for virulence; organisms lacking M protein are readily opsonized by complement via the alternate pathway. Organisms bearing M protein bind fibrinogen, fibrin, and their degradation products to form a dense coating on the organism's surface that **blocks complement deposition** (Fig. 12.3). The fibrinogen molecules bind to the outer halves of the M protein molecules, near the tips. Even in the absence of fibrinogen and its derivatives, M protein-bearing streptococci are poorly opsonized by the alternate pathway. M proteins bind factor H, a protein that inhibits the cleavage of the complement protein C3 converting without cleavage of C3, complement cannot be activated. The proximal halves of the M protein are the site of factor H binding. High concentrations of factor H may thus accumulate among the fibrillae, ready to pounce on any C3 convertase that forms on the surface of the streptococci.

Fortunately for the host, the body has devised a way around these antiopsonic defenses. The tips of the M protein molecules project past the fibrinogen coat, so that antibody to M protein can opsonize the organism. Antibody to M protein is the only antistreptococcal antibody definitely known to opsonize group A streptococci, and, once acquired, it protects the host against infection. Unfortunately for us, **nearly 100 different M proteins (serotypes) exist**, and anti-M antibody is type-specific. Therefore, repeated strep infections with different serotypes are possible. The carboxy halves of the M molecule are highly conserved from one serotype to another, but the amino terminal halves vary, especially at the tips, where the M protein binds opsonic antibody. This antigenic or serotypic variation provides a means for the organism to maintain itself in the human population. As more individuals become immune to a particular M protein, new variants then appear. M protein molecules contain blocks of amino acid sequence repeats that are only about 40 residues long; new epitopes can arise by recombination at a rate exceeding the usual random mutation rates.

Hyaluronic Acid Capsule

The hyaluronic acid capsule is another antiphagocytic structure on the streptococcal surface. It makes the organism slippery and interferes with the attachment of phagocytes. Paradoxically, Group A streptococci secrete a hyaluronidase that destroys this capsule in the course of tissue infections. The capsule also interferes with attachment to epithelial cells in vitro, yet these organisms can attach quite efficiently in vivo. These organisms shut off capsule production—or turn on hyaluronidase production—when it encounters epithelial surfaces. Streptococci recovered during outbreaks of acute rheumatic fever are usually heavily encapsulated. Hyaluronic acid is, at most, only weakly immunogenic, as it is a "self" antigen. What, then, is its role in the pathogenesis of rheumatic fever? Is its synthesis coregulated with that of a rheumatogenic antigen? These questions are as yet unanswered.

DAMAGE

Streptococci characteristically evoke an intense inflammatory response in tissues. The organisms elaborate many substances that can damage mammalian cells or activate phagocytes and lymphocytes, but their exact role in vivo is not known for at least two reasons: isogenic mutants are only just now becoming available, and good animal models for infections by these organisms are lacking. Recent interest has focused on the **streptococcal pyrogenic exotoxins (SPEs)** because of their likely involvement in streptococcal TSS.

The three streptococcal pyrogenic exotoxins (SPEs) A, B, and C belong to a larger family of pyrogenic toxins that includes the staphylococcal enterotoxins and staphylococcal TSS toxin (see Chapter 11, "*Staphylococcus*"). Although these proteins are structurally diverse, they share some sequence homology. SPEs have also been called "erythrogenic toxins" because they are responsible for the red rash of scarlet fever. Pyro-

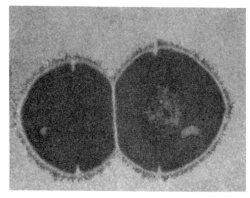
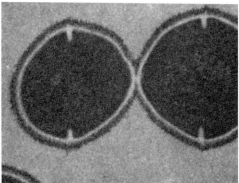

Figure 12.3. Group A streptococci. *Top panel*: Organisms as they appear after growth in broth culture. Note the fuzzy layer on the surface, which is made of M protein and LTA. The hyaluronate capsule is in a dehydrated and collapsed state because of the fixation process, and cannot be seen. *Bottom panel*: The same streptococci after brief immersion in plasma. Note the dense appearance of the fuzzy layer, which is produced by fibrinogen bound to the M protein. In this young culture, the chains are two or three bacterial cells long. Crosswalls are beginning to form in preparation for the next cell division.

genic exotoxins have a number of biological properties in common. They are T-cell mitogens (or, more accurately, **superantigens**; see below), and they enhance delayed hypersensitivity reactions and suppress antibody responses. SPEs potentiate the biological effects of Gram-negative endotoxin, and, like endotoxin, stimulate monocytes to release **tumor necrosis factor** and **interleukin-1**, the principal mediators of septic shock (see Chapter 63, "Sepsis"). The reappearance of severe shock-inducing streptococcal infections has been epidemiologically associated with the reappearance of SPE A in streptococcal isolates, much as in former days, when severe scarlet fever was mostly caused by streptococci that elaborated SPE A. However, not all isolates from invasive infections elaborate SPE A, and many strains elaborate SPE A without being invasive. Still, exotoxins such as SPE A and others are the most likely explanation for the streptococcal TSS. The search is on for pathogenetic factors common to these invasive strains, many of which seem to be genetically related.

ACUTE RHEUMATIC FEVER

The incidence of severe, life-threatening streptococcal infections may be increasing, but these infections are still relatively uncommon. Far more common is simple strep throat, which in most cases would resolve without treatment. Strep throat is unique, however, in that it is the only infection that may be followed by **acute rheumatic fever (ARF)**, which can be an extremely serious disease. ARF is a **nonsuppurative sequel** of group A streptococcal pharyngitis, as opposed to suppurative complications such as peritonsillar abscess. ARF manifests in most patients as **polyarthritis, carditis,** or both. Other manifestations include a neurological disorder known as Sydenham's chorea (St. Vitus's dance), subcutaneous nodules, and a distinctive serpiginous rash called erythema marginatum. All of these manifestations eventually resolve, except for carditis.

In the most severe cases, patients with acute rheumatic carditis die of intractable heart failure during the acute attack. More commonly, they survive and recover; but in some patients (generally those with more severe symptoms during the acute attack), cardiac damage progresses insidiously to severe **valvular scarring,** with both narrowing of the orifice (stenosis) and inability to close properly, resulting in back-flow (regurgitation). Valvular scarring creates a new set of complications, some of which are directly caused by impaired heart function, others by infection of the damaged valves by bacteria that find their way into the bloodstream (bacterial endocarditis; see Chapter 64, "Intravascular Infections").

Some Key Observations about Acute Rheumatic Fever

The following are key observations about ARF:

- Only group A streptococci cause ARF, and the pharynx is the only site of infection that is ever followed by ARF. Some group A serotypes are rheumatogenic, others are not.
- The streptococcal infection must evoke an immune response in the host in order to cause ARF. Carriage of the organism without an immune response, or symptomatic infection without an immune response (as sometimes occurs when patients are treated promptly, and even, on occasion, in untreated cases), does not result in ARF.
- ARF can be completely prevented by treating streptococcal pharyngitis with penicillin. Treatment can be delayed for as much as a week and still be effective, but it must continue until all infecting organisms are eradicated, which can only be reliably achieved with ten days of treatment. In fact, the main objective in giving penicillin to any patient with a sore throat is to prevent acute rheumatic fever.
- ARF can occur after asymptomatic infection; indeed, one-third or more of ARF patients cannot recall a sore throat. However, these patients' high titers of antibodies to various streptococcal antigens indicate a previous streptococcal infection.
- ARF itself does not respond to penicillin, nor is there convincing evidence of streptococcal cells, living, dead, or fragmented, in affected tissues.
- Once a person has had an attack of ARF, he or she remains highly susceptible to recurrences following subsequent bouts of streptococcal pharyngitis, each of which may cause further heart damage. These patients must take prophylactic antibiotics into adulthood, if not for life.
- Innate resistance to strep throat has not been demonstrated, but no more than 10% of people are susceptible to rheumatic fever.

Pathogenesis of Acute Rheumatic Fever

ARF is caused only by some strains of group A streptococci, and only when infecting the pharynx, and only in some humans. It is not surprising that the pathogenesis of this disease has baffled seven generations of investigators. The leading hypothesis for some years has been that ARF is an **autoimmune disease** evoked by the streptococcal infection. Streptococci possess a number of antigens that cross-react, that is, **share epitopes**, with human tissues, notably heart muscle and valvular connective tissue. Some of these epitopes are components of the M protein molecule. Antibodies to certain purified M proteins react with myosin, phosphorylase, and several other unidentified proteins in heart tissue, as well as with proteins in the brain and synovium. Furthermore, autoantibodies are found in the blood of persons with ARF. The existence of these antibodies may appear to be strong circumstantial evidence for humoral autoimmune disease, but, in fact, these antibodies are not likely to be the explanation for ARF. For one thing, autoantibodies are also found in persons who have had uncomplicated pharyngitis, although in lower titer. Another argument against a role for autoantibodies is that the latent period between pharyngitis and ARF is just as long in recurrent attacks as in initial attacks.

Current research on the pathogenesis of ARF is focused on the hypothesis that cellular autoimmunity, rather than humoral autoimmunity, is the pathogenetic mechanism, and that streptococcal antigens evoke **cross-reactive T cells**. For example, various streptococcal preparations, including fragments of M protein containing the heart cross-reactive epitopes, stimulate the production of cytotoxic T cells that react against cultured cardiac myocytes. Streptococcal **superantigens** (including the pyrogenic exotoxins and several other molecules, possibly including M protein) are another area of interest. Superantigens, like ordinary antigens, stimulate T-cell proliferation when bound to class II major histocompatibility complex (MHC) molecules on antigen-presenting cells (Chapter 7, "Induced Defenses"). However, instead of interacting with the antigen-binding groove on these cells, they interact with conserved regions of the V domain of the T-cell receptor. As a result of this binding, many lymphocytes are activated. An ordinary antigen might stimulate 1 in 10,000 lymphocytes; a superantigen stimulates as many as 1 in 5. The superantigen phenomenon could conceivably account for the breakdown of tolerance to self-antigens and the induction of autoimmunity; autoreactive T cells are among the clones stimulated.

ACUTE GLOMERULONEPHRITIS

Acute glomerulonephritis (AGN) is the other important nonsuppurative sequel of streptococcal infection. AGN is caused by only a few M serotypes and probably only certain strains within those serotypes. This disease differs from ARF in several ways. Unlike ARF, AGN may follow either pharyngitis or impetigo, and probably other streptococcal infections as well. In some outbreaks, the attack rate is as high as 40%, suggesting that susceptibility is common, if not universal. Recurrent attacks are rare, probably because the number of nephritogenic strains is so limited. AGN is not reliably prevented by penicillin treatment.

AGN results in hypoalbuminemia (because of a glomerular protein leak) and salt retention. Patients look pale, with puffy eyes and swollen hands and feet. Their urine contains high quantities of protein, leukocytes, and erythrocytes, so many that the urine may have a smoky or rusty appearance. The severity of AGN ranges from asymptomatic (detected only by urinalysis)

to acute renal shutdown, but most patients do well with treatment.

The pathogenesis of acute glomerulonephritis may involve an inflammatory response evoked by **immune complexes**: lumpy deposits of immunoglobulin G (IgG) and complement (C3) are found on the epithelial side of the glomerular basement membrane, and complement levels in the blood are depressed. The nature of the antigens involved is not known. Autoimmunity is a possibility, in that cross-reactions have been described between streptococcal antigens and glomerular tissue. Alternatively, streptococcal antigens could be deposited in the glomeruli, either before or after complexing with antibody. Several candidate antigens are currently under investigation.

DIAGNOSIS AND TREATMENT OF GROUP A STREPTOCOCCAL INFECTIONS

The diagnosis of group A streptococcal infections other than pharyngitis is straightforward. Impetigo and erysipelas can be diagnosed by sight: impetigo is a cluster of small vesicles on a pink base that break down to honey-colored crusts, and erysipelas is a raised, fiery red patch of skin with a sharply demarcated, rapidly advancing margin (see Fig. 61.1). Severe infections such as fasciitis and sepsis can be diagnosed by cultures of pus and blood. In such serious diseases, antibiotics active against streptococci should be started immediately, without waiting for the cultures to grow.

The diagnosis of pharyngitis, on the other hand, can be problematic. Strep throat cannot be distinguished from viral pharyngitis by physical examination, so definitive diagnosis requires **throat culture**. The results take 2 or 3 days to come back; therefore, the patient must either undergo (possibly unnecessary) penicillin treatment or return for a second visit. In addition, because of the high rate of asymptomatic carriage, 50% of positive cultures obtained at the peak of the strep season may not represent true infection. Currently (as in J.'s case), a test for the group A carbohydrate antigen is performed in the physician's office, which can be accomplished in less than an hour using a commercial kit. These kits use antigroup A carbohydrate antibodies in **latex agglutination tests or enzyme immunoassays**. Like cultures, these tests suffer from the carriage vs. infection problem, but at least the results are available before the patient goes home. The rapid tests are not as sensitive as a throat culture, so a negative result must be confirmed by culture.

Standard treatment for pharyngitis is a single injection of a slowly absorbed penicillin (benzathine penicillin), which produces detectable blood levels of penicillin for 3–4 weeks. Oral penicillin can be used, but it is less reliable because patients tend to stop taking it as soon as they feel better, which is not **sufficient therapy** to eradicate the organism and prevent ARF. Like diagnosis, treatment has its knotty issues. Penicillin is not 100% effective; should the patient be retested in 10 to14 days to make sure that the streptococci have been eradicated? If the organism is still present, does it represent persistent, dangerous infection or merely a harmless post-treatment carrier state? (Postinfection carriage is seen in many types of epithelial infections.) How should a patient whose treatment has failed be retreated, given that penicillin did not work the first time? Discussion of such issues is beyond the scope of this text. It is important to realize that strep throat is not a simple problem, and that hundreds of millions of dollars—and some lives—hang on the answers to these questions.

The diagnosis of ARF rheumatic fever depends on **evidence of a preceding streptococcal infection.** This evidence is best obtained by serological tests, of which three are in common use: antistreptolysin O, anti-DNAase B, and a commercial latex agglutination test (Streptozyme) which is made with a mixture of streptococcal antigens. The antistreptolysin O and anti-DNAase B tests are preferred for the diagnosis of ARF.

PREVENTION OF STREPTOCOCCAL INFECTIONS

The only way to prevent streptococcal infection is to take antibiotics, usually penicillin unless the patient is allergic to it. Preventive therapy is prescribed for household contacts of ARF patients, for closed populations (e.g., military recruits) to control and prevent outbreaks, and for persons who have had ARF, to prevent recurrences. The last group must take penicillin continuously, usually in the form of monthly injections of benzathine penicillin.

Clearly, a streptococcal **vaccine** would be desirable. One approach to strep A vaccine is to evoke the type-specific anti-M antibody that opsonizes streptococci of that serotype and protects against infection. A vaccine could, therefore, consist of purified M proteins of all the prevalent serotypes. However, the vaccine must exclude epitopes that cross-react with human tissues. Development of such a vaccine is laborious but technically feasible, and is, in fact, in progress. A second approach is to find an immunogen that protects against multiple serotypes, perhaps by evoking antibodies that block adherence to epithelial cells or the binding of fibrinogen. Such a vaccine would have to act at the mucosal level. Studies of this type of vaccine are also underway, but are at an early stage.

GROUP B STREPTOCOCCI

Most human group B streptococci inhabit the **lower GI and female genital tracts** and belong to the species *Streptococcus agalactiae.* Vaginal colonization is found in 20% or more of healthy women. This figure includes pregnant women, who may pass the organism to their babies during birth. (Other organisms transmitted this way include *Chlamydia trachomatis* and herpes simplex virus (Chapter 69, "Congenital and Neonatal Infections"). If the mother, and therefore the baby, lack protective antibody, the streptococci can invade the mucosae and, in some cases, enter the bloodstream. Group B streptococci are the leading cause of **neonatal sepsis and meningitis** (these two conditions generally appear together). Neonatal group B sepsis is a devastating disease: 10–20% of affected babies die, and one-third to one-half of the survivors have permanent brain damage. Group B streptococci also cause **cellulitis** and blood-borne infections such as **arthritis** and **meningitis** in adults, particularly elderly patients, diabetics, alcoholics, and, on occasion, parturient women. In fact, group B streptococci are the cause of such infections more frequently than are group A. Invasive group A infections, despite their notoriety, are still not all that common.

Unlike the hyaluronate capsule of group A streptococci, the **polysaccharide capsules** of group B streptococci are not host constituents and are, therefore, immunogenic. One serotype, III, accounts for over one-half of neonatal group B streptococcal infections. Anticapsular antibodies opsonize the organisms and protect against invasive disease. The best way to prevent neonatal disease would be to immunize the mother during pregnancy with capsular polysaccharides; her IgG antibodies would cross the placenta and protect the baby. Unfortunately, capsular polysaccharides are not sufficiently immunogenic to evoke an antibody response, and only about 60% of adults make antibodies to type III polysaccharide. Vaccines employing polysaccharide–protein conjugates analogous to *Haemophilus influenzae* vaccines (Chapter 44, "Vaccines") show promise and are currently under development.

OTHER PATHOGENIC STREPTOCOCCI

Other Large-colony Streptococci

The remaining human isolates of β-hemolytic streptococci that make large colonies on agar belong, for the most part, to groups C and G. Although these organisms are similar to group A streptococci and have been termed "pyogenes-like," they are recovered much less frequently. Like group A, they may be isolated from the normal human pharynx, vagina, GI tract, and skin. Both have M protein, and group C streptococci have a hyaluronic acid capsule. Both groups bind fibrinogen, secrete many of the same extracellular enzymes as group A streptococci, and cause similar types of infections including pharyngitis, cellulitis, and blood-borne infections. Both groups have been implicated in AGN, but neither has been known to cause ARF.

Minute-colony Streptococci

Minute-colony streptococci, so-named because the colonies are about the size of a pinhead, are part of the normal flora of the mucous membranes, particularly of the oropharynx. The taxonomy of these organisms is confusing; the designation *"Streptococcus milleri* group*"* is frequently encountered. These organisms may exhibit any of the three hemolytic patterns and belong to some of the same serogroups as large-colony streptococci. However, minute-colony streptococci are quite different from the other groups of streptococci. They are microaerophilic or anaerobic and are most noted for causing **abscesses** in soft tissues, lung, brain, and the abdominal cavity. Other organisms in addition to minute-colony streptococci are often found in these abscesses.

Group D Streptococci

Group D streptococci are, for the most part, α- or γ-hemolytic. They are divided into two groups, **enterococci** and **nonenterococci**. The enterococci have recently been assigned to their own genus, *Enterococcus*. As the name implies, they are part of the normal flora of the GI tract, as well as the genitourinary tract.

If a prize were ever awarded for being "the world's toughest pathogenic bacteria," enterococci would probably win it. These organisms can grow in salt concentrations sevenfold higher than normal tissue fluids, as well as in detergents, including bile. Unlike most other streptococci, they are merely inhibited, not killed, by penicillin, and they are resistant to cephalosporins. Often, treatment of infections such as endocarditis requires two antibiotics to achieve killing. The killing of enterococci by a combination of a cell-wall-active antibiotic such as penicillin and an aminoglycoside is the prototype of **antibiotic synergism.** Penicillin alone only arrests growth, and aminoglycosides such as gentamicin are ineffective except at very high concentrations, but combining these two antibiotics kills the organism. It is thought that the penicillin disrupts the cell wall sufficiently to allow the aminoglycoside to enter the cell and kill it. Unfortunately, many enterococci have become resistant to aminoglycosides even in the presence of penicillin. Even worse, in the 1980s, strains emerged that were resistant to penicillin and even to vancomycin, a cell-wall-active antibiotic that is the ultimate weapon against Gram-positives. **Vancomycin-resistant enterococci (VRE)** have been termed "the nosocomial pathogen of the 90s." Enterococci have been shown to transfer vancomycin-resistant plasmids to staphylococci in the laboratory. Currently, many staphylococci are sensitive only to vancomycin. When and if the transfer occurs in patients, it will "set infectious diseases back 60 years," in the words of recent commentators (Edmond et al., Ann Intern Med 1996;124:329).

Fortunately, enterococci are of low virulence. Usually they are recovered from mixed infections in which they seem to be "along for the ride" with other, more virulent organisms, such as Gram-negative bacilli and anaerobes. Enterococci are being recovered from hospitalized patients more frequently, probably because of the widespread use of cephalosporins, which suppress the competing flora. Bedsores, wounds, and intra-abdominal infections are particularly apt to yield enterococci. Most infections due solely to enterococci are urinary tract infections. Occasionally, however, enterococci cause much more serious disease, particularly endocarditis, which occurs in drug addicts and the elderly.

The **nonenterococcal** group D species that most commonly cause human disease is *Strepococcus bovis*. This organism does not grow in high salt concentrations, and most strains are killed by penicillin. *S. bovis* inhabits the GI tract. Bacteremia caused by this organism is strongly associated with colonic lesions, particularly tumors. Patients with otherwise unexplained *S. bovis* bacteremia are thoroughly investigated for colon cancer.

Viridans Streptococci

Viridans ("greening") streptococci are not specifically identified in most clinical laboratories, which report them simply as "non-β-hemolytic Streptococcus spp." or some such designation. They comprise a number of species inhabiting the normal oropharynx, where they make up 30–60% of the normal bacterial flora. Although in general they are of low virulence, they are the most common cause of **subacute bacterial endocarditis** which affects abnormal heart valves (see Chapter 64, "Intravascular Infections"). Part of the reason why these streptococci are the causes of this disease is simple opportunity: they frequently seed the bloodstream during tooth-brushing, chewing, and the like. In addition, the ability of viridans species to cause endocarditis has been correlated with the production of sticky dextrans, which may facilitate their adherence to platelet-fibrin thrombi that form on damaged valve surfaces. Dextran production is not present in all endocarditis-associated strains, however, and other adherence mechanisms undoubtedly exist. Viridans streptococci have emerged as an important cause of severe sepsis in immunocompromised patients, particularly in certain cancer centers.

The viridans streptococci also include the pathogens responsible for **dental caries**—the "mutans" group, consisting of *Streptococci mutans* and several closely related species. These organisms have surface proteins that bind to salivary glycoproteins deposited on teeth (the pellicle). They thrive on dietary sucrose, which they metabolize into sticky glucan polymers. This process involves the expression of a number of surface proteins, including glucosyltransferases involved in glucan synthesis. In some strains, these proteins mediate attachment of the organisms to the pellicle. (As aside, the notion of specific adherence of bacteria as the first step in pathogenesis, emphasized throughout this book, was first developed by researchers studying dental caries.) Sticky masses of bacteria build up on the tooth surface to form plaque. *S. mutans* is only one of approximately 200 species of bacteria that have been found in plaque, but in an environment well supplied with sucrose, it can amount to 50% or more of the bacteria present. Cavity formation results when the *S. mutans* (and also lactobacilli) ferment sugars to lactic acid, which demineralizes the tooth enamel. Many bacteria carry out lactic acid fermentation; a unique feature of both *S. mutans* and lactobacilli is that they remain metabolically active at low pH, and thus continually produce lactic acid.

Antibody to several of the adhesive surface proteins has been shown to protect against tooth decay in experimental situations, raising the possibility of a vaccine against dental caries. Unfortunately, some of these proteins elicit autoantibodies in experimental animals, including rheumatoid factors and heart-reactive antibodies. Vaccine development will, therefore, depend on the same sophisticated molecular dissection that is currently being used to develop a group A streptococcal vaccine.

SELF-ASSESSMENT QUESTIONS

1. What morphological and physiological properties distinguish the genus *Streptococcus*? What are the main groups within this genus?

2. What factors contribute to spread in streptococcal lesions?

3. Discuss the role of M protein in streptococcal pathogenesis.

4. What are the main diseases caused by the streptococci? How are they grouped by: (a) symptoms; (b) types of streptococci?

5. Discuss the immunological aftermath of suppurative streptococcal infections.

6. What are the problems in the microbiological diagnosis of streptococcal infections?

SUGGESTED READINGS

Bisno AL, Stevens DL. Streptococcal infections of skin and soft tissues. N Engl J Med 1996;334:240–245.

Bronze MS, Dale JB. The reemergence of serious group A streptococcal infections and acute rheumatic fever. Am J Med Sci 1996;311:41–54.

Schwartz B, Facklam RR, Breimen RF. Changing epidemiology of group A streptococcal infection in the USA. Lancet 1990;336:1167–1171.

Stevens DL. Streptococcal toxic-shock syndrome: spectrum of disease, pathogenesis, and new concepts in treatment. Emerging Infect Dis 1995;1:69–78.

Stollerman GH. Rheumatogenic streptococci and the return of rheumatic fever. Adv Intern Med 1990;35:125.

CHAPTER 13

Pneumococcus and Bacterial Pneumonia

GREGORY A. STORCH

Key Concepts

The pneumococcus:

- Is an α-hemolytic streptococcus;
- Is a frequent agent of pneumonias in adults as well as other localized infections, especially in children;
- Causes infections characterized by acute inflammation;
- Has a capsule that makes it resistant to phagocytosis;
- Occurs in many antigenic capsular types, some of which have been used to make a polyvalent vaccine.

The pneumococcus is the most frequent causative agent of acute bacterial pneumonia and one of the classic bacterial pathogens. Although it yields to antibiotic therapy, it remains a serious medical problem, especially in certain risk groups. Recently, antibiotic resistance has become widespread, increasing the difficulty of treating pneumococcal infections.

The pneumococcus, *Streptococcus pneumoniae*, is a Gram-positive coccus that belongs to the group of α-hemolytic streptococci. Its outstanding characteristic is an ample polysaccharide **capsule** that shields it from phagocytosis and which is highly antigenic. The capsule is the main virulence factor of the organism. The bacterium causes disease not by exotoxins but by eliciting a powerful inflammatory reaction.

CASE

Mr. P., a 58-year-old salesman who is a heavy smoker and an alcoholic, noted that he had nasal congestion and a low-grade fever. Two days later he abruptly developed a shaking chill, cough, and severe pain on the right side of his chest that worsened with breathing. The cough was productive of rust-colored sputum. When he was seen in the emergency room, he appeared acutely ill and had a temperature of 104°F. His respiratory rate was relatively rapid at 40/minute. His breathing was shallow, with little movement of the right side of the thorax. This pattern of breathing, in which the patient is reluctant to move one side of the chest due to pain, is known as "splinting."

The laboratory reported that his white blood cell count was 23,000/μL, indicative of leucocytosis (an increase in the number of circulating white blood cells). Twenty-three percent of the white cells were "band" forms, indicative of rapid leucocyte synthesis and mobilization. A chest x-ray revealed consolidation of the right upper lobe (Fig. 13.1). A Gram stain of the sputum showed many neutrophils and lancet-shaped Gram-positive diplococci (Fig. 13.2). Blood was obtained for culture, and treatment was begun with penicillin. Both the blood cultures and sputum cultures were positive for the pneumococcus, *S. pneumoniae*. Two days later Mr. P. was much improved, and, after eight more days on penicillin, he recovered completely.

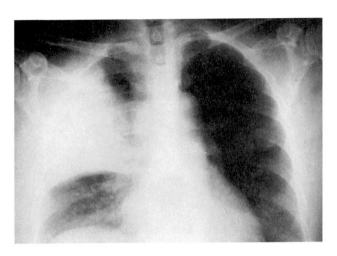

Figure 13.1. Chest x-ray showing homogeneous consolidation involving the right upper lobe. The air spaces of the lobe are filled with liquid.

Mr. P.'s case illustrates many of the classical manifestations of pneumococcal pneumonia: abrupt onset of severe symptoms, ill appearance of the patient, rust-colored sputum, homogeneous involvement of an entire lobe of the lung, leukocytosis, and rapid response to penicillin. **Bacteremia,** the presence of bacteria in the bloodstream, occurs in about 25% of the cases and is indicative of more severe illness. Pneumococcal pneumonia is a dramatic illness that can threaten the life of an affected patient who may have been well only a few days earlier. It was one of the most important causes of death in the pre-antibiotic era. Today, thanks to penicillin and other effective antibiotics, it is less often fatal. Nevertheless, it remains the most common form of bacterial pneumonia and may still be extremely serious. Even now, about 5% of all patients die from it, with fatality rates much higher in elderly or debilitated patients and those with bacteremia, even when they are treated with an appropriate antibiotic.

Many aspects of pneumococcal pneumonia have been carefully studied and merit attention. Perhaps the central motif is that the pneumococcus appears to cause disease by its mere existence: as far as is known, its presence alone elicits an acute inflammation that accounts for the major symptoms. It produces no powerful exotoxins. Other respiratory pathogens, especially *Haemophilus influenzae* type b and *Klebsiella pneumoniae,* also have a thick polysaccharide capsule and do not produce exotoxins. However, the pneumococcus differs from these Gram-negative bacteria in that it does not contain endotoxin.

THE PNEUMOCOCCI

The pneumococcus is classified in the genus *Streptococcus,* based on its morphology and purely fermenta-

tive energy metabolism. Like other "aerobic" streptococci, the pneumococcus is anomalous in its ability to grow in the presence of oxygen, a somewhat unusual feature of strictly fermentative bacteria. The placement of *S. pneumoniae* among the streptococci is supported by the high degree of DNA homology among these organisms.

Pneumococci are Gram-positive bacteria and commonly grow in pairs (diplococci) but may also form short chains. Like other Gram-positive bacteria, pneumococcal cells are surrounded by a cell wall composed of murein and more than a dozen glycopeptides. Recent studies suggest that the cell wall itself is responsible for stimulating much of the inflammatory response associated with pneumococcal infection. Exterior to the cell wall is a **polysaccharide capsule** that imparts a mucoid or "smooth" appearance to colonies on agar. (You may recall that in 1944 Avery, McCarty, and MacLeod demonstrated that an extract derived from smooth pneumococcal strains was able to transform "rough," unencapsulated strains to smooth strains. This experiment led the researchers to conclude that DNA is the carrier of genetic information.)

When a suspension of killed pneumococci is injected into a rabbit, the most abundant antibodies produced are ones directed against the capsular polysaccharide. Antisera against different strains of pneumococci react strongly with the strains used to produce the antiserum and only weakly or not at all with other strains. The existence of some 84 different **serotypes,** each reacting with its specific typing serum, has been established as a result of these experiments. The basis for antigenic difference among serotypes lies in the chemical structure of the capsular polysaccharide. Because the capsule prevents phagocytosis, nonencapsulated strains rarely if ever cause disease and are seldom found in nature. Antibodies to the capsule play a major role in protection

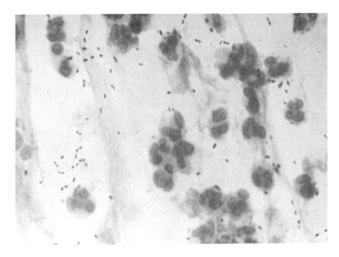

Figure 13.2. Gram stain of sputum revealing many neutrophils and "lancet-shaped" Gram-positive diplococci.

against subsequent infections by pneumococci of the same serotype.

The capsule is not the only pneumococcal component that provides protection against host defenses. Also important is the so-called **C-substance**, a choline containing teichoic acid that is part of the cell wall. The serum of most people contains a **nonantibody β-globulin**, called **C-reactive protein**, that reacts with the C-substance. The complex that results from this reaction activates the complement cascade, leading to the release of inflammatory mediators as well as to the opsonization of the organisms to enhance phagocytosis. Because levels of C-reactive protein are increased in the sera of patients with many inflammatory diseases, not just pneumococcal infection, it is referred to as an **acute phase reactant** (Chapter 6, "Constitutive Defenses"). These characteristics have led to the speculation that C-reactive protein is a primitive, nonspecific host defense mechanism against infection. The fact that all strains of pneumococci have the same C-substance has led to attempts to use this single component in a vaccine that would elicit protection against all serotypes. Unfortunately, this effort has not proved successful to date.

ENCOUNTER

Pneumococcal pneumonia is the most common form of **bacterial pneumonia** acquired in the community (as opposed to hospital-acquired pneumonias, see Chapter 59, "Respiratory System"). It is estimated that approximately 500,000 cases of this disease occur per year in the United States. The incidence is higher in certain subgroups, including children younger than 5 years, adults older than 40, African-Americans, and native Americans. Although the reason for this distribution is not known, poverty and a debilitated state of health are risk factors. Certain diseases also predispose to pneumococcal infections, including sickle cell anemia, Hodgkin's disease, multiple myeloma, HIV infection, and the absence of the spleen for any reason. Alcoholism is also an important risk factor. Pneumococcal infections are also distinctly seasonal, with the highest incidence occurring in the winter and early spring. Most cases are sporadic; however, outbreaks take place, particularly in residential institutions, army barracks, and work camps, where people are housed under crowded conditions.

The **reservoir** of *S. pneumoniae* is thought to be humans who harbor the organism, rather than animals or the inanimate environment. **Transmission** occurs directly from person to person. Interestingly, if the physician had asked Mr. P. whether he had been exposed recently to another person with pneumonia, the answer would probably have been no. Most people who harbor pneumococci experience no symptoms at all.

Colonization by pneumococci typically occurs in the **nasopharynx**. The outcome of colonization may be (1)

BOX 13.1. EXAMPLES OF ENCAPSULATED ORGANISMS

Bacteria

Streptococcus pneumoniae (pneumococcus)
Streptococcus pyogenes (some strains)
Staphylococcus aureus (some strains)
Neisseria meningitidis (meningococcus)
Neisseria gonorrhoeae (gonococcus, some strains)
Haemophilus influenzae
Klebsiella pneumoniae
Escherichia coli (some strains)
Bacteroides fragilis (some strains)

Fungi

Cryptococcus neoformans

clearance of the organisms, (2) asymptomatic persistence for several months (the **carrier state**), or (3) progression to disease. The outcome is determined by the intrinsic virulence of the colonizing strain and the efficiency of host defense mechanisms. Some serotypes of *S. pneumoniae* are more virulent than others. Certain serotypes cause severe disease, whereas others are commonly isolated from the nasopharynx of asymptomatic persons. The interval between colonization and the onset of disease is variable (and ordinarily undefinable in clinical practice), but there is some evidence to suggest that disease is most likely to occur shortly after colonization.

Several aspects of *S. pneumoniae* colonization have been elucidated by longitudinal studies in which nasopharyngeal cultures were obtained at regular intervals from healthy individuals. Pneumococci were recovered in as many as two-thirds of normal preschool children. In general, colonization is less common in adults, although contact with children increases its frequency. The results of one study that illustrates these points are shown in Table 13.1. One individual may become colo-

Table 13.1. Likelihood of Colonization with *S. Pneumoniae*

Group	Percentage with *S. pneumoniae* colonization
Preschool children	38–45
Elementary school children	29–35
Junior high school children	9–25
Adults with children at home	18–29
Adults without children at home	6

PARADIGM   ▪ ▪ ▪

The Bacterial Capsule as Defense Against Opsonization and Phagocytosis

The antiphagocytic capsule that characterizes virulent strains of pneumococcus is also found in a number of other extracellular pathogenic bacteria. Important examples of encapsulated bacteria are *Haemophilus influenzae* type b and *Neisseria meningitidis* (the meningococcus), which, together with the pneumococcus, are the most frequent causes of bacterial meningitis. Nonencapsulated pneumococci are readily opsonized and phagocytized; consequently, they are avirulent. Over ten thousand nonencapsulated pneumococci must be injected into the peritoneal cavity to kill a mouse, but only about 10 encapsulated bacteria—a thousandfold difference in virulence!

Compared with nonencapsulated bacteria, encapsulated pneumococci are not well recognized by the first line of humoral defense in the body, the alternative pathway of the complement system. One function of this system is to opsonize (i.e., make more tasty) the bacterial particles for subsequent phagocytosis. The unopsonized bacteria are virtually ignored by the neutrophils, the host's front line of defense in the bloodstream. Adding to the antidefensive nature of the capsule is that its constituent polysaccharide, which is hydrophilic relative to the surface of the phagocytic cell, is particularly resistant to phagocytosis.

If the capsule provides the pneumococcus with "stealth-like" capability, how is the host able to vanquish this formidable opponent? In the initial encounter, some binding of complement components does occur, so that the bacteria are at least partially opsonized. This degree of opsonization is inadequate to potentiate intravascular phagocytosis (or, in the case of the mouse peritoneal model, intraperitoneal phagocytosis), but it is sufficient to permit clearance by the macrophages of the spleen, the body's premier particle filter. This response assumes, of course, that the quantity of bacteria in the circulation is not too great, as sometimes occurs in severe, neglected pneumococcal pneumonia. Individuals who lack a spleen due to any cause (congenital, sickle cell anemia, posttraumatic or therapeutic splenectomy, etc.), are at grave risk of succumbing to overwhelming sepsis with these encapsulated bacteria, even with a small initial inoculum. Many asplenic patients are advised to keep available a supply of an antibiotic so that they can begin taking it at the first sign of an infection.

Within several weeks following an initial encounter with an encapsulated bacterium, the host develops anticapsular antibodies that protect against future encounters with that strain. Anticapsular antibodies are more efficient than the alternative complement pathway in opsonizing encapsulated bacteria. Even asplenic patients who have anticapsular antibodies are relatively well protected against bacteremia with that strain. For this reason, asplenic individuals should be immunized with pneumococcal vaccine, which contains a mixture of the most common serotypes of pneumococcal capsule.

EDITORS

---

nized many times, usually with different serotypes, and sometimes one individual may even be colonized by more than one pneumococcal serotype simultaneously. The extent to which colonization stimulates the immune response is not known. In one study, 50% of colonized children but only a few adults had antibodies to their homologous strain. It has been suggested that secretory IgA antibodies are important in determining whether or not colonization takes place after exposure.

Transmission from a sick person, or more commonly, from an asymptomatic carrier, is via **droplets** of respiratory secretions that remain airborne over a distance of a few feet. Infecting organisms may also be carried on hands contaminated with secretions. Transmission occurs readily within families and in closed institutions. Since healthy carriers outnumber symptomatic individuals, most of the links in the chain of transmission from person to person are invisible. In contrast, in a disease such as measles, the agent is also transmitted from person to person but asymptomatic colonization does not take place. In measles, each link in the chain is evident.

ENTRY

Most of the time, infections of the lung are prevented by elaborate mechanisms, including the tortuous pathway that air and inhaled particles must follow to reach the lungs, the **epiglottis** that protects the airway from aspiration, the **cough reflex**, the presence of a layer of sticky **mucus** that is continuously swept upward by the cilia of the respiratory epithelium, and **alveolar macrophages**. Ordinarily these mechanisms are highly effective in preventing progression from colonization to infection. However, a number of factors can interfere with these mechanisms, including loss of consciousness, cigarette smoking, alcohol consumption, viral infections, or excess fluid in the lungs.

How do these considerations relate to the case of Mr. P.? The source of the infecting organisms was certainly another individual who may have been entirely healthy. It is possible that Mr. P. had the misfortune to acquire one of the more virulent pneumococcal serotypes. His smoking and alcohol consumption may have depressed his defense mechanisms by weakening his cough reflex and decreasing the activity of alveolar macrophages.

SPREAD, MULTIPLICATION, AND DAMAGE

Pneumococci have a particular predilection for the human respiratory tract, but we do not know the reasons for this marked tropism. Besides the **lung**, they are also a major cause of infection at other sites in the respiratory tract including the paranasal sinuses and the middle ear. In addition, they are one of the three most common causes of bacterial **meningitis**, along with *Haemophilus influenzae* type b and the meningococcus. Finally, pneumococci may cause infection at other sites, such as the heart valves, the conjunctivae, the joints, or the peritoneal cavity.

Much of the information currently known about the pathogenesis of pneumococcal pneumonia is derived from studies carried out in the 1940s by W. Barry Wood and his colleagues. They produced pneumonia by injecting pneumococci suspended in mucin into the bronchi of anesthetized mice. Animals were sacrificed at various intervals and histological sections of the lungs were examined. Four zones of the pneumonic process were identified (Fig. 13.3). In the original study, all four zones were found simultaneously in different regions of the lung, with the first one located at the expanding edge of the involved area. Thus, the four zones correspond to four stages of the inflammatory process.

In the first stage the lung alveoli fill with **serous fluid** containing many organisms but few inflammatory cells. Recent studies suggest that components of the pneumococcal cell wall stimulate the outpouring of fluid and the subsequent inflammatory response. The fluid that fills the alveoli serves as a culture medium for the rapid multiplication of the organisms. This fluid also provides a rapid means of spread of the infection, both into adjacent alveoli through the pores of Kohn and to nearby areas of the lung via the bronchioles. Note that although this outpouring of fluids may have less severe consequences in some organs, in the lungs it threatens the basic function of that organ, namely gas exchange.

In the second stage, called **early consolidation**, the alveoli are infiltrated by neutrophils and red blood cells. Strong **chemotactic signals**, produced by the pneumococci and by the alternate pathway of **complement**, lead to the recruitment of large numbers of neutrophils. The stage is now set for the classic struggle between bacteria and phagocytes. On the one hand, pneumococci resist being taken up due to the presence of their capsule; on the other hand, if they are ingested by the neutrophils, they are rapidly killed. Clearly, the extent of successful phagocytosis determines the outcome of the infection. Fortunately, the immune system employs various mechanisms that make even the heavily encapsulated pneumococci more "digestible" to the neutrophils. If the patient has had previous contact with pneumococci of the invading serotype, he or she will have developed type-specific antibodies that interact with complement to op-

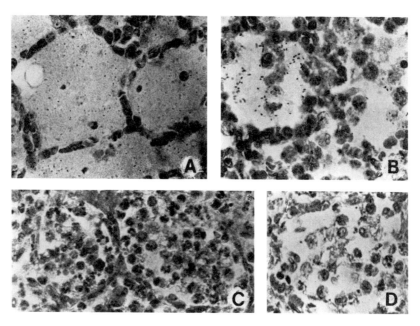

Figure 13.3. Four zones or stages of lung involvement in pneumococcal pneumonia. Pneumonia was induced in rats by intrabronchial installation of live pneumococci suspended in mucin. **A.** Alveoli filled with clear exudate (×430). **B.** Early consolidation. Organisms are plentiful, and some are engulfed by neutrophils (×430). **C.** Late consolidation. A closely packed cellular infiltrate is present and phagocytosis of organisms has occurred (×530). **D.** Resolution found at center of lesion. Macrophages are present, and the exudate is beginning to clear (×430).

sonize the organisms and facilitate their uptake. If the individual lacks specific immunity, the organisms may be opsonized by complement components, activated by the alternative pathway and possibly by the interaction of pneumococcal C-substance with C-reactive protein of the serum. Binding of complement components differs among pneumococcal serotypes, which may explain in part why some serotypes are more virulent than others.

In the case of our patient, Mr. P., neutrophils failed to contain the pneumococci early on, and the infection progressed to adjacent areas until it involved a whole lobe of his left lung. What accounted for his fever and ill appearance? We do not know. Although Mr. P.'s lung involvement was serious, the resulting impairment of gas exchange does not fully explain why the patient becomes so sick in this disease. It is likely that the systemic manifestations are due either directly to pneumococcal components in the circulation, or to products of the inflammatory response induced by the bacteria.

The third stage of pneumococcal pneumonia is called **late consolidation**. Here, the alveoli are packed with victorious neutrophils and only a few remaining pneumococci. On a macroscopic level, the affected areas of the lungs are heavy and resemble the liver in appearance, a state that early pathologists called **hepatization**. In the fourth and final stage, or **resolution**, neutrophils are replaced by scavenging macrophages, which clear the debris resulting from the inflammatory process. One of the remarkable aspects of pneumococcal pneumonia is that in most cases the architecture of the lung is eventually restored to its normal condition. This restoration is different from what takes place in many other forms of pneumonia, where recovery is accompanied by necrosis and normal lung tissue is replaced by fibrous scar tissue.

Pneumococcal pneumonia may lead to both local and distant complications. The most common local complication is **pleural effusion**, the outpouring of fluid into the pleura, that occurs in about one-quarter of all cases. Usually, the pleural fluid effused is a sterile exudate, stimulated by the adjacent inflammation. However, in about 1% of cases, pneumococci can be isolated from this site. Infection of the pleural space is called **empyema**, a condition that is treated by drainage of the infected fluid and administration of appropriate antibiotics.

Distant complications of pneumococcal pneumonia result from spread of the organisms via the bloodstream. In the early stages of pneumonia, the organisms may enter the lymphatic vessels draining the infected area of the lungs, pass into the thoracic duct, and from there into the bloodstream. Pneumococcemia can be documented by positive blood cultures in about 25% of all cases. However, pneumococcemia probably occurs much more often, at least transiently. When bacteremia is present, the organisms may cause infection at secondary sites, such as the meninges, heart valves, joints, or peritoneal cavity. Had Mr. P. not responded quickly to penicillin

therapy, the physician caring for him would have been on guard for such complications.

Host defenses against pneumococcal bacteremia depend largely on the **lymphoreticular system** to remove circulating bacteria from the bloodstream. **Humoral factors**, including antibodies, complement, and perhaps C-reactive protein, assist macrophages in the spleen, liver, and lymph nodes in carrying out their filtering function. The critical role of the spleen is demonstrated by the overwhelming bacteremia that sometimes strikes individuals whose spleens have been removed surgically, or whose splenic functions are compromised by another disease such as sickle cell anemia.

DIAGNOSIS

Pneumococcal pneumonia can often be suspected on clinical grounds. Although the astute physician may be able to make an educated guess, laboratory confirmation is essential. The first step is to perform a **Gram stain** of a specimen of sputum. If it contains neutrophils and more than ten lancet-shaped Gram-positive diplococci per oil-immersion field, the diagnosis of pneumococcal pneumonia is likely. In the case of Mr. P., the results of the Gram stain of sputum confirmed the clinical suspicion and justified the use of penicillin as initial therapy.

In Mr. P.'s case, final identification was made by culturing the sputum. The culture was performed by streaking the specimen on **blood agar** and **chocolate agar** (so called because of its appearance, due to its content of boiled blood). Pneumococcal colonies are surrounded by an area of α-**hemolysis**, familiar to those who have seen it. Since most streptococci normally present in the body are also α-hemolytic, pneumococci must be differentiated by other properties, e.g., their lancet shape, and their sensitivity to a compound called **optochin**. Because pneumococci are fastidious organisms with exacting growth requirements, they are not always cultured from sputum of patients with pneumococcal pneumonia. Thus, a negative sputum culture does not rule out pneumococcal pneumonia.

Unfortunately, the interpretation of a positive sputum culture is not always straightforward. A positive finding may indicate the cause of the patient's pneumonia, but it may also be the result of contamination of the sputum specimen as it passes through the mouth of a colonized individual. In this instance, a laboratory finding must be interpreted within the clinical context. In contrast, growth of *S. pneumoniae* from Mr. P.'s blood could be considered definitive proof of the etiology of the disease. In recent years, interest has increased in the use of specific antisera to detect the capsular antigen directly in sputum, blood, or urine, thus obviating the need for culture. Unfortunately, these techniques tend to be positive in no more than 50% of the cases of pneumococcal pneumonia.

PREVENTION AND TREATMENT

Penicillin revolutionized the treatment of pneumococcal pneumonia. Other antibiotics, such as erythromycin, are available for patients who are allergic to penicillin. Despite the dramatic effectiveness of penicillin, the mortality rate in pneumococcal pneumonia remains unacceptably high. Treatment fails for two reasons: First, pneumococcal infections sometimes progress rapidly and patients are already near death when they seek medical attention. Second, some patients are debilitated by other diseases and die from their combined effects. Recent work on the pneumococcal cell wall has suggested another possible explanation. Lysis of pneumococcal cells by penicillin releases cell wall breakdown products that stimulate an abrupt increase in inflammation. The ultimate effect of penicillin therapy is to cure the infection, but the short-term effect of increased inflammation may be deleterious to some patients.

In the past several years, the worldwide spread of antibiotic resistance in pneumococci has emerged as a major concern. Resistance to penicillin was essentially unknown from its introduction in the 1940s until its first recognition in Australia and New Guinea in the late 1960s. During the 1980s, antibiotic resistance became widespread in a number of European countries, and by the 1990s a major increase in antibiotic-resistant pneumococci in North America became apparent. Approximately three-fourths of the penicillin-resistant strains have only an intermediate level of resistance and can still be treated with penicillin or related drugs unless the infection occurs in the central nervous system, where the penetration of penicillin is poor. However, the remaining one-fourth of strains have high-level resistance and must be treated with other antibiotics. Unfortunately, the penicillin-resistant strains are sometimes also resistant to other unrelated antibiotics that might have served as alternatives.

Interestingly, the mechanism of penicillin resistance does not involve the production of β-lactamase, an enzyme that breaks down penicillin and accounts for most penicillin resistance among staphylococci. Instead, the resistant organisms have undergone changes in membrane proteins that bind penicillin. Called penicillin binding proteins, these proteins function as enzymes in cell wall murein synthesis. The genetic information encoding these altered proteins appears to have been acquired from other species of streptococci that may reside in the oropharynx. Available evidence suggests that the emergence of resistance to penicillin and other antibiotics is related to the overuse of antibiotics in our population.

What about a vaccine? A vaccine would be useful, especially for the members of the population who are at risk for pneumococcal pneumonia. However, the antigenic diversity of the pneumococcus is a significant barrier to developing a vaccine based on the polysaccharide capsular antigens. Nonetheless, most cases of pneumococcal pneumonia are caused by 12 to 18 serotypes. Accordingly, a vaccine based on these types was approved for use in 1977. It is recommended for the elderly and individuals with diseases that predispose them to pneumococcal infections. Unfortunately, patients with Hodgkin's disease or multiple myeloma, who are especially at risk, often do not make adequate antibodies in response to the vaccine. Likewise, young children, in whom pneumococcal infections are also important, also respond poorly to polysaccharide vaccines in general, including this one (see Chapter 44, "Vaccines and Antisera," for a discussion of vaccination of children against *H. influenzae*). For these reasons, the vaccine has yet to have a dramatic impact on the overall morbidity and mortality caused by this organism. Current research is directed at producing an enhanced pneumococcal vaccine by conjugating the pneumococcal polysaccharides to carrier molecules in order to increase their immunogenicity. A similar approach has been dramatically successful for *H. influenzae* type b. Concern about antibiotic resistance is spurring this research, and inclusion of the antibiotic-resistant serotypes in a conjugate vaccine is a high priority.

CONCLUSION

Pneumococcal pneumonia has evolved from one of the major infectious causes of death to a fairly frequent disease that usually yields to treatment. Certain risk factors can be clearly identified, but it remains unclear why some seemingly healthy people become affected. Pneumococci are frequent colonizers and it is not obvious why they cause disease in some individuals but not others.

Pneumococcal pneumonia begins locally as an acute inflammation that involves mainly the alveoli and spreads laterally to adjacent areas. It exemplifies the classical stages of inflammation: exudate formation, influx of neutrophils, and resolution via macrophages. The local pathological manifestations do not explain the high fever and other systemic signs of the disease.

The main virulence factor and principal antigen of pneumococci is a capsular polysaccharide. It has many antigenic varieties that subdivide this species into distinct serotypes. A polyvalent vaccine composed of the most common serotypes is currently available.

SELF-ASSESSMENT QUESTIONS

1. Discuss the epidemiological features of pneumococcal pneumonia.
2. What properties of pneumococci are thought to be relevant to their pathogenesis? Given that the pneumococcus can be transformed with DNA, what experiment would you suggest that may help elucidate the pathological features?

3. Describe the histopathological events in pneumococcal pneumonia.

4. What would be your main concerns in treating an elderly patient with this disease? What about the patient without a spleen?

5. Discuss the complications in the diagnosis of pneumococcal infections of different organs.

SUGGESTED READINGS

Applebaum, PC. New prospects for antibacterial agents against multidrug-resistant pneumococci. Microb Drug Res 1995;1:43.

Austrian R. Random gleanings from a life with the pneumococcus. J Infect Dis l975;131:474–484.

Breiman RF, Butler JC, Tenover FC, Elliott JA, Facklam RR. Emergence of drug-resistant pneumococcal infections in the United States. JAMA 1994;271:1831–1834.

Breimen RF, Spika JS, Navarro JJ, Darby CP. Pneumococcal bacteremia in Charleston Country, South Carolina. Arch Intern Med 1990;150:1401–1405.

Sims RV, Steinmann WC, McConville JH, King LR, Zwick WC, Schwartz JS. The clinical effectiveness of pneumococcal vaccine in the elderly. Ann Intern Med 1988;108:653–657.

Tuomanen EI, Austrian R, Masure HR. Pathogenesis of pneumococcal infection. N Engl J Med 1995;332:1280–1284.

CHAPTER 14

Neisseriae: Gonococcus and Meningococcus

PENELOPE J. HITCHCOCK

EDWARD N. ROBINSON, JR.

ZELL A. MCGEE

Key Concepts

Neisseria gonorrhoeae (the gonococcus):
- Are Gram-negative cocci.
- Cause gonorrhea which can lead to pelvic inflammatory disease (PID) in women and epididymitis in men.
- Can be carried asymptomatically by both men and women.
- Exhibit phase variation and antigenic variation.
- Can cause disseminated infections (serum-resistant strains).
- Infections are treated with antibiotics, although many strains are resistant to penicillins.

Neisseria meningitidis (the meningococcus):
- Are Gram-negative cocci.
- Cause septicemia and meningitis.
- Are heavily encapsulated and possess a hemolysin, which allows them to disseminate in the bloodstream, leading to disseminated intravascular coagulation (DIC).
- Can be prevented with vaccination with capsular polysaccharide, except for group B strains.

The Gram-negative cocci, in contrast with the great variety of pathogenic Gram-negative bacilli, contain only one genus of organisms that frequently cause disease. This genus, *Neisseria*, has two important species that are pathogenic for humans, *Neisseria gonorrhoeae*, the agent of **gonorrhea**, and *Neisseria meningitidis,* a major cause of **septicemia** and **meningitis**.

The gonococcus attaches to the mucosal epithelia of the male urethra or female cervix where it elicits a brisk inflammatory response. Ascent of the organism into the female upper reproductive tract results in infection and inflammation of the uterus and fallopian tubes, called **pelvic inflammatory disease (PID)**. This condition may result in scarring of the upper tract and adjacent organs and chronic pelvic pain. Tubal scarring can lead to **ectopic pregnancy** (development of the embryo in the fallopian tube rather than the uterus) and/or infertility. In men, ascent of the organism into the upper reproductive tract is less frequent but may cause **epididymitis**. Certain strains of gonococci can invade the bloodstream and can

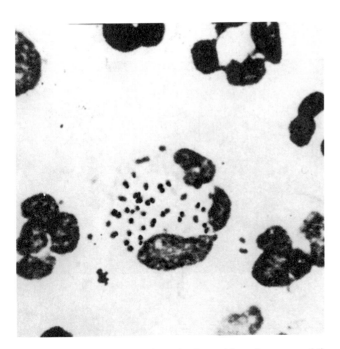

Figure 14.1. Gram stain of urethral pus. Note the neutrophil with gonococci on its surface.

cause skin lesions or arthritis. Individuals with complement deficiencies are predisposed to such systemic spread.

Meningococci are surrounded by a large capsule that endows them with the ability to withstand defense mechanisms in the bloodstream. This defense mechanism thus allows them to grow to high numbers in the blood. Meningococci also shed large amounts of outer membrane material. These membrane blebs contain lipopolysaccharide (**endotoxin**). The lipopolysaccharide/endotoxin induces the production and release into the bloodstream of potent biological mediators, such as tumor necrosis factor (TNF-α), that elicit the systemic signs of meningococcemia, disseminated intravascular coagulation, and shock. In addition, meningococci also have a predilection for the central nervous system (CNS). In the CNS, they can cause the serious complication bacterial meningitis.

■ CASE

Ms. P., a 14-year-old Hispanic female, came to the emergency room with an acutely painful abdomen. Her temperature was 101.3°F and laboratory tests indicated an elevated white blood cell count and sedimentation rate. The results of the urinalysis and a pregnancy test had not yet returned. Pelvic examination revealed a purulent cervical discharge. Samples of the discharge were taken for staining and culture. A Gram stain of the discharge revealed Gram-negative cocci in association with neutrophils (Fig. 14.1). Abdominal tenderness was apparent during the bimanual examination.

Ms. P. reported that her last menses was 4 days ago. When asked about her sexual behavior, she told the resident physician that she had intercourse for the first time 2 years ago. That relationship ended a few months ago, and she recently began "going steady" with a new friend. She and her partners have never used condoms or any other form of birth control.

Consider the following questions:

1. What test would you order for the cervical specimen? What do you expect to see when you examine the stained preparation?
2. Assume that Ms. P. has pelvic inflammatory disease (PID). How did she acquire the infection?
3. Is it significant that this patient has just finished menses?
4. If the patient has PID, what other causative organism, other than gonococci, should be considered?
5. If the patient has PID, would the proper use of male condoms have prevented the infection? Could any other forms of birth control and/or disease prevention have prevented transmission?
6. What other benefits would Ms. P realize if she and her partner used male condoms consistently and correctly? (See Chapter 66, "Sexually Transmitted Diseases," for additional discussion of PID.)

The gonococcus (*Neisseria gonorrhoeae*) usually causes an uncomplicated, localized **cervicitis** and **urethritis**. In addition, it may cause PID and disseminated gonococcal infection (DGI) (Table 14.1). About 800,000 new cases of gonorrhea occur every year in the United States. Of the infectious diseases that must legally be reported to the U.S. Public Health Service, gonococcal infections are the most frequent. Gonococcal infections and their complications are responsible for $1.0 billion per year in direct and indirect health care costs in the United States.

NEISSERIAE

The gonococcus and the meningococcus belong to the genus *Neisseria*, the main group of Gram-negative cocci associated with human disease. The neisseriae includes a number of nonpathogenic members that are often found in the bodies of healthy people, especially in the nasopharynx. One of these, recently renamed *Moraxella catarrhalis*, is emerging as an important cause of upper respiratory tract infections, especially in immunocompromised patients. Neisseriae are aerobes but can grow anaerobically. They have typical Gram-negative cell envelopes containing endotoxin. These organisms are fragile and do not survive for long outside of their human hosts. Virtually the only source of infection for Ms. P. is another infected person (not objects such as a toilet seat).

Table 14.1. Gonococcal Infections: Sites and Types

A. Lower tract infections
   1. Cervicitis
   2. Urethritis (male and female)
   3. Abscess formation in glands adjacent to the vagina, e.g., Skene's duct or Bartholin's glands

B. Upper tract infections
   1. Endometritis (uterine infection)
   2. Epididymitis
   3. Pelvic inflammatory disease (PID) (infection of the fallopian tube [salpingitis], the ovary, or adnexal tissues)

C. Other (nonreproductive tract) localized sites
   1. Proctitis (rectal gonorrhea)
   2. Pharyngitis
   3. Ophthalmia neonatorum (bilateral conjunctivitis in infants born of mothers infected with gonococci)
   4. Extension of the infection to areas contiguous with the pelvis causing peritonitis or perihepatitis (Fitz-Hugh and Curtis syndrome)

D. Disseminated gonococcal infection (DGI)
   1. Dermatitis–arthritis–tenosynovitis syndrome: fever, polyarthritis, and tenosynodermatitis (vesicles or pustules on a hemorrhagic base) caused either by immune complexes or by whole gonococci
   2. Monoarticular septic arthritis (one infected joint)
   3. Rarely, endocarditis (infection involves heart valves) or meningitis (infection of the central nervous system)

When initially cultured from patients, neisseriae grow best in an atmosphere with increased CO_2 (which can be provided by a "candle jar," a closed canister that uses a burning candle to convert O_2 to CO_2). A complex medium containing boiled blood, iron, and vitamins ("chocolate agar") is also required for optimal growth.

Substantial, albeit poorly understood, differences exist in the pathogenic potential of different strains of gonococci. Based on the characteristics of the bacterial outer membrane, a given strain may cause uncomplicated cervicitis or urethritis, complications such as PID, or disseminated gonococcal infection (DGI). Host factors (e.g., complement dysfunction) are also thought to be important in the severity and clinical presentation of the disease. Likewise, strains of meningococci differ in their pathogenic potential, which is associated with the presence or absence of certain outer membrane proteins.

Encounter and Entry

Gonococci are obligate human pathogens. They do not spontaneously infect other animals, cause disease in any convenient experimental animal, or reside free in the environment. It follows that humans must serve as the reservoir for these organisms. Both men and women may carry gonococci without demonstrating symptoms, although the prevalence of **asymptomatic carriers** is greater among women. Asymptomatic carriers of either sex are a major problem in the control of gonorrhea because, without symptoms, they are unlikely to be diagnosed or to receive treatment. Note that as part of its insidious pathogenic profile, the gonococcus has evolved to maximize its transmissibility. For this reason, it is important to culture and treat the known sexual contacts of a patient with this disease. Such "case-contact tracing" and treatment is especially important in PID because the male sexual partners of PID patients are more likely to be asymptomatic and may not seek therapy on their own. Thus, the cured PID patient may be discharged from the hospital only to return to an infected sexual partner and become infected again.

Once gonococci are introduced into the vagina or the urethral mucosa of either gender, they seek columnar epithelial cells of the distal urethra or cervix. There, they attach to the surface of the cells and multiply. Several surface structures of the organisms anchor them to the urethral or vaginal epithelial cells. Gonococci possess **pili** (Fig. 14.2) and other **surface proteins** that probably help them attach to host cells. Sophisticated genetic mechanisms enable the bacteria to control the presence or absence of these components (a phenomenon called **phase variation**, see "Paradigm") or to control their composition (**antigenic variation**). Pili and surface proteins are immunodominant, that is, they are "seen" by the immune system. However, they are also highly changeable, which makes them ineffective targets. It is not surprising that antibodies to these components do not protect against gonococcal infection.

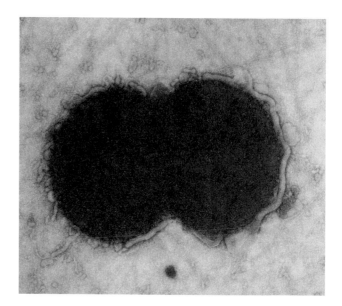

Figure 14.2. Transmission electron micrograph of *Neisseria gonorrhoeae*. Note the presence of pili, long thin strands of protein, emanating from the surface of the organisms.

PARADIGM

■ ■ ■

Alteration of Gene Expression by DNA Rearrangements

The basic strategies that pathogenic microbes employ in immune avoidance, subversion, or disruption are quite limited but have been found in highly unrelated species. In some cases, immune evasion involves activities or molecules that are expressed continuously. Examples include sialylation of lipopolysaccharide, production of IgA1 protease, and occupancy of an intracellular environment. In other cases, evasion of more specific host immune responses involves a variable process called **antigenic variation**. Antigenic variation results in changes in the composition or structure of predominant surface molecules. These changes allow an organism to avoid recognition by specific antibodies arising during the course of infection. This variability does not occur in response to specific antibodies. Rather, the changes are generated by genetic rearrangements that take place at a high frequency within the population. Consequently, new variants emerge by virtue of their selective escape from antibody-mediated immune mechanisms. In most cases, the repertoire of new antigenic types that can be expressed is so great that protective immunity rarely develops. Thus, chronic and repeated infection are hallmarks of diseases caused by these agents.

Antigenic variation occurs in microorganisms as diverse as African trypanosomes (which cause African sleeping sickness), *Borrelia* species (which cause relapsing fever), and *Neisseria gonorrhoeae*. In all of these microbes, antigenic variation results from the reassortment and recombination of duplicated gene segments. This mechanism is analogous (but not identical) to the way in which diversity is generated within immunoglobulins of animals.

Having evolved to grow exclusively within human hosts, gonococci are a paradigm for organisms that have evolved special mechanisms to adjust to life in immunocompetent individuals. Research into a **gonococcal vaccine** has involved a great deal of effort to understand the molecular mechanisms of gonococcal pilus antigenic variation. The gonococcal chromosome contains a single copy of the complete **pilin** gene (pilin is the structural protein that is polymerized to form pili). This gene is called *pilE*, for "pilin expression locus." In addition, the gonococcal chromosome contains 10 to 15 copies of variant-encoding pilin genes. All of these copies are truncated at their 5' ends and lack transcriptional promoter elements, as well as the sequences specifying the N-terminal part of pilin. These copies are called *pilS* loci, for "silent (nonfunctional) loci." Antigenic variation occurs when the genetic information from these nonfunctional alleles is transferred to the complete pilin gene locus by homologous recombination. In Figure 14.3 , this process is depicted as an antigenic switch from a *β*-pilin type to an *α*-type.

Pilin diversification depends not only on the mere number of *pilS* genes but also on the fact that small stretches of *pilS* sequence can be recombined into the expression locus resulting in chimeric pilin types. Such an event is depicted in Figure 14.3 as the formation of a *pilE* hybrid between the α- and γ-alleles. Note that the *pilS* alleles always act as donors of new genetic information but are not altered themselves by the process. In this way, a virtually infinite variety of pilin serotypes can be expressed using only a limited number of *pilS* alleles.

Another form of altered gene expression arising from DNA rearrangements is called **phase variation**. In this process, the expression of a particular gene product is turned on or off at high frequency. Oscillation between on and off states occurs by two basic mechanisms. One mechanism involves the site-specific **inversion** of a DNA segment which bears a transcriptional promoter. An example of this mechanism is the phase variation of type 1 fimbriae expression in *E. coli*. (Fig. 14.4). In the "on" state, the promoter element is oriented so that transcription of the fimbrial subunit gene, *fimA*, can take place. Inversion of the element (depicted in color) orients the promoter in a direction divergent to that of *fimA* (i.e., the "off" state). Analogous inversion systems control the expression of flagellar types in *Salmonella* and pilus expression in other Gram-negative pathogens.

The second mechanism of phase variation is associated with the somewhat unusual occurrence of short nucleotide repeats at the 5' ends of genes. Such repeats can readily be gained or lost as a consequence of strand misalignment during normal DNA replication and repair. Events of this sort, which occur at frequencies much higher than point mutations, disrupt the integrity of the gene's translational reading frame. *N. gonorrhoeae* employs this mechanism to change the expression of its virulence-associated Opa proteins. Multiple copies of complete *opa* genes (which each encode different Opa antigenic variants) are scattered throughout the genome. Each gene copy contains repeats of the sequence "CTCTT" within the 5' end of its reading frame. Gain or loss of these elements alters the translational reading frame of the gene and determines whether the intact protein can be made. An example (Fig. 14.5) shows a protein expressed from a gene carrying six copies of the element. If a CTCTT sequence is gained or lost within this stretch, the reading frame is altered and translation is terminated prematurely. In this way, gonococci can turn on or off the expression of any of its *opa* genes independently. A similar mechanism is known to control the expression of other gonococcal surface proteins and to oscillate expression of the biosynthetic genes for gonococcal lipopolysaccharide, resulting in its structural variability. Analogous phase variation mechanisms have been shown to operate in a number of important surface molecules in other Gram-negative pathogens. In each of these other instances, different repetitive elements are found. The only common feature is that the number of nucleotides of the repeat element is not three, nor is it divisible by three. Since the genetic code operates through trinucleotide codons, deletion or addition of a three base pair repeat would not change the reading frame.

The biological significance of phase variation remains somewhat unclear. Perhaps it represents a simplified form of antigenic variation. Gain or loss of the molecules controlled may have important functional consequences that are unrelated to the immune pressure. Nonetheless, the widespread distribution of this form of phase variation among microbes suggests that it is biologically significant and that pathogens find advantage in existing as heterogeneous populations.

J. MICHAEL KOOMEY

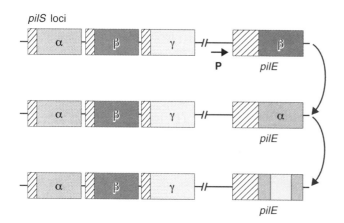

Figure 14.3. Antigenic variation of pili in *Neisseria gonorrhoeae*.

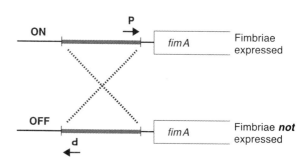

Figure 14.4. Phase variation of *E. coli* fimbriae by inversion of DNA segment containing a promoter.

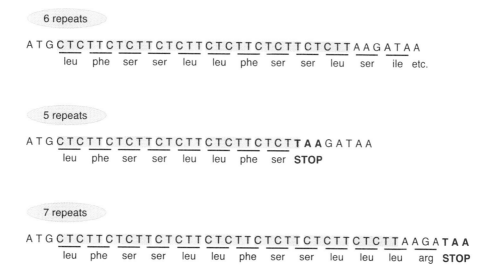

Figure 14.5. Representation of the phase variation mechanism of the gonococcal *opa genes*. The sequences have been modified and shortened in order to demonstrate the mechanism more succinctly.

Gonococci may or may not be taken up by neutrophils, depending on the type of outer membrane proteins they possess. Some of the outer membrane proteins are called colony opacity-associated proteins, or "**Opa proteins**." Organisms that lack these proteins are not engulfed by neutrophils. Gonococci lacking these Opa proteins are commonly associated with PID, DGI, and arthritis.

Spread and Multiplication

After colonizing the mucosal cell surface, gonococci multiply rapidly and are shed in large numbers into the

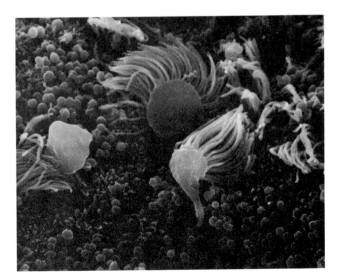

Figure 14.6. Scanning electron micrograph of human fallopian tube tissue 20 hours after infection with *Neisseria gonorrhoeae*. Note that gonococci attach almost exclusively to the surface of nonciliated cells. The damage occurs to the ciliated cells. Ciliated cells sloughed from the surface of the mucosa at the left and at the center, whereas intact ciliated cells are seen at the top and right of the photomicrograph.

genital secretions of infected men and women. Gonococci do not have flagella and are not motile. How they move up into the urethra or through the cervix is not known for certain, although they may be aided by urethral or uterine contractions.

Genital mucosal secretions contain three types of immunoglobulin G (IgG) and both IgA1 and IgA2. IgG found in secretions may reflect leakage of the antibody from serum onto the mucosal surface, whereas most of the IgA is actively secreted into the lumen of the genital tract. Gonococci produce an extracellular **protease** that specifically cleaves IgA1 in the hinge region. This property is also present in some other bacteria that inhabit mucosal epithelia, such as *Haemophilus influenzae* and certain streptococci. How this protease contributes to pathogenicity is not known. The protease may help the organisms escape phagocytosis by removing the Fc end of the immunoglobulin from gonococcus-bound IgA molecules. Because the Fc region is the portion recognized by phagocytes, the organisms may be less likely to be taken up by white blood cells when this portion is removed.

What we know about invasion of epithelial cells by gonococci is assumed from studies with in vitro organ culture of human fallopian tubes. Two types of cells comprise the epithelial mucosal surface of human fallopian tubes: ciliated cells and nonciliated cells. The nonciliated cells have fingerlike processes, called microvilli, on their luminal surface. When gonococci are incubated with fallopian tube sections, a number of events occur:

- **Attachment**—Gonococci attach to the nonciliated cells.
- **Ciliary stasis**—Motility of the ciliated cells slows and ultimately ceases. Ciliary activity is thought to be important in three ways: in transporting the egg from the ovary to the uterus; in moving the fertilized egg from the fallopian tube to the uterus; and in providing a flushing mechanism for clearing bacteria from the mucosal surface.
- **Death of ciliated cells**—Ciliated cells die and are selectively sloughed from the epithelial surface (Fig. 14.6). This step does not require intact organisms and can be elicited by gonococcal LPS or peptidoglycan fragments (parts of the cell wall).
- **Internalization**—The microvilli of nonciliated cells, acting as pseudopodia, engulf the bacteria. Gonococci are then internalized by these "nonprofessional" phagocytes by a process known as parasite-directed endocytosis.
- **Intracellular replication**—The organisms are transported to the interior of the cell within phagocytic vacuoles. These vacuoles coalesce to form larger vacuoles, within which gonococci multiply. Inside the nonciliated cells, gonococci are sheltered from antibodies, professional phagocytes, and antibiotics that do not enter human cells well.
- **Intracellular traffic**—The gonococci are transported to the base of the nonciliated cells where the bacteria-laden vacuoles fuse with the basement membrane.
- **Exocytosis**—The phagocytic vacuoles discharge their gonococci into the subepithelial connective tissue. From here, we presume, the organisms either cause local inflammation or enter blood vessels to cause disseminated disease.

Damage

Gonococci do not secrete exotoxins; thus, the damage is most likely caused by LPS and other components of the bacterial cell wall, such as peptidoglycan. Both LPS and peptidoglycan are known to induce the production of tumor necrosis factor-alpha (TNF-α) by a variety of human cells, and TNF-α has been shown to cause the sloughing of ciliated cells from human fallopian tube mucosa. In addition to death of ciliated cells, as demonstrated in the fallopian tube model, nonciliated epithelial cells containing gonococci may lyse, releasing cellular tissue factors that mediate inflammation. The inflammatory response in the male urethra is probably responsible for local symptoms such as pain on urination (dysuria) and urethral discharge of pus. It is noteworthy that these symptoms do not distinguish gonococcal urethritis from that caused by other genital pathogens, like the chlamydiae (Chapter 27, "Chlamydiae"). However, the urethral discharge in gonorrhea tends to be more copious, thick, and greenish yellow, and the pain is more intense. Women with gonococcal cervicitis are more often asymptomatic compared with men with urethritis.

Survival of gonococci in the bloodstream

Normal human serum is capable of killing circulating organisms of many Gram-negative species, including *N. gonorrhoeae*. (In contrast, Gram-positive bacteria are resistant to the bactericidal action of serum). This natural protective effect depends on complement activation and IgG and IgM antibodies. In the case of the gonococcus, the targets for antibodies are the lipopolysaccharide (LPS); the major outer membrane protein, called protein I; and other proteins exposed on the surface of the organisms. Thus, in order for gonococci to survive in the bloodstream, they must be able to evade this defense mechanism.

Strains of gonococci that are usually associated with disseminated infections are serum-resistant. These strains have different surface constituents than their serum-sensitive counterparts. In some serum-resistant gonococcal strains LPS is altered by the addition of a sialic acid molecule on the short, core carbohydrate chain. Because sialic acid is a surface component of red blood cells, it is believed that this modification camouflages the organisms and protects them from the antibodies responsible for serum killing. Serum-resistant strains are more sensitive to penicillin and have specific nutritional requirements. It is not clear whether these properties directly contribute to the ability of the organisms to disseminate or whether these properties are closely linked genetically.

Host factors also affect the outcome of gonococcal infections. For example, individuals deficient in the final components of the complement cascade (the membrane attack complex) are predisposed to recurrent systemic infections with both gonococci and meningococci.

The manifestations of disseminated gonococcal infection include pustular skin lesions with a surrounding red areola, inflammation of the tendons and joints (tenosynovitis), and/or frank infections of the joints (suppurative arthritis). Often, despite appropriate diagnostic attempts, cultures of blood, joint fluid, or skin lesion are sterile. Several plausible reasons can explain this phenomenon. First, gonococci may be present but in numbers too low to be detectable in culture. Second, the nutritional requirements of these organisms may be unusual, and it may not be possible to isolate them using normal culture conditions. Third, in cases of tenosynovitis, fragments of cell-wall peptidoglycan (murein) or perhaps immune complexes consisting of gonococcal antigens and host antibodies, rather than viable gonococci, may be deposited in synovial tissue and cause local inflammation. The latter possibility is supported by experiments in rats that show that purified gonococcal peptidoglycan, when injected into joints, induces arthri-

tis. If this phenomenom were to apply to humans, active joint infection need not be present at the site of intense inflammation.

Outcome of Gonococcal Infection

What is the outcome of gonorrhea? Data from the preantibiotic era suggest that symptoms of urethral infection in males usually subside in several weeks without treatment. However, repeated infections, if untreated, may lead to scarring and stricture of the urethra. Such sequelae of gonococcal infection are now relatively unusual, because most men seek medical attention once urethritis becomes apparent. Symptoms of cervicitis include cervical discharge (reported as vaginal discharge), bleeding, and pain. Paradoxically, local urogenital infections are asymptomatic in approximately 30% of women and are often heralded by the complications of the infection. Chronic fallopian tube inflammation can lead to scarring and stricture, resulting in such long-term sequelae as chronic pelvic pain; ectopic pregnancy; recurrent PIDs by chlamydiae, anaerobes, and other organisms; and infertility. For unknown reasons, disseminated gonococcal infections occur predominantly in women. Gonococcal arthritis is the most common type of joint infection in sexually active adults.

The outcome of gonococcal infection depends not only on the gender of the patient but also on the timeliness of medical attention. Prompt treatment decreases the risk of ascending or disseminated infection and the resulting sequelae.

Meningococcal Infection

Gonococci and meningococci are taxonomic cousins; the two organisms share about 80% of their DNA base sequences as measured by DNA hybridization, and both possess similar lipopolysaccharide (LPS) endotoxins. Both organisms can colonize mucous membranes without causing symptoms. (It is estimated that, in endemic areas, up to 10% of the population may be meningococcal carriers.) Both gonococci and meningococci cause purulent infections. Nevertheless, they usually cause a contrasting spectrum of diseases. Gonococci most often produce a localized inflammation and, even when the gonococci spread to the bloodstream, the infection is rarely lethal. In contrast, meningococcal infection of the bloodstream is a systemic and life-threatening disease. Why do these two species cause such different illnesses? It is probably significant that the meningococcus is heavily **encapsulated** and possesses a **hemolysin**, factors that may play a role in the pathogenicity of this organism.

Occasional epidemics of meningococcal meningitis occur, but the more usual outcome of exposure to the organism is colonization of the nasopharynx with no local symptoms or systemic consequences. The reason why some people develop disease and others do not is not easy to fathom. Based on organ cultures of nasal epithelium, the mechanism of penetration through mucous membranes appears to be similar for the meningococcus in the nasopharynx and the gonococcus in the fallopian tube. What is known, however, is that patients susceptible to meningococcal meningitis are deficient in bactericidal anticapsular antibodies. Individuals with capsule-specific antibodies, presumably produced in response to past colonization, resist the ability of the meningococcus to invade the bloodstream. These observations were instrumental in developing the currently used protective vaccines that are made of purified capsular material.

If they are not killed by normal serum factors in the bloodstream, meningococci multiply rapidly, reaching blood titers that are among the highest known for any bacterium. It is possible, for example, to observe the organisms directly on a smear of the buffy coat of blood (the layer containing the white cells when whole blood is centrifuged). Other bacterial septicemias rarely result in bacteria visible in buffy coat stains.

The entry of meningococci into the bloodstream can lead to a devastating disease, **purpura fulminans** caused by **disseminated intravascular coagulation** (DIC) with skin manifestations (petechiae and ecchymoses), meningitis, shock, and death. These systemic signs are the direct result of the ability of the meningococcus to survive and multiply in the bloodstream. DIC is accompanied by shock, fever, and other responses to endotoxin mediated by TNF-α and interleukin-1. In meningococcal sepsis and meningitis, the likelihood of death or neurologic damage is proportional to the elevation in serum and cerebrospinal fluid TNF-α concentrations. Because TNF-α is a chemical mediator of our defense system, this observation gives weight to Lewis Thomas' observation, "Our arsenals for fighting off bacteria are so powerful . . . that we are in more danger from them than from the invaders. We live in the midst of explosive devices. We are mined."

As mentioned above, meningococcal disease is effectively prevented by vaccination with capsular polysaccharide. A notable exception is disease caused by group B meningococci. The capsule of group B strains contains a polymer of sialic acid that is not immunogenic and does not elicit protective antibodies.

In contrast, when gonococci reach the bloodstream of most individuals, they are usually killed by host defense mechanisms. Even the serum-resistant strains do not grow appreciably in the circulation, although they may survive long enough to reach other organs. Although gonococcal meningitis and endocarditis have been reported on rare occasion, gonococcal bacteremia is seldom fatal.

Diagnosis

Finding neutrophils containing Gram-negative diplococci in cervical or urethral secretions is generally presumptive evidence of gonococcal infection. It is also a good reason why medical students should learn how to perform and interpret Gram stains. Positive microscopic findings justify beginning antibiotic therapy before the results of cultures are known. Thus, the Gram stain of urethral exudate of men is more sensitive than the Gram stain of cervical exudate in women. A cervical Gram stain may be negative, despite a positive culture result. A positive Gram stain of cervical secretions is confirmatory evidence of active gonorrhea in a symptomatic woman, but routine Gram stain of asymptomatic women's secretions is not clinically useful.

Because the social implications of gonorrhea can be as serious as the medical consequences, the physician must confirm the clinical findings by culturing or using genetic probes. It is also important to monitor how the laboratory identifies these organisms. There are three reasons to culture: (a) to be completely certain of the identity of the infecting microorganism, (b) to identify infection in asymptomatic individuals, and (c) to deal with public health and legal ramifications. Another important reason for culture, i.e., to rule out antibiotic resistance, is not presently an issue. Currently, resistance to the current drugs of choice for gonococcal infections, such as the broad-spectrum antibiotic, ceftriaxone, has not been reported.

Gonococci grow on several kinds of media that allow presumptive identification within a day. The most commonly used medium is called "chocolate agar" because it contains heated blood and has the appearance of milk chocolate. Special varieties of this medium are known as Thayer-Martin medium and Martin-Lewis medium; each contains different antibiotics to inhibit other bacterial species and yeasts. Specimens taken from the cervix, urethra, and other sites that contain bacteria should always be cultured on chocolate agar with antibiotics (e.g., Thayer-Martin or Martin-Lewis medium) to inhibit the normal flora. It is noteworthy that an occasional strain of gonococci is sensitive to the antibiotics used in the Thayer-Martin medium. For this reason, fluids that are normally sterile (e.g., cerebrospinal fluid, blood, synovial fluid) should be cultured on chocolate agar without antibiotics to allow recovery of these antibiotic-sensitive gonococcal strains.

A nucleic acid based detection test for the gonococcus using urine specimens has been recently approved for clinical use. The test uses a highly sensitive nucleic acid amplification method called the ligase chain reaction (see Chapter 55, "Diagnostic Principles"). It has proved to be as sensitive and specific as culture, but has the advantage of requiring only a urine sample, not invasive sampling (i.e., urethral or cervical swabs). The disadvantages of this test are its cost and the technical sophistication required to perform it.

All members of the genus *Neisseria* and related genera possess an oxidative enzyme that makes the colonies turn purple when flooded with a so-called "oxidase reagent."

If a Gram-negative diplococcus is oxidase-positive, it is a member of *Neisseria* or a close relative. To distinguish *N. gonorrhoeae* from the other species of this genus, the microbiological laboratory determines the pattern of fermentation of various sugars. Unlike other neisseriae, gonococci utilize glucose but not maltose or sucrose, and meningococci utilize both glucose and maltose.

Treatment

A relatively high proportion of gonococci now bear a plasmid that encodes a β-lactamase, an enzyme that destroys penicillins. Gonococci bearing the resistance plasmids can cause serious locally invasive diseases such as PID as well as disseminated gonococcal infections. As a consequence of this widespread penicillin resistance, the recommended initial therapy for gonorrhea is no longer penicillin, but a β-lactamase-resistant cephalosporin, ceftriaxone, given intramuscularly. Single-dose oral therapy is effective and offers the distinct advantage of observed therapy (i.e., no treatment failures due to lack of compliance and no injection required). Both ciprofloxacin and cefixime are available for this purpose, but gonococci resistant to ciprofloxacin are being reported with increasing frequency.

Prevention

Despite effective antimicrobials and active public health measures, an estimated 800,000 cases of gonococcal infections occur annually in the United States, including 450,000 reported cases. Prevention efforts must be based on a multipronged approach that includes:

- Behavioral interventions including condom use and decreasing the number of sexual partners;
- Early diagnosis and treatment;
- Partner notification;
- Screening and case-finding;
- Vaccine development and utilization.

Attempts at vaccine development have proved to be difficult because gonococci, as solely human pathogens, have a long-standing and sophisticated relationship with their host. These organisms have managed to survive the host's immune response, as discussed in the paradigm section, by antigenic variation, phase variation, and the occupation of protective intracellular environments.

A new approach to prevention is being actively pursued. Topical microbiocides for intravaginal and intrarectal use are being developed to safely and effectively prevent sexually transmitted diseases, including HIV. These products will inactivate pathogens in cervical and vaginal secretions and in ejaculate, thus providing bidirectional protection. Ideally, these products would not be inherently spermicidal, but they could be formulated with or without spermicidal activity. Either product could be used to prevent infection, no matter what a person's contraceptive choices might be.

CONCLUSION

The mode of transmission as well as the biological properties of gonococci combine to give them a unique set of characteristics. The strong adhesins of gonococci allow them to enter the genital tract of humans. They are able to traverse epithelial cells and either cause local inflammation or disseminate to other parts of the body. Meningococci have an outstanding ability to survive in the bloodstream and to cause systemic infections that often have disastrous consequences.

Gonococci and meningococci are found only in human beings, some of whom act as asymptomatic carriers. In principle, effective vaccines should prevent new infections or control and prevent disease. It is hoped that such vaccines will be available soon.

SELF-ASSESSMENT QUESTIONS

1. What are the microbiological distinguishing features of the gonococci? How do they differ from meningococci?
2. Starting with an infected male partner, discuss the events that lead to gonococcal pelvic inflammatory disease.
3. What are three approaches to prevent gonorrhea?
4. Why is it difficult to make an effective vaccine against the gonococcus?
5. Discuss the serious clinical consequences of gonorrhea.

SUGGESTED READINGS

Britigan BE, Cohen MS, Sparling PF. Gonococcal infection: a model of molecular pathogenesis. N Engl J Med 1985;312: 1683–1694.

Dillon JR, Yeung KH. Beta-lactamse plasmids and chromosomally mediated antibiotic resistance in pathogenic *Neisseria* species. Clin Microbiol Rev 1989;2 (Suppl):S125–S133.

Figueroa JE, Densen P. Infectious diseases associated with complement deficiencies. Clin Microbiol Rev 1991; 4:359–395.

McGee ZA, Pavia AT. Is the concept, "agents of sexually transmitted disease" still valid? J Sex Transm Dis 1991;18: 69–71.

Stephens DS. Gonococcal and meningococcal pathogenesis as defined by human cell, cell culture, and organ culture assays. Clin Microbiol Rev 1989;2 (Suppl):S104–S111.

Swanson J, Koomey M. Mechanisms for variation of pili and outer membrane protein II in *Neisseria gonorrhoeae.* In: Berg D, Howe M, eds. Mobile DNA. Washington, DC: American Society for Microbiology, 1989; 743–761.

CHAPTER 15

Bacteroides and Abscesses

FRANCIS P. TALLY

Key Concepts

Bacteroides:
- Are strict anaerobic Gram-negative rods that play a causative role in abscess formation.
- Are members of the normal flora of the gut and oral cavity.
- Includes *Bacteroides fragilis*, a bacterium that can withstand short exposure to oxygen; has a nontoxic lipopolysaccharide and a capsule; and produces several enzymes such as a neuraminidase, proteases, and lipases that may play a role in its pathogenicity.

Abscess formation in the peritoneal cavity:
- Begins when the colon wall is breached by a ruptured bowel, a ruptured appendix, or abdominal surgery and a large number of bacteria enter the peritoneal cavity.
- Is caused by a mixture of facultative and strict anaerobes (including *Escherichia coli*, *B. fragilis*, clostridia, and anaerobic streptococci); as infection proceeds, facultative anaerobes use up the available oxygen, and strict anaerobes become dominant.
- Is treated with surgical drainage and antibiotics; a combination of antibiotics or antibiotics sensitive to both facultative anaerobes and strict anaerobes is necessary.

Spillage of microbe-laden materials, such as the contents of the intestine or the oropharynx, into deep tissues often results in infections caused by a mixture of bacteria. Examples are **peritonitis** caused by a ruptured appendix, or a **pulmonary abscess** due to aspiration of oropharyngeal bacteria. From such sites it is usually possible to isolate many different combinations of infecting bacteria. These infections are exceptions to a "one germ–one disease" concept. That is, they are polymicrobial rather than monomicrobial.

The bacteria involved in these infections include **strict anaerobes** and **facultative anaerobes** (such as Enterobacteriaceae), probably interacting in complex metabolic ways. This chapter focuses on one of the most frequently involved genera, the *Bacteroides*. These strictly anaerobic Gram-negative rods are common members of the normal oral and gut flora. However, the main pathogen of the genus, *Bacteroides fragilis*, has special pathogenic attributes. One of these properties may be its antiphagocytic capsule. But other pathogenic properties remain to be elucidated.

CASE

Ms. A., an 18-year-old college freshman, was admitted to the hospital with diffuse abdominal pain, diarrhea, and nausea without vomiting. Her pain was localized to the right side of the abdomen. Physical examination revealed tenderness in the lower quadrant of her abdomen, principally over McBurney's point. She received a cephalosporin antibiotic and was taken to the operating room where her ruptured appendix was removed. Cultures of the peritoneal cavity in the neighborhood of the appendix grew a mixture of bacteria, typical of those found in stool. On the second day after the operation her temperature spiked to 38.6°C. Blood cultures obtained preoperatively grew *Escherichia coli*.

Humans, Health, and History

The famous magician Houdini died of peritonitis. Houdini was known for his astounding feats of escape while enchained and enclosed in containers submerged in water. He possessed amazing physical strength and could control many muscles, including, it is said, some normally not under voluntary control. His fame was the cause of his demise. Houdini received an unexpected blow to his abdomen from a bystander intent on testing his legendary muscular powers. The magician's large intestine ruptured, and he died a few days later. Had Houdini lived today and been in the hands of a competent physician who treated him with antibiotics and surgical repair, he would have had a good chance of surviving.

Ms. A. improved postoperatively and completed a 7-day course of cephalosporin. Since she had no further symptoms and her blood cultures were negative, the antibiotic was stopped. However, 36 hours later her temperature was 38.8°C and she felt diffuse pain over the site of the appendectomy. A CAT scan of her abdomen revealed a retroperitoneal abscess. Cultures obtained after drainage of the abscess grew *B. fragilis*. She was again treated with antibiotics (this time a mixture of gentamicin and clindamycin to treat, respectively, the Gram-negative aerobes and the anaerobes) for 8 more days and had an uneventful recovery.

Several questions are raised by Ms. A.'s case:

1. How did the two episodes of her disease differ with regard to pathogenesis and to the kind of bacteria involved?
2. How did anaerobic bacteria survive in oxygenated tissue? Why did they survive the first course of antibiotic treatment?
3. How do the organisms involved, specifically *B. fragilis*, cause damage?
4. Was Ms. A. treated properly?

No other place in the body is more prone to contamination by a large number of endogenous bacteria than the peritoneal cavity. The resulting intra-abdominal sepsis dramatically illustrates what happens when microorganisms are introduced in large numbers into the wrong place. The spillage of a few milliliters of intestinal content into the peritoneal cavity delivers many billions of bacteria to a customarily sterile site. Left untreated, peritonitis is often fatal, as in the case of Houdini. Indeed, in the pre-antibiotic era, perforation of the colon was a medical catastrophe. Currently, the mortality rate is lower but still significant, between 1% and 5%. In addition, the diagnosis and management of these cases is far from simple. The physician who is not aware of the need for proper antibiotics and supportive therapy may well lose a patient to this disease.

Two points should be emphasized. First, intra-abdominal infections typically result in **biphasic diseases**, as in the case of Ms. A. They start with an acute inflammation and progress to the formation of localized abscesses. Second, of the hundreds of species contained in the colonic inoculum, a few are most commonly isolated from abscesses. *B. fragilis* is found in the majority of cases and is the most important of the anaerobic bacteria associated with abscess formation. Seldom found alone, it is typically cocultured with a variety of other bacteria.

The largest number of intra-abdominal infections are caused by the rupture of infected appendices or intestinal diverticula, the abnormal outpouchings of the colon. In the U.S. there are over 250,000 cases of appendicitis and some 350,000 cases of diverticulitis a year. Of these infections, about 15% perforate and result in peritonitis and many produce abscesses as a late complication. The prevalence of diverticula increases with aging and so does diverticulitis as the cause of intra-abdominal infection.

INTRODUCTION TO THE *BACTEROIDES* AND OTHER STRICTLY ANAEROBIC BACTERIA

Bacteroides are strict anaerobic, Gram-negative rods, which are present in large amounts in the large intestine of humans and other vertebrates. They number 10^{11} or more per gram of feces, and are the dominant organisms along with anaerobic streptococci. The *Bacteroides* group comprises many species (Table 15.1), of which *B. fragilis* and *Bacteroides thetaiotamicron* are the most prominent pathogens. Among *Bacteroides*, *B. fragilis* is a minor component, usually present in concentrations of 10^8 or 10^9 per gram of feces. The reason why this species becomes dominant in deep tissue infections is discussed below.

Two other frequently isolated genera of anaerobic Gram-negative rods were originally classified as *Bacteroides*. Unlike the *Bacteroides*, however, *Porphyromonas* and *Prevotella* form characteristically pigmented colonies on blood agar. *Prevotella melaninogenica*, named for its production of a black pigment, is commonly found in the human gingival flora and is often associated with periodontal diseases. Although this

Table 15.1. The Major Clinically Significant Nonspore-forming Anaerobic Bacteria

Group	Genus	Typical species	Typical diseases
Gram Negative			
Rods	*Bacteroides* (*fragilis* group)	*fragilis, distasonis, thetaiotamicron*	Intra-abdominal infections
	Fusobacterium	*nucleatum, necrophorum*	Oral, dental, pleuropulmonary infections
	Porphyromonas	*asaccharolytica, gingivalis*	Oral and dental infections
	Prevotella	*bivius, disiens melaninogenicus*	Pelvic infection
			Oral, dental, and pleuropulmonary infection
Gram Positive			
Rods	*Actinomyces*	*israeli*	Actinomycosis (lumpy jaw)
	Propionibacterium	*acnes*	Infections of prosthetic devices
Cocci	*Peptostreptococcus*	*magnus, asaccharolyticus, anaerobius*	Intra-abdominal, soft tissue, bone and joint infections

organism is also found in other sites, it is most commonly associated with infections of oral origin, including aspiration pneumonia (Chapter 59, "Respiratory System") and rather serious infections following human bites. In contrast, *Prevotella bivius* and *Prevotella disiens* are common vaginal flora associated with pelvic infections and peritonitis. Table 15.1 includes the major strict anaerobes of clinical significance, except the clostridia which are described in Chapter 20, "Clostridia."

Bacteroides are not killed by short exposure to oxygen, although they do not grow in its presence. *B. fragilis* is among the most oxygen-resistant species within the genus. This is because these bacteria contain **superoxide dismutase**, which detoxifies oxygen radicals, and **catalase**, which breaks down hydrogen peroxide. The *Bacteroides* obtain energy by fermentation of carbohydrates. They can use complex polysaccharides such as mucins present in the colon, which may be why they are present in large numbers in feces.

The outer membrane of *B. fragilis* contains a nontoxic **lipopolysaccharide**. In this way, it is different from that of the typical endotoxins of most Gram-negative bacteria. For example, the lipopolysaccharide of *Fusobacterium necrophorum*, another common oral Gram-negative strict anaerobe, is distinctly toxic. Another virulence factor is a polysaccharide **capsule**, which protects *B. fragilis* from phagocytosis and is probably involved in attachment to mesothelial cells and in abscess formation.

B. fragilis also produce several enzymes that may be involved in pathogenesis, including a **neuraminidase, lipase**, and **proteases**. Neuraminidase cleaves terminal sialic acid from host carbohydrates, allowing *B. fragilis* to use these carbohydrates as an energy source in the absence of free glucose. In one animal model, mutant *B. fragilis* that failed to make neuraminidase were less able to produce abscesses. Periplasmic enzymes, such as **li-**

pases and **proteases**, may also play a role in pathogenesis, but these roles have not been definitely documented. Like the staphylococci, streptococci, and pseudomonads, *B. fragilis* probably has multiple virulence factors that act in concert.

ENTRY, SPREAD, AND MULTIPLICATION

The colon wall can be breached as a result of blunt trauma, a ruptured bowel, a penetrating wound, or abdominal surgery. In the case of Houdini, a sudden impact caused the colon literally to explode. In Ms. A.'s case, obstruction of outflow from the appendix led to inflammation and eventually to perforation. Whatever the mechanism, the number of organisms contaminating the peritoneal cavity is enormous when the colon wall is breached. Nevertheless, phagocytes are mobilized rapidly to the infected site and, up to a point, dispose of large numbers of bacteria. Because of the large number of phagocytes that migrate to the site of peritoneal contamination, the minimal infecting dose that results in disease in humans is possibly quite high, perhaps several milliliters of intestinal content, judging from experiments with laboratory animals.

Organisms that enter the peritoneal cavity find themselves first in a liquid environment that could, in principle, lead to their dissemination throughout the cavity. However, the omentum and the loops of the small intestine drape themselves around areas of inflammation and serve to contain the infection. Although this takes time, the abscesses that eventually develop are usually well localized. Lymphatic drainage and the effect of gravity also influence the location of abscesses. These factors likely influenced the location of Ms. A.'s abscess at a retroperitoneal site even though the original bacterial spill was near her appendix.

Because the bacterial inoculum is potentially diverse,

a large number of factors are involved in determining which species become dominant in the infection. Many intestinal bacteria can grow in the peritoneal fluid, which is not particularly antibacterial. The first line of defense is most likely the rapid mobilization of phagocytic cells. Thus, bacteria that eventually survive and grow must be quite resistant to phagocytosis. In fact, many survivors are encapsulated. One major reason for the predominance of *B. fragilis* may be that it is one of the members of the genus *Bacteroides* with the largest capsule.

Prior to spillage of colon contents, the peritoneal cavity is well oxygenated, and highly oxygen-sensitive anaerobes are killed. After spillage of colonic contents, the first organisms that become numerically dominant are facultative anaerobes, especially *E. coli*. However, many of the less oxygen-sensitive strict anaerobes survive and can be isolated from both the fluid and surface of mesothelial cells. Eventually, the site of infection becomes increasingly anaerobic, in part because facultative anaerobes metabolize what oxygen is present and in part because the site becomes increasingly avascular. The surviving strict anaerobes then take over. Animal studies have documented that this need for synergy between various microorganisms is required for abscess formation. The inoculation of a single species of intestinal bacteria seldom leads to infection, while infection by a mixture of facultative and strict anaerobes produces acute inflammation and abscess formation.

In peritoneal abscesses, the dominant *B. fragilis* is often accompanied not only by facultative anaerobes but also by other strict anaerobes, such as clostridia or anaerobic streptococci (i.e., *Peptostreptococcus*).

DAMAGE

If the peritoneal defenses are unable to eradicate spilled intestinal contents, an abscess usually develops. The areas of inflammation become walled-in and surrounded by a thick, fibrous collagen-containing capsule. Inside this capsule are live and dead white blood cells, bacteria, and cell debris. In general terms, these abscesses resemble those caused by the staphylococci (Chapter 11).

Intra-abdominal abscesses exact a high toll on the host because they can extend to nearby sites, with resultant necrosis of adjacent tissue. In addition, they serve as reservoirs from which the organisms enter the bloodstream. The resulting bacteremia may produce septic shock or cause metastatic infections at distant sites. The reasons for shock are not known, since the lipopolysaccharide (LPS) of these organisms is nontoxic. Vigorous intervention with antibiotics helped Ms. A. overcome her bacteremia.

OTHER *BACTEROIDES* INFECTIONS

In addition to *B. fragilis*, other species of this genus are also found in abscesses of the female genital tract, usually owing to contamination with the vaginal flora. Here the infecting organisms ascend through the cervix, the uterus, and fallopian tubes to reach the vicinity of the ovaries. The resulting infection is known as **pelvic inflammatory disease** (PID) (see Chapter 66, "Sexually Transmitted Diseases"). Tubo-ovarian abscesses occasionally complicate PID. The most common agent of this disease is not *B. fragilis*, but *Prevotella bivius*, a common inhabitant of the human vagina.

DIAGNOSIS

Proper chemotherapy of mixed bacterial infections requires the determination of the bacterial species involved and their antibiotic sensitivity. Specialized techniques are required for growing members of the genus *Bacteroides* and other anaerobes. In general, these techniques involve limiting the exposure of the specimen to oxygen, because even oxygen-tolerant strains may eventually be killed. Clinical specimens must be protected from air using special collecting devices and transported to the laboratory without delay. The most convenient way to handle and culture clinical specimens is with the use of an incubator in the form of a glove box, a device in which the atmosphere can be made anaerobic by flushing with a mixture of inert gases (Fig. 15.1). This equipment is specialized and costly and not all hospital laboratories are equipped with it. It is possible, however, to carry out anaerobic microbiological work with smaller but less convenient glass jars.

TREATMENT

Localized purulent infections such as abscesses usually require dual therapy, namely, drainage of the contents and administration of antibiotics. Additionally, the anatomical defect that allowed spillage from the intestine must be repaired. Thus, a combined medical and surgical approach is often necessary in cases of intra-abdominal infections.

In the past, antibacterial therapy was difficult because *B. fragilis* is resistant to many common antibiotics. Fortunately, several agents have excellent activity against this organism (metronidazole, clindamycin, β-lactam–β-lactamase inhibitor combinations, and imipenem). It must be kept in mind, however, that the target in these infections is seldom a single bacterial species but a mixed flora with different sensitivities. For this reason, a combination of antibiotics or an antibiotic effective against both aerobes and anaerobes is usually given. The need for using more than one drug, or a drug with a broad spectrum of activity, is demonstrated in the animal ex-

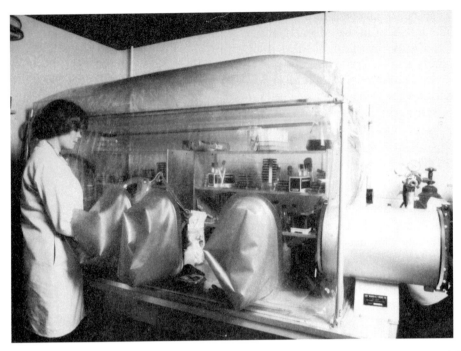

Figure 15.1. An anaerobic glove box used for the culture of strictly anaerobic bacteria. This device is used for large-scale work and for experimentation. Note the port on right, which is used to introduce and remove material from the chamber. It has two doors (not visible) and can be independently flushed free of oxygen.

Table 15.2. Antimicrobial Therapy of Experimental Peritonitis*

Treatment regimen	Acute mortality (%)	Abscess formation in survivors (%)
Untreated	37	100
Gentamicin alone	4	98
Clindamycin alone	35	5
Gentamicin and clindamycin	7	6

* A gelatin capsule containing fresh rat feces was placed in the peritoneal cavity of normal rats. The drugs were administered at the same time.

periment summarized in Table 15.2. Both mortality rate and abscess formation are significantly reduced only when the combination of antibiotics is used. Gentamicin presumably reduces the mortality due to the aerobe (*E. coli*), and clindamycin prevents abscess formation by *B. fragilis*. In the case of Ms. A., the cephalosporin first administered was effective against *E. coli* but not against *B. fragilis*. Her second treatment recognized the need for an appropriate choice and she also received clindamycin, an effective drug against this organism.

Bacteroides cells possess sophisticated genetic systems that transfer genes for drug resistance. Plasmids and transposons can be transferred between *B. fragilis* and *E. coli*; although genes from *B. fragilis* are not efficiently expressed in *E. coli* and vice versa, this transfer may be important in the epidemiology of drug resistance. Drug resistance has therefore become a significant problem in the treatment of infections by *B. fragilis*.

CONCLUSION

Bacteroides fragilis is a versatile pathogen that colonizes the human large bowel. It possesses special virulence characteristics because it emerges from a numerically inferior position in the normal intestinal flora to become a dominant pathogen in normally sterile tissue. Left for future work is the elucidation of the roles of specific virulence factors. Among the many questions that may be asked: Is the capsule alone sufficient to resist phagocytosis? Do the various enzymes secreted by the organisms participate in damage? How do they do it? What is the role of the capsule? Although the diseases caused by *B. fragilis* can be cured, the organisms still present challenges to therapy and, above all, to prevention. Unfortunately, no way presently exists to prevent these infections.

SELF-ASSESSMENT QUESTIONS

1. What are the major medical problems caused by *B. fragilis*? Why was *Bacteroides* not implicated in many of these conditions until recently?

2. What are *Bacteroides*? Describe their major structural, physiological, and ecological properties.

3. What do we know about the pathophysiology of *B. fragilis* infections? (*Clue*: Not much.)

4. What are the special therapeutic and diagnostic problems of these infections?

SUGGESTED READINGS

Finegold SM. Anaerobic bacteria: general concepts. In: Mandell GL, Bennett JE, Dolin R. Principles and practice of infectious diseases. 4th ed. New York: Churchill Livingstone, 1995.

Finegold SM, George WL. Anaerobic infections in humans. San Diego: Academic Press, 1989.

Gorbach SL, JG Bartlett. Anaerobic infections. N Engl J Med 1974;290:1177–1184; 290:1237–1354; 290:1289–1294.

Hentges DJ. The anaerobic microflora of the human body. Clin Inf Dis 1993 16 (Suppl 4):S175.

Lorber B. *Bacteroides*, *Prevotella*, and *Fusobacterium* species (and other medically important anaerobic gram-negative bacilli). In: Mandell GL, Bennett JE, Dolin R. Principles and practice of infectious diseases. 4th ed. New York: Churchill Livingstone, 1995.

Tally FP, Ho JL. Management of patients with intraabdominal infection due to colonic perforation. In: Current clinical topics in infectious diseases. New York: McGraw-Hill, 1987.

Enteric Bacteria: "Secretory" (Watery) Diarrhea

GERALD T. KEUSCH

DAVID W.K. ACHESON

Key Concepts

Enteric bacteria that cause secretory diarrhea:
- Include members of Enterobacteriaceae and Vibrionaceae.
- Are usually transmitted to humans in contaminated food and water.
- Face formidable defenses in the gastrointestinal tract; they adhere to the epithelial cells of the GI tract via pili (fimbriae) or surface adhesins.
- May elaborate toxins (*Vibrio cholerae*, enterotoxigenic *Escherichia coli*) that reduce sodium absorption and increase chloride secretion of the intestinal cells, which leads to watery diarrhea.
- Can be treated with oral rehydration therapy.

Diarrhea, usually no more than a bothersome brief illness in industrialized nations, is one of the leading causes of infant and childhood mortality in developing countries. Diarrheal diseases kill over 5 million children yearly and contribute to malnutrition and growth retardation in those who survive these illnesses. For these reasons, diarrheal disease control is a major goal for the World Health Organization.

Watery diarrhea is caused by the loss of electrolytes and fluids from the small intestine. An extreme example is cholera, which can cause fatal dehydration in hours, usually in small children. "Traveler's diarrhea" is a generally milder form of watery diarrhea. It most commonly affects adults. Infections of the intestinal tract can lead to local tissue damage or inflammation and cause **bloody diarrhea** or **dysentery**. These infections are discussed in Chapter 17, "Invasive and Tissue-damaging Enteric Bacterial Pathogens."

Bacteria, viruses, and protozoa that cause diarrheal disease are grouped together as **enteric pathogens**. Several traits endow these agents with the ability to cause secretory diarrhea, and these virulence factors vary in their mode of action. The array of factors particular to each organism determines the characteristics of the clinical illness.

CASES

Mr. D., a 33-year-old blood group O, fully immunized, rather nervous accountant who is taking H$_2$ blockers for ulcer disease; his 29-year-old healthy wife; and their 10-month-old baby boy returned from a 2-week trip to South America. The next morning Mr. D. passed a semisolid stool, which was quickly followed by a large watery bowel movement. Within an hour he passed another large watery stool, now opaque gray–white in color. He vomited several times and became slightly sweaty. When soon thereafter Mr. D. passed another large watery stool, he called his physician, who advised him to go to the emergency room. On presentation, Mr. D. was afebrile but had a rapid heart rate with a feeble pulse and low blood pressure. He complained of muscle cramps and dizziness. All of these signs and symptoms were consistent with significant loss of extracellular fluids. Laboratory studies showed a normal leukocyte count, a slightly elevated level of serum sodium, normal serum potassium level, and an elevated blood urea nitrogen level, likewise consistent with dehydration.

A diagnosis of cholera was suspected. Mr. D. was immediately given 2 liters of fluid intravenously and then started on oral rehydration solution. His stool volumes progressively diminished over 48 hours and the patient was discharged. Because of the suspected diagnosis, special media were used and the stool culture grew *Vibrio cholerae*, strain O1 E1 Tor. Mrs. D., a native South American, had two loose bowel movements on the second day of her husband's illness. Her stool culture grew only *Escherichia coli*.

Two weeks later, baby D. stopped feeding and developed watery diarrhea. His rectal temperature was 38°C. His parents brought the infant to the pediatrician. The baby had signs and symptoms of dehydration, with an estimated fluid loss of approximately 7% of body weight, and was admitted to the hospital. Neither leukocytes nor red blood cells were seen in the stool. Baby D. was rehydrated with an oral rehydration solution. His fever abated and appetite returned although the diarrhea persisted. The preliminary laboratory report stated that the stool cultures contained "normal fecal flora"; 2 days later, the laboratory identified "enteropathogenic *E. coli*" by serological tests. Baby D. improved and was discharged after 4 days, having lost 1 lb in weight. One month later, he returned to his normal growth curve.

The following questions arise:

1. Why did the physicians caring for Mr. D. think of cholera?
2. Are all enteric bacteria capable of causing disease or are some more frequently pathogenic than others? Which enteric pathogens cause diarrhea and where do they come from?
3. What are the clinical manifestations caused by enteric pathogens? Why do the organisms cause different intensity of symptoms in individuals?
4. What factors are involved in colonization? What factors are involved in causing symptoms?
5. What is the proper therapy for watery diarrhea?
6. Can these diseases be prevented?

Mr. D. and his son developed two different secretory diarrheal diseases. Mr. D had acquired cholera during travel; baby D. was infected with an enteropathogenic *E. coli* (EPEC), probably acquired after returning home. Among the most common bacterial pathogens in the United States are strains of *E. coli* present in the intestine of humans or animals. Other important causes of watery diarrhea include *Shigella sonnei* and *Salmonella*, which are discussed in Chapter 17 ("Invasive and Tissue-damaging Enteric Bacterial Pathogens"). In addition, viruses

(most commonly rotavirus) or protozoa (*Giardia, Cryptosporidium,* or *Cyclospora*) can also cause watery diarrhea.

Most diarrhea episodes can be traced to a specific pathogen; however, clinical laboratories do not routinely use all available diagnostic methods. The predominant isolate under aerobic culture conditions, *E. coli*, cannot usually be classified as either pathogenic or nonpathogenic strains by the usual laboratory studies. As many as 40% of patients under 2 years of age have rotavirus (see Chapter 37, "Rotaviruses") and many preschool children in day care will be infected with *S. sonnei* or protozoa (see Chapter 51, "Intestinal and Vaginal Protozoa").

Although infants in the United States may have 1–2 readily treated diarrhea episodes per year, infants and children in developing countries may have 5–10 or more. Many of these infants and children advance to life-threatening dehydration. Limited access to medical care in some countries means that many potentially treatable cases will end in death.

ENTERIC PATHOGENS: ENTEROBACTERIACEAE AND VIBRIONACEAE

Most of the bacteria that cause diarrheal disease belong to a large family of Gram-negative rods, the **Enterobacteriaceae**. Some belong to the **Vibrionaceae** (Tables 16.1 and 16.2). The Enterobacteriaceae include members of the normal flora of the intestine as well as frank pathogens. Members of both families may cause a wide spectrum of disease including diarrhea, urinary and respiratory tract infection, sepsis, and meningitis. The members of the Enterobacteriaceae are differentiated on the basis of serological and metabolic properties (see Tables 16.1 and 16.2). The family Vibrionaceae also includes many nonpathogenic species as well as organisms that cause epidemic cholera, sporadic diarrhea, and local skin or bacteremic infections.

Cholera is the paradigm of secretory diarrhea and is caused by *V. cholerae,* a member of the Vibrionaceae. One particular serological type, *V. cholerae* O1, has been responsible for yearly epidemics in the Indian subcontinent for centuries and, for at least the last two centuries, periodic global pandemics. It is named "O1" because it contains a **lipopolysaccharide** (LPS) antigen that belongs to the O1 serogroup. The O1 group contains two biotypes, the "classical" and "El Tor types." Until 1961, the El Tor type was considered an avirulent commensal when it was found to cause the seventh recorded pandemic in the early 20th century. Beginning in Indonesia, El Tor cholera rapidly spread in Asia, reaching Europe and Africa in the early 1970s and Latin America in 1991. Although the disease rapidly disappeared from Europe, it has become endemic in Africa and Latin America (Fig. 16.1).

Table 16.1. Main Genera of Pathogenic Enterobacteriaceae and Vibrionaceae

Genus	Main Reservoirs	Principal Diseases
Enterobacteriaceae		
Escherichia	Ileum and colon of vertebrates	Diarrhea, dysentery, urinary tract infections, septicemia, neonatal meningitis, others
Shigella	? Human colon	Diarrhea, dysentery
Salmonella	GI system of animals, and humans	Diarrhea, bloody diarrhea, typhoid (enteric) fever, aortitis, osteomyelitis, other focal infections
Proteus	? Colon of vertebrates, ? water, ? soil	Urinary tract infections, septicemia, pneumonia
Klebsiella, Enterobacter, Serratia, Citrobacter	? Colon of vertebrates, water, sewage	Pneumonia, septicemia—special problems in debilitated or immunocompromised patients
Yersinia	Rodents, pigs, water	Plague, bloody diarrhea, diarrhea, pseudoappendicitis and mesenteric adenitis syndrome
Vibrionaceae		
Vibrio (*alginolyticus, vulnificus*)	Marine water ecosystems	Watery diarrhea—certain species associated with phytoplankton; can cause skin infections or septicemia
Campylobacter	GI system of animals	Diarrhea, bloody diarrhea septicemia (certain species only)

Table 16.2. Gram-negative Rods That Cause Diarrhea, Bloody Diarrhea, and Dysentery

	Diarrhea	Bloody Diarrhea	Inflammatory Diarrhea/ Dysentery Ileitis	Colitis
Enterobacteriaceae				
ETEC	+			
EPEC	+		±	
EAggEC	+			
EIEC		+		+
EHEC		+		+
Shigella		+	±	+
Nontyphoidal *Salmonella*	+	±	+	±
Salmonella typhi			±	
Yersinia enterocolitica	+	+	+	
Others	+			
Vibrionaceae				
Vibrio cholerae	+			
Vibrio parahemolyticus	+	+	±	±
Campylobacter jejuni	+	+	±	+

Abbreviations: ETEC = enterotoxigenic *E. coli*; EPEC = enteropathogenic *E. coli*; EAggEC = enteroaggregative *E. coli*; EIEC = enteroinvasive *E. coli*; EHEC = enterohemorrhagic *E. coli.*

A small endemic focus of cholera exists along the Gulf Coast of the U.S., known since 1973, and a few cases of cholera occur yearly due to eating shellfish harboring the organism. In the United States, cholera is transmitted primarily by eating contaminated raw or partially cooked shellfish harvested from this area of the Gulf of Mexico. Cholera rarely occurs in other areas of the United States because of the high level of environmental sanitation and protected drinking water supplies.

In contrast to *V. cholerae*, which is never a member of the normal human flora, *E. coli* is the most abundant **facultative anaerobe** in normal human feces. However, it is outnumbered by at least 1000:1 by **strict anaerobes** such as *Bacteroides.* Most fecal *E. coli* are avirulent and do not cause disease; some human strains have been cultivated in the laboratory for so long that they have lost the ability to colonize humans. These strains include *E. coli* K12, the strain that occupies center stage in molecular biology and gene cloning and is no doubt the best understood cellular form of life.

E. coli is an umbrella designation for a number of rather varied pathogenic and nonpathogenic strains. There are at least five distinguishable groups of *E. coli* now known to cause enteric disease (Table 16.3). With one exception (the sorbitol nonfermenting *E. coli* serotype O157:H7), routine stool cultures cannot distinguish pathogenic from nonpathogenic *E. coli.* The problem in distinguishing "bad" *E. coli* from "good" *E. coli* is that all strains share the same basic taxonomic and biochemical features, although they may have different virulence factors. How then are these strains distinguished? The classic way is to determine the antigenic reactivity of the **O** antigen of the outer membrane lipopolysaccharide. There are 173 different *E. coli* O antigens. These O antigens may associate with the 60 different H antigens. This association allows for a vast number of combinations. In addition, some strains have a capsular polysaccharide antigen called K. Determining the combination of O and H antigens helps identify certain virulent clones (Table 16.3). Similar tests are also used to distinguish different cholera vibrios and the over 2300 distinct *Salmonella* serotypes.

ENCOUNTER

Some enteric pathogens are well adapted to the external environment and only incidentally cause disease.

The cholera vibrio is a normal inhabitant of coastal estuarine waters, where it lives in close association with phytoplankton. Humans are incidentally infected when they enter this ecosystem or when the organisms contaminate drinking water or food. Seasonal increases in the vibrio population also occur. High temperatures or algal blooms increase the likelihood of vibrio transmission to humans. If the organisms reach the drinking water and food supplies, epidemic spread can occur. Note that inducing diarrhea can be viewed as an evolutionary mechanism that facilitates the dispersal of the organisms and their transfer to new hosts.

Certain enteric pathogens (for example *Salmonella*) are seldom found in the environment but are usually associated with humans or animals. Although these or-

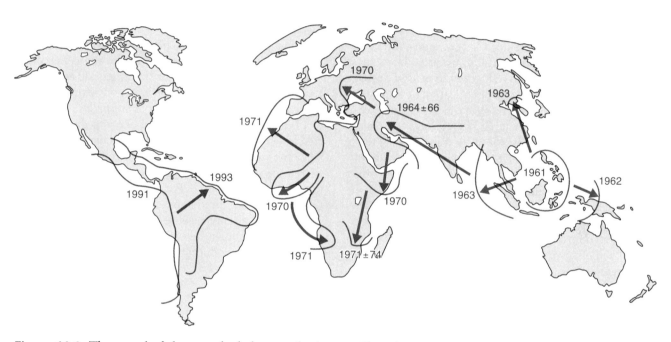

Figure 16.1. The spread of the seventh cholera pandemic from Southeast Asia. This pandemic was caused by the El Tor biotype of *V. cholerae*, which has a higher asymptomatic carriage rate than the classical biotype. In the 1990s, a new type has emerged from El Tor by acquiring a novel lipopolysaccha- ride antigen, i.e., O139 instead of O1. Prior infection with El Tor provides no immunity to *V. cholerae* O139 "Bengal". Infections with this new strain appeared in Bangladesh in the 1990s and have spread to India and other countries; this may represent the beginning of the eighth pandemic of cholera.

Table 16.3. Classification of Pathogenic *E. coli* and Representative Serotypes

Group	Symptoms	Epidemiology
Enterotoxigenic (ETEC)	Watery diarrhea (travelers' diarrhea)	Worldwide, adults and children
Enteropathogenic (EPEC)	Watery diarrhea	Infants <1 year of age
Enteroaggregative (EAggEC)	Watery diarrhea, persistent diarrhea	Infants <6 months of age, ? AIDS patients
Enteroinvasive (EIEC)	Bloody diarrhea	Uncommon, often foodborne
Enterohemorrhagic (EHEC)	Bloody diarrhea, hemorrhagic colitis, hemolytic–uremic syndrome, thrombotic thrombocytopenic purpura	Western nations

ganisms display considerable host specificity, species barriers are often crossed. The diseases caused in humans by animal-specific strains are called **zoonoses** (see Chapter 70, "Zoonoses").

The route for transmission of enteric pathogens is from feces to mouth; however, many intermediary vehicles intervene, characterized as the 7 "F's": feces, food, fluids, fingers, flies, fomites (inanimate objects), and fornication. The number of organisms required to cause disease (**inoculum size**) is probably better known for enteric bacteria than for most other organisms. Experimental infections have been induced in human volunteers who agreed to drink buffered solutions containing a known number of living bacteria. A few hundred *Shigella dysenteriae* type 1 are sufficient to cause disease in many volunteers. In contrast, 1,000–10,000 *Shigella flexneri* and over 100 million enterotoxigenic *E. coli* are required to cause the same attack rate. A direct consequence of a small infective dose is that, under the same conditions, *Shigella* are generally transmitted from person to person, because small inocula are readily passed by fingers or objects after contact with stool or soiled diapers. It is more difficult to directly transfer an infectious dose of enterotoxigenic *E. coli* because transmission requires a visible lump of feces! It is more likely that large numbers of *E. coli* enter humans when they ingest contaminated food or water in which the organisms have already multiplied.

Despite the high standards of modern hygiene, we are nevertheless in constant contact with enteric bacteria. Feces are an approximate 20% suspension of bacteria in water. Each day, we are in contact with and ingest fecal microorganisms to a greater or lesser extent, depending on our age (which determines behavior) and the state of environmental sanitation. Because potential pathogens are so common, why do not we get diarrhea every day? The answer to this question requires an understanding of the mechanisms of pathogenesis of these diseases and host defenses, both specific and nonspecific.

ENTRY

Having arrived at the mouth, microorganisms face a perilous journey along the alimentary canal to their final destiny. The gastrointestinal tract is a tube lined with differentiated epithelial cells that keep bacteria "outside" the body and deliver them to the environment through the anus. The journey is perilous because the microorganisms face host defenses and hostile conditions. They are subjected to wide variation in pH, from less than 1 in the stomach to 9 or higher near the ampulla of Vater, where they are bathed in bicarbonate-buffered pancreatic juice. In the small intestine, they are smothered in mucus; rolled up in sticky polysaccharide balls; and kneaded, squeezed, and swept distally toward the anus by **peristaltic motions** of the bowel unless they

find a way to hold on. Throughout the journey, they encounter soluble proteins such as lysozyme, proteases, lipases, and secretory IgA immunoglobulins, as well as bile salts and phagocytic and lymphoid cells. If they pause in the large intestine, they meet the populous normal flora that resists implantation by new species, in part by previous occupancy of adhesion sites on the gut wall and in part by producing inhibitory substances (e.g., bacteriocins).

The efficiency of these host defenses is the reason why the infectious dose of most noninvasive enteric pathogens is high and that disease is not common. Some conditions, however, may be advantageous to the pathogen. For example, pathogens mixed with food are protected from stomach acid, and the infectious dose is therefore diminished. In some patients, gastric acid secretory capacity can be seriously impaired by intrinsic disease (pernicious anemia), infections such as *Helicobacter pylori* (gastritis), prior surgery (gastric resection, diversions, or transections of the vagus nerve), or antiulcer drugs that inhibit or buffer gastric acid. These patients are at greater risk for infection with acid-sensitive bacteria like *V. cholerae* or *Salmonella*.

In the case, Mr. D. was more likely to develop clinical cholera upon exposure to the organism for two reasons: first, he was an ulcer patient receiving H_2 blockers to reduce gastric acid secretion, and second, he was blood group O positive. For unknown reasons, O-positive persons are predisposed to develop more severe cholera, presumably because certain oligosaccharides on cells or in secretions enhance binding of the organism, or cholera toxin production, or cause other altered responses of the mucosa.

SPREAD AND MULTIPLICATION

Cholera vibrios have several features that may help them reach the epithelial surface of the small intestine. Their flagellum make them actively mobile, and they produce a protease that hydrolyses mucus. They colonize the site by adhering to the epithelial surface. **Adherence** is not a simple feat because the surfaces of both microbe and host are negatively charged (for optimal adherence, the surfaces should not be mutually repulsive). Vibrios often have specific adhesins at the end of their **pili** or **fimbriae** to increase the distance between the host cell surface and the bacterium and diminish the electrostatic repulsion. A complex system of macromolecular assembly involves synthesis of appendage proteins, chaperones to deliver them to the bacterial cell surface, and usher proteins to assist in proper assembly. Adherence is typically accomplished by binding of sugar-binding proteins (i.e., the bacterial adhesins) to carbohydrates present in glycoproteins or glycolipids (i.e., the cell receptors) on one or the other interacting cell, much like other specific **receptor-ligand binding** events.

Among the enteric bacteria, the most important adhesins are pili or fimbriae (see Chapter 2, "Normal Microbial Flora" and Chapter 3, "Biology of Infectious Agents"), although examples of nonpilus adhesins are known as well. Virtually all Gram-negative bacteria possess type-1, or **common pili**. These pili are protein rods that help these bacteria stick to the mucosal surfaces of the gastrointestinal tract. Common pili have a special affinity for mannose-containing proteins and lipids in mucosal membranes. Despite their frequency, common pili are rarely involved in adherence of pathogenic microorganisms, which are endowed with more specialized adhesins. For example, cholera bacilli use a specific adherence pilus, called the toxin coregulated pilus (TcpA). It is so named because its synthesis is switched on by the same regulatory system that switches on the production of cholera toxin (Fig 16.2).

After adhering via their pili to receptors on intestinal brush border membranes, neither the cholera vibrios of Mr. D. or the *E. coli* of the baby will invade the mucosa. They will readily multiply because the resident flora at the level of the jejunum and upper ileum is scanty and thus there is little competition.

DAMAGE

Vibrio cholerae and Enterotoxigenic *E. coli*

Mr. D.'s diarrhea was caused by colonization of the small bowel by organisms that survived their passage across the stomach. If we had examined the small bowel mucosa, no visible damage would have been noted. Instead, the pathology occurs at the biochemical level, that is, the increase in **adenylate cyclase** activity caused by cholera toxin. In the small intestine, but not in the outside environment, cholera bacilli make **cholera toxin**; the specific pilus protein TcpA; and several accessory virulence genes. It is now known that the gene for cholera toxin is within a bacteriophage integrated into the chromosome, that the flanking accessory virulence genes are actually the phage genes, and that TcpA serves as the phage receptor on the surface of the organism. Nature is conservative and creative!

How do cholera bacilli "know" that they are in the small intestine? A number of their virulence genes, including that for cholera toxin and TcpA are activated together by a single master switch gene designated *toxR*, which is triggered by the change in environment from salt water to the human intestine. The cholera bacilli detect the change in environment by sensing the reduction in free iron in the host. By switching on the virulence genes only when the Y are in a host, these pathogens do not waste energy making products not required outside of the host. The switching occurs rapidly once the signal is perceived. **Sensory mechanisms** of this sort that coordinate regulation of virulence are a common theme in

bacterial pathogens (see "Paradigm" in Chapter 19, "*Bordetella pertussis*").

Once it is made, cholera toxin binds to a cell surface receptor (the GM1 ganglioside), is internalized within a vesicle, and is routed to the basolateral membrane of the intestinal epithelial cell. Here, the specific target of the cholera toxin, the G_S regulatory protein of the adenylate cyclase complex is located. Cholera toxin is an enzyme capable of modifying G_S by ADP-ribosylation (the transfer of the ADP-ribosyl moiety of nicotinamide adenine dinucleotide [NAD] to substrate proteins; see Chapter 9, "Damage"). The modification of G_S protein results in permanent activation of adenylate cyclase and an increase in intracellular **cyclic AMP**. Increased concentra-

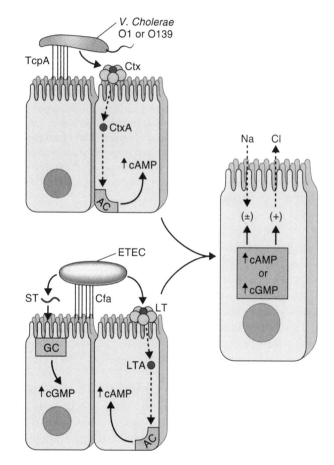

Figure 16.2. The pathogenesis of cholera and ETEC infections. The organisms colonize the mucosal surface via microbial adhesins, the **toxin coregulated pilus** (*TcpA*) of *V. cholerae* and the **colonization factor antigen** (*Cfa*) of enterotoxigenic *E. coli*. **Cholera toxin** (*Ctx*) or **labile toxin** (*LT*) binds to receptor, is taken up in vesicles, and is transported to the basolateral membrane to the **adenylate cyclase** (*AC*) complex. The toxins **transfer ADP-ribose** to the **GTP-binding protein** of AC, elevating **cyclic-AMP**. ETEC also produce a heat-stable (*ST*) toxin which binds to the membrane guanylate cyclase (*GC*) and increases cyclic GMP levels (c-GMP). Both c-AMP and c-GMP reduce Na^+ absorption in villus cells and increase Cl^- secretion in crypt cells, leading to **watery diarrhea**.

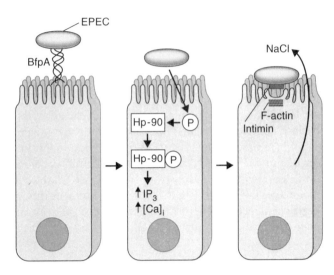

Figure 16.3. The pathogenesis of EPEC. First, the organism attaches to the small bowel epithelial cell via a **bundle-forming pilus** (*BfpA*). This binding sets in motion signal-transducing events involving **phosphorylation** of a major epithelial cell protein, Hp-90; **activation** of phospholipase C; increases in **inositol triphosphate** (*IP$_3$*) and **calcium** (*[Ca]$_i$*); and damage to the microvilli. In a third stage, **intimin** mediates intimate adherence, and a 39 kDa protein causes **polymerization of actin** and other host cytoskeletal proteins and **rearrangements of the cytoskeletal structure**. Together these form the characteristic EPEC pedestal with the intimately adherent organism (the **attaching and effacing** lesion).

tions of cyclic AMP inhibit sodium absorption by small bowel villous cells and increase chloride secretion by crypt cells. Because the amount of NaCl in the gut lumen is increased, water is retained by osmotic force and the unabsorbed isotonic fluid is excreted as diarrheal stool. In a case of cholera, such as Mr. D.'s, the volume of water lost can be so prodigious that the patient is rapidly dehydrated, may go into shock, and, if not quickly treated, may die.

In endemic regions of Asia, Africa, and Latin America, cholera occurs primarily in children less than 10 years old, because older adolescents and adults are usually protected by acquired immunity. During epidemics in previously cholera-free areas, all age groups are susceptible. This age-specific pattern is typical of endemic vs. epidemic infections. Mortality is caused by electrolyte and water losses, and therefore with proper fluid replacement no patient should die of cholera. Without therapy, as in the past, as many as 50% of patients are likely to die.

Related to cholera are infections due to **enterotoxigenic *E. coli*** (ETEC). These strains produce one or both **enterotoxins**, called **LT** and **ST**, both of which act by changing the net fluid transport in the gut from absorption to secretion. LT is structurally similar to cholera toxin and activates the adenylate cyclase–cyclic AMP

system in the same manner and for the life of that cell (Chapter 9, "Damage"). However, cholera is usually more serious as it leads to the secretion of much greater amounts of liquid stools. In neither disease is the intestinal mucosa visibly damaged; the watery stool does not contain white or red blood cells and no inflammatory process occurs in the gut wall. ST interacts with and activates the **guanylate cyclase** of intestinal cells which leads to an increase in **cyclic GMP** and altered sodium and chloride transport, much like LT and cholera toxin. However, effects on guanylate cyclase are turned off if the toxin is washed away from the cell. Toxins related to cholera or ST toxins have also been found in a number of other diarrheal pathogens such as *Salmonella*, *Campylobacter*, *Yersinia*, *Aeromonas*, and most recently, the enteroaggregative *E. coli*.

Enteropathogenic *E. coli*

Baby D. was infected with an enteropathogenic *E. coli* (EPEC), one of a small group of specific serotypes originally recognized because they cause outbreaks of diarrhea in the newborn nursery (Table 16.3). This kind of diarrhea is caused by complex mechanisms that do not appear to involve secreted toxins. Much is known about the molecular basis of the steps involved. In step one, the organisms adhere to target epithelial cells in a relatively distant ("nonintimate") manner. Binding is via a so-called bundle-forming pilus (Fig. 16.3). In step two, the bacteria attach more closely, cell **actin** is polymerized immediately beneath the organism and alters the shape of microvilli, a rearrangement known as "effacement" of the plasma membrane. Actin polymerization is associated with several biochemical events: activation of a host cell tyrosine kinase which phosphorylates a host cell protein, Hp-90; mobilization of calcium from intracellular stores; increase in phospholipase C activity; and release of inositol phosphates and diacylglycerol. In step three, the "intimate" contact between the bacteria and epithelial cells is mediated by a number of new bacterial proteins (a protein called intimin and a secreted 39 kDa protein that is essential although its function is unknown). Together with additional secreted proteins, the EPEC organism attaches within 10 nm of the broad, flat pedestal created by altered cytoskeletal proteins which results in the characteristic **attaching and effacing EPEC lesion**. How does this lesion cause diarrhea? We still do not know. The production of enterotoxins is not involved. Diarrhea may be related to the widespread signal transduction events that occur during bacterial binding, together with direct damage to the absorptive surface.

OTHER INFECTIONS CAUSED BY VIBRIOS AND *E. COLI*

In late 1992, a remarkable event occurred. For the first time, epidemic cholera due to a non-O1 *V. cholerae* strain was detected in South India, rapidly spreading to Bangladesh and neighboring countries in Asia and displacing the resident O1 strain. Individuals immune to O1 *V. cholerae* were not immune to the new strain, O139 *V. cholerae*. Thus a new epidemic began that involved all ages in the endemic countries of Asia, not just younger children as before. This event is an example of the continuing emergence of new disease pathogens with extended virulence.

The appearance of the new strain was traced to a mutation of V. *cholerae* El Tor, which conferred the expression a previously unknown lipopolysaccharide (LPS) somatic antigen, O139. This mutation required a large deletion in the O1 LPS biosynthetic genes and the insertion of a new segment of DNA for the O139 antigen. Where did the new gene come from? We do not know, although evidence points to a genetic exchange with other bacteria in the environment. In addition, the organism acquired at least one new gene involved in making a capsule, an unusual feature in *V. cholerae* O1. The new organism has since traveled to Europe and the United States, suggesting that a new pandemic, the eighth recorded, may be under way. In 1995, however, the classic O1 vibrio displaced O139 as the dominant cholera organism in Dhaka, Bangladesh, whereas O139 has persisted in nearby Calcutta, India. The ultimate fate of O139 cannot yet be predicted.

Other marine vibrios lacking the characteristic virulence attributes of *V. cholera*, such as *Vibrio parahemolyticus*, cause a bloody diarrhea associated with ingestion of sushi or raw shellfish, especially in Japan. Other vibrio species, such as *V. vulnificus* or *V. alginolyticus*, are often acquired through an injury or a break in the skin and may cause severe subcutaneous and invasive illnesses.

EPEC and ETEC strains of *E. coli* represent only the earliest described diarrhea-causing *E. coli* species (Table 16.3). The repertoire is already large and consists of a veritable alphabet soup of pathogenic groups: EPEC, ETEC, EIEC (enteroinvasive), EHEC (enterohemorrhagic), EaggEC (enteroaggregative), and possibly more waiting in the wings. Each is associated with identifiable genetic traits and characteristic epidemiology, and causes distinctive conditions. EIEC and EHEC are discussed in (Chapter 17, "Invasive and Tissue-damaging Enteric Bacterial Pathogens." EAggEC autoagglutinate (aggregate) in tissue culture and are associated with diarrhea in children who are less than 6 months of age, often persisting for weeks with marked nutritional consequences. Recent data suggest that EAggEC is also the agent of persistent diarrhea in some adults with HIV infection.

Other *E. coli* involved in invasive disease in infants and young children, and which cause bacteremia and systemic diseases such as meningitis or urinary tract infections in children and adults, are discussed in Chapters 59 ("Respiratory System") and 61 ("Skin and Soft Tis-

sue"), respectively. In every case, specific virulence factors are critical in determining the nature of the resulting disease. Many of these factors are known; others are being investigated. Still others remain to be discovered.

DIAGNOSIS

Mr. D. was diagnosed with cholera because his physician knew about the ongoing epidemic in the country Mr. D. visited and alerted the laboratory to use special media not routinely employed. On the usual media for bacterial diarrhea, *V. cholerae* is similar to commensals in its sugar fermentation patterns and will not be picked for further diagnostic studies. On special media, however, the distinctive *V. cholerae* colonies are easily identified. Further analysis of the isolate at the Centers for Disease Control and Prevention in Atlanta, Georgia, revealed it to be genetically identical to the epidemic Latin American and not to the Gulf Coast endemic strain. This information indicated that Mr. D.'s was an imported case and constituted no threat to the local population. The case was not attributed to contaminated seafood that could cause a local outbreak, nor was excretion of viable organisms a problem because of the effective water sanitation in Mr. D.'s home town.

The stool from baby D. was grown on both cholera-selective media (because of the father's diagnosis), as well as other media designed for both selection and differentiation of possible pathogens. By incubating the culture in air, the numerically dominant strict anaerobes in normal feces were eliminated. The media used permit the growth of enteric bacteria and not others by inclusion of inhibitors, such as dyes (e.g., eosin and methylene blue, as in the so-called EMB agar) or bile salts (as in MacConkey agar), which selectively inhibit growth of Gram-positives. Because these media are not especially rich, they also exclude fastidious Gram-negatives (such as *Haemophilus influenzae*).

The diagnosis of baby D. was not as simple as Mr. D.'s diagnosis. All the pathogenic groups of *E. coli* described look alike on agar plates and under the microscope, as do most other enteric Gram-negative rods. They must be further classified on the basis of their biochemical and nutritional properties, such as which sugars they ferment and other biochemical reactions. Because some of the classical intestinal pathogens, like *Salmonella* and *Shigella*, do not ferment lactose, inclusion of this sugar in the medium, together with a colored pH indicator, allows rapid selection of possible lactose nonfermenting pathogens, as lactose-fermenting colonies turn a distinctive color due to the production of acid. The lactose negatives are picked for further determinative work. Other pathogens cannot be selected by this method and must be sought by different techniques. Probes and polymerase chain reaction (PCR) primers are available for most of the virulence genes of these organisms, and their action can be detected in tissue culture. However, none of these tests is clinically used today for specific diagnosis. The only serological reagents currently available commercially are antisera directed against most EPEC somatic O antigens; it remains difficult to carry out complete serotyping, a much more important marker for clones of pathogenic *E. coli*. In the case of the remaining member of the family, Mrs. D., it is likely that she had an ETEC infection, but no lab studies were carried out.

TREATMENT AND PREVENTION

The therapeutic needs for the D. family members were to replace electrolyte and fluid losses and correct metabolic imbalances. Luckily, "secretory" diarrheas are usually self-limiting and terminate without specific antibiotics, as long as the patient is well-hydrated and prevented from going into shock. Mr. D. was so severely dehydrated that he required intravenous fluids. Baby D. did well with only an oral electrolyte–glucose solution designed to enhance a physiological sodium and glucose cotransport system in the small bowel epithelial cell. Mrs. D. had such a mild and self-limited disease that no specific therapy was needed.

Oral rehydration is a simple form of therapy, which if universally applied could save the lives of millions of children every year throughout the developing world. Effective solutions can be made in the community by mixing salt, table sugar, and water. Unfortunately, it not easy to ensure that such a simple solution is available in every country and household. Experience has shown that practical problems occur in ensuring that the solution is made correctly and that adequate amounts are given at the right time. The key is education of mothers, caretakers, and medical practitioners. Much effort is now being devoted to determining how to teach this methodology. Given access to isotonic replacement fluids, no should succumb to cholera. Mortality rates in cholera epidemics exceeding 1% point to a lack of public health resources and/or inappropriate case management by inexperienced clinical personnel.

Considerable efforts have been devoted to **vaccine** development for cholera. The challenge has been twofold: (a) to identify and prepare protective antigens; and (b) to find a way to present the antigen in a way that leads to a local immune response in the intestine. So far, partial success has been achieved using live oral vaccines with attenuated genetically engineered strains or killed cholera vibrios given by mouth. With the exception of a first-generation live oral cholera vaccine, it is important to note that no vaccines for secretory diarrhea pathogens have become available for routine use. Application of molecular genetics should lead to a new generation of vaccines in the coming years, including both live and purified nonviable antigen preparations.

CONCLUSION

Diarrhea is not only the trivial bother that besets all of us occasionally. It is a major cause of infant death in the developing world. Symptomatic treatment by fluid replacement requires widespread educational effort.

In every instance, local defenses of the gastrointestinal tract must be overcome for disease to occur. The efficacy of these defense mechanisms is best demonstrated by the relative rarity of intestinal infections in developed countries, despite the fact that the gut is a tube open to the exterior. Disease is seen when the load of pathogens in the environment and their opportunity for transmittal are high and when predisposing causes like malnutrition, which impair host defenses, are present as well.

SELF-ASSESSMENT QUESTIONS

1. What are the main defenses of each segment of the gastrointestinal tract against microorganisms?
2. Which are the main types of bacteria that cause intestinal infections? What distinguishes them in the laboratory?
3. Explain the main virulence factors of each group of intestinal pathogens.
4. How many types of disease do different strains of *E. coli* produce?
5. How would drugs effective against bacterial diarrhea and dysentery differ?
6. What issues should be considered in the prevention of intestinal bacterial infections?

SUGGESTED READINGS

Behrens RH. Diarrhoeal disease: current concepts and future challenges. The impact of oral rehydration and other therapies on the management of acute diarrhoea. Trans Roy Soc Trop Med Hyg 1993;87(Suppl 3):35–38.

Besser RE, Feikin DR, Eberhart-Phillips JE, Mascola L, Griffin PM. Diagnosis and treatment of cholera in the United States. Are we prepared? JAMA 1994;272:1203–1205.

Cantey JR. *Escherichia coli* diarrhea. Gastroenterol Clin North Am 1993;22:609–622.

Guerrant RL. Lessons from diarrheal diseases: demography to molecular pharmacology. J Infect Dis 1994;169: 1206–1218.

Kaper JB, Morris JG Jr, Levine MM. Cholera. Clin Microbiol Rev 1995;8:48–86.

Mekalanos JJ, Sadoff JC. Cholera vaccines: fighting an ancient scourge. Science 1994;265:1387–1389.

Wachsmuth IK, Blake PA, Olsvik O, eds. *Vibrio cholerae* and cholera: molecular to global perspectives. Washington, DC: American Society for Microbiology, 1994.

Waldor MK, Mekalanos JJ. Lysogenic conversion by a filamentous phage encoding cholera toxin. Science 1996;272: 1910–1914.

CHAPTER 17

Invasive and Tissue-damaging Enteric Bacterial Pathogens: Bloody Diarrhea and Dysentery

GERALD T. KEUSCH

DAVID W. K. ACHESON

Key Concepts

The main invasive enteric pathogens are:

- *Shigella*, which cause dysentery and bloody diarrhea. *Shigella* is closely related to enteroinvasive *Escherichia coli* (EIEC).
- Enterohemorrhagic *E. coli* (EHEC), which cause hemorrhagic colitis. The most common serotype is O157:H7.
- *Salmonella*, which can cause nontyphoidal gastroenteritis and typhoid fever; typhoid fever is a systemic infection of mononuclear phagocytes sometimes characterized by relapses and the carrier state caused by bacterial survival in the gallbladder.

This chapter describes a group of intestinal pathogens that cause structural damage to the distal portions of the intestine, most commonly the large bowel. These organisms invade and damage the mucosa, leading to **bloody diarrhea** or **dysentery**. Dysentery is characterized by the frequent passage of stools (often more than 30 per day) that typically contain a small volume of blood, mucus, and pus. Other symptoms include cramps and pain caused by straining to pass stool (Table 17.1).

These serious, sometimes life-threatening infections frequently require antibiotics. The use of antibiotics causes problems in some developing countries where antibiotic resistance is common and effective new drugs are either unavailable or too expensive. Rehydration therapies so useful in secretory diarrhea have little impact on dysentery.

This chapter focuses on *Shigella*, the prototypic invasive enteric pathogen and the closely related **enteroinvasive** *Escherichia coli* (**EIEC**). These organisms will be contrasted with other tissue-damaging pathogens, including *Salmonella* and **enterohemorrhagic** *E. coli* (**EHEC**). We also include the agent of typhoid fever, *Salmonella typhi*, because it too enters the host by crossing the intestinal mucosa. However, typhoid fever, a systemic infection of mononuclear phagocytes, is a unique syndrome.

■ CASE 1

Shigella Dysentery

Infant V., a 22-month-old girl living in a low-income area in a Texas city near the Mexican border, became febrile, lost her appetite, and developed watery diarrhea. By the next day

---

Table 17.1. Definitions of Clinical Types of Intestinal Infection

---

Secretory or watery diarrhea
Stools: copious, watery, no blood, no pus
Tissue invasion: absent
Site: small intestine
Examples: *Vibrio cholerae, E. coli* ETEC strains

Dysentery
Stools: scant volume, blood, mucus, pus
Tissue invasion: present
Site: large intestine
Examples: shigellae, *Entamoeba histolytica* (leukocytes absent in stool)

Hemorrhagic colitis
Stools: copious, like liquid blood, no leukocytes
Tissue invasion: absent
Site: large intestine
Example: *E. coli* EHEC strains

Bloody watery diarrhea
Stools: copious, liquid, bloody or blood-tinged, pus (sometimes)
Tissue invasion: present
Site: ileum, colon
Examples: salmonellae, *Campylobacter jejuni, Yersinia enterocolitica*

---

her diarrhea had abated, but her parents noticed mucus and that her stools were blood-tinged. The number of stools and the bloody appearance increased, and the baby began to vomit. The parents brought the child to a hospital emergency room. Her temperature was found to be 40°C. Shortly after arrival, she had a generalized seizure. Physical examination revealed a sick-looking, somnolent infant with mild dehydration and hyperactive bowel sounds. Laboratory results showed leukocytosis and a mild decrease in serum sodium and glucose. The child was given fluids and an antibiotic. Several days later, *Shigella flexneri* grew from her stool culture. No further seizures occurred, and over the next few days, the dysentery subsided. The child had lost 2 lb in weight, however, but caught up to her growth curve 2 months later.

The following questions arise:

1. What is the likely source of the shigellae?
2. How did these organisms enter into V.'s intestinal tract?
3. What bacterial properties were involved in producing the bloody diarrhea?
4. How should this disease be treated?

The classic causes of **dysentery** are bacteria of the genus *Shigella* but also include the **ameba**, *Entamoeba histolytica* (Chapter 51, "Intestinal and Vaginal Protozoa"). Approximately 15,000–20,000 cases of **shigellosis** are reported to the U.S. Centers for Disease Control and Prevention (CDC) each year. Since fecal cultures are infrequently obtained, it is estimated that the real number of cases is at least tenfold greater. Children under five are 10 times more likely to contract this disease than the rest of the population. Severe and fatal cases are uncommon in industrialized countries.

THE SHIGELLAE

The genus *Shigella* consists of **four species**, which are distinguished serologically by the **O antigen** of their lipopolysaccharide (LPS). These are named *S. dysenteriae* (serogroup A), *S. flexneri* (group B), *S. boydii* (group C), and *S. sonnei* (group D). Each of these groups is further subdivided into subgroups. *S. dysenteriae* type 1 (which is now encountered primarily in developing countries) causes the most serious illness (dysentery), while *S. sonnei*, the predominant isolate in industrialized countries, causes the mildest one (watery diarrhea). *Shigella* cannot be readily distinguished from *E. coli* by DNA hybridization and are actually differentiated pathogenic clones of *E. coli*.

Encounter

Shigellae are highly host-specific, causing natural infections in humans and only occasionally in other higher

---

Humans, Health and History

The known history of shigellosis has followed an interesting course. Following its original description in 1898, *S. dysenteriae* was the major isolate until replaced by *S. flexneri* after World War I, which itself was supplanted by *S. sonnei* in industrialized countries following World War II. Beginning in 1969, however, epidemic *S. dysenteriae* reappeared in Latin America, Asia, and Africa. The reasons for these changes in prevalence over time are not known. *S. flexneri* has recently increased again in the U.S. among young adult males, apparently due to homosexual practices, but not in the rest of the population.

primates. Encounter is most commonly by direct person-to-person contact, although transmission through food or water contaminated with feces also occurs. In contrast to cholera and enterotoxigenic *E. coli* (ETEC) and enteropathogenic *E. coli* (EPEC) strains (Chapter 16, "Secretory Diarrhea"), the inoculum needed for *Shigella* infection is very small—a few hundred to a few thousand organisms. The small size of the effective inoculum allows the organisms to be easily transmitted from one person to another.

Entry, Spread, and Multiplication

How do shigellae survive in the stomach? These organisms are relatively acid-resistant during certain phases of their growth, significantly more so than many other enteropathogenic bacteria. The organisms sense the acid environment and adapt to it because they possess a global regulatory system of genes whose expression requires a **sigma factor** of **RNA polymerase** (called RpoS) that is made only in the stationary phase of growth. When exposed to acid, the organisms survive but are less able to invade cells, at least in cell culture. Once they reach the small bowel (an alkaline or neutral environment) and begin to grow again, their acid resistance is repressed and the invasive phenotype is restored. Acid resistance is also enhanced by anaerobiosis, the condition the organisms later encounter in the colon. It is likely, therefore, that when shigellae are excreted in the stool, they express the acid-resistance phenotype. This phenotype is useful because when they are subsequently ingested by a new host, they are already prepared to survive passage through the stomach. Thus, acid resistance may well contribute to the shigellae's success as pathogens.

Once past the stomach, the organisms pass through the small bowel and enter the colon. Bacterial multiplication occurs mainly in the intracellular environment of the intestinal epithelial cell. Invasion and survival of shigellae within gut cells is a complex process that involves multiple genes present on both a large virulence plasmid and the chromosome. This is an interesting story and makes a good model for understanding the invasive properties of other enteric bacteria. Several steps are involved:

1. The shigellae **approach the mucosal surface** by an as yet unknown mechanism (they have no flagella and are nonmotile). Intestinal epithelial cells are resistant to invasion by *Shigella* at their luminal surface, although they are susceptible at their **basal surface**.
2. How do the shigellae reach the lower portion of the intestinal cells? By stealth, first entering specialized **M cells** , antigen-sampling cells that overlie the lymphoid follicles (Fig. 17.1). Invasion of M cells depends on several plasmid-encoded outer membrane proteins (**invasion plasmid antigens**, or IpaB, C, D).

3. The bacteria are now released into the **lamina propria**, where they are ingested by macrophages. As a result, the macrophages release interleukin-1 (IL-1), causing a marked **inflammatory response** with recruitment of neutrophils (the process can be inhibited by IL-1 antagonists or by antibody to CD18, a surface determinant that mediates migration of neutrophils in inflammation). This initial inflammatory response to small numbers of invading shigellae markedly increases the subsequent invasion and is essential to cause clinical illness; the host leukocytic response is thus a key part of pathogenesis. The invading organisms are now near the "back door," the susceptible basal surface of the epithelial cells.
4. The shigellae must now prod the epithelial cells to ingest them. Mucosal epithelial cells are not "professional phagocytes" and usually do not take up particles. Thus entry requires major reorganization of actin and cytoskeletal elements, just as occurs in regular phagocytosis. These changes are elicited by bacterial factors.
5. Once inside the epithelial cells, the organisms rapidly escape the **phagosomal vesicle**, assisted by a microbial protein that lyses the phagosome membrane. They then enter the cytoplasm where they multiply.
6. Having successfully invaded an epithelial cell, how do the organisms now infect other epithelial cells? Rather than starting over from the intestinal lumen, they instead invoke a particular example of **molecular parasitism** that involves appropriating elements of the host cell's cytoskeleton. As they multiply, the shigellae make a protein called **IcsA** (for "intracellular spread") at one pole of the rod-shaped organisms. IcsA is an ATPase that causes polymerization of host cell **actin** (see Fig. 8.1). The deposition of actin bundles near one end of the bacterium (the "rear") propels the organisms forward. The force exerted is strong enough to push the organism and the overlying cell membrane into a fingerlike projection that pokes into the adjacent cell (see Figs. 8.1 and 17.1). The bacterium is now surrounded by two cell membranes, one from the old (previously invaded) cell and one from the new cell. When these membranes lyse, the organism is released in the cytoplasm of the new host cell and the process can begin again. In this manner, **cell-to-cell invasion** occurs without the need to reenter the extracellular milieu. Could this explain why circulating antibodies have little effect on the disease? What about cell-mediated immunity?

Damage

When a sufficient number of contiguous invaded cells die and slough off, the result is a surface erosion in the gut wall, or an **ulcer**. Neutrophils that accumulate in

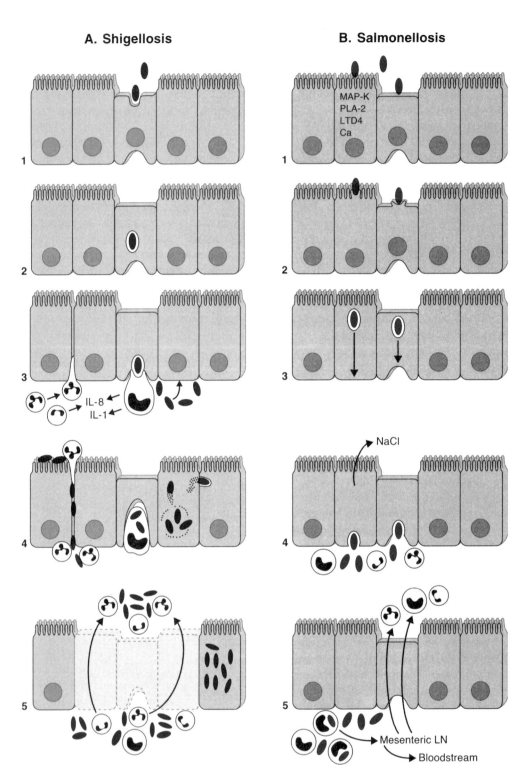

A. Shigellosis

B. Salmonellosis

Figure 17.1. Invasion strategies of *Shigella* compared with Salmonella in the intestinal epithelium. Shigellae (**A**) are unable to invade intact epithelial cells from the luminal surface. Instead, they initially enter the mucosa overlaying intestinal lymphoid follicles via specialized M cells (*1*). Having transited through the M cells (*2*), some bacteria enter underlying macrophages (*3*). There, the *ipaB* gene product is transferred to the macrophage via a type III secretion mechanism (see paradigm) and induces release of the cytokine IL-1b. A cascade of additional cytokines generates an influx of polymorphonuclear leukocytes (*3*) which migrate through the mucosa and cause separation of tight junctions between columnar epithelial cells (*4*). This separation subsequently permits the organisms to penetrate the disturbed epithelium. Once in the lamina propria, shigellae can invade the basal surface of epithelial cells (*3*). Internalized bacteria escape from phago-

somes and travel from an infected cell to adjacent ones, using a mechanism that depends on actin and other host cytoskeletal proteins (*4*). Cell death results in a focal ulcer and exudation of inflammatory cells into the lumen, along with red blood cells to produce the dysentery stool (*5*). In *Salmonella* infection (**B**), organisms approach the mucosal surface (*1*), where they induce MAP-kinase, PLA-2 activity, production of LTD4, and mobilization of intracellular Ca^{++} (*2*). These events induce surface ruffles (*3*, and see Fig. 17.3), leading to uptake of organisms within host cell membrane bounded vesicles (*4*). These mediators result in electrolyte accumulation in the lumen (*4*) and an inflammatory exudate (*5*), to produce the diarrhea of *Salmonella* gastroenteritis. Bacteria are taken up by macrophages in mesenteric lymph nodes and some escape to the bloodstream, resulting in transient bacteremia (*5*).

PARADIGM ■ ■ ■

Bacterial/Host Communication Using Specialized Secretion Mechanisms

Microbes have evolved a variety of mechanisms for secretion of proteins into the environment. Often this ability allows them to survive within a host because the secreted molecules aid in microbial survival or dissemination. The challenge for microbes is how to transmit water-soluble proteins across their own and the host's lipid membranes. Complex and incompletely understood mechanisms operate in these processes. In Gram-negative cells, toxins typically are delivered extracellularly in a two-step process. The toxin is first secreted into the periplasmic space, where the toxin assembles into its final quaternary structure. In a second step, the toxin is transferred across the outer membrane, apparently without unfolding. Translocation across the outer membrane may require a dedicated protein pore through which the toxin, but not other proteins, may pass. Once extracellular, toxins secreted in this fashion gain access to the host cell by first binding to host surface molecules. This process of extracellular secretion is known as the **general secretion pathway**, or, sometimes, **type II secretion**, and is the subject of intense study.

Another mechanism for transmitting proteins from the microbe to the host cell that has received a great deal of attention in recent years is called **contact-dependent** or **type III secretion**. In contrast to the process described above, in this system there is no detectable periplasmic form of the protein being secreted. In some examples of type III secretion, there is no detectable extracellular form. Rather, the secreted protein is delivered directly from the microbe into the host cell by a process that has been likened to injection with a syringe.

Type III secretion systems have been studied in a wide range of pathogens, including some that cause disease on animals and plants. Examples are *Yersinia* (responsible for mild diseases such as food poisoining as well as the more notorious and life-threatening plague), *Shigella*, and the enteropathogenic *E. coli* (EPEC). The type of molecule delivered into the host cell differs in each case. In the case of *Yersinia*, type III secretion is used for translocation of toxin molecules that disrupt the monocyte signaling pathways, thereby eliminating an arm of the immune system. For *Shigella*, the system is used to transfer proteins that cause the host cell to take up the microbe. Host cell invasion by shigellae is the first step in its eventual intracellular survival and cell-to-cell spread. How type III systems function is the focus of much current research. Each system that has been studied consists of several proteins that are genetically conserved, i.e., share sequence similarity and, therefore, are likely to have similar functions. In fact, many of the proteins of the secretion system of one organism may functionally replace those of another. Some of the conserved proteins appear to form a pore within the host cell membrane, through which other proteins may pass into the cytosol of the host. In addition, in the *Yersinia* type III system, an outer membrane protein has biochemical and sequence similarity to the proposed outer membrane pore of the type II system described above. This suggests that the protein of the two systems may share common functions.

In these days of rapidly diminishing antibiotic choices, the possibility that type III secretion systems may prove useful targets for antimicrobial drug design has captured the imagination of investigators. Another possibility for exploiting type III secretion lies in the notion of using suitably engineered microbes to deliver therapeutic molecules into eukaryotic cells with the same efficiency that they currently deliver toxins and invasion proteins. Both of these fanciful possibilities will likely be much closer to reality after more basic research is done to fully define how type III secretion can so efficiently accomplish the challenging task of moving proteins across membranes.

VICTOR DARITA

---

large numbers in the mucosa are shed in the stool, where they are easily detected by light microscopy.

The bloody and pus-containing stools and the pain associated with bowel movements (**tenesmus**) are characteristic of *Shigella* dysentery. Despite the ulcers and the inflammatory response, bacteremia is uncommon, except for *S. dysenteriae* type 1 infection. Bacteremia is most often encountered in poorly nourished infants in developing countries, and is promoted by defects in host defenses associated with malnutrition, such as depressed complement activity.

One species, *S. dysenteriae* type 1 produces in addition **Shiga toxin,** a cytotoxin that kills intestinal epithe-lial and endothelial cells. Shiga toxin is an enzyme that irreversibly inactivates the mammalian 60S ribosomal subunit, and thereby stops protein synthesis. Shiga toxin acts in a complex way. First, Shiga toxin targets the sodium-absorptive villus cell and decreases sodium absorption, which leads to an excess of fluid in the lumen. Second, effects of the toxin on mucosal endothelial cells contribute to the bloody diarrhea that follows.

Experimental infections in monkeys have shown that strains with inactivated Shiga toxin gene still cause disease but with much less damage to the mucosa and less bleeding. Thus, both invasion and toxin production are important in pathogenesis, which may explain why the highly toxigenic *S. dysenteriae* type 1 causes the most severe clinical illness of all *Shigella* species. *S. flexneri* also causes severe illness, dysentery, and bloody diarrhea, despite its lack of the genes for Shiga toxin.

It is curious that *S. sonnei* uses the same mechanisms of invasion as *S. dysenteriae* type 1 and *S. flexneri*, but only rarely causes the dysentery syndrome; most commonly, it leads to a self-limited watery diarrhea. The basis for these differences is not understood, but is probably related to the fact that these organisms do not induce as intense an inflammatory response and do not make Shiga toxin.

Diagnosis

When patients develop bloody diarrhea or dysentery, *Shigella* must obviously be included in the list of possible causes. In some parts of the world, up to 50% of patients with bloody diarrhea or dysentery are **culture-positive** for *Shigella*. In contrast, this diagnosis may escape consideration in the mild watery diarrhea caused by *Shigella sonnei*, which grossly resembles that of other pathogens such as ETEC, EPEC, or even rotavirus. The presence of leukocytes in diarrheal stool is a simple indicator of an invasive pathogen, and their detection provides immediately useful diagnostic information.

The specific diagnosis of shigellosis relies on culturing the organisms. Because shigellae rapidly die off when excreted in stool, isolation rates depend on rapid processing of the stool sample, by either streaking directly onto isolation agar or, in field studies, into a transport medium to maintain viability until the sample can be processed. As with other enteric bacteria, media have been designed to detect the lactose-negative phenotype characteristic of *Shigella*. A rapid presumptive diagnosis can be made by suspending suspicious colonies in saline and carrying out agglutination reactions with antisera to group antigens of *Shigella*. Additional information is provided by testing for biochemical and fermentation patterns, which allow genus and species identification.

Now that many genes characteristic of *Shigella* and EIEC strains have been cloned and sequenced, it has become possible to identify the organism more rapidly by looking for specific genes using **DNA probes** or **amplification methods** such as polymerase chain reaction (PCR) (see Chapter 55, "Diagnostic Principles"). These methods can be used on stool samples or environmental samples such as food or water for quick diagnosis or to trace transmission routes. They are likely to come into increasing and widespread use in the future, but because of cost and lack of facilities, they are not in general use at present.

Therapy and Prophylaxis

Shigellosis does not usually cause severely dehydrating diarrhea, thus, intravenous fluids are rarely needed to treat this infection. Oral fluids usually suffice to correct the mild to moderate degree of dehydration and

electrolyte abnormality. In more severe cases that involve bloody diarrhea or dysentery and high fever, the use of effective antibiotics reduces the duration of illness and the period of infectivity to others. Reducing the infective period is particularly important because the small inoculum needed for infection with *Shigella* frequently results in transmission to other household members.

The use of antibiotics is complicated by the ease with which the organisms acquire **antibiotic resistance;** it is not pure chance that transferable antibiotic resistance was first discovered in *Shigella*. The problem is greatest in developing countries where multiresistant *S. dysenteriae* type 1 is most commonly found, and where cost and availability of the newest antimicrobials are limiting factors. The most reliably effective drugs at present are the **fluoroquinolones.** Use of these drugs in patients under 17 years of age is not approved by the Food and Drug Administration because animal toxicity studies suggest that younger patients may be at risk of cartilage and joint damage. Some new β-lactam and cephalosporin antibiotics are also effective. To make educated empiric decisions on which drug to use, clinicians should be aware of the drug susceptibility pattern of pathogens encountered in their own community and institutions.

No vaccine for shigellosis has been licensed, but many candidates are under study using virulence molecules as candidate antigens. These are being altered and packaged in different ways; the goal is to produce living attenuated vaccines that can be administered by mouth and immunize the gut itself. There is also renewed interest in the possibility of using nonliving antigens for the same purpose. Various gene fusions and chemically conjugated vaccine antigens are being made and tested in experimental systems. Ultimately, however, these vaccines must be tested in humans, since no animal model truly mimics human shigellosis.

ENTEROHEMORRHAGIC *E. COLI*

◼ CASE 2

Enterohemorrhagic *E. coli* Disease

Mr. R., an 85-year-old resident of a nursing home, was awakened by the onset of severe abdominal cramps, primarily in the right lower quadrant of the abdomen. Later that morning, he had a watery diarrhea every 15–30 minutes, initially with small amounts of visible blood. Later that day, bright red stools consisting of what seemed to be pure blood appeared. He was nauseated but did not vomit. When seen the next morning by the physician on call, he did not have a fever. However, clinical examination of the abdomen revealed tenderness over the colon.

Because of the clinical findings, Mr. R. was hospitalized. Frankly bloody stools continued. A barium enema revealed edema of the ascending and transverse colon with areas of spasm. Routine stool cultures were negative for *Salmonella* and *Shigella*. However, **sorbitol nonfermenting** *E. coli* were subsequently identified by the State Public Health Laboratories as serotype O157:H7, an EHEC strain. The patient was treated with intravenous fluids and gradually recovered over the next 7 days. By the time he was discharged back to the nursing home, his stool was negative for this particular *E. coli* strain.

The day before he became ill, Mr. R. was visited by his 2 1/2-year-old granddaughter. They all shared a fast-food hamburger lunch. Two days after Mr. R. fell ill, the baby developed watery diarrhea. The diarrhea increased over the next 2 days and then became tinged with blood. When the baby began to vomit and the urine output appeared to diminish, the parents brought the baby to the pediatrician. She was somewhat pale, lethargic, with a fluctuating level of consciousness. The laboratory reported a significant decrease in platelets and red blood cells, many of which looked abnormal. The diagnosis of diarrhea-associated hemolytic–uremic syndrome (HUS) was made, and the child was hospitalized. A stool culture was negative. The baby was treated conservatively, and no antibiotics were given. No hypertension developed, the renal failure and hemolytic anemia did not progress, and dialysis was not performed. She was discharged 1 week later with no further diarrhea and improvement in the blood count.

The following questions arose:

1. What is the likely source of the organisms that caused these diseases?
2. Why do only certain strains of *E. coli* cause the clinical manifestations seen in these cases?
3. By what mechanisms does the etiological agent responsible cause these diseases?
4. What are the principal therapeutic concerns in such cases?

The enterohemorrhagic *E. coli* (**EHEC strains**) include a number of *E. coli* serotypes that can cause a characteristic **nonfebrile bloody diarrhea** known as **hemorrhagic colitis**. The most commonly identified serotype in the U.S. is O157:H7. It is estimated that EHEC strains cause at least 20,000–40,000 infections yearly in the U.S. Approximately 250–500 deaths are caused by the **hemolytic-uremic syndrome (HUS)**, a complication of hemorrhagic colitis consisting of a particular form of hemolytic anemia, thrombocytopenia, and renal failure. These deaths occur most commonly in young children, and are now the most frequent cause of acute renal failure in children in the U.S. EHEC produce one or two related but antigenically distinguishable toxins that share the same enzymatic specificity and binding site as Shiga toxin of *S. dysenteriae* type 1. These constitute a family of protein toxins; the *E. coli* versions are known as Shiga toxins 1 and 2 (also called Shigalike or Vero toxins). Less often, **bloody watery diarrhea** is due to other pathogens, including in the U.S. *Shigella*, *Salmonella*, *Campylobacter jejuni*, or more uncommonly, *Yersinia enterocolitica*.

Encounter

We know the most about *E. coli* O157:H7 because the organism can be easily identified in the clinical laboratory. These strains have a convenient distinguishing laboratory characteristic, the inability to ferment sorbitol. However, their real prevalence compared to other EHEC serotypes has not been determined. O157:H7 clearly causes both outbreaks and sporadic disease, primarily as a zoonosis that is transmitted from animals to humans. Undercooked hamburger is the principal vehicle, but other food vehicles have been described. Ground water may become contaminated in the vicinity of cattle farms and transmit infection as well. The organism appears to be acid-resistant and the estimated infectious dose is tiny, approximately 50 organisms per gram of hamburger. Person-to-person transmission in day care centers, as in *Shigella* infections, has been documented.

Entry, Multiplication, and Damage

Once past the stomach, EHEC colonize the terminal regions of the bowel where they remain confined to the surface of the gut mucosa and multiply locally. They do not invade the bloodstream. EHEC possess a homologue of the EPEC *eae* gene complex (Chapter 16, "Secretory Diarrhea") that mediates the same dramatic rearrangements of actin and cytoskeletal elements that leads to a characteristic **attaching and effacing** lesion of the brush border (see Fig. 17.2). EHEC's production of Shigalike toxins may be responsible for a local cytokine response in the colonic mucosa. It is currently believed that pro-

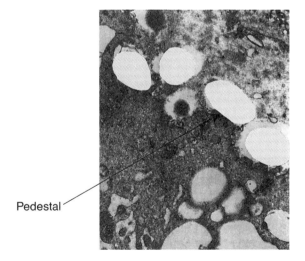

Pedestal

Figure 17.2. Electron micrograph of colon from monkey infected with a O157:H7 EHEC strain isolated from a human with hemorrhagic colitis. This animal developed bloody diarrhea. Note the attaching bacteria and the altered epithelial cell membrane beneath them showing intimate attachment and "pedestal" formation. This attaching and effacing lesion is associated with EHEC and EPEC expressing the *eae* gene complex (original magnification, ×28,526). Four bacteria are artificially colored.

fuse bleeding is caused by the interaction of inflammatory cytokines and Shigalike toxins, which damages blood vessels in the lamina propria.

The major complication of EHEC, which occur in approximately 5% of severe clinical cases, is damage to small blood vessels. When this occurs predominantly in renal glomeruli, usually in small children, HUS results. When the target is the brain, commonly in older adults, the syndrome is called thrombotic thrombocytopenic purpura. Because these conditions are also complications of infection by Shiga toxin–producing *S. dysenteriae* type 1, it is difficult to escape the conclusion that the toxin is required to cause these clinical pictures. HUS resulting from EHEC is the most common cause of acute renal failure in children in the U.S. It is estimated that as many as 5–10% of HUS-affected children will die promptly, and an unknown number may require dialysis or, eventually, a renal transplant. Shiga toxin is cytotoxic, suggesting that direct damage to glomerular endothelial cells may be the initiating factor of these diseases. Endothelial cell products (including von Willebrand factor, plasminogen activator inhibitor, prostacyclin, nitric oxide, and others) may mediate local pathophysiology leading to platelet thrombi, the characteristic feature of the disease.

Diagnosis

The classic syndrome of hemorrhagic colitis is sufficiently characteristic to be recognized clinically (see the case, above). Less severe bloody diarrhea is not so revealing, and diagnosis depends on detecting the organism in stool. Culture methods using sorbitol–MacConkey agar identify just O157:H7 but miss the occasional sorbitol-positive O157:H7 and other EHEC strains which, like most *E. coli*, ferment sorbitol. An enzyme immunoassay to detect Shiga toxins 1 and 2 is commercially available to detect toxin or any toxin-producing organisms in stool and is both highly sensitive and specific. Newer methods using PCR to detect specific DNA have been described, but are not yet in use.

Therapy

Treatment for EHEC infections is controversial. Some clinicians have suggested that antibiotic therapy may increase the likelihood of the hemolytic–uremic syndrome based on the possibility that antibiotics help release of Shiga toxins and LPS from dying or dead organisms and increase the exposure of the host to their effects. No proof for this hypothesis exists, but the reason for this notion may be that patients with more severe diarrheal disease are more likely to be treated with antibiotics, and will thus fare worse than patients with less severe disease, with or without the drugs. Fluid therapy is relatively simple because EHEC do not typically cause large volume losses and severe dehydration. The major challenge is to treat complications of EHEC by support-

ive measures, including dialysis for renal failure if needed. Thrombotic thrombocytopenic purpura usually responds rapidly to exchange transfusion, for unknown reasons.

NONTYPHOIDAL *SALMONELLA* AND TYPHOID FEVER: INTRODUCTION TO THE AGENTS

■ CASE 3

Typhoid Fever

Ms. J., an Asian exchange student in the U.S., returned home for a 3-month visit. Near the end of her visit, she cared for her aunt who had high fevers and some diarrhea. Three weeks later, when back in the U.S., Ms. J. had a shaking chill and fever to 38.5°C, with headache, muscle pain, and loss of appetite. The fever continued and progressively increased over the next several days. When seen at the Student Health Service, she appeared ill and confused. Her abdomen was diffusely tender and her liver and spleen were enlarged, although she did not have jaundice. In spite of the high fever, her pulse was relatively low at 90 beats per minute. The white blood cell count was low, only 3000, with a moderate monocytosis. An astute clinician made the presumptive diagnosis of typhoid fever, and therapy with cephtriaxone was initiated and continued for 14 days.

Admission blood cultures subsequently grew *Salmonella typhi*, thus confirming the diagnosis. The fever gradually abated over the next 3 days, and Ms. J. made an uneventful recovery. However, 6 weeks later, all of her symptoms recurred, including a maximum fever of 38.5°C. *S. typhi* was again isolated from blood culture and was found to still be sensitive to trimethoprim–sulfamethoxazole. She was treated again for 2 weeks with the same drug with a rapid response. She experienced no further recurrence.

A number of questions arose:

1. Do the same salmonellae cause diarrhea, dysentery, and typhoid fever?
2. Can the epidemiology of typhoid fever be distinguished from that of other salmonelloses?
3. Why were organs other than those of the digestive system involved in Ms. J.'s disease?
4. Why is it particularly important to treat cases of typhoid fever with antibiotics?

There are four clinical syndromes, plus the carrier state, associated with the genus *Salmonella*:

- **Gastroenteritis** (nausea, vomiting, and diarrhea, caused mainly by serovars *S. enterica* subspecies *enterica*). This disease resembles some of those described in Chapter 16, "Secretory Diarrhea."
- **Focal infection of vascular endothelium** (caused by serovars *choleraesuis* and *typhimurium*).

- **Infections of particular organ systems** (e.g., osteomyelitis in sickle cell disease patients most commonly due to serovar *typhimurium*).
- **Typhoid fever** (caused mainly by serovars *typhi* and *paratyphi* A and B).

Some salmonellae are specific to animals and do not cause human disease; some, such as *typhi* and *paratyphi* A or B are human-specific and cause typhoid fever. A large number can cross host species. These are the most common causes of *Salmonella* diarrhea.

The genus *Salmonella* is vast, comprising over 2300 serological varieties (**serovars**), and growing. The main antigens of *Salmonella* that distinguish its serovars are **somatic (O)**, **flagellar (H)**, and **capsular (K)**. Individual isolates express more than one O and H antigen at a time, and each strain is defined by a particular combination. The tremendous diversity of the genus is due to the ability of *Salmonella* to undergo **antigenic variation**, the ability to create mosaics of genes for their antigens through recombination, alterations in length, gene duplications, and point mutations. Only two species of *Salmonella* are now recognized, *Salmonella enterica* and *S. bongori*. *S. enterica* consists of six subspecies, each of which contains multiple serovars (Table 17.2). Most human pathogens are grouped within a subdivision of *S. enterica* called subspecies *enterica* (subsp. I). However, it is still clinically useful to sort serovars into groups designated by the letters A, B, C, etc. Serogrouping is usually the first information available from the clinical laboratory regarding a *Salmonella* isolate, and provides a tentative clue to identification of the organisms likely to be involved.

Encounter

Salmonellae are common members of the normal flora of many animals, including chickens, cattle, and reptiles (e.g., pet turtles). The strains that cause **gastroenteritis** are usually transmitted by chicken meat, eggs, and dairy products. Unless care is taken in poultry farms, chicken eggs often become contaminated, both on their surface and within. Outbreaks are most frequent in summer months and are often related to contaminated egg or chicken salads. **Typhoid fever**, on the other hand, is traceable to a human carrier (such as the infamous Typhoid Mary), although the routes of transmission often involve contaminated water or food. It is interesting that, because its host range is strictly limited to humans, *S. typhi* could potentially be eradicated, whereas organisms that colonize many other species can not.

Like other enteric pathogens, salmonellae must travel from feces, whether human or animal, to the mouth. Significant changes and adaptations in the organisms are required for survival of this trip. The organism must use it genetic potential for attachment, replication, and sur-

Table 17.2.   Classification and Serogroup of Some Human Pathogenic Salmonellae

Species	Group	Serovar
S. enterica	A	*paratyphi* A
	B	*typhimurium*
		derby
		heidelberg
	C1	*cholerasuis*
		infantis
		virchow
	C2	*muenchen*
		newport
	D1	*dublin*
		enteritidis
		typhi
S. bongori		

vival. In addition, it must be able to disperse in the environment and infect new hosts.

Entry

Salmonellae are more acid-sensitive than shigellae, and therefore have a predilection for individuals who produce little or no stomach acid (hypo- or achlorhydria). A relatively large inoculum is required to infect human volunteers with normal gastric acid secretion (10–100 million organisms), but the inoculum size is reduced 10- to 100-fold when bicarbonate is given along with the inoculum. Salmonellae also sense the acid environment of the stomach and at low pH express at least 40 proteins of possible importance in pathogenesis. The organisms that successfully escape being killed in the stomach pass through the small bowel to the distal ileum and colon. There, like shigellae, they penetrate the mucosal barrier (see Fig. 17.1). It is not known with certainty whether entry involves the M-cell surface, the apical membrane of the gut epithelial cells, or the tight junction between cells. Contact of salmonellae with cells in culture induces a dramatic "ruffling" of the plasma membrane, a visual harbinger of cytoskeletal rearrangements that lead to uptake of the organisms within phagocytic vesicles (Fig. 17.3). Hence, the entry of salmonellae into cells is another example of microbe-directed phagocytosis.

In contrast to the shigellae, which must escape to the cytoplasm to multiply intracellularly, salmonellae remain within vesicles for many hours. Salmonellae are unusually resistant to the lysosomal contents of cells or to the antibacterial peptides made by intestinal epithelial cells called cryptins. The bacteria-containing vesicles eventually travel to the basal membrane, and the organisms are released into the lamina propria. For salmonellae, then, gut epithelial cells are not the main habitat for

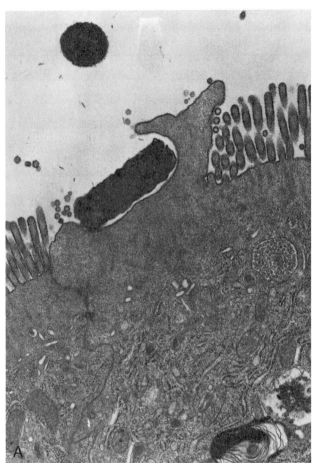

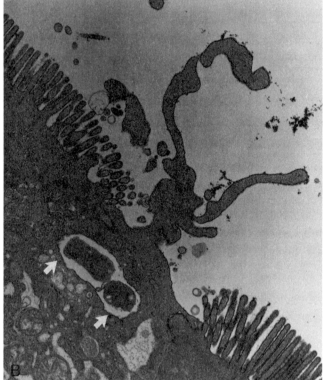

Figure 17.3. Ruffling of host cell membranes during intracellular *Salmonella* infection. A mouse pathogenic *Salmonella* (var. *typhimurium*) was inoculated into ligated loops of mouse ileum and samples for electron microscopy taken after 30 minutes. At this time, the bacteria were associated exclusively with M cells. **A.** A bacterium in contact with an M cell and the initial phase of a ruffle response on the M-cell surface. **B.** Pronounced ruffling. Two bacteria (*arrows*) are seen in a vesicle inside the M cell. Original magnification, ×12,000.

multiplication but rather barriers to be crossed. After the alterations in the brush border are reversed, the gut cells are apparently not harmed.

Spread and Multiplication

The pathogenesis of salmonellosis is shown schematically in Fig. 17.4. After salmonellae reach the lamina propria, they often enter the bloodstream and may be recovered in blood cultures early in the course of the disease. They normally do not cause sustained **bacteremia** because they are rapidly taken up by the phagocytic cell system and are effectively killed. Exceptions to this rule include some serovars (*typhimurium, enteritidis,* and *dublin*), which spread systemically more often than the others, and frequently cause focal systemic infections. Clinical conditions that impair mononuclear cells enhance susceptibility to *Salmonella* bacteremia. For example, patients with sickle cell anemia have a tenfold higher incidence of invasive salmonellosis. A marked in-

crease in incidence and severity of infection is observed as well in patients with AIDS, leukemia or lymphoma, and chronic granulomatous disease.

In typhoid fever, passage of the organisms into the small bowel is followed by invasion across the mucosa and their rapid uptake by mononuclear cells in regional lymph nodes. An initial bacteremia carries them to the liver and spleen. The hallmark of typhoid-causing serovars is their ability to survive and grow within these cells (Fig. 17.2), in contrast to the gastroenteritis-causing salmonellae. This systemic spread is clinically silent and brief. As the organisms multiply in macrophages of liver, spleen, and mesenteric lymph nodes, patients are also clinically asymptomatic. When the number of intracellular organisms reaches a threshold, they are released into the bloodstream, initiating a continuous bacteremia characteristic of typhoid fever. This event signals the start of clinical illness, manifested by daily high fevers that continue for 4–8 weeks in untreated cases. This second bacteremia leads to invasion of the **gallbladder**, **kidney**, and reinvasion of the **gut mucosa**, especially at the Peyer's patches. At this stage, the organism can be isolated not only from blood, but also from stool and urine (Fig. 17.5). Uptake of organisms by monocyte/macrophages in bone marrow makes this site a useful source of culture material when other sites are negative, as the organisms may be actually enriched at this site.

Damage

The interaction of **gastroenteritis-producing** salmonellae with epithelial cells activates the inflammatory response and results in damage to the intestinal mucosa. Here too, the interaction of the organisms with the host cells is complex. One of the first events in this interaction is the assembly of **nonpili appendages** within 15 minutes of contact between the organism and the host cell. In *typhimurium*, the best studied serovar, at least 14 genes of an operon called *inv* are involved. By 30 minutes, ruffles form on the host cell, and the bacterial appendages disappear (Fig. 17.3). To be pathogenic, salmonellae must not only assemble the appendages, but also be able to shed them; thus *invA* or *E* mutants that assemble appendages but never lose them are avirulent, as are *invC* or *invG* mutants that never assemble these structures.

Many biochemical events are activated by signals during invasion. Activation of the mitogen-activated protein kinase (MAP kinase) may be the first signal. MAP kinase is linked to a receptor on the cell surface. Binding of the organisms leads to activation of phospholipase A_2 (PLA_2), release of arachidonic acid, production of prostaglandins and leukotrienes, and a sharp increase in intracellular calcium concentration. These events certainly underlie the induction of ruffles and subsequent bacterial uptake, but a number of the mediators involved are also capable of altering **electrolyte** transport and causing diarrhea. As yet, the mechanism by which fluid secretion is induced by *Salmonella* remains uncertain. Invasion induces the production of inflammatory cytokines, such as IL-8, leading to local leukocyte infiltration. This ability to invade and cause inflammation is known to be necessary but not sufficient to cause diarrhea in experimental animals. Thus, additional traits need to be expressed. It is known that the disease is dependent on transepithelial signals, probably cytokines, elicited by the organism to recruit neutrophils. Evidence also exists that some salmonellae produce a cholera toxin–like molecule that alters electrolyte and fluid transport.

A distinctive feature critical to typhoid fever is the ability of the organism to survive and multiply within macrophages. This feature is controlled by microbial and host genes. The microbial contribution has been studied in *typhimurium* infection of mice. It is of inter-

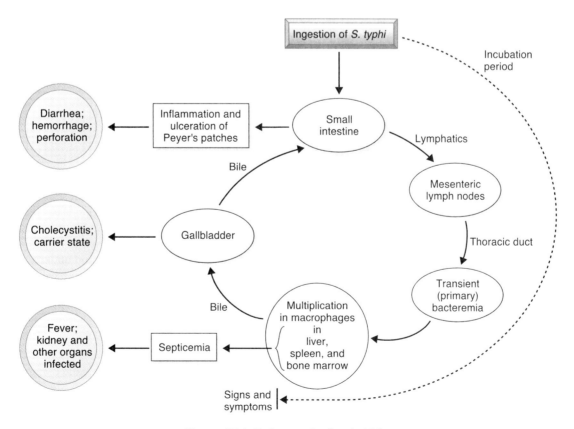

Figure 17.4. Pathogenesis of typhoid fever.

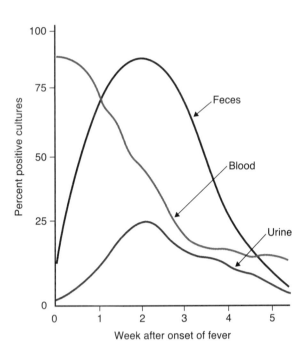

Figure 17.5. The isolation of typhoid bacilli from various sources in the course of untreated typhoid fever. The late rise in positive stool cultures is caused by secondary invasion of the gut by organisms from the gallbladder.

est that this organism typically causes a typhoidlike syndrome in mice and diarrhea in humans, whereas the human typhoid bacillus is not a mouse pathogen. Virulence in *typhimurium* is regulated by a **two-component regulator/signal system** consisting of two genes, PhoP/PhoQ. Mutations in these genes lead to decreased microbial survival in macrophages, increased sensitivity to acid pH and mammalian antimicrobial peptides, and, consequently, to attenuation of virulence. This system is similar to a number of other bacterial two-component systems. It permits the organism to sense environmental signals and adapt in response by modifying the expression of a whole repertoire of genes. These include at least 20 genes that are either activated or repressed. For all of them, the response is mediated by binding of transcriptional regulators to enhancer DNA sequences.

Invasive nontyphoidal salmonellae (such as serovar *dublin*) possess a virulence plasmid that shares a conserved 8 kb region of DNA containing *spv* (for *Salmonella* plasmid *v*irulence) genes. This region encodes genes that are turned on when salmonellae enter eukaryotic cells. Other plasmid genes encode resistance to complement by blocking assembly of the terminal attack complex on the cell surface, thus enabling the organisms to resist this host defense mechanism.

In addition to these microbial factors, host genes also regulate survival of salmonellae within macrophages. These genes were initially identified as a locus on mouse chromosome 1. It was subsequently found that the same

locus was involved in resistance to at least two other facultative intracellular pathogens, the protozoan *Leishmania* and the attenuated vaccine strain for tuberculosis, BCG. The human homologue of this gene was later identified on chromosome 2 and found to be part of a family of at least three genes that control a natural macrophage-specific membrane transport protein. How these genes affect the early killing of intracellular pathogens is not yet clear, but mechanisms distinct from those in activated macrophages appear to be involved. Recent studies have shown this locus is also linked to the genes for the interleukin-1 receptor and for susceptibility to type 1 diabetes in mice and the IL-8 receptor gene cluster in humans.

Invasion of the gallbladder by typhoid bacilli may be temporary or may result in the long-term colonization that characterizes the **typhoid carrier state**, especially in the presence of gallstones. Occasionally, acute necrotizing cholecystitis may result. Typhoid bacilli survive well in gallstones and can be recovered from the center of a stone; viable organisms may still be obtained after dipping stones in antibiotics. Gallstones are a source of prolonged asymptomatic carriage and excretion of the organism in stool.

The source of secondary gut invasion may be bacteria from the bloodstream during the prolonged secondary bacteremia or bacteria shed in the bile that penetrate M cells. Such secondary reinvasion leads to severe bleeding and/or perforation attributable to the marked inflammatory response induced in the Peyer's patches. We do not know why the invasion of the gut at this stage results in more extensive damage to the intestinal mucosa than the primary invasion, but severity could be immunologically mediated. Invasion of liver, spleen, and kidney can result in hepatitis, splenitis that makes the spleen prone to rupture, or glomerulonephritis. The clinical prognosis is much worse when these events occur.

Endocarditis and **vascular infection** are caused by specific *Salmonella* serovars capable of adhering to endovascular surfaces. *S. choleraesuis* and *S. typhimurium* adhere well to endothelial cells and may cause aortitis or endocarditis. These conditions are difficult to treat and often require surgical intervention. *S. typhimurium* also causes osteomyelitis in individuals with hemoglobinopathies (e.g., sickle cell anemia), trauma, and underlying bony abnormalities. Despite its predilection to cause continuous bacteremia, *S. typhi* only rarely adheres to vascular epithelia and is an uncommon cause of endocarditis.

Diagnosis

Salmonellosis is generally diagnosed in the laboratory by culture on selective media and a combination of serological and biochemical tests to identify individual serovars. The salmonellae are nonlactose fermenters, and the same media used for shigellae allow them to be selected for further testing as well. Most clinical laboratories can identify *S. typhi* and determine the O-serogroup for other isolates (A–E for human *Salmonella*) and deduce the most likely serovars, but they are not usually equipped for more detailed diagnoses. Further identification is most useful for epidemiological purposes and usually requires the assistance of a State Public Health Laboratory or the Centers for Disease Control and Prevention.

Typhoid fever is not recognized in the asymptomatic incubation period. The specific diagnosis is usually made by blood culture, which becomes positive early in the course of clinical illness (see Fig. 17.5). Isolation of *S. typhi* is helped by their resistance to bile salts (the organisms survive in bile itself within the gallbladder). *S. typhi* is one of just three organisms that produce a capsular antigen called Vi, an antiphagocytic virulence factor.

Typhoid fever can also be diagnosed by **serology**. A rising titer or a single very high anti-O antigen titer is suggestive. The Vi antigen also elicits an antibody response; however, because other organisms also produce the same antigen, this response is suggestive but not definitive for *S. typhi*. These tests rely on **agglutination** of the organisms by antibodies present in patient sera. In a positive test, the bacteria make clumps visible to the naked eye. The highest dilution of serum that results in agglutination is the antibody titer.

Therapy and Prophylaxis

In the past, *Salmonella* **gastroenteritis** was not usually treated with antibiotics, because such drugs did not shorten the duration of the disease. Instead, they prolonged carriage of the organisms in the stool. This is not the case with new fluoroquinolones, which both eradicate the organism and decrease the period of illness. A concern exists that excessive use of fluoroquinolones will select for resistance and that they may no longer be effective in the future.

Systemic nontyphoidal *Salmonella* infections require antimicrobial therapy. A number of drugs may be used, depending on antibiotic resistance patterns. Prevention of salmonellosis relies on avoiding potentially contaminated water or foods that contain raw eggs or unpasteurized milk or milk products, or cooking these foods enough to kill the organisms. Preventive measures are especially important for people with diminished gastric acid or an immunodeficiency disease, such as HIV infection. However, it is neither easy nor foolproof. Considerable work is currently under way to develop attenuated vaccine strains for immunization.

The morbidity and mortality from typhoid fever have been significantly reduced by antibiotic therapy. Most cases in the U.S. are now imported. It must be remembered that therapy does not eradicate the organism. Oddly, the relapse rate is higher in treated individuals, possibly because early therapy aborts immune responses

necessary for preventing relapse. Without effective cell-mediated immunity, surviving bacteria can multiply to the point where they again cause clinical symptoms. Progress has been made in developing a **typhoid vaccine** in the past few years. A live oral attenuated *S. typhi* strain, rendered avirulent by a mutated enzyme for galactose metabolism, is able to penetrate the mucosal M cells. However, the bacteria cannot survive because the enzymatic defect results in the accumulation of galactose, which is ultimately toxic to the bacteria. Thus, natural immunity can develop while the organism self-destructs. Even better vaccines using strains engineered with deletions in aromatic pathway genes may be in the wings. A purified Vi polysaccharide vaccine induces protection in older children and adults, and a Vi–protein conjugate vaccine is being developed to immunize infants too young to respond to the polysaccharide alone. These vaccines have an efficacy of 60–80%.

Typhoid carriers are a public health concern because they are often asymptomatic shedders; they not only carry the organism but constantly spread them via their feces. Treatment of typhoid carriers has been difficult but also represents a social imperative. Since there was no successful treatment in her day, Typhoid Mary was jailed. Today, the recommended course of action is prolonged antibiotic therapy (a new fluoroquinolone may be the most effective form), with removal of the gall bladder if gallstones are present.

CONCLUSION

Bacterial pathogens may damage the intestinal mucosa and lead to bloody and/or inflammatory enteritis. Damage results from the invasion or intimate interaction with the surface of the intestinal mucosa, the elicitation of an inflammatory response alone or in concert with the production of cytotoxins that alter gut epithelial cells or endothelial cells, or production of bacterial protein toxins. Multiple genes encoded by chromosomal or plasmid DNA are required for virulence. The inflammatory response may not only be a response to injury, but, as in the example of *Shigella*, is required for pathogenesis.

Watery diarrhea is indistinguishable on the clinical level whether caused by nontyphoidal *Salmonella*, ETEC strains, certain *Shigella* species, or rotavirus. Shigellae and, on occasion, certain salmonellae may produce frankly bloody diarrhea or dysentery. The noninvasive EHEC typically cause nonfebrile grossly bloody diarrhea known as hemorrhagic colitis. These organisms share virulence traits with EPEC and *Shigella*. The differences in clinical manifestations can be ascribed to the specific virulence factors these organisms express, but this extrapolation is less than perfect.

Typhoid bacilli are highly human-specific organisms that enter the host via the fecal–oral route and invade the intestinal mucosa. However, unlike nontyphoidal *Salmonella*, they produce typhoid fever, a fundamentally different infection in which the organism behaves as an intracellular pathogen of mononuclear phagocytes. Both microbial and host genes affect this interaction. The identification of these genes has yielded new information about the basic pathogenic mechanisms involved.

SELF-ASSESSMENT QUESTIONS

1. Describe the steps in pathogenesis of shigellosis and typhoid fever.

2. What are the distinguishing characteristics of EHEC (enterohemorrhagic *E. coli*) strains and the diseases they cause?

3. Describe the systemic and local manifestations of typhoid fever. How does typhoid fever differ from *Salmonella* gastroenteritis?

4. Describe the properties of typhoid bacilli that help explain the complex cycle of typhoid fever and distinguish these organisms from nontyphoidal salmonellae.

5. Given the route of transmission of *Shigella*, *Salmonella*, and the enterohemorrhagic *E. coli*, what precautions can be taken to lessen the risk of infection with these organisms?

6. Which, if any, of these infections is likely to represent a problem in AIDS patients?

SUGGESTED READINGS

Acheson DWK, Donohue-Rolfe A, Keusch GT. The family of Shiga and Shiga like toxins. In: Alouf JE, Freer JH, eds. Sourcebook of bacterial protein toxins. New York: Academic Press, 1991.

Bliska JB, Galan JE, Falkow S. Signal transduction in the mammalian cell during bacterial attachment and entry. Cell 1993;73:903–920.

Eckmann L, Kagnoff MF, Fierer J. Intestinal epithelial cells as watchdogs for the natural immune system. Trends Microbiol 1995;3:118–120.

Lindberg AA, Pal T. Strategies for development of potential candidate Shigella vaccines. Vaccine 1993;11:168–179.

Moors MA, Portnoy DA. Identification of bacterial genes that contribute to survival and growth in an intracellular environment. Trends Microbiol 1995;3:83–85.

CHAPTER 18

Pseudomonas aeruginosa: Ubiquitous Pathogen

DEBBIE S. TODER

Key Concepts

Pseudomonas aeruginosa:

- Is a ubiquitous opportunistic pathogen found in soil and water.
- Has minimal nutritional requirements and survives in a variety of environments.
- Is a frequent cause of nosocomial (hospital-acquired) infections.
- Is an important pathogen in individuals with cystic fibrosis, burns, and diabetes.

Pseudomonads inhabit the soil and water; contact with healthy humans is widespread but usually insignificant. However, these organisms are important **opportunistic pathogens** that cause a variety of infections in immunocompromised patients, such as burn victims, cancer patients, and children with cystic fibrosis. Pseudomonads have flexible nutritional requirements and are capable of using a wide variety of carbon and nitrogen sources to grow in diverse environments.

Because of this adaptability and their intrinsic and acquired resistance to many common antibiotics, pseudomonads find the hospital environment accommodating. Equipment that requires a wet, body-temperature environment, such as dialysis tubing and respiratory therapy equipment, is particularly susceptible to contamination by *Pseudomonas*. In the hospital, *Pseudomonas aeruginosa* can be cultured from hand washing sinks, hand creams, and even certain cleaning solutions. Although few healthy humans are colonized with *P. aeruginosa*, admission to the hospital increases the carriage rate.

CASE 1

R., a 4-year-old Caucasian boy on maintenance chemotherapy for acute lymphocytic leukemia (now in remission),

was brought by his parents to the emergency room because of fevers as high as 41°C over the preceding 24 hours. In the emergency room, he was alert but ill-appearing and preferred to sit on his mother's lap. His skin was pale, his breath and pulse were rapid, and he was in mild respiratory distress with clear lung fields. Despite his fever, his extremities were cool and clammy. A central venous catheter had been surgically implanted because of many intravenous medications he required. The site where the catheter entered the skin was intact and dry without any redness.

Blood analysis revealed that he had a white blood count of $300/\text{mm}^3$, of which only 30% were neutrophils (an absolute neutrophil count of 90, normal being >1000). A third-generation cephalosporin (ceftazidime) and an aminoglycoside (tobramycin) were started intravenously. Within the next hours, R.'s status deteriorated, with worsening respiratory distress, requiring intubation and mechanical ventilation, and circulatory failure requiring fluid therapy and drugs to increase his blood pressure. He was tentatively diagnosed with shock probably due to sepsis (bacterial infection of the bloodstream).

The initial blood cultures were positive for *P. aeruginosa*, but those obtained during fevers the second and third days of hospitalization were negative. R. gradually improved and he was gradually weaned from the drugs used to increase his blood pressure and from ventilatory support. His next course of cancer chemotherapy was delayed be-

Table 18.1. Relationship between Selected Predisposing Factors and Varieties of *Pseudomonas* Infections

Predisposing factor	Type of infection
Local breach of the immune system	
Cystic fibrosis	Pneumonia, chronic recurrent
Trauma	Osteomyelitis
IV Drug abuse	Endocarditis, septic arthritis, osteomyelitis
Neurosurgical operations	Meningitis
Surgical operations	Pneumonia
Tracheostomy	Pneumonia
Intravenous lines	Cellulitis, suppurative thrombophlebitis
Corneal injury	Panophthalmitis
Kidney stones	Urinary tract infection
Catheterization	Urinary tract colonization and urinary tract infection
Systemic	
Neutropenia	Septicemia, pneumonia, abscesses
Diabetes	Malignant otitis externa
Premature infants and neonates	Septicemia, meningitis, enteritis
Both systemic and local	
Burns	Burn wound infection, septicemia

cause his blood counts remained low, but these did improve and this therapy was continued.

The following questions arise:

- What was the main predisposing factor for R.'s illness?
- Where did *P. aeruginosa* come from? How did it gain entry into R.'s bloodstream?
- What caused the symptoms of the infection?
- What other sites could become infected in such a patient?

In this case, R.'s impaired host defenses, a consequence of his cancer and treatment, put him at increased risk for infection. Although it did not play a role in this case, an indwelling catheter in the bladder or a vein, or an endotracheal tube increases risk by serving as a portal for infection.

As in this case, *P. aeruginosa* generally causes disease in humans only when a local or systemic breach occurs in the immune system (Table 18.1). Local lesions are often seen in people with corneal abrasions, burns, and surgical wounds. *P. aeruginosa* also causes osteomyelitis following a puncture wound (typically with a nail) of the foot. *P. aeruginosa* infects chronic cutaneous ulcers in persons with impaired local circulation, such as diabetics. Once the organism has gained entry, dissemination through the bloodstream and sepsis are possible. Patients with severe defects in immunity, such as those induced by malignancies, diabetes, or chemotherapeutic or other immunosuppressive agents are at greatest risk from systemic pseudomonal infections. In-

fections in these patients are most often caused by bacteria with which they are colonized. Therefore, acquisition of *P. aeruginosa* and other Gram-negatives in the hospital is an important problem.

■ CASE 2

The parents of Z., a 2-year-old girl with a chronic cough, became alarmed because her cough worsened over a week's time and her color "became poor" with coughing. Her parents are unable to remember when she was last cough-free and state that she sometimes spits out yellow–green mucus after forceful coughing, most often on arising in the morning.

On examination, Z. was an alert but pasty and pale-looking child with increased respiratory effort and rapid breathing. On inspiration, crackles were heard throughout the lung fields. Her extremities showed moderate clubbing with mild cyanosis. A chest x-ray (Fig. 18.1) showed increased (abnormal) interstitial and peribronchial markings. By gagging the child with a sterile swab, a specimen of the green mucus was obtained and sent for Gram stain and culture.

Based on the history, physical examination, and x-ray, a tentative diagnosis of cystic fibrosis was made. Intravenous ceftazidime and tobramycin were administered while awaiting the results of a sweat chloride test (diagnostic of cystic fibrosis) and sputum culture. The sputum Gram stain showed many Gram-negative bacilli. In culture, these bacteria were initially described as non–lactose-fermenting Gram-negative rods and then identified as *P. aeruginosa*. Z. gradually improved and, after 2 weeks of therapy, her x-ray (Fig. 18.2) showed improvement.

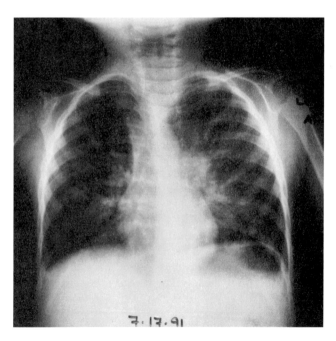

Figure 18.1. Chest x-ray of a patient with *P. aeruginosa* infection, showing interstitial and peribronchial markings.

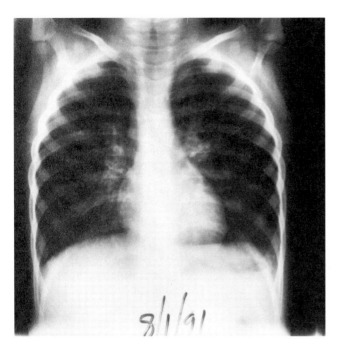

Figure 18.2. Chest x-ray of the same patient as shown in Fig. 18.1, after 2 weeks of intravenously administered ceftazidime and tobramycin.

The following questions arise:
- How does *P. aeruginosa* infection differ between the two cases?
- Do the same strains of *Pseudomonas* infect patients with cystic fibrosis and others?
- What was the route of entry of the organism in this case?
- Do antibiotics help in such a case?

This case illustrates an early episode in the course of *P. aeruginosa* infection in cystic fibrosis. Bronchopulmonary *P. aeruginosa* infection in this disease is characterized by exacerbations and remission. Although the organism is probably never completely eradicated, antipseudomonal antibiotic therapy leads to a decrease in the number of organisms in the sputum and improved pulmonary function.

Interestingly, antibiotics with little in vitro antipseudomonal activity often appear to improve the clinical status of patients with cystic fibrosis. It is possible that these antibiotics downregulate the production of virulence factors by *P. aeruginosa* in the cystic fibrosis lung. In vitro, subinhibitory concentrations of antibiotics have been shown to have this effect. The behavior and appearance of *P. aeruginosa* is different in the cystic fibrosis lung than in other infections; mucoid strains are associated almost exclusively with this disease. The polysaccharide responsible for the mucoid phenotype does not, by itself, cause tissue destruction, but it may enable the organisms to evade host defenses and persist in the lung.

Pseudomonas infection in cystic fibrosis is unique because of its exceptionally chronic course; affected individuals may become infected in childhood and, despite continued infection live, with ongoing therapy, into the fourth or fifth decade of life. Although the infection is never cleared and lung function progressively declines, *Pseudomonas* sepsis virtually never occurs in cystic fibrosis.

THE PSEUDOMONADS

The members of the genus *Pseudomonas*, colloquially called the pseudomonads, belong to a large group of aerobic nonfermenting, actively motile Gram-negative rods. About one-third of clinical isolates are pigmented and produce characteristic green or blue–green colonies colored by the water-soluble pigment pyocyanin. Colonies on agar plates have a characteristic fruity or grapelike odor, which is sometimes noticed near wounds or other sites that are heavily colonized with these organisms.

Medically, the most important species of this genus is *P. aeruginosa*, but others may also infrequently cause disease. A large number of cell-associated and secreted molecules participate in the pathogenesis of *P. aeruginosa* infections (Table 18.2). As discussed in Case 2, some strains associated with cystic fibrosis make a polysaccharide capsule consisting of a compound called alginate that gives colonies a distinctive mucoid phenotype.

Pseudomonads are rapidly growing, robust organisms that can persist in marginal environments. Consequently, they are difficult to eradicate from contaminated areas, e.g., hospital rooms, clinics, operating rooms, and medical equipment such as respiratory support devices. They may even survive in some antiseptic solutions used to disinfect instruments and endoscopes.

These organisms do not carry out fermentations; rather, they obtain energy from the oxidation of sugars. Nevertheless, many strains can grow anaerobically using nitrate as a terminal electron acceptor. Pseudomonads have minimal nutritional requirements, needing only acetate and ammonia as sources of carbon and nitrogen. These simple needs are met by a large number of organic compounds, so they grow well on simple media, including nutrient agar and the media used for enteric bacteria. Being nearly omnivorous makes them popular candidates for industrial and environmental uses, such as cleaning up toxic wastes. The first patent awarded for a genetically engineered bacterium was for a pseudomonad designed to clean up petroleum spills because it is able to oxidize hydrocarbons.

Most pseudomonads (except *P. mallei*) are motile, with one or several polar flagella. In this, they differ from *Escherichia coli* and other enterobacteriaceae, which have flagella all around the cell. In fact, pseudomonads are taxonomically quite distant from the enterobacteriaceae. Most pseudomonads produce indophenol oxidase, an enzyme that renders them positive in the oxidase test frequently used in diagnostic microbiology. They share this characteristic with the neisseriae; few other clinically important bacteria are oxidase positive.

Table 18.2. Virulence Factors of *P. aeruginosa*

Product	Location	Mechanism of action	Possible contribution to virulence
Pili	Polar	Adherence	Colonization
Lipopolysaccharide	Outer membrane	Lipid A is biologically active portion	Simulates release of vasoactive peptides activates clotting; fibrinolytic complement systems
Flagellum	Polar	Motility	Dissemination
Exotoxin A	Secreted	ADP-ribosylation of EF-2	Tissue damage
Exoenzyme S	Secreted	ADP-ribosylation of several proteins (not EF-2)	Tissue damage
Elastase	Secreted	Cleavage of elastin, collagen, immunoglobulins, complement components, etc.	Tissue damage
Alkaline protease	Secreted	Proteolysis	Tissue damage
Phospholipase C (heat-labile hemolysin)	Secreted	Hydrolysis of phospholipids, especially in eukaryotic membranes	Tissue damage, obtaining inorganic phosphate
Heat-stable phospholipase	Secreted	Hydrolysis of phospholipids especially in eukaryotic membranes	Tissue damage, obtaining inorganic phosphate

Pseudomonads are resistant to many commonly used antibiotics, including first- and second-generation penicillins and cephalosporins, tetracyclines, chloramphenicol, and vancomycin. The aminoglycosides, fluoroquinolones, and some newer β-lactams are usually effective. Because the resistance pattern among *Pseudomonas* strains varies from hospital to hospital and changes from year to year, the proper choice of antibiotics for empiric therapy of hospital-acquired infection must be based on continuous surveillance of drug sensitivity.

ENCOUNTER AND ENTRY

Because *P. aeruginosa* lives in the water and soil, it can be found on vegetables and living plants as well as in water taps, drains, and other wet surfaces. Humans may ingest the organism from such sources. Splashed water from a contaminated sink or droplets suctioned from a colonized endotracheal tube may spread the organisms. If present in large enough numbers, pseudomonads may enter the skin, possibly through insignificant abrasions. Infections involving the hair follicles (folliculitis) may occur as a result of bathing in contaminated hot tubs. The temperature in hot tubs favors *Pseudomonas* reproduction: a hot tub can contain up to 100 million organisms per milliliter! Such large inocula may overwhelm normal defenses and result in infections in immunocompetent people.

P. aeruginosa does not adhere well to normal intact epithelium. In vitro, pili act as adhesins to buccal and tracheal epithelial cells. Animal models of adherence that involve injury of epithelium before exposure to the organisms have proven informative. Influenza virus, endotracheal intubation, and treatment with chemicals have been used to damage airway epithelium. Piliated strains adhered better to damaged tracheal epithelium than did otherwise identical nonpiliated strains. These models are attractive because they take into account the clinical observation that *Pseudomonas* infections occur when the immune system—local or systemic—is breached. Similar studies have investigated burn wound infections and corneal infections. Infection of the cornea occurs when it has been injured (e.g., abrasion often associated with contact lenses).

While appropriate animal models have been developed to study the pathogenesis of human infections such as corneal and burn wound infections, developing an animal model of the chronic, persistent lung infection seen in cystic fibrosis is more difficult. When *Pseudomonas* are instilled intratracheally in an animal, the organisms are either cleared or the animal dies of acute pneumonia. To overcome this problem and establish experimental chronic infection, bacteria are embedded in agar beads before instillation. Histological changes resembling those seen in cystic fibrosis lung infection then occur. Such a model is useful for studying therapeutic interventions or, by the use of isogenic strains, the role of specific bacterial gene products. Unfortunately, the artificial introduction of the organisms in agarose beads does not allow the study of encounter or entry.

Recent advances in the molecular biology of cystic fibrosis have allowed new approaches to examination of the initial encounter between *P. aeruginosa* and the cystic fibrosis host. Cystic fibrosis respiratory cells in monolayer bind more *P. aeruginosa* than do those of normal cells. Binding is decreased in cystic fibrosis cells that have been "rescued" by a normal copy of the gene for the cystic fibrosis transmembrane conductance regulator (CFTR). CFTR dysfunction may affect binding by decreasing sialylation of surface glycolipids; *P. aeruginosa* binds to these asialoglycolipids. Because the transgenic mice with the ion transport defect of cystic fibrosis have more severe gastrointestinal disease than do humans, survival of the experimental mice was not initially good enough to allow study of lung disease. Recently, CF mice with a "leaky" mutation—a small amount of normal CFTR mRNA is made—have been shown to develop lung disease in response to exposure to bacterial pathogens.

SPREAD AND MULTIPLICATION

Pseudomonads are typical extracellular pathogens. Their growth in tissue depends largely on their ability to resist ingestion by neutrophils. Many strains possess an antiphagocytic polysaccharide slime layer and make cytolytic exotoxins. Nonetheless, the low frequency of pseudomonad infections in healthy persons shows that the phagocytes usually have the upper hand. Patients with reduced numbers of circulating neutrophils, like the individual in Case 1, are at high risk for *Pseudomonas* infection .

What determines whether colonization, local infection, or systemic infection occurs after contact with *Pseudomonas*? The use of isogenic strains of *Pseudomonas* in animal models has allowed the role of a given gene product to be studied. Animals are infected with strains differing only in one gene, and thus any pathogenic differences can be attributed to the product of this gene. In a burned mouse model, strains deficient in a number of extracellular products (toxin A, elastase, or exoenzyme S, see Table 18.2) persist in the wound but do not disseminate. Strains lacking flagella are also less virulent than wild-type strains. Tissue damage by toxins and proteases may facilitate flagella-mediated mobility and invasion.

P. aeruginosa employs several strategies to obtain scarce nutrients during infection. Obtaining iron is vital and difficult; virtually all of the iron in human serum is tightly bound to transferrin. *P. aeruginosa* produces iron-binding compounds or siderophores, which compete with transferrin for iron. Interestingly, in a retrospective study, leukemic patients who became bacteremic with *P. aeruginosa* had more decreased total iron-binding capacity than a group of patients who became colonized but not infected. Iron limitation increases the production of two extracellular products of *P. aeruginosa*, elastase and exotoxin A. In turn, these proteins may damage tissue or create conditions (e.g., lower pH) that make iron more accessible to the organisms. When another necessary nutrient, phosphate, is limited, *P. aeruginosa* increases production of phospholipase C. This enzyme hydrolyzes phospholipids from host cell membranes to release phosphate in an available form.

To survive in the host, *Pseudomonas* must not only obtain nutrition but must also be able to evade host defenses. In the bloodstream, the organisms do not usually survive and only cause sepsis in immunocompromised patients, such as in Case 1. Neutrophils are clearly involved in curbing the proliferation of the organisms, as seen by the increased incidence of *Pseudomonas* sepsis in persons with severe neutropenia.

In cystic fibrosis (Case 2), the organisms colonize an environment that is deficient in normal defenses. In this disease, ion transport across the respiratory epithelium is abnormal due to a defect in CFTR, the cystic fibrosis transmembrane conductance regulator. As described above, binding ability for *P. aeruginosa* is increased in the CF respiratory epithelium. Persistence of the organism may be attributable, in part, to dehydration of respiratory secretions resulting in impairment of the mucociliary system, which normally rids the lungs of inhaled particles and bacteria. Phagocytes function normally in cystic fibrosis and high levels of antibodies to pseudomonal antigens are found in most chronically infected patients. Some evidence show, however, that these antibodies may be defective in their function, specifically in their ability to opsonize *Pseudomonas*. The mucoid exopolysaccharide (also called alginate) produced by pseudomonads in chronic infection of the cystic fibrosis lung may shield the organism from the immune system. Strains that produce alginate secrete less of the proteases and toxins than do nonmucoid cells. Such mucoid strains also grow more slowly. These apparent disadvantages and the high energy cost to the cell of producing alginate must be offset by improved survival tactics in the cystic fibrosis lung. The switch to mucoidy is under complex regulation, involving at least two negative regulators and an alternative sigma factor (see Suggested Readings).

DAMAGE

Like other Gram-negatives, *P. aeruginosa* can cause hypotension and shock, as in Case 1, probably due to lipopolysaccharide, also known as endotoxin (see Chapter 9, "Damage"). The organisms also elaborate a wide variety of exotoxins that can cause local inflammation, tissue destruction, and abscess formation (see Table 18.2). As discussed above, the organisms may damage local tissue in order to obtain nutrients; in this case, damage allows the organism to persist. Damage may also be necessary for dissemination; as mentioned previously, strains lacking exotoxins or elastase persist locally in burn wounds but fail to disseminate.

Epidemiological and animal studies demonstrate the

importance of various virulence factors (see Table 18.2). The mechanism of action of some of these factors is fully known; for most, it is not. Exotoxin A is a toxin of the group that inactivates host target proteins by modifying them through the addition of an adenosine–ribose–diphosphate moiety of nicotinamide, a process known as ADP-ribosylation (Chapter 9, "Damage"). The *Pseudomonas* exotoxin A resembles diphtheria toxin in that the target protein is a factor involved in host cell protein synthesis, elongation factor 2, or EF-2. In vivo, this activity contributes to morbidity and mortality, as demonstrated by EF-2 depletion in the liver of infected mice.

Other *Pseudomonas* products, such as elastase, have multiple biological activities; determining which of these are most important in vivo has proven difficult. Elastase cleaves not only elastin but also collagen, which results in direct damage to tissues. This enzyme may increase susceptibility to tissue damage by neutrophil elastase because it cleaves the α1-proteinase inhibitor and other proteinase inhibitors. In addition, *Pseudomonas* elastase also cleaves components of the immune system including complement and immunoglobulins. Another enzyme secreted by this organism, an alkaline protease, inhibits the activities of γ-interferon. Recently, a second protease has been shown to cleave elastin. Like alginate, the production of secreted virulence factors is highly regulated. Full expression of elastase requires a transcriptional activator (LasR) and a diffusible molecule. This regulatory system may allow the cells to communicate and respond to conditions of substrate limitation caused by increased bacterial density.

The outcome of *Pseudomonas* infection depends on the nature and severity of the infection, the state of host defenses, and the promptness and efficacy of treatment. A high-grade bacteremia in a neutropenic patient carries a 50–70% mortality rate. *Pseudomonas* endocarditis likewise carries a high mortality rate, up to 50%.

DIAGNOSIS, PREVENTION, AND TREATMENT

P. aeruginosa is easily cultured and identified by the clinical microbiology laboratory. Knowledge of prevailing patterns of susceptibility and resistance in a given hospital allows for empiric therapy while awaiting culture and sensitivity results. Because this bacterium is relatively resistant to most antimicrobials, serious infec-

tions are usually treated with two antibiotics in combination to achieve an additive or synergistic effect. The ability to develop and acquire antibiotic resistance contributes to the success of *Pseudomonas* in the hospital environment as does the resistance of the organism to many commonly used disinfecting agents. Attention to infection control measures may allow prevention of some *Pseudomonas* nosocomial infections.

CONCLUSION

P. aeruginosa is a paradigm of an opportunistic environmental pathogen. It is abundant in our environment and causes diseases mainly in patients who have impaired defenses. Occasionally, if the inoculum size is very large, it overcomes the defenses of healthy persons. Prevention and treatment of *Pseudomonas* infection in patients debilitated by major underlying diseases is an important goal in modern medicine.

SELF-ASSESSMENT QUESTIONS

1. Describe the microbiological characteristics of the pseudomonads.
2. What are the main clinical syndromes of *P. aeruginosa* infections?
3. What types of patients are most often infected?
4. Describe some of the virulence factors of these organisms.
5. List some of the therapeutic problems encountered in pseudomonad infections.

SUGGESTED READINGS

Deretic V, Schurr MJ, Boucher JC, Martin DW. Conversion of *Pseudomonas aeruginosa* to mucoidy in cystic fibrosis: environmental stress and regulation of bacterial virulence by alternative sigma factors. J Bacteriol 1994;176:2773–2780.

Imundo L, Brasch J, Prince A, Al-Awquati Q. Cystic fibrosis epithelial cells have a receptor for pathogenic bacteria on their apical surface. Proc Natl Acad Sci 1995;92:3019–3023.

Passador L, Cook JM, Gambello MJ, Rust L, Iglewski BH. Expression of *Pseudomonas aeruginosa* virulence genes requires cell-to-cell communication. Science 1993;260:1127–1130.

Poole K. Bacterial multidrug resistance—emphasis on efflux mechanisms and *Pseudomonas aeruginosa*. J Antimicrob Chemother 1994;34:453–456.

Bordetella pertussis and Whooping Cough

ARNOLD L. SMITH

Key Concepts

Bordetella pertussis infection:
- Causes whooping cough, or pertussis, a disease that causes characteristic paroxysmal cough in infants.
- Can be prevented with DPT, a vaccine containing *B. pertussis* antigens, along with diphtheria and tetanus antigens.
- Is extremely contagious.
- Involves several virulence factors, including adhesins and toxins.

The agent of whooping cough, *Bordetella pertussis*, is found on epithelial cells of the trachea, bronchi, and bronchioles of patients. These **Gram-negative coccobacilli** make powerful toxins that penetrate tissues, kill cells, immobilize the ciliary elevator, and cause the accumulation of thick mucus in the airway. The characteristic **"whooping" cough** is due to sensitization of cough receptors in the trachea by a toxin and to the patient's effort to expectorate the accumulated mucus and cell debris. Killed whole *B. pertussis*, added to diphtheria and tetanus toxoids, yield the **"DPT vaccine"** which is given to infants. The pertussis component of the vaccine is responsible for some of its rare side effects. New pertussis vaccines are **"acellular,"** consisting of inactivated toxins and adhesins.

■ CASE

Eight weeks after her birth, P. was taken to her family doctor for a checkup and her first baby shot. The immunization was postponed for a month because she had a slight cold and a runny nose. The cold may have been acquired from one of her three siblings or her grandfather who lived with the family, all of whom had had colds recently. Subsequently, P. began sneezing and coughing. Any loud noise would bring on a coughing spell. P.'s mother became concerned when P. turned blue after a series of coughing spells that ended with vomiting. Later, during an examination of the infant by a physician, P. had a series of "barky" coughs, after which she vomited and could not catch her breath. Her mother was told that P. had whooping cough and needed to be hospitalized.

The laboratory report showed an elevated white blood cell count in her blood, chiefly due to a large increase in the number of lymphocytes. A nasopharyngeal specimen contained *B. pertussis* by fluorescent antibody detection, the causative agent of whooping cough.

P.'s mother wanted to know the following:
- How dangerous is whooping cough?
- Why was the physician sure of the diagnosis?
- Where did P. catch the "bug?"
- Will antibiotics make her better?
- When can she get her baby shots?

If you had to answer these questions, you would have to know something about:
- The epidemiology of *B. pertussis*.
- How the infection causes disease.
- The pros and cons of vaccination.
- How whooping cough is diagnosed.

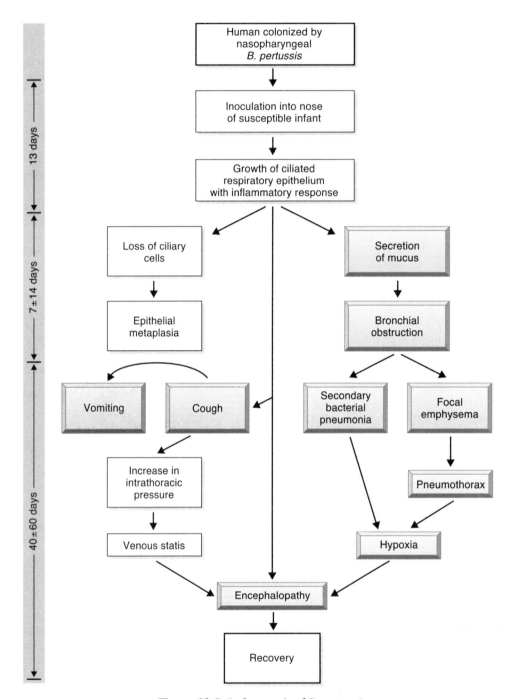

Figure 19.1. Pathogenesis of *B. pertussis*.

Whooping cough, or **pertussis,** is a severe childhood disease that has been nearly eradicated due to vaccination. The vaccine used to contain killed *B. pertussis*, the "P" in DPT, which is very effective in preventing the disease. In recent years, the number of infants who have not received the vaccine has increased. As a result, the number of cases of whooping cough in the U.S. has risen sharply. In 1981, the childhood incidence of whooping cough was 0.5/100,000 population. This number increased threefold to 1.5/100,000 children by 1985. In 1993, 5000 cases of whooping cough in the U. S. were confirmed, the highest number since 1967!

Whooping cough is an important disease for four reasons:
1. Adults with mild disease, indistinguishable from a cold, are the reservoir.
2. It is highly communicable among susceptible infants less than 1 year of age.
3. It is life-threatening in infants with underlying cardiac or pulmonary disease.
4. It can lead to neurological sequelae.

The pathogenesis of whooping cough is shown diagrammatically in Fig. 19.1. The local manifestations of whooping cough are those of **tracheitis** and **bronchitis**, with accumulation of mucus, inflammatory cells, bacteria, and dead epithelial cells in the airway lumen. The **mucociliary elevator** is impaired by damage to the ciliary epithelial cells and the cough is more easily triggered due to sensitization of cough receptors. The intense straining against the closed vocal cords (i.e., the Valsalva maneuver) in an effort to expel the mucus and debris in the lower airway, can lead to hemorrhages in the brain, conjunctiva, and beneath the tongue. The result is the violent cough that gives the disease its name. In addition, infants with whooping cough have systemic manifestations, such as low-grade fever, malaise, and lymphocytosis. Feeding may precipitate a coughing attack in infants precluding adequate oral intake, leading to dehydration.

BORDETELLA PERTUSSIS

Bordetella are small, Gram-negative, strictly aerobic coccobacilli that belong to a group of nutritionally fastidious organisms that includes the genus *Haemophilus*. *Bordetella* grow in complex media containing blood, which fulfill their nutritional requirements, plus other additives to neutralize fatty acids and other inhibitory compounds. *Bordetella* are also very sensitive to chemical and physical agents in the environment and do not survive outside the body for appreciable periods of time.

B. pertussis has specific adhesins that permit them to attach to epithelial cells of the respiratory tract. They also manufacture exotoxins that penetrate into host cells and ultimately produce the signs and symptoms of the disease. As with other Gram-negatives, *B. pertussis* possesses **endotoxin**, which is probably responsible for the fever and perhaps for some of the other signs of the disease as well.

ENCOUNTER

B. pertussis are thought to be exclusively human pathogens because they neither survive in the environment, nor are they known to infect other animal species. Their reservoir is suspected to be older adults with chronic bronchitis or bronchiectasis, or young adults with symptoms of a mild upper respiratory tract infection; they are rarely recovered from the nasopharynx of healthy persons. The failure to recover *B. pertussis* may be due to their ability to enter respiratory epithelial cells of carriers. The turnover of epithelial cells would then make the sequestered bacteria available for transmission. The organisms are exceptionally contagious and may infect upward of 90% of the members of a nonimmune family exposed to the organism.

Not all people will recognize that they have been infected because the classic symptoms of whooping cough are dependent on the state of immunity. Young infants have whooping, paroxysmal cough with vomiting and respiratory distress. In people older than 15 years, the disease may be indistinguishable from a mild "viral" upper respiratory tract disease without cough. This milder manifestation of *B. pertussis* disease may be attributed to host resistance due to previous immunization or infection. It becomes important, then, for the physician treating a baby like P. to take a complete history of all family members and to alert them to the possibility that they may contract or have whooping cough. In addition, the epidemiology of this disease is not always clear because vaccination records for childhood diseases are often poorly kept.

ENTRY

B. pertussis enter the trachea and bronchi by inhalation. The organisms attach to the cilia of epithelial cells of the large airways and are seldom found anywhere else (Fig. 19.2). Whooping cough is entirely a superficial infection, which means that the organisms do not invade tissue but remain on the mucosal surface: other important bacterial diseases with this characteristic include diphtheria and cholera. *B. pertussis* shows a strong **tissue tropism** for the ciliated epithelial cells of the respiratory tract. The reason for this tropism is not clearly understood, but it may be due to the specific interaction between pertussis adhesins and receptors on the cilia of these cells. *B. pertussis* has specific adhesins for ciliated respiratory epithelial cells as well as adhesins for phagocytic cells. **Filamentous hemagglutinin** (**Fha**) is a surface structure without a distinct organization that mediates binding to the galactose residues of ciliated cell glycolipids called **sulfatides**. Another ciliated cell glycolipid, lactosylceramide, is the target

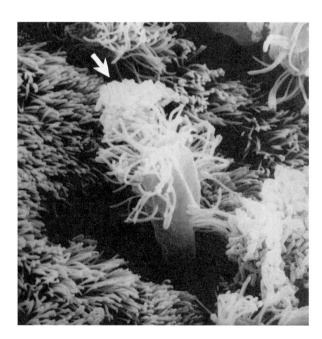

Figure 19.2. *B. pertussis* adhering to dilated respiratory epithelial cells seen in the scanning electron microscope. Note the clump of bacteria attached to the partially extruded epithelial cell (*arrow*).

PARADIGM   ■ ■ ■

Regulation of Virulence Properties

Microbial factors that affect normal host physiology and thereby result in disease are often under rigorous control by the microorganism. It is not advantageous to a microbe to produce a toxin or an invasion protein, for example, if a host environment lacks the proper receptor for such factors. Consequently, microbes have evolved sophisticated regulatory systems to control expression of virulence factors and thereby optimize their effectiveness.

One of the most widely observed schemes used by bacteria to control virulence factors production is a two-component regulatory system. In this system, two gene products interact to control the transcription of other genes whose expression is presumed to be required in a specific host environment (Fig. 19.3). The two factors that make up this system are a sensor protein with kinase activity (called BvgS in *Bordetella pertussis* for *Bordetella virulence genes*) and a response regulator (BvgA in *B. pertussis*) that activates transcription after being phosphorylated by the sensor kinase. A single bacterial species may have several such systems that allow the microbe to adapt to a variety of environments it may encounter, ranging from systems that respond to the level of available nitrogen to those that control the response to changes in the osmolarity of the growth environment.

Sensor kinase and response regulator proteins contain conserved domains that are important for the basic function of each type of protein. It is therefore possible to identify genes encoding potential two-component systems by sequence analysis tools that can recognize the conserved domains. A single microbe may have several two-component systems, each of which controls a specific trait; *E. coli*, for instance, may contain as many as 50 different two-component systems. Because of the modular nature of these proteins and the conservation of functional domains, cross-regulation—in which a response regulator of one system is phosphorylated by the sensor kinase of another two component system—has been observed.

Two-component systems that regulate a variety of phenotypes in pathogenic microbes have been identified (see Table 19.1). The prevalence of these highly conserved systems in a wide variety of species has generated interest and some limited success in designing new classes of broad-spectrum antimicrobials that can block these systems.

The possibility that strains of pathogenic bacteria with mutations in specific two-component systems may be good candidates for vaccine use has also been tested. The rationale for this approach is that some two-component systems may regulate gene expression only during certain stages of microbe interaction with a human host. Mutants deficient for such systems might still survive within the host long enough to elicit an immune response before becoming growth-limited due to the mutation. *Salmonella typhi*, the agent of typhoid fever, was mutated by deletion of the *phoP/phoQ* two-component system that regulates survival of this organism within macrophages. When tested in human volunteers, a single dose of the resulting strain, Ty800, induced greater intestinal and humoral immune responses than did four doses of the approved oral typhoid vaccine strain Ty21a. This work establishes a precedent for studying the use of two-component mutants as vaccines against other important pathogens.

VICTOR DIRITA

Table 19.1. Examples of Two-component Regulatory Systems in Pathogenic Bacteria

Organism and manifestation	Sensor/regulator	Signals	Regulated virulence properties
Bordetella pertussis— whooping cough	BvgS/BvgA	Mg^{+2}, SO_4-$2'$ temperature	Pertussis toxin, adenylate cyclase toxin/hemolysin, filamentous hemagglutinin
Pseudomonas aeruginosa— lung infections in cystic fibrosis patients	PilS/PilR ??/A1gR	?? ??	Pilus colonization factor, alginate biosynthesis; mucoidy
Salmonella—gastroenteritis, typhoid fever, bacteremia	PhoQ/PhoP	Mg^{+2}	Macrophage survival, invasion of epithelial cells, resistance to cationic peptides
Staphylococcus aureus— abscesses	AgrC/AgrA	Peptide Pheromone	Exoprotein production, including activation of hemolysins, proteases, and toxins and repression of coagulase and protein A
Enterococcus faecalis— urinary, biliary, cardiovascular infections	VanS/VanR	Vancomycin	Enzymes for vancomycin resistance

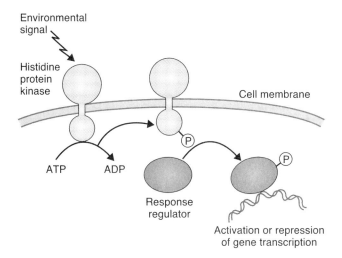

Figure 19.3. The two-component regulatory system for signal transduction. The sensor/transmitter is activated by a signal to become an active protein kinase capable of phosphorylating a response regulator. In the phosphorylated form, the regulator protein acts on DNA to either allow or prevent the expression of a specific set of genes.

for binding of an adhesin, the bacterial cell-associated **pertussin** toxin. When secreted, pertussin also functions as a toxin, by a mechanism similar to that of cholera toxin, by ADP-ribosylating Gi protein bound to the inner membrane of the host cell (see Chapter 9, "Damage"). In addition to Fha, other surface components, a protein called **pertactin** and **pili** (or fimbriae) also facilitate binding of *B. pertussis* to mammalian cells. The possession of multiple, if not redundant, mechanisms for adherence emphasizes the importance of this step in the infectious process.

SPREAD AND MULTIPLICATION

The first stages of whooping cough result in a mild inflammatory response in the submucosa, which is manifested clinically by infrequent coughing, a runny nose, and a low-grade fever. At this so-called **catarrhal stage**, the organisms multiply rapidly and spread to contiguous mucosa of the lower respiratory tract. Within a few days, masses of bacteria are entrapped in the cilia and thick mucus. The epithelium remains intact, but the submucosa beneath it becomes increasingly inflamed and the peribronchial lymph nodes enlarge. Reactive hyperplasia in the lymph nodes indicates that bacteria, their toxins, or other products are transported to those sites from their superficial origin in the bronchial lumen. Destruction of respiratory epithelial cells, which also evokes subepithelial inflammation, may also occur in prolonged infections.

Approximately 3 weeks after entry of the organisms, the cough becomes intense and uncontrollable. At the end of a series of coughs, deep inspiration and a "forced" expiration, the "whoop" occur. In infants with poor systemic oxygenation, either from chronic pulmonary disease (such as bronchopulmonary dysplasia) or congenital heart disease, the decreased cardiac output (due to the increased intrathoracic pressure) can cause severe systemic hypoxia and death. This cough persists with varying severity for another 2 months. It results from attempts by the body to clear the airways of the large amount of material that accumulates on the epithelium when the mucociliary elevator is impaired and sensitivity of the cough receptors increases.

DAMAGE

B. pertussis has an impressive array of virulence factors (Table 19.2). One of its most important, pertussis toxin, resembles cholera toxin in that it affects **cyclic AMP metabolism**. It is also an A-B toxin, consisting of an A (active) subunit and a B (binding) domain composed of five nonidentical subunits (Chapter 9, "Damage"). The toxin attaches to host cells via the B domain allowing the A fragment to enter and act in the cytoplasm. *B. pertussis* has two mechanisms to increase intracellular **cAMP**. The first mechanism resembles that of cholera toxin, diphtheria toxin, and *Pseudomonas aeruginosa* exotoxin A. These toxins are **ADP-ribosyl-transferases**: they split the nicotinamide portion from NAD and attach the remaining ADP-ribose (adenosine-diphosphoribose) to specific host cell proteins (Chapter 9, "Damage"). One of these target proteins is **G-protein**, which is involved in the regulation of adenylate cyclase. ADP-ribosylation of this enzyme results in an increase in cAMP, which inhibits several functions of neutrophils, such as chemotaxis and the oxidative burst. The second cAMP-enhancing mechanism that *B. pertussis* uses is the secretion of an extracellular adenylate cyclase. This enzyme enters the host cells and increase their content of cyclic AMP. Why *B. pertussis* has two mechanisms to increase intracellular cAMP is not certain. It must be important to the bacterium, as *B. pertussis* adenylcyclase requires mammalian calmodulin to become active. Adenylcyclase is actually a **bifunctional molecule** with the amino terminus binding to erythrocytes while the carboxyl terminus has the catalytic activity.

Local damage is probably caused by another toxin, a **tracheal cytotoxin**, which kills ciliated cells specifically and leads their extrusion from the epithelium. Curiously, this exotoxin is not a protein, but **consists of a peptidoglycan fragment**, 1,6 anhydromuramic acid-N-acetylglucosamine tetrapeptide (Fig. 19.4). A similar compound is made by gonococci (Chapter 14, "Neisseriae") and acts in an analogous fashion by killing ciliated epithelial cells in the fallopian tubes. It is likely that tracheal cytotoxin is not the only one involved in local damage. *B. pertussis* also produces a **heat-labile toxin** that can inflict cytotoxicity on nucleated human cells. Thus, there are many mechanisms by which the organism can inflict local damage.

Table 19.2. Major Toxins and Virulence Factors of *B. pertussis*

Name	Chemical nature	Site of action	Biochemical activities	Physiological effects
Pertussis toxin	Protein	Local and systemic	ADP-ribosylates protein	Impairs neutrophil chemotaxis, phagocytosis, and bactericidal activity; encephalopathy; lymphocytosis; hypoglycemia
Adenylate cyclase	Protein	Local	Converts ATP to cAMP	Histamine sensitization mimics pertussis toxin activity on neutrophils; increases capillary permeability leading to edema
Tracheal cytotoxin	Murein	Local	?	Kills ciliated respiratory epithelial cells; adjuvant
Endotoxin	Lipopolysaccharide	Systemic	?	Fever; adjuvant
Pili (fimbriae)	Protein	Local	?	Facilitating adherence to respiratory epithelium
Filamentous hemagglutinin	Protein	Local	?	Binds bacteria to cilia
Hemolysin	?	Local	?	Cytotoxic for respiratory epithelium

Given the nature of the local damage, is it likely that antibodies will have a significant effect on the cause of the disease? Preexisting antibodies produced by previous infections or by vaccination prevent the disease, especially if they are of the IgA type. However, once the disease is established, antibodies may play a lesser role. When the exotoxins have entered their target cells, they become impervious to antibodies.

DIAGNOSIS

Whooping cough is an uncommon disease in countries where the DPT vaccine is widely used. Although the clinical signs and symptoms are ususally quite distinctive, neither clinicians nor the laboratory are always alert to this particular diagnosis. It is also important to remember that laboratory diagnosis of *B. pertussis* is difficult because the number of organisms decreases as the severity of symptoms increases. Thus, *B. pertussis* can be cultured only from a small number of patients.

To culture *B. pertussis*, a small swab is placed in the posterior wall of the pharynx, which usually makes the patient cough. The swab is often treated with a drop of penicillin solution to kill other normally occurring bacteria that are sensitive to this drug (to which *B. pertussis* is intrinsically resistant). The swab is then applied to the surface of a plate containing a medium called **Bordet-Gengou**, which is incubated for 2–3 days. Positive identification of the organisms may then be carried out using specific antisera.

PREVENTION AND TREATMENT

The traditional **vaccine** against pertussis consists of a killed suspension of *B. pertussis* cells mixed with puri-

fied diphtheria and tetanus toxoid proteins (DPT). DPT is administered to infants at 2, 4, and 6 months of age. The side effects associated with the use of DPT vaccine have been attributed largely to the pertussis component and not to the other two. The vaccine can produce three types of complications.

Fever, malaise, and pain at the site of the injection are seen in about 20% of the infants inoculated. This complication is commonly seen with vaccines prepared from whole bacteria that contain murein, Gram-negative lipopolysaccharide (LPS), and other substances that elicit an inflammatory response. **Convulsions** occur in about one in 2000 children vaccinated. This number may not represent the true incidence. A small number of children, about one in 30,000, suffer from spontaneous convulsions called idiopathic seizures and some children

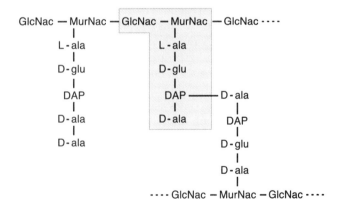

Figure 19.4. Portion of cell wall murein that corresponds to the structure of tracheal cytotoxin. *GlcNac,* N-acetylglucosamine; *MurNac,* N-acetylmuramic acid; *meso-DAP,* meso-diaminopimelic acid; *ala,* alanine; *glu,* glutamic acid.

will have seizures with fever due to any cause. Serious central nervous reactions occur rarely, at an estimated rate of one in every 110,000 children vaccinated. What would the number of these complications be in similar populations that do not receive the vaccine? Such a comparable population does not presently exist in countries where the vaccine is widely used.

In assessing the risks of using the DPT vaccine, the potential for a severe complication should be weighed against the undisputed benefits of the vaccine in nearly eradicating whooping cough. Many epidemiologists are convinced that vaccination should be widespread. In fact, all states in the U.S. have laws requiring children to be immunized against pertussis. Vaccination is required prior to enrollment in school or, in some areas, in day care centers. Because of the minor adverse reactions, such as fever and irritability probably due to the LPS in the whole cell vaccine, vaccines consisting of Fha, pertussis toxoid, fimbriae (Fim 2 and Fim 3), and pertactin in various combinations have been developed. The efficacy of these **acellular vaccines** compared with DPT in nonimmune children has been variable. Current pertussis vaccine recommendations consist of initial immunization with the whole cell vaccine, but booster shots with the acellular vaccine. Development of an acellular vaccine to replace the "P" in DPT is ongoing.

CONCLUSION

There is much to be learned from the specific aspects of the pathogenesis of the causative agent. *B. pertussis* is a superficial pathogen, which does not penetrate into deep tissues. It produces a series of powerful toxins, most of which function to counteract the defense mechanisms of the lower respiratory tract. The disease it produces, whooping cough, can be virtually eliminated by vaccination.

SELF-ASSESSMENT QUESTIONS

1. Discuss the aspects of whooping cough that can be directly attributed to the location of the organisms in the body.
2. How does *B. pertussis* cause systemic symptoms, given its superficial location?
3. Describe the activity of the main toxins of *B. pertussis*.
4. Discuss the pros and cons of the pertussis component of the DPT vaccine.

SUGGESTED READINGS

Hewlett EL. Pertussis: current concepts of pathogenesis and prevention. Pediatr Infect Dis J 1997;16:S78–84.

Miller JF, Mekalanos JJ, Falkow S. Coordinate regulation and sensory transduction in the control of bacterial virulence. Science 1989;243:916.

Salyers AA, Whitt DD. Whooping cough (*Bordetella pertussis*). In: Salyers AA, Whitt DD. Bacterial pathogenesis. Washington, DC: ASM Press, 1994; 157–168.

Tuomanen E. Adherence of *Bordetella pertussis* to human cilia: implications for disease prevention and therapy. In: Leive L, ed. Microbiology 1986. Washington, DC: American Society of Microbiology, 1986;59–64.

Wilson R, Read R, Thomas M, Rutman A, Harrison K, Lund V, Cookson B, Goldman W, Lambert H, Cole P. Effects of *B. pertussis* infection in human respiratory epithelium in vivo and in vitro. Infect Immun 1991;59:337.

Clostridia

SHERWOOD L. GORBACH

Key Concepts

Clostridia:
- Are Gram-positive, anaerobic, spore-forming rods responsible for several unrelated diseases including pseudomembranous colitis, botulism, tetanus, gas gangrene, and cellulitis.
- Often cause disease due to the production of toxins.
- Include pathogens such as *C. difficile*, which is associated with the use of antimicrobial drugs; botulism (caused by *C. botulinum*); tetanus (caused by *C. tetani*); and gas gangrene (caused by *C. perfringens*).

Clostridia are strict Gram-positive rods responsible for several unrelated diseases with different clinical manifestations. These include **pseudomembranous colitis** (an inflammatory disease of the colon); **botulism**; **tetanus**; soft tissue infections including muscle invasion (**gas gangrene**) and cellulitis (an infection of subcutaneous connective tissue); and food poisoning. Many of the clostridial diseases are serious and life-threatening. All are caused by exotoxins secreted by the clostridia. In the case of botulism, the disease is acquired by eating toxin-contaminated food; the clinical symptoms are produced by the toxin without colonization and invasion by the organism.

CASE

An 81-year-old man was hospitalized with a history of 38.5°C fevers for the preceding 5 days. Because of confusion and inability to care for himself, he had been a resident of a local nursing home for 3 years. However, he had been able to dress himself and move about the wards until a week before his hospital admission, when he complained of weakness and could not get out of bed. Except for a urinary tract infection 4 weeks previously, for which he was treated

with a 10-day course of ampicillin, he had experienced no recent illness.

On physical examination, he was resting comfortably in bed but appeared confused and rather unhappy about his change of surroundings. His temperature was 39°; other vital signs were normal. There were no localized physical findings; abdominal examination was unremarkable.

As the house staff and attending physician pondered the diagnostic possibilities at the bedside the next morning, their deliberations were interrupted by the staff nurse, who informed the group that the patient had passed two loose bowel movements during the night. Indeed, the attending physician's olfaction, perhaps heightened by the new information, now recognized the occurrence of another such event, no doubt triggered by deep palpation of the patient's abdomen.

A stool specimen was sent to the laboratory, which within 24 hours yielded a positive result for the toxin of *Clostridium difficile*. Specific treatment for antibiotic-associated diarrhea caused by *C. difficile* was begun with oral metronidazole. The patient became afebrile within 36 hours, and he returned to his nursing home without further laboratory investigations within 72 hours.

A number of questions arise:
1. Where do the causative organisms come from?
2. Is the history of previous treatment with ampicillin pertinent to *C. difficile* infection?

3. What is the role of the spores of *C. difficile* in the disease process?
4. What caused the patient's symptoms?

C. difficile is an anaerobic, Gram-positive, spore-forming rod first identified in 1935. As the name implies, it has fastidious growth requirements. Although isolated occasionally in blood cultures and in wounds, it went unrecognized as a cause of diarrheal disease until 1977, when it was identified as the organism responsible for a severe ulcerating disease of the large bowel known as **pseudomembranous colitis** (**PMC**; "pseudomembranous" refers to the yellowish plaques composed of fibrin with a few cellular elements that overlay the ulcerations in the colonic mucosa.) Since then, the organism has been linked to a spectrum of intestinal disorders associated with antibiotic treatment, ranging from an asymptomatic carrier state, to mild or moderate diarrhea, to fulminating, life-threatening PMC.

The organism is harbored in the large intestine of humans, where it tends to remain in a dormant state in low numbers. It can also be found in environmental sources, particularly hospitals. Under adverse conditions, the organism reverts to its highly resistant spore form. The spores can be cultured from the floor, bedpan, and toilet in a hospital room occupied by a patient with *C. difficile*, as well as from the hands and clothing of medical and nursing personnel. The mode of transmission is via the spore form, which is extremely difficult to eradicate from the environment. *C. difficile* is currently the major cause of diarrhea acquired in a hospital. In nursing homes, where patients tend to stay for prolonged periods, 20–30% of the residents are asymptomatic carriers of *C. difficile*.

A remarkable feature of *C. difficile* diarrhea is its association with antimicrobial drugs. Most symptomatic patients have received an antimicrobial agent in the recent past. Virtually all antimicrobial drugs have been implicated; however, the most common antimicrobial drugs associated with *C. difficile* diarrhea are cephalosporins, ampicillin, and clindamycin. (This order reflects the frequency of use of the drugs in clinical practice; actually, clindamycin is associated with a higher incidence of disease per administration.)

The risk associated with use of a particular antimicrobial drug is not necessarily related to its in vitro activity against *C. difficile*, but rather to the relative resistance of the spore form of *C. difficile* to almost all antimicrobial drugs. The sequence of events in antibiotic-associated *C. difficile* diarrhea begins with suppression of normal flora by the antimicrobial drug, with persistence of the spore form of *C. difficile*. Clindamycin suppresses the most common type of bacteria in the flora, the anaerobic bacteria; this suppression may explain the strong association of its use with *C. difficile* diarrhea. *C. difficile* is either present already in the flora or is acquired from the hospital environment during antibiotic treatment. In response to the throat posed by the antibiotic, the organism enters into its spore state. At some time during or after antibiotic administration, the spores germinate and the vegetative form of *C. difficile* grows in large numbers, producing its toxins. When toxin production achieves a critical level in the large bowel, diarrhea begins.

Like other toxin-related gastrointestinal infections (notably, diarrhea caused by *Vibrio cholerae* and toxigenic *Escherichia coli*), bacterial invasion of the bowel wall is not found in *C. difficile* diarrhea. Instead, the organism produces its toxins in the intestinal lumen, and the toxins cause damage to the epithelial lining of the bowel wall. The major toxins are designated A and B. **Toxin A** causes both fluid production and damage to the mucosa of the large bowel, and it is responsible for the clinical disease. **Toxin B** is a cytotoxin that causes abnormalities in tissue-culture systems. The standard laboratory test that diagnoses the disease uses this property to detect toxin in the feces.

THE CLOSTRIDIA

The genus *Clostridium* is composed of **Gram-positive, spore-forming anaerobic rods** that live in soil and in the intestine of animals. Production of protein toxins by at least 14 of these clostridial species is associated with a range of diseases, including botulism, tetanus, gas gangrene, food poisoning, diarrhea, and PMC. The toxins responsible for botulism and tetanus are **neurotoxins**, whereas those causing gas gangrene and intestinal infections are **cytotoxins**; that is, they cause direct damage to cells. **Botulism** is caused by preformed botulinum toxin in contaminated food; thus, the *C. botalinum* organism itself need not be present in the victim. In tetanus and PMC, the organisms are ensconced in the host, either in a wound (in the case of tetanus) or in the bowel lumen (in PMC). However, the organism itself does not invade the tissues; it merely produces toxins that cause the disease. The organism that causes gas gangrene has dual virulence factors of toxin production and tissue invasiveness. Clostridia can also produce **suppurative wounds and tissue abscesses**, in which the organism acts as a simple invader, without systemic signs of toxin production (Table 20.1).

In addition to the 30 clostridial species encountered in human infections, there are another 50 or more species found in the environment, particularly in soil and in animal wastes. Clostridia are highly active metaboli-

Table 20.1. Major Clostridial Diseases

	Toxin production	Tissue invasiveness
Botulism		
Botulinum food poisoning	+	−
Infant botulism	+	−
Wound botulism	+	±
Tetanus	+	±
Pseudomembranous colitis	+	±
Gas gangrene	+	+
Suppurative wounds and abscess	−	+

cally and many strains have important industrial uses. Clostridial fermentation of crude substrates produces useful chemicals such as alcohols and acetone, and some species are used in the production of fermented foods and cheese. The clostridia used for these purposes, like most members of the genus, are not ordinarily pathogenic.

BOTULISM AND *C. BOTULINUM*

Encounter

Clostridium botulinum spores found in soil or marine sediments contaminate meats, vegetables, and fish. Because the spores are relatively heat-resistant, they survive food processing and canning when the temperatures are insufficiently high. Under anaerobic conditions, such as that found in canned foods, the spores germinate and release potent toxins. Proteolytic enzymes produced by some strains of the organism cause spoilage of the food; however in many cases, the food has a normal appearance and taste. Even an experimental nibble of such food can contain enough toxin to cause lethal disease.

Damage

C. botulinum produces eight immunologically distinct neurotoxins (types A, B, C[α], C[β], D, E, F, and G). Human cases are associated mostly with types A and B, and occasionally with type E, which is formed in fish products. As the interest in home canning and prepared foods has increased, cases of food-borne botulism have risen concomitantly. Among the most potent poisons known, botulinum toxins are proteins of 150 kilodaltons that can be crystallized to a white powder of unknown taste. One microgram is sufficient to kill a large family, and 0.4 kg could kill all the people on earth.

Botulism is an intoxication caused by the ingestion of a preformed **neurotoxin**. Botulinum toxin prevents the release of the neurotransmitter acetylcholine, thereby interfering with neurotransmission at **peripheral cholinergic synapses**. The clinical disease, which occurs within 12 to 36 hours after ingestion, is characterized by a flaccid paralysis of muscle. Cranial nerves are affected first, particularly those involving the eyes, producing diplopia (double vision) and blurred vision. Difficulty swallowing is an early sign. The paralysis descends, and striated muscle groups weaken, especially those in the neck and extremities, with subsequent involvement of respiratory muscles. The toxin does not act by directly killing cells, nor does it produce systemic signs of fever or sepsis. Patients generally succumb to paralysis and respiratory failure.

Infant botulism is a rare form of paralytic disease occurring in infants between 3 and 20 weeks of age. It produces a generalized hypotonic ("floppy") state. The infant's cry becomes feeble and the suck reflex weakens. In this disease, *C. botulinum* colonizes the large intestine, where it produces toxin. Infant botulism differs from the classic botulinum food poisoning in the following ways: the toxin is not found in food but rather is produced in the infant's intestinal tract; the condition has a slow onset, probably because the toxin is absorbed more slowly from the large intestine; and the disease has a favorable outcome in the majority of cases, without specific treatment.

Wound botulism is another rare form of the disease in which a traumatic wound is contaminated by spores of *C. botulinum*. Toxins are produced at the wound site; they are absorbed into the tissues and cause a severe neurological disease similar to that of food-borne botulism.

Treatment and Prevention

Specific **antitoxin** is available for types A, B, and E intoxication. The trivalent antitoxin should be administered as soon as possible to bind any circulating toxin. Because this antitoxin is acquired from horses, a high incidence of hypersensitivity reactions is associated with its use. The most important aspect of treatment is supportive care, which is necessary to maintain respirations and other vital functions. Patients should be given parenteral nutrition. The illness may last for many weeks, and individual muscles may be paralyzed for months or even permanently. With good supportive care, the mortality from botulism is currently 25%.

Botulism can be prevented by proper canning methods. Although the spores are heat-resistant, the toxins are heat-labile, and terminal heating of contaminated food can kill *C. botulinum* spores. As a result of improvements in the canning industry, outbreaks associated with commercial foods are quite rare, and most cases of botulism are now associated with home canning.

TETANUS AND *C. TETANI*

Tetanus, which is caused by *C. tetani*, is a tragic disease, not only because of its severity, but because it can be completely prevented by appropriate immunization. Indeed, prevention of tetanus by active immunization has been one of the triumphs of modern bacteriology. Experience with tetanus in the two World Wars of this century demonstrated beyond doubt the benefits of the tetanus toxoid vaccine. Universal immunization of the American forces in World War II virtually eliminated this disease as a complication of traumatic injuries in soldiers. In developing countries where immunization is not widely practiced, tetanus remains a serious public health problem.

Encounter, Entry, Spread, and Multiplication

C. tetani is ubiquitous in the gastrointestinal tract of humans and animals and in soil samples. Because of their resistance to environmental conditions, tetanus spores contaminate wounds of trauma victims.

Most cases of tetanus are associated with a **traumatic wound**. Tissue necrosis, anoxia, and other bacterial contaminants in the wound provide an optimal environment for germination of tetanus spores and production of toxin. Neonatal tetanus results from contamination of the umbilical cord at the time of delivery, either through unsanitary procedures or local customs of wrapping the cord in dung or mud.

Damage

The major toxin, known as **tetanospasmin**, accounts for all the symptoms of tetanus. Tetanospasmin is a 150-kilodalton protein molecule composed of a heavy chain and a light chain held together by a disulfide bridge. Like other A-B two-chain toxins, the individual heavy and light chains are nontoxic. The complete toxin attaches to peripheral nerves in the region of the wound, where it is transmitted to **cranial nerve nuclei** either through intraspinal transmission among involved motor neurons or bloodstream delivery of toxin to other neuromuscular junctions. The major action of tetanus toxin is **inhibition of neurotransmitter release and normal inhibitory input**, thereby causing the lower motor neuron to increase resting tone, and producing the characteristic **reflex spasms** (see Chapter 9, "Damage"). Several types of neurotransmitters are blocked, including GABA (γ-aminobutyric acid). Clinically, the disease presents as a **spastic paralysis**. Generalized tetanus, responsible for about 80% of cases, usually begins with trismus or "lockjaw". Trismus is caused by tetanic spasm of the masseter muscles and prevents opening of the mouth. The disease typically descends, initially involving the neck and back muscles, progressing to produce board-like rigidity of the abdominal musculature, eventually causing stiffness of the extremities. Individual muscle groups spasm, leading to a generalized spasm that is characterized by a tonic seizure, adduction of the arms, arching of the neck and back, extension of the legs and clenching of the fists (Fig. 20.1). Death usually results from respiratory failure caused by paralysis of chest muscles.

Treatment and Prevention

The treatment of tetanus is mainly a physiological exercise in preventing complications. Antitoxin should be given at the earliest possible moment, but it is often a futile gesture because any toxin that has been produced is already irreversibly fixed to the nerve cells. Antibiotic treatment, particularly penicillin G, is directed at the organism because it may continue to produce toxin in the wound. In addition, surgical debridement of the involved wound should be performed to eliminate the environmental niche of the organism.

Prevention of tetanus is achieved through immuniza-tion. Active immunization should be carried out in all infants and children and in pregnant women who have not been previously immunized. The vaccine consists of **tetanus toxoid**, a form of the toxin that has been inactivated in formalin but retains its antigenicity. Tetanus toxoid is the "T" of the DPT vaccine given to infants and children. Passive immunization in the form of human globulin is administered to people with a "tetanus-prone wound." Because the disease itself does produce a sufficient antibody reaction for subsequent protection, it is necessary to immunize tetanus patients with the toxoid as well. Antibodies are insufficiently produced during the disease state because the amount of toxin present in the patient is too small to be immunogenic. It is a tribute to the enormous potency of tetanus toxin that such a small amount is still sufficient to produce severe symptoms.

CLOSTRIDIA THAT CAUSE TISSUE INFECTIONS AND *C. PERFRINGENS*

Traumatic wounds are commonly contaminated with clostridial spores other than those of *C. botulinum* and *C. tetani*. These other clostridial spores are widespread in soil. In contrast to *C. tetani* and *C. botulinum*, which have little or no invasive properties, these other clostridia in wound infections cause local damage in addition to systemic effects. The major pathogen of wound infections, *C. perfringens*, produces a variety of toxins that act both locally and systemically. The more common form of clostridial wound infections is a localized cellulitis that can usually be cured with surgical management and antibiotics. More severe trauma can be associated with gas gangrene, a necrotizing, gas-forming process of muscle associated with systemic signs of shock.

Encounter, Entry, Spread, and Multiplication

C. perfringens and a variety of other clostridia are found in soil and in the intestinal tract of many animals. In wartime, 20–30% of wounds are contaminated by these organisms. The physiological condition of the

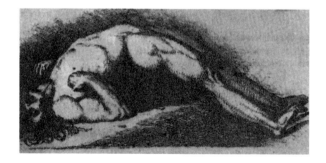

Figure 20.1. Advanced tetanus may lead to opisthotonos, the bending backward of the body caused by spastic paralysis of the strong extensors of the back. This classic painting of a British soldier wounded in 1809 in the Napoleonic Wars portrays this condition, as well as "sardonic smile" and lockjaw, caused by spasms of facial muscles.

wound site is critical in allowing the organism to germinate and to produce its toxins. The proper conditions are a low oxidation-reduction potential (anaerobic conditions), compromised blood supply, calcium ions, and the availability of various peptides and amino acids. All of these conditions are characteristic of damaged tissue.

Damage

C. perfringens produces 12 toxins, but the α-toxin, a **lecithinase** that damages cell membranes, is the toxin responsible for gas gangrene. A zinc-metallophospholipase, it interacts with eukaryotic cell membranes and **hydrolyzes phosphatidylcholine and sphingomyelin**, leading to cell death. Because the muscle tissue is destroyed (myonecrosis), it no longer reacts to stimuli. It grows black and gangrenous (Fig. 20.2). Abundant gas is produced by the organism, resulting in crepitus, which can be palpated as small gas bubbles under the skin. Systemically, the patient develops fever, sweating, low blood pressure, and decreased urinary output. The patient generally succumbs to shock and renal failure within a few days of onset.

Treatment and Prevention

Treatment of gas gangrene involves surgical removal of the involved muscle, which may necessitate extensive resection and even amputation of the affected limb. Antibiotics such as penicillin are administered to control the wound infection, but they are ineffective without adequate surgical debridement and drainage. Antitoxin, which is produced in horses, has had a negligible effect in this disease, and it is not recommended for treatment. Oxygen administered under high pressure (hyperbaric) is used in centers with appropriate chambers. Hyperbaric oxygen inhibits production of the α-toxin and suppresses growth of the organism in tissue. Milder forms of clostridial wound infection, without evidence of myonecrosis or systemic effects, can be managed with more conservative surgical intervention and appropriate antibiotics.

Prevention of gas gangrene and other clostridial wound infections involves prompt and appropriate attention to traumatic injuries. Under war conditions, front-line hospitals and evacuation facilities have ameliorated the damage caused by gunshot and shrapnel. Trauma units, now available in most American cities, have reduced the incidence of clostridial soft tissue infections by initiating prompt attention to injured wounds.

CONCLUSION

The pathogenic clostridia have a broad spectrum of colonization and invasiveness. In botulism, the organisms do not invade the body at all; in tetanus, they barely set up household in tissues; and in clostridial gangrene, they have considerable invasive capacity.

The toxins of tetanus and botulism both act on the nervous system, and both are extraordinarily potent. They differ, however, in the way that they enter the body and in the details of their mode of action. These toxins cause serious disease without killing their target cells, whereas those involved in wound infection and pseudomembranous colitis are generally cytolitic.

SELF-ASSESSMENT QUESTIONS

1. Discuss the properties of clostridia that explain their ecology.
2. What elicits pseudomembranous colitis? Who is at risk for this disease?
3. Why is ingesting botulinum toxin more dangerous than ingesting tetanus toxin? Why is infant botulism usually a mild disease?
4. Contrast the mode of action of tetanus and botulinum toxins on the nervous system.
5. We are usually immunized against tetanus early in life. Why aren't we immunized against the other clostridial infections?

SUGGESTED READINGS

Gorbach SL. *Clostridium perfringens* and other clostridia. In: Gorbach SL, Bartlett JG, Blacklow NR. Infectious diseases. 2nd ed. Philadelphia: WB Saunders, 1997.

Gorbach SL. Gas gangrene and other clostridial skin and soft tissue infections. In: Gorbach SL, Bartlett JG, Blacklow NR. Infectious diseases. 2nd ed. Philadelphia: WB Saunders, 1997.

Hart GB, Lamb RC, Strauss MB. Gas gangrene. J Trauma 1983;23:991.

Smith LD, Williams BL. The pathogenic anaerobic bacteria. 3rd ed. Springfield, IL: Charles C Thomas, 1984.

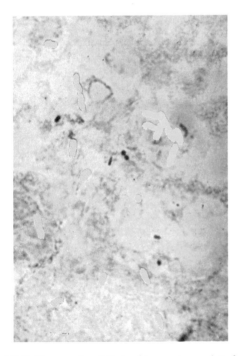

Figure 20.2. Gram stain of *C. perfringens* in exudate from gas gangrene. Note absence of neutrophils.

Legionella: Parasite of Cells

N. CARY ENGLEBERG

Key Concepts

Legionella:
- Are aerobic Gram-negative bacilli.
- Invade human macrophages.
- Have fastidious growth requirements and must be grown on special media.
- Cause waterborne infections such as Legionnaires' disease (legionellosis) and Pontiac fever.

Legionnaires' disease:
- Is caused by *Legionella pneumophila*.
- Affects only a minority of people exposed to the infectious agent. These people usually have risk factors such as smoking, advanced age, or pulmonary disease.
- Is cleared by a cell-mediated response.
- Causes damage in the lungs due to a vigorous host response to the infectious agent.
- Is difficult to diagnose, thus necessitating treatment based on suspicion alone.
- Is treated with antibiotics known to penetrate infected cells (erythromycin and tetracycline).
- Can be prevented by regularly checking institutional water systems for the presence of *L. pneumophila*.

The legionellae are aerobic Gram-negative bacilli that parasitize protozoa in the environment and are opportunistic invaders of human phagocytic cells. These bacteria are found in a variety of natural aquatic habitats and occasionally inhabit human-made water distribution systems. They are fastidious organisms, and their isolation from water or from infected tissues requires special culture media. Humans acquire *Legionella* by inhalation. When the organisms are deposited in the air spaces of the lungs, they may produce a severe form of pneumonia called **Legionnaires' disease** or **legionellosis**. Because this infection is often associated with contaminated water systems, large outbreaks of Legionnaires' disease may occur in institutions such as hospitals and hotels.

CASE

Mrs. R., a 57-year-old female, was admitted to the hospital with a high fever and altered mental status. Eight days earlier, she had developed a "flulike" illness with fever, anorexia, malaise, headache, and muscle aches. These symptoms were followed by a cough that became progressively worse but was productive of only scanty, clear sputum. Five days before admission, she saw a local physician who ordered a chest x-ray. The x-ray showed a small left upper lobe infiltrate consistent with pneumonia. She was treated with oral cephalexin (a first-generation cephalosporin antibiotic). Her fever and chills increased steadily, and she became confused and lethargic. Mrs. R.'s past medical history was unremarkable, but she had smoked one pack of cigarettes a day for 40 years.

On admission, her temperature was 104°F, her heart rate was 88 beats/minute, and she was cyanotic. The white cell count was 13,700/mm³, and the patient was severely hypoxic. A Gram stain of the sputum showed numerous neutrophils but no bacteria. A chest x-ray showed extension of the left upper lobe infiltrate and a new right middle lobe infiltrate.

The patient was intubated and placed on mechanical ventilation in the intensive care unit (ICU). She was given broad-spectrum antibiotics, including a high-dose of erythromycin. Shortly after admission, her blood pressure dropped precipitously, and she required vasopressive agents. After a stormy ICU course, the patient began to improve slowly and eventually recovered. Respiratory secretions, obtained by aspiration through the endotracheal tube, were negative for *Legionella pneumophila* by direct fluorescent antibody microscopy, but a culture of the specimen grew the organism after 3 days of incubation.

The case of Mrs. R. raises several questions:

1. How did Mrs. R. acquire *L. pneumophila*, and why wasn't anyone in her family or workplace also infected?
2. Why was the diagnosis of Legionnaires' disease so difficult to make in this case?
3. Why did Mrs. R.'s pneumonia worsen during treatment with an antibiotic that can efficiently kill *L. pneumophila* growing in the laboratory?

FAMILY LEGIONELLACEAE

L. pneumophila does not grow on routine bacteriological media. Instead, a special medium that meets the peculiar nutritional needs of this organism is required. The bacterium requires high levels of the amino acid, cysteine, as well as supplements of inorganic iron for optimal growth. In addition, the concentration of sodium must be kept low, and activated charcoal is added to absorb inhibitory substances in the media.

Once microbiologists learned how to grow *L. pneu-*

mophila in the laboratory, related organisms were isolated from human and environmental sources. Thirty separate species have been identified within the genus *Legionella*, and they comprise the only genus in the family Legionellaceae. DNA–DNA hybridization studies indicate that the Legionellaceae have no close relatives among known bacteria.

In nature, the Legionellaceae are found in ponds, lakes, and hot springs, where they feed on organic matter generated by photosynthetic algae and other plant life. Like other bacteria in these environments, they are fed upon by **protozoa**. However, legionellae actually profit from ingestion by protozoans and, instead of being killed and digested like other bacteria, they grow to large numbers inside these unicellular organisms.

Encounter

The source of the 1976 Philadelphia outbreak was never identified, but investigations of numerous later outbreaks established a link between the occurrence of Legionnaires' disease and the colonization of plumbing systems with *L. pneumophila*. In hospitals or hotels where epidemics have occurred, the *L. pneumophila* strain isolated from respiratory cultures of patients can also be found in tap water, in swabs taken from faucets or shower heads, or in sediment from hot water tanks. In some respects, *Legionella* is particularly well-adapted to these environments. The bacterium grows at temperatures up to 46°C and tolerates much higher temperatures, and it is relatively chlorine-resistant compared to enteric bacteria. Given the strict nutritional requirements of this organism, it is not surprising to find it in association with other microorganisms, such as protozoa, which may provide essential nutrients to support their growth.

Legionnaires' disease is nearly always a primary pulmonary infection and is never transmitted from person to person. Instead, humans acquire the infectious agents from an environmental source, usually a water distribution system colonized with the microorganism (Fig. 21.1). In the laboratory, *L. pneumophila* in water

---

Humans, Health and History

An Outbreak of Legionnaire's Disease

Legionella was unknown as a bacterial species until 1976, when a highly publicized outbreak of what became known as Legionnaires' disease occurred among attendees of an American Legion convention in Philadelphia. In all, 182 attendees became ill, and 29 died. For an uncomfortable period after the convention, the cause of the epidemic remained obscure. Eventually, researchers from the Centers for Disease Control discovered the bacterial pathogen by inoculating lung tissue from patients into the peritoneal cavity of guinea pigs. They discovered that the agent could be grown in egg yolks and eventually in supplemented artificial media. Soon after the bacterium (*L. pneumophila*) was isolated, culture and serological methods were developed to facilitate the clinical diagnosis of Legionnaires' disease, and species of *Legionella* were recognized as a significant cause of pneumonia in many parts of the world.

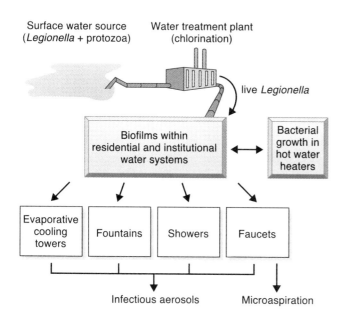

Figure 21.1. Sources of legionellae for human disease.

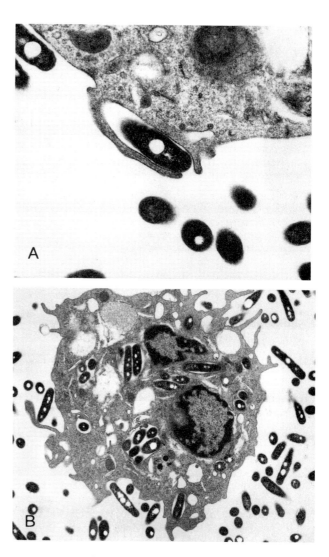

Figure 21.2. Electron micrographs. **A.** Uptake of *L. pneumophila* by a macrophage. **B.** *L. pneumophila* begin to multiply within membrane-bound phagosomes within the host macrophage.

aerosols can infect guinea pigs and produce an illness similar to Legionnaires' disease. Showers, humidifiers, water fountains, respiratory therapy equipment, or evaporative cooling towers associated with central air conditioning systems may produce similar aerosols that can transmit *H. pneumophila* to humans. An alternative mode of entry is by microaspiration of bacteria from the oropharynx or mouth into the lower pulmonary airways, during or after the ingestion of contaminated water or ice. The circumstances of Mrs. R.'s exposure are unknown, but if water was the source, she may have acquired the infection at home, at work, or at any place where running water is available.

In outbreak situations, only a minority of exposed individuals actually become infected. In these uncontrolled situations, the risk of infection depends not only on the size and amount of the inhaled inoculum, but also on the susceptibility of individual hosts. Although not much is known about the infectious inoculum that leads to *L. pneumophila* outbreaks, several **host factors** are known to predispose individuals to infection. These include cigarette smoking, advanced age, chronic pulmonary disease, and immunosuppression (e.g., transplant patients, patients on corticosteroid therapy). Mrs. R. may have been particularly susceptible to infection due to her significant smoking history. Although we do not know the source of her infection, it is possible that other less susceptible individuals were exposed to the same source as Mrs. R. but did not become infected.

Entry

In the air spaces of the lung, *Legionella* are ingested by resident **alveolar macrophages.** These phagocytic cells, which normally function as a front line of defense against invaders, fail to kill or even inhibit the growth of *L. pneumophila* in the lung (Fig. 21.2). In laboratory experiments, *L. pneumophila* actually grows faster in cultures with human macrophages than in artificial media. Several lines of evidence suggest that phagocytosis and intracellular growth are essential events in the pathogenesis of Legionnaires' disease.

L. pneumophila are ingested spontaneously by phagocytic cells; the molecular mechanism that triggers phagocytosis is unknown. However, in the presence of serum, the bacteria bind complement to a major outer membrane protein, a porin. The organisms are resistant to complement-mediated lysis, but the presence of surface-bound C′3 enhances uptake by phagocytic cells by several orders of magnitude.

PARADIGM   ■ ■ ■

Intracellular Parasitism

To grow in phagocytic cells, pathogens must be able to outmaneuver their hosts. They must evade the antimicrobial defenses of these cells, and they must satisfy their nutritional requirements by competing successfully with the host cell for essential intracellular nutrients. To meet these necessities, bacterial and eukaryotic pathogens have evolved different intracellular lifestyles (Fig. 21.3). As the figure suggests, phylogenetically unrelated organisms may share a common strategy for intracellular survival and growth. However, the precise mechanisms and virulence factors that mediate these events in different species are usually very different and have evolved independently.

The ability to survive phagosome–lysosome fusion may involve adaptation of the pathogen's surface, its metabolism, or both. Gram-negative enteric organisms with smooth lipopolysaccharide, such as salmonellae, are less susceptible to killing by lysosomal contents than are "rough" mutants that lack the long polysaccharide chains on their surface. Similarly, mycobacteria may be protected by the waxy nature of their surfaces. The leishmaniae are adapted to the hostile environment of the acidified phagosome because they possess metabolic enzymes that function well at low pH.

For organisms that multiply in the host cell cytoplasm, escape from the phagosome is essential to their survival. *Listeria monocytogenes*, a Gram-positive bacillus that causes septicemia and meningitis, is a case in point. After ingestion by most cells, *L. monocytogenes* secretes a pore-forming cytotoxin, called **listeriolysin O**, that disrupts the phagosomal membrane, releasing the bacterium into the cytoplasm. The cytoplasm is a desirable location for the bacterium, since it provides nutrients and protects the bacterium from attack by cellular killing mechanisms. Mutant *L. monocytogenes* that do not produce this cytotoxin cannot escape the phagosome; they neither grow nor survive in the host cell. How do these organisms travel from cell to cell? *L. monocytogenes* promptly divide and then begin to move within the cytosol. Their motility depends on the presence of a bacterial protein called **ActA**. This protein catalyzes the polymerization of cellular actin on the surface of the bacterial cell at one of its poles. The polymerized actin forms a growing scaffold that pushes the bacteria through the cytoplasm. Eventually, the organisms are pushed outward onto the plasma membrane, make contact with a neighboring cell, and prompt ingestion. This process results in the direct spread of the infection to adjacent host cells (see also Chapter 8, "The Parasite's Way of Life").

The legionellae and several other unrelated pathogens remain within an endosome after ingestion. These organisms owe their survival to inadequate responses of both **oxidative** and **nonoxidative intracellular killing mechanisms** of the phagocytes. Typically, the respiratory burst and the resulting production of microbicidal oxygen derivatives is blunted or absent in these organisms. Likewise, the acidification of the phagosome and the fusion of the phagosome with lysosomes, which exposes the ingested organism to toxic lysosomal contents, does not occur. Some pathogens, such as *L. pneumophila*, form replicative endosomes that associate with cellular organelles (e.g., rough endoplasmic reticulum), but other pathogens occupy featureless intracellular vacuoles.

Regardless of the mechanism involved, intracellular parasitism has consequences in clinical medicine. Intracellular organisms are less accessible both to the host immune response and to antimicrobial agents. Recovery from infection may require a cell-mediated immune response that inhibits or kills intracellular organisms. Such a response generally takes longer to mount than an antibody response. As a result, therapy for these infections generally lasts longer and relapses, presumably resulting from the reemergence of surviving intracellular organisms, are more common than in most extracellular infections. In selecting optimal antimicrobial therapy, the capacity of drugs to penetrate infected host cells must be considered. Antibiotics that penetrate poorly into host cells are generally less useful in treating these infections.

N. CARY ENGLEBERG

Multiplication and Spread

After ingestion, the normal acidification of the **phagosome** and fusion with **lysosomes** does not occur. Instead, the phagosome associates first with other cellular organelles (e.g., smooth vesicles, mitochondria) and later with the rough endoplasmic reticulum. Within the resulting **specialized endosome**, bacterial multiplication proceeds until the host cell is literally packed with bacteria (Fig. 21.2). Eventually, the cell dies and ruptures, releasing bacterial progeny that initiate the cycle in other cells.

Several mutations of *L. pneumophila* genes are known to impair the ability of the organism to grow within phagocytic cells. There are at least two large gene clusters on the chromosome that encode functions required for proper trafficking of the phagosome and avoidance of lysosomal fusion. Disruption of certain genes, designated as "*dot*" (for *d*efect in *o*rganelle *t*rafficking), results in bacterial mutants which are ingested normally but promptly fuse to lysosomes. Several of the *dot* gene products are localized within the cell envelope, raising speculation that they and other proteins encoded

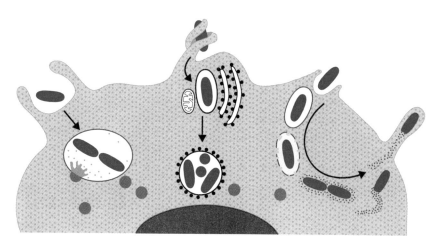

Figure 21.3. Three lifestyles of intracellular pathogens. Left: *Salmonella* spp. enter a cell by generating a membrane ruffling or "splash." The result is a large phagosome that may fuse with lysosomes; however, the bacterium survives and eventu- ally grows within the phagolysosome. **Center:** intracellular life cycle of *Legionella pneumophila.* **Right:** intracellular survival, growth, and motility of *Listeria monocytogenes.*

in these clusters may assemble to form a functional complex that protects the *L. pneumophila* phagosome and allows it to become a site for bacterial replication. These gene clusters may be examples of "pathogenicity islands" (see Chapter 4, "Genetics of Bacteria").

The host may be able to inhibit the intracellular growth of *L. pneumophila* by nonspecific immune mechanisms. Upon contact with the organism, macrophages secrete **tumor necrosis factor-alpha** (TNF-α), which inhibits intracellular growth of the bacteria. Secretion of TNF-α suggests that normal cells in normal hosts may be able to limit *L. pneumophila* without ever inducing a specific immune response, which may in turn explain the resistance of most humans to Legionnaires' disease.

Once infection is established, however, a specific immune response is required to clear the infection. Experience with animal infections suggests that specific antibodies may play a role in containing *L. pneumophila* infection but that recovery from infection requires a **cell-mediated immune response.** Antibodies produced during infection may bind to the bacterial surface and enhance uptake of the bacteria by neutrophils. Although *L. pneumophila* are not efficiently killed by neutrophils, they cannot grow in these cells. In contrast to the humoral response, the cellular immune response limits the growth of *L. pneumophila* in macrophages. By cellular immune processes described in Chapter 7, *Legionella*-immune lymphocytes proliferate and secrete **cytokines** after contact with cells presenting *Legionella* antigens with Class II histocompatibility molecules. One of the most important of these cytokines, γ-**interferon,** is known to suppress the growth of *L. pneumophila* within macrophages by inducing these cells to limit the availability of **iron** to the intracellular bacteria. Limiting this

essential nutrient and eliminating the intracellular niche as a site for multiplication may constitute the critical functions of the immune system in controlling *L. pneumophila* infection.

Damage

Macrophages infected with *L. pneumophila* release cytokines that may contribute to the influx of blood monocytes and neutrophils into the air spaces of the lung. As nodular areas of infection enlarge, they become visible as infiltrates on chest x-rays. These areas typically develop into microabscesses and may coalesce to form cavities. The bronchi and bronchioles are not affected. During full-blown infection, *L. pneumophila* can be isolated from the blood or from a variety of organ tissues.

Much of the local damage produced by the infection is attributable to a vigorous host inflammatory response. Some debate surrounds the role of bacterial products. For example, *L. pneumophila* possesses a lipopolysaccharide endotoxin that is weakly toxic, and it also produces an extracellular protease that has cytolytic and hemolytic activity. Conflicting evidence exists about the potential role of the protease. Although the purified protease can damage the lungs of experimental animals, protease-deficient mutants of *L. pneumophila* are as virulent as wild-type strains.

Illness in humans usually begins with "flulike" complaints, as in the case of Mrs. R. Virtually all patients with Legionnaires' disease have **fever,** and they typically develop clinical features of pneumonia: **cough, shortness of breath,** and sometimes **chest pain.** Patients rarely have the grossly purulent (thick yellow or green) sputum associated with bacterial bronchopneumonias. Watery diarrhea is present in 25–50% of patients with Legionnaires' disease, and nausea, vomiting, or abdominal pain may also be present. **Blood oxygen levels** may be low and may contribute to mental status changes, as seen in Mrs. R.'s case. Typically, blood cell counts show only moderate elevation of total leukocytes, without a preponderance of neutrophils. In many patients, other laboratory tests suggest dysfunction of the kidneys or liver. None of these clinical features is sufficiently specific to establish the diagnosis of Legionnaires' disease, because any of them can occur in association with other pneumonias.

Diagnosis

The laboratory diagnosis of Legionnaires' disease may be difficult. The bacteria are not present in large numbers in the sputum, and they stain poorly. The Gram stain usually shows abundant neutrophils and no stainable bacteria. Several **rapid diagnostic techniques** have been used to make a prompt diagnosis of Legionnaires' disease. They include examination of sputum by direct **fluorescent antibody staining** (DFA), hybridization with a **DNA probe**, or detection of *L. pneumophila* serogroup 1 antigen in the urine by **enzyme immunoassay**. Although these tests may be useful in guiding the initial therapy of the patient, none of them is sufficiently sensitive or specific to be relied upon as the sole method of diagnosis. Culture is the most specific way to diagnose the infection, although 3–5 days of incubation may be required before *Legionella* colonies can be identified. Culture is more sensitive when specimens are taken directly from the lower respiratory tract and are treated to limit the growth of normal flora.

Because the laboratory diagnosis of Legionnaires' disease is imperfect and occasionally untimely, it is necessary to treat patients for this potentially fatal disease on suspicion alone. As a case in point, Mrs. R. was recognized as having a severe, atypical pneumonia that progressed in spite of treatment with an oral cephalosporin antibiotic. In the absence of an alternative diagnosis, she was treated with an antibiotic that is known to be effective in Legionnaires' disease, pending the results of the culture. This clinical decision may have saved her life.

Treatment and Prevention

Legionellae grown in culture are sensitive to most antibiotics. However, successful antibiotic therapy requires drugs that can penetrate infected cells, such as erythromycin and tetracycline. As in Mrs. R.'s case, it is not unusual for the patient's condition to worsen while receiving penicillin or cephalosporin because these antibiotics penetrate eukaryotic cells poorly.

Prevention of Legionnaires' disease is presently practiced at an institutional level. In hospitals, hotels, and other large buildings where cases have occurred, water systems are checked regularly for *Legionella*. If found, the systems are flushed and decontaminated by super-

heating of the water to 60°C, ultraviolet irradiation, or treatment with copper and silver ions.

Protective immunity has been induced in guinea pigs by injection of **vaccines** containing various bacterial protein fractions or by inhalation of a live, mutant strain of *L. pneumophila* that cannot grow intracellularly. Immunization of humans, particularly those with one of the high-risk conditions mentioned above, may be possible in the foreseeable future.

OTHER LEGIONELLAE AND *LEGIONELLA*-ASSOCIATED DISEASES

In addition to *L. pneumophila*, several other species of *Legionella* cause human disease. In general, these species also cause water-related infections, and they produce clinical features comparable to Legionnaires' disease. Prominent among these species is *L. micdadei*, formerly known as the Pittsburgh Pneumonia Agent before its relationship to *L. pneumophila* was established.

Certain legionellae have also been associated with an illness called Pontiac fever. This illness was first recognized during a 1968 outbreak at the county health department building in Pontiac, Michigan. In this outbreak, 95% of the departmental employees became ill with fever, muscle aches, headache, and dizziness that resolved spontaneously within 2–5 days. The cause of this flulike illness was not identified at the time, but serum samples from patients and lung tissue from guinea pigs exposed to the building air were frozen for future reference. After the identification of *L. pneumophila* 9 years later, the frozen specimens were retested. The Pontiac patients were found to have increased titers of specific *Legionella* antibodies, and the guinea pig lungs yielded growth of *L. pneumophila* in culture.

Like Legionnaires' disease, Pontiac fever is an airborne disease, but here the similarity ends. Unlike Legionnaires' disease, Pontiac fever typically affects a high proportion of exposed individuals, and it affects healthy, as well as high-risk, individuals. It does not produce pneumonia and is never fatal. It may not be an infection at all, but rather a manifestation of hypersensitivity. Why the same bacteria produce such different clinical syndromes is still a mystery.

CONCLUSION

The legionellae produce an airborne infection of the lungs that results in a life-threatening pneumonia. Infection depends on the capacity of the bacterium to grow within phagocytic cells of the host. Treatment and immune mechanisms are beneficial insofar as they can affect the bacteria that occupy the intracellular niche.

SELF-ASSESSMENT QUESTIONS

1. Discuss the ecology of *L. pneumophila* and its relation to the epidemiology of legionellosis.

2. Why does legionellosis tend to manifest in outbreaks?

3. Contrast pneumonia due to *Legionella* with that due to pneumococci (Chapter 13, "Pneumococcus and Bacterial Pneumonia").

4. Why don't all of us come down with legionellosis, given the widespread occurrence of the organisms?

5. What other pathogenic bacteria are acquired from the water supply routes other than ingestion?

SUGGESTED READINGS

Edelstein PH. Legionnaires' disease. Clin Infect Dis 1993;16: 741–749.

Engleberg NC, Brieland JK. Legionella; infection and immunity. In: Delves PJ, Roitt I, eds. Encyclopedia of immunology. 2nd ed. London: Academic Press, 1998.

Fraser DW, Tsai TR, Orenstein W, et al. Legionnaires' disease: description of an epidemic of pneumonia. N Engl J Med 1977;297:1189–1197.

Salyers AA, Whitt DD. Legionnaires' disease. In: Saylers AA, Whitt, PA, eds. Bacterial pathogenesis; a molecular approach. Washington, DC: ASM Press, 1994;301–306.

CHAPTER 22

Helicobacter pylori: Pathogenesis of a "Slow" Bacterial Infection

RICHARD M. PEEK JR.

MARTIN J. BLASER

Key Concepts

Helicobacter pylori:

- Is a recently discovered bacterium that is the causative agent of most gastric and duodenal ulcers.
- Colonizes the mucus gel layer overlying the gastric mucosa because it produces urease, which converts urea to ammonia and increases the pH locally.
- Is extremely common and probably infects up to half of the world's population.
- Causes clinical disease in only 5–10% of infected individuals.
- Is associated with adenocarcinoma of the stomach.
- Can be detected by histologic examination, culture, rapid urease testing, serologic testing, and urease breath tests.
- Is treated with a combination of antibiotic and acid-reducing drugs.

INTRODUCTION

Helicobacter pylori is a Gram-negative bacterium that resides in the mucus gel layer overlaying the gastric mucosa. Marshall and Warren first identified curved bacilli adjacent to the gastric epithelium of patients with chronic gastritis in 1983. Since then, a strong link has been established between *H. pylori* and a diverse spectrum of gastroduodenal diseases, including chronic gastritis, gastric and duodenal ulceration, gastric adenocarcinoma, and non-Hodgkin's lymphoma of the stomach. This bacterium colonizes the stomach for years or decades, not days or weeks as is usually the case for bacterial pathogen. The longevity and

persistent low-grade gastric inflammation with gradual progression to disease both suggest that *H. pylori* should be considered a prototypic "slow" bacterium. In this sense, *H. pylori* resembles the spirochetes of syphilis and Lyme disease and the leprosy bacillus, all of which can cause low-grade but continuing infection. Recent insights into *H. pylori* pathophysiology are beginning to answer perplexing questions raised by the bacterium's unique ecological niche. For example, how does an organism that colonizes over half of the world's population lead to overt clinical disease in only 5–10% of infected individuals? And how does *H. pylori* infection lead to such divergent clinical sequelae?

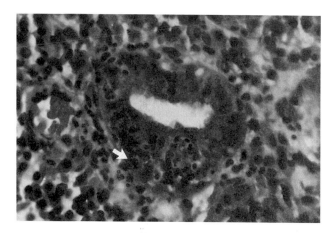

Figure 22.1. Hematoxylin and eosin stain of *H. pylori*-associated gastritis. Numerous neutrophils, lymphocytes, and plasma cells are present in the lamina propria. In addition, the gland in the center of the figure is infiltrated with neutrophils (*arrow*) and lymphocytes.

CASE

Mr. C., a 45 year-old man, was evaluated for recurrent burning epigastric pain. Seven years earlier, he had noted abdominal pain which often awakened him from sleep, was associated with nausea, and improved with meals. He was initially treated with cimetidine to reduce the production of gastric acid for 8 weeks, and his symptoms resolved. However, 4 months later, the symptoms recurred. On endoscopy, a 1-cm duodenal bulb ulcer was seen. The patient was once again given cimetidine. However, four times in the ensuing 6 years, an ulcer and the burning epigastric pain recurred. Mr. C.'s mother and one of his two siblings also had a history of peptic ulcer disease.

Another endoscopy showed that an ulcer was still present. Biopsies of two sites were taken for histologic examination and culture. These specimens showed chronic active gastritis with elevated numbers of neutrophils and mononuclear leukocytes in the lamina propria and the glandular epithelium (Fig. 22.1). Curved, rod-shaped bacteria were identified on the mucosal surfaces of all biopsies, and cultures grew *H. pylori*.

This time, in addition to acid reduction therapy, Mr. C. received a course of a bismuth salt, tetracycline, and metronidazole. Repeat endoscopy 6 weeks after completion of therapy showed healing of his ulcer, and biopsies showed resolution of the gastritis. No *H. pylori* were found on histologic examination or culture. Mr. C. remained symptom-free, with no further therapy after 6 months.

This case raises a number of questions:

1. Was *H. pylori* the cause of Mr. C.'s 7-year bout of recurrent duodenal ulceration?
2. What features permit *H. pylori* to colonize the stomach when other bacteria are usually killed there?
3. What bacterial (and/or host) factors allow an infection with specificity for gastric epithelium to cause disease at an anatomically distinct site such as the duodenum?
4. How can *H. pylori* infection be detected in patients with disease?
5. How can *H. pylori* be eliminated from the stomach?

HELICOBACTER PYLORI

H. pylori is the prototypic species of the genus *Helicobacter*. These organisms are Gram-negative curved or spiral bacteria that live in the mucus layer above the gastric epithelium. They have multiple flagella at one pole. They are nutritionally fastidious bacteria and **microaerophilic**, i.e., they grow ideally in an atmosphere of reduced oxygen (about 5%).

H. pylori are robust producers of **urease,** which catalyzes the hydrolysis of urea into ammonia and carbon dioxide. Other *Helicobacter* species, e.g., *Helicobacter mustelae*, *Helicobacter muridarum*, and *Helicobacter nemastrinae*, have been found in the stomachs of other mammals; all are strongly urease-positive, suggesting that ammonia production is an important conserved survival mechanism for helicobacters in the acidic gastric environment.

ENCOUNTER, ENTRY, AND MULTIPLICATION

H. pylori is one of the most common infections of humans. It affects up to half of the world's population; however, prevalence of the infection may be declining in the developed world. The specific mode of transmission of *H. pylori* is not known. Direct person-to-person spread is most likely since *H. pylori* has not been cultured from animal reservoirs (with the possible exception of cats). Also, persons who have greater contact with human feces and secretions, such as adults living in institutions and children in orphanages, have high infection rates. *H. pylori* is thought to be spread by either the fecal–oral or the oral–oral route and has been cultured from the stools of infected children. This organism has also been cultured from **dental plaque** and detected in saliva using polymerase chain reaction (PCR). Thus, transmission by either of these two routes may occur.

Two ingestion experiments by human volunteers and several outbreaks of accidental infection have provided clues into the initial events that occur during acute *H. pylori* infection. A self-inoculation experiment conducted by an investigator from Australia resulted in acute, severe gastrointestinal symptoms and persistent gastritis. The fasting gastric pH on day 5 following ingestion was 1.2 (in the normal range of 1–2) and was accompanied by intense inflammation in the gastric antrum. By day 8, however, the fasting gastric pH rose

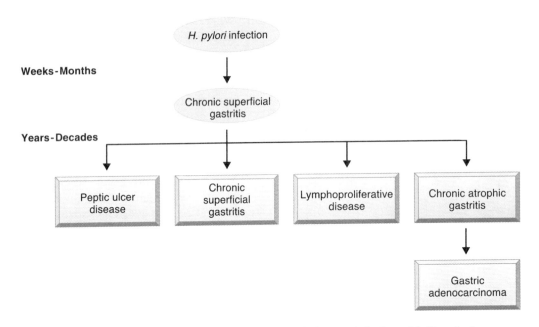

Figure 22.2. Diversity of clinical consequences following infection with *H. pylori.*

to 7.6. Along with acute symptoms, specific immunoglobulin M (IgM) antibodies peaked early, and significant titers of both IgA and IgG developed later. These findings suggest that ingestion of the organisms is followed by a period of intense bacterial proliferation and gastric inflammation with concomitant **hypochlorhydria**, which may last for weeks. Ultimately, the inflammatory response is reduced to a low-level stable state and the host mounts a humoral immune response that is ineffective in eliminating *H. pylori* (but may control induction of inflammation). Normal gastric pH is also restored, and most infected persons remain asymptomatic for years or for life.

DAMAGE

Essentially all persons who become infected with *H. pylori* develop **chronic superficial gastritis** involving the antrum and the fundus. The gastritis persists throughout their lifetime whether or not they have gastrointestinal symptoms. Long-term pathologic outcomes vary between infected persons (Fig. 22.2). Some persons develop **ulceration**. In others, however, the inflammatory process is associated with permanent loss of epithelial glands, termed **atrophic gastritis**, which occurs over a course of decades. Atrophic gastritis is a well-recognized risk factor for **gastric cancer**.

H. pylori pathogenesis is complex, in keeping with the ability of the organism to cause a variety of clinical manifestations. *H. pylori* has evolved mechanisms to ensure a prolonged existence within its host; for example, although both humoral and cellular recognition of *H. pylori* occur the organism can evade immunologic clear-

ance. In addition, *H. pylori* has evolved properties, such as making a **less potent endotoxin** than most Gram-negatives, that lessen mucosal inflammation and injury. This observation suggests that it may be beneficial for the long-term survival of the bacteria to minimize damage to its host.

H. pylori infection is invariably associated with chronic gastric inflammation, which may serve as a means for the organism to obtain a constant source of nutrients. In this model, *H. pylori* releases **inflammatory effector molecules** that induce tissue inflammation, which causes **release of nutrients** that sustain the *H. pylori* population. One potential marker of inflammation is CagA, a protein of 120–140 kDa which is found in 60–70% of strains. Serum and mucosal antibodies to CagA are present in about 90% of all patients with duodenal ulceration, and expression of CagA *in vivo* is highly correlated with peptic ulcer disease and duodenitis. *H. pylori* isolates that are positive for CagA (**cagA$^+$** strains) induce higher degrees of inflammation and damage in the gastric mucosa than *cagA$^-$* strains. In addition, mucosal levels of **interleukin-8 (IL-8)**, a potent chemoattractant and neutrophil-activating peptide, are significantly higher in persons with harboring *cagA$^+$* rather than *cagA$^-$* strains. The high levels of IL-8 may explain the link between these **cagA$^+$** strains and peptic ulcer disease.

Some *H. pylori* strains also secrete a **cytotoxin** (encoded by *vacA*) that induces **vacuolation** of cells in culture. *H. pylori* clinical isolates that produce the cytotoxin are associated with peptic ulcer disease and increased infiltration of the gastric antrum by neutrophils. Intragastric administration of this purified toxin to mice results in epithelial cell erosions and degeneration.

The mechanism of ulcer development due to *H. pylori* infection is not well understood. Continuous inflammation within the gastric mucosa may be sufficient to lead to mucosal breakdown, erosive gastritis, and ultimately to ulceration. A more perplexing question concerns the development of duodenal ulcers. *H. pylori* is found only in association with gastric epithelium; how then can this infection lead to disease in the duodenum? The answer most likely involves the development of gastric tissue in the duodenum, a phenomenon well known in patients with high acid secretion (as in a condition called the Zollinger-Ellison syndrome). *H. pylori* infection results in downregulation of **somatostatin-producing D-cells**, which in turn leads to inappropriately elevated **gastrin levels** and enhanced gastric acid secretion. *H. pylori* can then populate these regions of gastric metaplasia, establish infection, cause inflammation and, in concert with elevated gastric acid levels, ultimately lead to ulceration at this site.

H. pylori infection is also associated with development of **adenocarcinoma of the stomach**. The sequential progression of chronic superficial gastritis to chronic atrophic gastritis, through intestinal metaplasia to dysplasia, and then finally to invasive adenocarcinoma, is lengthy. Progression to adenocarcinoma may take some 15–20 years after onset of superficial gastritis. Specifically, how does adenocarcinoma occur? Enhanced cell proliferation secondary to chronic *H. pylori* infection may increase the likelihood of DNA damage in response to environmental mutagens such as **N-nitrosamines** or **inflammation-related free radicals**. These environmental mutagens are associated with reduced concentrations of ascorbic acid in gastric juice, an important defense mechanism against oxidative DNA damage (Fig. 22.3). The risk of gastric cancer may also be related to certain strain characteristics of *H. pylori*. Infection with a *cagA*$^+$ (as opposed to a *cagA*$^-$) strain has been associated with a twofold increase in risk of gastric adenocarcinoma, perhaps due to the heightened inflammatory response that develops after infection with a *cagA*$^+$ strain.

In addition to gastric adenocarcinoma, persons infected with *H. pylori* have an increased risk of developing **non-Hodgkin's lymphoma of the stomach**. Although little is known about the specific factors involved, the ongoing, local chronic inflammatory process initiated by *H. pylori* is likely to be important. Thus, the seemingly divergent diseases of peptic ulceration and gastric cancer may both be related to *H. pylori* infection. In its early stages, the infection can induce sufficient inflammation to disrupt mucosal integrity, alter the acid homeostasis within the stomach, and lead to ulcers. In its later stage, it may promote the development of neoplasm on a pathologic background of atrophic gastritis.

DIAGNOSIS

Several techniques are currently available to detect *H. pylori* infection. They can be classified as either invasive or noninvasive. All of these tests are quite sensitive and specific (Table 22.1), and the choice of which test to select depends on the laboratory resources available and the clinical situation, i.e., diagnosing infection versus documenting eradication.

Invasive methods involve obtaining gastric tissue specimens by endoscopy and include **histologic examination**, microbiological **culture**, and **rapid urease test-**

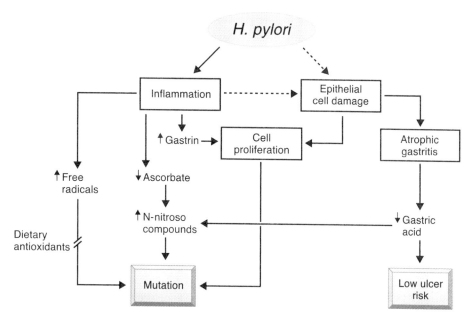

Figure 22.3. Potential mechanisms of carcinogenesis following infection with *H. pylori*.

Table 22.1. Diagnosis of *Helicobacter pylori*

Method	Specimen	Sensitivity
Invasive tests		
Urease test of biopsy	Mucosal biopsy	High
Histology, Giemsa stain	Mucosal biopsies (2)	Very high
Culture of biopsy	Mucosal biopsy	High
Noninvasive tests		
Serology (ELISA)	Serum	High
Urea breath test	Breath sample	Very high
Tests used in research		
Culture of stool	Stool sample	Low to medium (30–50%)
Polymerase chain reaction	Stool sample, gastric juice, biopsy of stomach	High

ing. Most pathologists initially utilize the Giemsa stain because it is sensitive and inexpensive; the Warthin-Starry stain is more sensitive but more difficult to standardize (Fig. 22.4). Detection of *H. pylori* by culture is less reliable than other available methods due to the fastidious growth of the organism. Biochemical confirmation of *H. pylori* includes positive tests for urease, catalase, and oxidase. A rapid urease test determines urease activity in gastric biopsy sample. When a biopsy containing *H. pylori* is placed onto indicator media, ammonia is produced from urea, the pH increases, and the indicator turns red. The rapid urease test is less expensive than either histology or culture and is the method of choice when endoscopy is used.

Noninvasive tests include **serology** and **urea breath tests**. Serologic tests measure the circulating antibodies directed toward a variety of *H. pylori* antigens and are very sensitive and specific for primary diagnosis of *H. pylori* infection. However, serological methods have limited utility in assessing posttreatment *H. pylori* status because titers fall gradually; it may be 6 months before a sufficient decrease is observed. Urea breath testing involves ingestion of radioactive carbon-labeled urea; if *H. pylori* (or other urease-containing gastric bacteria) are present, urea is metabolized to ammonia and bicarbonate, and radioactive carbon dioxide is detected in breath samples. The urea breath test is a convenient method to document *H. pylori* eradication, since it does not require endoscopy and is easy to perform.

TREATMENT

On the basis of a large body of data indicating that *H. pylori* is the major cause of peptic ulcer disease, a 1994 NIH consensus conference found that "all patients with gastric or duodenal ulcers who are infected with *H. pylori* should be treated with antimicrobials regardless of whether they are suffering from the initial presentation of the disease or from a recurrence."

An ideal treatment for *H. pylori* would be inexpensive, safe with minimal side effects, simple, effective, and short in duration. In addition, treatment should not induce significant resistance. All regimens used to date fall short of these parameters. Several factors that limit the effectiveness of therapy for *H. pylori* include: (1) rapidly developing bacterial resistance to metronidazole, quinolones, and macrolides; (2) reduced availability of certain drugs, such as amoxicillin, in stomach acid; and (3) patient noncompliance following side effects or the burden of ingesting multiple pills for 7–10 days.

In general, antisecretory agents (e.g., H_2 blockers, proton-pump inhibitors) combined with antimicrobial agents relieve ulcer symptoms and promote ulcer healing. In addition, the gastric pH is raised by these agents which, in turn, increases the efficacy of such antibiotics as **amoxicillin** and **clarithromycin**. Finally, **proton-pump**

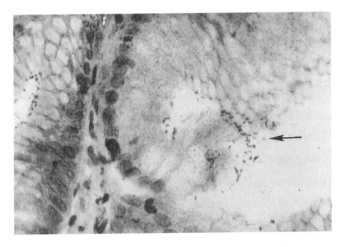

Figure 22.4. Warthin-Starry stain of *H. pylori*. *H. pylori* stain black selectively because they are impregnated with silver and are therefore easily detectable in biopsy specimens. Numerous bacteria can be seen within the lumen of a gastric gland (*arrow*).

inhibitors may have a direct suppressive effect on *H. pylori*. Several large, multicenter eradication trials have documented that eradication rates of over 90% can be achieved with 1-week therapies consisting of a proton pump inhibitor and two antibiotics (usually including clarithromycin and/or **metronidazole**). Fixed combinations of anti-*H. pylori* agents in a single pill are being marketed which will make the treatment easier to swallow. In conclusion, although a recommendation for a standardized treatment regimen does not exist at this time, it is becoming the standard of care that all patients with gastric or duodenal ulceration who are infected with *H. pylori* receive therapy to reduce the recurrence rate of peptic ulceration.

PREVENTION

The potential to prevent *H. pylori*-associated disease with a vaccine is exciting. It is likely to be most appropriately applied in areas where childhood infection is endemic. To develop an effective vaccine against *H. pylori*, the factors important for its virulence must be identified, characterized, produced on a large scale, and then administered in an immunologically relevant way. In mice, an oral vaccine consisting of *H. pylori* urease prevented chronic infection by the related species *H. felis*. Interestingly, infected mice that received an oral treatment with recombinant urease were able to eliminate a chronic *H. felis* infection and also developed protection against subsequent *H. felis* challenge. Thus, therapeutic vaccination may be possible.

CONCLUSION

H. pylori infects over half of the world's population, but in most individuals the infection is clinically silent. Transmission is probably via fecal–oral and/or oral–oral routes. *H. pylori* infection is a virtual necessary condition for the development of peptic ulceration in the absence of drug-induced disease. The infection is also linked with gastric adenocarcinoma and non-Hodgkin's lymphoma of the stomach. Several excellent diagnostic tests are currently available, and effective therapeutic regimens now exist. The overwhelming evidence linking peptic ulcer disease to *H. pylori* infection indicates that ulcer patients who are infected should receive antimicrobial therapy directed toward *H. pylori* to decrease ulcer recurrence. In the future, vaccines may not only provide a means to prevent *H. pylori* infection but may possibly offer a therapeutic intervention.

SELF-ASSESSMENT QUESTIONS

1. Discuss the evidence that indicated that the gastric ulcer of Mr. C., the patient in this case, was due to infection by *H. pylori*.
2. How does *H. pylori* withstand the acidity of the stomach?
3. How does *H. pylori* induce the acute changes in the gastric mucosa?
4. How may *H. pylori* infection lead to stomach cancer?
5. Why is a vaccine against *H. pylori* likely to be of limited use?
6. Discuss the main diagnostic tools in determining if a gastric ulcer is due to *H. pylori*.

SUGGESTED READINGS

Blaser MJ. *Helicobacter pylori*: its role in disease. *Clin Infect Dis* 1992;15:386–391.

Brown KE, Peura DA. Diagnosis of *Helicobacter pylori* infection. Gastroenterol Clinics North Am 1993;22:105–115.

Hopkins RJ, Morris JG, Jr. *Helicobacter pylori*: the missing link in perspective. Am J Med 1994;97:265–277.

Marshall BJ. *Helicobacter pylori*. Am J Gastroenterol 1994; 89:S116–S128.

Marshall BJ, Warren JR. Unidentified curved bacilli in the stomach of patients with gastritis and peptic ulceration. Lancet 1984;1:1311–1315.

chapter 23

Mycobacteria: Tuberculosis and Leprosy

JOHN K. SPITZNAGEL

"The captain of all the men of death that came against him to take him away, was the Consumption, for it was that that brought him down to his grave."

JOHN BUNYAN (1628–1688)

Key Concepts

Tuberculosis:
- Is caused by *Mycobacterium tuberculosis*, a slow-growing, acid-fast obligate aerobe that invades host macrophages.
- Is transmitted by inhalation or ingestion.
- Can take two forms: primary tuberculosis, a usually mild disease; and secondary tuberculosis, a disease caused by reactivation of dormant organisms.
- Elicits a cellular immunity that usually halts the progress of the disease.
- Damage in the primary form includes the formation of granulomas followed by caseation; in immunocompetent patients, the lesions heal spontaneously; immunocompromised patients may proceed to miliary (disseminated) tuberculosis.
- Damage in the secondary form is caused by a delayed-type hypersensitivity reaction to reactivated organisms.
- Is diagnosed by a tuberculin skin test and microscopic and culture tests.
- Is treated with a combination of antibiotics (in order to thwart drug resistance) for 6 months.

Leprosy:
- Is caused by *Mycobacterium leprae*.
- Takes two forms: tuberculoid (a self-limiting disease) and lepromatous (the malignant form).

Tuberculosis conjures up the image of a contagious, chronic, severe disease of the lungs that is often fatal without treatment. Tuberculosis is not a single disease, but rather one that varies in its manifestations de-pending on many factors: history of previous exposure, nutrition, presence of other infections, and immunological competence. Infection of otherwise healthy persons without previous exposure results in a mild, **self-limiting** disease in about 97% of cases, depending on age. Most of the remaining 3% develop clinical tuberculosis well after their initial infection with tubercle bacilli. In these individuals, the latent bacteria present in their tissues reemerge years or even decades later. This so-called **secondary tuberculosis** produces the classic illness that we associate with tuberculosis. The damage incurred in these infections is due in small part to direct effects of the bacteria on the host tissues and in large part to the hypersensitivity reactions of the now sensitive host to products of the bacteria. Tubercle bacilli persist in tissues for long periods, in part because of their **intracellular location** in macrophages. In contrast, persons with depressed immunity, such as those with HIV infection or AIDS, may succumb rapidly, dying of **severe systemic disease** in as few as 4 weeks from the time of diagnosis.

We first discuss tuberculosis in the immunocompetent host and then describe how it affects persons with HIV infection and AIDS. Finally, we briefly discuss **leprosy**, a mycobacterial disease that affects several million persons worldwide, although it is a rare disease in the U.S.

CASE

Ms. C., a 24-year-old African-American schoolteacher and housewife, had recently lost more than 10% of her weight, had night sweats, and felt feverish. She had a cough that produced greenish sputum flecked with blood. Her physician suspected that she might have pulmonary tuberculosis and administered a tuberculin skin test. Forty-eight hours later, Ms. C. showed a strong positive skin reaction, with thickening of the skin and redness at the injection site. The physician referred her to the local health department, where the diagnosis of tuberculosis was confirmed by a chest x-ray (Fig. 23.1) and the presence of "acid-fast bacilli" in a stained smear of her sputum. A careful history revealed that between the ages of 10 and 12 years, she had

lived with an aunt, now deceased, who was said to have had tuberculosis. Given the symptoms, the tuberculin test results, and the radiological and laboratory findings, Ms. C. undoubtedly suffered from tuberculosis.

Ms. C. became worried about her health and wondered about her ability to continue working in school. She and her husband had planned to have a baby soon, but she thought that "pregnancy and new babies do not mix well with tuberculosis." Her physician reassured her that she stood a good chance of being cured. Effective antibiotics could be taken by mouth, although she had to take them for many months. Once treatment was initiated, she could resume her teaching and, in time, plan a pregnancy.

Relevant questions include:

1. How could Ms. C. have contracted tuberculosis in today's world? Did she get it from her aunt?
2. Did she later develop clinical signs and symptoms from this possible early contact with tubercle bacilli?
3. Why did it take so long for Ms. C. to show signs of an active tubercular infection?
4. What pathobiological events account for her current signs and symptoms? Why did she have fevers, weight loss, cough, bloody sputum, a "positive" skin reaction, and an abnormal chest x-ray?
5. What is the risk that Ms. C. will pass the disease to her husband? Her students? Others?

Tuberculosis has been one of the great afflictions of humankind. It has, however, yielded dramatically to improvements in living standards and is generally responsive to chemotherapy. Today, however, tuberculosis still ranks as a major infectious cause of death in the world. The World Health Organization estimates that over 60 million cases and 3 million deaths occur worldwide due to tuberculosis each year.

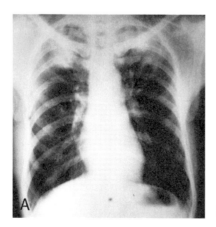
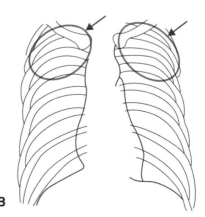

Figure 23.1. Pulmonary tuberculosis. A. Chest radiograph of a young adult with recent cough and loss of weight showing bilateral upper lobe shadowing. Although this x-ray is from a patient different from the one described in the text, the abnor-

malities shown here are similar to those seen in the x-rays of the case patient. **B.** The areas most affected are circled in the drawing.

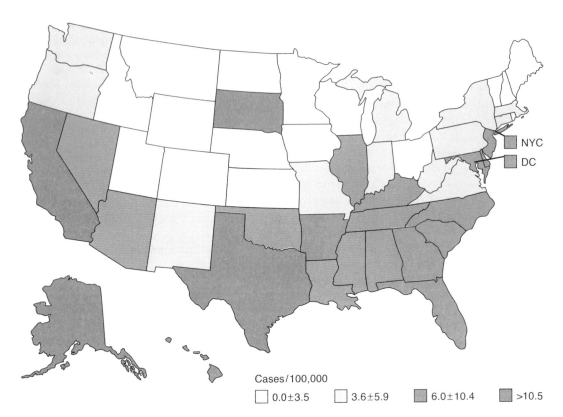

Cases/100,000
☐ 0.0±3.5   ☐ 3.6±5.9   ▨ 6.0±10.4   ▪ >10.5

Figure 23.2. Rates of tuberculosis in the United States, 1994.

The incidence of tuberculosis is rising at alarming rates in the United States, coincident with the increase in AIDS cases, increased immigration, and relaxed preventive measures. For over a century, a steady decline in the number of cases occurred; from 1953 the decrease was 5–6% annually in the U.S. However, the numbers of cases of tuberculosis rose by 3% to 6% from 1986 to 1990, with the greatest increases occurring in the large cities of the U.S. (Fig. 23.2). The increase is particularly significant in minority populations (Fig. 23.3).

In the last century, tuberculosis was a topic of myths. The disease was thought to afflict sensitive, passionate people and to endow them with a pale, languid look that was celebrated in literature and opera (e.g., Shelley's "The Sensitive Plant," Verdi's *La Traviata*, Puccini's *La Boheme*). It was not until the end of the last century, when the cause of the disease was elucidated by Robert Koch, that the myth of the "consumptive passion" was dispelled.

MYCOBACTERIUM TUBERCULOSIS

Tubercle bacilli belong to a distinctive genus, *Mycobacterium*, which includes several closely related species (Table 23.1) of **obligate aerobes** whose growth is facilitated by CO_2. Species other than *M. tuberculosis* were first called "atypical mycobacteria" because they only partially resembled the tubercle bacillus; they are

now known to cause a variety of diseases. Also included in this genus is the agent of leprosy, *Mycobacterium leprae*. Many of the mycobacteria are harmless organisms, some of which live on the human body without causing disease (e.g., the smegma bacillus), or in the environment, especially the soil.

Distinguishing Characteristics

The genus has three distinguishing characteristics: **acid-fastness**, unusual **resistance to drying and chemicals**, and **slow growth**.

Acid-fastness—mycobacterial hallmark

Mycobacteria have the unusual ability to retain basic dyes when treated with acid solutions. The reason for this **acid-fastness** is that mycobacteria surround themselves with unique acidic waxes, long-chain branched hydrocarbons. The main wax, called **mycolic acid**, is a β-hydroxy fatty acid linked covalently to the cell wall murein. The waxes of mycobacteria are important in pathogenesis, as will be discussed later.

The waxy barrier drastically affects the permeability properties of these organisms. Common stains do not penetrate mycobacteria. Thus they fail to take up the dyes used in the Gram stain and, therefore, cannot be labeled Gram-positive or Gram-negative. It is possible, however, to stain them using special techniques. One is to melt the wax temporarily by heating a smear of the bacteria while it is covered with a saturated solution of a basic, red dye, such as fuchsin. Alternatively, one can add a detergent to the stain. The stained smear is then treated with 3% hydrochloric acid in ethanol, which decolorizes nearly all organisms except for the mycobacteria. The smear is then counterstained with a blue dye to provide a contrasting background. Mycobacteria appear as slender, red rods over a background of blue. Fluorochrome dyes for fluorescence microscopy are now more commonly used. The fluorescent-dyed bacteria are more easily detected than are the fuchsin-dyed bacteria.

Resistance of mycobacteria to chemical agents and drying helps them survive both in the body and in the exterior environment. Thus, they are unusually resistant to killing by phagocytes. Since they are also highly **resistant to germicides,** preparations used as general disinfectants for surfaces must be tested by the manufacturer for their power to kill mycobacteria (mycobactericidal disinfectants usually contain iodine or strong detergents). The mycobacteria's **resistance to drying** also contributes to

their potential for transmission. The wax coating does not, however, help them withstand heat. For instance, they are killed during **pasteurization** of milk (e.g., heating to 60°C for 30 minutes).

Slow growth

Mycobacteria grow very slowly. The generation time of the tubercle bacilli is about 13 hours on the best laboratory media. Other mycobacteria grow faster than the tubercle bacilli, but still considerably more slowly than common bacteria. It is possible that slow growth results from inability to transport nutrients rapidly across the wax layer. Slow growth causes delays in diagnosis by culture; laboratory cultures of clinical material must be incubated for up to 8 weeks. It also greatly delays testing the drug sensitivity of clinical isolates. This delay has tragic consequences for AIDS patients infected with drug-resistant tubercle bacilli and their contacts. The patient may die without receiving the most effective drugs, and contacts may contract drug–resistant tubercle bacilli.

Not all mycobacteria can be grown in artificial media. The leprosy bacillus has so far resisted cultivation outside the body of humans or a few animals. The inability to grow these bacteria under routine laboratory conditions continues to impede leprosy research. However, their DNA can readily be cloned into other bacteria and used for research. Much effort is being expended to develop rapid diagnostic methods for both the tubercle and leprosy bacilli, using DNA probes and nucleic acid amplification (see Chapter 57, "Digestive System").

ENCOUNTER AND ENTRY

It is likely that Ms. C. contracted tuberculosis by breathing aerosols or dust particles containing tubercle bacilli. Most likely, bacteria-laden droplets were produced by her aunt's frequent coughing bouts. In fact, airborne transmission of tuberculosis is an efficient means to spread the disease for at least two reasons. First, untreated tuberculosis leads to the formation of open pulmonary lesions that contain large numbers of bacteria. Coughing spreads the organisms from such lesions into the environment. Second, because tubercle bacilli are highly resistant to drying, they become part of so-called **droplet nuclei,** the products of dried aerosols. Such particles are especially infectious because they remain suspended in air for hours, and they are the ideal size for bypassing the mucus blanket of the airways and reaching the alveoli. These two characteristics account for the epidemiology of tuberculosis: it is widespread in crowded areas, primarily among young children who are repeatedly exposed to the organisms.

The inoculum size of tubercle bacilli required to cause infections is usually high. The number of bacilli in a patient's sputum is directly related to the likelihood that ex-

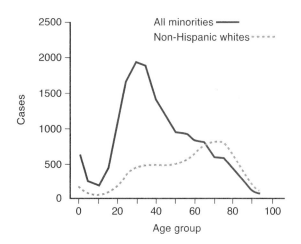

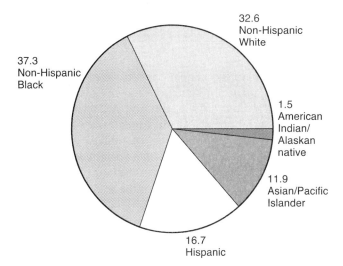

Figure 23.3. The incidence of tuberculosis by age and ethnicity in the United States, 1989.

Table 23.1. Characteristics of Mycobacteria of Major Clinical Importance[a]

Species	Reservoir	Virulence for Humans	Main Disease Caused	Case-to-Case Transmission	In Vitro Growth Rate	Optimum Growth Temperature (°C)
M. tuberculosis	Human	+ + +	Tuberculosis	Yes	S	37
M. bovis	Animals	+ + +	Tuberculosis	Rare	S	37
Bacillus Calmette-Guerin (BCG)	Artificial culture	±	Local lesion	Very rare	S	37
M. kansasii	Environment	+ +	Tuberculosis-like	No	S	37
M. scrofulaceum	Environment	+	Lymphadenitis	No	S	37
M. avium-intracellulare	Environment; birds	+	Tuberculosis-like	No	S	37
M. fortuitum	Environment	±	Skin abscesses	No	F	37
M. marinum	Water, fish	±	Skin granuloma	No	S	30
M. ulcerans	Probably environment; tropical	+	Severe skin ulcerations	No	S	30
M. leprae	Human	+ + +	Leprosy	Yes	None	Not applicable

[a] This table omits many essentially saprophytic mycobacteria. S = slow; F = fast.

posed family members will contract the disease. The location of the organisms in the body depends largely on the site of entry. For example, infection of the lungs (which is most prevalent in countries such as the U.S.) results from **inhalation** of the bacteria. Infection of the intestine or the tonsils is usually due to **ingestion** of the organisms, because tubercle bacilli may be acquired by drinking unpasteurized milk from infected cows. Cattle suffer from a disease similar to human tuberculosis, caused by bovine strains of mycobacteria, *Mycobacterium bovis*.

SPREAD, MULTIPLICATION, DAMAGE

Tubercle bacilli do not produce exotoxins or endotoxin. The severe manifestations of tuberculosis are linked to host reactions to the organisms. Damage is caused by uncontrolled, progressive, chronic inflammation, and by organisms living within macrophages. It follows that infection has different manifestations in a "virgin" host than in a person who has been infected previously. Tuberculosis has two major forms:

Primary tuberculosis is the disease of persons who are infected for the first time. It is usually mild and often asymptomatic. Occasionally, however, the primary disease progresses to systemic disease, such as tuberculous meningitis, miliary tuberculosis, or both (see below). In these cases, the immune reaction fails to develop.

Secondary tuberculosis is usually caused by the reactivation of dormant organisms within the body. This form is the distinctive presentation of tuberculosis, a chronic disease associated with extensive tissue damage, often progressing to death if untreated.

Primary Tuberculosis

Shortly after Ms. C. inhaled tubercle bacilli as a child, she may have developed flulike symptoms of lower respiratory tract infection or she may not have had any symptoms. She probably developed an acute localized pulmonary inflammation that was soon followed by a chronic inflammatory response.

Primary tuberculosis is characterized by a sequence of pathobiological steps (Fig. 23.4). Tubercle bacilli are ingested by and multiply within resident pulmonary alveolar macrophages (Fig. 23.5). Later, they infect nonresident macrophages that collect in the area. Loaded with mycobacteria, newly arrived cells migrate through the lymphatics to the **hilar lymph nodes**, where an immune response develops, dominated by T-helper cells, (CD4+ cells) (Fig. 23.6). Inflammation will now be present in several places—at the original site of infection, along lymphatic channels, and in the regional lymph nodes. The development of inflammation takes about 30 days. Despite their slow growth, the mycobacteria will have multiplied substantially by this time.

At this stage of the infection, the **tuberculin skin test** (discussed in detail below) is usually positive and a **chest x-ray** reveals growing opacities in the lung. The immune defenses curb the proliferation of the organisms and retard their local spread, while macrophages, activated by T cells, begin to kill the organisms or to slow their growth. A number of tubercle bacilli will have already disseminated throughout the body (see Fig. 23.6). In the tissues, especially in the hilar lymph nodes, the organisms are contained in **tubercles**, small granulomas consisting of **epithelioid cells**, **giant cells**, and **lymphocytes**.

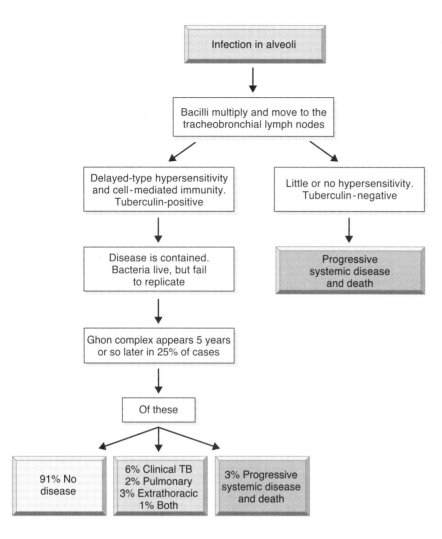

Figure 23.4. The various courses of untreated primary tuberculosis.

Figure 23.5. Tubercle bacilli enter through the respiratory tract.

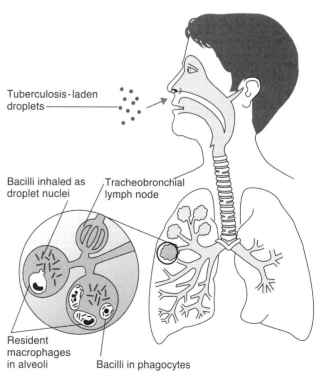

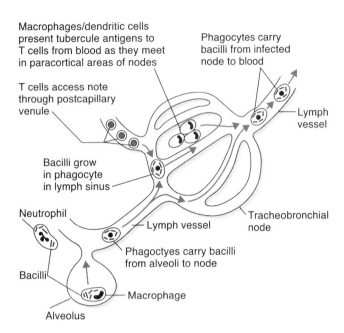

Macrophages/dendritic cells present tubercule antigens to T cells from blood as they meet in paracortical areas of nodes

Phagocytes carry bacilli from infected node to blood

T cells access note through postcapillary venule

Lymph vessel

Bacilli grow in phagocyte in lymph sinus

Neutrophil

Lymph vessel

Tracheobronchial node

Phagoctyes carry bacilli from alveoli to node

Bacilli

Macrophage

Alveolus

Figure 23.6. Tubercle bacilli multiply in phagocytes and spread to lymph nodes and the circulation.

Granuloma formation is caused in part by one of the waxes of the organisms known as **cord factor** (because it prompts growth of the organisms in ropelike arrangements). Direct injection of cord factor into tissue results in granulomas indistinguishable from those caused by tubercle bacilli. With time, the centers of the tubercles become necrotic and advance to form cellular masses of cheesy debris, called **caseous material**, or **caseation**.

Primary tuberculosis may take two courses (see Fig. 23.4). In people who are otherwise healthy, the lesions heal spontaneously and become **fibrotic** or **calcified**. These lesions usually persist for a lifetime and can be seen years later in chest x-rays as radiopaque nodules. The presence of a calcification in the peripheral lung along with one or more calcified hilar nodes suggests prior infection with *M. tuberculosis*. In contrast to healthy individuals, immunocompromised persons, such as those with HIV infection, may fail to contain the primary infection, and organisms may invade the bloodstream. Bloodborne organisms can then localize and cause disease in almost any individual organ of the body. Or, they can disseminate and cause a potentially fatal infection known as **miliary tuberculosis**. In this disease, tubercles are found in many organs, including the liver, spleen, kidneys, brain, and meninges. Caseation and cavitation are less frequent than in secondary tuberculosis. The term *miliary* is derived from the resemblance of the tubercles to grains of millet (bird seed).

How is primary tuberculosis halted? Clearly, the original cellular response fails to curb the multiplication of the organisms. With time, however, cellular immunity to the organisms develops. Macrophages that become acti-

vated by lymphokines produced by CD4+ T lymphocytes now inhibit the intracellular growth of the tubercle bacilli. Although antibodies appear in the circulation, humoral immunity does not play a major role in the immune response to tuberculosis because of the intracellular location of the organisms. Antibodies are also unhelpful in diagnosis.

Although activated macrophages usually kill intracellular bacteria, they cannot always destroy the exceptionally hardy tubercle bacilli. Intracellular organisms may, however, be kept in check for long periods of time. An uneasy equilibrium is reached: some macrophages kill the organisms; others are themselves killed and release their bacterial contents; and still others harbor dormant bacteria for long periods of time. Immunological processing of killed bacteria leads to continued antigenic stimulation.

The involvement of macrophages has its price. Two **cytokines** produced by these cells, interleukin-1 and tumor necrosis factor (Chapter 6, "Constitutive Defenses of the Body"), contribute to the symptoms of the disease. Among its various activities, **interleukin-1** acts as the mediator of the fever experienced by tuberculosis patients. **Tumor necrosis factor** interferes with lipid metabolism and leads to severe weight loss. In response to the carbohydrates, lipids, and proteins of the tubercle bacilli, macrophages also produce a plethora of other cytokines, such as IL6, IL-10, IL-8, granulocyte–monocyte colony stimulating factor, and transforming growth factor-β which result in a complex modulation of the immune responses. In particular, increased production of IL-10 may suppress the immune response and promote the progression of the disease. The net effects of these complex events are the local pathological manifestations of tuberculosis, including caseation necrosis and fibrosis with calcification.

Delayed-type hypersensitivity and the tuberculin reaction

Immunological reactivity to tuberculosis can be demonstrated by the **tuberculin skin test**. The test is carried out by injecting proteins made by tubercle bacilli, which are known as **tuberculin**. The material commonly used is not an isolated protein molecule, but a mixture known as **PPD**, "purified protein derivative." A positive reaction— reddening and thickening of the skin 2 to 3 days after inoculation—indicates cellular immunity to tubercle bacilli. The most important criterion for a positive test is the thickening and hardening (induration) of the skin at the site of injection which represents infiltration of the area by mononuclear phagocytes and T cells.

This **delayed-type hypersensitivity reaction** reflects the local events that take place in the infected tissue. Depending on the site of the reaction, delayed-type hypersensitivity may account for diverse manifestations, e.g., pleurisy with effusion (the sometimes massive accumulation of exudate in the pleural cavities), or the sudden inflammation of the meninges. Surprisingly few tubercle bacilli are present in the pleural fluid or in the cerebrospinal fluid during these infections, but they are able to cause a severe inflammation as the result of a local tuberculin reaction. Likewise, the number of inflammatory cells is also very small. Aspects of the pathogenesis of tuberculosis are depicted in Figure 23.4.

Secondary Tuberculosis

Secondary tuberculosis usually becomes noticeable 1 or 2 years after the primary disease, probably because it takes that long to develop full-blown delayed-type hypersensitivity. Years after acquiring primary tuberculosis, some people (such as Ms. C.) develop the chronic, progressive symptoms that characterize tuberculosis (see Fig. 23.4). The flare-up can sometimes be blamed on impairment of immune function; clearly, any compromise of the T-cell-macrophage immune system may render a person abnormally vulnerable to the reactivation of latent mycobacteria. Of course, reinfection with externally acquired tubercle bacilli could lead to the same manifestations. Certain infections, such as measles, are known to transiently depress cell-mediated immune responses, and predispose patients to reactivation of tuberculosis. It is likely that other common agents have similar effects but are less clinically evident. Patients who receive corticosteroids for inflammatory diseases, undergo cancer chemotherapy, or are infected with HIV may reactivate tuberculosis. In other cases, the precipitating cause of reactivation of the disease is not known.

Subtle depression of the immune system due to severe stress and hormonal or other causes may go undetected. Ms. C. did not suffer from malnutrition, which has also been shown to elicit reactivation disease. A contributing factor in her case may be that dark-skinned persons are more susceptible to the disease (see Fig. 23.3). The existence of genetic factors is inferred from the high incidence of clinical disease in persons with a specific histocompatibility type, HLA-Bev15. The disease may reactivate in older people as a result of the poorly understood loss of immune competence that occurs with aging.

The most common location of secondary tuberculosis is the **apex of the lungs,** because the greater level of oxygenation at this site may give the highly aerobic tubercle bacilli an edge in growth. Lesions slowly become necrotic, caseate, and eventually merge into larger lesions. With time, the caseous lesions liquefy and discharge their contents into bronchi. This event has several serious consequences. It results in a well-aerated **cavity** in which the organisms actively proliferate. The discharge of caseous material also distributes the organisms to other sites in the lung, which can lead to a rapidly progressive **tuberculous pneumonia** known historically as "**galloping consumption.**" In addition, the bacteria-

laden contents of caseous lesions are coughed up and become a source of environmental contamination. Because inflammation of the surface of the bronchi causes increased mucus secretion and stimulation of the cough reflex, patients cough up sputum. Destruction of tissues results in **bloody sputum**.

What accounted for the various symptoms of Ms. C.? Her fever, weight loss, and night sweats may have been due to the release of interleukin-1 and tumor necrosis factor from the many macrophages involved. Her sputum probably included mucus from inflamed bronchi and material from caseous lesions. Bronchial inflammation may have been caused by a local tuberculin reaction, due to the protein from tubercle bacilli in the caseous material. At this time, Ms. C. became infectious and able to transmit tuberculosis to others.

Range of Manifestations of Tuberculosis

Tuberculosis is insidious. Most people are unaware of their initial encounter with the organisms; however, a small proportion of persons, particularly the very young, the very old, and those with immunocompromising diseases, do not develop sufficient cellular immunity in time to contain the organisms and therefore develop disseminated tuberculosis (see Fig. 23.4). This rampant infection is different from secondary reactivation tuberculosis (although it sometimes occurs in these patients).

Although it is most commonly localized in the lung, secondary infection may affect the genitourinary or gastrointestinal tracts, the testicles, the fallopian tubes, the ovaries, or the skin, in other words, almost any organ. Tuberculosis of bone is especially debilitating when it involves the spine, which may collapse as the result of tissue destruction, resulting in lifelong disability. It is impossible to predict which organs the infection will affect because the organisms are able to colonize practically any site of the body.

In view of the damage caused in tuberculosis by the immune responses of the host, one may well ask which is worse: the severe cell-mediated immune response to the disease and its resulting damage, or no immune response to tuberculosis at all. Without cellular immunity and delayed hypersensitivity, caseation necrosis would not develop. However, the tubercle bacilli would proliferate unchecked. The result could be, for example, miliary tuberculosis, a disease that can kill much more rapidly than chronic pulmonary tuberculosis. Historically, much evidence has accumulated to show that the cell-mediated immune response is protective. With the emergence of HIV infection in the population, it has been shown that selective destruction of CD4+ T cells leads to rapid progression of tuberculosis. In addition, these patients fail to develop the lesions typically associated with secondary tuberculosis. Thus, the immune response serves to contain the disease, even if it eventually causes a great deal of damage. In fact, the body relies on three defensive strategies. One involves the antimicrobial action of activated macrophages. The second consists of walling off and containing the lesion by fibrosis and calcification. The third, which may be called "self-debridement," consists of attempts by the body to expel the caseous material through the tracheobronchial tree or other ducts. In short, defense mechanisms allow a large proportion of patients with tuberculosis to curb progression of the disease for life. Some, because of evident immune compromise or for undefined idiosyncratic features of their immune systems, fail to deal with the organisms. They develop clinical disease, and many die of tuberculosis.

DIAGNOSIS

Tuberculin Skin Test

The tuberculin skin test is the most important tool for diagnosing latent or clinically undeclared tuberculosis. This test is especially useful in places such as the U.S. where tuberculosis has become rare and where less than 1% of children and young adults now give a positive test. The test is much less useful in regions where a high proportion of the population is tuberculin-positive or has received the BCG vaccine (see below). A positive test in the wake of an earlier, negative test indicates recent exposure to tubercle bacilli, which constitutes a call for therapeutic intervention. Medical personnel are definitely at risk, especially when exposed to infectious patients. Medical students should be tested at intervals for tuberculin reactivity.

Certain caveats exist regarding this test. Patients who are immunocompromised (e.g., patients with AIDS) may not have a positive reaction. Such people are said to be **anergic** or unresponsive. Anergy can be ruled out by a delayed hypersensitivity reaction to a control skin test. Antigens for these control tests are proteins from microorganisms to which exposure and hypersensitivity are virtually ubiquitous among adults (e.g., *Candida*, mumps). A positive tuberculin test result may also be caused by cross-reactive immunity to mycobacteria other than the tubercle bacillus. Thus, a person infected with atypical mycobacteria may give a positive tuberculin test. This caveat is especially important because mycobacteria of this group are usually treated differently than tuberculosis.

Microscopic and Cultural Diagnostic Tests

The initial diagnostic approach includes a careful history, direct examination of sputum or exudates, and a chest x-ray (see Fig. 23.1). Direct examination of sputum is especially important, because the infectiousness of a patient depends on the presence of tubercle bacilli in the sputum. The acid-fast or fluorochrome stains are rapid and sensitive; however, in the future, more sensitive methods of rapid diagnosis may become generally available. Such methods are particularly useful in the diagnosis of tubercular meningitis, and include the detection of a tubercle bacillus–specific antigen and a lipid, **tuberculostearic acid**, in the cerebrospinal fluid.

The only rigorous diagnostic method is the cultivation of the organisms. Culture may be crucial when microscopic examination is negative. Although sputum from a patient with active tuberculosis may have too few organisms to be detected microscopically, it may give rise to a positive culture. The problem is that it usually takes 3 to 8 weeks before a positive culture can be read with assurance. Radiometric culture techniques accelerate the diagnosis by early detection of radioactive CO_2 released by organisms metabolizing ^{14}C-labeled palmitic acid. Results may be obtained in as few as 7–14 days. This time may also be shortened by coupling culturing with the **polymerase chain reaction** (PCR, Chapter 57, "Digestive System"). Finally, if growth of tubercle bacilli occurs, it is important to test them for antibiotic sensitivity. Overall, the entire process may take six or more weeks.

What other infections resemble tuberculosis? Table 23.1 shows that they are numerous. They mainly consist of those caused by the atypical mycobacteria, the most common of which are *Mycobacterium avium* complex (MAC) and M. kansasii. Disease caused by these organisms tends to be less severe and more indolent, but it can also lead to disability and even death. Both are important complications in AIDS patients with low CD4+ counts. Other diseases that must be included in the differential diagnosis are those caused by actinomycetes, *Nocardia*, and systemic fungi (see Chapter 50, "Blood and Tissue Protozoa").

TREATMENT

We now have excellent therapeutic resources against tuberculosis; they include several highly effective drugs that can be administered by mouth to ambulatory patients, such as **rifampin, isoniazid (INH), pyrazinamide,** and **ethambutol**. These drugs are relatively inexpensive (by the standards of affluent countries) and work well in patients with normal immune systems if taken for 6 months. Treatment quickly renders the patient noncontagious, provided the tubercle bacilli are sensitive to the drugs in the combination used. Thirty years of clinical investigation have confirmed the importance of multiple drug therapy due to the ease with which tubercle bacilli become resistant to antimycobacterial drugs. Chromosomal mutations yield levels of resistance up to 1000-fold greater than the wild type, and arise in one of every 10^6 to 10^7 bacteria. A tuberculous cavity may contain as many as 10^{11} bacteria. Not surprisingly, drug-resistant mutants appear more frequently in patients with multiplying tubercle bacilli. Unfortunately, drug-resistant organisms which frequently arise in certain underdeveloped countries are now becoming more prevalent in the developed countries.

The solution? Give at least two drugs. The chance that one organism will become resistant to two drugs simultaneously is infinitesimally small (Chapter 5, "Biological Basis for Antibacterial Action"). However, this simple measure can be too costly in poor countries. Moreover, patient compliance is often hard to ensure. Once resistant strains begin to circulate in a population, any newly diagnosed patient's organisms may be resistant. In such a case, the patient may remain infectious while receiving drug therapy. Because instituting therapy is an urgent matter, it is advisable to start it before the results of cultures are obtained, as long as the clinical findings (history, examination, x-ray), a positive smear, and a positive tuberculin test suggest the disease. In areas where resistant strains occur, therapy is typically initiated with four or more drugs at once.

Another reason for multiple drug therapy is that some of the agents used act synergistically. For example, INH acts on intracellular mycobacteria, while rifampin works both on intra- and extracellular organisms, including slow-growing strains. Administered together, these drugs are much more effective than either one given alone. Recent experience suggests that drug-sensitive, pulmonary tuberculosis can be treated successfully with INH and rifampin for 6 months in addition to pyrazinamide for the first 2 months.

AIDS AND MYCOBACTERIAL INFECTIONS

Tuberculosis is again becoming a major problem partly due to the global epidemic of AIDS pandemic. The incidence of tuberculosis among AIDS patients is 500 times higher than that of the general population. In the U.S., increased immigration from developing nations and relaxed tuberculosis control measures have also contributed significantly to the resurgence of the disease. Of the many infections associated with AIDS, tuberculosis stands out, because it spreads easily by the respiratory route. An individual with latent *M. tuberculosis* is likely to reactivate infection after becoming infected with HIV. Moreover, an individual with AIDS who becomes infected with *M. tuberculosis* is more likely to develop rapidly disseminated disease.

AIDS patients with tuberculosis are likely to develop **extrapulmonary disease**, involving the lymph nodes, the bone marrow, the genitourinary tract, and the central nervous system. Patients with AIDS react like the small group of people in Figure 23.4 who develop rapidly advancing or miliary tuberculosis soon after primary infection. Blood cultures are likely to be positive for tubercle bacilli in these patients. The reason for these manifestations is the depletion of CD4$^+$ T cells which, with the associated loss of macrophage function, leads to the impairment of cell-mediated immunity. These patients

respond to treatment as do other tuberculosis patients. With effective therapy, sputa readily become negative for viable tubercle bacilli and the disease progress is arrested. On the other hand, the unfortunate patient with AIDS who acquires multidrug-resistant tuberculosis is likely to develop disease that is persistent and usually fatal.

Because of their diminished cell-mediated immunity, AIDS patients are susceptible to another type of mycobacterial infection caused by MAC. These organisms are often found in water and soil and are harmless to most immunocompetent individuals. Before the AIDS epidemic, MAC was rarely described as a cause of pneumonia, and disseminated infections with this organism were virtually unheard of. Today, almost 8% of AIDS patients have disseminated MAC infections, up from 5% just 2 years ago. Systemic infections with MAC normally involve multiple organs, where the organisms may reach densities of 10^{10} per gram of tissue. Patients with disseminated MAC infections may experience a nonspecific chronic illness with fever, malaise, and wasting, or they may have organ-specific manifestations, such as diarrhea with involvement of the intestine or abdominal pain from involvement of the liver, spleen, and retroperitoneal lymph nodes.

MAC infections are more difficult to treat than those caused by *M. tuberculosis*, because these organisms are inherently resistant to most antibiotics, including isoniazid and pyrazinamide. Current therapy for these infections consists of combinations including the newer macrolides, such as **clarithromycin**, **rifabutin** (a rifampin-like rifamycin), **ethambutol**, **clofazimine** (an antileprosy drug), or **fluoroquinolones**, such as ciprofloxacin. However, more research is needed to understand the pathogenesis of MAC infections and their innate resistance to the antituberculosis antibiotics.

PREVENTION

The history of tuberculosis strongly suggests that it can be effectively controlled by sanitary measures and improved standards of living. In disadvantaged parts of the world, other measures must be taken. Currently, an effective vaccine made from killed organisms does not exist. The immunology of tuberculosis tells us why: by and large, killed vaccines produce circulating antibodies, which are of limited importance in this disease. To elicit a cell-mediated immune response, antigens must be present for long periods. The most effective vaccines of this type are those that contain live organisms that can persist in the body for prolonged periods without producing progressive disease.

Currently a live mycobacterial vaccine, known as **BCG**, or **Bacille Calmette-Guerin**, after its French discoverers is available. It consists of a bovine strain of tubercle bacilli that lost its virulence during prolonged cultivation in vitro, and is believed to be incapable of reverting to a virulent form. BCG is used in parts of the world where tuberculosis is endemic and where other preventive measures are not generally available. In addition, the safety and immunogenicity of the BCG vaccine make it a potential carrier for protective antigens from other pathogenic organisms. Genes for such antigens are being cloned into BCG in an effort to produce a "multi-vaccine" which can protect against a number of different infectious diseases. These developments are discussed in Chapter 45, "Introduction to the Fungi and the Mycoses" on the poxvirus.

Administration of BCG vaccine causes the recipient to "convert" to tuberculin-positive. In fact, this conversion is a criterion for successful immunization. In the U.S., it has become standard practice to screen regularly for tuberculin conversion and to administer INH to selected persons who have converted to a positive reaction. Such treatment is called **chemoprophylaxis**. The rationale for using only one drug in this situation is that such individuals carry significantly fewer than the 10^7 organisms needed for spontaneous drug resistance to develop. To preserve tuberculin conversion as a screening test for new tuberculosis cases, BCG is not used in the U.S. or other countries with a low incidence of tuberculosis.

Because tuberculosis is communicable, and not everyone with the disease is aware that they can infect others, it is a dangerous public health hazard. It is estimated that 10–15 million asymptomatic infected persons live in the U.S. today. Greater than 90% of the current cases of tuberculosis are believed to come from this group. Consequently, Ms. C. and her contacts should be followed. Because her husband had a positive tuberculin test and a negative chest x-ray, he was placed on prophylactic treatment with INH. The students who came in contact with Ms. C. were tested with tuberculin. Two pupils in her class were tuberculin-positive and were also started on INH prophylactically. The rest of the class remained tuberculin-negative and were retested several months later.

CONCLUSION

Tuberculosis is one of the best studied examples of a human disease caused by facultative intracellular pathogens. An essential point to remember about tuberculosis is that the major lesions of the established disease are due to the hypersensitivity developed from previous exposure to the organism. Thus, manifestations of the disease are different during the first and subsequent encounters.

The tubercle bacillus, because of its unusual waxy envelope, grows slowly and is a highly successful parasite, and it usually does not affect the life of its victim for many years. When it causes extensive damage to the lungs, it ensures its spread from the body into the environment and increases its chances of infecting other people. In the recent past, the availability of modern antitubercular drugs appeared to promise elimination of tuberculosis. Now the immunity impairment caused by HIV infection, combined with the increasing incidence of drug resistance, is making the elimination of *M. tuberculosis* more difficult to achieve.

MYCOBACTERIUM LEPRAE

Leprosy caused by *M. leprae* shares some of its pathobiological features with tuberculosis but differs in its clinical manifestations. The contrast in the social response to the two diseases could not be greater or more paradoxical. Because lesions found in leprosy are far more visible, the victims of this disease were vehemently shunned, even though these individuals are much less infectious than patients with tuberculosis! Tuberculosis, the more "sociably acceptable" of the two diseases, is actually far more contagious. Leprosy is rare in the U.S. today, but it is still important worldwide. An estimated 2 million people have leprosy, mainly in tropical Third World countries, where the disease causes economic loss and human misery.

The epidemiology of leprosy is not well understood. Clearly, it is a communicable disease. It appears that infected persons must live in close contact with potential victims for long periods to transmit the disease. One source of infection is that victims of lepromatous leprosy tend to shed bacilli from their nasal septa; it is not known if other routes of transmission exist.

M. leprae has been studied less extensively than the tubercle bacillus because it cannot be cultivated in vitro. This organism was one of the first found to be associated with a human disease. G. A. Hansen discovered *M. leprae* in lesions of leprosy patients in 1873 and, hence, leprosy is often called **Hansen's disease**. The first successful propagation of the leprosy bacillus in the laboratory did not occur until 1960, when it was discovered that *M. leprae* could grow in the footpads of mice. Even then, the yields of the organisms are low. In 1970, it was found that *M. leprae* causes a systemic infection in the nine-banded armadillo, where it grows to more than 10^{10} bacilli per gram of infected tissue. This finding revolutionized leprosy research because, for the first time, sufficient quantities of the organisms were available for basic research on the proteins, nucleic acids, lipids, and carbohydrates of *M. leprae*. Today, many genes encoding important antigens of this organism have been cloned and expressed in *Escherichia coli*, providing novel reagents for the analysis of the host response in this disease.

Leprosy bacilli grow best at low temperatures. Accordingly, they appear to multiply most rapidly in the skin and in the appendages of human hosts. There are two polar forms of leprosy, **tuberculoid** and **lepromatous**. Intermediate forms occur as well.

Tuberculoid Leprosy

Tuberculoid leprosy is often charaterized by red blotchy lesions with anesthetic areas on the face, trunk, and extremities. It causes palpable thickening in peripheral nerves in response to bacillary growth in the nerve sheaths. Patients with these signs and symptoms are usually sensitive to the *M. leprae* equivalent of tuberculin, prepared from infected tissues. In contrast to the lepromatous form, patients with tuberculoid leprosy have an active cell-mediated immune response to *M. leprae*, and nerve damage is thought to be mediated by these T-cell responses. It is difficult to find any acid-fast bacilli in a tuberculoid lesion.

Tuberculoid leprosy is analogous to secondary tuberculosis in that this form of leprosy provokes vigorous cell-mediated immunity and exaggerated allergic responses. The prognosis with tuberculoid leprosy tends to be better than with lepromatous leprosy. In some cases, tuberculoid leprosy is a self-limiting disease; it may, however, progress to the lepromatous form.

Lepromatous Leprosy

M. leprae, like *M. tuberculosis* and MAC, survives and multiplies within macrophages. These mycobacteria have an arsenal of defenses that they use to escape killing by phagocytes. For instance, phenolic glycolipid, a surface lipid of *M. leprae*, has been implicated as a defense against oxidative killing by macrophages. To exert their maximal killing potential, macrophages must be activated. Activation of macrophages is mediated by cytokines that are produced by CD4+ T cells. In lepromatous leprosy, it appears that *M. leprae* is able to reduce or to suppress the number of specific T cells produced by the host that can activate the infected macrophages and provide cell-mediated immunity. Lepromatous leprosy is likewise associated with diminished delayed hypersensitivity to **lepromin**. This lack of cellular immunity is associated with the presence of enormous numbers of *M. leprae* in the cooler areas of the skin and in superficial nerves. Loss of eyebrows and thickened and enlarged nares, ears, and cheeks, results in a lionlike appearance (**leonine facies**). Both skin and nerves may be involved. With time, the loss of local sensation leads to inadvertent, traumatic lesions of the face and extremities. These lesions may become secondarily infected, eventually resulting in bone resorption, disfigurement, and mutilation.

Thus, lepromatous leprosy is the malignant form of the disease; it is analogous to systemic progressive (miliary) tuberculosis, where the organisms grow profusely. In both diseases, the cell-mediated immune response is weak. It is not clear why cell-mediated immunity is decreased in leprosy patients; the infecting organisms may themselves play a role in this immunosuppression. Recent evidence has shown that persons belonging to the histocompatibility haplotype HLA-DR3 are more susceptible to tuberculoid leprosy, and those with the HLA-MT1 class are more susceptible to lepromatous leprosy.

The prognosis of leprosy patients has dramatically improved with the introduction of effective drugs, such as **dapsone**, rifampin, and clofazimine. Paradoxically, some of these drugs cause such effective destruction of the organisms that the antigens released lead to a distressing inflammation called **erythema nodosum leprosum**. Recent evidence suggests that BCG vaccination can protect against *M. leprae* infection, and major trials are under way comparing the efficacy of BCG alone and BCG mixed with armadillo-derived, heat-killed *M. leprae* preparations.

SELF-ASSESSMENT QUESTIONS

1. Which attributes of mycobacteria are attributable to their waxy coat?
2. List the steps of an acid-fast stain.
3. Describe the properties of mycobacteria that contribute to their encounter with humans.
4. Which property of tubercle bacilli is most likely to account for tissue damage in primary tuberculosis in tuberculin-negative individuals?
5. Cell-mediated immunity in tuberculosis is responsible for tissue damage. On balance, is this type of immune response good or bad for the host?
6. How does tuberculosis affect a patient with AIDS compared to the patient without AIDS?
7. What accounts for the differences in the response of AIDS patients to tuberculosis compared with non-AIDS patients?
8. What are the differences and similarities in the immune response to leprosy and tuberculosis?
9. What steps are usually taken in the microbiological diagnosis of tuberculosis? What problems are encountered with each step? Why are serological techniques not usually employed?

SUGGESTED READINGS

American Thoracic Society. Treatment of tuberculosis and tuberculosis infection in adults and children. Am J Respir Crit Care Med 1994;149:1359–1374.

Barnes PF, et al. Tuberculosis in patients with human immunodeficiency virus infection. N Engl J Med 1991;324: 1644–1649.

Bloch AB, et al. Nationwide survey of drug-resistant tuberculosis in the United States. JAMA 1994;271:665–671.

Bloom BR. Learning from leprosy: a perspective on immunology and the Third World. J Immunol 1986;137:110.

Bloom BR, ed. Tuberculosis. Washington, DC: ASM Press, 1994.

Bloom BR, Murray CJL. Tuberculosis; commentary on a reemergent killer. Science 1992;257:1055–1063.

Colditz, et al. Efficacy of BCG vaccine in the prevention of tuberculosis. JAMA 1994;271:698–702.

Huebner RE, Castro KG. The changing face of tuberculosis. Annu Rev Med 1995;46:47–55.

Iseman MD. Treatment of multidrug-resistant tuberculosis. N Engl J Med 1993;329:784–791.

Syphilis: A Disease with a History

EDWARD N. ROBINSON, JR.

PENELOPE J. HITCHCOCK

ZELL A. MCGEE

Key Concepts

Syphilis:
- Is caused by the spirochete *Treponema pallidum*.
- Is characterized by three stages: primary syphilis, in which the organism is localized to a chancre, or skin lesion; secondary syphilis, in which the organism disseminates to distant sites; and tertiary syphilis, in which the immune response to the organisms leads to the destruction of tissue.
- Can be transmitted from mother to fetus (congenital syphilis).
- Is initially diagnosed by tests such as Venereal Disease Reference Laboratory Test (VDRL); positive results should be confirmed with more specific tests.
- Is readily treated with penicillin.

The agent of syphilis, *Treponema pallidum*, can be transmitted from an infected mother to her fetus and may cause congenital syphilis; it has often occupied center stage in the history of medicine. A recent resurgence of syphilis in select populations within the United States has once again focused attention on this ancient infectious disease. Syphilis is a multistage disease, and each stage has a dramatically different clinical presentation. The first two stages (**primary and secondary**) manifest as acute and subacute disease respectively, whereas **tertiary syphilis** is a chronic disease that lasts many years.

T. pallidum, a **spirochete,** cannot be cultured in artificial media. It does not produce toxins. In fact, it is not known how *T. pallidum* causes disease. Nevertheless, scientific observations are beginning to elucidate why the organism is able to escape the immune system and how it induces disease. Fortunately, *T. pallidum* remains **sensitive to penicillin,** which is why the disease is easily treatable today.

CASE

Mr. B., a 24-year-old homosexual man, came to the clinic with fever, swollen lymph nodes, and spotty discolorations of his skin, most notably on the palms of his hands and soles of his feet. He had recently noted a penny-sized, gray, translucent lesion on the inner aspect of his lower lip. The physician recognized the "macular rash" on the palms and soles and the lesion on his lip as characteristic of secondary syphilis. Mr. B. reported that he engages in oral sex as well as anal-receptive intercourse.

A scraping of Mr. B.'s lip lesion was examined under a dark-field microscope; it revealed the presence of large numbers of corkscrew-shaped spirochetes. The laboratory reported "positive serology," indicating the presence of the characteristic serum antibodies to *T. pallidum*. These laboratory findings confirmed the diagnosis of secondary syphilis. Because his sexual behavior put him at high risk of other sexually transmitted diseases, Mr. B. consented to a serum test for the presence of antibodies to the human immunodeficiency virus (HIV). He was serologically negative for HIV at that time. Mr. B. was treated with a course of penicillin, and his lesions and symptoms abated. He was considered cured, as his syphilis serologic titers (the level of antibodies in serum) declined over months.

Humans, Health and History

History of Syphilis: "For One Small Pleasure I Suffer a Thousand Misfortunes"

The route of the global spread of syphilis is a controversial subject that is not likely to be resolved. One view is that Christopher Columbus brought the syphilis agent back to Spain from the New World. Although the first documented outbreaks of syphilis occurred in Europe shortly after Columbus's return, this point does not prove the American origin of the disease.

The spread of syphilis through Europe was rapid and, for the first few decades, it was accompanied by a high mortality rate. In 1494, King Charles VIII of France invaded Italy with an army of mercenaries from many countries, including Spain. Because the mercenaries initially saw little fighting, much of the campaign was spent consorting with female camp followers. Soon, however, the French army devastated the attacking forces. In returning to their home countries, the mercenaries carried syphilis to all of Europe. What the defending army was unable to accomplish, syphilis did.

Understandably, no country wanted to claim syphilis as its own:

"The Italians called it the Spanish or the French disease; the French called it the Italian or Neapolitan disease; the English called it the French disease; the Russians called it the Polish disease. And . . . the first Spaniards who recognized the disease called it the disease of Espaniola, which meant, at that time, the disease of Haiti."

Interestingly, it was the poet Fracastorius who gave the disease the name by which we know it today. Fracastorius' poem, *Syphilis Sive Morbus Gallicus*, published in 1530, assigned a nonpolitcal name to the "venereal pox," that of the shepherd Syphilos. Ambroise Paré, in 1575, referred to it as "Lues Venerea," the lover's plague.

During the 16th and 17th centuries, many clinical manifestations of syphilis were observed and catalogued. One of the most puzzling aspects of the disease is that within a few years of its emergence, it ceased to be a rapid killer and acquired the complex clinical manifestations that today characterize the disease (Fig. 24.1). The change in the organism's virulence, from high to moderate, supports the notion that the most successful pathogens do not kill their host. In fact, the less severe the symptoms, the less likely the pathogen will be eliminated. The epitome of this principle is the organism that causes asymptomatic disease, since the host is neither diagnosed nor treated. An organism that goes undetected is able

to reproduce, and it is this ability and not the ability to cause disease that is the main selective force in nature. *T. pallidum* is particularly successful as a human parasite because it possesses, among others, the following traits: spread by sexual transmission, efficient transmission from one adult to another (horizontal transmission), a long infectious period, transmission from mother to child (vertical transmission), long persistence in the host, and usually, lethality only after decades of infection.

In general, sexually transmitted diseases do not "travel alone." Thus, early physicians found it difficult to separate the manifestations of one disease—for instance, gonorrhea—from another (syphilis) because one person might have both diseases simultaneously. Many physicians who studied these diseases thought that they were separate entities. Unfortunately, however, John Hunter confused the issue for six decades. In 1767, Hunter, in a courageous but ill-conceived experiment, placed onto his skin pus taken from the urethra of a man with gonorrhea. A chancre developed. Undoubtedly, Hunter had taken pus from a man co-infected with both *Neisseria gonorrhoeae* and *T. pallidum*. It was not until 60 years later that Philippe Ricord correctly distinguished the two diseases. Ricord also recognized the **stages of syphilis** (**primary, secondary,** and **tertiary**).

One of the medical profession's most ignoble episodes began in the 1930s, and it involved syphilis. Syphilis research conducted in a manner that is now considered reprehensible was carried out in 1932 in Macon County, Georgia (the so-called **"Tuskegee experiment"**) and continued for decades thereafter. Under the auspices of the U.S. Public Health Service, physicians withheld treatment from several hundred black men infected with syphilis. In an attempt to document the natural course of the disease, a progression well-known from previous medical studies, doctors allowed these men to develop the cardiac and neurological impairments that are the hallmark of tertiary syphilis. Penicillin was available and known to be effective against syphilis during part of the trial.

The incidence of syphilis has changed in recent decades. Between 1947 and 1965, a dramatic decline in the cases of syphilis was reported in the United States. However, from 1986 through 1990, the nation experienced a syphilis epidemic. Although the incidence has since fallen, it remains at an unacceptably high level. Primary syphilis rates were higher among men than women, however, the increased rate of syphilis in the women was accompanied by a parallel increase in rates of congenital syphilis.

Historically, homosexual males have been a significant reservoir of syphilis in the U.S. Rectal intercourse results in the localization of the syphilitic chancre, the primary lesion, in the rectal mucosa. Because this location is hidden from sight and chancres are usually painless, the rectal chancre is often overlooked by both patient and physician. With changing sexual behavior dictated by the fear of AIDS, e.g., reduced number of sexual partners and increased use of condoms, the incidence of syphilis among homosexual males has decreased dramatically. Currently, the syphilis epidemic is focused in regions of the Southern United States and among heterosexuals, people of low socioeconomic status, and users of drugs, especially crack cocaine. The reasons for the decline in cases over the last few years are unknown, but may be due to improved contact tracing and treatment of sexual partners, changing sexual practices among those at highest risk, or simply the expected fluctuation in the epidemic curve of any infectious disease.

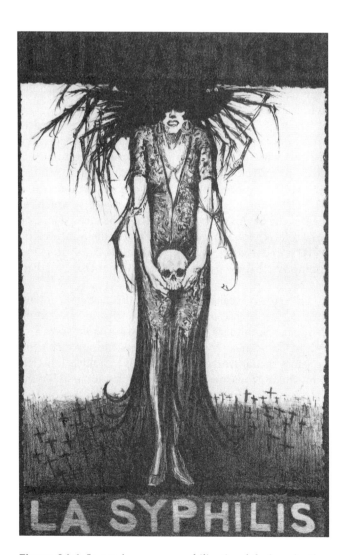

Figure 24.1. In previous years, syphilis stirred the imagination to extremes of gloom and hysteria. This French illustration ascribes to syphilis a degree of mortality that has not been seen since the advent of serological testing and penicillin therapy in this century.

TREPONEMA PALLIDUM

The agent of syphilis is a **spirochete,** a type of bacteria with a highly characteristic appearance. Spirochetes are helical, slender, and relatively long cells (Fig. 24.2). They are widespread in nature but only a few cause disease in humans and animals. The principal human spirochetoses are syphilis, Lyme disease (Chapter 25, "Lyme Disease"), relapsing fever (caused by members of the genus *Borrelia*), and leptospirosis (due to *Leptospira*). The syphilis treponeme has some close relatives that cause other diseases (e.g., **yaws, pinta, bejel**) that are found mostly in tropical countries. The latter diseases pose a medical problem in the United States primarily because these patients, who may have acquired the diseases in a tropical country, develop positive specific and nonspecific serologic tests for syphilis, and these tests may remain positive throughout the patients' life.

T. pallidum is so thin (0.1–0.2 μm) that it cannot be seen by standard microscopic techniques. It can be visualized by special stains (silver impregnation or immunofluorescence) or with special lighting (**dark-field microscopy**). When observed in a freshly prepared wet mount using a dark-field microscope, it exhibits a characteristic **corkscrew-like movement and flexion.** The organisms resemble Gram-negative bacteria in that they have an outer membrane, which, although lipid-rich, does not contain lipopolysaccharide. Unlike the flagella of other bacteria, which protrude freely into the medium, those of spirochetes are contained within the periplasm.

The amount of information regarding the mechanisms by which *T. pallidum* causes disease has been limited both by the **inability to cultivate the organisms serially in artificial media** and by the **lack of a suitable animal model.** In artificial media, these bacteria can be kept alive for only short periods of time (a few divisions at most). To bypass these constraints, research efforts

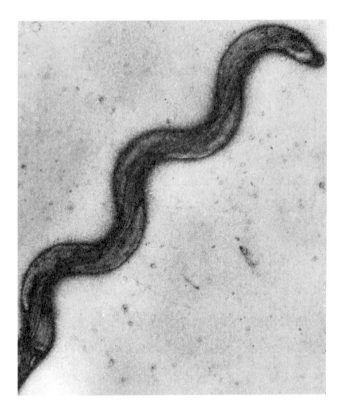

Figure 24.2. Electron photomicrograph of *T. pallidum*, negatively stained. At the dark end of the organism are the insertion points of the periplasmic flagella (ropelike contractile structures), which enable the organisms to engage in their typical corkscrew-like motility.

have focused on producing and characterizing specific proteins of *T. pallidum* using genes cloned into *Escherichia coli* vectors.

ENCOUNTER, ENTRY, SPREAD, AND MULTIPLICATION

T. pallidum is sensitive to drying, disinfectants, and heat (as low as 42°C). Therefore, they are unlikely to be acquired by means other than personal contact. The two major routes of transmission are **sexual** and **transplacental**. Sexual exposure to a person with an active chancre carries a high probability of acquiring syphilis.

The organisms enter a susceptible host through the mucous membranes or the minute abrasions in the skin surface that occur during sexual intercourse. Once in the subepithelial tissues, the organisms replicate locally in an extracellular location (Fig. 24.3). In culture, they adhere to cells by their tapered ends and probably stick to cells in tissue by the same means. Not all of them stick, and many are soon carried through lymphatic channels to the systemic circulation. Thus, even if the initial manifestation of the disease consists of an isolated skin lesion, syphilis is a systemic disease almost from the outset.

Treponemes can cross the placental barrier from the bloodstream of an infected mother and cause disease in the fetus. It is not known how the organisms cross this barrier. Chapter 69, "Congenital and Neonatal Infections," provides a general discussion of this issue.

DAMAGE

Primary Syphilis

Initially, neutrophils migrate to the area of inoculation and are later replaced by lymphocytes and macrophages. The result of the battle between the locally replicating treponemes and the cellular defenses of the host is the lesion of primary syphilis, the **syphilitic chancre** (Fig. 24.4). The chancre is painless. The time between the initial introduction of the organisms and the appearance of the ulcer depends on the size of the inoculum. The larger the size of the inoculum, the earlier the chancre appears. This lesion heals spontaneously within 26 weeks, but by this time the spirochetes have spread through the bloodstream and may cause lesions in other parts of the body. These diverse lesions comprise the cluster of findings that characterize "secondary syphilis," such as that manifested in Mr. B.

The syphilitic chancre and other genital ulcer diseases are associated with increased risk of HIV transmission. Patients who have genital ulcers are estimated to have a three- to fivefold increased risk of acquiring HIV infection. Furthermore, recent studies have demonstrated that HIV can be isolated from genital ulcers, which increases the likelihood of transmitting the virus. The possible role of genital ulcers in facilitating the transmission of HIV underscores the importance of recognizing and promptly treating primary syphilis, chancroid, or herpes.

Three to six weeks after the ulcer heals, the secondary form of the disease occurs in about 50% of infected individuals. **Secondary syphilis** is the systemic spread of the infection and represents the replication of the treponemes in the lymph nodes, the liver, joints, muscles, skin, and mucous membranes distant from the site of the primary chancre. The signs and symptoms of secondary syphilis may be so varied and involve such different tissues and organs, that the disease has been called "the Great Imitator." The rash and other manifestations of secondary syphilis resolve within weeks to months, but one-fourth of affected individuals experience a recurrence within approximately 1 year or so (Fig. 24.3).

Do cytokines play a role in secondary syphilis? When penicillin therapy of syphilis results in fever and sometimes shock (the so-called **Jarisch-Herxheimer reaction**), the clinical events strongly suggest the release of interleukin-1 (IL-1), which causes fever, and the release of tumor necrosis factor/cachectin (TNF-α), which causes shock; see Chapter 6, "Constitutive Defenses," and Chapter 7, "Induced Defenses." If this hypothesis is cor-

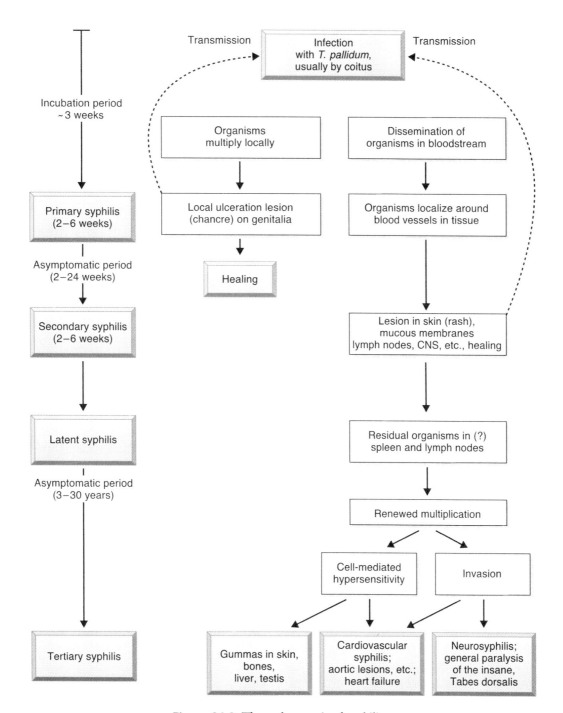

Figure 24.3. The pathogenesis of syphilis.

rect, as is suggested by recent evidence showing that anti-TNF-α antiserum prevents the Jarisch-Herxheimer reaction, which molecules do the spirochetes release to stimulate the production of these potent cytokines? This biphasic course of the disease is puzzling for several reasons. Why does the primary chancre heal? (We do not even understand how spirochetes kill so many epidermal cells to create a chancre.) Why do the defense mechanisms that are so successful in resolving the primary chancre fail to function systemically during secondary

syphilis? How does the organism survive in the body for long periods of time? Where are the organisms located, intracellularly or extracellularly? What is the role of the specific immune response in the disease process? We do not have answers to these questions or to others regarding other aspects of syphilis. It remains one of the more fascinating and puzzling of infectious diseases.

The mechanisms whereby treponemes evade host defenses over a period of years are not well understood. Recently, it has been demonstrated that *T. pallidum* con-

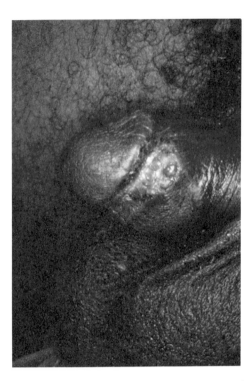

Figure 24.4. Chancre of the penis. The chancre is the first manifestation of syphilis in some patients. The lesion is painless and, on dark-field examination, has many motile, "corkscrewing" spirochetes, thus confirming the diagnosis of syphilis.

tains 100-fold fewer membrane-spanning proteins than the outer membrane of typical Gram-negative bacteria. This finding suggests that, in the case of *T. pallidum*, antibodies against surface proteins may not play their usual antimicrobial role. In addition, when the organism is isolated from tissues, it has been found to be coated with plasma proteins, which may play a protective role.

Tertiary Syphilis

The mystery deepens with the resolution of the secondary stage. In about one-third of individuals, the organisms disappear and the person is spontaneously cured. In the remaining individuals, the treponemes remain latent for years without causing signs or symptoms (see Fig. 24.3). In about one-half of this group, the manifestations of tertiary syphilis eventually develop, sometimes years or even decades after the primary infection.

In adults, **tertiary syphilis** is responsible for a majority of the morbidity and mortality associated with the disease. Fortunately, tertiary syphilis is uncommon in the U.S., where routine serological screening identifies most cases before this stage develops. The hallmark of tertiary syphilis is the **destruction of tissue caused by a response to the presence of treponemal antigens.** This change manifests as **vasculitis** and **chronic inflammation.** Soft masses, or **gummas**, composed of few tre-

ponemes and inflammatory cells, are lesions that commonly destroy bone and soft tissue ("late benign syphilis"). However, they may also involve vital organs, such as the liver. In cardiovascular syphilis, vasculitis involves the arteries supplying the thoracic aorta. Destruction of the elastic tissue in the aorta media leads to dilatation of the wall and **aortic valve insufficiency** or to the formation of aortic aneurysms with resultant **rupture of the aorta.** The central nervous system may also be involved, either by direct invasion of the parenchyma by treponemes or by brain infarction caused by vasculitis.

The clinical findings of **neurosyphilis** can be subtle. The severity of signs and symptoms depends on the location of the lesions. Involvement of the dorsal columns of the spinal cord results in loss of position sensation, a classic condition known as **tabes dorsalis.** It often manifests as a staggering, or **ataxic gait.** In turn, the loss of position sensation causes trauma in the knee and ankle joints, which results in bone overgrowth. Misalignment of the knee or occasionally the ankle, can also occur in the so-called "**Charcot's joint.**" A generalized involvement of the brain leads to impaired motor function (paresis) as well as to gradual loss of higher integrative functions and personality changes. This clinical picture is known as **general paresis** or paralysis of the insane. A physical sign of neurosyphilis is the **Argyll-Robertson pupil:** the pupil only reacts to light when an object is moved from far to near the eye. If untreated, neurosyphilis may be fatal.

The lesions of tertiary syphilis usually contain few or no treponemes. What then accounts for the presence of lesions in the tissues? Researchers have demonstrated that the immune system likely plays a deleterious role in the development of the syphilitic lesions. Human cells exposed to treponemes in culture elaborate intercellular adhesion molecules (ICAMs), which facilitate the chemotaxis and attachment of inflammatory cells. Does this mobilization of inflammatory cells contribute to the disease? Further elucidation of this complex process awaits more research.

Congenital Syphilis

Although serological tests are available that can detect latent forms of syphilis, antibiotics are safe and inexpensive, and the causative organisms remain sensitive to antibiotic therapy, about several thousand babies are born with congenital syphilis in the U.S. each year (the exact figures are hard to come by). This number actually underrepresents the problem, as the majority of infected fetuses likely die in utero. The manifestations of congenital syphilis are varied, and include life-threatening organ damage, silent infections, congenital malformations, and developmental abnormalities. Congenital anomalies include **premature birth, intrauterine growth retardation,** and **multiple organ failure** (e.g., central nervous system infection, pneumonia, and enlargement of the liver and spleen). The most common manifestations of syphilis become evident at about 2 years of age and include **facial and tooth deformities** (the so-called **Hutchinson's incisors** and **"mulberry" molars**). Other less common manifestations include **deafness, arthritis, and "saber shins."** Congenital syphilis is especially tragic because it is completely preventable by penicillin therapy of women with a positive serological test for syphilis early in pregnancy. Prevention of congenital syphilis is one reason why prenatal care is essential.

DIAGNOSIS

Before this century, physicians relied on the clinical sign and symptoms of the disease to make a diagnosis of syphilis. Therefore, only individuals with obvious skin or mucosal lesions were considered to have syphilis and, thus, received therapy. Patients with asymptomatic or latent syphilis were undiagnosed and, therefore, untreated. Early in this century, Wassermann, Neisser, and Bruck discovered that the sera of patients with syphilis have antibodies that react with normal human tissue. The tissue component was found to be a lipid present in the membranes of mitochondria, called **cardiolipin**. Why patients with syphilis form these curious antibodies is not known. In fact, these antibodies are produced in patients with other diseases as well; **biological "false-positive" tests** for syphilis occur in patients with hemolytic anemia, systemic lupus erythematosus, leprosy, narcotics abuse, and aging.

The original test of Wassermann and colleagues led to the development of more rapid and reproducible tests. Several variations exist and are known by their eponyms (e.g., the Venereal Diseases Reference Laboratory test, **VDRL**, or the Rapid Plasma Reagin, **RPR**). Although nonspecific, these tests are cheap and easy to perform, which makes them suitable for initial screening of large numbers of serum samples, as in premarital "blood tests." However, their relative lack of specificity makes it necessary to test all positive samples by more specific, technically demanding, and expensive tests directed against treponemal antigens. One such **treponeme-specific test** is the Fluorescent Treponemal Antibody test or (**FTA**), an indirect fluorescent antibody test (see Chapter 55, "Diagnostic Principles").

TREATMENT—"ONE NIGHT WITH VENUS, THE REST OF LIFE WITH MERCURY"

Two major advances in the diagnosis and management of syphilis have occurred during the 20th century: the development of serological tests for diagnosing syphilis and the use of penicillin for treating the disease. Fortunately for Mr. B. and for the rest of the world, the organisms are still exquisitely sensitive to penicillin.

Before penicillin, treatment depended on an arsenic-containing compound synthesized by Ehrlich early in this century (it was the first effective synthetic chemotherapeutic agent). This compound was called "606," in recognition of 605 previous failures in that laboratory. Before the introduction of penicillin, therapy consisted of the tedious, expensive, and dangerous administration of arsenic and **mercury or bismuth** for a minimum of 2 months and as long as 2 or 3 years. An alternative therapy was the induction of high fevers in individuals with neurosyphilis. The basis of the therapeutic use of fever was the known heat sensitivity of *T. pallidum*. Fever first was induced by the production of erisypelas (streptococcal skin infections). However, when the streptococcal infections spread to and killed others who did not have syphilis, this method was abandoned. Subsequent efforts focused on malaria as the fever-inducing agent. Deaths were not unexpected, especially when the extremely virulent and deadly *Plasmodium falciparum* was inadvertently used instead of the more innocuous *Plasmodium vivax*.

Currently, the treatment of all stages of syphilis relies on the continued sensitivity of *T. pallidum* to **penicillin**. The optimal strengths, and types of penicillin (aqueous, procaine or benzathine penicillin) and duration of therapy for each stage are not known. Reports of treatment failures following accepted and standard regimens of penicillin have surfaced with increasing frequency. Treatment failure is believed to be due to lack of penetration of penicillin into the central nervous system harboring treponemes or the lack of immunity in patients infected with HIV. These failures have caused tremendous uncertainty. Some experts recommend intensified treatment of later stages of syphilis and of individuals coinfected with HIV. Although cases of treatment failure are dramatic, they are difficult to interpret without knowing how many individuals are successfully managed by the same regimen. Without further evidence to justify major changes in the approach to syphilis treatment, current recommendations by the Centers for Disease Control and Prevention have remained conservative.

CONCLUSION

From the mid 1980s to the mid 1990s, the largest single-year increase in infectious syphilis in more than a quarter of a century was reported in the U.S. During this period, the incidence of congenital syphilis also increased. In addition, genital ulcer diseases, such as syphilis, increase the risk of HIV transmission, contributing to the epidemic of AIDS.

Several factors are fueling the syphilis epidemic: drug use, a decline in socioeconomic and educational levels among groups at risk, and limited access to health care, due in part to the overburdening of health care facilities by the AIDS epidemic.

Among all the sexually transmitted diseases, syphilis is one of the easiest to control for the following reasons:

- The cases are clustered. Most of the current increase is occurring in low-income, minority heterosexuals and their children.
- Good diagnostic tests are available. These tests are inexpensive and give accurate, fairly rapid results.
- Treatment is available. An inexpensive antibiotic, penicillin, is effective for primary and secondary syphilis in single doses. Furthermore, antibiotic resistance is not a problem.

The solutions to the recent epidemic, therefore, involve social, behavioral, and biomedical research efforts. Our inability to prevent and to control syphilis speaks to our shortcomings in biomedical research as well as in societal programs and service delivery. To paraphrase Winston Churchill's comment on Russia, syphilis is "a riddle wrapped in a mystery inside an enigma." Whether we will be able to deal effectively with this enigma remains to be seen.

SELF-ASSESSMENT QUESTIONS

1. What is the likely role of antitreponemal antibodies in each of the three stages of syphilis?
2. What explains the resolution of primary syphilis and the emergence of the secondary stage?
3. In what ways does tertiary syphilis appear to be an autoimmune disease?
4. During which stage of syphilis is a patient most contagious?
5. What would it take to make syphilis disappear from the face of the earth?
6. If you were involved in syphilis research, what problems would you tackle?

SUGGESTED READINGS

Austin SC, Stolley PD, Lasky T. The history of malariotherapy for neurosyphilis: modern parallels. JAMA 1992;268: 516–519.

Blanco DR, Miller JN, Lovett MA. Surface antigens of the syphilitic spirochete and their potential as virulence determinants. Emerging Inf Dis 1997;3:11–20.

Cox DL, Chang P, McDowall AW, Radolf JD. The outer membrane, not a coat of host proteins, limits antigenicity of virulent *Treponema pallidum*. Infect Immun 1992;60: 1076–1083.

Larsen SA, Steiner BM, Rudolph AH. Laboratory diagnosis and interpretation of tests for syphilis. Clin Microbiol Rev 1995;8:1–21.

Quétel C. History of syphilis. Baltimore: Johns Hopkins University Press, 1992.

Rolfs RT. Treatment of syphilis, 1993. Clin Infect Dis 1995; 20(Suppl 1):S23–38.

CHAPTER 25

Lyme Disease

ALLEN C. STEERE

JOHN M. LEONG

Key Concepts

Borrelia species:

- Are spiral-shaped spirochetes.
- Are transmitted to humans by tick bites.
- Cause Lyme disease and relapsing fever.
  Lyme disease is caused by *Borrelia burgdorferi*. A multiphased disease, it is treated with antibiotics.
  In Stage 1 (acute, local) the skin is affected at the site of the tick bite (erythema migrans lesion).
  In Stage 2 (disseminated) the central nervous system, the skin, and other systems are affected.
  In Stage 3 (chronic) the joints and the central nervous system are affected; the organisms are not usually found in the lesions, but their DNA can sometimes be detected.

Lyme disease, or **Lyme borreliosis,** is a recently recognized illness caused by the tick-borne spirochete, *Borrelia burgdorferi.* Prior to the recognition of this disorder, *Borrelia* species were only known to cause an illness called **relapsing fever.** Although it differs from syphilis in the mode of transmission, Lyme disease and syphilis are similar in their multisystem involvement, occurrence in stages, and mimicry of other diseases (Fig. 25.1).

As with syphilis, Lyme disease usually begins with localized infection of the skin. In Lyme disease, a characteristic expanding skin lesion called **erythema migrans** usually occurs at the site of the tick bite (Stage 1). Within several days to weeks, the spirochete may spread to other sites (Stage 2), particularly to other skin sites, the nervous system, joints, heart, or eyes. Symptoms change and are typically intermittent during this stage of the illness. After months to years, sometimes following long periods of latent infection, the spirochete may cause chronic infection (Stage 3), most commonly of the joints, nervous system, or skin.

■ CASE

Mr. T., a 27-year-old male resident of Connecticut, developed joint and muscle pains and an expanding erythematous skin lesion on his left leg on July 5. Three days later, he experienced severe headache, neck stiffness, photophobia, and mild thought disturbances. A week thereafter, multiple secondary annular skin lesions appeared followed by right-sided facial palsy. Blood analysis revealed a high titer of IgM antibodies against *B. burgdorferi,* but the IgG response to the spirochete was negative. Mr. T.'s signs and symptoms resolved or improved within several weeks.

Two months after the first symptoms, Mr. T. had severe neuritic pain on the skin of his abdomen within the distribution of the T8 through T11 dermatomes. This symptom

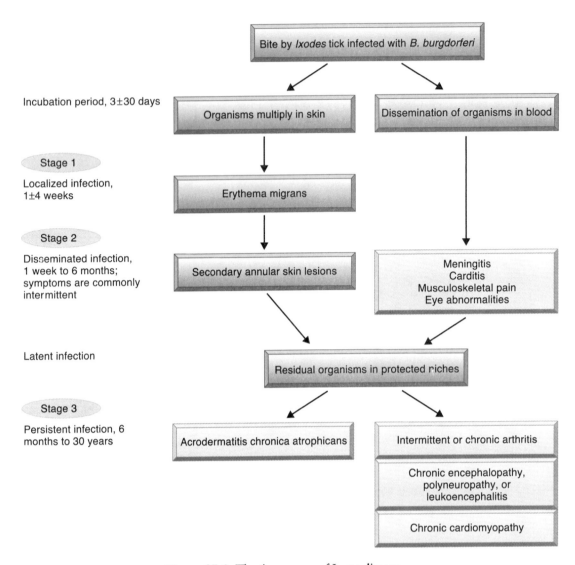

Figure 25.1. The time course of Lyme disease.

was followed by intermittent joint pains, which occurred in one joint at a time for several days, followed by longer pain-free periods. During the second year of illness, Mr. T. had a sudden onset of severe swelling of first one knee and then the other. Synovial fluid analysis revealed numerous white cells, and his antibody response was high for IgG and low for IgM. His immunogenetic profile showed that he had HLA-DR4 and HLA-DR2 specificities. The swelling of the knees remained for about one year, but then subsided.

Seven years after disease onset, Mr. T. began to notice that he was forgetful, lethargic, somnolent, and had hearing impairment in the left ear. He still had a markedly elevated IgG antibody titer to *B. burgdorferi*, but no detectable IgM antibody. Spinal fluid analysis showed elevated total protein and evidence of intrathecal antibody production to the spirochete. He was treated with intravenous ceftriaxone for 30 days. His memory deficit and fatigue improved within the following several months.

INTRODUCTION TO BORRELIA

Borrelia species, along with the leptospiras and treponemes, belong to the spirochetes (Fig. 25.2). Like all spirochetes, the borrelias consist of a protoplasmic cylinder surrounded first by a cell membrane and by an outer membrane that is only loosely associated with the underlying structures. Flagella are contained between the two membranes. Borrelias are longer and more loosely coiled that the other spirochetes, and many of their outer membrane proteins are encoded by genes located on plasmids, a feature unique to this genus. This arrangement may be advantageous to the organism in making antigenic changes in these proteins. The borrelias are fastidious and grow best at 33°C in a complex liquid medium (called Barbour–Stoenner–Kelly medium).

Humans, Health and History

Lyme Disease

Lyme disease was first described in 1975 as a distinct entity due to a geographic clustering of children in Lyme, Connecticut, who were thought to have juvenile rheumatoid arthritis. The rural setting of the case clusters and the identification of the characteristic erythema migrans as a feature of the illness suggested that the disorder was transmitted by an arthropod. It soon became apparent that Lyme disease was a multisystem illness that affected primarily the skin, nervous system, heart, and joints. Epidemiologic studies implicated certain *Ixodes* ticks as vectors of the disease. Further epidemiologic features of the disease are described in Chapter 56, "Epidemiology."

In addition to providing clues about the cause of the disease, erythema migrans helped link Lyme disease in the United States to certain syndromes in Europe. Early in this century, several European investigators described the characteristic expanding skin lesion of erythema migrans, which they attributed to *Ixodes* tick bites. Many years later, it was recognized that erythema migrans was often followed by a chronic skin disease (acrodermatitis chronica atrophicans) which had already been described as a separate entity. In the 1940s, a neurologic syndrome was described in Europe (called Bannwarth's syndrome, meningopolyneuritis, or meningoradiculitis). This syndrome was sometimes preceded by an erythema.

These various syndromes were linked conclusively in 1982, when the causative agent, a previously unrecognized spirochete now called *B. burgdorferi*, was isolated from *Ixodes dammini* ticks. The spirochete was then recovered from patients with Lyme disease in the United States, as well as from individuals with erythema migrans, Bannwarth's syndrome, or acrodermatitis in Europe. The patients' immune responses were linked conclusively with this organism. Although regional variations exist, the basic outlines of the disease are similar worldwide, and its most common name is Lyme disease or Lyme borreliosis.

Whereas the various clinical manifestations of syphilis were brought together as a single entity in the 19th century, the many manifestations of Lyme disease were not recognized as parts of a single entity until the 1980s. In both diseases, the causative spirochete may survive for years and, after long periods of latency, may cause slowly progressive disease, particularly of the nervous system. And in both diseases, the mechanisms of spirochetal attachment and survival and the ways in which the organism damages host tissues are incompletely understood.

Why has Lyme disease become a major concern in certain parts of the world? The most obvious reason is the recent recognition of a disease that has escaped definition in the past. However, Lyme disease is now causing **focal epidemics** as it spreads in the northeastern and upper midwestern United States. These epidemics are thought to be due to a large increase in the number of deer and, by extension, the deer ticks, that transmit this disorder in these parts of the country. At the same time, rural areas where deer and the deer tick live have become increasingly populated by susceptible suburbanites who have never been exposed to the spirochete.

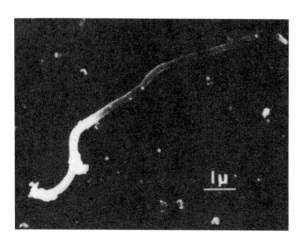

Figure 25.2. Scanning electron micrograph of *Borrelia burgdorferi*.

Of the *Borrelia* species, *B. burgdorferi* is the longest (20 to 30 μm) and narrowest (0.2 to 0.3 μm), and it has the fewest flagella (7 to 11). All isolates of *B. burgdorferi* examined to date carry four to nine different plasmids. These include the typical supercoiled variety, but also an unusual type of **linear plasmid** that has not been found in other prokaryotic organisms. One of these small linear plasmids (49 kb) codes for the two major outer-surface proteins. These outer-membrane proteins may undergo antigenic variation during the course of the disease, but this variation seems to be minor as compared with that of relapsing-fever borrelias.

ENCOUNTER AND ENTRY

Lyme disease spirochetes are transmitted by certain ticks that normally feed on mice and deer. The deer hosts provide the nearly ideal "Club Med Cruise" environment for the adult activities of dining, meeting, and mating, with an opportunity for travel included. While in the midgut of the tick, the spirochetes are in a dormant, nonreplicating state attached to midgut epithelial cells. When the tick feeds on a mammalian host, the spirochetes are exposed to a higher temperature and to the contents of mammalian blood. This exposure, which leads to changes in the expression of outer-surface proteins, alters the manner in which borrelias interact with host cells. The organisms now replicate, invade the gut wall, and spread throughout the tick, including to the salivary glands. From this site, they are injected into the skin of the mammalian host.

SPREAD AND MULTIPLICATION

In humans, the spirochete usually first causes localized infection of the skin at the site of the tick bite. Several days later, the organisms spread within the skin and within days to weeks, they disseminate to many sites, particularly to other skin sites, the nervous system, musculoskeletal tissues, the heart, or eyes. The bacterial properties that allow the spirochete to cause infection in a variety of tissues are still being defined. Bacterial spread within the host is probably facilitated by the spirochete's ability to bind human plasminogen and urokinase-type plasminogen activator to its surface. Plasmin, the activated form of plasminogen, is a potent protease that could promote tissue invasion.

Once the spirochete has reached different tissues, adherence to host cells at these sites promotes colonization. In vitro studies have demonstrated that *B. burgdorferi* may adhere to many different cell types, and to date, two different bacterial binding mechanisms have been identified. The first attachment step involves binding to several protein receptors that belong to the integrin family. Integrins mediate attachment of mammalian cells to extracellular matrix proteins. *B. burgdorferi* binds to a **platelet-specific integrin receptor** and to the ubiquitiously expressed receptors for the extracellular matrix proteins, **vitronectin** and **fibronectin**. A second pathway for cell attachment is mediated by host cell sugars. *B. burgdorferi* binds to **glycosaminoglycans**, which are long, linear, highly sulfated polysaccharides that are linked to a protein core. The spirochetes also recognize sugar structures present in glycolipids such as **galactocerebroside** which are found on the surface of oligodendroglia in the brain. These cells are likely to be affected in Lyme encephalopathy; thus, these attachment mechanisms may contribute to the tissue tropism of the organism. Finally, despite a vigorous host immune response, the spirochete can sequester itself in certain tissues, sometimes for years. The mechanisms that promote long-term survival of the organism are still unknown.

DAMAGE

Stages 1 and 2

Local spread of *B. burgdorferi* in the skin results in a pathognomonic skin lesion, **erythema migrans** (Stage 1, Fig. 25.1). **Disseminated infection** (Stage 2) is often associated with characteristic symptoms that affect the skin, nervous system, and musculoskeletal sites, including secondary annular skin lesions, excruciating headache, mild neck stiffness, and migratory pain in joints, bursae, tendons, muscle, or bone. The triad of early neurologic abnormalities is **meningitis**, **cranial neuritis**, and **radiculoneuritis**. Cardiac involvement may result in fluctuating degrees of atrioventricular block or myopericarditis. **Eye abnormalities** include conjunctivitis, iritis, choroiditis, or panophthalmitis. The spirochete has been detected in or recovered from most of these tissue sites during this stage of the illness.

B. burgdorferi is not known to produce direct damage to these tissues or to elaborate toxins. Rather, it seems to damage tissue by persisting at these sites and elicit an immune response that causes "bystander" injury to the host. In vitro, the organism is a potent inducer of the proinflammatory cytokines **tumor necrosis factor** (TNF) and **interleukin-1** (IL-1) from peripheral blood mononuclear cells. Histologically, all affected tissues show an infiltration of lymphocytes and macrophages, and sometimes plasma cells. Plasma-cell precursors are large and can resemble immunoblasts or Reed-Sternberg cells. Some degree of vascular damage, including mild vasculitis or hypercellular vascular occlusion, may be seen in multiple sites, suggesting that the spirochetes or immune complexes may have been present in and around blood vessels.

Stage 3

Months after disease onset, patients in the United States usually begin to have brief attacks of **arthritis**, especially in the knee. Although the pattern varies, episodes of arthritis often become longer during the second and third years of illness, and in a small percentage of patients, chronic arthritis begins during this period (Stage 3, Fig. 25.1). The onset of prolonged episodes of joint involvement usually coincides with the development of IgG reactivity to *B. burgdorferi* surface proteins called OspA and OspB. As with a number of rheumatic diseases, chronic Lyme arthritis appears to have an immunogenetic basis. The majority of patients with chronic arthritis have HLA-DR4 specificity and IgG antibody reactive to OspA. In these patients, arthritis typically does not respond to antibiotic therapy. Their T-cell lines preferentially recognize OspA, whereas those from patients with treatment-responsive arthritis rarely recognize this spirochetal protein. Although *B. burgdorferi* DNA can usually be detected in the joint prior to antibiotic therapy, it has not been detectable after prolonged courses of antibiotics. Thus, in genetically susceptible people, *B. burgdorferi* appears to trigger an immune response that may continue after the apparent eradication of the spirochete from the joint, perhaps owing to the presence of cross-reactive antigens.

Chronic neurologic involvement, affecting either the peripheral or central nervous system, may also occur in Lyme borreliosis, sometimes following years of latent infection. *B. burgdorferi* DNA has been detected in cerebrospinal fluid in patients with Lyme encephalopathy as much as 27 years after disease onset, a finding that is analogous to the persistence of spirochetal DNA in tertiary neurosyphilis. However, the features of late neurologic involvement differ in the two diseases. In Lyme disease, the most common form of chronic central nervous system involvement affects memory, mood, or sleep, sometimes with subtle language disturbance.

Another example of prolonged latency followed by persistent infection in Lyme borreliosis is a late skin manifestation called **acrodermatitis chronica atrophicans**, which has been observed primarily in Europe. This skin lesion usually begins insidiously with bluish-red discoloration and swollen skin on an extremity. The lesion's inflammatory phase may persist for many years or decades, and it gradually leads to atrophy of the skin. *B. burgdorferi* has been cultured from such lesions as much as 10 years after their onset.

DIAGNOSIS

Except for erythema migrans skin lesions, it is generally not possible to culture *B. burgdorferi* from patients' specimens, and it is often difficult to visualize the spirochete in histologic sections. Recently, detection of *B. burgdorferi* DNA in joint fluid by polymerase chain reaction (PCR) has shown promise as a substitute for culture in patients with Lyme arthritis. However, current PCR methods lack sufficient sensitivity to detect spirochetal DNA in cerebrospinal fluid in patients with neuroborreliosis. Consequently, serologic testing by enzyme-linked immunosorbent assay (ELISA) and Western blot is currently the most practical laboratory method used in diagnosis.

As with syphilis, the specific immune response in Lyme disease may be delayed, and patients with Stage 1 infection are often seronegative. After the first several weeks of infection, particularly if the spirochete disseminates, most patients become seropositive. As with other serologic tests, false-positive and false-negative results may occur. Immunoblotting is a helpful technique in sorting out false-positive results. In a small percentage of patients, antibiotic therapy during the first several weeks of infection seems to abort the specific humoral immune response, but a few spirochetes may survive in sequestered sites.

TREATMENT AND PREVENTION

The treatment of Lyme disease is guided by the stage and manifestation of the disease. In contrast with the agent of syphilis, *B. burgdorferi* is only moderately sensitive to penicillin, and consequently, this drug is used less frequently. The duration of therapy is generally 10 to 30 days and is guided by the clinical response. For patients with arthritis, a month or longer course of doxycycline or amoxicillin is often curative. Intravenous therapy is generally necessary for patients with objective neurologic involvement, and the third-generation cephalosporin drugs (e.g., ceftriaxone or cefotaxime) are used most often for this purpose.

In an experimental mouse model, vaccination with recombinant OspA has been shown to be protective. This vaccine is currently undergoing phase III efficacy trials in human subjects. At present, the best mode of preventing Lyme disease is by minimizing the frequency of tick bites using protective clothing and insecticides.

A COMPARISON OF VARIOUS SPIROCHETOSES

The spirochetoses that affect humans in the United States in addition to Lyme disease include **syphilis, relapsing fever,** and **leptospirosis** (Table 25.1). Except for syphilis, these are animal diseases that only incidentally affect humans when they are bitten by *Borrelia*-infected ticks, or when they come in contact with animal urine contaminated with leptospires. The initial phases of these infections have many similarities to Lyme disease including the possible presence of fever, headache, muscle pain, meningitis, photophobia, malaise, or fatigue. However, each disease also has unique clinical features. Relapsing fever is associated with intermittent episodes of high fever, which are thought to occur due to variation of the major antigen, a variable protein of the spirochete. Leptospirosis has a predilection for the kidney. Both Lyme disease and syphilis may occur in stages over a period of years and typically cause neurologic abnormalities late in the illness. However, the actual neurologic syndromes are different. In each of these diseases, diagnosis is usually made by recognition of a characteristic clinical picture with serologic confirmation. Spirochetes are susceptible to a wide range of antibiotics.

Table 25.1. Main Features of the Spirochetoses

Name of disease	Causative agent	Mode of transmission	Unique clinical aspects
Lyme disease	*Borrelia burgdorferi*	Ticks of the *Ixodes ricinus* complex	Erythema migrans, recurrent arthritis
Relapsing fever	*Borrelia recurrentis, B. hermsii*, others	Human body louse, ticks (*Ornithodorus*)	Recurrent high fever
Syphilis	*Treponema pallidum*	Sexual contact	Chancre, tabes dorsalis, aortitis
Leptospirosis	*Leptospira* sp.	Contact (urine) with infected animals	Jaundice, renal involvement

CONCLUSION

Lyme disease is a potentially dangerous and insidious disease that can be readily treated if diagnosed in time. It has three stages that have features in common with those of syphilis. Physicians and other health personnel must be alert to the possibility of this disease among people living in affected areas, especially those who are frequently out of doors.

SELF-ASSESSMENT QUESTIONS

1. What is the likely role of antitreponemal antibodies in each of the three stages of syphilis?
2. How would you explain the resolution of primary syphilis and the emergence of the secondary stage?
3. In what ways does tertiary syphilis appear to be an autoimmune disease?
4. During which stage of syphilis is a patient most contagious?
5. What would it take to make syphilis disappear from the face of the earth?

SUGGESTED READINGS

Dattwyler RJ, Luft BJ. *Borrelia burgdorferi*. In: Gorbach SL, Bartlett JG, Blacklow NR, eds. Infectious Diseases, 2nd ed. Philadelphia: Saunders, 1998; 1937–1946.

Steere AC. Lyme disease. N Engl J Med 1989;321:586–596.

Steere AC. Lyme disease. In: Isselbacher KJ, Braunwald E, Wilson JD, Martin JB, Fauci AS, Kasper DL, eds. Harrison's principles of internal medicine. 13th ed. New York: Mc Graw-Hill, 1994;745–747.

CHAPTER 26

Cat Scratch Disease, Bacillary Angiomatosis, and Other Bartonelloses

DAVID H. WALKER

Key Concepts

Bartonella species:

- Include *Bartonella henselae*, which causes cat scratch disease (in immunocompetent persons) and bacillary angiomatosis (in immunocompromised persons); *Bartonella quintana*, which causes trench fever and bacteria and blood vessel tumorlike proliferations; and *Bartonella bacilliformis*, the agent of Oroya fever and verruca peruana.
- Are transmitted by a cat scratch or bite (*B. henselae*), the bite of a louse and possibly contaminated intravenous paraphernalia, or other arthropods (*B. quintana*), or the bite of sandflies in South America (*B. bacilliformis).*
- Cause different diseases in immunocompetent persons and immunocompromised persons.
- Are diagnosed by culturing the organisms, microscopic examination of biopsies using special stains, or the detection of specific antibodies in blood.

Bartonella species cause important infections of both immunocompetent and immunocompromised persons, with remarkably different consequences depending on the state of host defenses. *Bartonella henselae* is the major cause of both **cat scratch disease**, a prevalent, self-limited infectious lymphadenitis transmitted by the scratch or bite of a healthy-appearing infected cat, and **bacillary angiomatosis**, cutaneous and visceral tumorlike blood vessel proliferations seen principally in people with acquired immune deficiency syndrome (AIDS). South American bartonellosis, caused by *Bartonella bacilliformis*, is transmitted by sandflies and results in a febrile illness with severe anemia, **Oroya fever.**

■ CASE

Two brothers, M. and J., became ill after having been scratched by a new kitten given to them by an aunt. M. is 5 years old and has been healthy all of his life. He developed a 6-mm cutaneous papule on the right hand where the kitten had scratched him 1 week before. After another week, he developed numerous enlarged lymph nodes in the right axilla. Acute and convalescent sera collected by M.'s pediatrician showed an eightfold rise in titer of antibodies to *B. henselae*. M.'s lymph nodes returned to normal size and consistency over a 3-month period without antimicrobial treatment.

J. is 3 years old. Unlike M., he acquired infection with

the human immunodeficiency virus (HIV-1) congenitally from his mother and now has AIDS. J. developed three painless, red skin lesions that resembled tumors. Biopsy of the largest of these skin lesions revealed proliferation of small blood vessels and numerous colonies of small bacteria. A diagnosis of bacillary angiomatosis was made. The lesions resolved after a month of continuous treatment with oral erythromycin. However, another crop of similar lesions developed 3 weeks after discontinuing the antibiotic. With the recurrence, J. also developed fever and chills. Blood cultures for *Bartonella* were obtained, and J. was treated with intravenous erythromycin until his fever resolved. Oral erythromycin was continued thereafter. His skin lesions disappeared on treatment, but he died of other complications of AIDS 4 months later. After 2 weeks of incubation, his blood culture grew *B. henselae.*

A number of questions arise:

1. Why did J. develop a different disease than M. when both were infected with the same organism, *B. henselae*?
2. Why did M. get well without treatment while J. suffered a relapse despite treatment with an appropriate antibiotic?
3. What was the source of the infections?
4. By what route(s) did the organisms travel to the skin papule, the lymph nodes, and the pseudoneoplastic skin lesions?

Cat scratch disease is a significant infection in the U.S., with more than 20,000 cases occurring annually. M. developed the typical clinical features and self-limited course of cat scratch disease, whereas J. developed a more indolent and relapsing disease in the context of AIDS. In addition to cat scratch disease and bacillary angiomatosis, there are two other medically important *Bartonella* infections (Table 26.1).

In parts of Peru, Ecuador, and Colombia, a skin disorder called "Peruvian wart" (**verruca peruana**) has been recognized since pre-Colombian times. The indolent angioma-like lesions of this condition resemble those seen in the case of J. In late 19th-century Peru, an epidemic of fever and anemia (**Oroya fever**) occurred among railroad construction workers. A Peruvian medical student at the time, Daniel Carrión, demonstrated that the lesions of verruca peruana contained an infectious agent that is also responsible for Oroya fever. He had himself injected with material from a skin lesion and unfortunately died of the acute febrile illness. His legacy was the important discovery that the two seemingly disparate diseases have a common etiology. We now know that in the natural course of infection, the febrile illness occurs first and may resolve to be followed months later by the skin lesions. In honor of the medical student whose autoexperiment permitted this connection to be recognized, the disorder was renamed "Carrión's disease." The etiologic agent of Carrión's disease, *Bartonella bacilliformis* was observed in 1913 by its discoverer, Alberto Barton, to infect red blood cells during the acute stage of infection. Blood infection leads to extreme anemia because of massive destruction of the red blood cells by the mononuclear phagocytes.

In the Northern Hemisphere, **trench fever**, caused by *B. quintana*, was one of the major causes of morbidity in World War I. This disease has appeared again in new forms in people with AIDS and in homeless persons. Immunocompromised persons are particularly susceptible to this infection, which may manifest as febrile bacteremia or tumorlike proliferations of blood vessels in the skin and visceral organs, indistinguishable clinically or pathologically from *B. henselae* bacillary angiomatosis. Homeless persons in Europe and North America have been found to have *B. quintana* infections of the bloodstream and cardiac valves. The chronic bacteremia of this infection may extend for months beyond clinical recovery. Originally, the trench fever bacterium was believed to be a kind of rickettsia. In 1961, cell-free cultivation of this etiologic agent on blood agar demonstrated that it was not an obligate intracellular bacterium. For many years, the trench fever agent was called *Rochalimaea quintana* in honor of the Brazilian microbiologist da Rocha-Lima. However, contemporary molecular tools revealed that this bacterium, now known as *Bartonella quintana*, is a close relative of *Bartonella bacilliformis*.

ENCOUNTER AND ENTRY

Bartonella henselae is introduced into human skin by a scratch or bite from a cat with a nonapparent, prolonged infection. Transmission from cat to cat occurs via fleas. In contrast, *B. quintana* infections during World War I were transmitted by the human body louse. In the present day, many affected individuals do not have lice. Other possi-

Table 26.1. Etiology and Epidemiology of *Bartonella* Infections

Organisms	Diseases	Reservoir in nature	Transmission
B. henselae	Cat scratch disease, bacillary angiomatosis	Cats	Cat scratch or bite, cat flea
B. quintana	Trench fever, bacillary angiomatosis	Human	Louse feces, (? other)
B. bacilliformis	Oroya fever (anemic), verruca peruana	Humans, rodents?	Sandfly bite

PARADIGM   ■ ■ ■

New Methods and the Discovery of New Etiologic Agents

Ever since microscopy, microbial cultivation, and animal inoculation led to the concept that living things invisible to the naked eye could cause diseases, advances in technology have led to the discovery of new infectious agents. Cell culture has enabled the discovery of viruses and other etiologic agents which cannot be cultivated on agar or in broth. Electron microscopy has allowed visualization of viruses and bacteria for which effective methods of growth had not been developed.

Recently, the application of molecular methods, particularly polymerase chain reaction (PCR) amplification and sequencing of DNA derived from the infectious agent, has led to discovery of previously undetermined or undiscovered etiologic agents of infectious diseases. The major causative agent of bacillary angiomatosis, *Bartonella henselae*, was initially identified using this approach. Classic serologic, epidemiologic, and ecological investigations later revealed that it also causes cat scratch disease.

Other uncultivable pathogens, including the agents that cause **human granulocytic ehrlichiosis** and **Whipple's disease,** have been identified by DNA analysis. Human granulocytic ehrlichiosis is a newly recognized, life-threatening disease, whereas Whipple's disease has been known since 1907. In both instances, scientists obtained affected tissues from patients and used the PCR to amplify a gene known to be present in all bacteria, namely, **16S ribosomal DNA (16S rDNA)**. The amplified DNA was sequenced and compared against the 16S rDNA sequences of other known bacteria stored in computerized data banks. Because certain variations in the 16S rDNA sequence are known to reflect the evolution of species, scientists can identify the closest relatives of the unknown pathogen even when an exact match is not available from the data bank.

Similarly, to identify the culprit causing the deadly, acute respiratory disease outbreak of 1993 in the Four Corners area of New Mexico, Arizona, Colorado, and Utah, researchers used a variation of this method. Based on serology, investigators suspected a Hantavirus-like agent. Consequently, researchers added a reverse transcription step to convert viral RNA in patient samples into DNA. Then, primers for conserved Hantavirus sequences were used for PCR. These studies revealed that the etiologic agent was indeed a novel strain of Hantavirus. Many of the riddles of newly emerging and poorly understood infectious diseases will surely yield to the study of genomic sequences by ever-improving methods.

N. CARY ENGLEBERG

---

ble, but unproven, modes of transmission of *B. quintana* include contaminated intravenous drug paraphernalia or other arthropods. Lastly, *B. bacilliformis* is transmitted through the bite of *Lutzomyia* **sandflies,** which imbibe the blood of an infected host, amplify the quantity of organisms, and then transmit the bartonellae by feeding on a new susceptible host. Humans may be the only reservoir of *B. bacilliformis* infection, but other bartonellae infect rodents and felines in endemic areas.

SPREAD, MULTIPLICATION, AND DAMAGE

In cat scratch disease, *B. henselae* causes a small papule at the site of inoculation. The organism then spreads via the lymphatic vessels to the regional lymph nodes where bacterial proliferation and a vigorous mixed **granulomatous** and **suppurative** host response occurs. This response typically limits the infection, and very few bacteria are found in infected lymph nodes (Fig. 26.1). In some persons, however, particularly people with AIDS, the host response is insufficient to control the infection. The bartonellae multiply freely and disseminate in large numbers via the bloodstream, often manifesting clinically as sepsis or as localized infection of the skin, liver,

and other viscera. In infections of skin and other organs, the bacteria secrete substances that stimulate proliferation of small blood vessels, resulting in the lesions of **bacillary angiomatosis** (Fig. 26.2). *B. quintana* has been found to cause an indistinguishable angioproliferative illness in people with AIDS, although the source of infection and mode of entry are not always clear.

Bartonella bacilliformis attaches to the erythrocyte, deforms the cell membrane as it enters the cell, and then multiplies within the erythrocyte cytoplasm. **Massive anemia** can then ensue from greatly enhanced erythrophagocytosis. Host defenses are also altered by this process. The pathogenesis of the typical chronic nodular skin lesions is similar to that of bacillary angiomatosis.

DIAGNOSIS

Bartonella infections can be diagnosed by cultivation of the organisms from blood or skin lesions; however, growth is slow and routine cultures are often discarded before organisms are detected. Alternatively, the diagnosis of *B. henselae* or *B. quintana* infection may be made by detection of specific antibodies in patients with suspicious clinical signs and symptoms. Bartonellae can also be detected in biopsies with the use of special silver

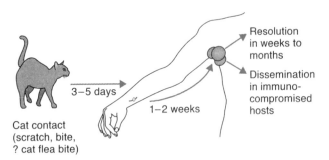

Figure 26.1. Acquisition and courses of infection with *Bartonella henselae.*

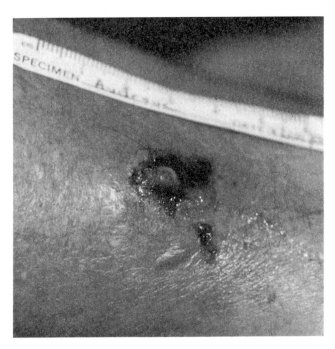

Figure 26.2. A lesion of bacillary angiomatosis on the forearm of an AIDS patient.

staining methods. In people with AIDS, biopsies of these lesions are often performed to rule out the similar-appearing, malignant angiomatous lesion, Kaposi's sarcoma. Likewise, *B. bacilliformis* can be visualized diagnostically in Romanowsky-stained smears of peripheral blood of patients with Oroya fever.

TREATMENT

In cat scratch disease, the course of illness is only marginally affected by antibiotic treatment. Although various antibiotics (rifampin, ciprofloxacin, trimethoprim–sulfamethoxazole, or gentamicin) have been tried, there is no established, effective antimicrobial therapy. The drug of choice for bacillary angiomatosis or bacteremia due to either *B. henselae* or *B. quintana* is **erythromycin**; doxycycline and azithromycin also produce good results. Unfortunately, relapses requiring repeated or long-term maintenance treatment occur in patients with inadequate host defenses. For *B. bacilliformis* infection, **chloramphenicol** is usually given in the acute febrile stage (Oroya fever) because of the frequency of complications due to *Salmonella* superinfection. **Rifampin** is used for the much less serious verrucous stage.

CONCLUSION

The bartonellae belong to a large and heterogeneous group of fastidious Gram-negative bacilli. Decades of confusion passed before they were assigned a logical taxonomic home based on nucleic acid homology of evolutionarily conserved genes. The species that cause human disease, *B. henselae*, *B. quintana*, and *B. bacilliformis*, may produce angiomatous skin lesions, sepsis, or visceral organ infection depending upon the circumstances of infection and the immune status of the host. When bartonellae proliferate in tissues or blood, treatment with an antibiotic is effective and warranted. In lymphadenopathic cat scratch disease, a vigorous host response limits its bacterial growth but also produces lymphadenitis, which is the hallmark of the disease. Antimicrobial therapy is of minimal, if any, value in this setting.

SELF-ASSESSMENT QUESTIONS

1. What different diseases are caused by the bartonellae?
2. What similar lesion can be observed in infections caused by *Bartonella henselae*, *B. quintana*, and *B. bacilliformis*?
3. Speculate on possible reasons why the number of bacteria in tissues is small in cat scratch disease and large in bacillary angiomatosis.
4. What is different about the epidemiology of *B. henselae* and *B. quintana*, and how do these differences reflect the different life cycles of the organisms?

SUGGESTED READINGS

Adal KA, Cockerell CJ, Petri WA. Cat scratch disease, bacillary angiomatosis, and other infections due to *Rochalimaea*. N Engl J Med 1994;330:1509–1515.

Brenner DJ, O'Connor SP, Winkler HH, Steigerwalt AG. Proposals to unify the genera *Bartonella* and *Rochalimaea*, with descriptions of *Bartonella quintana* comb. nov., *Bartonella vinsonii* comb. nov., *Bartonella henselae* comb. nov., and *Bartonella elizabethae* comb. nov., and to remove the family *Bartonellaceae* from the order *Rickettsiales*. Int J Syst Bacteriol 1993;43:777–786.

Regnery R, Tappero J. Unraveling mysteries associated with cat-scratch disease, bacillary angiomatosis, and related syndromes. Emerg Infect Dis 1995;1:16–21.

Relman DA, Loutit JS, Schmidt TM, Falkow S, Tompkins LS. The agent of bacillary angiomatosis: an approach to the identification of uncultured pathogens. N Engl J Med 1990; 323:1573–1580.

Schultz MG. Daniel Carrión's experiment. N Engl J Med 1968;278:1323–1326.

CHAPTER 27

Chlamydiae: Genital, Ocular, and Respiratory Pathogens

PRISCILLA B. WYRICK

JANE E. RAULSTON

Key Concepts

Chlamydiae:

- Include *Chlamydia trachomatis*, a sexually and vertically transmitted bacterium that causes genital tract infections; *Chlamydia pneumoniae*, which may be an almost universal pathogen of humans; and *Chlamydia psittaci*, an avian pathogen that can be transmitted to humans.
- Are obligate intracellular pathogens that act as energy parasites within the host cell.
- Cause damage by evoking both a cellular and humoral immune response.
- Can be treated with antibiotics that are able to enter host cells.

Few other pathogenic bacteria are better adapted for survival and persistence in the human body than the chlamydiae, and none other are more widespread. In addition, chlamydiae infect members of many other species of mammals and birds. Chlamydiae's ability to produce inapparent infections in these hosts is unexcelled, and individuals may be infected for long periods of time without apparent harm. It is estimated that 10% to 20% of the human population of the world is infected with *Chlamydia* at any one time, and this figure is increasing. These organisms achieve a balanced relationship with their host: on the one hand, they rarely kill it; on the other, they have a remarkable ability to evade the human immune mechanisms. Another distinguishing feature of chlamydiae is that they are true **obligate intracellular bacteria**: they grow only inside animal cells.

Members of the species *Chlamydia trachomatis* are the most common agents of sexually transmitted bacterial infections and are the leading cause of preventable blindness in the world. By remaining localized in the genital tract for prolonged periods, chlamydiae may eventually produce serious and costly complications. One major reason that these infections are so common is that they often cause no initial symptoms or, at most, a mild **cervicitis** or **urethritis** with minimal exudate and pain. Additionally, it is speculated that every adult person has experienced pneumonia caused by *Chlamydia pneumoniae*, and that a significant percentage of these individuals have associated complications such as coronary artery disease. Another species, *Chlamydia psittaci*, can be transmitted from birds to pet bird owners, farmers, and veterinarians to cause pneumonia, arthritis, and bloodstream infections.

▋ CASE

A 23-year-old male, Mr. C., saw a physician because of a purulent discharge from his penis. The diagnosis of gonorrhea was made (see Chapter 14, "Neisseriae") and he was given ceftriaxone (a cephalosporin) by intramuscular injection. He improved initially, but over the previous 3 days he noticed a milder but persistent urethral discharge and pain on urination. Worried that he might not have been cured, he went to a sexually transmitted disease (STD) clinic for evaluation. He reported having no sexual intercourse since his last visit. His latest sexual partner, Ms. G., accompanied him to the clinic, although she had no complaints of pain, vaginal irritation, or discharge.

On physical examination, Mr. C. had a small amount of clear urethral discharge. Ms. G. was found to have a greenish discharge emanating from the mouth of her cervix. Her cervix was inflamed and bled easily when a swab was used to remove adherent secretions. Gram stains of the secretions from both Mr. C. and Ms. G. revealed numerous neutrophils, but no evidence of Gram-negative diplococci, whose presence would indicate the presence of gonococci.

Mr. C. was told that he had "postgonococcal urethritis," a condition often caused by *C. trachomatis*. This diagnosis was confirmed by finding the organisms in a smear of pus treated with fluorescent antibodies. The incubation time of infections with chlamydiae is generally longer than with gonococci. The ceftriaxone therapy may have eradicated the gonococci in Mr. C., but did not eradicate the chlamydiae, probably because chlamydiae are intracellular and neither penicillins nor cephalosporins penetrate human cells adequately. Therefore, Mr. C. may have experienced the overlapping manifestations of two infectious agents acquired simultaneously. Ms. G. was told that she had "mucopurulent cervicitis," the female counterpart of gonococcal and chlamydial urethritis.

Mr. C.'s original treatment did not follow the current recommendations of the U.S. Public Health Service, which take into account that about 45% of the cases of gonorrhea have coexisting chlamydial infections. The recommended treatment of uncomplicated gonorrhea is the administration of both a cephalosporin for the gonococcus and a tetracycline for the chlamydiae. At the clinic, both patients were treated with tetracycline and were strongly advised to return after finishing therapy to ensure that they had no evidence of either infection.

Mr. C. did not return to the clinic for a checkup, but Ms. G. did. Upon examination, a cervical discharge was noted. Marked tenderness of the left adnexa was found both by direct palpation and by moving the cervix back and forth. This finding strongly suggested salpingitis, inflammation of the fallopian tubes, and pelvic inflammatory disease (PID). A cervical swab was taken and placed into a transport medium for chlamydial culture. Ms. G. reported that she had not been feeling ill but had remembered the doctor's advice about coming in for a checkup. When she showed the doctor her bottle of pills, there were 10 left—her explanation for the leftovers was that "she may have missed a few doses."

A number of questions arise:

1. What are chlamydiae and what diseases do they cause?
2. How frequent are these infections?
3. How do chlamydiae cause disease?
4. How are these infections diagnosed? How are they differentiated from gonorrhea?
5. What is the best treatment and prophylaxis?
6. What are the chances that Ms. G. will have another episode of PID?
7. Is it likely that she will have permanent or serious damage from this disease?

CHLAMYDIAE

Chlamydiae are small (0.2 to 0.8 μm in diameter) in comparison with typical bacteria such as *Escherichia coli*. Their chromosome is approximately 1,000 kB in size, which can encode for approximately 600 proteins. They are Gram-negative in architecture and composition, with a lipopolysaccharide-containing outer membrane and a cytoplasmic membrane. Chlamydiae do not possess murein (peptidoglycan), the classic bacterial cell wall component. This absence of murein is intriguing because the organisms carry the genes for murein synthesis and penicillin-binding proteins. A distinct layer located just beneath the outer membrane can be seen by freeze-fracture electron microscopy, suggesting a structure analogous to murein.

The chlamydiae parasitize the host cell for nutrients and energy. Thus, they depend on the host for adenosine triphosphate (ATP). This inability to manufacture their own ATP and thus the energy to drive biosynthetic reactions is one of the major reasons chlamydiae cannot grow in cell-free laboratory media and are obligate intracellular pathogens. The chlamydiae are therefore **energy parasites**.

Presently, there are four designated species of the genus *Chlamydia*; *C. trachomatis* and *C. pneumoniae* cause disease in humans while *C. psittaci* and *C. pecorum* are primarily animal pathogens. Some strains of *C. psittaci* are highly infectious in humans and often cause devastating human disease. *C. trachomatis* is currently divided into three strains based on the type of disease syndrome observed. Some of these strains include human pathogens that, besides STDs, cause lymphogranuloma venereum (LGV) and trachoma.

Entry, Multiplication, and Spread

The reproduction of chlamydiae is characterized by a unique developmental cycle (Fig. 27.1). In the extracellular environment, chlamydiae exist in a transit form called the **elementary body (EB)**. Within cells, chlamydia exist in a reproductive form called the **reticulate body (RB)**. The first step in the chlamydial developmental cycle is the entry of EBs into epithelial cells of the conjunctiva, respiratory tract, gastrointestinal tract, or genital tract. EBs ensure their uptake into host cells using a variety of strategies, such as masquerading as nutrients, growth factors, or hormones and binding to specific re-

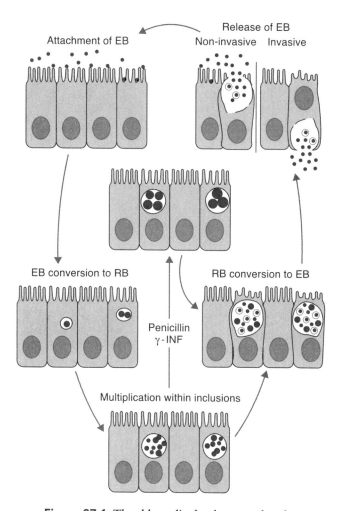

Figure 27.1. The chlamydia developmental cycle.

ceptors. The organisms are then internalized by the **re-ceptor-mediated endocytosis** pathway (Figs. 27.2 and 27.3).

Following its uptake by the host cell, the EB is rapidly incorporated into an endocytic vesicle. The EB modifies the vesicle in two ways: it maintains the pH above 6.2 and prevents the vesicle from fusing with lysosomes. In some species, such as *C. psittaci*, the EB-containing vesi-

cles develop separately, whereas in other species, such as *C. trachomatis*, they fuse with one another to form a single developing microcolony within the Golgi-perinuclear network.

The spherical, small (0.2 μm diameter) infectious EB then changes into a larger (0.8 μm diameter) intracellular, metabolically active organism. RBs synthesize macromolecules using metabolites and energy from the host, grow, and divide by binary fission (Fig. 27.2B). The organisms develop slowly within the vesicle, taking 2 to 3 days to complete a single developmental cycle. As the number of progeny chlamydiae increases, the vesicle membrane expands (with the help of added Golgi-derived lipids) to accommodate about 200–1,000 organisms. Such microscopically visible membrane-bound structures are called **inclusions** (Fig. 27.2C).

It is believed that RBs obtain their nutrients from the host cell using a unique device. On the surface of chlamydiae are 18–23 hollow tubes arranged in a hexagonal array (Fig. 27.3B) that protrude from the chlamydial cytoplasm into the host cell cytoplasm. These structures are thought to act as "drinking straws" (Fig. 27.3C). These structures allow the procaryotic chlamydiae to feed from their eukaryotic host without having to leave the confines of their protective inclusion vacuole.

RBs are fragile and do not survive well outside their host cells and thus they can infect new epithelial cells. In order to perpetuate the infectious process, the RBs must transform themselves back into infectious EBs before escaping from the host cell. Numerous disulfide bonds cross-linking three major outer membrane proteins are formed to help provide rigidity and stability for the EBs. Gradually, the EBs leave their host cell to infect a fresh cell. Alternatively, if the chlamydiae have reproduced within the host cell to very high numbers, the host cell is depleted of nutrients and lyses, releasing ruptured inclusions. The fragile RB die, and fewer mature EB are left to continue the infection.

Damage

The different chlamydial species and the diseases they cause are listed in Table 27.1.

Table 27.1. Chlamydial Diseases in Humans

Species	Biovariant	Serovariant	Disease syndromes
Chlamydia trachomatis	Trachoma	A–C	Trachoma, conjunctivitis
		D–K	STDs: urethritis, epididymitis, prostatitis, proctitis; cervicitis, endometritis, salpingitis, PID, ectopic pregnancy, infertility, arthritis; infant conjunctivitis, and pneumonia
	LGV	L1–L3	Lymphogranuloma venereum
Chlamydia pneumoniae			Pneumonia, upper respiratory disease, cardiovascular disease, arthritis
Chlamydia psittaci			Psittacosis, abortion, heart tissue damage, arthritis

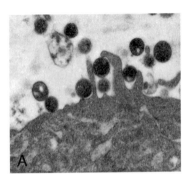
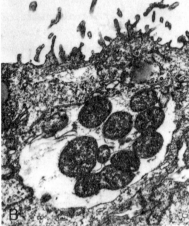
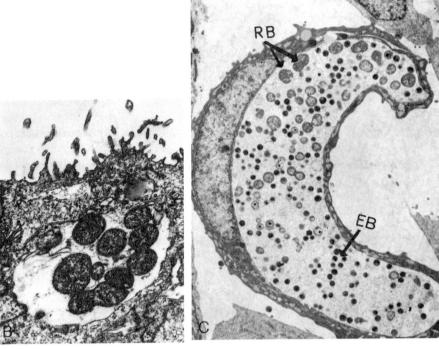

Figure 27.2. A. The infectious process is initiated by attachment of infectious EB to the microvilli of epithelial cells. **B.** Metabolically active RB of genital *C. trachomatis* contained in an early developing inclusion. **C.** A late, mature *C. trachomatis* inclusion containing many RB and EB.

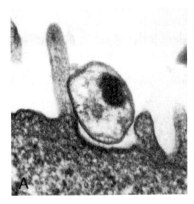
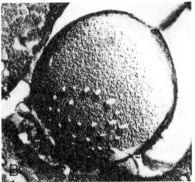
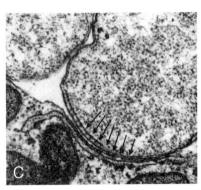

Figure 27.3. A. Entry of EB by receptor-mediated endocytosis in a clathrin-coated pit. **B.** The surface projections on EB. **C.** The projections on RB insert through the inclusion membrane into the host cell cytoplasm.

Infection of the reproductive organs

How do chlamydiae damage their hosts? Direct inoculation of fallopian tube in vitro cultures with *C. trachomatis* produces only mild salpingitis that heals with minimal scarring. In vivo, however, the infection produces severe salpingitis, adhesions, scarring, and tubal occlusions. These observations support the belief that the immune response is an important component in the pathogenesis of the chlamydial disease process. In an animal model, repeated inoculation of the eye with a chlamydial heat shock protein (hsp60) induces intense inflammation in the conjunctiva, with large numbers of infiltrating macrophages and lymphocytes. High titers of antibodies to hsp60 are found in patients with trachoma and in women with tubal scarring following chlamydial pelvic inflammatory disease (PID). These antibodies react with the portion of the heat shock protein that is unique to chlamydiae, suggesting the proteins are made by the organisms. Thus, the process of scarring following chlamydial infections may be due to a delayed-type hypersensitivity response to specific chlamydial antigens, such as hsp60. In other words, damage is produced by the host's own immune response to the infection.

Chlamydial infections may be acute, as in the case of Mr. C., or they may become chronic. The infections are often inapparent over a long period of time, sometimes months or years. Cultured cells growing in the laboratory can tolerate rather large loads of chlamydia progeny (as many as 500–1,000 per host cell), but mucosal epithelial cells in vivo may not produce as many infectious chlamydiae so rapidly. Also, the presence of cytokines, such as γ-interferon, may induce a persistent state, with the altered RB growing even more slowly. The location of the organisms during the silent periods is not known. Infected patients mount an antibody response, but it is probably ineffective in combating the organisms in their intracellular habitat. However, inflammation and scarring occur even in asymptomatic individuals, possibly triggered by secreted chlamydial lipopolysaccharide.

Pregnant women with *C. trachomatis* genital infections may transmit the organisms to their babies during birth. Some evidence suggests that intra-amniotic infection with chlamydiae may occur during the late stages of pregnancy. Newborn infants may develop **conjunctivitis** and **pneumonia**. Left untreated, some babies with chlamydial pneumonia develop a chronic respiratory disease syndrome.

Other chlamydial diseases

Some strains of *C. trachomatis* cause **trachoma**, an inflammation of the conjunctiva followed by vascularization and scarring of the cornea that may lead to blindness. Inflammation interferes with the flow of tears, an important defense mechanism against many bacteria. Scarring causes the eyelid to turn inward allowing the eyelashes to continually abrade the cornea. Abrasion leads to ulceration and complications of secondary bacterial infections. The combination of these processes leads to blindness.

Other highly invasive strains of *C. trachomatis* cause a sexually transmitted disease called **lymphogranuloma venereum** (LGV). LGV is found predominantly in developing countries. Following initial exposure and the formation of primary genital lesions, the organisms quickly penetrate through the genital mucosae and become systemic. The typical presentation is a regional lymphadenopathy in the areas draining the genital tract.

A recently designated species, *C. pneumoniae*, is perhaps the most prevalent chlamydial pathogen in the human population. In the United States and Europe, seroepidemiological studies indicate that 50% of the population have been infected with *C. pneumoniae* by 20 years of age, and this figure rises to 80% in older adults. As the percentage of adult infections continues to rise, it is thought that everyone will develop antibodies to *C. pneumoniae* sometime in their lifetime. Many of these infections cause acute upper respiratory illness or are asymptomatic. However, chronic **respiratory infec**-

tions with *C. pneumoniae* are associated with progressive and detrimental disease syndromes such as asthma, cystic fibrosis, and lung cancer. Perhaps the most far-reaching aspect of infection with *C. pneumoniae* is an association with **atherosclerosis**. Extensive studies continually reveal that these organisms can be directly observed in anywhere from 40% to 100% of atherosclerotic heart lesions. It is not yet clear how *C. pneumoniae* participates in the cardiovascular disease process, but it is hoped that antimicrobial treatment directed toward these organisms may produce favorable effects.

C. psittaci is primarily an animal pathogen, but humans can become infected as well. Certain avian strains of *C. psittaci* are transmitted to humans by the inhalation of fecal dust aerosols, leading to a respiratory, "flu-like" syndrome called **psittacosis**. Cases of heart valve damage in people who own diseased pet birds have also been reported. Ovine abortion strains of *C. psittaci* are known to cause abortion in pregnant women exposed to infected sheep during lambing. Thus, the impact of *C. psittaci* on human health is probably underestimated.

Finally, a well-recognized link exists between most pathogenic species of chlamydiae and arthritic disease syndromes. Chlamydial DNA has been detected in the synovial fluid of patients with **reactive arthritis** and **undifferentiated oligoarthritis**. The contribution of the chlamydiae to arthritic disease processes is not yet clear.

Diagnosis

It is common to find patients with multiple sexually transmitted infections; in the United States, gonorrheal and chlamydial infections often coexist. It is important to differentiate the chlamydiae from other pathogens, since some antibiotic drugs are inefficient in eradicating these intracellular bacteria. Confirmation of chlamydial infection in patients has been somewhat difficult, since the "gold standard" for many years has been to isolate the organisms using cell culture techniques. However, false-negative results arise due to sampling variations, collection of inadequate specimens (exudate rather than epithelial cells), or improper specimen handling. In addition, the question remains whether chlamydiae that persist in the body may be noninfectious for in vitro cell cultures.

Fortunately, DNA technology has entered the picture. Amplification kits, one involving a polymerase chain reaction (PCR), the other a ligase chain reaction (LCR), have greatly improved the sensitivity and specificity of chlamydial detection. One additional bonus is that these DNA amplification methods are over 90% effective in chlamydial diagnosis using urine specimens from men. DNA methods are often preferable to the standard culture procedure which requires an invasive and uncomfortable intraurethral swabbing.

Other popular methods available for chlamydial detection include (1) fluorescent antibody staining of patient specimens with microscopic evaluation (Fig. 27.4),

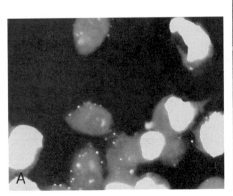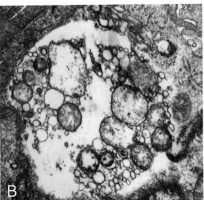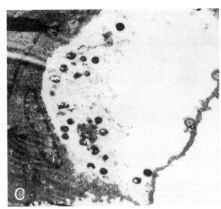

Figure 27.4. A. Fluorescent micrograph of chlamydial inclusions (blue) in infected genital epithelial cells. **B.** Disruption of protein synthesis by antibiotic action on growing RB damages the RB. **C.** Residual EB remaining in an inclusion in an antibiotic-exposed infected epithelial cell.

and (2) an enzyme-linked immunoassay (EIA). These tests have been available longer than the DNA amplification methods and are also used to accompany culture diagnosis to counter false-negative results.

Treatment

The metabolically active RB forms of chlamydiae are the chemotherapeutic targets for antichlamydial therapy. To be effective, an antimicrobial agent must penetrate four membrane layers: (1) the host cell plasma membrane; (2) the inclusion membrane; (3) the chlamydial outer membrane; and (4) the chlamydial cytoplasmic membrane. In addition, because these organisms grow very slowly, bactericidal concentrations of antibiotics must be maintained over an extended period of time to ensure complete eradication of chlamydiae. The standard drugs of choice include the tetracyclines, macrolide antibiotics (e.g., erythromycin), and sulfonamides. Figures 27.4 B and C illustrate that although antibiotics destroy RBs, they have no apparent effect on EB particles, which may continue to perpetuate the infectious cycle. Therefore, antibiotics often require 2 to 4 doses per day for at least 7–10 days; noncompliance of patients with these regimens is a major problem contributing to the predominance of these infections in society.

A new macrolide derivative, called azithromycin, has shown remarkable efficacy against all chlamydial pathogens examined to date. The chemical structure of erythromycin was modified to enhance tissue penetration and long-term maintenance of intracellular bactericidal concentrations. Clinical studies confirm that azithromycin is effective when provided in only one or two doses. The longevity of azithromycin in tissues is anticipated to resolve many of the problems for patients who do not adhere to standard dose regimens with the other antimicrobial compounds.

A question currently under investigation in research laboratories concerns the fate of residual chlamydial

Table 27.2. Who Should Receive Antichlamydial Therapy?
Patients with any of the diseases listed in Table 27.1.
Patients with gonorrhea
All of their sexual partners
Neonates born to women with untreated chlamydial infections

antigens following antimicrobial therapy. As shown in Figure 27.4, empty chlamydial envelopes are often observed following in vitro exposure of RB to antibiotics. This issue is not trivial, since much of the damage resulting from chlamydial infection is immune-mediated.

In the laboratory, infected cell cultures exposed to penicillin produce still enlarged, but viable, RB forms which are unable to mature into infectious EB until the drug is removed from the growth medium. Similar large, abnormal forms are also observed when chlamydia-infected cultures are exposed to γ-interferon. These research studies raise the question of whether such chlamydial forms may be induced in vivo and serve as a source of persistent infection.

Antichlamydial therapy should be administered not only to the infected patient but also to all sexual partners. Treatment of sexual partners is crucial for women, since repeated infection or reexposure to chlamydial organisms greatly enhances the incidence of serious complications such as PID, ectopic pregnancy, and infertility. Pregnant women and infants born to infected mothers should also receive antichlamydial therapy; in these instances, the macrolide antibiotics are the drugs of choice. Finally, patients with any of the other disease syndromes outlined in Table 27.2 should receive antimicrobial therapy.

CONCLUSION

Chlamydiae are insidious pathogens. They sequester themselves inside host cells in vesicles that protect them from the array of hostile armaments the host cell reserves for invading pathogens. The infected person mounts both a humoral and a cell-mediated response, but sometimes the response is destructive. Serious complications can occur, some of which are life-threatening. It is important for researchers to discover how chlamydiae behave inside host cells in order to know what pathways can be exploited to interrupt the disease process. Perhaps we might be able to devise even more rational approaches to prevent infection.

SELF-ASSESSMENT QUESTIONS

1. How do RB differ from EB? What is an inclusion? What are the stages of the chlamydial developmental cycle? How are their energy requirements met?
2. How do chlamydiae cause disease?
3. Why are asymptomatic chlamydial infections a public health problem? What are the possible complications for women?
4. What diagnostic tests are used to identify chlamydiae?
5. Awareness of sexually transmitted chlamydial infections alters the therapeutic strategy for all sexually transmitted diseases. Why? How does it alter them?

SUGGESTED READINGS

Beatty WL, Byrne GI, Morrison RP. Repeated and persistent infection with *Chlamydia* and the development of chronic inflammation and disease. Trends Microbiol 1994;2:94–98.

Hackstadt T, Rockey DD, Heinzen RA, Scidmore MA. *Chlamydia trachomatis* interrupts an exocytic pathway to acquire endogenously synthesized sphingomyelin in transit from the Golgi apparatus to the plasma membrane. EMBO J 1996;15:964–977.

Kuo CC, Grayston JT, Campbell LA, Goo YA, Wissler RW, Benditt EP. *Chlamydia pneumoniae* in coronary arteries of young adults (15–34 years old). Proc Natl Acad Sci USA 1995;92:6911–6914.

Schachter J. The intracellular life of *Chlamydia*. Curr Top Microbiol Immunol 1988;138:109–139.

Toye B, Laferriere C, Claman P, Jessamine P, Peeling R. Association between antibody to the chlamydial heat-shock protein and tubal infertility. J Infect Dis 1993;168:1236–1240.

Wyrick PB, Davis CH, Knight ST, Choong J, Raulston JE, Schramm N. An in vitro human epithelial cell culture system for studying the pathogenesis of *Chlamydia trachomatis*. Sex Trans Dis 1993;20:248–256.

CHAPTER 28

Rocky Mountain Spotted Fever and Other Rickettsioses

DAVID H. WALKER

Key Concepts

Rickettsiae:
- Are obligate intracellular bacteria (i.e., cannot be grown on artificial media).
- Are usually arthropod-borne.
- Cause several severe diseases: Rocky Mountain spotted fever (*Rickettsia rickettsii*), typhus (*Rickettsia prowazekii, Rickettsia typhus, Rickettsia tsutsugamushi*), and others.
- Have a predilection for vascular endothelia, and thus cause blood vessel damage and bleeding in various organs; in the skin, vascular damage results in rashes.
- Cause infections that can be treated with antibiotics that penetrate host cells.

Rickettsiae comprise a large collection of bacteria that can only grow inside eukaryotic cells. Together with the chlamydiae, the rickettsiae are the principal medically important **obligate intracellular bacteria**. The other defining characteristic of these organisms is their **epidemiology**. Most rickettsioses are **zoonoses**, infections that are transmitted from animals to humans and are spread, mainly through arthropod vectors (ticks, mites, fleas, lice, and chiggers).

The most important rickettsiosis in the U.S., **Rocky Mountain spotted fever**, is a serious, life-threatening disease. In common with many other species of rickettsiae, the causative agent invades vascular endothelial cells, causing generalized vascular damage. Another important rickettsiosis is **Q fever**, which often manifests as pneumonia. Other rickettsioses have played important roles at other times in history, and some have appeared to emerge anew in people with AIDS.

CASE

L., a 9-year-old girl, was taken to her pediatrician on May 31, two days after the onset of 40.5°C fever, severe headache, and muscle pains. The next day she developed nausea, vomiting, and abdominal pain and was admitted to the hospital for observation for possible appendicitis. On the second day following admission, an erythematous rash consisting of 2- to 4-mm macules (areas of discoloration) appeared on her wrists and ankles. Within 24 hours of its onset, the rash involved the arms, legs, and trunk, and many of the lesions had become maculopapular (discolored and raised) with petechiae (dark red spots caused by bleeding in the skin). A serological test for Rocky Mountain spotted fever and cultures of the blood, cerebrospinal fluid (CSF), and urine were negative. L. became stuporous and had edema in her face and extremities.

Treatment with intravenous doxycycline was begun for the suspected diagnosis of Rocky Mountain spotted fever. Within 72 hours, L. was alert and afebrile. She was sent home after 4 days in the hospital with instructions to take oral doxycycline for three more days. By the time of her discharge from the hospital, the rash had faded remarkably.

Table 28.1. Etiology and Epidemiology of the Principal Rickettsioses   *Dogs – principal host? reservoir*

Rickettsial agent	Disease	Reservoir in nature	Transmission	Geographic distribution
R. rickettsii	Rocky Mountain spotted fever	Ticks (transovarian transmission)	Tick bite	North and South America
R. conorii	Boutonneuse fever	Ticks (transovarian transmission)	Tick bite	Southern Europe, Africa, and Asia
R. prowazekii	Epidemic typhus Recrudescent typhus	Humans, flying squirrels Humans	Louse feces None	Potentially worldwide Potentially worldwide
R. typhi	Murine typhus	Fleas and rats	Flea feces	Worldwide, especially tropics and subtropics
R. tsutsugamushi	Scrub typhus	Chiggers (transovarian transmission)	Chigger bite	Asia, Oceania, and North Australia
Ehrlichia chaffeensis	Human monocytic ehrlichiosis	Deer?	Tick bite	North America
C. burnetii	Q fever	Cattle, sheep, goats, other livestock, cats	Aerosol from infected birth products and ticks	Worldwide

L. lived in a mobile home on the outskirts of Burlington, North Carolina and played after school in the nearby high grass and weeds. Her mother had removed several ticks from her body nearly every day during the month of May before she became sick. When L. returned to her pediatrician at the end of June, she was completely recovered. A serum sample was collected and sent along with one collected during the acute phase of her hospitalization to the state public health laboratory in Raleigh. A dramatic rise in titer of antibody to *Rickettsia rickettsii* was detected in the convalescent sample.

A number of questions arise:

• What caused the rash, stupor, and gastrointestinal symptoms?

• Why was the serological test for Rocky Mountain spotted fever negative in the hospital?

• Assuming that rickettsiae were circulating in the blood, why were the blood cultures negative?

• How did a girl from an eastern state get "Rocky Mountain" spotted fever?

Characteristics of the rickettsioses are shown in Table 28.1. The classic rickettsiosis, epidemic typhus, has been one of the most important infectious diseases due to its devastating effects on humanity. This disease influenced the outcome of most European wars between 1500 and 1900. During and immediately after World War I and the Russian Revolution, 30 million persons suffered from epidemic typhus, and 3 million of them died. The human body louse transmits *R. prowazekii* by depositing its feces on the skin. With the discovery of effective insecticides, in World War II, delousing interrupted the transmission of epidemic typhus and greatly reduced its incidence.

The most common rickettsiosis in the U.S. is **Rocky Mountain spotted fever**. It affects approximately 600 people annually, especially in the **eastern and southern states**

rather than in the Rocky Mountains, where it was first described. This disease can be extremely serious and, if untreated, has a **mortality rate of about 20%**. Because the disease responds well to certain antibiotics, especially in the early stages, a speedy diagnosis is essential.

The typhus group and spotted fever group of diseases are characterized by **disseminated vascular infection**. Injury in the lungs, central nervous system (CNS), and other systemic microcirculation may cause neurological signs, seizures, coma, acute respiratory failure, shock, and acute renal failure.

Q fever differs significantly from the typhus and spotted fever infections in that it has an acute form, manifested mainly as pneumonia, and a chronic form, in which the heart valves are usually affected. The causative agent, *Coxiella burnetii*, grows in the macrophages in the lung, liver, bone marrow, and spleen, where it stimulates granuloma formation. In one kind of rickettsiosis (ehrlichiosis), the organisms grow in white blood cells.

THE RICKETTSIAE

Rickettsiae are **small Gram-negative rods** that have an outer membrane and a thin murein layer (Figure 28.1). However, they are not readily stainable by the Gram method. DNA homology studies reveal that spotted fever and typhus rickettsiae are relatively closely related to other strict intracellular parasites, the *Ehrlichia* and *Bartonella*. In contrast, *C. burnetii* is more closely related to *Legionella* and only distantly related to the other rickettsiae. Spotted fever and typhus rickettsiae have lipopolysaccharides that are antigenically distinct for each group.

Rickettsiae are highly adapted to the intracellular

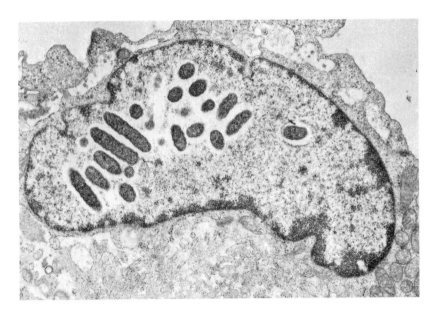

Figure 28.1. Electron micrograph of a thin section of a human endothelial cell infected with *R. rickettsii*, the etiological agent of Rocky Mountain spotted fever. The rickettsiae are the dark, rod-shaped bacteria in the nucleus, about the same size as the mitochondria and smaller than most other bacteria. These rickettsiae have invaded the nucleus. Although *R. rickettsii* organisms usually occupy the cytoplasm and few enter the nucleus, their presence in this location is characteristic of spotted fever rickettsiae and would be most unusual for other rickettsiae, *Mycobacteria, Salmonella, Legionella,* etc.

niche, where they propagate by binary fission with a generation time of 8–10 hours. Rickettsiae thrive in the high potassium environment of the eukaryotic cytosol and have specific membrane transport systems for acquiring ATP, amino acids, and other metabolites from the host cell. Unlike chlamydiae, rickettsiae are not strict energy parasites, as they are also able to synthesize at least some of their required ATP. Rickettsiae are also capable of **independent metabolism** (e.g., tricarboxylic acid [TCA] cycle and electron transport system) and **use their own biosynthetic machinery** to make proteins and other complex components. However, they cannot be cultivated on artificial medium and, in the laboratory, they must be grown in animals, embryonated eggs, or cell cultures.

ROCKY MOUNTAIN SPOTTED FEVER

Encounter and Entry

R. rickettsii are transmitted from tick to tick by the transovarian route and usually cause little harm to this host. Note that the ticks involved in Rocky Mountain spotted fever (*Dermacentor* species) are different from the *Ixodes* involved in Lyme disease (Chapter 25, "Lyme Disease"). When wild animals are bitten by *Dermacentor* ticks, they become transiently infected and a transient reservoir of the rickettsiae. Thus, this disease cannot be eradicated by public health measures. Risk of transmission can be reduced by the use of tick repellents and protective clothing. Individuals may prevent this illness by removing ticks from the skin before the bacteria are inoculated, usually between 6 and 24 hours after attachment. For a discussion of insect-borne diseases, see "Paradigm," Chapter 33, "Arthropod-borne Viruses." The 1994 distribution of cases of the disease in the U.S. is shown in Figure 28.2.

Spread, Multiplication, and Damage

Signs and symptoms of Rocky Mountain spotted fever begins an average of 1 week after an infected adult tick inoculates *R. rickettsii* into the skin while taking a blood meal. The rickettsiae spread throughout the body via the bloodstream. Upon encountering **vascular endothelial cells**, rickettsiae attach to the cell membrane and induce these cells to engulf them (Fig. 28.3 and Table 28.2). Once inside the cells, rickettsiae **rapidly escape from the phagosome into the cytosol**, presumably by lysis of the phagosomal membrane by a phospholipase.

Ensconced in the cytosol, *R. rickettsii* multiply and spread to other endothelial cells through long cellular

Table 28.2. Cellular and Subcellular Locations

Rickettsial	Host target cell	Cellular location
Rickettsia	Endothelium	Cytosol
Coxiella	Macrophages	Phagolysosome
Ehrlichia	Leukocytes	Cytoplasmic endosomal vacuole

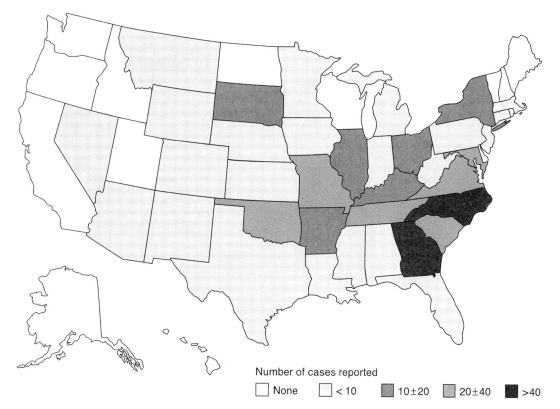

Figure 28.2. Cases of Rocky Mountain spotted fever in the U.S., by state, 1994.

Number of cases reported

☐ None   ☐ < 10   ◼ 10±20   ◼ 20±40   ◼ >40

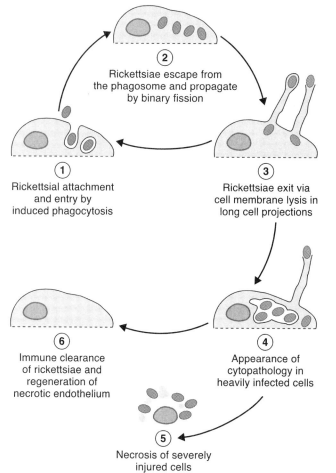

Figure 28.3. Sequence of rickettsia–host cell interactions in Rocky Mountain spotted fever.

① Rickettsial attachment and entry by induced phagocytosis

② Rickettsiae escape from the phagosome and propagate by binary fission

③ Rickettsiae exit via cell membrane lysis in long cell projections

④ Appearance of cytopathology in heavily infected cells

⑤ Necrosis of severely injured cells

⑥ Immune clearance of rickettsiae and regeneration of necrotic endothelium

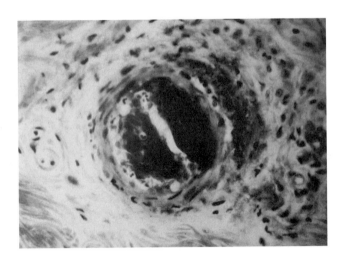

Figure 28.4. Severe injury to the arterial endothelium and media resulted in red blood cell extravasation and a thrombus plugging the vascular lesion.

projections of the cell membrane. This phenomenon is described in more detail in Chapter 17 ("Invasive and Tissue-damaging Enteric Bacteria"). **Injury to the host cell** correlates with the quantity of bacteria accumulated intracellularly. The subcellular target of injury appears to be the cell membrane. Although the mechanism of damage to this structure is not known, it may be due to the action of phospholipase, protease, or free radical–induced membrane lipid peroxidation.

The effects of damage to foci of contiguous endothelial cells are visible in the skin where dilation of the blood vessels first produces a pink rash. Later, leakage of red blood cells results in **hemorrhagic spots**, from which the name of the disease is derived (Fig. 28.4). Within the blood vessels of the brain, lung, heart, liver, and other visceral organs, these pinpoint hemorrhages lead to encephalitis, pneumonitis, cardiac arrhythmia, nausea, vomiting, and abdominal pain.

Even before the introduction of the effective antimicrobial treatment, 75% of patients with Rocky Mountain spotted fever survived. **Clearance** of intracellular rickettsiae from the endothelium is achieved though the concerted effects of the immune system with important contributions by cell-mediated immunity, particularly T lymphocytes and their cytokines, such as γ-interferon and tumor necrosis factor. Males, older individuals, alcohol abusers, and patients are more likely to die from this disease.

Similar diseases are caused by antigenically related organisms. The geographic distribution of these diseases coincides with a population of infected ticks (e.g., in Southern Europe, Africa, and Asia—boutonneuse fever and Israel spotted fever; in Australia—Queensland tick typhus; in northern Asia—another tick typhus) or mites (in North America, Europe, and Asia— rickettsialpox).

A substantial number of people become infected while traveling in southern Europe or Africa, where their activities expose them to ticks. Upon returning to North America or northern Europe, they seek medical attention for what is recognized by the astute physician as boutonneuse fever. The prevalence of antibodies to spotted fever group rickettsiae among healthy subjects in the affected countries suggests that many infections are not diagnosed.

TYPHUS GROUP FEVERS

The classic epidemic disease, **typhus fever**, is spread among humans by the body **louse** and is associated with high mortality and dramatic epidemics. In the U.S., the human disease is not seen except for cases of **recrudescent typhus** (Brill-Zinsser disease), which is due to reactivation of the agent, *R. prowazekii*. This agent can remain latent in the body for years or even decades after recovery from epidemic typhus or zoonotic typhus acquired from flying squirrels. Recrudescent typhus was described in the late 1800s in New York City among immigrants from eastern Europe, where epidemics of typhus were notorious. It is presumed that typhus epidemics can be ignited from a patient with recrudescent typhus and body lice, which spread the infection to other persons. Absence of epidemic typhus in developed countries today is an effect of the socioeconomic conditions and low prevalence of human body lice. Where war, natural disasters, and famine occur, epidemic typhus often followed; thus this disease is associated with crowding, poverty, and "lousy" sanitary conditions. It is foolish to believe that epidemic typhus could never return.

The reservoir of the epidemic typhus rickettsiae is not only human beings but also flying squirrels and their fleas and lice. The infection has been transmitted from this source to humans in the eastern U.S. Could an epidemic of typhus arise from one of these cases if it occurred among a louse-infested population? Possibly.

A more prevalent and widely dispersed rickettsiosis is **murine typhus**. This endemic disease is caused by *R. typhi*, which is transmitted in a natural cycle between rats and rat fleas. Humans become infected by the deposition of infected flea feces on their skin. Murine typhus occurs throughout the tropics and subtropics and was an important problem in the southern U.S. until the development of insecticides and intense rat control efforts.

Scrub Typhus

Scrub typhus is a disease of major importance in parts of the world distant from the everyday lives of Americans and Europeans. However, during World War II and the Vietnam War, Americans and Europeans came into contact with the ecological conditions in the South Pacific, Burma, and China. As a result, *R. tsutsugamushi* infected 18,000 soldiers in World War II and was one of the major causes of undiagnosed febrile illness among soldiers in Vietnam. The indigenous populations of endemic areas in many countries of Asia are continuously exposed to the agent of this infection. In a study in rural Malaysia, scrub typhus was the most frequent reason for febrile hospitalization.

Several factors exacerbate the problem of scrub typhus. The organisms exist in a variety of **antigenic types**, and immunity to one strain wanes over a period of a few years and to other strains after a few months. Subsequently, the patient becomes fully susceptible to reinfection. To make matters worse, clinical diagnosis is difficult because rash and eschar (a dry scab), considered the textbook hallmarks of the disease, are absent in the majority of cases. In many endemic areas, medical care is suboptimal, and laboratory diagnosis is virtually nonexistent. Scrub typhus is a neglected disease that, from time to time, rivets the attention of missionaries, the military, and medical examination committees.

Other Rickettsioses

Q fever is short for "Query Fever," referring to its unknown etiology when it was first described. The etiologic agent, *C. burnetii*, stands apart from other rickettsiae, and the disease differs from other rickettsioses in its clinical manifestations, pathological lesions, and epidemiology. Extracellularly, the organisms are much more resistant than the other rickettsiae to the many deleterious effects of the environment. Resistance may be due to the formation of a **sporelike structure** that has been observed by electron microscopy. Consequently, this agent does not require the protection afforded by a living vector but may also be transmitted via aerosols. Q fever is distinctly zoonotic, and the main reservoirs are infected sheep and other animals. The organisms are present in large amounts in the placenta and fetal membranes and are spread in copious numbers during birthing of ewes. The disease is most often seen among sheep farmers, veterinarians, and workers in laboratories that use sheep for experimentation.

The kind of disease produced by *C. burnetii* varies from acute pneumonia to chronic endocarditis. **Acute infection** may be asymptomatic or associated with nonspecific influenza-like febrile illness, atypical pneumonia, or granulomatous hepatitis. **Chronic infection** is usually diagnosed in patients with a long course, cardiac valvular infection, and negative routine blood cultures for bacteria. The pathogenic mechanisms appear to be largely immunopathological with T-lymphocyte-mediated granulomas in self-limited disease and an immune complex–mediated component in some cases of chronic illness.

Previously unrecognized infectious diseases continue to be described; two different human diseases caused by *Ehrlichia* species are among the newest to be discovered. *Ehrlichia chaffeensis* is transmitted by the Lone Star

tick. It infects mainly monocytes and macrophages, hence the disease it causes is called human monocytic ehrlichiosis. Another ehrlichial organism is closely related to pathogens of horse, sheep, cattle, goats, and deer (*Ehrlichia equi*) and seems to be transmitted by the same *Ixodes* tick as Lyme disease. This agent infects mainly neutrophils and is the cause of human granulocytic ehrlichiosis. Most cases are clinically similar to Rocky Mountain spotted fever and are characterized by fever, headache, and often, severe multisystem involvement, but with a lower incidence of rash. The spectrum of severity is quite broad and ranges from asymptomatic to fatal. Patients with *E. chaffeensis* often have reduced numbers of circulating leukocytes as well as low platelet counts. More than 400 cases of human ehrlichiosis have been documented since the first recognized case in 1986. Human granulocytic ehrlichiosis is diagnosed much more readily than human monocytic ehrlichiosis because the organisms are visible more often in circulating leukocytes.

DIAGNOSIS OF RICKETTSIOSES

The clinical diagnosis of rickettsioses is difficult, particularly when the patient first visits a physician and treatment is most effective. At the time of presentation during the first three days of illness, only 3% of patients with Rocky Mountain spotted fever have the classic triad of fever, rash, and history of tick bite. In contrast to most infectious diseases, laboratory studies are seldom helpful in establishing a diagnosis of rickettsiae disease in the acute stage of the illness. Very few laboratories attempt to isolate rickettsiae because of the technical requirements for inoculation of antibiotic-free cell culture, animals, or embryonated hen's eggs at the correct stage of development. In addition, the handling of these agents is notoriously hazardous.

For these reasons, the diagnosis of most rickettsioses requires considerable diagnostic acumen by physicians. Laboratory confirmation of rickettsioses is usually achieved in the convalescent stage by demonstrating a fourfold or greater rise in the titer of antibodies to specific rickettsial antigens. The only rickettsial disease that can be expected to have diagnostic levels of antibodies at the time the patient seeks medical attention is chronic Q fever. The serological methods usually employed are indirect fluorescent antibody assay, latex agglutination, and complement fixation (see Chapter 55); and newer methods are currently being developed. An archaic test that is still in use in some laboratories is the Weil-Felix test. This test relies on the agglutination of certain strains of the enteric bacterium, *Proteus vulgaris*, which shares cross-reactive antigens with certain rickettsiae. The results of the Weil-Felix test are nonspecific and insensitive, yet many hospitals persist in using it despite the availability of better methods.

Despite the fact that it is now antiquated, it is worth recounting how the Weil-Felix test was put to a humanitarian use by two Polish physicians in World War II. These physicians were aware that the occupying Germans did not send people suspected of having epidemic typhus to labor camps. Ingeniously, these doctors inoculated the population of several villages with an innocuous vaccine consisting of killed *P. vulgaris*. The high Weil-Felix titer of these people's serum was taken by the German medical staff to indicate that these villages were hotbeds of epidemic typhus. The inhabitants were spared, thanks to the microbiological stratagem of the two physicians.

TREATMENT

Rickettsial diseases generally respond well to antimicrobial agents that enter host cells and are active in the intracellular environment. Most of these diseases respond to oral or intravenous therapy with doxycycline, tetracycline, or chloramphenicol, each of which has its advantages and disadvantages under particular circumstances. Fluoroquinolone antimicrobial drugs are becoming the treatment of choice for some rickettsioses. Penicillins, aminoglycosides, and other antimicrobials do not affect the course of rickettsial diseases. Sulfa drugs actually seem to exacerbate both spotted and typhus fevers.

CONCLUSION

Although rickettsial infections are not common in the U.S., some of these diseases can be life-threatening. They must be diagnosed promptly, and antibiotic therapy must be instituted with due speed. The most devastating disease caused by these organisms, epidemic typhus, has receded in importance as a result of louse control but could emerge among the homeless in the U.S. or populations of eastern Europe, such as Bosnia when living conditions there deteriorated.

Rickettsiae are delicate organisms (except that which causes Q fever) but are well adapted to intracellular life and to passage from reservoir to host via arthropods. Their localization in blood vessels causes vascular injury with increased permeability and hemorrhages, sometimes with severe consequences.

SELF-ASSESSMENT QUESTIONS

1. What epidemiological features are shared by all rickettsioses but not necessarily by Q fever?
2. Describe three characteristics of rickettsiae that set them apart from other groups of bacteria.
3. What are the characteristics of the pathogenesis of Rocky Mountain spotted fever?
4. How could one study pathogenic properties of rickettsiae even though they cannot be grown in cell-free media?

SUGGESTED READINGS

Hechemy KE, Paretsky D, Walker DH, Mallavia LP. Rickettsiology: current issues and perspectives. Ann NY Acad Sci 1990;590.

Marrie TJ. Q fever. Vol I. Boca Raton, FL: CRC Press, 1990.

Walker DH. Biology of rickettsial diseases. Vols I and II. Boca Raton, FL: CRC Press, 1988.

Walker DH, Barbour AS, Oliver JH, Lane RS, Dumler JS, Dennis DT, Persing DH, Azad AF, McSweegan E. Emerging bacterial zoonotic and vector-borne diseases. Ecological and epidemiological factors. JAMA 1996;275:463–469.

Winkler HH. Rickettsia species (as organisms). Ann Rev Microbiol 1990;44:131–153.

Zinsser H. Rats, lice and history. Boston: Little, Brown, 1935; Bantam edition.

CHAPTER 29

Mycoplasma: Curiosity and Pathogen

GREGORY A. STORCH

Key Concepts

Mycoplasma:
- Are the smallest organisms capable of growth on cell-free media.
- Lack a rigid cell wall.
- Usually require sterols for growth.
- Species that cause human disease include *Mycoplasma pneumoniae, Mycoplasma hominis,* and *Ureaplasma urealyticum.*

M. pneumoniae:
- Causes pneumonia limited to the respiratory mucosa that lines the airways.
- May cause mild hemolytic anemia due to production of a cold hemagglutinin IgM antibody.
- Is usually diagnosed by it clinical features.
- Is treated with erythromycin or tetracycline.

M. hominis:
- Are transmitted through sexual contact as well as vertically.
- Cause pelvic inflammatory disease, chorioamnionitis, and postpartum fever.
- Have been isolated from the central nervous system of newborns.

U. urealyticum:
- Are transmitted through sexual contact as well as vertically.
- Cause urethritis.
- Are associated with chronic lung disease in very low-birth-weight premature infants.
- Cause pelvic inflammatory disease, chorioamnionitis, and postpartum fever.
- Have been isolated from the central nervous system of newborns.

The mycoplasma belong to a highly distinct group of bacteria that lack a cell wall and require sterols for growth. Most of the species associated with the human body are innocuous. One species, however, is a common cause of pneumonia, while others cause infections in the genitourinary tract of adults and in the respiratory tract and central nervous system of newborn infants. These or-ganisms are sensitive to broad-spectrum antibiotics that inhibit functions other than cell wall synthesis.

CASE

Michelle, a 7-year-old who previously had been in good health, developed fever, headache, and a dry cough. Her

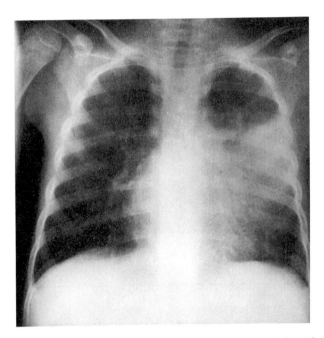

Figure 29.1. Chest x-ray reveals an infiltrate in the left mid-lung field.

12-year-old brother had had similar symptoms 2 weeks earlier. Over the next 2 days, her temperature increased and the cough worsened, producing small amounts of clear sputum. Her physician noted that she appeared slightly pale and had a temperature of 39.3°C and a respiratory rate of 40 per minute. Scattered rales (abnormal respiratory sounds) were heard through the stethoscope over the left posterior lung.

Her white blood cell count was in the normal range, 8600 per microliter with a normal differential. She was slightly anemic (hematocrit of 29%) and had an increased number of reticulocytes. A Gram stain of her sputum revealed only a few neutrophils and no bacteria. Her chest x-ray showed an infiltrate of the left midlung field (Fig. 29.1). A test to detect so-called cold hemagglutinins was positive. This finding and the clinical picture allowed the tentative diagnosis of **primary atypical pneumonia** caused by *Mycoplasma pneumoniae*. Michelle was treated with erythromycin and made an uneventful recovery.

A number of questions arise:
1. How did Michelle acquire the organism?
2. What are the distinguishing features of the mycoplasma?
3. What is known about the pathogenic properties of these organisms?
4. How is a definitive diagnosis made?
5. What can Michelle's family do to avoid spreading the organisms to other family members?

Mycoplasma pneumoniae is a common cause of pneumonia in children and young adults. As in Michelle's case, the illness usually has a less abrupt on-

set and a milder course than pneumococcal pneumonia. A rather imprecise term, "walking pneumonia," probably includes mycoplasma infections. Occasional cases may be quite severe, especially in individuals with *sickle cell disease*. Headache and cough are prominent clinical features. Before the etiology of this disease became known, it was referred to as "primary atypical pneumonia" to distinguish it from "typical" cases of lobar pneumonia (usually caused by pneumococci). Clinicians knew that patients with typical pneumonia responded to penicillin, while those with atypical pneumonia did not.

THE MYCOPLASMA

The mycoplasma have a number of unusual features:

- They are the smallest organisms capable of growth on cell-free media. They are classified with the bacteria because, in general, they have the structure and composition of procaryotes.
- They are unique among the bacteria in that they lack a rigid cell wall (no murein) and can assume a variety of shapes. This characteristic has important implications for antibiotic therapy, because many commonly used antibiotics (especially the β-lactams) act by inhibiting cell wall murein synthesis, and thus are ineffective against mycoplasma.
- Their cell membrane contains **sterols**, which, with some exceptions, must be supplied in the medium in order to support their growth.
- Mycoplasma are common in nature and capable of living in unusual environments, such as hot springs and the acid outflows of mining wastes.

Only three species are known to cause human disease (Table 29.1): *Mycoplasma pneumoniae*, a common cause of respiratory disease, and two organisms that ac-

Table 29.1. Common Mycoplasmas and Diseases They Cause

Organism	Disease	Site
M. pneumoniae	Primary atypical pneumonia	Respiratory tract
M. hominis	Pelvic inflammatory disease, other	Genitourinary tract
U. urealyticum	Urethritis	Genitourinary tract
M. genitalium	?Urethritis	Genitourinary tract
M. fermentans	??HIV cofactor	?
M. salivarium, M. orale	None	Mouth, oropharynx
Others (less common)	None	Genitourinary tract, oropharynx

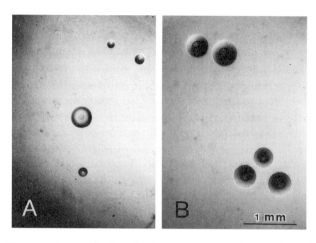

Figure 29.2. Colonies of *M. pneumoniae*. Note their small size and "fried egg" appearance, especially in B.

count for some cases of infections of the genitourinary tract, *Mycoplasma hominis* and *Ureaplasma urealyticum*. The latter two organisms can also be isolated from many newborns, especially from the respiratory tract and central nervous system. Other species are commonly found as part of the normal human flora but have not been linked to disease. On the other hand, different species cause a number of severe diseases in domestic animals. Mycoplasmas have also been implicated in the pathogenesis of acquired immunodeficiency syndrome (AIDS), a subject that is being vigorously investigated.

Mycoplasmas can be readily cultivated in the laboratory, although most species require special media that contain sterols. *M. pneumoniae* grows slowly, and several weeks may be required for colonies to become evident. The colonies are much smaller than those of the common bacteria and have a dense center which gives them a fried egg appearance (Fig. 29.2). *M. hominis* can be grown on the blood agar plates used in all clinical microbiology laboratories. However, this organism is probably often undetected because its very small colonies may not be noted unless the culture plate is examined under a dissecting microscope.

Mycoplasma pneumoniae

Encounter and entry

Infected humans constitute the only known **reservoir** of *M. pneumoniae*. Patients become ill following exposure to the respiratory secretions of persons harboring the organism. In contrast to the pneumococcus, prolonged asymptomatic colonization with *M. pneumoniae* is uncommon. In most cases the source of the infection is not recognized because most mycoplasma infections are mild. *M. pneumoniae* infections are moderately contagious, and spread within household or residential institutions is sometimes observed. In these situations, an interval of 2 to 3 weeks between cases is sometimes discerned.

Mycoplasma infection begins with the binding of mycoplasma organisms to the respiratory epithelium. Microscopic studies of *M. pneumoniae* have revealed a specialized terminal attachment structure. A special protein is found in this structure and is thought to mediate attachment of the organisms to a receptor on the respiratory epithelium. Monoclonal antibodies to this protein inhibit the attachment of *M. pneumoniae*.

Spread, multiplication, and damage

The pathogenesis of *M. pneumoniae* infection differs markedly from that of the other forms of pneumonia, such as that caused by the pneumococcus or *Legionella pneumophila*, mainly because its involvement is largely limited to the respiratory mucosa that lines the airways. There is no evidence of involvement of the lung alveoli. An infiltrate of mononuclear cells surrounds infected bronchi and bronchioles. The pattern of involvement is that of a **bronchopneumonia** rather than a lobar process.

In experimentally infected tracheal organ cultures the organisms line up along the mucosa, with the terminal attachment structure in contact with the epithelium (Fig. 29.3). Mycoplasma infection is not highly destructive of tissue, but ciliary function is impaired in cells with mycoplasma bound to their exterior. This impairment is thought to result from local elaboration of **tissue-toxic substances**, probably including hydrogen peroxide. The main cells in the inflammatory response elicited by *M. pneumoniae* are **lymphocytes**, with very few neutrophils. Some immune-compromised patients with mycoplasma infection do not have visible pulmonary infiltrates, suggesting that the immune response may play a role in causing the manifestations of disease.

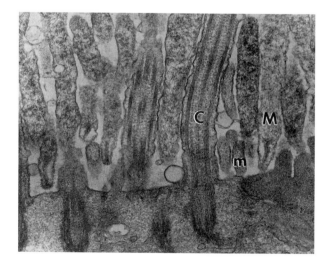

Figure 29.3. Transmission electron photomicrograph of a hamster tracheal ring infected with *M. pneumoniae*. Note the orientation of the mycoplasma via their specialized tiplike organelle which permits close association with the respiratory epithelium (×50,000). *M, Mycoplasma; m,* microvillus; *c,* cilia.

The clinical manifestations of *M. pneumoniae* infections are generally limited to the respiratory tract, but other organs are occasionally involved. Michelle, the patient described above, had a mild **hemolytic anemia**, which was caused by an antibody stimulated by mycoplasma. This IgM antibody binds to red blood cells and at reduced temperatures, causes them to agglutinate (stick together). These antibodies are called **cold hemagglutinins**, which are detectable in about 50% of severe mycoplasma infections. Only a small number of these patients actually experience clinically significant hemolysis. The reason why *M. pneumoniae* infection stimulates the production of cold agglutinins is not known.

Unusual complications of *M. pneumoniae* infections include **encephalitis** and other central nervous system complications. Some patients develop a rash known as **erythema multiforme**. The pathogenic mechanisms that account for these complications are not yet known.

Diagnosis

Culturing mycoplasma takes a week or more and requires special media and experienced personnel. Consequently, the diagnosis of mycoplasma pneumonia is usually suspected from clinical features and confirmed by serologic tests. However, an undesirable feature of serologic testing is that it requires convalescent phase serum, which becomes available long after therapeutic decisions about the patient must be made. Thus, *M. pneumoniae* is an attractive target for the development of rapid diagnostic tests that do not involve culture, such as immunoassays to detect mycoplasma antigens or nucleic acid amplification techniques to enable the detection of specific mycoplasmal nucleic acids.

In contrast to pneumococcal pneumonia, sputum production is scanty and the sputum nonpurulent. The peripheral blood usually does not show the leukocytosis and marked increase in young leukocyte forms characteristic of pneumococcal infection. The chest x-ray in mycoplasma pneumonia is highly variable, but most commonly reveals a patchy infiltrate suggestive of bronchopneumonia.

Cold hemagglutinins can be rapidly demonstrated at the bedside: blood drawn from the patient into a tube containing an anticoagulant will look clumpy when placed in an ice bucket. The clumps disappear when the tube is again warmed.

PREVENTION AND TREATMENT

No vaccine is currently available to prevent mycoplasma infections. Treatment with erythromycin or tetracycline is effective, although it should be remembered that *M. hominis* is uniformly resistant to erythromycin.

GENITAL MYCOPLASMAS

In epidemiology and pathogenesis, the infections caused by the genital mycoplasmas, *U. urealyticum* and *M. hominis*, differ considerably from infection by *M. pneumoniae*. These organisms are common residents of the genitourinary tract, especially of sexually active people. They are almost certainly transmitted through sexual contact and are also commonly transmitted vertically, from mother to newborn infant during pregnancy and birth. Not surprisingly, most of the diseases caused by these organisms affect the genitourinary tract of newborns. *U. urealyticum* is clearly established as the cause of urethritis and *M. hominis* as that of pelvic inflammatory disease (Chapter 66, "Sexually Transmitted Diseases"). Both organisms can cause chorioamnionitis (inflammation of the fetal membranes) and postpartum fever. Spontaneous abortion and premature delivery have been linked to these organisms, although this association has not been definitively proven. Several provocative studies have demonstrated an association between *U. urealyticum* and chronic lung disease in very low-birth-weight premature infants. Both organisms have also been isolated from the spinal fluid of newborn infants. This association is confusing because some of these infants have evidence of central nervous system inflammation, but others do not. It is possible that, at least in some cases, mycoplasmas are innocent bystanders in the central nervous system, whereas in other cases, they are responsible for disease.

CONCLUSION

Mycoplasmas call attention to themselves because they lack a cell wall, many require sterols for growth, and they make characteristic small colonies on agar. These organisms show a marked tropism for mucous membranes and produce characteristic clinical manifestations.

M. pneumoniae is unequivocally responsible for a common form of pneumonia in humans. Other mycoplasmas are commonly found in the genitourinary tract of adults and in the respiratory tract and the central nervous systems of newborn infants. In these settings, the presence of these organisms is not uniformly associated with disease. Our knowledge about the mycoplasmas and their role in disease is still in flux. The association of mycoplasmas with a wide variety of clinical symptoms in animals suggests that the full extent of their role in human disease may not yet be fully appreciated.

SELF-ASSESSMENT QUESTIONS

1. What distinguishes the mycoplasma from other bacteria?
2. Discuss the pathophysiology of mycoplasma pneumonia.
3. Compare the epidemiology of pneumonia due to mycoplasma with that due to pneumococci or legionella.
4. Why do you think it has been difficult to definitely establish the role of mycoplasma in certain diseases?

SUGGESTED READINGS

Levin S. The atypical pneumonia syndrome. JAMA 1984;251: 945–948.

Taylor-Robinson D. Infections due to species of *Mycoplasma* and *Ureaplasma*: an update. Clin Inf Dis 1996;23:671–682.

Strategies to Combat Bacterial Infections

FRANCIS P. TALLY

O ver the last two centuries, health and longevity of people living in developed countries have taken a quantum jump forward. We take it for granted that we, our relatives and our acquaintances, have survived infancy and will reach old age. Disease is the exception and premature death relatively uncommon. Two interrelated factors have contributed to this increased life expectancy: improvement in nutrition and control of infectious diseases. Initially, the most important factors in reducing the incidence of infectious disease were preventive measures, largely purification of the water supply and control of human wastes and disease vectors. Later, in the last 100 years, these measures were joined by medical intervention: vaccination and antimicrobial therapy. Preventive measures, not therapy, have played the greatest role in the control of infectious diseases.

This chapter discusses the strategies that have been developed for prevention and therapy of infectious diseases. The emphasis here is on bacteria, but the same principles apply to all other infectious agents.

Note: Antiviral strategies are discussed in Chapter 43, "Strategies to Combat Viral Infections, " and antibacterial and antiviral vaccination in Chapter 44, "Vaccines and Antisera".

THERAPY

Despite the great advances in preventive medicine in the last century, until recently little could be done to treat patients with infectious diseases. The medical literature up to about 1930 is full of vivid descriptions of gruesome infections by streptococci, staphylococci, and clostridia. The dawning of the age of antimicrobial therapy, with the introduction of the sulfonamides in the 1930s, allowed physicians to finally cure many of these fatal infections. Here is a description of the first time penicillin was used clinically:

> "The time had now come to find a suitable patient for the first test of the therapeutic power of penicillin in man . . . . In the septic ward at the Radcliffe Infirmary (Oxford, England) there was an unfortunate policeman aged 43 who had a sore on his lip four months previously, from which he developed a combined staphylococcal and streptococcal septicaemia. He had multiple abscesses on his face and orbits: he also had osteomyelitis of his right humerus with discharging sinuses, and abscesses in his lungs. He was in great pain and was desperately ill. There was all to gain for him in a trial of penicillin and nothing to lose. Penicillin treatment was started on 12 February 1941, with 200 mg (10,000 units) intravenously initially and then 300 mg every three hours . . . . Four days later there was striking improvement, and after five days the patient was vastly better, afebrile and eating well, and there was obvious resolution of the abscesses on his face and scalp and in his right orbit."

Unfortunately, this first clinical trial of a β-lactam antibiotic ended abruptly because the total supply of the drug was exhausted by the 5-day course of treatment, despite efforts to recover the drug from the patient's urine. The patient died 4 weeks later.

Although the experiment ended tragically, it served to demonstrate the efficacy and superiority of the new therapy over any that was available until that time. Today, it has become increasingly difficult to prove the superiority of new antibiotics over those already in use. In assessing new drugs, pharmaceutical companies must carry out complex and expensive trials that include laboratory work, experimental animals, and lengthy clinical studies. The practicing physician may often find it difficult to evaluate such intricate studies.

The selection of the most appropriate drug to treat a particular infection is also not a simple matter. For example, the β-lactam imipenem may be thought to be a true "wonder drug" because it has the widest antibacterial spectrum of any antibiotic presently available and is resistant to inactivating β-lactamases. However, there are specific infections for which penicillin (which has neither of these desirable properties) is far preferable. For example, because of its broad spectrum, imipenem may wipe out other members of the normal bacterial flora and lead to colonization by resistant species. In addition, imipenem is far more expensive. Thus, pharmacokinetic properties of the drugs, their cost, and many other properties must also be considered. The selection of an appropriate drug involves the following criteria:

- Which pathogens are causing the infection? If their identity cannot be determined at this time, what are the likely possibilities?
- What antibiotics are they susceptible to?
- Will the drug penetrate the site of infection and will it work under the conditions at that site?
- What is the toxicity of the drug to the patient?
- What is the effect of the drug on the microbial ecology? Will its use lead to the emergence of broadly based antibiotic resistance, and thus pose a threat to the patient being treated and to other infected patients in the community?
- Are other host factors relevant to the proposed therapy?

Note that in many cases the proper conclusion may be that the patient should not to be treated with antimicrobial drugs at all because the benefit of such treatment is not likely to outweigh its drawbacks.

THE INFECTING ORGANISMS

The proper choice of an antimicrobial drug depends on the identification of the infecting organisms. Consider, for example, patients with recurrent urinary tract infection. Often the infection is caused by *Escherichia coli*, but it may be due to group D streptococci, *Pseudomonas aeruginosa,* or one of the other Enterobacteriaceae, such as *Klebsiella, Enterobacter,* or *Serratia.* These organisms have differing susceptibilities, and the determination of their antimicrobial susceptibility is mandatory.

Note that physicians treating urinary tract infections for the first time usually do not wait for the result of laboratory cultures and drug susceptibility testing. Such shotgun treatment is often instituted on presumption of the causative agents. In such cases, physicians must take into account factors pertinent to the individual patient and the local environment, especially recent experience with similar cases and the antibiotic susceptibility pattern in their hospital or community. Other situations that require empirical therapy are those in which an adequate sample of in-

fected material for direct analysis or culture cannot be obtained. The treatment of recurrent infections, however, may be postponed until culture and susceptibility data become available.

The drawbacks of "shotgun" antibiotic therapy are:

- Failure to "cover" the pathogen
- The synergistic toxicity of multiple drugs
- Possible antagonism between drugs
- Increased likelihood of superinfection by resistant bacteria or fungi
- Increased cost of therapy

Obviously, these disadvantages are minimized when the identity of the infection agent can be determined. In general, the more rapid the diagnosis, the sooner proper therapy can be instituted. Much effort is directed toward the development of rapid diagnostic methods, but most still require one or several days. (For details, see Chapter 55, "Diagnostic Principles".)

ANTIBIOTIC SUSCEPTIBILITY

Different kinds of bacteria differ in their antibiotic susceptibility. Gram-positive bacteria, possibly because they lack an outer membrane, are generally more susceptible than Gram-negative bacteria, usually because they are more permeable to many of the classical antibiotics. For example, streptococci and pneumococci are generally about one thousand-fold more susceptible to penicillin G than *E. coli.* However, the exceptions are too numerous to make these generalizations very useful. Much depends on the presence of antibiotic-resistant strains in a particular environment. Nationwide and local monitoring of resistant strains is helpful in providing general guidelines, but basically, each individual isolate should be tested for susceptibility.

The importance of microbial drug resistance is illustrated by the catastrophic outbreaks of chloramphenicol resistance that occurred in Mexico in the late 1960s and the early 1970s with *Shigella* dysentery and subsequently with *Salmonella* infection. During the initial epidemics, it was not recognized that the reason patients failed to respond to chloramphenicol was that the bacteria had become resistant. Rather, it was thought that the disease was caused by a protozoan parasite. A similar scenario occurred 2 years later in outbreaks of typhoid fever caused by *Salmonella typhi* that was also chloramphenicol-resistant. It is estimated that more than 30,000 people died in each of these outbreaks because they were treated with chloramphenicol alone.

Two fundamental shifts occurred in the 1990s in the spectrum of antibiotic resistance among clinically important pathogens. First, antibacterial resistance, which first appeared among Gram-negative bacteria, has be-

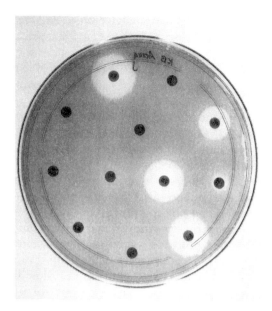

Figure 30.1. The disc diffusion method for determining antibiotic susceptibility. Bacteria were uniformly seeded on the surface of a nutrient agar plate, and filter paper discs containing different antibiotics were placed at intervals over the surface. After incubation, susceptibility to some of the antibiotics is indicated by clear areas around the discs. The diameter of the clear area depends on the extent of diffusion of the drug throughout the agar. Resistance to other antibiotics is indicated by growth (turbidity) up to the edge of the discs.

come widespread in medically important Gram-positive bacteria. These include methicillin-resistant *Staphylococcus aureus*, vancomycin-resistant enterococci, and penicillin-resistant *Streptococcus pneumoniae*. Organisms such as *S. aureus* and *S. pneumoniae*, which were among the most frequent killers in the preantibiotic era, are becoming increasingly serious clinical problems. Second, antimicrobial-resistant organisms have spread from hospitals into the community and now affect children in day-care centers and elders in nursing homes.

It is extremely important that drug resistance be monitored on a nationwide and local basis, and that the information be made readily available to medical personnel. The simplest and most widely used assay for microbial susceptibility is to place a disk containing an antibiotic on an agar plate inoculated with the organisms. As the antibiotic diffuses into the agar, it inhibits bacterial growth up to the limit of the effective concentration (Fig. 30.1). This test is not, however, a truly quantitative technique, because many factors influence the diffusion of the drug. Quantitative techniques require the use of dilutions of the drug in liquid media. These techniques provide an estimate of the **minimum inhibitory concentration**, or **MIC**, a parameter that is used to ascertain whether an effective antibiotic concentration is attainable in body fluids.

STATIC VERSUS CIDAL DRUGS

The minimum inhibitory concentration (MIC) tells us the **bacteriostatic** concentration of a drug, but not the **bactericidal** one. The two concentrations are not usually the same: most agents that are bactericidal are bacteriostatic at lower concentrations. The **minimum bactericidal concentration** (**MBC**) is determined by subculturing the tubes or microtiter plates that have no visible growth into antibiotic-free media. This subculturing allows the bacteria whose growth was inhibited in the first culture but which are still alive to replicate. This technique is time-consuming and has some technical problems. It may, however, yield important information because bactericidal and bacteriostatic drugs are often equally effective. For example, in patients with endocarditis and meningitis, the outcome with bactericidal drugs is frequently more satisfactory. Bactericidal drugs tend to be superior in immunocompromised patients, especially those who are neutropenic.

MULTIPLE DRUG THERAPY

The use of combinations of antibiotics (usually two drugs) is clearly needed in a number of clinical situations. As discussed in Chapter 5, "Biological Basis for Antibacterial Action," when drugs are combined, three results are possible:

1. **Synergism,** in which the two drugs in combination work better than one. An example is the use of trimethoprim and sulfamethoxazole for *E. coli* and *Shigella* enteric infections. The two drugs work on folate metabolism, but inhibit different steps (Chapter 3, "Biology of Infectious Agents"). Synergistic action may also be indirect, for example, by one drug preventing the inactivation of another, as in the case of inhibition of β-lactamases by clavulanic acid.

2. **Antagonism,** an undesirable effect that may lead to treatment failure. An example is the combination of penicillin and any of a number of protein-synthesis inhibitors (chloramphenicol, tetracycline) for the treatment of pneumococcal meningitis. The fatality rate among patients treated with this drug combination has been shown to be significantly higher than with penicillin alone. For unknown reasons, antagonism that can be readily demonstrated between two drugs in vitro often fails to manifest with the same pair of drugs in clinical situations.

3. **Indifference,** in which each drug acts independently of the other.

There are various indications for combined therapy, e.g.,:

- To prevent the emergence of resistant organisms, e.g., in tuberculosis, in which combination therapy has proven particularly effective.

Table 30.1. Physicochemical Conditions That Affect the Activity of Antimicrobial Agents

	Decrease	Increase
Low pH	Aminoglycosides Some β-lactams (porin changes) Erythromycin	Tetracycline Chloramphenicol
Low redox potential	Aminoglycosides	Metronidazole
High divalent cation concentration	Aminoglycosides Tetracycline (Ca++)	

- To treat severe infections caused by organisms that are relatively drug-resistant, such as *P. aeruginosa* (See Chapter 18, "*Pseudomonas aeruginosa*").
- To treat polymicrobial infections such as intra-abdominal abscesses, in which each organism may be susceptible to different drugs.
- As initial empiric therapy to "cover" multiple potential pathogens.
- To treat usually fatal infections, such as may be caused by *P. aeruginosa* (see Chapter 18, "Pseudomonas").

In other instances, the reason for multiple therapy may be more subtle. For instance, the use of several drugs may allow a lower dosage of each one, which may prevent problems of toxicity. It may also be necessary in order to achieve drug synergy for the treatment of severe, recalcitrant infections, such as endocarditis or bacteremia in a granulocytopenic patient.

LOCAL FACTORS AND PHARMACOKINETICS

Tissue inflammation occurs early in many infections which changes the environment in which an antibiotic is to work. If the infection is not controlled, cell death and tissue necrosis change conditions even further. In an abscess caused by staphylococci or a mixed anaerobic–aerobic flora, the environment becomes anaerobic and the pH may drop as low as 5.5. Antibiotics must be selected for their ability to function under these conditions. As shown in Table 30.1, the efficacy of aminoglycosides is diminished at low pH or in the presence of a high concentration of divalent cations.

The pharmacokinetic factors that should be considered in the choice of drugs include (1) absorption, (2) distribution in tissues, and (3) excretion. The **absorption** profile of a drug dictates its route of administration. The most convenient route is usually by mouth, and this route is used with highly absorbable antibiotics such as the quinolones or chloramphenicol. Many antibiotics,

such as vancomycin, the aminoglycosides, and the newer β-lactams are not absorbed via the gastrointestinal tract and must be given by parenteral injection. A major exception to this rule is the use of nonabsorbable antibiotics to treat infections limited to the GI tract. A good example is the use of oral vancomycin to treat *Clostridium difficile*–induced diarrhea or colitis (Chapter 20, "Clostridia"). Also, drugs cannot be given orally if the patient is vomiting or in shock, because absorption becomes unreliable.

Distribution of drugs takes place via the circulation and is followed by entry into tissues by passive diffusion. The diffusion and polarity properties of antibiotics are relevant here, as they are with all drugs. Some antibiotics bind to plasma proteins, which has a good and a bad side. On the one hand, protein binding limits the amount of unbound drug that is available for diffusion. On the other hand, the drug remains available for a much longer time.

The barriers that the drug must cross are a vital consideration. Drugs that cross the blood-brain barrier most readily are nonpolar at neutral pH. These factors are critically important because of the seriousness of infections of the central nervous system. Note, however, that the permeability properties of the blood–brain barrier may become modified during infection. Two other organs with important barriers are the eye and the prostate, and infections at each of these sites require careful selection of drugs. Infections of the interior of the eye may require direct injection of drugs into the tissue. Similar considerations about the placental barrier are discussed in Chapter 69, "Congenital and Neonatal Infections." Some drugs can efficiently penetrate host cells, a property that may be important in the treatment of intracellular infections, such as those caused by chlamydiae or legionellae. Erythromycin or rifampin are examples of drugs that effectively cross host-cell membranes.

Lastly, consideration must be given to the speed of **excretion** of the drug. Most drugs are excreted by the kidney. Certain drugs (e.g., chloramphenicol, erythromycin, lincomycin) are excreted by the liver via the biliary tree. Some of the newer cephalosporins are excreted via both liver and kidneys. This pattern of excretion can be used to advantage in infections of the urinary tract or the biliary tree. However, the level of renal or hepatic function must be taken into account because an effective drug level may only be reached if the excretion mechanisms are working properly.

Antibiotic Toxicity

Antibiotics, like all drugs, have toxic side effects as well as beneficial properties. Toxicity is sometimes so severe that it limits the general usefulness of some of them. For example, chloramphenicol is associated with cases of fatal aplastic anemia and is used only in life-threatening infections, such as meningitis with ampicillin-resistant *Haemophilus influenzae*. As with all drugs, toxicity is generally dose-dependent. An overview of the main types of toxic manifestations is provided below. Practicing physicians need more detailed information and must constantly update it.

Allergy

Antimicrobial agents may be recognized as foreign substances by the immune system, resulting in sensitization of some individuals. The most common antibacterial drugs associated with severe allergic reactions are the penicillins, cephalosporins, and sulfonamides. A likely reason why penicillins lead this list is that they readily bind to proteins and function as haptens to elicit IgE antibody responses. The most severe reactions result in immediate hypersensitive responses: hives, angioneurotic edema, and anaphylactic shock. These complications may be fatal. Mild to fairly severe allergic reactions include rash, urticaria (hives), lymphadenopathy, asthma, and fever. In some cases, fever may confuse the clinical picture, because it may be attributed to the infection and not to the drug. Previous history of drug sensitivity often dictates the choice of other agents. If a history of allergy is questionable, the patient may be skin-tested with the drug in question.

Other Systemic Reactions

All major organs of the body may be affected by toxicity from antimicrobial drugs. The most frequent reactions involve the **gastrointestinal tract**, ranging from mild distaste to perforation of the colon. Gastrointestinal distress and diarrhea are the most common reactions and often require discontinuation of the drug. These manifestations are often due to a direct stimulatory effect of the drugs on the sympathetic nervous system. However, diarrhea may be caused by changes in the intestinal flora. This form of toxicity usually occurs late in the course of treatment and may manifest only after treatment is stopped. About a third of the cases of antibiotic-associated diarrhea have been associated with the toxin produced by *Clostridium difficile* (see Chapter 20, "Clostridia"). The spectrum of diseases caused by this organism ranges from the trivial and self-limiting diarrhea to a severe and life-threatening pseudomembranous colitis.

The **liver** is the major site of drug metabolism and is frequently affected. Many drugs induce mild alterations of function of the hepatic parenchyma, usually manifested by an increase in the serum level of certain transaminases. Some drugs affect biliary excretion. Most of these manifestations are mild and reversible, although cases of liver failure have been reported in pregnant women treated with tetracycline.

The **kidney** is also a frequent site of adverse reactions, resulting in decreased renal function. These reactions are caused by three general mechanisms: (1) immunological damage to the glomeruli which blocks filtration, (2) damage to the tubules, and (3) obstruction of the collecting system by crystals of the drug. These reactions are an important problem because many drugs are excreted via the urinary tract. An unrecognized decrease in renal function may result not only in ineffective levels in the urine but also in toxic serum levels of the drug. The aminoglycosides are the most important class of drugs that cause these side effects. They also cause eighth cranial nerve toxicity (deafness and imbalance). The frequency of these toxic reactions is so high that frequent monitoring of renal function and blood levels of the drug is required during aminoglycoside therapy.

Other organs that are sometimes affected by antimicrobial agents include the **skin**, which may be affected by allergic reactions. More serious skin reactions include exfoliative dermatitis and a disease known as Stevens-Johnson syndrome, which leads to the formation of bullae, large vesicles on the skin, and inflammation of the eyes and mucous membranes. The **hemopoietic system** may be adversely affected, leading to decreased production of red and white blood cells in the bone marrow. Furthermore, peripheral red and white blood cells may become immunologically sensitized, resulting in their hemolysis or sequestration by fixed macrophages. The circulatory system, central nervous system (CNS), musculoskeletal system, and the respiratory tract can also be affected by antibiotics. Most of these reactions are specific to individual drugs. Information about the reactions caused by specific antibiotics is made available to physicians in reference manuals published periodically, which should be consulted before prescribing medication.

Interactions with Nonantimicrobial drugs

Antimicrobial drugs sometimes interact with other medications a patient may be taking. The drugs may interact directly or by affecting an enzyme that influences their pharmacology. The drugs most commonly involved are anticoagulants and anticonvulsants. An example follows.

▮ CASE

A 67-year-old woman with recurrent thrombophlebitis and pulmonary embolism had been asymptomatic on an oral anticoagulant (warfarin), which maintained her clotting or prothrombin time at 24 seconds, twice the normal value. She had been recently diagnosed with pulmonary tuberculosis and was placed on isoniazid and rifampin. Several days later she required hospitalization for recurrence of her thrombophlebitis. Laboratory evaluation revealed that her prothrombin time was only 2 seconds above normal, despite taking the same amount of warfarin. Her physician then learned that rifampin induces the liver to make a warfarin-inactivating enzyme. Rifampin was stopped and the

Table 30.2. Some Examples of Interaction of Antimicrobial Agents with Other Drugs

Antimicrobial Agent	Interacts with	Effect
Aminoglycosides	Anesthetics	Neuromuscular blockade (additive)
	Ethacrynic acid	Ototoxicity
Ampicillin	Oral contraceptives	Decreases gastrointestinal absorption
	Antacids	"
Erythromycin	Terfenadine	Fatal cardiac arrhythmias
	Digitalis	Increases concentration and toxicity
	Theophylline	Increases activity
	Cyclosporine	"
Rifampin	Anticoagulants	Decreases activity
	Digitoxin	"
	β-blockers	"
	Oral contraceptives	"
	Ketoconazole	"
	Corticosteroids	"
Isoniazid	Ketoconazole	Decreases absorption
Sulfonamides	Anticoagulants	Increases activity
	Methotrexate	"
Tetracyclines	Digitalis	Increases concentration and toxicity
	Oral contraceptives	Decreases gastrointestinal absorption
Amphotericin B	Digitalis	Decreases potassium concentration, enhances digitalis toxicity
Imidazoles	Cyclosporine	Increases activity (immunosuppression)

patient was treated with intravenous heparin to raise her clotting time.

This case is an example of the numerous interactions that occur between drugs. The potential consequences may be catastrophic for the patient, particularly if the therapy affected is life-saving, as in the case above. Imagine if the patient had required anticoagulation therapy to prevent clotting on an artificial heart valve. An opposite effect, prolongation of clotting time, may also occur with sulfonamides and metronidazole and lead to massive gastrointestinal bleeding. A list of prominent adverse drug interactions that involve antimicrobial agents is presented in Table 30.2. The severity of such complications cannot be overestimated and the message must not be lost on the practitioner.

PROPHYLACTIC USE OF ANTIMICROBIAL DRUGS

Soon after the introduction of effective antibacterial agents in the 1930s, it became clear that they could be used not only to treat infections but to prevent them as well. However, prophylaxis is a complex and controversial subject because the use of antibiotics to prevent infections carries risks as well as benefits. Antimicrobial drugs may be used prophylactically for two purposes:

- To prevent the acquisition of exogenous pathogens. An example is the administration of antibiotics to persons who are exposed to patients with menigo-

coccal infections. The meningococcus spreads rapidly among susceptible individuals, but antibiotics such as rifampin can usually forestall its clinical manifestations. Likewise, the antituberculous drug, isoniazid, is given to persons who are at high risk of acquiring tuberculosis, such as the children living in the same quarters as a patient with pulmonary tuberculosis (see Chapter 23, "Mycobacteria").

- To prevent commensal organisms from spreading from their usual residence to normally sterile sites of the body. The use of antibiotics to prevent postoperative infections after certain high-risk surgical procedures also falls in this category. An example is the administration of antibiotics to patients with damaged heart valves who are at risk of acquiring endocarditis. The drugs are used to prevent bacteremia and infection of damaged heart valves when such patients undergo dental or major or minor surgical procedures (see Chapter 12, "Streptococci").

The risks involved in antibiotic prophylaxis must be clearly understood. They include allergy or other toxic reactions to the drugs, selection of resistant mutants, and masking or delaying the diagnosis of the infection. The following criteria should be met for the prophylactic use of antibiotics:

- A surgical or medical intervention carries a significant risk of microbial contamination. Significant risk occurs when the surgeon crosses a tissue plane that contains a rich microbial flora, such as the colon or the oral cavity. In these areas, the risk of infection is unacceptably high and the administration of prophylactic antibiotics is necessary. Antibiotic prophylaxis should also be used when the risk of infection is low but its outcome is potentially disastrous, for instance in surgery for the implantation of heart valve or hip prostheses. Antibiotic prophylaxis is not indicated when the risk of infection is low and the outcome trivial, such as a hernia operation.

- The antibiotics used prophylactically should be directed against the most likely pathogens. Previous studies should suggest which infectious agents are likely to be involved and what drugs they are probably susceptible to. In operations involving the colon, antibiotics should cover the prime pathogens in the intestine. When surgery crosses the oral mucosa, prophylactic antibiotics with a narrow spectrum are indicated, because most of the bacteria in the oral cavity are susceptible to penicillin.

- A suitable concentration of the drug must be achievable at the right time in the relevant tissues. Studies in experimental animals (which have also been confirmed in randomized human studies) have shown that prophylactic antibiotics are of no value if given after surgery is completed. However, their effectiveness could be readily demonstrated if they are given just prior to surgery and adequate tissue levels are achieved. It makes sense that a drug should be present in the body when the wound is likely to be contaminated; once the wound is closed, it rapidly becomes impermeable to exogenous bacteria.

- Antimicrobial drugs should be used for a short time to minimize the emergence of drug resistance. Indications for the prophylactic use of antibiotics are expanding with the occurrence of new diseases, new drugs, and new therapeutic methods. The above guidelines should be applicable in the development of new indications.

SUGGESTED READINGS

Gold HS, Moellering RC. Antimicrobial-drug resistance. N Engl J Med 1996;335:1445–1454.

Handbook of antimicrobial therapy. The Medical Letter. Published yearly.

Hessen MT, Kaye D. Principles of selection and use of antibacterial agents. Inf Dis Clin North Am 1995;9:531–545.

Moellering RC. Principles of anti-infective therapy. In: Mandel GL, Bennett JE, Dolin R. eds. Principles and practice of infectious diseases. 4th ed. New York: Churchill Livingstone, 1995.

Sande MA, Mandel GL. Antimicrobial agents. General considerations. In: Gilman AG, Goodman LS, Rall TW, Murray F, eds. Pharmacological basis of therapeutics. 7th ed. New York: Macmillan, 1985.

Review of the Main Pathogenic Bacteria

These charts are intended to review the general features of the main human pathogenic bacteria. Included are the organisms of greatest medical relevance.

Many of the bacteria that cause relatively uncommon diseases were not included. Complete this chart as a method of reviewing this subject matter.

Organism	Gram Reaction, Morphology, Other Distinguishing Traits	Common Habitat and Mode of Encounter	Main Pathogenic Mechanism(s)	Typical Disease(s)	Relevant Chapters
Staphylococcus aureus					11, 61, 62, 73
Staphylococcus epidermidis					11, 67
Group A sreptococci					12, 61, 64
Other β-hemolytic streptococci					12, 69
α-Hemolytic streptococci					12, 64
Pneumococcus (S. pneumoniae)					13, 59
Meningococcus (Neisseria meningitidis)					14, 58
Gonococcus (N. gonorrhoeae)					14, 66
Haemophilus influenzae					58, 65
Bacteroides spp.					15, 61
Escherichia coli					16, 57, 60, 69, 73
Shigella spp.					17, 57
Klebsiella pneumoniae					16, 59, 67
Proteus spp.					16, 60
Vibrio cholerae					16, 57
Salmonella spp.					17, 57
Pseudomonas aeruginosa					18, 63, 67
Bordetella pertussis					19, 59

Organism	Gram Reaction, Morphology, Other Distinguishing Traits	Common Habitat and Mode of Encounter	Main Pathogenic Mechanism(s)	Typical Disease(s)	Relevant Chapters
Other enterics (*Enterobacter, Citrobacter, Serratia, Campylobacter, Yersinia*)					16, 57
Helicobacter pylori					22, 57
Clostridium difficile					20
C. botulinum					20
C. tetani					20
C. perfringens and others					20, 73
Legionella pneumophila					21
Mycobacterium tuberculosis and others					23, 59, 68
M. leprae					23
Treponema pallidum					24, 66
Borrelia burgdorferi					25, 66
Bartonella henselae					26
Chlamydia trachomatis					27, 66
Rickettsia spp.					28
Ehrlichia spp.					28
Mycoplasma spp.					29, 59

The following charts refer to pathogenic characteristics of bacteria. Complete these charts as a method of reviewing this subject matter.

Capsulated Bacteria of Medical Importance

Genus and Species		
1.	6.	
2.	7.	
3.	8.	
4.	9.	
5.		

Medically Important Strict Anaerobes

Genus and Species		
1.	6.	
2.	7.	
3.	8.	
4.	9.	
5.	10.	

Typically Pyogenic (pus-producing) Bacteria

Genus and Species		
1.	4.	
2.	5.	
3.	6.	

Major Bacterial Toxins

Genus and Species		
1.	4.	
2.	5.	
3.	6.	

Viruses

CHAPTER

31

Biology of Viruses

BERNARD N. FIELDS[1]

Key Concepts

Viruses:

- Are obligate intracellular parasites that use the host cell's machinery to replicate.
- Contain a nucleic acid core surrounded by a protein capsid; the capsid of some viruses is surrounded by an envelope.
- Are absorbed into host cells by first binding to receptors on the host cell; the virus then enters the particles by receptor-mediated endocytosis or crossing the host cell membrane via coated pits or fusion with the host cell membrane (enveloped viruses).
- Have single- or double-stranded RNA or DNA, which, following the adsorption of the virus into the host cell, is then translated inside the host cell to make viral proteins.
- Assemble new virus particles within the host cell, which are then released during cell lysis (nonenveloped viruses) or by budding (enveloped viruses).

Viral infection:

- Can be lytic, latent, or chronic.
- Can be acquired from other humans or from the environment; direct contact routes include sexual contact and vertical transmission and environmental routes include respiratory (aerosols), gastrointestinal (fecal-oral contamination), and transcutaneous (inoculation).
- Is often characterized by an incubation period; the virus replicates within the host.
- Can spread via nerves to the nervous system and via the blood to many organs. Many viruses spread via multiple pathways.
- Is curtailed within the host primarily through cell-mediated immunity.
- Can be diagnosed through culturing in cell cultures, embryonated eggs, or animals and immunocytochemical staining and identification of virus particles or antigens in tissue specimens.

The fundamental difference between viruses and all other infectious agents is in their mechanism of reproduction. Unlike cellular forms of life, viruses do not simply divide. Virus replication is carried out by the host cell machinery, which synthesizes multiple copies of the viral genome and viral proteins. These viral constituents assemble spontaneously within the host cell to form progeny virus particles. Viruses have no means to produce energy and contain a few enzymes at most. Thus, viruses are totally dependent on host cells; they are **obligate intracellular parasites**. Viruses are important pathogens of virtually all forms of life, including humans and other animals, plants, fungi, and bacteria. Because they are relatively amenable to study, viruses play a key

[1]Deceased

role as models in molecular biology. A description of viruses that infect bacteria, the **bacteriophages**, can be found in Chapter 4, "Genetics of Bacterial Pathogenesis."

Viruses are small, although the largest ones (e.g., the smallpox virus) are barely visible with the light microscope and fall within the lower size range of bacteria (e.g., the mycoplasmas or chlamydiae). Viruses vary in volume over a 1000-fold range and in structure from relatively simple to very complex (Fig. 31.1). The nucleic acid of a virus is either DNA or RNA, never both.

STRUCTURE AND CLASSIFICATION OF VIRUSES

A virus particle, called a **virion,** contains a **core** of either DNA or RNA surrounded by a protein shell and, in some cases, by a lipid envelope. The smallest viral genomes encode three or four proteins, the larger genomes more than 50 structural proteins and enzymes. The number of proteins encoded may be greater than predicted from the size of its nucleic acid because of the economic arrangement of some viral genomes; thus, the same stretch of nucleic acid may contain multiple open reading frames and/or overlapping regions that can be transcribed into several distinct mRNAs. Genetic researchers have determined the nucleotide sequence of part or all of the genomes of many viruses.

The viral nucleic acid is surrounded by a **capsid,** a single or double protein shell. Together, the nucleic acid and the capsid are referred to as the **nucleocapsid.** Capsids are composed of smaller repetitive subunits

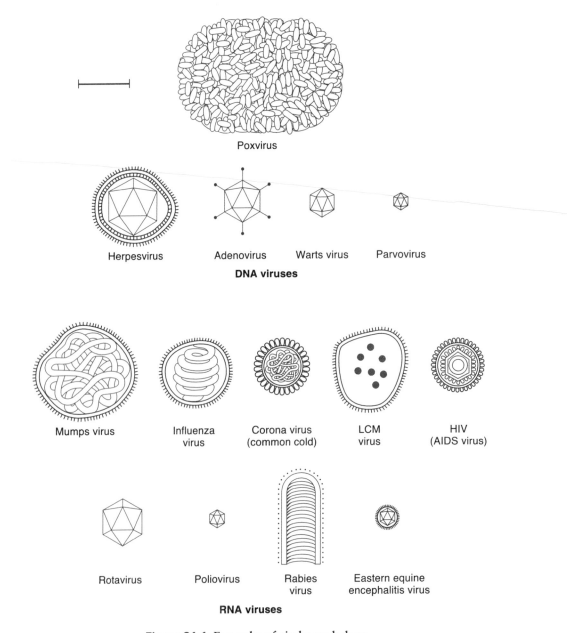

Figure 31.1. Examples of viral morphology.

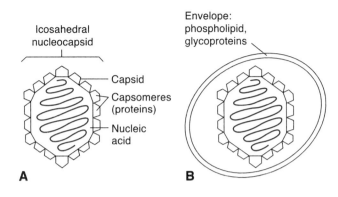

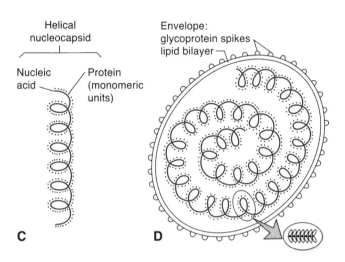

Figure 31.2. Basic viral forms. A. Icosahedral, nonenveloped; **B.** Icosahedral, enveloped; **C.** Helical, nonenveloped; **D.** Helical, enveloped. Inset depicts the nucleic acid–protein association.

(**capsomers**) arranged in symmetric patterns. The repeating subunits of viral proteins self-assemble into mature virions.

Capsomers are arranged in two fundamental patterns of capsid structural symmetry, **icosahedral** and **helical**. Viruses with icosahedral symmetry contain a defined number of structural subunits (20 triangular faces and 12 vertices), whereas this number varies in viruses with helical symmetry. Viruses with icosahedral symmetry generally follow simple principles of geometric organization (Fig. 31.2). In these viruses, the nucleic acid is usually condensed and is geometrically independent of the surrounding capsid structure. Retroviruses such as HIV, the virus that causes AIDS, have a mixed symmetry: icosahedral in the capsid, and helical in the nucleic acid core. Some of the largest viruses, such as the smallpox virus, have even more complex structural patterns.

Human viruses with helical symmetry invariably have RNA genomes. A general feature of these viruses is that the protein subunits of the capsid are bound in a regular, periodic fashion along the RNA. In sharp contrast to the loose interactions in viruses with icosahedral symmetry, this close interaction imposes constraints on viral assembly.

Many viruses possess an **envelope** that surrounds the nucleocapsid (see Fig. 31.2). These viruses are called **enveloped viruses**; viruses without an envelope are called **nonenveloped viruses**. The viral envelope is composed of virus-specific proteins plus lipids and carbohydrates derived from host cell membranes, e.g., the nuclear membrane, endoplasmic reticulum, Golgi apparatus, or plasma membrane. In some cases, the viral-specific envelope proteins include a **matrix protein** (**M protein**) that lines the inner side of the envelope and is in contact with the nucleocapsid (Fig. 31.3). Viral-specific glycoproteins may protrude from the outer surface of the envelope, forming structures known as **spikes**. Certain viruses contain surface glycoproteins that agglutinate red blood cells (**hemagglutinins**) by binding to receptors on the red cell surface.

A large number of viruses carry out **virion-associated enzymatic activities**, depending on the strategy used for replication of their nucleic acid. The viral enzyme that makes virus-specific mRNA, which is required for the synthesis of all viral proteins, may be an RNA-dependent RNA polymerase (**RNA transcriptases**) or a DNA-

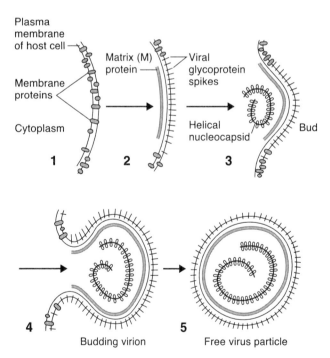

Figure 31.3. Viral budding through the cytoplasmic membrane. *1.* The host cell plasma membrane seen early in infection. *2.* Viral encoded M protein molecules become associated with the plasma membrane. Viral glycoprotein spikes are incorporated in the membrane. *3.* The viral nucleocapsid is assembled near the membrane and budding begins. *4.* Budding continues with further insertion of viral spikes in the membrane. *5.* Budding is completed, releasing a free virion.

Table 31.1. Classification of Viruses

Family	Example	Nucleic acid polarity or structure	Genome size, kilobases or kilobase pairs	Envelope	Capsid symmetry
RNA Viruses					
Single-stranded					
Picornaviridae	Poliovirus	(+)	7.2–8.4	No	I
Togaviridae	Rubella virus	(+)	12	Yes	I
Flaviviridae	Yellow fever virus	(+)	10	Yes	I
Coronaviridae	Coronaviruses	(+)	16–21	Yes	H
Rhabdoviridae	Rabies virus	(−)	13–16	Yes	H
Paramyxoviridae	Measles virus	(−)	16–20	Yes	H
Orthomyxoviridae	Influenza viruses	(−) segments[a]	14	Yes	H
Bunyaviridae	Hantavirus	Three circular (−) segments	13–21	Yes	H
Arenaviridae	Lassa fever virus	Two circular (−)	10–14	Yes	H
Retroviridae	HIV	Two identical molecules (+)	3–9	Yes	I-capsid H-nucleocapsid (probable)
Double-stranded					
Reoviridae	Rotaviruses	10–12 segments[b]	16–27	No	I
DNA Viruses					
Single-stranded					
Parvoviridae	Human parvovirus B-19	ss (+) or (−)	5	No	I
Mixed strandedness					
Hepadnaviridae	Hepatitis B	ds with ss portions	3	Yes	Unk
Double-stranded					
Papovaviridae	JC virus	Circular	8	No	I
Adenoviridae	Human adenoviruses		36–38	No	I
Herpesviridae	Herpes simplex virus		120–220	Yes	I
Poxviridae	Vaccinia	Covalently closed ends	130–280	Yes	Complex

[a] Influenza C = 7 segments.
[b] Reovirus, orbivirus = 10 segments; rotavirus = 11 segments; Colorado tick fever = 12 segments.
Note: (+) message sense; (−) anti-message sense; I = icosahedral; H = helical; Unk = unknown.

dependent RNA polymerase. Retroviruses contain an RNA-dependent DNA polymerase known as **reverse transcriptase.** Some viruses have mRNA processing enzymes such as "capping enzymes" which modify viral mRNAs at their 5 end by adding a methylguanosine cap, or enzymes that polyadenylate the 3 end of viral mRNA. Additional virally encoded enzymes include protein kinases, nucleoside triphosphate phosphatases, endonucleases, and RNAses. Certain viruses, such as the influenza viruses, have enzymes on their surface (e.g., neuraminidase) that are involved in the attachment to host cells.

The principal viruses that cause disease in humans belong to about a dozen different families containing hundreds of kinds. Each kind often contains a number of individual strains which differ in virulence and antigenic properties (serotypes). Viruses are classified using a combination of genetic, physicochemical, and biological factors. These include the type and structure of the viral nucleic acid (single- or double-stranded RNA or DNA), the nature of virion ultrastructure (including size, type of capsid symmetry, and the presence or absence of an envelope), as well as their strategy for genome replication (Table 31.1, Fig. 31.4). In many instances, electron-micrographic studies provide sufficient information to identify both the family and the genus to which a virus belongs. Subdivisions within these major taxonomic groups are usually based on immunologic, cytopathologic, pathogenetic, or epidemiologic features. The current classification of viruses will probably be revised as increased knowledge of their nucleic acid sequences permits assessment of the degree of their genetic relatedness.

VIRAL REPLICATION

The steps in viral replication include infection of a susceptible cell, reproduction of the nucleic acid and proteins, and assembly and release of infectious progeny. The structural and genetic diversity of viruses is reflected in the variety of replicative strategies employed by viruses.

Attachment and Penetration

The first stage of viral infection of target cells begins with adsorption of the virus particles and ends when the first infectious progeny viruses are formed. During this

stage, called the **eclipse period**, a dramatic drop occurs in the amount of infectious virus that can be recovered from disrupted cells.

The first step in the attachment of viruses to host cells is **adsorption**, an initially reversible step resulting from random collisions between virions and target cells. Approximately one in 10^3 to 10^4 such collisions leads to tighter binding. Although attachment requires appropriate ionic and pH conditions, it is largely temperature-independent and does not require energy. The next step involves the specific binding of viral proteins to receptors on the host cell surface. The virion structure that mediates cell attachment has been identified for a number of viruses. For enveloped viruses, the viral attachment protein is typically one of the spikes inserted on the outer surface of the viral envelope, such as the hemagglutinin of influenza viruses. Some enveloped viruses,

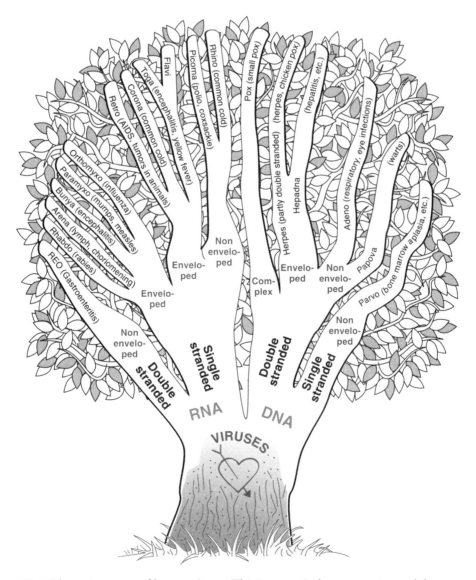

Figure 31.4. The main groups of human viruses. This is a practical representation and does not represent phylogenetic relationships.

such as the herpesviruses and vaccinia, have more than one type of cell attachment protein. In nonenveloped viruses, surface peptides often function as viral attachment proteins.

The nature of the cellular receptors for animal viruses has been determined in only a few specific cases. Even when the specific receptor is still unknown, it has been possible to identify "families" or classes of cellular receptors using competition binding studies. Viruses of the same species but different serotypes may compete for the same receptors of the same class (e.g., poliovirus serotypes 1, 2, 3) or different classes (e.g., human rhinovirus 2 and 14). Viruses from different families may also compete for the same class of receptor. Binding studies suggest that approximately 10^4 to 10^6 viral binding sites (receptors) are present per cell.

Once adsorption has occurred, the entire virion or a substructure containing the viral genome and virion polymerases must be translocated across the plasma membrane of the host cell. The rate of penetration depends on the nature of the virus, the type of host cell, and environmental factors such as temperature. Some nonenveloped viruses such as poliovirus undergo a process of receptor-mediated endocytosis (**viropexis**) and appear in the cytoplasm within endocytic vesicles (endosomes). Other nonenveloped viruses probably cross the plasma membrane directly and appear free in the cytoplasm without endocytic vesicles.

Enveloped viruses use at least two strategies for penetration. The first is exemplified by Semliki Forest virus. This virus binds to specific cell-surface receptors which then aggregate at distinct sites on the plasma membrane (**coated pits**) and are internalized by receptor-mediated endocytosis. The virions subsequently appear inside clathrin-coated vesicles within the cell cytoplasm (Fig. 31.5). The viral envelope then fuses with the endosomal membrane, releasing the viral nucleocapsid into the cytoplasm. A second mechanism for penetration of en-

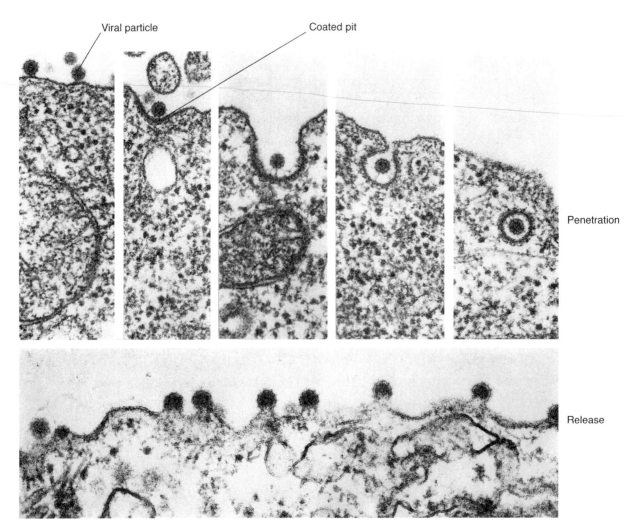

Figure 31.5. Penetration and release of an enveloped virus (Semliki Forest virus). The top five thin sections show stages in adherence of the virus to clathrin-coated pits and the gradual invagination of the membrane carrying the virus into the interior within a clathrin-coated endosome. The bottom section shows the release of the virus by budding from the membrane.

veloped viruses is exemplified by paramyxoviruses (e.g., Sendai virus), in which the viral envelope fuses directly with the cell plasma membrane and the viral nucleocapsid is discharged free into the cytoplasm.

The next step in viral replication is **uncoating**, the process of removing or disaggregating part or all of the viral capsid in order to make the viral genome accessible to the host cell's transcription and translation machinery. In many viruses, penetration and uncoating occur simultaneously. Certain viruses undergo an alteration in capsid structure leading to a loss of an internal protein as they are translocated across the plasma membrane. Structural alterations associated with loss of this protein may facilitate entry of the viral nucleic acid into the cytoplasm.

Nonenveloped viruses may induce *fusion of lysosomes with the endosome,* leading to removal of their capsids by lysosomal enzymes. In certain reoviruses, endosomal proteases sequentially remove the outer capsid proteins to produce a "subviral particle." During this process, the viral transcriptase becomes activated. Uncoating of poxviruses, such as vaccinia, takes place in two steps: first, the outer protein coat is degraded by endosomal enzymes; second, the remaining nucleocapsid is degraded, liberating the viral DNA.

Macromolecular Synthesis

The synthesis of all viral macromolecules first requires the translation of viral messenger RNA (mRNA) into virus-specific proteins. How is viral mRNA made? Viruses that contain double-stranded DNA synthesize mRNA in the same way as the host cell, using a DNA-dependent RNA polymerase. RNA viruses, however, must make their mRNA from RNA, which involves a different mechanism. A number of strategies have evolved to synthesize viral mRNA by transcription of viral genomes as well as for the translation of this mRNA into protein (Fig. 31.6). These variations are described in detail in chapters on individual virus groups (Chapters 32 to 42).

Single-stranded positive polarity RNA viruses

The simplest translation strategy is for the nucleic acid of the virion to function directly as mRNA. Examples of viruses that use this approach are the picornaviruses (e.g., poliovirus) and togaviruses (e.g., Eastern equine encephalitis virus). By convention, the genomes of these viruses are said to have positive (+) **strand polarity.** Upon entry into the host cell, the mRNA is translated to produce the various viral proteins. In certain viruses, such as poliovirus, cellular ribosomes bind to the mRNA to form large polyribosomes that produce a single large polyprotein. This large precursor molecule is then cleaved in a series of proteolytic steps to produce the proteins of the core and the capsid. Note that this unusual arrangement results in the synthesis of equimolar amounts of each viral protein.

In these viruses, how is the viral RNA synthesized? Here, a **virally encoded RNA polymerase** known as **transcriptase** synthesizes a complementary (-) **strand** RNA using the genomic RNA as template. In turn, the newly synthesized RNA serves as template for the synthesis of more genomic (+) strand RNA. The new genomic RNAs may serve either as mRNAs or as precursor RNAs for progeny virions.

Single-stranded negative polarity RNA viruses

The RNA of negative-strand viruses does not carry coding sequences for proteins; only its complementary strand does. Therefore, these viruses must use a different strategy to make mRNA. Here the genome is replicated via a (+) single-stranded RNA intermediate, which then serves as a template to synthesize more (-) single stranded genomic RNA. Mammalian cells do not possess enzymes that use RNA as templates for making RNA. Viruses that use this strategy must therefore contain an RNA transcriptase in their virion, which is introduced into the host cells during infection.

Some (-) single-stranded RNA viruses (e.g., influenza viruses) have **segmented genomes** consisting of more than one RNA molecule. RNA replication results in a unique mRNA for each viral protein rather than a single large polycistronic mRNA molecule. The presence of multiple mRNAs allows the synthesis of each viral protein to be regulated independently, thus allowing for the production of different amounts of individual virally encoded proteins. Other viruses have evolved a particularly economic way of using a given amount of genetic information: A single region of genomic RNA may have multiple reading frames, each of which is transcribed into unique mRNAs, which are in turn translated into distinct proteins.

Double-stranded RNA viruses

As with DNA, the information contained in double-stranded RNA must first be copied into a (+) single strand of RNA to act as mRNA. Because of its double-strandedness, the virion RNA cannot function directly as mRNA (even though it contains a [+] strand). Viruses with double-stranded RNA genomes, such as the reoviruses, contain a virally encoded RNA-transcriptase that transcribes (+) single-stranded RNAs from the (-) strands of the viral genome. The double-stranded RNA genome is always found as segments, each of which results in a unique mRNA.

RNA viruses that replicate via a DNA intermediate

The retroviruses (such as HIV) contain (+) single-stranded RNA but employ a unique replicative strategy using a DNA intermediate. Viral (+) single-stranded

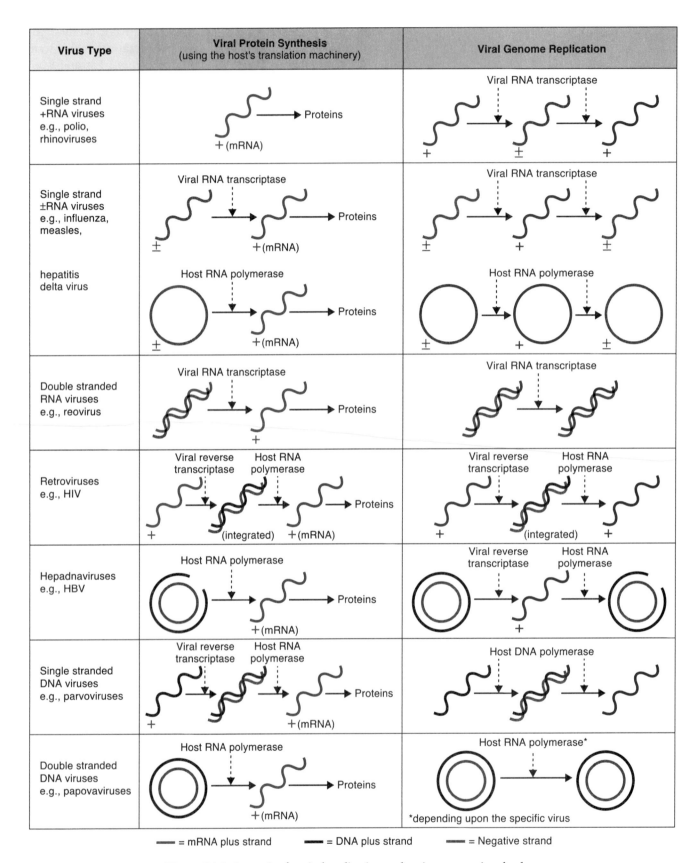

Figure 31.6. Strategies for viral replication and main enzymes involved.

RNA serves as a template for a virion RNA-dependent DNA polymerase (reverse transcriptase). The DNA is then integrated into host chromosomal DNA, where it may reside for a long time. In this regard, integrated retroviruses resemble the prophages of lysogenic bacteriophages. Like the chromosomal DNA, transcription of the integrated viral DNA is carried out by the host cell RNA polymerases.

DNA viruses

In general, DNA-containing viruses make mRNA using strategies similar to those of eukaryotic cells. In cells infected with papovaviruses (e.g., warts viruses), adenoviruses, and herpesviruses, transcription of viral DNA into mRNA occurs in the nucleus of the host cell and depends on host cell enzymes. In the case of papovaviruses (e.g., the oncogenic monkey virus called SV40), the initial proteins produced after infection are called **T antigens** (**tumor antigens**). Because they are the first viral proteins to be synthesized, T antigens are also called **early proteins**. Some T antigens enhance DNA replication by binding near the site of initiation of DNA replication. Subsequently, mRNAs encoding the capsid polypeptides (**late proteins**) are transcribed. In SV40 virus, the early mRNAs are derived from only one of the two viral DNA strands (referred to as the **E** or **Early** strand), and the late mRNAs from the other (the **L** or **Late** strand). Adenoviruses also have early and late genes, but they are intermixed along both strands of the viral DNA rather than on separate strands.

The individual mRNAs for both early and late proteins often correspond to sequences of viral DNA (**exons**) separated by spacer sequences, called **introns**. The products of transcription are RNA molecules with sequence the same as that of the DNA. These immature mRNA molecules are then extensively cut and spliced, which removes the intervening introns. In many viruses, mRNAs are synthesized from overlapping regions of the viral DNA. This redundancy reduces the amount of viral DNA needed to encode some viral proteins and is another example of genetic economy among the viruses.

Poxviruses are the most structurally intricate of the animal viruses, and their replicative cycle is correspondingly complex. The initial steps of transcription and translation occur in the host cell cytoplasm; hence, these viruses cannot use the host RNA polymerases, which are localized in the nucleus. Consequently, poxviruses carry their own DNA-dependent RNA polymerase to initiate transcription. One of the virus-encoded early proteins is responsible for a second stage of uncoating in which the viral DNA is made fully accessible for transcription and replication. Replication, transcription, and later viral assembly all occur in virus-initiated "factories" within the host cell cytoplasm. Early proteins include a number of enzymes (e.g., a DNA polymerase and a thymidine kinase), as well as some structural proteins. As infection

proceeds, DNA replication begins, the synthesis of the early nonstructural proteins ceases, and the synthesis of late proteins takes place. Many of the late proteins are structural proteins, but other late proteins include enzymes and proteins that appear to play a role in viral assembly.

Assembly of Progeny Virions and Release from the Host Cell

Once replication of the viral genome and synthesis of the viral proteins are complete, intact virions are assembled and released from the host cells. Assembly of the nonenveloped viruses and the nucleocapsid of enveloped viruses often proceed by the self-assembly of viral capsomers into crystal-like arrays. Once the capsid is formed, it becomes filled with the viral nucleic acid to make a viable virion (Fig. 31. 7).

Nonenveloped virions are usually released when the cell lyses. Events leading to cell disruption include inhibition of the synthesis of host cell macromolecules and lipids, disorganization of the host cell cytoskeleton, and alteration of host cell membrane structure. Membrane disruption may result in increased cell permeability and the release of proteolytic enzymes from lysosomes. The host cell's failure to replenish energy-rich substrate molecules inhibits the function of ion transport pumps and disturbs transport of essential nutrients and cellular waste products.

Enveloped viruses are typically released from infected cells by budding. This process may or may not be lethal to the cell. In all cases, virus-specified proteins inserted

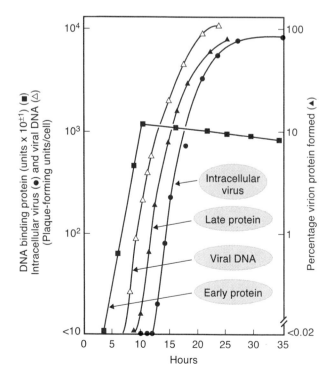

Figure 31.7. Adenovirus replication in cell culture.

into host cell membranes displace some of its normal protein components, which results in the restructuring of the membrane. Viral capsids may then bind to virus-specified matrix proteins lining the cytoplasmic side of these altered patches of membrane (see Fig. 31.3). In the smallest enveloped viruses, the togaviruses, the capsids bind directly to intracytoplasmic domains of viral proteins inserted in the host cell membrane, rather than to matrix proteins.

Defective Viruses and Virioids

Certain viruses cause disease even though they cannot replicate autonomously. In order to replicate, such **defective viruses** (e.g., the hepatitis delta virus) require coinfection with a "helper" virus. Infection with the delta virus is dependent on a coincident infection with hepatitis B virus (HBV) and does not occur in its absence. Coinfection with HBV and the delta virus frequently results in fulminant hepatitis, apparently by allowing the derepression and increased multiplication of HBV. Conversely, the defective adeno-associated human parvoviruses do not significantly alter the disease caused by the helper adenovirus alone. Defective viruses can only be detected by searching for their antigens using specific nucleic acid probes, or inducing their replication by the addition of helper viruses.

Recently researchers have discovered a new class of infectious agents, the **virioids**. Virioids (along with prions, see below) are the smallest known agents of disease. Virioids cause disease in plants and consist of naked, covalently closed circles of single-stranded RNA less than 300–400 nucleotides in length. In spite of this very small size, virioids replicate without the help of viruses. How they replicate and cause disease remains unknown.

PRIONS

Prions are transmissible agents that appear to defy the central tenet of biology. They are widely believed to consist of "infectious proteins," rather than nucleic acid containing viruses or microorganisms. How, then, would they transmit genetic information? The question has great clinical as well as biological importance because prions cause a number of fatal neurologic diseases, such as Creutzfeld-Jakob disease (CJD) and kuru in humans (see Chapter 34, "Paramyxoviruses"), scrapie in sheep, and more recently, bovine spongiform encephalopathy (BSE or "mad cow disease") in cattle.

There is considerable evidence—including sensitive chemical analysis and physical measurements—to suggest that prions do not contain nucleic acids. Instead, they consist of a single protein which is almost certainly the transmissible agent of disease. An understanding of the biological nature of prions came from the finding that the prion protein (called PrP^{sc}) has the same amino acid sequence as a normal cellular protein of unknown

function (PrP^c), which is encoded by a cellular gene. These two forms of PrP differ only in their folded conformation. In the PrP^{sc} conformation, the protein is highly resistant to digestion with proteolytic enzymes, protein denaturing reagents, and high temperature. It appears that the two forms of the protein, PrP^{sc} and PrP^c, can combine to make dimers. The PrP^{sc} form can function as a template, "teaching" the PrP^c form to assume the PrP^{sc} conformation. Once PrP^{sc} is formed, this process of conversion is continuous and ongoing as more PrP^c is synthesized in neural tissue. Therefore, the transmissible agent (prion) does not transmit primary sequence information but rather the ability to function as a template for improper molecular folding.

Prion-infected material can be transmitted by direct inoculation into the CNS, by percutaneous exposure, or by ingestion. In the case of kuru, the disease was transmitted and sustained by ritualistic cannibalism of human brains among certain New Guinea natives. Similarly, a recent epidemic of "mad cow disease" (BSE) in Great Britain was attributed to the practice of refeeding offal from slaughterhouses (including neural tissues from slaughtered cows) to younger cattle as a source of protein. Transmission of CJD to humans has been associated with grafting of human tissues (e.g., corneal transplants, dura mater grafts) and with treatment with human pituitary gland extracts. In addition, cases of a novel form of the human disease ("new variant CJD") have appeared in Great Britain in the wake of the "mad cow" epidemic. It is widely believed that these novel human infections were acquired by eating meat from cattle infected with BSE.

In all prion diseases, the accumulation of nondegradable PrP proteins in the brain and spinal cord eventually results in neurological degeneration. The diseases caused by prions are referred to as **transmissible spongiform encephalopathies**, because of the telltale pathological alterations, readily seen spongy cavitations in the brain. With minor variations, all of the prion diseases manifest this pathology, since all of the known diseases are associated with aberrantly folded PrP. Fortunately, these human diseases are very rare and transmission of prions from animals to humans occurs with less efficiency than between animals.

THE PATHOBIOLOGY OF VIRAL DISEASES

The signs and symptoms of disease are the culmination of a series of interactions between the virus and the host. After encountering a host cell, a virus must be able to enter it, undergo a period of primary replication, and then spread to its final target tissue. Once a virus reaches its target organs, it must then infect and successfully replicate in a susceptible population of host cells.

Three possible outcomes follow infection of a host cell by a virus: lytic infection, latent infection, or chronic infection (Fig. 31.8). In a **lytic infection,** the virus undergoes multiple rounds of replication. This replication results in the death of the host cell, which is used as a factory for virus production. The number of viral particles produced in a single cell during lytic infection varies from a few with some viruses to thousands with others. Examples of lytic infections are those caused by polio or influenza viruses.

At the opposite end of the spectrum is a **latent infection,** which does not result in the immediate production of progeny virus. Latent infections, which are usually caused by DNA viruses or retroviruses, reflect the persistence of viral DNA either as an extrachromosomal element (as with some herpes viruses), or an integrated sequence into the host cell (as with the retroviruses). During cell growth, the genome of the virus is replicated along with the chromosomes of the host cell. An example of latent infection is that produced by herpes simplex virus type 1 (HSV-1). Upon **reactivation** of the herpes simplex virus, fever blisters or cold sores result. In the cases of a retrovirus, latent infections may result in **transformation** of the cell, a cancerous state.

A **chronic infection** differs from a lytic and a latent infection in that virus particles continue to be shed after the period of acute illness has passed. It is marked by a slow release of virus particles without death of the host cell and any other overt injury. This kind of infection is usually associated with RNA viruses. The amount of virus produced is usually lower than in lytic infections, and the viruses are often altered ("mutated") from the original ones. Chronic infections are associated with a defective host immunity that is too weak to rid the body of the infection. Often, chronic infections do not result in overt disease. Hepatitis B virus causes a persistent infection in the liver that may lead to chronic hepatitis and even liver cancer.

Encounter and Entry

Transmission of a virus from an infected host to a susceptible individual may occur in a variety of ways. The source of human-to-human transmission of viruses are acutely ill individuals, or chronic carriers; pregnant women can also transmit viruses to fetuses. Transmission may be accomplished by direct contact, such as sexual contact (as in AIDS) or via the environment. Environmental spread may involve fecal-oral contamination (as in the diarrhea caused by rotaviruses), aerosols (as in chickenpox), or direct inoculation via infected needles or blood products (as in hepatitis B). Animal-to-human transmission usually takes place via the bite of the diseased animal itself (as in rabies) or via the bite of an insect vector (as in viral encephalitis).

For most viruses, it is not known how many particles are required to initiate a respiratory infection. For influenza A, adenovirus, or coxsackie A21 virus, as few as 10 particles may suffice. In other cases, the number is likely to be considerably larger.

The respiratory route

Respiratory infection takes place by means of aerosol droplets, nasal secretions, or saliva. Respiratory aerosolization usually occurs via coughing or sneezing. A sneeze may generate up to 2 million aerosol particles, and a cough up to 90,000. The fate of these particles depends both on ambient environmental conditions (e.g., humidity, wind currents) and particle size. Small particles remain airborne longer and may escape the filtering action of the nose, which traps particles larger than 6 μm in diameter. The number of viral particles aerosolized sometimes varies even for different strains of the same virus. Aerosolization is not the only possible route of respiratory transmission. Epstein-Barr virus (EBV) is typically spread by saliva during kissing. A critical pathway of spread for rhinoviruses that cause the common cold, is, surprisingly, not via aerosols but from hands to eyes, nose, or mouth—a cycle that can be interrupted by hand washing.

Entry via the respiratory route requires that the virus overcome a formidable series of host defenses. In the lung, immunologic defenses include secretory IgA, natural killer (NK) cells, and macrophages. Nonspecific glycoprotein viral inhibitors are present in tracheobronchial mucus. Ciliated respiratory epithelial cells continually sweep mucus up from the lower respiratory tract into the upper respiratory tract, where it is usually swallowed.

The gastrointestinal route

Gastrointestinal transmission occurs when viruses shed in feces contaminate food or water, which is then ingested by a susceptible individual ("fecal-oral spread"). Stool-tainted hands, resulting from poor personal hygiene, provide another vehicle of spread for enteric viruses. The high incidence of enteric virus infections in infant day care centers and institutions for the mentally impaired reflects the difficulty of maintaining hygiene in these settings.

Gastrointestinal transmission is limited to those viruses that can withstand the internal environment of the gastrointestinal tract. The harsh acidic environment

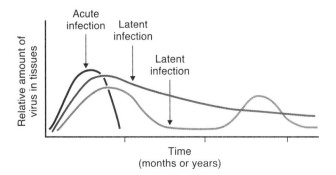

Figure 31. 8. The three types of viral infections.

of the stomach inactivates acid-labile viruses such as rhinoviruses. Bile salts, present in the lumen of the small intestine, can destroy the lipid envelope of many viruses and may account for the fact that entry via the gastrointestinal route is limited largely to nonenveloped viruses. Proteolytic enzymes and secretory IgA also contribute to host antiviral defenses in the gastrointestinal tract. Certain proteolysis-resistant viral capsid proteins allow some viruses to withstand digestion in the gut.

In some enteric viruses, passage across the mucosal barrier of the gut is mediated by a specific population of cells overlying Peyer's patches known as **microfold (M)** cells. These cells, and perhaps their analogs in bronchial lymphoid tissue, appear to facilitate transport of some viruses, including reoviruses and possibly enteroviruses, across the small intestine.

The transcutaneous route

The stratum corneum of the skin provides both a physical and biological barrier against the entry of viruses. Some viruses overcome the skin barrier by direct inoculation via insect or animal bites or via mechanical devices such as needles.

In viral diseases in which the vector is an insect or an infected animal, the disease cycle may be complex. For example, dengue fever is characterized by a continuous cycle between humans and infected mosquitoes. Dengue viruses multiply in the gut of a mosquito, spread to its salivary glands, and are injected into a human during the mosquito's blood meal. Viral replication within the host leads to a high-titer level of viruses in the bloodstream (**viremia**) which is sufficient to allow the viruses to be picked up by an uninfected mosquito during biting. In other arthropod-borne virus infections, the human being is a "dead-end host" because the degree of viremia in infected individuals is insufficient to transmit the infection to a new group of insect vectors. Examples of this type of cycle are found in the togaviruses, such as various equine encephalitis viruses. The normal animal reservoirs for these *arbo*-*borne* viruses (*arbo*viruses) include small birds and mammals. Horses, like humans, are usually dead-end hosts, although in Venezuelan equine encephalitis, horses may be a reservoir of virus.

Some arbovirus infections do not require a viremic vertebrate intermediate host. The virus is passed in transovarian fashion to the progeny of an infected tick or mosquito or by sexual transmission between male and female mosquitoes. Transovarian transmission may allow survival of arthropod viruses through the winter months.

Iatrogenic inoculation (induced by medical or diagnostic procedures) sometimes allows the entry of a large number of viruses. Hepatitis B virus (HBV), cytomegalovirus (CMV), and human immunodeficiency virus (HIV) may all be present in contaminated blood products used for transfusion. Infected corneal transplants, instruments used in neurosurgical procedures, and pituitary tissues used to prepare growth hormone have been implicated as causes of Creutzfeldt-Jakob disease. Iatrogenic inoculation may be purposeful and benevolent, as in the case of parenteral vaccination using live attenuated virus (e.g., the measles or Sabin polio vaccines).

The sexual route

Sexual transmission with entry across the genitourinary or rectal mucosa is important for herpes simplex virus type 2 (HSV-2), CMV, hepatitis B virus, and HIV. Often, the virus spreads to other organs of the body but in some viruses, e.g., HSV-2, lesions are often found near the site of entry.

Endogenous and exogenous viruses

Most viral diseases result from exposure to **exogenous** virus. However, some viral diseases result from the reactivation of an **endogenous** virus which has been latent within specific host cells. Examples of infections caused by reactivated endogenous viruses include shingles (herpes zoster), progressive multifocal leukoencephalopathy (caused by JC or BK papovaviruses), recurrent labial and genital herpes (herpes simplex virus), and some types of cytomegalovirus infections.

In the majority of viral diseases, transmission of viruses occurs between members of a susceptible host population (**horizontal spread**). **Vertical spread** of infection occurs when the fetus becomes infected in utero through virus carried in the germ cell line, virus infecting the placenta, or virus in the maternal birth canal. Rubella virus, cytomegalovirus, herpes simplex virus, varicella-zoster virus (VZV), and hepatitis B virus can all produce vertically transmitted congenital infections.

Multiplication and Spread

For some viruses, the processes of entry, primary replication, and tissue tropism all occur at the same anatomic site. Examples of this type of viral infection include the upper and lower respiratory infections caused by the rhinoviruses, ortho- and paramyxoviruses; the enteritis caused by rotaviruses; and the dermatologic lesions induced by human papillomavirus (warts). Other viruses enter at one site and, to produce disease, subsequently spread to a distant area, such as the central nervous system. In these diseases, it is useful to distinguish between primary viral multiplication near the entry site and secondary multiplication at the eventual target organ or tissue. Enteroviruses enter via the gastrointestinal tract and spread to the CNS to produce meningitis, encephalitis, and/or poliomyelitis. Measles virus and varicella virus enter the body through the respiratory tract but then spread to produce skin disease (exanthem) and often generalized organ involvement. Neural, hematogenous, and lymphatic pathways are all used by viruses to spread to target tissues.

A great deal of viral replication may occur before any signs or symptoms of clinical illness are detectable. This **incubation period** varies from a few days (influenza), to weeks (measles, varicella), to months (rabies, hepatitis), to years (prions). Viral infection does not always lead to overt clinical disease. The percentage of those infected who develop overt disease ranges from 100% (rabies, measles) to 0 (BK, JC papovaviruses. For many viral infections, symptomatic disease is less common in children than in adults (e.g., EBV mononucleosis, paralytic poliomyelitis, hepatitis A virus infection).

Neural spread

Examples of agents that spread via nerves include the rabies virus, herpes simplex virus, chickenpox (varicella-zoster) virus, and the scrapie agent of sheep. The herpes simplex virus apparently enters the nerves via receptors located primarily near synaptic endings rather than on the nerve cell body. Rabies virus accumulates at the motor end plate of the neuromuscular junction (NMJ) and may utilize the acetylcholine receptor (AChR) or a closely related structure to enter the distal axons of motor neurons. Rabies virus also infects muscle and spreads via motor and sensory nerves to the spinal cord.

The kinetics of neural spread for rabies, herpes simplex, and polio strongly suggest that these agents use intraneuronal mechanisms involved in fast axonal transport. The scrapie agent of sheep appears to spread slowly along neural pathways and may be an example of movement via slow axonal transport. Infection of Schwann cells may provide another "neural" pathway to the CNS. Neural spread is important not only for entry into the CNS but also for spread within the CNS and from the CNS to the periphery (as in herpetic infections).

The olfactory pathway represents a special category of neural spread. The rod processes of olfactory receptor cells lie exposed in the olfactory mucosa and are the only place in the body where the nervous system is in direct contact with the environment. Experimental, intranasal or aerosol inoculations of rabies virus, herpes simplex virus, poliovirus, and some togaviruses have led to CNS infection via the olfactory route. This route may provide a pathway to the CNS in humans for rabies, and possibly other viruses in circumstances where high-titer aerosols are present, such as in caves occupied by large numbers of rabid bats or in accidental laboratory-acquired infections. The olfactory route of spread might explain the localization of herpes simplex virus in the orbitofrontal and medial temporal cortex in cases of herpes simplex encephalitis.

Hematogenous spread

Hematogenous spread is an important mechanism for many viruses. A period of primary replication usually precedes the initial viremia and may be asymptomatic or result in prodromal symptoms. For enteric viruses, primary replication occurs in Peyer's patches and peritonsillar lymphatic tissue. For respiratory viruses, primary replication takes place in epithelial or alveolar cells; for many enteroviruses and togaviruses, in skeletal muscle. In some cases virus travels via the lymphatic system, from the site of initial multiplication to regional lymph nodes before entering the bloodstream. The initial (primary) viremia often disseminates the virus to tissues such as the spleen and liver where continued multiplication in parenchymal cells leads to an amplified secondary viremia. Growth in endothelial cells may help sustain the viremic phase in some togavirus infections. Sustained secondary amplification of the viremia is required if a virus is to overcome clearance by lymphoreticular cells.

Blood-borne virus particles may travel free or in association with cellular elements. Hepatitis B virus, picornaviruses, and togaviruses all travel free within plasma; Colorado tick fever virus and Rift valley fever virus are associated with red blood cells; Epstein-Barr virus, cytomegalovirus, rubella, and human immunodeficiency virus are lymphocyte- or monocyte-associated.

Multiple pathways for spread

Some viruses use different pathways of spread at different stages in the infectious cycle. Varicella-zoster virus disseminates to the skin by the hematogenous route to produce "chickenpox," then spreads centripetally along nerves from the skin to neurons in the dorsal root ganglion where it remains latent. Reactivation results in centrifugal spread of virus down sensory nerves to their skin dermatome and the production of "shingles" (zoster). Neural spread of virus presumably accounts for recurrent episodes of oral and genital infection caused by the herpes simplex virus. Poliovirus is an example of a virus capable of spreading by both hematogenous and neural routes. The hematogenous route is generally accepted as the primary pathway to the CNS, although the virus may spread to the CNS via autonomic nerves in the gut. Axonal transport may play a role in the spread of poliovirus within the CNS.

HOST FACTORS IN DEFENSE AND DAMAGE

A large number of constitutive and induced host defenses are involved in viral infections. The age and genetic make-up of the host have important implications for the outcome of certain viral infections. Newborns, for example, are particularly susceptible to severe disseminated herpes simplex virus infections. In contrast, many of the exanthematous illnesses, poliovirus infection, and Epstein-Barr virus infection are typically more severe in older individuals than in children. In mice, specific genes help determine susceptibility to certain viral infections, acting through effects on the immune system, interferon production, or viral receptors. Inadequate host nutritional status may increase susceptibility to infections such as measles, perhaps by depressing cell-mediated immunity. This association accounts for the high mortality associated with measles in some developing countries. The host may also influence viral infections in other ways that are still poorly understood. Stress may trigger recurrent fever blisters (herpes labialis). Strenuous exercise may have an adverse effect on the course of polio.

The most important induced defense mechanism against viral infections is usually cell-mediated immunity. Patients with defective cell immunity but normal antibody-forming capacity often recover poorly from viral infections. Conversely, patients who lack antibodies but have normal cell-mediated immunity responses do not ordinarily suffer abnormally from viral diseases. Phagocytosis by neutrophils does not play as important a role in viral as in bacterial infections. Macrophages, on the other hand, are often involved in viral containment as well as in the spread of viruses in the body.

The Antibody Response

Most viruses are sufficiently antigenics to stimulate the immune response. Viruses contain a large number of foreign proteins, each of which may contain multiple antigenic sites. In addition, although the amount of viral antigenic material may initially be quite small, it is amplified during viral replication. However, antibodies do not usually play a primary role in terminating acute viral infections but are very important in preventing reinfection. In some cases, antibodies may themselves be implicated in the pathogenesis of disease (e.g., in dengue fever).

The immunogenicity of viruses depends on the nature of the virus itself and on a variety of host factors. The prions responsible for neurological degenerative diseases such as kuru and Creutzfeldt-Jakob disease do not appear to provoke any detectable immune response in the host. The route of viral infection may also play a role in immunity. In experimental influenza infections, intravenous inoculation is more immunogenic than intraperitoneal inoculation, which in turn exceeds the subcutaneous route.

Antibodies that protect the host by destroying the infectivity of virus are called **neutralizing antibodies**. These antibodies are usually directed against epitopes present on viral proteins located on the surface of the virus particle. The binding of neutralizing antibodies to virus is generally a reversible reaction. Neutralizing antibodies reduce viral infectivity by possibly inhibiting various steps of the replication cycle such as attachment, penetration, or uncoating of virus. In addition, such antibodies may produce aggregation of virions, accelerate viral degradation in vesicles, or enhance viral opsonization and subsequent phagocytosis. In poliovirus infec-

tion, binding of neutralizing antibodies appears to induce a conformational rearrangement of the viral outer capsid which blocks viral uncoating but not attachment.

Complement

Viruses can trigger the activation of both the alternative and classic pathways of complement in the absence of an antibody response. Activated complement components (e.g., C3b) may act as opsonins to enhance phagocytosis of viruses (Chapter 6, "Constitutive Defenses"). Activation of the alternative complement pathway, in combination with antibody, may lead to lysis of enveloped viruses or virus-infected cells. Although the complement system plays a role in the protection against viral infection in animals, human complement deficiency is not typically associated with an increase in the frequency or severity of viral illnesses. Thus, this system is not likely to play as important a role in defending against viral as against bacterial infections.

Cell-mediated Immunity

Cell-mediated immunity is ordinarily a major factor in both the termination of viral infections and the pathogenesis of these diseases. Because of the viral intracellular habitat, infected cells are susceptible to the action of lymphocytes that recognize viral antigens on their surface (Chapter 6, "Constitutive Defenses"). Virus-infected cells can be lysed by several types of lymphoid cells through both the antibody-independent and the antibody-dependent pathways.

Independent of antibody, cytotoxicity by **natural killer (NK) cells** provides one of the earliest host defenses against viral infection (peak activity at 2 to 3 days) and precedes the appearance of antibody (7 days), cytotoxic T lymphocytes (CTL), and delayed type hypersensitivity (DTH). Natural killer cells are large granular lymphocytes that bind to infected cells and then secrete cytotoxic molecules contained in azurophilic granular vesicles. These cells do not represent a specific virus-induced defense mechanism although they are activated nonspecifically by virus-induced interferons (see below).

Antibodies participate in the lysis of infected cells via **antibody-dependent cell-mediated cytotoxicity (ADCC**, Chapter 7, "Induced Defenses"). In ADCC immune responses, virus-specific antibody bound to antigens on the surface of infected cells interacts with receptors for the Fc portion of IgG on the surface of the NK cells. Binding of IgG to the Fc receptor activates the NK cells and results in target cell killing. Macrophages, lymphocytes, and neutrophils also have Fc receptors and may also participate in ADCC.

Cytotoxic T lymphocytes (CTLs) constitute a specific virus-induced defense mechanism because they must be activated by antigen presented by macrophages or other antigen-presenting cells. Lysis of infected cells mediated by CTLs is typically restricted to class I histocompatibility antigens, although examples of class II-restricted

CTLs have been described (Chapter 7, "Induced Defenses"). In contrast to neutralizing antibodies, which typically recognize epitopes on intact viral surface proteins, CTLs recognize protein fragments derived from both the viral surface and internal proteins. The pathways by which these peptides are processed, appear on the surface of infected cells, and interact with major histocompatibility complex (MHC) antigens are subjects of active investigation.

Virus-induced Immunopathology

Immunological injury results from cell lysis elicited by one or more of the mechanisms described above. Such damage is seen in children immunized with inactivated measles virus vaccine who experience severe disease when later infected with the same virus. The role of cell-mediated immunity is dramatically illustrated in mice infected with the virus that causes lymphochoriomeningitis. When mice are inoculated intracerebrally with the virus, normal mice die within about a week. However, mice whose cell-mediated immunity has been suppressed by irradiation survive even though virus multiplication is unaffected.

Virus-induced immunopathology may also result from antibody production. Viruses may combine with virus-specific antibodies to form circulating immune complexes to cause a variety of lesions. Immune complexes become trapped in basement membranes at a variety of sites including the skin, the kidney, the choroid plexus, and the walls of blood vessels. Accumulation of immune complexes results in tissue injury by attracting and activating a variety of inflammatory mediators. In addition, virus stimulation of B lymphocytes may induce cross-reacting antibodies to normal host structures that contain antigenic regions similar to those of the virus (**molecular mimicry**).

Interferons

In addition to the usual humoral and cellular defense mechanisms, viral infections elicit an inducible defense mechanism, the **interferons**. These are proteins encoded by the host cells whose synthesis is induced by viruses and other agents. Interferons inhibit viral replication indirectly by inducing the synthesis of cellular proteins that minimize viral replication. The discovery and practical applications of interferons are discussed in Chapter 43 on antiviral strategies.

There are three main kinds of interferons (see Table 43.2), called α, β, and γ. Leukocytes produce more than a dozen α-("leukocyte")interferons that share about 70% amino acid sequence homology. β-("fibroblast") interferon is produced by fibroblasts and epithelial cells and has 30% homology to α-interferons. Immune, or γ-interferon is usually induced by the activation of T cells by specific antigens, but can also be induced by other compounds, including bacterial endotoxin.

Interferons are induced by both active and inactivated viruses, by double-stranded RNA, and by a number of other compounds. The amount of interferon produced varies with different viruses. All interferons act at extremely low concentrations and are generally most active in cells of the species in which they are induced ("species-specific"), presumably because of variation in the nature of the interferon receptor. Interferon production appears to involve a derepression of cellular genes induced by the presence of viral nucleic acid in the host cell cytoplasm. This results in the rapid production of mRNAs for interferon and subsequent interferon synthesis.

Newly produced interferon is released into extracellular fluid and then binds to a specific receptor on adjacent cells. Consequently, interferon tends to act locally rather than systemically. Binding of interferon to a receptor leads to a complex series of events. A protein kinase is synthesized which phosphorylates a protein-synthesis initiation factor. In the phosphorylated form, this factor cannot participate in the formation of the protein-initiation complex, thus leading to inhibition of viral protein synthesis. In addition, an induced 2,5-oligoisoadenylate synthetase produces 2,5-oligoadenylates, which in turn activate a cellular endonuclease (RNase L) that degrades viral mRNA. Interferons also increase the activity of NK cells, CTLs, and cells involved in ADCC reactions. The relative importance of each of these activities in creating the interferon-induced antiviral state is not established.

Diagnosis of Viral Diseases

A reasonably accurate diagnosis of some viral illnesses, such as measles, can be made on clinical grounds alone. In other cases the best that can be done clinically is to identify the group of viruses that are the likely pathogens. More definitive diagnosis is often necessary because some of the available antiviral agents have an activity that is limited to certain types of viruses only. Definitive diagnosis requires the isolation of the virus in animals or in tissue culture, identification of the virus or detection of virus-specific antigens or viral nucleic acids in tissues or body fluids, or demonstration of specific serologic responses. Appropriate specimens must be obtained for diagnostic studies during a suitable phase of the illness. Specimens must be rapidly transported and adequate clinical information must be provided to the diagnostic laboratories.

Isolation of virus from clinical specimens is done in cell cultures, embryonated eggs, and animals such as suckling mice. Cell culture techniques involve the use of primary cultures of cells prepared from organs of freshly killed animals (e.g., monkey kidney cells); of human diploid cell lines; and continuous (heterodiploid) cell lines such as HeLa, HEp-2, BHK-21, and Vero. Some viruses grow better on certain cell lines than others. Inoculation into the amniotic cavity or the allantoic cavity of embryonated chicken eggs is useful for the isolation of influenza virus. Intraperitoneal and intracerebral inoculation into neonatal mice may be necessary for isolation of Coxsackie A viruses and may help in the isolation of many arboviruses, rabies virus, arenaviruses, and orbiviruses. Adult mice or guinea pigs are used to isolate lymphocytic choriomeningitis (LCM) virus. Identification of the agent responsible for prion diseases such as kuru and Creutzfeldt-Jakob disease may require intracerebral inoculation of higher primates, such as chimpanzees.

Once cell cultures have been inoculated, the specimens are examined for distinctive patterns of **cytopathic effect** (CPE). Viruses such as that of herpes simplex and many enteroviruses produce early CPE, whereas CPE due to CMV, rubella, and some adenoviruses may take weeks. Cultured cells are examined for cell lysis and vacuolization. The presence of syncytia suggests HSV, respiratory syncytial virus, measles, or mumps virus. Cytomegaly is seen with HSV, varicella-zoster virus, and CMV.

Immunocytochemical staining of cell cultures to detect viral antigens using fluorescein or enzyme-conjugated specific antiviral antibodies may aid in the detection and identification of many viruses. Ortho- and paramyxoviruses (influenza, parainfluenza, measles, mumps) may be detected by the ability of infected cultures to adsorb certain red blood cells (**hemadsorption**).

Identification of virus particles or antigens in tissue specimens provides another important method of viral diagnosis. Skin scrapings from the base of vesicles help identify HSV or VZV. Similar techniques may help identify CMV-infected cells in urine sediment or measles-infected cells in scrapings from characteristic spots in the mouth (Koplik spots). In some cases, examination of specimens by electron microscopy (EM) is of diagnostic value, but only when viruses are present in high concentrations. Using special techniques as few as 10^4 particles per milliliter may be detected. The use of specific antisera to aggregate virus in prepared stool specimens facilitates EM detection of rotaviruses, hepatitis A virus, and the Norwalk agent. EM examination of brain biopsy specimens may allow identification of herpes simplex encephalitis and prion diseases.

A fourfold or greater increase in the antibody titer to a specific viral agent in a patient's acute and convalescent (3 to 4 weeks later) sera is usually considered diagnostic of acute infection. A single serum specimen is only occasionally useful in viral diagnosis. A number of different types of antibodies including neutralizing, complement-fixing, and hemagglutination-inhibiting antibodies are routinely assayed (see Chapter 55, "Diagnostic Principles," for details on these techniques). The time course of these antibody responses and their sensitivity and specificity differ greatly.

Restriction enzyme analysis of the genomes of DNA viruses (e.g., herpes simplex virus, cytomegalovirus) and oligonucleotide fingerprinting of ribonuclease-cleaved genomes of RNA viruses (e.g., influenza, dengue fever, en-

teroviruses) are valuable in epidemiologic studies and in establishing the origin of certain types of viral isolates. In situ hybridization and the polymerase chain reaction technique (or other nucleic acid–amplification methods) may enable the detection of even single copies of virus genomes in tissue samples or cells from body fluids. Some of these extremely sensitive methods are becoming commercially available and may help revolutionize rapid viral diagnosis.

Treatment and prevention of viral diseases are discussed in further detail in Chapters 43 ("Strategies to Combat Viral Infections") and 44 ("Vaccines and Antisera in the Prevention and Treatment of Infections") and in the chapters on the individual viruses.

SELF-ASSESSMENT QUESTIONS

1. Why are viruses not considered to be cellular forms of life?

2. How do viruses with icosahedral and helical symmetry differ in the connection between their nucleic acid and capsid?

3. Draw from memory a sketch of a typical nonenveloped and enveloped virus.

4. Why is the nucleic acid of (—) strand RNA viruses noninfectious?

5. Name three ways in which the mRNA of animal viruses resembles that of eukaryotic cells.

6. Why are the DNA-containing poxviruses not able to use the DNA replicative machinery of the cell?

7. Name two strategies used by viruses to make economic use of the information in the genome.

8. Define lytic, latent, and persistent viral infections.

9. Name three ways used by viruses to spread in the nervous system.

10. Viruses spread through the blood in three different ways. Name them.

11. How do antibodies contribute to immunopathology in viral diseases?

12. Why are live attenuated viral vaccines usually more effective than killed vaccines? Give two general reasons.

13. How does the activity of NK cells differ from that of CTL cells in viral infections?

14. Discuss how interferons differ from antibodies in their origin, specificity, and mode of action in viral infections.

15. Name four methods by which viruses may be detected in clinical specimens.

SUGGESTED READINGS

Fields BN, Knipe DM, Howley PM, eds. Virology. 3rd ed. Philadelphia: Lippincott-Raven, 1996.

White DO, Fenner F. Medical virology. 3rd ed. New York: Academic Press, 1986.

CHAPTER 32

Picornaviruses: Polio Virus, Other Enteroviruses, and the Rhinoviruses

CODY MEISSNER

GREGORY A. STORCH

Key Concepts

Picornaviruses:
- Are a family of small RNA viruses.
- Include the enteroviruses, rhinoviruses, and the hepatitis A virus.

Enteroviruses:
- Derive their name from their natural habitat, the gastrointestinal tract.
- Include polioviruses, coxsackievirus, and the echoviruses (now known as numbered enteroviruses).

Polioviruses:
- Are positive-strand viruses that can cause either asymptomatic infection or flaccid paralysis.
- Replicate quickly in the intestine and can be shed in the feces weeks to months after infection.
- Can spread from the gastrointestinal tract to the central nervous system.
- Can be prevented with either a killed vaccine (Salk) or a live, attenuated vaccine (Sabin).

Rhinoviruses:
- Cause the common cold.
- Are distinguished into over 100 serotypes, which prevent development of an effective vaccine.
- Can be transmitted person-to-person through contamination or aerosols.
- Bind to specific receptors on respiratory epithelial cells.
- Probably cause damage by mechanisms other than viral-induced cytopathology.

The picornaviruses (pico = small, rna = RNA-containing) are a family of small RNA viruses consisting of two major groups: (a) the **enteroviruses**, which include **poliovirus** and other pathogens, and (b) the **rhinoviruses**, which are among the most common agents of the common cold. The **hepatitis A virus** is a member of a separate group of picornaviruses. In this chapter, the enteroviruses and the rhinoviruses will be treated separately.

CASE

An Outbreak of Poliomyelitis

In October 1972, 11 of 130 students attending a private school in Greenwich, Connecticut came down with paralytic poliomyelitis. Three weeks elapsed between the first and the last case. Nine of the 11 cases were boys 12 to17 years of age, and all were members either of the football or the soccer team. The clinical history of these patients was similar: they reported "flulike" symptoms, fever up to 39°C, sore throat, and muscle pains. These symptoms lasted 13 days. Two to three days afterward, they complained of stiff neck, increased muscle pain, and fever up to 41°C. These symptoms were followed by flaccid paralysis of the legs that varied in intensity from relatively minor to totally incapacitating. During the first 3 weeks of October, 17 other students were seen at the school infirmary with nonspecific complaints that suggested an acute viral syndrome.

Poliomyelitis was diagnosed by serological studies based on a rising titer of antibodies to type 1 poliovirus, but not types 2 and 3. The diagnosis was confirmed by the isolation of type 1 virus from the feces and throat washings of patients with paralytic disease. More than 50% of the students of the school had received no oral polio vaccine because of religious convictions. A small number of day students at the school lived at home, where they interacted with friends from surrounding towns in activities that included swimming classes at the local YMCA. Paralytic disease did not occur among nonmembers of the school. An immunization survey of the public schools revealed that more than 95% of the students had been vaccinated.

Several questions are raised by this outbreak:
1. Where did the virus come from and how did it spread among the students?
2. What caused the illness among the 17 students who complained of nonspecific signs and symptoms?
3. Why did the disease not spread to all the students or to the community outside of the school?
4. How does poliovirus cause paralysis and the other symptoms of the disease?
5. What could have been done to halt further spread of polio in the school?

POLIOMYELITIS

Poliomyelitis is no longer a common disease in the U.S., although it continues to be important in some developing countries. Paradoxically, its dreaded consequences, paralysis and death, are more common in unvaccinated individuals living in countries with a high standard of sanitation (see Fig. 54.1). We emphasize polio because it serves as a good model for understanding the epidemiology and pathogenesis of viral infections because of its tropism, its well-understood and comparatively simple replication cycle, and the relative ease with which it can be studied in the laboratory. Furthermore, several related viruses (other enteroviruses) continue to cause important diseases in the U.S.

Humans, Health and History

Polio and Age

Poliomyelitis is an ancient dreaded disease. An Egyptian stone slab from about 1350 B.C. shows a young priest with the typical withered leg of a polio survivor (Fig. 32.1). In the prevaccine era of the early 1950s, about 21,000 paralytic cases per year occurred in the U.S. The figure is now less than 30 cases a year—a striking testimony to the efficacy of the polio vaccine. The virtual elimination of this disease from this country and much of Europe is one of the spectacular triumphs of medical research.

Within the last 100 years, poliomyelitis has undergone major changes in disease incidence and age distribution. Before the 1900s, most infections occurred in infants. Few developed paralytic disease because, in infants, the virus is not as neurotropic and is more likely to confine its replication to the alimentary tract. Poor standards of sanitation and crowding facilitated transmission of virus, particularly among children in the first year of life. Infection, symptomatic or not, confers lifelong immunity and, if widespread, pre-vents large outbreaks from taking place in older persons.

Around the turn of the century, the situation changed when improved living conditions limited circulation of the virus. As unexposed children without immunity grew older, they entered an increasingly larger pool of susceptible individuals. Introduction of poliovirus into this population resulted in more frequent infections later in life, resulting in devastating epidemics of paralytic disease. These epidemics occurred because older persons are more likely to develop paralytic disease when infected by poliovirus. In a sense, polio became a disease of affluent societies. Polio, then, is an example of an infection in which changes in the severity of disease are due to changes in the host, rather than in the infectious agent. Underdeveloped countries of the world continue to experience the endemic pattern of poliovirus infection early in life, even today.

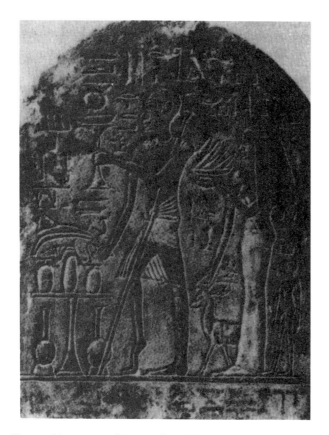

Figure 32.1. An early case of paralytic polio? This Egyptian stele depicting the typical paralysis of a polio victim dates from the 18th dynasty (1580–1350 B.C.)

ENTEROVIRUSES

Polioviruses belong to a heterogeneous group of viruses called the **enteroviruses**, which derive their name from their natural habitat, the gastrointestinal tract. Enteroviruses belong to the picornavirus family (Fig. 32.2). There are six major groups of enteroviruses. The most notorious member of this group is poliovirus, and more is known about its molecular biology and mechanism of pathogenesis than the other members of this group. Polioviruses are divided into three antigenic types; most epidemics are caused by **type 1**. Other enteroviruses include **coxsackievirus**, first isolated during a polio outbreak in Coxsackie, New York, and **echovirus** (enteric cytopathic human orphan virus). Echoviruses were so named because initially they could not be linked to any human disease, having been isolated from feces of individuals who had no symptoms. This distinction has been dropped for newly discovered enteroviruses, and they are now simply assigned a number, e.g., enterovirus 70.

Hepatitis A was originally classified as enterovirus type 72 because of its similarities to other enteroviruses. As more information has been acquired about this virus's differences in nucleotide sequences, poor growth in cell culture, and resistance to conditions that inacti-

vate other picornaviruses, it has become clear that hepatitis A should be classified in a separate genus.

Encounter and Entry

Enteroviruses are secreted in large amounts in stool. In the outbreak at the school in Connecticut, the likely source of contamination was a single individual who shed high titers of virus from his or her gastrointestinal tract. A summer or early fall outbreak is typical of countries in temperate climates; in the tropics, the diseases caused by these agents are endemic and occur throughout the year. The major portal of entry is the mouth, and the transmission is primarily from person-to-person via the fecal-oral route.

Spread and Replication

Soon after ingestion, enteroviruses replicate in the lymphoid tissue of the pharynx and the intestine. They may then spread throughout the body via the bloodstream (Fig. 32.3). In most cases, the infection does not proceed further; enteroviruses are either contained in the **Peyer's patches** of the small intestine or are kept in check soon after the onset of **viremia**. With poliovirus, the distinction between infection and disease is particularly important.

When viremia persists, distant sites become seeded as the viruses localize in their target organs. Their tropism is due to the presence of specific receptors on the membranes of target cells. All three types of poliovirus share similar receptors. Research has shown that saturation of binding sites with an excess of type 1 virus blocks the binding of types 2 or 3. Binding of coxsackie or other enteroviruses remains unaffected, indicating different binding sites for these related viruses.

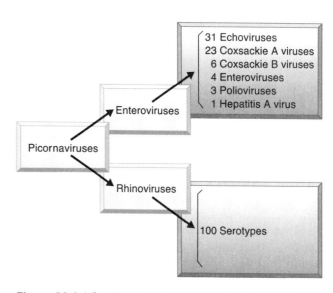

Figure 32.2. The Picornavirus family includes the genera *Rhinovirus* and *Enterovirus* with many different clinically important species.

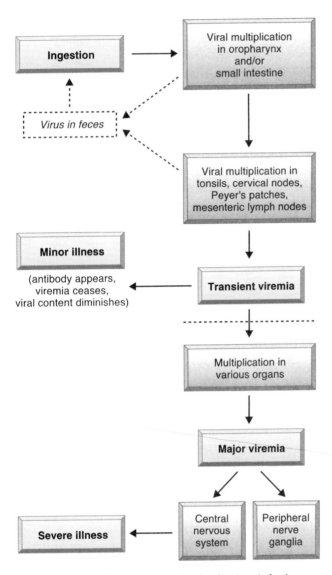

Figure 32.3. The pathogenesis of poliovirus infection.

Replication of poliovirus is better understood than that of the other enteroviruses, in part because they reproduce rapidly and yield high titers in cell culture. Polioviruses are a prototype of **positive-strand viruses**, meaning that their **genomic RNA** can act directly as messenger RNA (mRNA). The first step in replication cycle is uncoating, which, oddly enough, begins while the virions are still extracellular. Once the virions are taken up by the host cell, uncoating is completed and genomic RNA is released into the cytoplasm, where replication and assembly take place. Poliovirus RNA is single-stranded and, as is typical of eukaryotic mRNAs, has a **poly (A) tract** at the 3′ end on the genome. A viral protein called **VPg** is attached to the 5′ end. This protein is not essential for infectivity, but may be involved in packaging the genome in the virion and in priming poliovirus RNA synthesis.

Synthesis of poliovirus proteins has been studied ex-

tensively and has revealed several unexpected facts. A single long polypeptide, a **polyprotein**, is synthesized in the cytoplasm using the host cells' protein synthesizing apparatus. A series of post-translational cleavage reactions cuts the polyprotein into four **structural proteins** and about seven **nonstructural proteins** (Fig. 32.4). After this processing, the structural proteins assemble to make the capsid. It is not known why poliovirus translates its messenger RNA into a polyprotein, but this mechanism allows each protein to be made in equal amounts. Several of these proteins are **proteases** involved in the stepwise cleavage of the polyprotein; one is an **RNA-dependent RNA polymerase**; and the others are structural constituents of the virions.

The RNA-dependent RNA polymerase responsible for poliovirus RNA replication is an unusual enzyme not found in eukaryotic cells (whose RNA is made from DNA templates) and is accordingly encoded by the viral genome. The enzyme makes complementary negative strands of RNA, which, in turn, serve as templates for additional positive-strand copies of the genome. As the structural viral proteins accumulate, increasing amounts of viral RNA are encapsidated into mature virions. The viral particles are then released as the host cell is destroyed.

Under optimal conditions of cell culture, roughly 1000 infectious virus particles are released per cell. A complete cycle of replication, from viral attachment to the release of progeny virus, is completed within about 10 hours, which is unusually rapid for animal viruses. Other enteroviruses follow a similar scheme of replication.

Damage

Poliovirus is a typically lytic virus and its replication is accompanied by destruction of infected host cells. Enterovirus infections typically have 2- to 5-day incubation periods. The viruses may continue to replicate in the intestine and be shed in the stool for weeks or months after all symptoms are gone. In the school outbreak, virus continued to circulate and to infect new students for some time. This ability to replicate weeks or months after infection explains the onset of symptoms in different students over a 3-week period.

Polioviruses spread from the gastrointestinal tract to the central nervous system, where they replicate in the neurons of the gray matter of both brain and spinal cord. Virus travels via the bloodstream, although spread along neural pathways is also possible. The characteristic **flaccid paralysis** of limb muscles occurs when **anterior horn cells** of the spinal cord are destroyed. The most severe form of disease is **bulbar poliomyelitis**, the paralysis of the respiratory muscles resulting from involvement of the **medulla oblongata**. This type of polio led to the development of "iron lungs," cumbersome predecessors of modern respirators that made patients inhale and exhale by external changes in pressure. The mortality rate in paralytic cases of poliomyelitis is 23%.

Why is infection by enteroviruses, and poliovirus in particular, often so mild or asymptomatic? Apparently, many factors are at work. They include the size of the viral inoculum, the concentration of viruses in the blood, the virulence of individual virus strains, and the presence of circulating antibodies. The same virus may cause different illnesses in different individuals. In the school outbreak described above, one strain of virus caused a spectrum of disease. Among the host factors involved, physical exertion and trauma correlate with increased risk of paralysis. These factors may explain, in part, the observation that 9 of the 11 students affected were actively participating in football and soccer. Another predisposing factor for bulbar poliomyelitis is tonsillectomy, perhaps because of lowering of titers of antipolio antibodies in the nasal secretions of immunized persons. Circulating antibodies may play an important role in controlling infections resulting from enteroviruses, as seen in patients with hypogammaglobulinemias, who have difficulty in resolving infections by echovirus.

DISEASES CAUSED BY OTHER ENTEROVIRUSES

The most frequent diseases caused by enteroviruses in the U.S. are due to coxsackievirus (Table 32.1). They cause a large number of illnesses, differing somewhat between those caused by group A and group B. Both cause so-called **aseptic meningitis**, a term used for nonbacterial meningitis. In addition, group A viruses cause **herpangina**, a fever of sudden onset with vesicles or ulcers on the tonsils and palate. Group B viruses also in-

fect other organs, particularly the heart. In general, echoviruses produce similar diseases (see Table 32.1).

Most of these infections are not sufficiently unique to allow diagnosis on clinical grounds alone. For example, the skin rashes (exanthem) due to coxsackievirus and echovirus are indistinguishable. One important exception is **hand, foot, and mouth disease**, a readily identifiable febrile illness that produces blisters in the palate, hands, and feet. It is usually caused by a specific type of coxsackievirus, **type A16**.

During the viremic phase, these enteroviruses infect any of several organs and do not exhibit the same tropism for cells of the central nervous system as poliovirus. During the period of hematogenous spread, virus may localize in the heart (**myopericarditis**), the respiratory tract (**pleurodynia**), the mucous membranes (**hemorrhagic conjunctivitis**), or the gastrointestinal tract (**hepatitis**). Infected newborns are at particular risk for severe disease unless they have acquired enough protective antibodies from their mother. Their own immune system may be insufficiently developed to curtail an enterovirus infection. Neonates may acquire coxsackievirus or echovirus by transplacental passage of the virus near term, from contact with maternal fecal material during birth, or from conventional person-to-person passage.

An interesting association between enterovirus infection and **juvenile onset diabetes** has been suggested, based on several pieces of evidence. It has been proposed that an initial coxsackie or echovirus infection may be a starting point for a series of events leading to an autoimmune destruction of beta cells in genetically predisposed individuals. Additional work is necessary to confirm or refute the role of enteroviruses as a possible cofactor in the etiology of diabetes.

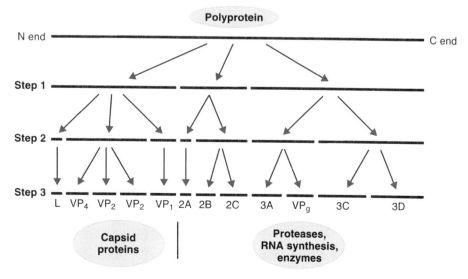

Figure 32.4. The synthesis of poliovirus polyprotein and its subsequent cleavage into structural proteins and virus-encoded enzymes.

Table 32.1. Major Enterovirus Diseases[a]

Disease	Polio	Coxsackievirus Type A	Coxsackievirus Type B	Echovirus	Enterovirus
Asymptomatic infection	+	+	+	+	+
Viral meningitis	+	+	+	+	+
Paralytic disease	+	+	+	+	−
Febrile exanthems (rash)	−	+	+	+	+
Acute respiratory disease	−	+	+	+	+
Myopericarditis	−	+	+	+	−
Orchitis	−	−	+	+	−

[a] The more recently identified enteroviruses are identified by number (i.e., enterovirus type 68).

Diagnosis and Therapy

Because diseases caused by enteroviruses are seldom sufficiently characteristic to enable a diagnosis on purely clinical grounds, it may be helpful to take into account certain epidemiological features. A person who becomes ill with symptoms of viral meningitis in the summer or early fall during a community-wide outbreak of coxsackievirus is likely to be a victim of that agent.

During endemic months, when enteroviruses circulate in a community, they can be readily isolated from throat washings or fecal specimens from symptomatic as well as asymptomatic persons. In this setting, recovery of an enterovirus from the throat or feces of an ill person does not prove that the symptoms are due to an enterovirus, as many asymptomatic people have enteroviruses in their stool. Definitive proof requires isolation of the virus from the involved site, such as cerebrospinal or pericardial fluids. Serological tests are not practical because related enteroviruses do not share common antigens.

At present, there is no therapy for infections by enteroviruses, with the possible exception of the administration of γ-globulin to immune-compromised patients suffering from severe echovirus or coxsackievirus infections.

Prevention

A disease caused by an agent whose only reservoir is human beings is a candidate not only for control but for elimination. The best example is smallpox, which appears to have been erased from the face of the earth, except for stocks of the virus maintained under secure conditions. Polio may be a candidate for this sort of medical success.

The issues surrounding polio vaccination merit close examination. Vigorous efforts to develop an effective polio vaccine go hand in hand with seminal developments in virology, mainly the use of cell cultures to study viral multiplication. The **killed Salk vaccine** was introduced in 1955 and led to a precipitous decline in the incidence of both paralytic and nonparalytic disease (Fig. 32.5). In 1961, the **oral, live, attenuated Sabin vaccine** was introduced in this country and it soon replaced the Salk vaccine. Considerable controversy surrounded the introduction of a live vaccine after the killed vaccine had already demonstrated its effectiveness. A comparison of the two vaccines is shown in Table 32.2.

The original arguments continue to form the basis for the use of the live vaccine (Fig. 32.6). Antibody production by the killed vaccine is not always long lasting and is slow to develop. Repeated booster shots are necessary. Perhaps most important, the immune response elicited by the live, attenuated vaccine closely resembles that brought about by natural poliovirus infection. The live, attenuated vaccine is administered orally, resulting in an active infection in the intestine and stimulating the local formation of secretory antibodies. In contrast, the killed vaccine is administered by injection and produces immunity in the circulation but not in the intestine (Fig. 32.6). Thus, a recipient of the killed vaccine, while protected from symptomatic disease, could still propagate and spread the virus.

Because immunization rates in this country never approach 100%, the live vaccine would reduce the number of individuals who may act as reservoirs for poliovirus. Contacts of individuals given the live, attenuated vaccine may be asymptomatically infected, regardless of their immunization status. In most instances, this contact produces a booster response in already immunized individuals. In the infrequent setting where the vaccine strain spreads to nonimmunized persons, the community may benefit from the increased number of immune individuals. However, spread of live virus by this means is not without harm; at least half of the few cases of paralytic poliomyelitis in the U.S. today are thought to be due to the virus used in the live vaccine. During replica-

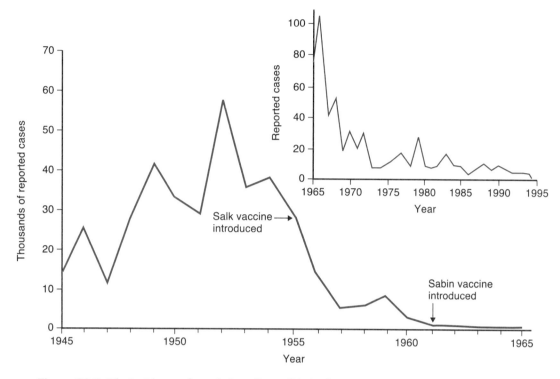

Figure 32.5. The incidence of paralytic poliomyelitis in the U.S. 1951–1982. Reported cases per 100,000 population.

Table 32.2. The Poliovirus Vaccines

	Advantages	Disadvantages
1. Inactivated vaccine (Salk)	a. Cannot undergo genetic mutation to increased virulence.	a. Fails to elicit gut immunity b. Requires parenteral administration c. Expensive d. Some lots have inadequate antigenic potency e. Confers immunity only after four boosters f. Stringent control of production required to ensure inactivation
2. Live, attenuated vaccine (Sabin)	a. Relatively inexpensive and easily administered b. Induces both systemic and local immunity c. Maintains potency without refrigeration d. Prepared in human cells, eliminating risk of latent viruses found in monkey kidney cells e. Induces herd immunity	a. Can mutate to more virulent strain b. Less reliable in tropical climates

tion in the gut of vaccine recipients, the vaccine strain may very rarely back-mutate to a less attenuated, more virulent strain before it is passed on to contacts. At least some of the individuals who develop vaccine-associated disease are immune-deficient. It should be emphasized, however, that the risk of developing polio from the vaccine strain is extraordinarily small, about one case of paralytic polio per 2.6 million doses distributed. Also, at times, the live vaccine has been found to contain con-

taminating viruses from the monkey cells used for cultivation.

The live vaccine should not be used in certain circumstances. Generally, immunocompromised individuals should not receive any live vaccine, including the Sabin vaccine. In some underdeveloped countries, the live, attenuated vaccine has not resulted in an acceptable antibody response. One reason for vaccine failure seems to be interference from other enteroviruses already repli-

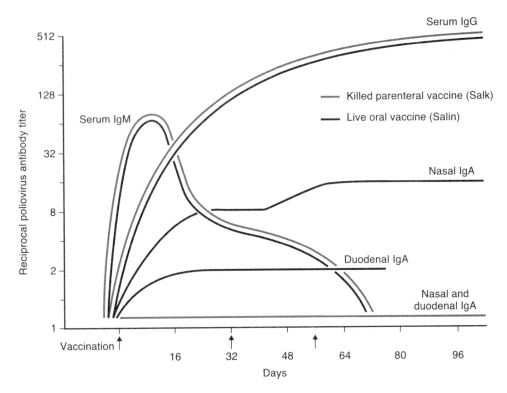

Figure 32.6. The antibody response to the live and killed poliovirus vaccine. The levels of serum IgG, as well as nasal and duodenal IgA are compared as a function of time after vaccination.

cating in the intestine. For this reason, the live vaccine is given to children in five doses, which minimizes the likelihood of other enterovirus replicating at the time of vaccination.

Conclusion

Enteroviruses commonly cause infections in human beings. Although readily communicable, only rarely do they cause severe disease. Illnesses caused by enteroviruses may be highly tissue-specific (polio) or can affect many organs (coxsackievirus and echovirus infections). These diseases are often difficult to distinguish clinically, and their presumptive diagnosis is often based on the epidemiological picture. The success in eradicating polio with vaccination is providential, as there is no other known way to control this disease.

HUMAN RHINOVIRUSES AND THE COMMON COLD

The human rhinovirus remains the agent most closely linked to the common cold. Along with the enteroviruses (poliovirus, coxsackie A and B viruses, echoviruses, and hepatitis A virus), the rhinoviruses comprise the Picornaviridae family. Unlike other respiratory viruses, such as influenza, parainfluenza, or respiratory syncytial virus, rhinoviruses have no lipid envelope surrounding the viral nucleocapsid. As is also true for the entero-

viruses, antigenic diversity is a striking characteristic of the rhinoviruses, with nearly 100 serotypes recognized to date. (Any two rhinovirus isolates are considered to be of different serotypes if their infectivity is not neutralized by the same antiserum.) Although some cross-reactivity exists among different serotypes, the extent of antigenic diversity has caused pessimism about the prospects for a rhinovirus vaccine.

Differences in the rhinoviruses and enteroviruses help explain why they cause disease in certain sites of the body. Enteroviruses are more resistant to gastric acidity (stable at pH 3.0) and to bile. Rhinoviruses replicate best at 33°C, a temperature found in the nose, while enteroviruses prefer the core body temperature, 37°C. Also, rhinoviruses are acid-labile and are readily inactivated by gastric secretions. These features may help explain why rhinoviruses seldom cause pneumonia and enteroviruses are an infrequent cause of the common cold.

■ CASE

The Common Cold

Ms. C., a 28-year-old woman, realized she was getting a cold when she noticed a scratchy feeling in the throat, sneezing, nasal discharge, low-grade fever, and malaise. The symptoms worsened, reaching a peak after 48 hours. Within several days, her nasal discharge thickened and was slightly yellowish, and then subsided over the next several days. All of her other symptoms resolved completely within about 7 days of onset. She thought that she acquired the illness from her 7-year-old child, who had had similar symptoms a few days earlier.

Encounter

Rhinovirus infections are very common. The average person experiences approximately one such infection per year, and school-age children and those in contact with them may experience many more. These infections occur most commonly in the fall and spring. Multiple serotypes circulate simultaneously but, over time, different serotypes predominate.

Infected humans, particularly children, are the only known reservoir for these viruses. The mode of transmission has been the subject of intense experimental study. One series of experiments demonstrated that

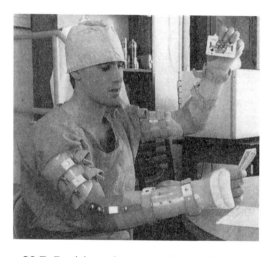

Figure 32.7. Participant in an experiment designed to study the mode of transmission of rhinoviruses. The arm braces worn by the subject allowed normal poker playing but prevented the wearer from touching any part of his head or face.

transmission may occur if individuals touch their nose or eyes after their hands became contaminated with rhinovirus (either from contaminated nasal secretions or environmental objects). In recent experiments, susceptible volunteers played poker with persons who had symptomatic rhinovirus infection, and became infected even if they were restrained from touching their face (Fig. 32.7). This suggests that rhinovirus infection may be transmitted by **aerosols** as well as by direct inoculation. The effective production and dispersal of aerosol droplets during a sneeze is shown in Figure 32.8.

Entry, Spread, and Multiplication

In experimental studies, even a small inoculum of rhinovirus suffices to initiate an infection. The first step in infection is the binding of the virus to specific receptors on respiratory epithelial cells. Recently, researchers were surprised to find that most of the diverse rhinovirus serotypes bind to the same receptor. The remaining serotypes bind to a second receptor. The major group receptor was found to be a well-known molecule designated **ICAM-1 (intercellular adhesion molecule-1)**. ICAM-1 is a member of the immunoglobulin supergene family and is known to play an important role in cell adhesion processes in the immune response. Thus, the human rhinoviruses join a small but possibly growing number of viruses whose receptors are molecules with known cellular functions. Other examples are rabies virus and the acetylcholine receptor (Chapter 35, "Rabies"), HIV and the CD4 molecule (Chapter 38, "Human Retroviruses"), and the Epstein-Barr virus and the receptor for complement component C3 (Chapter 41, "Herpes").

An interesting finding concerning the interaction between rhinovirus and its receptor is that expression of ICAM-1 on the cell surface is increased by certain inflammatory mediators that may be relevant in rhinovirus infection. This finding suggests that rhinovirus-

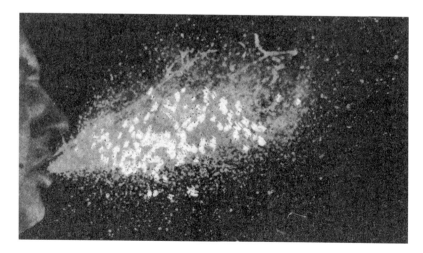

Figure 32.8. Droplet dispersal following a sneeze by a patient with a cold; note strings of mucus.

induced inflammation may facilitate the entry of the virus into nearby uninfected cells and, thus, spread the infection.

Detailed structural studies of rhinoviruses have revealed that the part of the virus that binds to the cellular receptor is located within a cleft or "canyon" on the surface of the virion. Neutralizing antibodies are thought to prevent infection by binding to the virions at sites near the canyon, making it impossible for the binding site on the virus to come in contact with the cellular receptor. The detailed molecular scheme of rhinovirus replication within the infected cell is similar to that described for poliovirus.

Rhinoviruses are thought to spread in respiratory epithelium by local extension. In experimental colds, the **posterior nasopharynx** is the site of the most intense infection. Neither viremia nor infection at sites outside of the respiratory tract is known to occur in these infections.

Damage

The nose of a patient with a cold becomes engorged with blood (**hyperemic**) and **edematous**. The thin nasal discharge contains large amounts of serum proteins. As the cold progresses, the discharge becomes **mucopurulent** and contains many cells, especially **neutrophils**. Respiratory epithelial cells are also present, some of which contain rhinovirus antigens, indicating that they are infected by the virus. If a biopsy of the mucosa were to be performed early in the course of a cold, it would reveal edema of subepithelial connective tissue with relatively small numbers of inflammatory cells. In contrast to some other viral respiratory infections, particularly influenza, only minimal histopathological changes would be observed, even in areas where viral antigens are present.

How does rhinovirus infection produce its characteristic disease manifestations? In general, there is a correlation between the severity of the cold correlates with the amount of rhinovirus that can be recovered. Large amounts of virus are found without tissue destruction, however, indicating that disease manifestations must be produced by mechanisms other than viral-induced cytopathology. Further support for this notion comes from the finding that nasal secretions of persons with a cold contain large amounts of the vasoactive substance **bradykinin**. In addition, it is thought that direct stimulation of nerve endings in the nasal mucosa produces some of the manifestations of the cold.

Despite the discomfort resulting from the events occurring in the nose, most rhinovirus infections are mild and have few other consequences. The most common complications are **sinusitis, otitis media,** and exacerbation of **chronic bronchitis** or **asthma**. Rarely, more severe infections with probable lower respiratory tract involvement may occur, especially in compromised hosts such as premature infants with chronic lung disease. Sinusitis or otitis media complicating a cold is usually a result of bacterial infections that develop because the normal draining of the sinuses or the middle ear is blocked.

Prevention and Treatment

Some degree of immunity to rhinovirus infection does develop. Infected people generate immunity effective against viruses of the same serotype. This immunity may be due, at least in part, to antibodies found in nasal secretions. It is reasonable to speculate that antirhinovirus antibody, particularly of the IgA class, might exert a protective effect by blocking the binding of the virus to the cell receptor.

A vaccine to prevent the common cold does not yet appear feasible, not only because of the serological diversity of these viruses, but also because rhinoviruses account for no more than 50% of colds. Nevertheless, several novel approaches to prophylaxis are currently being explored. One is the use of **recombinant α-interferon** administered by nasal spray. In recent studies, this spray was effective in preventing colds if used just after the first cold occurred in a family. An earlier approach of using interferon nasal sprays throughout the cold season was not successful because the nasal symptoms produced by long-term interferon administration were as bothersome as those of a cold (Chapter 43, "Strategies to Combat Viral Infections"). Other chemotherapeutic agents are also under study. New approaches of this kind may finally lead to progress in controlling the widely experienced miseries of the common cold.

SELF-ASSESSMENT QUESTIONS

1. Discuss the changes in severity and incidence of polio in the U.S. in the last 100 years.
2. What diseases do the enteroviruses cause? What are their common clinical features?
3. Discuss the replication cycle of poliovirus.
4. What are the issues associated with vaccination against polio?
5. Discuss how the eradication of smallpox may help us eradicate polio.
6. Describe features of the attachment of rhinoviruses to human cells.
7. Describe the pathogenesis of rhinovirus infection.

SUGGESTED READINGS

CDC. Progress toward global poliomyelitis eradication, 1985–1994. MMRW 1995;44:273.

Evans AL. Viral infections of humans. 2nd ed. New York: Plenum, 1982;182–251.

Melnick JL. Current status of poliovirus infections. Clin Microb Revs 1996;9:293.

CHAPTER 33

Arthropod-borne Viruses

CODY MEISSNER

Key Concepts

Arboviruses:

- Are viruses that are transmitted by an arthropod vector.
- Cause zoonoses; these diseases only accidentally affect humans.
- Are often named after the disease they cause or the place where they have been found (i.e., LaCrosse, Semliki Forest, Rift Valley fever).
- Cause encephalitis, dengue fever, and yellow fever.
- Are diagnosed by isolation of the virus or rise in antibody titer; diagnosis on clinical grounds is difficult.
- Cannot be treated, although vaccines against many arboviruses can prevent infection.

The arthropod-borne **viruses** (**arboviruses**) are a varied group of agents that cause a wide range of illnesses, from mild influenza-like infections to encephalitis or hemorrhagic fevers. These diseases are more prevalent in the tropics than in the temperate regions of the world because they follow the distribution of the **mosquitoes** and flies involved in their transmission. The principal diseases in this group are dengue, yellow fever, and a large number of encephalitides. Some of these diseases can be prevented with vaccination, but effective therapeutic measures are not available for this group of viruses.

CASE 1

In the summer before he was to enter medical school, Mr. R. spent the month of July sunning himself on the beaches of Maryland. The weather was particularly hot and wet. His favorite spot was a pond in a wooded area where he could watch horses from a nearby farm. One afternoon, he suddenly became lethargic and fatigued and went home to bed. That evening he was awakened for supper by his father but felt confused and was not hungry. By 10 PM, he

had a fever of 40.7°C and refused to answer questions. Four hours later, his father had difficulty rousing him and brought him to the emergency room of a local hospital. Several hours after admission, Mr. R. was unable to respond to simple commands. His condition gradually deteriorated, and he experienced periods of increasing stupor and paralysis of the limbs. He lapsed into coma 2 weeks after admission and died 2 weeks after that.

Serum samples obtained from Mr. R. showed an eightfold rise in antibody titer against Eastern equine encephalitis (EEE) virus. At autopsy, examination of his brain showed disseminated small foci of necrosis in both the gray matter and the white matter. EEE virus was isolated from brain tissue by intracerebral inoculation of suckling mice at the state laboratory. A diagnosis of EEE virus was made on the grounds of the laboratory data and the clinical signs and symptoms.

Several questions arise:

1. Where and how did Mr. R. acquire the virus?
2. How common is this disease? What circumstances predispose to the disease?
3. What other viruses cause similar diseases?

4. What measures could Mr. R. have taken to prevent the disease?

Eastern equine encephalitis (EEE) is an often fatal but fortunately rare disease. In the United States, a total of 178 cases occurred between 1955 and 1985. The virus causing EEE is found among **marsh birds** that live in the fresh water swamps of the Atlantic and Gulf states and in regions around the Great Lakes. This disease is rare in humans because the mosquitoes that transmit it among marsh herons and egrets do not usually bite humans. Only when people-biting mosquitoes become involved are humans at risk. The likelihood that a person infected with this virus manifests clinical disease ranges from about 1 in 4 in children to as low as 1 in 50 in adults. However, the fatality rate among those who have symptoms is very high, 50–80%. In children, mental retardation occurs in as many as half the survivors.

▇ CASE 2

Amelia, a 7-year-old girl, was at summer camp in Wisconsin when she fell from the upper level of a bunk bed. She was found by her counselor on the floor experiencing a generalized seizure which lasted 6 minutes. The next day she became increasingly lethargic and vomited several times. She was admitted to a local hospital with a temperature of 102. Examination of the spinal fluid revealed 5 red blood cells and 725 white blood cells/mm^3 with 47% lymphocytes, indicating an inflammatory reaction in the central nervous system. No antibiotic or antiviral agent was administered. Thirty-six hours after admission, Amelia became afebrile and was discharged. She returned to camp in good condition.

Acute and convalescent blood specimens obtained 2 days and 5 weeks after onset of illness showed a change from no detectable antibody to LaCrosse virus to a titer of 1:128, indicating a significant rise in specific antibody. Attempts to isolate a virus from a spinal fluid specimen were unsuccessful.

LaCrosse virus is one of the most common causes of central nervous system infection due to members of the **California encephalitis virus group.** The spectrum of illness due to viruses in this group ranges from mild febrile illness to aseptic meningitis and fatal encephalitis. Cases occur chiefly in the east-central states in children under 10 years of age. The majority of symptomatic infections are associated with mild signs of meningoencephalitis. In contrast to EEE, the case fatality rate is less than 1%. Focal or generalized seizures occur in up to 60% of cases. Symptoms generally resolve completely after a few days. Diagnosis of infection by California encephalitis virus is nearly always made by serologic evaluation, as virus is rarely isolated from spinal fluid. Efforts to prevent the disease have focused on elimination of the breeding sites of the mosquitoes involved in its transmission, such as discarded cans, bottles, and tires.

ARBOVIRUSES

Arboviruses are a large group of viruses that share two characteristics: transmission by arthropod vectors, and an RNA genome (Table 33.1). More than 100 different members are known to infect humans. Many cause **encephalitis** while others produce **yellow fever, hemorrhagic fever,** or **dengue fever,** diseases characterized by internal hemorrhages, severe joint and muscle pain, and skin rashes. Arboviruses are often named after the disease they cause or the place where they have been found (e.g., LaCrosse, Semliki Forest, Rift Valley fever, Colorado tick fever, Venezuelan equine encephalitis, West Nile fever, etc.). They are diseases of wild and domesticated animals; humans are only accidentally infected. Vectors include mosquitoes, ticks, and flies. Some diseases that are not transmitted by an arthropod vector are caused by viruses that are biochemically similar to members of this group. For example, the virus that causes rubella (German measles) belongs to the same group as EEE virus, although it is transmitted directly from person to person.

The members of two main families of arboviruses (**Togaviridae** and **Flaviviridae**) have enveloped virions that contain a **single-stranded positive-sense RNA genome.** The RNA serves as messenger RNA and is transcribed directly into large proteins. These proteins are then cleaved to make both regulatory proteins and the structural proteins of the virion. Members of another important family (**Bunyaviridae**) contain a **single-stranded negative-sense genome** and carry an RNA transcriptase in their virions. The envelope contains surface glycoprotein spikes that it acquires as the virions bud through the cytoplasmic membrane. The lipid-containing envelope appears to be essential for viral integrity because treatment with detergents or lipid solvents inactivates these viruses. Many enveloped viruses are also sensitive to drying, suggesting that arthropod transmission may constitute a protective mechanism from detrimental environmental factors.

ENCOUNTER

The natural life cycle of the viruses that cause EEE and other encephalitides is from bird to bird, via the bite of mosquitoes (Fig. 33.1). It is not known if the virus survives the winter in cold climates or if it is reintroduced each year by migrating birds. As its name implies, horses acquire EEE, but they seldom play a role in the development of human infection. The virus is present in the horses' blood for so short a time that it is unlikely the horse would be bitten by a mosquito during the viremic phase. Like humans, horses do not participate in the

Table 33.1. Important Human Arboviruses

Genus and example	Main disease manifestations	Primary vector	Major geographic distribution
Togaviridae Family			
Alphavirus			
Eastern equine encephalitis	Encephalitis	Mosquito	Eastern U.S., Caribbean
Western equine encephalitis	Encephalitis	Mosquito	Western U.S., Canada, Mexico, Brazil
Venezuelan equine encephalitis	Encephalitis	Mosquito	Central and South America, Texas, Florida
Many others	Fevers, encephalitis	Mosquito	Africa, Asia, Central and South America
Flaviviridae Family			
Flavivirus			
St. Louis encephalitis	Encephalitis	Mosquito	North America
Japanese B encephalitis	Encephalitis	Mosquito	Japan, East Asia
Dengue	Fevers, hemorrhages (sometimes)	Mosquito	All tropics
Yellow fever	Hemorrhagic fever	Mosquito	Africa, Central and South America
Many others	Encephalitis	Mosquito, tick	Worldwide
Bunyaviridae Family			
Bunyavirus			
California	Encaphalitis	Mosquito	North America
Rifts valley	Fever	Mosquito	Africa
Others	Fevers	Mosquito, flies	Worldwide
Reoviridae Family			
Orbivirus			
Colorado tick fever	Fever	Tick	North America

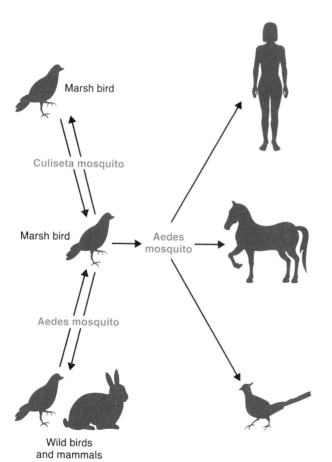

Figure 33.1. Life cycle of the EEE virus. The complete cycle takes place between wild birds by the bite of *Culiseta* mosquitoes and between wild birds and wild mammals via *Aedes* mosquitoes. One-way spread to humans, horses, and pheasants takes place by the bite of *Aedes* mosquitoes.

normal life cycle of the virus. However, they are important **sentinel animals**. When horses become infected, they alert the human population that the virus has escaped its normal biological boundaries and is a threat to humans.

Some time must pass before a mosquito that has acquired the virus can transmit it. Mosquitoes do not become sick with the virus, and once infected, they can spread it for the rest of their lives (one season). The normal vertebrate hosts of the virus (birds) are also relatively unaffected, thus permitting a stable life cycle. The frequency of encounter is dictated by humans' proximity to both the animal reservoir and the insect vector.

ENTRY, SPREAD, AND MULTIPLICATION

EEE virus gains access to humans via the bite of an infected mosquito. Virus-containing saliva is introduced into the capillary bed as the mosquito's proboscis penetrates the skin and endothelial cells of the capillary wall.

The virus localizes in the vascular endothelium and the lymphatic cells of the lymphoreticular system, where replication occurs. A **primary viremia** is induced as the virus is liberated from these infected cells. This period is of short duration, and about the time when Mr. R.'s symptoms first appeared, the virus had probably already been cleared from his blood.

DAMAGE

In many instances, infection by EEE and related viruses does not progress past the stage of replication in the vascular endothelium. If viremia does occur in a patient without a protective antibody titer, the virus may localize elsewhere, primarily in the central nervous system. The clinical manifestations seen in Mr. R's case are consistent with damage to various parts of the brain, as subsequently confirmed at autopsy.

It is not known how EEE virus crosses the blood–brain barrier or why penetration into the brain occurs in only

---

PARADIGM ■ ■ ■

Arthropod-borne Infections

Many of the infections described in this text are acquired by exposure to arthropods. Nearly any arthropod that uses humans as a source of nutrition can also be a vector for infection, including mosquitoes, ticks, biting flies, fleas, lice, and other blood-feeding bugs. Viruses, bacteria, protozoa, and helminths are among the infectious agents that may be transmitted. Although the routes of transmission are varied and complex, a few general principles apply to all arthropod-borne diseases.

- In nearly all instances, the infectious agent must infect the vector and multiply or develop before the arthropod becomes an effective transmitter of infection. The agent must be able to infect both the vector and human hosts. Arboviruses, for example, are well adapted to grow in insect, as well as mammalian, cells. Alternatively, agents that do not infect arthropods are rarely, if ever, transmitted by passive or transient contamination of the arthropod's mouthparts. Consequently, a bloodborne virus such as HIV that cannot replicate in arthropods is not spread by this means.
- The geographical distribution of an arthropod-borne infection is largely determined by the habitat requirements of the vector. The ambient temperature, humidity, altitude, and presence of certain flora and fauna are factors that may determine whether a specific vector will survive in a specific locale. Some disease control measures are designed to eliminate a vector's habitat (e.g., draining standing water to prevent mosquito breeding). On the other hand, manipulations of the environment may have an opposite, unforeseen effect (e.g., felling of

trees creates stump holes where water may pool, providing optimal conditions for mosquitoes to breed).
- The feeding behavior of the vector often determines the epidemiology of an arthropod-borne infection. As with arboviruses, high local incidence of malaria is often associated with mosquito species that prefer to bite humans rather than animals. Similarly, ticks survive year-round in temperate climates, but they bite only during warmer seasons. As a result, early Lyme disease, Rocky Mountain spotted fever, and ehrlichiosis occur almost exclusively in the spring and summer.
- Human conditions or behaviors, such as some occupational or recreational activities, lead to greater contact with certain arthropods. Diseases transmitted by fleas and lice are commonly associated with impoverished conditions or wars. Mosquito-borne diseases tend to flourish in communities where humans do not have mosquito netting or other means to protect themselves from exposure, particularly at night.
- Arthropods shuttle infectious agents from animals with which humans would otherwise have no direct contact. For example, arboviruses may be carried from wild birds to humans even though the human host has no exposure to the avian source. In this and other cases, carriage by an arthropod spreads the infection and expands the potential host range.

N. CARY ENGLEBERG

some infected persons. Damage to brain and cerebellar tissue appears to be due largely to vascular involvement. Small hemorrhages are seen throughout these organs, with little preferred localization. Neurons are severely affected and many die, leading to extensive necrosis.

DISEASES CAUSED BY OTHER ARBOVIRUSES

In the U.S., two other encephalitides closely related to EEE, called **St. Louis encephalitis (SLE)** and **western equine encephalitis (WEE)** are seen. Of these, SLE is the most common, having caused about 5000 cases between 1955 and 1985. Occasionally, SLE occurs in epidemics, including one in 1975 that resulted in some 1800 cases. Fortunately, it is a milder disease than EEE. **Japanese encephalitis** was relatively common in the Far East, but its spread has been stemmed by the use of a killed virus vaccine administered to pigs and children. The vaccine is available in the United States and is given to travelers at risk for exposure.

The arbovirus disease of greatest historical importance is **yellow fever**. It has caused fearsome and extensive epidemics in Africa and the Americas. Despite the presence of suitable vectors and hosts, yellow fever has never taken hold in Asia. The devastating impact of yellow fever on the U.S. Army in Cuba during the Spanish-American war led Walter Reed to his classic investigation into the etiology of the disease. His success in identifying a filtrable agent as the cause of yellow fever was the first proof that viruses cause human disease. Control of the disease is achieved by vaccination and by control of the vector, the mosquito *Aedes aegypti.*

Yellow fever continues to be a serious disease in much of western Africa and the Americas, where the mosquito vector has not been eradicated. An epidemic in central Nigeria in 1986 caused nearly 5000 deaths within the first 3 weeks. African monkeys, which remain asymptomatic after infection, are the reservoir in parts of Africa. In contrast, the virus may cause devastating epidemics in monkeys of Central and South America. As a consequence, outbreaks of yellow fever in monkeys continually move from one region of that continent to another. Symptoms of yellow fever in humans range from none to several and include high fever, chills, headache, myalgia, and vomiting. The disease is fatal in 50% of the cases. In some patients, an improvement in symptoms is followed by jaundice, hemorrhagic complications, and renal failure.

Dengue fever is another arbovirus disease transmitted by the same mosquitoes. It is the **most prevalent human disease caused by arboviruses** and is found in tropical and subtropical regions of much of the world. Fortunately, it does not cause significant mortality. Clinical manifestations include sudden onset of fever, headache, pain behind the eye, and lumbosacral pain, often followed by a generalized rash. The incubation period may last up to 7 days, and North American travelers to endemic areas may become sick several days after returning home. This disease differs from other arbovirus infections in that it is not a zoonosis but is transmitted by mosquitoes directly from person to person.

There are four serotypes of dengue virus, any combination of which may circulate in a given population. Although dengue virus infection results in solid, protective immunity against the infecting serotype, there is only partial cross-reactivity with other serotypes. In fact, antibodies generated against one serotype may not only fail to neutralize another viral serotype, they may actually enhance infection by providing an efficient means of viral uptake by permissive phagocytic cells (i.e., via opsonization). This situation is called **immune enhancement**. In immune enhancement, a virus is bound by non-neutralizing antibody and forms an infectious immune complex that readily enters macrophage cells. The result of immune enhancement is an increased viral load. At least in the early stages of illness, enhanced disease with hemorrhagic complications, **dengue hemorrhagic fever (DHF)**, or even shock, i.e., **dengue shock syndrome (DSS)** may occur. Persons with partial immunity due to prior dengue infection or newborns with maternal antibody are at risk for these severe complications.

In the Far East, where multiple dengue serotypes have historically circulated, the full clinical spectrum of dengue, DHF, and DSS occurs. Until recently, only dengue serotype 2 circulated in the Americas, and as a result, DHF and DSS were uncommon in the Western hemisphere. Unfortunately, with the relaxation of mosquito control programs and the importation of Asian dengue viruses, the American situation has changed. Serogroup 1 and serogroup 3 viruses have caused outbreaks in Central and South America associated with large numbers of dengue cases and frequent DHF. Hopefully, efforts to manufacture an effective vaccine against all four serogroups will soon succeed and permit some measure of control over this growing problem.

DIAGNOSIS

Diagnosis of diseases caused by any arbovirus on clinical grounds alone is difficult because of the paucity of specific findings on physical examination. Proof of the etiology requires either isolation of the virus or demonstration of a rise in antibody titer during the illness. The EEE virus cannot usually be isolated from the blood of an infected person because the viremic phase is brief. Isolation of the virus from tissues such as brain should be attempted only in laboratories with appropriate containment facilities because of the danger of infection to laboratory workers.

TREATMENT AND PREVENTION

Lack of specific therapy for these diseases increases the emphasis on prevention. In endemic regions, community surveillance programs should be established to **follow the density of vectors** (i.e., mosquitoes) during the appropriate season of the year. At appropriate times, **personal protection against mosquitoes** should be emphasized (e.g., the use of repellents and bed nets). In parts of the U.S., the appearance of even a single case of viral encephalitis often causes great concern in the population and among public health workers. Widespread **aerial spraying of insecticides** is sometimes carried out, but not without considerable controversy. Because arboviruses cannot spread from infected patients directly, person-to-person contact is not a concern.

Vaccines against many of the arboviruses that cause encephalitides are either available or under development. Vaccination is an important consideration for travelers to areas where yellow fever is endemic. A live attenuated vaccine induces good immunity for at least 10 years.

SELF-ASSESSMENT QUESTIONS

1. What are the main disease types caused by the arboviruses?
2. How does the mode of transmission of arboviruses affect their geographic distribution and seasonal pattern?
3. How do positive-strand viruses differ from negative-strand viruses?
4. What is the relationship among humans, horses, and birds in the epidemiology of arbovirus encephalitides?
5. Why is it important in the U.S. to notice if horses suffer from viral encephalitis during the summer months?

SUGGESTED READINGS

Hayes EB, Gubler DJ. Dengue and dengue hemorrhagic fever. Pediatr Infect Dis J 1992:11:311–317.

Lanciotti RS, Lewis JG, Gubler DJ, Trent DW. Molecular evolution and epidemiology of DEN-3 virus. J Gen Virol 1994; 75:65–75.

Pan American Health Organization. Dengue and dengue hemorrhagic fever in the Americas: guidelines for prevention and control of dengue and dengue hemorrhagic fever in the Americas. Washington, DC: Pan American Health Organization, 1994; scientific publication no. 548.

Rigau-Perez JG, Gubler DJ, Vorndam AV, Clark GG. Dengue surveillance—United States, 1986–1992. In: CDC surveillance summaries (July). MMWR 1994;43 (no. SS-2):7–11.

Shaio MF, Cheng SN, Yuh YS, Yang KD. Cytotoxic factors released by dengue virus-infected human blood monocytes. J Med Virol 1995;46:216–223.

Whitley RJ. Viral encephalitis. N Engl J Med 1990;323: 242–250.

CHAPTER 34

Paramyxoviruses: Measles, Mumps, Slow Viruses, and the Respiratory Syncytial Virus

STEPHEN E. STRAUS

GREGORY A. STORCH

The family of viruses known as Paramyxoviridae (Table 34.1) includes several medically important pathogens that possess particular affinities for infecting and damaging **respiratory tract** and **central nervous system** tissue. For example, the genus *Paramyxovirus* within this family consists of the **mumps** and **parainfluenza** viruses. Prior to development of live attenuated mumps vaccine recommended for infants at age 12–15 months, mumps was recognized as a common cause of epidemics of glandular inflammation (salivary, pancreas, testes) and associated meningoencephalitis. The current lack of an effective vaccine for the parainfluenza viruses leaves those viruses as major causes of childhood croup (laryngotracheitis) that appear in epidemic waves each fall.

This chapter focuses primarily on members of two other genera of the Paramyxoviridae family, the **measles virus** and the **respiratory syncytial virus** (RSV). RSV is the major cause of serious respiratory infection in young infants. It has been chosen for detailed description as an example of an important viral pathogen that has eluded serious attempts to develop an effective vaccine. Before getting into the reasons for that, we begin with a more optimistic story, that of measles.

▊ CASE

Ms. M., an aspiring journalist, took ill just before crucial college midterm examinations. She had looked forward to a relaxed spring break after these examinations, but now her ability to take them seems in doubt. She feels miserable, has fever, a runny nose, cough, a blotchy rash, and is told by the health service physician that she might have measles.

"That's absurd," she thinks, "Only little kids get measles and I think I had it as a child."

Her rash appeared first on the neck and head, then spread to the trunk and extremities during the next few days. At first, the rash was composed of discrete, reddish lesions that blanched on pressure. They then quickly merged together and became increasingly brownish.

If you were the university health service physician, it would be your responsibility to make a definitive diagnosis, despite Ms. M.'s protestations, and to take several steps to ensure that if it were measles, she would not contribute to the further spread of the illness on campus. What must you know?

1. Given the current rarity of the disease in the U.S., is it reasonable to consider measles as a probable diagnosis?
2. What information can be gleaned from the medical history of the patient, her physical findings, and laboratory tests to confirm or rule out the diagnosis of measles?
3. Could Ms. M. have had measles previously and now have it again?
4. What other illnesses are associated with rashes, and could any of them be Ms. M.'s problem?
5. What complications might Ms. M. or others experience from this illness?
6. How can transmission of measles to others be prevented?

These and other issues are addressed in this chapter.

Table 34.1. The Classification of Paramyxoviruses	
Family	
Paramyxoviridae	
Genus	
Pneumovirus	Respiratory syncytial virus
Paramyxovirus	Mumps virus, parainfluenza virus
Morbillivirus	Measles, canine distemper virus

History and Epidemiology of Measles

The history of measles is one of the most interesting, colorful, and generally underappreciated of all of the infectious diseases. Except for plague, cholera, typhus, and smallpox, measles has perhaps had the greatest impact on people, on the successes or failures of their explorations, their colonization attempts, their military campaigns, and their ability to survive to old age. Curiously, among the general public, these facts are little known. The availability of an effective vaccine has so reduced the incidence of measles in developed nations that we have been quick to forget that it is among the most spectacularly contagious of human infections, one that is still a major killer of children in underdeveloped countries.

Measles is an ancient disease. A Moslem physician of the 10th century, Rhazes, is credited with its first recorded accounts. Numerous epidemics swept across Europe through the Middle Ages and the Reformation period. Measles accompanied European explorers and immigrants to isolated new lands where the indigenous populations were susceptible to the disease. Among the most dramatic and informative effects of measles in totally susceptible populations was that of the 1851 epidemic in the Faroe Islands neighboring Greenland. Within 6 weeks, all but five of the 4000 inhabitants of the affected region contracted measles! Similar epidemics were responsible for decimating the Hawaiians and other isolated native populations upon their first contact with infected Europeans.

The study of measles made a natural progression from the field to the laboratory. In a model of early scientific investigation, Home demonstrated in the mid-18th century that measles could be transmitted by exposure to blood of infected individuals. These findings were confirmed in 1905 and extended several years later through studies of experimental transmission to monkeys. In 1954, Enders and Peebles reported successful growth of measles virus in cultured cells. This paved the way for studies of the molecular biology of measles virus and for the important development of an effective, live, attenuated measles virus vaccine.

MEASLES VIRUS

The disease is caused by the measles virus, a *Morbillivirus* of the paramyxovirus family (Table 34.1). The members of this virus family are pleomorphic, meaning that they have a variety of different shapes. The viral genome, composed of **RNA**, is contained within a helical nucleocapsid that is surrounded by a lipid bilayer **envelope** (Fig. 34.1). The surface is studded with **glycoproteins** that project from the envelope surface.

Measles virus has a **single-stranded, nonsegmented RNA** genome with **negative sense** (Fig. 34.2). Individual mRNAs, transcribed from the parental RNA, are translated into measles proteins. Important measles virus envelope glycoproteins include **hemagglutinins**, whereas those in the related mumps viruses have both **hemagglutinin** and **neuraminidase** activity (Fig. 34.1). These proteins are named after easily identified biological properties and are more fully described in the chapter on influenza virus (Chapter 35).

Measles virus possesses an additional glycoprotein known as the **F** (for "fusion") **protein**, which endows the virus with the ability to cause **membranes to fuse** together. Presumably, the F glycoprotein participates in fusion of the infecting virus to the host cell membrane. Secondarily, its expression on the surface of infected cells during viral replication causes fusion of adjacent cells. This results in one classic hallmark of measles virus infection, namely, the formation of **giant cells**, or **syncytia** (Fig. 34.3). (Discussion of a related RSV protein follows in the sections emphasizing that virus.) Measles virus also contains an M (for "matrix") protein on the inner surface of the viral envelope. This protein is said to participate in the proper envelopment of assembling nucleocapsids and to be required for spread of infectious progeny virions to adjacent cells. Other internal proteins, a large protein (L) and the polymerase (P) are believed to participate in transcription and genome replication. Measles replication is manifested not only by formation of syncytia, but also by the appearance of **eosinophilic inclusions** in the cytoplasm and the nucleus.

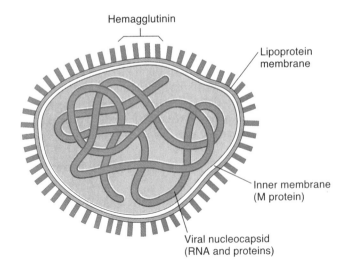

Figure 34.1. Schematic diagram of measles virus.

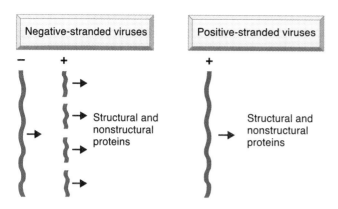

Figure 34.2. Transcription and translation of proteins by negative-stranded and positive-stranded RNA viruses.

These inclusions are aggregates of proteins that take up the eosin (red) stain commonly used in staining tissue slices.

ENCOUNTER

What do you need to know to consider further if Ms. M. has measles or to discount that possibility? First, did she ever have measles or has she been vaccinated? Before vaccination programs were initiated in this country, measles occurred primarily in 5- to 6-year-old children, and Ms. M. may have been too young to remember her early childhood diseases. A parent or an older sibling might recall; a simple phone call could be of help with her history. Because even these histories commonly prove unreliable, it would be more useful to obtain evidence of proper childhood vaccination, a fact widely solicited today by university health services from newly accepted applicants. Second, we would want to ask whether Ms. M. has recently been in contact with anyone who has this disease; however, patients may not be aware of measles exposure until a cluster of cases is recognized.

The infection is **extremely contagious**, maximally so during the 2- to 3-day period prior to the appearance of the rash. Experiments done with virus-containing aerosols have shown that the disease can be acquired through **inhalation**. Therefore, Ms. M.'s exposure may have involved a seemingly innocuous encounter in an elevator, a bus, or anywhere. For instructive purposes, let us assume that other cases of measles have recently been recognized among individuals at Ms. M.'s university.

SPREAD AND MULTIPLICATION

Measles virus is inhaled during exposure to individuals with measles. It is believed that the virus replicates in **respiratory epithelial cells** and, about 3 days later, **spreads through the bloodstream** to infect distant body

sites, including the lung and lymphoid tissues of the tonsils, lymph nodes, gastrointestinal tract, and spleen. After a few more days, a second, larger wave of virus is released from these sites into the bloodstream, producing maximal symptoms and skin involvement. Infections such as measles, that involve multiple replicative cycles and spread from the site of inoculation to local and then to distant sites typically have incubation periods of at least 10–14 days. Infections that manifest themselves at or near the site of inoculation (e.g., herpes simplex and influenza) and do not disseminate characteristically have short incubation periods (2–7 days).

DAMAGE

Most of the pathology associated with measles infection can be attributed directly to **viral invasion** and **cytopathic destruction** of tissues. It seems likely, however, that some of the features of the disease are attributable to damage inflicted by the **host immune responses** to the

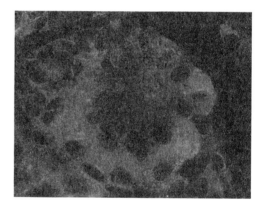

Figure 34.3. Giant cell (syncytium) formation in measles pneumonia.

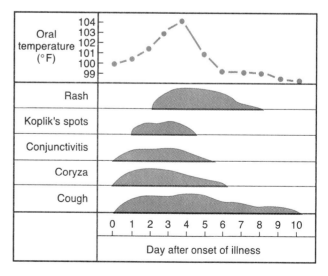

Figure 34.4. Signs and symptoms of measles infection.

virus. Measles causes the classic viral **enanthem** (lesions on mucous membranes) in the mouth called **Koplik's spots**, as well as a diffuse **exanthem** (external lesions), the typical measles rash (Fig. 34.4). Biopsies of measles lesions show viral antigens and particles in the tissues, but the most prominent finding is an intense inflammatory response with edema and mononuclear infiltration. **Immunodeficient children** occasionally fail to develop a rash during measles infections, which suggests that the inflammatory response may be a major cause of tissue damage in the mucocutaneous lesions.

Both the **humoral and the cellular immune** responses modulate the outcome of acute measles infection. Administration of measles-specific globulin to susceptible individuals shortly after exposure to the virus will ameliorate the infection. The cellular immune response, however, is probably the major determinant of protection against severe measles infection and reinfection. **Patients with agammaglobulinemia** tolerate measles well, whereas those with congenital or acquired cellular immune deficits, such as those associated with acute leukemia, are prone to severe or fatal infection. Virus replication and spread are intense and unbridled, leading to fulminant pneumonia, respiratory failure, and death.

Measles infection itself stresses and further decreases cellular immunity. During measles infections, patients are at an increased risk of reactivating herpes simplex infections and tuberculosis, and transiently losing their delayed hypersensitivity response to tuberculin and to other antigens.

How Does the Host Respond to Measles?

Acute measles virus infection is **nearly always symptomatic** and is inevitably accompanied by **immune responses** in immunocompetent people. IgM antibodies circulate within 1 week of development of the rash and persist for several weeks or months. IgG antibodies can be detected in serum shortly after the IgM antibodies; they peak within a few weeks and gradually decline, although they persist for life. Secretory IgA antibodies are detectable in nasal secretions. A measles-specific lymphocyte-mediated immune response can be demonstrated in acute infection. So can interferon, whose levels wane rapidly with convalescence. Cellular immunity and protection from reinfection persist for life; thus, Ms. M. probably had neither the vaccine nor the disease in childhood.

DIAGNOSIS

The clinical manifestations of measles usually follow a **stereotyped pattern** illustrated in Figure 34.4. Mounting fever over three to four days, rash beginning on the third or fourth day, and **"the three c's"** (cough, coryza [runny nose], and conjunctivitis) occur in most cases. With a known exposure, and certainly with the classic

"measly" or **morbilliform appearance** (Fig. 34.5), a tentative diagnosis of measles can be made on clinical grounds with some confidence. There are, however, more precise means of establishing the diagnosis, and it is appropriate to employ such tests whenever the appearance or the history is in doubt.

The definitive diagnostic tool is **virus isolation**. The virus can be recovered from nasopharyngeal secretions, blood, or urine any time after the onset of symptoms and until the second or third day of rash. The procedure is expensive, slow, and not routinely available, so that most physicians appropriately resort to serodiagnostic studies.

Serum collected at the time when rash is present (the acute phase) already contains measurable **IgM antibodies** to measles antigens but may have little or no IgG antibody to the virus. The rapid evolution of an immune response to viral proteins results in a **rise in antimeasles IgG level**, so that the quantity of such antibodies would be greater 24 weeks after the onset of the illness. By then, most measles infections have resolved. Several serological methods are applicable, but the most widely used tests involve hemagglutination inhibition or an enzyme immunoassay (ELISA test, see Chapter 55). Recently, **tests for measles IgM antibodies** have become available and can be used to diagnose measles from a single blood sample obtained early in the illness.

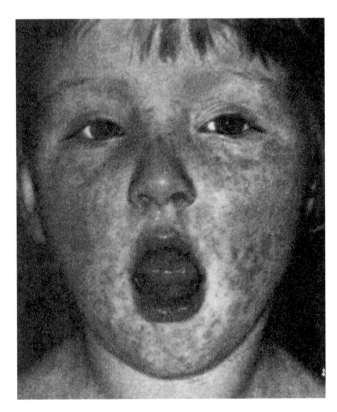

Figure 34.5. A child with measles, showing classic rash and a runny nose.

As the health service physician, you can confirm Ms. M.'s diagnosis by collecting serum to test for measles IgM antibodies. Alternatively, you could store serum during her first visit to your office and ask her to return about 2 weeks later to have another serum specimen drawn. At that time, you would submit both specimens for testing. A typical confirmatory result might be an eightfold rise in hemagglutination inhibition (HAI) titer, from 1:8 to 1:64, between the samples. These numbers mean the following: in the first sample there was already a sufficient quantity of measles antibody to be detectable in the assay when the serum was diluted eight times, but not more; in the convalescent serum specimen, there was so much more measles antibody that it could still be detected in serum that had been diluted 64-fold.

Complications

As implied above, immunologically competent individuals experience few complications, although the course of measles infection tends to be more severe in adults than in children. It is important to be aware that even in children, **measles is not benign**. The infection itself is prostrating. The most common complications involve **superinfections** of the middle ear and the lung, primarily with pneumococci, staphylococci, or meningococci. Injury to respiratory tract tissues may render a patient more susceptible to bacterial superinfection. **Pneumonia** is the major reason for hospitalization in measles cases. It can be especially severe if the pneumonia is caused by the virus itself (giant cell pneumonitis) rather than by superinfecting bacteria.

About 1 in 1000 children with measles experience **neurological complications**. In general, these symptoms appear several days after resolution of the rash and consist of fever, headache, irritability, confusion, and seizures. Most patients survive this meningoencephalitis, but permanent sequelae include deafness, mental retardation, and seizure disorders.

Death from measles, which is rare in developed countries, stems largely from pulmonary and central nervous system complications. In developing nations, measles remains a major killer, felling tens of thousands of infants each year and making measles a major priority of international health programs. There are several reasons for the remarkable prevalence of measles in children of the Third World. First, even though there is an effective vaccination for the single strain of measles virus that circulates around the world, unchanged from year to year, vaccination is expensive and beyond the meager public health resources of many countries. Second, because the vaccine is a live one, it is stable only when stored in the cold, necessitating a "cold chain," the unbroken series of refrigerated containers for shipment and storage until it reaches the ultimate consumer. This, too, is a barrier to use in developing nations. Third, modern diagnostic and therapeutic tools are often not available to limit evolving

complications. Finally, and most importantly, the infants of these regions frequently lack the immunological resources to combat the measles virus and other complicating pathogens. Malnutrition impairs cellular immune defenses (Chapter 74) and poor hygiene favors bacterial superinfection of the skin and respiratory tract (Chapter 71).

PREVENTION

Assuming that our patient, Ms. M., has measles, she may already have exposed others to her virus, at school or elsewhere. Is it possible to break the cycle of the infection in her community? Yes. We noted above that immune serum globulin can modify measles infection. This is appropriate for exposed individuals who are at risk of complicated infection, including infants who are less than 1 year old and especially children with leukemia or other disorders associated with substantial impairment of cellular immunity.

Of greater value, however, is the **measles vaccine**. A number of different ones have been developed. The first one, a killed virus vaccine, provided limited protection and sometimes modified rather than prevented the disease associated with subsequent exposure to measles virus. The resulting **atypical measles syndrome** has many clinical features that differ from those of classic measles. Atypical measles occurs in young adults and adolescents and is difficult to diagnose because the exanthem has a highly variable appearance and pleuropulmonary complications are frequent.

Antibodies that neutralize virus infectivity are required to **limit the spread of measles virus** to uninfected cells. Many antibodies can be induced by viral proteins but fail to inactivate the virus. The killed measles vaccine induced little antibody to the F (fusion) protein but high levels of antibody to the hemagglutinin. Inasmuch as antibody to the F protein is required to prevent cell-to-cell spread of measles virus, the killed vaccine provided only partial protection against infection.

A **live attenuated virus vaccine** is well tolerated and confers durable immunity. Measles vaccine is usually administered together with those against mumps and rubella, all consisting of attenuated live viruses (see Chapter 44). Use of this vaccine, supported by laws in most states requiring that children must be vaccinated before attending school, brought about a dramatic decrease in the incidence of measles in the United States (Fig. 34.6). However, in the early 1990s, measles epidemics recurred. Some outbreaks occurred in high school and college age individuals, probably resulting from the combined effects of inadequate immunization (for example, immunization at too young an age), lack of immunization, and occasional vaccine failure. Other outbreaks occurred in pre-school age children in inner cities, resulting from delays in normally recommended

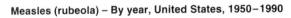

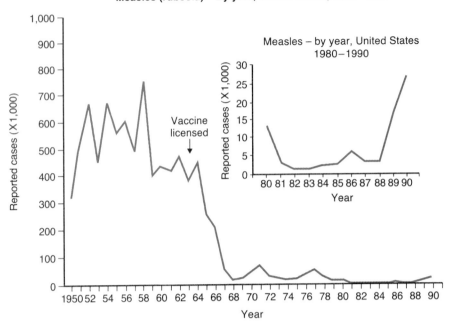

Figure 34.6. Reported cases of measles in the U.S., 1950–1990, showing the profound decline in measles incidence since the introduction of the vaccine, and the recent resurgence of the disease.

immunizations. In response, public health officials made a dramatic change in the use of measles vaccine, recommending that all individuals born after 1956 receive two doses of measles vaccine. The year 1956 was chosen because it had been found that most individuals born before that year were immune as the result of natural infection. In addition, efforts to deliver vaccine to young children were increased. These measures were successful in reducing the incidence of measles to record low levels. It is now evident that the eradication of measles is feasible, although major international efforts will be required.

As the university health service physician, your responsibilities extend well beyond diagnosing and caring for Ms. M. You are obliged to report her infection to state health authorities who track measles outbreaks. More importantly, you would need to see that all possible efforts are made to institute a campus-wide search to identify Ms. M.'s potential contacts and others who may be susceptible to measles. If evidence of preexisting immunity cannot be obtained, vaccination is required.

SUBACUTE SCLEROSING PANENCEPHALITIS AND THE SLOW VIRUS INFECTIONS

A process known as a **slow virus infection** consists of the gradual appearance of disease months or years after a virus enters the body. It is to be distinguished from chronic viral infections such as that associated with hepatitis B virus (see Chapter 41) in which the disease pro-

gresses steadily after exposure. It is also different from recurrent viral infections like zoster (see Chapter 40), in which the virus can remain dormant for decades before reactivating.

A slow virus infection is unrecognized and undetectable for a long time, until it produces a slowly progressive disorder, one that is characteristically fatal. The best studied slow virus infections of humans involve central nervous system degeneration and include **kuru, Creutzfeldt-Jakob disease** (CJD), and **subacute sclerosing panencephalitis** (SSPE). Kuru and CJD are caused by "unconventional agents," meaning that their exact nature has been hard to define. They are now widely thought to be caused by **prions**, misfolded protein molecules that have a remarkable ability to cause the misfolding of nascent proteins of the same kind.

SSPE is caused by a kind of measles virus, and is the best understood of the slow virus infections. Although rare, SSPE has captured the attention of the scientific and medical communities. It is a slowly progressive, unrelenting and untreatable, degenerative, neurological disorder that is characterized by scarring and demyelination of many areas of the brain. Death usually occurs within 2 years of onset. The incidence of SSPE diminished in parallel with the decrease in measles cases that followed the introduction of the measles vaccine (Fig. 34.6).

SSPE occurs several years after the initial measles infection and is less likely to occur in individuals who received live measles vaccine. The remarkable aspect of the pathogenesis of SSPE is its association with an altered measles virus. How or why the alteration occurs in the virus is unknown but, presumably, it results from a spontaneous mutation. Using special techniques, the virus can be recovered from the brains of some affected patients, but its pattern of replication in brain, cultured cells, or experimental animals is altered. It appears that the measles M protein, normally involved in virus assembly, is not expressed normally; thus, the release of infectious progeny virus is impaired.

RESPIRATORY SYNCYTIAL VIRUS INFECTION

A cousin of the measles virus, RSV, causes an infection that is well known to all physicians who care for young children. Its most characteristic clinical manifestation is **bronchiolitis**, the inflammation of the terminal bronchioles. Because of its extensive morbidity and significant mortality (approximately 4500 deaths per year in the U.S.), RSV infection is a major candidate for vaccine development. Efforts to make an effective human vaccine have all failed so far.

▮ CASE

A 4-month-old infant boy developed a nasal discharge, low-grade fever, and was fussy. The next day, the parents called the pediatrician because he was having difficulty breathing. On examination, he had an obvious nasal discharge and was breathing 60 times per minute with mild nasal flaring and rib retractions. Auscultation of the lungs revealed scattered rales (crackles) and wheezes. A chest x-ray revealed hyperexpansion and patchy infiltrates in the lungs. The baby was admitted to the hospital, where treatment consisted of oxygen, humidified air delivered via a mist tent, fluids, and suctioning of secretions. He began to improve after 48 hours and was discharged home, where the symptoms gradually resolved over the next 7 days. A fluorescent antibody stain of nasal secretions performed on the day of admission was positive for respiratory syncytial virus antigen, and 3 days later, a culture was reported as positive for that virus.

THE RESPIRATORY SYNCYTIAL VIRUS (RSV)

RSV also has a **single-stranded, nonsegmented RNA genome** that is of **negative sense**. The entire genome has been cloned and sequenced. **Ten genes and their corresponding proteins** have been identified. Unlike measles virus (or the influenza or parainfluenza viruses), no hemagglutinin activity has been identified. Two virally specified surface glycoproteins are prominent. One of them, the large glycoprotein, designated **G**, is responsible for the initial binding of the virus to the host cell; the other, the fusion protein, designated **F**, permits fusion of the viral envelope with the host cell membrane, leading to entry of the virus. The F protein also induces fusion of membranes of the infected cells. RSV gets its name resulting from the formation of syncytia, or multinucleated masses of fused cells.

In comparison to the rhinoviruses or the influenza viruses, isolates of RSV display less antigenic heterogeneity; however, recent studies have defined two distinct groups, A and B, as well as subgroups within each group. Both groups A and B circulate concurrently and have been detected in many locations throughout the world. The relationship of this antigenic diversity to the immunology or pathogenesis of RSV infection is not yet known, although recent evidence suggests that, of the two groups, infections caused by the group A viruses may be more severe.

ENCOUNTER AND ENTRY

The epidemiology of RSV infection has been extensively studied. The virus has been found in **every part of the world** where it has been sought. In temperate areas, it causes a highly **seasonal disease**, with epidemics every winter and essentially disease-free summers. Infection occurs in early childhood almost universally. Most infections lead to symptomatic illness, but no more than 1% are severe enough to require hospitalization. The mortality rate for hospitalized cases is less than 5%, but is higher in patients at risk, especially those with congenital heart disease, bronchopulmonary dysplasia related to prematurity, neuromuscular disease, or immune deficiency.

The only known source of RSV is infected humans who shed the virus in nasal secretions. As in the case of the rhinoviruses, transmission is thought to occur when secretions containing virus contaminate the hands of individuals. Small-particle airborne transmission plays, at most, a minor role in transmission. In a classical experiment, volunteers in close physical contact with RSV-infected infants were more readily infected than those who remained 6 feet away (Table 34.2).

Table 34.2. Transmission of Respiratory Syncytial Virus

Volunteers:	Cuddlers[a]	Touchers[b]	Sitters[c]
Exposed	7	10	14
Infected	5	4	0
Incubation time	4 days	5.5 days	

[a] Close contact with infected infant.
[b] Self-inoculation after touching surfaces contaminated with infants' secretions.
[c] Sitting over 6 feet from infected infant.

SPREAD, MULTIPLICATION, AND DAMAGE

Infection proceeds **downward along the respiratory mucosa** starting from the initial site of inoculation. **Cell-to-cell transmission** of virus may be important in this process. It is possible that **aspiration** of virus-contaminated secretions accelerates the process. **There is no clinically significant spread to distant sites.**

Severe RSV infection results in one of two somewhat overlapping clinical syndromes: (a) **bronchiolitis and (b) pneumonia.** The child with bronchiolitis has difficulty breathing and there is functional evidence of obstruction of the airways that resembles asthma. Breathing is very noisy, with wheezing. As illustrated in the case history, the chest x-ray reveals hyperexpansion of the lungs, resulting from trapped air; it may also show streaky infiltrates, usually in both lungs. In the child with pneumonia, pulmonary infiltrates are more prominent. Wheezing and hyperexpansion may also occur, but less prominently than in bronchiolitis. In either syndrome, the airways are inflamed and edematous.

Tissue sections from fatal cases show **necrosis of the epithelial cells** that line the small bronchioles. There is also **infiltration of lymphocytes** among the mucosal epithelial cells and evidence of increased mucous secretion. The underlying elastic and muscle fibers are not affected. In cases of pneumonia, alveolar involvement consisting of **swelling of the alveolar lining cells and interstitial inflammation** accompanies bronchiolar involvement.

Bronchiolitis can be distinguished from asthma because bronchiolitis usually occurs in infants 2–8 months of age in whom bronchial smooth muscle is incompletely developed. Thus, smooth muscle contraction may be less important in bronchiolitis than in asthma. If an individual bronchiole is completely obstructed, the portion of the lung ventilated by it may collapse. If obstruction is incomplete, a ball-valve effect may occur, leading to hyperexpansion of the distal lung. The entire process is associated with mismatches in ventilation and perfusion of the lung, and results in decreased oxygenation, along with the increased work of breathing.

In most cases, the infection is successfully controlled by the immune system, and recovery begins after several days; however, in the severe cases that occur in children compromised by other diseases, there may be **respiratory failure**, and the child may die unless mechanical ventilation is provided. There is considerable concern that severe bronchiolitis in infancy may be associated with chronic lung disease in later life. Infants with bronchiolitis are more likely to have episodes of wheezing as they grow older, but any relationship between bronchiolitis in infancy and chronic lung disease in adulthood remains conjectural.

Doubts have been raised about the role of the immune system in protecting against RSV infections. First, most individuals experience multiple infections with RSV, indicating that immunity is incomplete. Second, infants are often infected at a time when they still have serum-neutralizing antibody from their mothers. Despite these negative findings, there is now evidence that the immune system provides protection. Most importantly, children with both congenital and acquired immune deficiencies suffer prolonged and severe RSV infection. Infants with high levels of serum antibody against RSV are less likely to develop lower respiratory tract involvement than infants with lower levels. Finally, in experimental animals, the administration of monoclonal antibodies to RSV glycoproteins or inoculation with vaccinia virus genetically engineered to express these antigens prevents lower respiratory tract involvement (although not usually nasal infection).

Do immune mechanisms contribute to the clinical manifestations of RSV infection? This is hinted by its resemblance to asthma, a process that involves the immune-mediated release of bronchoconstricting inflammatory mediators. Increased levels of histamine and IgE antibody directed against RSV have been found in nasal secretions from children with RSV bronchiolitis. Another hint that the immune system might contribute to RSV disease derives from an experience in the 1960s with an experimental killed RSV vaccine. Children given this vaccine not only were unprotected against RSV infection, but actually developed more severe disease following natural exposure to RSV! It is now known that the killed vaccine elicited only a partial antibody response against the virus, much the same as described above for early measles vaccines. The responses were sufficient to permit immune-mediated damage to tissues once exposure to the infection had occurred, but not sufficient to limit virus growth and spread.

PREVENTION AND TREATMENT

Because RSV infection is so prevalent and accounts for considerable morbidity, this virus is an important **candidate for vaccine development.** For a number of years there was understandably little activity in this area, for fear of repeating the experience with the earlier vaccine. Recently, interest in an RSV vaccine has been renewed, and promising results have been reported by cloning DNA copies of the viral genes. By using individual genes cloned into vaccinia virus vectors (Chapter 42), it has been possible to show that the immune response associated with either the F or G glycoprotein can protect small mammals, such as the mouse and the cotton rat, against RSV challenge. The immune response to F tends to be broad, whereas that to G tends to be specific for the RSV group (A or B) used to induce the immune response. Ongoing work is evaluating the use of vaccines composed of the F and/or G glycoproteins that have been produced by cloning RSV genes into expression vectors. One approach of particular interest has been to produce a chimerical protein composed of the extracellular domains of both F and G.

A different immunologic strategy is called **passive protection**, and involves the **administration to high-risk infants of preparations of immune globulins** with activity against RSV. This approach is appealing because it gets around the problem that newborn infants (especially those who are premature) may not respond adequately to a conventional vaccine. One avenue being explored is the use of antibodies prepared from the blood of adults with high levels of anti-RSV antibodies. A different approach involves the use of "humanized" monoclonal antibodies which contain the antigen recognition site of a mouse monoclonal antibody combined by genetic engineering with the immunoglobulin structure of a human immunoglobulin. Ongoing clinical trials are investigating the efficacy and safety of these approaches.

In the area of treatment, an antiviral drug called **ribavirin** is available to treat severe RSV infection (Chapter 43). Although the drug is active against RSV in the laboratory, its actual clinical utility is controversial. It is given by aerosol and partly because of expense is generally reserved for very severe RSV infections occurring in infants whose condition is already compromised, especially by chronic lung disease resulting from immaturity or from congenital heart disease.

SELF-ASSESSMENT QUESTIONS

1. What peculiar effects do measles and RSV have on tissue cells?
2. Describe the replication cycle of measles virus.
3. Discuss the role of the immune responses to Paramyxoviridae.
4. What problems are associated with vaccination against measles and RSV?
5. How could we eradicate measles from the face of the earth?

SUGGESTED READINGS

Bellini WJ, Rota JS, Rota PA. J Inf Dis 1994; 170(Suppl.):S15.

Griffin DE. Curr Top Microbiol Immunol 1995;191:117.

Hall WR, Hall CB. Atypical measles in adolescents: evaluation of clinical and pulmonary function. Ann Intern Med 1979; 90:882–886.

McIntosh K, Chanock RM. Respiratory syncytial virus. In: Fields BN, Knipe DM, et al. Virology. 2nd ed. New York: Raven Press, 1990:1045–1072.

Norby E, Oxman MN. Measles virus. In: Fields BN, Knipe DM, et al. Virology. 3rd ed. New York: Raven Press, 1996.

Rabies

GEORGE M. BAER

Key Concepts

Rabies:
- Is a zoonosis caused by the rabies virus, transmitted to humans by the bite of an infected wild or domesticated animal.
- In developing countries, is mainly a disease of dogs; in developed countries, of wild animals.
- Has a variable incubation period ranging from several weeks to about one year.
- Is spread from the site of the bite through nerves to the central and peripheral nervous systems; the virus then travels back to peripheral sites.
- Signs and symptoms include Negri bodies in neurons, difficulty swallowing, increased muscle tone, and hydrophobia.
- Is diagnosed with fluorescent antibody assay of skin biopsies early in the disease.
- Is prevented by vaccination of wild and domesticated animals.
- Is treated in humans with local wound treatment, passive administration of antibody, and vaccination.

Rabies is a disease that has instilled terror in human society—and with good reason. Virtually, all people who are bitten by a rabid animal and develop symptoms die, and many of the symptoms are visible and frightening. In developed countries, the disease in dogs has been controlled with canine vaccines, and, consequently, human rabies cases are rare. Surveillance in these countries is still important, because the rabies virus is still commonly found in a variety of wild animals (including **foxes, skunks, raccoons, and insectivorous bats**). A limited number of countries are free of the disease, mainly islands such as England, Australia, Japan, Taiwan, and most of the small Caribbean islands. The disease is still common in many developing countries, where canine rabies persists and thousands of people are vaccinated after being bitten by potentially rabid animals, mainly dogs.

This chapter will discuss the distribution of rabies in various parts of the world and the animal species involved, as well as the multiplication and spread of virus in those animals, the diagnosis of the disease, and treatment of persons exposed (including the crucial question: to treat or not to treat).

CASE 1

As Mr. V., a 38-year-old dock hand, was walking home in suburban Seattle, Washington, he was suddenly attacked by an average-size brown dog, which bit him on the right calf. The dog only let go when hit repeatedly with a lunch box. The dog then ran away. Mrs. V. cleaned her husband's many punctured wounds when he got home. Both Mr. and Mrs. V. were concerned about rabies and called the state health department. An official told them that no cases of rabies in dogs had been reported in Washington in decades, and only two cases of rabies had been reported in any terrestrial animal. Only bats had been reported rabid in the last decade. The couple was told not to worry about rabies in the dog.

Mr. V. asked his family doctor the following questions:
1. Should he be treated for rabies exposure?
2. If he had been bitten by a bat that then flew away, would the treatment have been different?
3. Did he consult the proper advisors in seeking rabies treatment recommendations?

CASE 2

Mr. R., a 22-year-old phlebotomist, was bitten on the right index finger by a bat while exploring a cavern in Mercedes, Texas. Despite urging from friends, he did not obtain medical care for the bite. Forty-eight days later, he complained of weakness in his right hand and went to the emergency room; based on a history of a puncture wound with a catfish fin earlier in the week, he was treated with an antibiotic and tetanus toxoid.

Several days later, Mr. R. was admitted to the intensive care unit of a hospital with a preliminary diagnosis of encephalitis or tetanus because of intermittent episodes of rigidity, breath holding, hallucinations, and difficulty swallowing. He was intubated because he had uncontrollable oral secretions. At that time, Mr. R.'s supervisor from work reported to the hospital authorities the history of the bat bite. Serum, cerebrospinal fluid (CSF), and skin samples were taken for laboratory workup, but all of the specimens were negative for rabies antigens. Despite supportive therapy, Mr. R.'s condition deteriorated and he died 4 days later after the severity of his earlier symptoms increased, followed by coma and respiratory failure.

Postmortem samples of brain tissue were positive for rabies by the fluorescent antibody test. The rabies variant isolated was identified serologically as identical to those found in Mexican freetail bats. Because of numerous possible contacts he had with people—family, friends, coworkers, and medical personnel while sick (and immediately before), rabies postexposure prophylaxis was begun for 67 of 105 possible contacts.

The following questions arise:
1. Is this a "typical" case of rabies in the U.S.?
2. What treatment would Mr. R. have received had he gone to the hospital when he was bitten?
3. What would have been the chances of success if Mr. R. had been treated for rabies?
4. How many cases of human rabies have there been in the U.S. in the last decade?
5. How many persons are immunized in the U.S. each year?
6. Were Mr. R.'s symptoms typical of human rabies cases?

Humans, Health and History

Rabies

It is not surprising that a disease transmitted by the bite of many kinds of animals was recognized in antiquity. In the Eshnunna Code, dated from the third millennium B.C., it is written:

"If a dog is mad and the authorities have brought the fact to the knowledge of its owner; if he does not keep it in, and it bites a man and causes his death, then the owner shall pay . . . 40 shekels of silver. If it bites a slave and causes his death he shall pay 15 shekels of silver."

Definite evidence that saliva was infective came in the early 19th century when a German scientist (Zinke) demonstrated that saliva from a rabid dog painted on wounds of a dachshund's leg caused the disease. Pasteur delineated the role of the central nervous system in rabies in 1881 when he injected rabbits intracerebrally (rather than intramuscularly) with a suspension of brain taken from a rabid cow and reproduced the disease. Pasteur produced the first rabies vaccines by passing infectious spinal cord material (he did not know it was a virus) through a series of rabbits. The now infected spinal cords were partially inactivated by drying over potash for various periods of time. Pasteur's first rabies vaccination injection consisted of cords dried for 14 days. Subsequent injections used cords dried for shorter periods of time, until the last injection employed fully virulent cord suspensions.

Pasteur's early studies of vaccine efficacy were performed on dogs, but the results from these studies led to the triumphant use of a spinal cord ("Pasteur") vaccine in humans in July 1885. Over the next few decades, the original vaccine underwent many changes, including chemical inactivation of the virus. Early vaccines were prepared from virus growing in nervous system tissue. Regrettably, these vaccines resulted in postvaccinal demyelination and tissue destruction in 34% of vaccinated individuals. Today, safe and effective vaccines are produced from inactivated viruses grown in non-neural tissue culture. Recombinant and subunit rabies vaccines are also being tested.

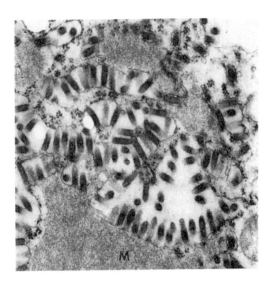

Figure 35.1. Neuron of a dog inoculated with rabies virus. This ultrathin section of a cell shows randomly spaced viral matrices (*M*) and virions (*arrow*) budding from the endoplasmic reticulum membranes; original magnification, ×62,560.

RABIES

The rabies virus is known to infect dozens of mammalian species, including humans. The reason for this unusually broad host range is not known. The viruses are bullet-shaped and fairly large compared to most other viruses (approximately 180 nm in length by 75 nm in width (Fig. 35.1). The rabies virus contains an **external glycoprotein (G) coat,** located immediately outside a **peripheral matrix (M) protein.** The infectious component of the virus is the **helical ribonucleoprotein (RNP) core,** an **unsegmented single-stranded RNA** tightly encased in the **major N protein.** Because the genome of this virus is of **negative polarity,** the virions contain an **RNA-dependent viral RNA transcriptase.** The replication cycle of rabies viruses takes place entirely in the cytoplasm of infected cells and results in the formation of numerous viral particles. Masses of nucleocapsids accumulate in the cytoplasm to form inclusions called **Negri bodies** that can be seen in stained preparations or by immunofluorescence (Fig. 35.2).

Resistance to rabies infection has long been correlated with the presence of neutralizing antibody, and the relationship between those antibodies and protection has been well established in a variety of animal species. Many of the viruses in this group elicit the formation of antibodies that protect against other members of the group.

ENCOUNTER

From 1990 to 1994, 14 human rabies deaths were reported in the U.S. These cases are either imported or associated with exposures to wild animals or to unidenti-

fied animals. Over 30,000 cases of animal rabies occur yearly worldwide, of which nearly 90% are in wild animals. Although most rabies cases in the U.S. are found in wild animals, most humans from areas of endemic rabies are vaccinated for exposure to dogs and cats that are either rabid or have escaped examination and observation.

Rabies epidemiology varies greatly from country to country. In almost all of Africa, Asia, and Latin America, rabies has been and continues to be a disease of dogs which account for over 90% of human cases and 90% of human rabies deaths. Where canine rabies persists, human rabies remains common, and millions of persons are vaccinated annually for exposures to rabid animals, mostly dogs. Worldwide, an estimated 33,000 people die of rabies every year and most of these cases occur in developing countries. In much of the developed world, where rabies in dogs has been controlled, the disease primarily affects a variety of wild animals and the animals they bite. In Western Europe, for instance, the red fox is the primary transmitter of rabies, and most cases are found in that species; in the U.S. and Canada, rabies is carried by skunks, raccoons, foxes, and insectivorous bats. For the past two decades, a zone of raccoon rabies in Northern Virginia has extended concentrically at a rate of ~25 miles per year to involve much of the Northeastern U.S. In some locations, as many as half of the trapped raccoons are rabid. It is crucial to monitor the exact location of rabid animals within each state through state health departments or federal health agen-

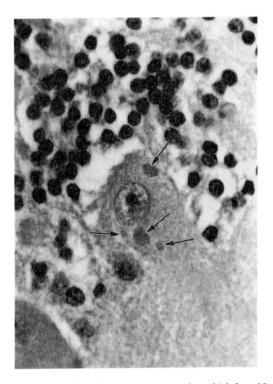

Figure 35.2. Negri bodies in a neuron of a rabid dog. Hematoxylin–eosin; original magnification, ×560.

PARADIGM ■ ■ ■

What Determines How a Virus Spreads in the Body?

To produce systemic illness, a virus must spread from its site of entry and primary replication to distant target tissues. This aspect of viral pathogenesis is exemplified by neurotropic viruses that enter the body through a number of different portals (e.g., respiratory, gastrointestinal, or urogenital) and then spread to reach the central nervous system (CNS). The two principal pathways of spread to the CNS are through the bloodstream and the nerves. Most neurotropic viruses (e.g., arboviruses, enteroviruses, measles virus, and mumps virus) reach the CNS by hematogenous spread. Others (e.g., rabies virus and herpes simplex virus) reach the CNS by the neural route. Almost nothing is known about the viral genes and proteins or the cellular mechanisms responsible for determining which pathway will be used by viruses to spread within the infected host.

In an attempt to determine which viral genes are involved in the mode of spread, a study has been carried out with reoviruses that, in the laboratory, cause infections of the CNS of newborn mice. **Reovirus type 3** infects neurons and produces a lethal necrotizing encephalitis after intracerebral inoculation. **Type 1**, on the other hand, infects ependymal cells and produces hydrocephalus. These differences suggest that type 3 is transported via nerves to and within the CNS, whereas type 1 utilizes a non-neural pathway.

To investigate whether reovirus types 1 and 3 use different pathways of spread to the CNS, Tyler and coworkers took advantage of the fact that the motor and sensory neurons innervating the hindlimb and forelimb footpads are located in different regions of the spinal cord. If type 3 spreads via nerves, it should appear preferentially in the region of the spinal cord containing the neurons innervating the skin and musculature at the site of viral inoculation. If type 1 spreads through the bloodstream, it should appear in all regions of the spinal cord in equivalent amounts and with similar kinetics. When type 3 and type 1 were injected into the forelimb and hindlimb footpads of neonatal mice, type 3 appeared first, and in much higher titer, in the region of the spinal cord innervating the injected limb. In contrast, type 1, after either hindlimb or forelimb inoculation, appeared at essentially the same time and in equivalent titer in all regions of the spinal cord. These results support the hypothesis that type 3 spreads through nerves and type 1 spreads via the bloodstream to reach the CNS.

To confirm these results, the spread of types 1 and 3 from the hindlimb to the spinal cord was studied after section of the sciatic nerve. Since the sciatic nerve is the principal neural pathway from the hindlimb to the spinal cord, its section should completely prevent the spread of virus from the hindlimb through nerves but should not affect its capacity to spread through the bloodstream. As predicted, sciatic nerve section completely inhibited the spread of type 3 to the spinal cord but had no significant effect on the spread of type 1.

Genetic analysis has shown that a single viral-encoded protein is responsible for determining the pattern of spread of reoviruses. Passive immunization of mice with antibodies directed against the type 3 protein, but not against the type 1 protein, inhibits the neural spread of type 3. It is not yet known how this protein determines the tropism of the two types of reoviruses for neurons and ependymal cells, respectively. It is likely that a combined genetic, biochemical study of animal model systems will help elucidate the mode of spread of viruses in the body.

MOSELIO SCHAECHTER

---

cies because this information will assist in deciding whether to recommend treatment for persons bitten by animals. If a given species has not been reported to be rabid in an area (e.g., terrestrial animals in the Pacific Northwest), treatment of persons exposed to those animals in that area is usually unnecessary. If a person is bitten by a bat, however, the situation is different, because rabid bats have been found in those states. Some animal species are almost never diagnosed as rabid, including rodents (mice, rats, hamsters) and lagomorphs (rabbits and hares).

Approximately 20,000 persons are vaccinated against rabies in the U.S. each year. Only a small number of persons who are vaccinated are known to have actually been bitten by a rabid animal.

The bite of a rabid animal does not necessarily result in rabies. Contrary to popular beliefs, humans are quite refractory to the rabies virus. The incidence of disease after the bite of a known rabid dog is about 15%, although this figure rises considerably with severe bites on the face and head.

The problems of encounter with the rabies virus are very different from those in other virus diseases, inasmuch as the location and time of possible virus entry (by bite) are known. Questions that are particular to rabies include:

- Did a bite or break of the skin occur?
- Has rabies been reported in the state or region where the bite occurred?
- Was the biting animal rabid? Is it available for laboratory diagnosis or did it escape?

- Is the species known commonly to carry the virus?
- Is the biting animal a dog or cat that can be observed? (If so, the period of presymptomatic virus transmission is a maximum of 10 days; if a person has been bitten by a dog 11 days before it gets sick, no treatment is needed.)

SPREAD AND MULTIPLICATION

After rabies viruses enter the body through a bite, the **incubation period** can last up to 12 months and, rarely, years. The length of this period depends on the size of the viral inoculum and the length of the neural path from the wound to the brain. Thus, severe bites on face and head tend to result in a shorter incubation period.

Studies in experimental animals have shown that, during the incubation period, the virus remains at or close to the bite. It is not known exactly where the virus resides during that period, nor the factors that stimulate the virus to advance to the peripheral and central nervous systems. When the virus eventually reaches the peripheral nerves, it quickly advances to the spinal ganglia, spinal cord, and brain. The virus moves passively within the **axoplasm of peripheral nerves** to the central nervous system.

From the brain, the virus often returns to the periphery using the same axoplasmic route as used for centripetal movement. A favored peripheral site is the highly innervated **submaxillary salivary glands**, but the virus is found in many other tissues. In approximately 25% of dogs, the virus never reaches these glands or any exit route. The levels of virus in the salivary gland tissue of rabid animals may be 1000 or more times the level found in the brain, suggesting that the virus replicates at this site as well. The location in the salivary glands helps explain the transmission of virus from one animal to another.

DAMAGE

A surprisingly limited amount of histopathological change occurs in the CNS of animals or humans dying of rabies. Neurons of infected animals and humans contain typical intracytoplasmic inclusions, the Negri bodies. These inclusions are highly pathognomonic, that is, indicative of the specific disease, and in the case of rabies may be the only such sign. In some cases, limited perivascular cuffing and limited neuronal necrosis may also occur. These limited histopathological changes are in striking contrast to the marked symptoms seen in human rabies.

Symptoms usually start with **difficulty in swallowing** and **increased muscle tone. Hydrophobia**, contractions of the muscles involved in swallowing, is sometimes elicited by the mere sight of liquid. Eventually, patients develop signs of extensive damage to the CNS, progress

to coma, and die. Rabies virus can be detected in and isolated from almost all tissues in the body.

DIAGNOSIS

Until 1960, rabies diagnosis in suspect animals was limited to the detection of Negri bodies in Ammon's horn and cerebellum (the inclusions are found in approximately 75% of positive cases), and inoculation into mice of specimens from brains without Negri bodies. These diagnostic tests resulted in the immediate diagnosis of some positive cases but a delayed diagnosis of the rest. Usually, a period of 24 weeks elapsed until the inoculated mice either died of rabies or survived.

In 1960, the **fluorescent antibody technique** in which brain impressions are stained with a fluorescein-tagged antibody, was introduced. Diagnosis can also be made in persons with encephalitis by fluorescent staining of skin biopsies of the nape of the neck where many hair follicles are found (the infected nerve network around hair follicles fluoresces) during the early encephalitic period. This technique has become the diagnostic procedure of choice early in the disease. Neutralizing antibodies are found in the serum and CSF later in infection, usually 8 to 10 days after the encephalitic symptoms appear.

PREVENTION

Vaccination of Animals

Rabies is a zoonosis, a disease transmitted to humans by animals. To that end, the best protection against the disease can be achieved by the elimination of the disease in dogs (and cats) by requiring **vaccination of pets** by law, thereby creating a barrier to animal-to-animal transmission (either dog-to-dog or wild animal-to-dog). An additional approach is to vaccinate wild animals. Vaccination of red foxes has been performed successfully on a mass scale in Europe by dropping baited oral vaccines from airplanes. A similar strategy is being used to vaccinate stray dogs in several developing countries. Unfortunately, an effective vaccine for raccoons, the major reservoir in the Northeastern U.S., is not yet available.

Postexposure Treatment of Humans

Once the decision to treat has been made, human treatment consists of three steps: (1) **local wound treatment**, (2) **passive administration of antibody** (antiserum or immunoglobulin), and (3) **vaccination.** Superficial wounds can be washed with soap and water; deep wounds should be flushed and swabbed with quaternary ammonium compounds or other viricidal substances. The passive antibody administered in developed countries is **human rabies immune globulin (HRIG)** collected from immunized persons and administered as soon as possible after rabies exposure; one-half is infiltrated at the bite site and one-half is administered intramuscularly.

Vaccination with modern tissue culture vaccines consists of a series of five doses, all administered intramuscularly in the deltoid region, 1 mL each, over a 4-week period. The most common vaccines are prepared with several kinds of human or monkey cells in culture from which the virus is purified. All individuals given such treatment have developed the expected level of antibodies. When the combination of globulin and vaccine has been properly applied in a timely fashion, no treatment failures have been noted, and complications are rare. It is interesting that chloroquine, a drug used for antimalarial prophylaxis, inhibits or suppresses antibody development in vaccine recipients. This fact must be taken into account when administering preexposure rabies vaccine in areas where malarial prophylaxis may also be in use.

CONCLUSION

The decision not to vaccinate Mr. V. was based on sound epidemiological principles, specifically the absence of reported rabies cases in the main species affected in other parts of the region (raccoons and skunks, in this case). In the case of Mr. R., on the other hand, treatment was not administered, with disastrous consequences. The main point in rabies control, is control of the disease in the animals that bite people. Because the prime offender is the dog, canine vaccination is essential in rabies zones.

SELF-ASSESSMENT QUESTIONS

1. How does the epidemiology of rabies vary in developed and developing countries?
2. What are the issues that should be considered in treating a person who has been bitten by an animal whose health status is unknown?
3. What are the general features of the rabies virus?
4. What is the most effective treatment strategy for a person bitten by a rabid animal?

SUGGESTED READINGS

Expert Committee on Rabies. 8th Report. Geneva: World Health Organization,1988.

Fishbein D. Human rabies. In: Baer GM, ed. The natural history of rabies. Boca Raton, FL: CRC Press, 1991.

Meslin FX, Fishbein DB, Matter HC. Curr Top Microb Immunol 1994;187:1.

Rabies Prevention United States, 1991. Recommendations of the Advisory Committee on Immunization Practices (ACIP). Centers for Disease Control, U.S. Public Health Service. Immunization Practices, U.S. Public Health Service, 1991.

Tyler KL, McPhee DL, Fields BN. Distinct pathways of viral spread in the host determined by reovirus S1 gene segment. Science 1986;233:770–774.

Influenza and Its Virus

STEPHEN E. STRAUS

Key Concepts

Influenza:

- Is caused by enveloped RNA viruses belonging to the Orthomyxovirus. Three strains (A, B, and C) infect humans.
- Epidemics and pandemics are the result of the virus' ability to undergo antigenic reassortments, leading to significant changes in viral antigens (notably, hemagglutinin and neuraminidase). The antigenically rearranged strains are usually of animal origin.
- Causes significant mortality in the elderly and individuals with underlying cardiopulmonary disease. Complications include bacterial superinfections and Reye's syndrome.
- Can be prevented by vaccination. A vaccine is prepared annually from strains most likely to emerge in the coming season.
- Can be treated or prevented with amantidine (A strains only), rimantidine, and other drugs.

Influenza (the "flu") ranks among the major epidemic diseases in developed countries. On several occasions in our history it has spread throughout the world, causing **pandemics**. In healthy adults, it is a relatively mild disease; however, it contributes significantly to the mortality of the elderly and of persons with underlying respiratory and cardiac problems.

The main reason why influenza has not been eradicated is that the viruses have the ability to change their main antigens, **hemagglutinin** and **neuraminidase**. Thus, previous exposure or vaccination does not ensure adequate immunity against newly emerging strains of the virus. Up-to-date vaccines, containing different combinations of antigens, are administered yearly to persons at risk. Several drugs are effective in the treatment of this disease.

Influenza viruses are enveloped and belong to the **Orthomyxovirus** group. Their RNA genome is divided into **eight segments of negative polarity**.

■ CASE

When Ms. I., a healthy 49-year-old schoolteacher, was told by her doctor that she probably had influenza, she recalled with concern the early winter of 1957. It seemed as if her entire family had developed the flu. With all of the coughing, chills and aches, it was hard to get any sleep. Everyone had to take turns getting out of bed to get aspirin or fluids for the ones who were the weakest. Schools were closed for several days during the flu outbreak because so many teachers and students had become ill. But the most upsetting recollection was the death of her grandfather. He was a smoker and had mild heart trouble, but basically he was quite sound. And he got the flu. His illness began as it did in the rest of the family although he coughed and spit a bit more. One night his fever increased and he started to get very short of breath. He was rushed to the hospital but died in 2 days despite antibiotics and oxygen.

Every so often the news reports indicate that a new strain of flu has gotten a foothold in the United States, this one apparently from the Far East. Ms. I. is apprehensive about the possible effects of a new Asian flu, and particularly, that her aging parents, who live downstairs from her, may be vulnerable. Ms. I. has had 4 days of runny nose, mild sore throat, and cough, not much different from many colds she has had over the years, but the amount of fever, muscle aches, and fatigue were bad enough for her to consult the family doctor. He did not carry out laboratory tests but based a tentative diagnosis on the clinical picture and on a bulletin he received from the State Board of Health about the presence of the new flu strain in the area. If Ms. I. had a typical course, he predicted that she would feel sick for 4–7 days, but the fatigue and dry cough could last for days or even weeks thereafter. Because Ms. I. visits so often with her parents, they were advised to come in to get a flu shot and several weeks of pills of a drug called amantadine.

This chapter will explain why the 1957 influenza epidemic was so severe. Ms. I. probably also asked several other thoughtful questions, including:

1. How do new influenza strains arise?
2. Why are people susceptible to repeated influenza infections?
3. What makes some strains of influenza more dangerous than others?
4. Why do Ms. I.'s parents need a flu shot when they have had one before?
5. What will the amantadine do for her parents and why shouldn't she take it also?

Beyond the classic presentation of influenza (such as that in Ms. I.'s case) lies an entire spectrum of pulmonary complications that are more likely to develop in certain settings: during pregnancy, in the elderly, and in any individual with congenital or acquired cardiopulmonary diseases. A few such individuals are at risk for the development of either primary influenza pneumonia, a devastating virus infection of the lung parenchyma, or more typically, secondary bacterial pneumonia.

Influenza has many imitators. Similar, but less severe respiratory illnesses caused by other viruses are all commonly called the "flu." Gastrointestinal symptoms such as cramping, nausea, vomiting, and diarrhea are not prominent features of influenza (except in children), and thus the term "intestinal flu" is a total misnomer.

Influenza Viruses

Influenza virus structure

Influenza viruses belong to the family **Orthomyxoviridae** and include three types, A, B, and C, that were originally defined serologically. Infection with one serotype affords no protection against the other types. Over the years of study important structural, epidemiologic, and clinical differences among the three types were defined, as summarized in Table 36.1.

Influenza A viruses are among the best studied of human RNA viruses. The entire amino acid sequence and the three-dimensional structure of their proteins are known, as are the sequences of all the RNA segments of representative strains of each viral serotype. Surprisingly, the influenza A virus genome consists of **eight discrete segments** of single-stranded **RNA of negative polarity** indicating that, in order to be used for protein synthesis, the RNA must be transcribed into translatable messages.

Influenza viruses are enveloped (Fig. 36.1). The viral envelope is covered with **spikes**, or **peplomers**, which in the cases of influenza A and B strains are composed of two different proteins, the **hemagglutinin** and the **neuraminidase**. Influenza C viruses have a single protein with both hemagglutinin and neuraminidase activity. Each of the influenza serotypes can be further subdivided into strains on the basis of subtle yet important

Humans, Health and History

Influenza

Epidemics of brief illness with fever, cough, and severe weakness were described by Hippocrates in the 5th century B.C. and reported repeatedly throughout the Middle Ages. Since 1173, over 300 outbreaks of influenza-like illness have been recorded at an average interval of 2.4 years. The development of intercontinental travel and commerce led to the first known **pandemic** (global epidemic) of influenza, which occurred in 1580 and originated in Asia, spreading to Europe and later to the Americas. Twenty-two pandemics of influenza illness have been recorded since the early 18th century; the most dramatic of these was the Great Spanish influenza pandemic of 1918–1919 in which over 20 million died worldwide.

Influenza is an Italian word reflecting an old belief that the illness was caused by the "influence" of atmospheric factors. An infectious etiology for influenza was not seriously espoused until the end of the last century when a bacillus, now known as *Haemophilus influenzae,* was recovered from the sputum of patients with this syndrome. The viral etiology of influenza was finally proven in 1933, when the contagious component in patient secretions was shown to pass through porcelain filters fine enough to exclude bacteria. The virus was first grown in the laboratory in 1940 (in fertilized chicken eggs), and by 1950 the three serologic types of influenza known to infect people were recognized.

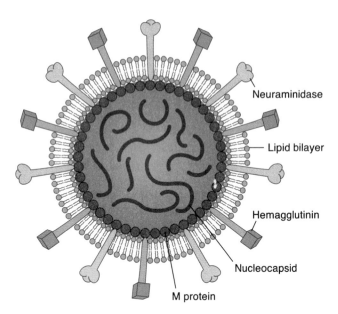

Figure 36.1. The structure of influenza virus detailing its surface proteins and segmented genome.

Table 36.1. Comparison of Influenza, A, B, and C Viruses

	A	B	C
Severity of illness	+ + + +	+ +	+
Animal reservoir	Yes	No	No
Spread in humans	Pandemic	Epidemic	Sporadic
Antigenic changes	Shift, drift	Drift	Drift
No. of RNA segments	8	8	7
No. of surface glycoproteins	2	2	1

differences, i.e., the composition of their viral surface antigens. Matrix proteins line the inner aspects of the viral envelope while other internal proteins, polymerases and the nucleoproteins, are associated with the viral RNA.

How do influenza viruses replicate?

Many biochemical and molecular aspects of the replication cycle of influenza virus have been elucidated. Influenza infection starts with the binding of the viral **hemagglutinin** to N-acetylneuraminic acid components of various host cell surface **glycoproteins** or **glycolipids**. After binding to these receptors, the viruses are drawn into the cell by receptor-mediated endocytosis. The endosome containing the virus fuses with an acidic lysosome. The acidic milieu alters the conformation of the viral hemagglutinin, uncovering peptide sequences that

stimulate **fusion of membranes**. The result is that the viral membrane fuses with the phagolysosomal membrane, releasing the nucleocapsid into the cytoplasm for further uncoating and replication.

Replication of influenza viruses is set in motion within an hour after infection and begins with **RNA transcription** that uses the infecting RNA genome as the direct template. This cannot be carried out by any known host cell enzymes and requires a **viral RNA-dependent RNA polymerase** activity provided by components of the infecting viral core (polymerase proteins PB1 and PB2). The transcripts made are of positive polarity and serve as **messengers** for protein synthesis. Each mRNA transcript is longer than the parental negative strands because after transcription its 5' end is "capped" by the addition of methylated nucleotides, and its 3' end is **polyadenylated**. The mRNA is then used for the synthesis of viral proteins.

Some of the details of the post-transcriptional **modification** of influenza mRNAs have been elucidated. Unlike the situation with most RNA viruses, replication of influenza virus takes place in the **nucleus**. This is necessary, because the influenza virus, unlike many other negative-stranded RNA viruses, lacks capping and methylating enzyme activities. In a remarkable and unique feat of **molecular parasitism**, influenza viruses evolved the means to "steal" the methylated caps plus 10 to 13 of the first nucleotides from the 5' ends of cellular mRNAs that had been previously synthesized and modified in the nucleus.

Ultimately, 10 transcripts are synthesized from the eight genomic RNAs and translated in the cytoplasm into seven structural and three nonstructural proteins (Table 36.2). How are the special RNA molecules destined for packaging into progeny virions made? Appar-

Table 36.2. Influenza Virus RNA Segments and Their Protein

RNA Segment	Protein	Function and location in virion
1	Polymerase-B2	RNA synthesis; core protein
2	Polymerase-B1	RNA synthesis; core protein
3	Polymerase-A	RNA synthesis; core protein
4	Hemagglutinin	Attachment to cell surface
5	Nucleoprotein	RNA synthesis; core receptor
6	Neuraminidase	Release of virus from cell envelope
7	Matrix-1, matrix-2	Scaffolding protein; transmembrane ion channel
8	Nonstructural-1, nonstructural-2	Regulates splicing of mRNA Unknown

ently, two viral proteins (polymerase PA and the nucleoprotein NP) facilitate the transcription of a special set of RNAs, identical in length to the infecting strands. These full-length positive strands are neither capped nor polyadenylated and therefore cannot direct protein synthesis. Instead, they are copied directly, again, to yield RNAs of negative polarity that are suitable for incorporation into new virus particles.

Influenza Virus Hemagglutinin and Neuraminidase

The hemagglutinin and neuraminidase of these viruses are two of the best studied of all viral proteins, and seem to be the most important determinants of influenza virulence. After the virus invades the host cell, these proteins migrate to the cell membrane to assemble in patches on the outer surface of the cell membrane, dis-

placing cellular membrane proteins that usually reside there. Their three-dimensional conformation has been determined by x-ray crystallography. Each of the 400 or so hemagglutinin spikes of a virion is composed of three identical polypeptides. Each spike has a hydrophobic end, which is embedded in the lipid envelope, and a hydrophilic end, which projects outward. The hemagglutinin attaches to a cell membrane receptor and antibodies directed against it neutralize virus infectivity. Some of the hemagglutinin sequence is highly conserved among diverse strains of each viral type, but specific regions vary greatly, allowing serologic discrimination between virus types. These antigenic differences between hemagglutinin determine the extent of cross-reactive immunity, and therefore the severity of disease in partially immune hosts.

The other peplomer, the neuraminidase protein,

PARADIGM   ■ ■ ■

Viral Evolution

Viral evolution depends on the same forces that determine evolution in cellular organisms: **genetic variability** and **selection**. What characterizes evolution among the viruses is the high degree of their variability, which is particularly marked among the ones with an RNA genome. RNA viruses are especially variable because RNA molecules are intrinsically unstable, the enzymes that replicate RNA (including reverse transcriptase) have relatively low **fidelity**, and the **genomes** of certain of them are **segmented**. Notice that arrangement into segmented genomes allows the segments to be rapidly reassorted among the progeny viruses, which is reminiscent of the reassortment of chromosomes in higher cells. Contrast this with unimolecular genomes, which undergo genetic change either by mutation or genetic recombination, which are intrinsically more infrequent. The high frequency with which new serotypes of influenza viruses arise almost every year can be explained by their segmented genome.

It is not possible to sort out the importance of each of the myriad factors operating on viral selection, but we can count among the more obvious ones the production of antibodies, cellular immunity, and interferons, both in the circulation and in tissues. Because of the importance of antibodies in neutralizing viruses and impeding their growth, it can be expected that the greatest variability will be seen in the antigens recognized by antibodies. In fact, the most evident viral antigens, such as those in the envelope of the enveloped viruses, tend to be more strain-specific than the proteins of the capsomere or those contained within the capsid.

Other selective forces may be attributed to the special environment of certain viruses. Take, for example, the rhinoviruses of the common cold or the influenza viruses, both of which reside on the respiratory epithe-

lium, and are highly variable even for RNA viruses. In their usual environment, these viruses become exposed to IgA antibodies, which make reversible complexes with their antigens, and are less apt to neutralize the viral infectivity. Because these antibodies only partially impair viral growth, they allow a large population of virions to accumulate, thus increasing the probability that mutations will arise. Among the mutants, some may be even less sensitive to mucosal antibodies and will be therefore selected. Viruses found in the bloodstream, on the other hand, are effectively neutralized by circulatory IgG and will not replicate in sufficient numbers for mutants to accumulate. These expectations are generally borne out because RNA viruses found in the circulation, such as measles and mumps, show considerably less antigenic variation than the influenza viruses.

Besides viral mutations that result in resistance to the immune response, those that impart resistance to antiviral chemotherapeutic agents are also of clinical interest. The prevalence of **drug-resistant mutants** is becoming an increasingly serious problem with the greater use of certain antiviral drugs. For example, drug-resistant herpes simplex viruses frequently arise in immune-compromised patients after prolonged therapy with acyclovir. Also clinically important are **attenuated mutants**, which have decreased virulence but can multiply in the host. Some of these mutants may be sufficiently stable and antigenically reactive to be used in live vaccines, as for example in the polio or yellow fever vaccines. The stability of these attenuated viruses and their lack of reversion to virulence is probably due to the fact that they differ from the virulent parents by many bases in their nucleic acids.

MOSELIO SCHAECHTER

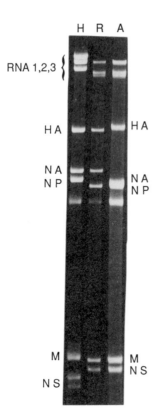

Figure 36.2. Genetic reassortment of influenza viral RNA segments. In this study, human (*H*) and avian (*A*) strains of influenza virus were used together to infect cells in culture. A recombinant (*R*) strain of progeny virus was derived. Each individual segment makes a separate band in gel electrophoresis. The recombinant strain contains some human and some avian RNA segments.

looks like a square-topped, mushroom-like projection from the cell surface. Each peplomer is composed of four identical peptides with a hydrophobic foot embedded in the viral envelope, and a stalk with a hydrophilic head that projects outward. As with the hemagglutinin, variable domains of the neuraminidase are important for serotyping and immune recognition. The neuraminidase is important for releasing the virus from the infected cell by removing receptors for the hemagglutinin on the cell surface. Antibodies to neuraminidase decrease the efficiency of virus spread in both culture and tissues. Neuraminidase is assayed for by the addition of red blood cells to an influenza virus suspension. The red cells agglutinate but then elute spontaneously at 37°. Disaggregation is due to the neuraminidase, which cleaves the bonds that form between the viral hemagglutinin and the N-acetylneuraminic acid on the red blood cell surface.

A third envelope-associated protein, a **matrix protein,** attaches to the inner aspect of the viral membrane, perhaps recognizing the presence of transmembrane viral polypeptides. It might be considered a **"scaffolding"**

protein on which viral nucleocapsids are constructed. As new copies of the viral genome are synthesized, they assemble together with the polymerase proteins and nucleoprotein at the inner cell membrane sites coated with the matrix protein. The virus gradually takes shape by the evagination of the altered cell membrane around the developing viral core. Ultimately, a new particle buds off from the cell surface.

Antigenic Variation Among the Influenza Viruses

To fully understand the features of influenza epidemiology, one must understand the virus's remarkable capacity for **antigenic change**. While many other viruses remain nearly identical year after year, influenza virus strains vary—sometimes slightly and sometimes enormously—from one year to the next. Variety is the way of life among these viruses.

Changes actually occur in several of the viral proteins, but the most noticeable ones take place in the two outer envelope proteins, **hemagglutinin** and **neuraminidase**. The strains of virus involved in any given outbreak are identified by the serologic properties of the two proteins. Slight variations in either protein are said to represent **antigenic drift**. A major change in the neuraminidase or hemagglutinin is termed **antigenic shift**.

Antigenic drift takes place in nature by changes in small discrete and highly variable domains of the proteins, presumably through random point mutations in the nucleic acid and selection of strains that escape neutralization by the antibodies of the host. Major antigenic shifts are believed to result from an entirely different process, involving the exchange of genes from different virus strains. To understand this process, it is useful to recall that influenza virus contains a multisegmented genome. If a cell is infected simultaneously with two or more different influenza viruses, the RNA segments from each parental strain become shuffled and are dealt out to the progeny in random order (Fig. 36.2). Each developing virus particle encapsidates some segments from both parental strains. This process of **genetic reassortment** occurs with very high frequency. Successful reassortants in nature are ones that escape neutralization in the serum of hosts that had previously been infected with antigenically similar viruses.

These mechanisms would be of no epidemiologic relevance unless different influenza strains actually arose. What evidence exists that these processes occur in nature? What is the origin of the different connecting strains? First, we know that human influenza A strains are similar to animal influenza strains. In the laboratory, human and animal strains reassort readily to generate hybrid progeny. Second, human influenza A strains have been recovered from animals in the field. The influenza virus strain associated with the great 1918–1919 Spanish pandemic apparently became adapted to infect swine, because pigs were later found to be infected with viruses related to the 1918 human strains. Third, strains recovered from wild ducks and horses are antigenically similar to strains later recovered during human epidemics. Thus, it is believed that animals provide a reservoir from which new genetic variants of human influenza virus can be drawn. The largest and most extensive animal reservoir is in birds.

To understand how different strains arise, imagine a cell that is **coinfected** with a human and an avian influenza A virus. The hybrid that arises may contain the avian hemagglutinin and neuraminidase genes but the remainder of the genes may be of the human virus type. Such a hybrid virus has no problem replicating efficiently in human cells. If humans had never been exposed to the avian hemagglutinin and neuraminidase antigens, such a hybrid virus would not be recognized by the immune system and could spread rapidly in the population. The possible result: an epidemic, possibly a pandemic.

ENCOUNTER

With these molecular features as a background, it is possible to comprehend the complex pattern of influenza infection over the ages. Over a century ago, it was recognized that some epidemics of the disease are associated with higher than usual mortality from cardiopulmonary disease. This allows the tracking and recognition of types of influenza that are epidemic from year to year. The Centers for Disease Control tabulates the total cardiopulmonary mortality for each week in each region of the United States. Almost every winter the expected mortality increases. When deaths in a region of the country exceed the expected level by a certain amount, an influenza epidemic is suspected in that region (Fig. 36.3). More precise characterization and proof of the onset of an epidemic are then based on the recovery and antigenic typing of virus strains at sentinel clinics in the region.

Through these surveillance mechanisms we have learned that influenza infection occurs in the United Stated on an annual basis, typically beginning in the fall and generally terminating in the late winter. In most years the influenza outbreaks are mild and sporadic, but every few years more severe epidemics develop. Pandemics (causing disease worldwide) appear less frequently; in this century they arose in 1918, 1957, and 1968.

Thus, influenza may be **endemic** (present but causing relatively few cases), **epidemic** (affecting many people in one area) or **pandemic**. Why does this illness have three different patterns? The answer lies in the distribution of immunity in the population. Individuals who have been infected in the past with a specific strain of influenza virus become immune to that strain. If the same strain were to be reintroduced the next year it would cause disease mainly among those who missed the earlier outbreak. For that year, influenza would be endemic. When antigenic drift occurs in the circulating influenza strains,

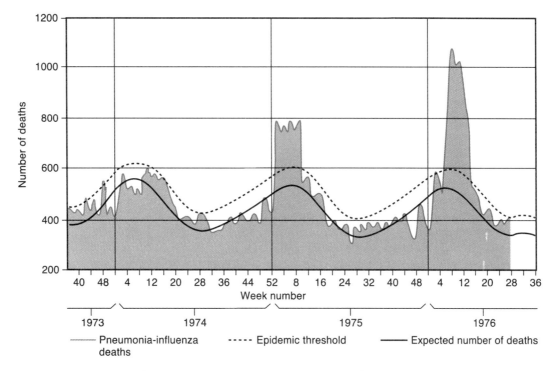

Figure 36.3. The rate of death from respiratory disease in the U.S. from 1973 to 1976. A higher than expected rate of respiratory deaths indicates the occurrence of influenza epidemics.

Table 36.3. Major Antigenic Shifts in Influenza A Strain in Recent Years

Year	Strain Designation[a]	Common Name
1947	H1N1	Spanish
1957	H2N2	Asian
1968	H3N2	Hong Kong
1976	H1N1 (swine)	Swine
1977	H1N1	USSR

[a] H, hemagglutinin; N, neuraminidase.

the differences are sufficient to permit epidemics, because illness occurs even among those who developed some immunity from earlier infections. Major antigenic shifts, however, lead to pandemics. Since nearly the whole population is susceptible, many are likely to be infected.

The strains that cause illness each year are identified by the serologic properties of their neuraminidase and hemagglutinin. A uniform classification scheme has been adopted internationally for these antigens. New influenza strains are named by their type, city or country of first isolation, strain, year of recovery, and hemagglutinin and neuraminidase subtypes. An example is the A/Victoria/3/75/H3N2. Thirteen different hemagglutinin (Hl–H13) and nine different neuraminidase subtypes (Nl–N9) have been recognized in viruses recovered from humans, swine, horses, and birds. Table 36.3 lists the influenza A virus strains associated with the most serious pandemics in this century. The influenza pandemic of 1957 led to the demise of Ms. I.'s grandfather because this virus was antigenically quite different from the earlier H1N1 virus.

Table 36.4 shows how minor and major antigenic changes can be measured and how these findings are reflected in the virulence of a circulating influenza A strain. In this example, stored sera collected from a large group of individuals in 1968 and 1972 were tested for their levels of antibodies directed against influenza A hemagglutinin. Prior immunity existing in 1972 to new H3 strains limited the spread and impact of the virus but an epidemic still occurred among those with partial immunity and those (particularly children) who missed the 1968 pandemic.

ENTRY

Influenza can be transmitted to the nasopharynx of susceptible individuals by **inhalation** of large-particle aerosols, but the major vehicle for transmission is **small-particle aerosols** liberated during sneezes or coughs. Experimental observations suggest that small droplets are

capable of reaching the terminal bronchioles and alveoli. A single infectious dose of virus contained within such a small droplet may be sufficient to induce disease. It is possible that the virus may also be transmitted from hand to nose after touching virus-bearing objects. In general, young children are the most efficient transmitters of the infection, spreading it among their friends and to their families. Thus, in 1957 Ms. I. may have been the index case for influenza in her family, having brought it home from school. And, in an ironic way, she now suffers from influenza that she probably acquired from her own pupils.

SPREAD, MULTIPLICATION, AND DAMAGE

Influenza viruses primarily infect upper and lower respiratory tract epithelial cells. Viral multiplication leads to lysis of these cells and to the release of viral antigens and destructive cellular enzymes. The host responds with an influx of **macrophages** and **lymphocytes**, followed by an outpouring of **humoral mediators of inflammation**, including interferon. This response helps to clear superinfecting bacteria and fungi, to inhibit virus replication, and to destroy virally infected epithelial cells. Release of **interleukin-1** from macrophages results in fever, while **interferon** probably causes the diffuse muscular aches and fatigue that is characteristic of influenza (which is one of the reasons for the limited therapeutic use of interferon). The inflammatory mediators provoke **vasodilation** and **edema**. In the nose this results in stuffiness and rhinorrhea. In the tracheobronchial tree the irritation caused by the debris and the host responses stimulates mucus production. The remaining undamaged ciliated epithelium and the cough reflexes help propel the mucus and debris upward. In areas where extensive destruction of epithelium has occurred superinfecting bacteria—especially virulent encapsulated ones—can gain a foothold, leading to secondary bacterial bronchitis or pneumonia.

The role of **cellular immune responses** in influenza is

Table 36.4. Antigenic Drift in Influenza A Strains[a]

Year sera collected	Mean hemagglutination inhibition antibody titer to		
	H2	H3[68]	H3[72]
1968	1:100	<1:10	<1:10
1972	1:100	1:80	1:30

[a] Each serum was tested against three influenza A virus strains: a strain containing an H2 type of hemagglutinin similar to that associated with the prior 1957 pandemic, the H3-containing strain associated with the 1968 pandemic, and the similar but slightly different H3-containing strain associated with the 1972 epidemic.

not known. Patients with cellular immune impairment are not at substantially increased risk for severe influenza infections. The **humoral responses** to the viral outer envelope proteins seem more important. The example in Table 36.4 shows that the presence of **neutralizing antibody** to hemagglutinin will protect against or limit infection. Antibody to the neuraminidase seems to modify the spread of virus through the respiratory tract and can prevent illness. Thus, in an individual with partial immunity to neuraminidase the disease may be restricted to the upper respiratory tract.

The bacterial superinfection that complicates influenza infection is confined, typically to a single pulmonary lobe and involves pneumococci, staphylococci, or *Haemophilus influenzae*; hence, the incorrect attribution of the cause of this disease a century ago to *H. influenzae*. These pneumonias present as recurrent fever and progressive purulent cough in an individual whose initial symptoms of influenza appeared to be on the wane. Bacterial pneumonia and cardiac failure account for most of the increase in mortality associated with influenza each year. The demise in 1957 of Ms. I.'s grandfather was probably the result of bacterial superinfection. The cumulative effects of a lifetime of insults to the respiratory tract from pollution, smoking, and prior infections gradually degrade one's ability to counter the growth of bacteria in influenza-damaged airways.

Influenza is also a major cause of disease in children. It is an important cause of **croup**. Infection in the upper respiratory tract results in an inflammatory response and local swelling sufficient to obstruct the eustachian tubes and the openings of the facial sinuses. Stasis of fluid proximal to the obstruction provides fertile ground for bacterial growth. Thus, otitis and sinusitis are common complications of influenza, especially in children.

Rare but serious complications of influenza that are less frequent than bacterial pneumonia include **primary influenza pneumonia** and **Reye's syndrome**. The former is a rare process in which extensive viral and later bacterial destruction of small airways and alveoli occur. Clinically, this pneumonia is suspected when fulminant multilobar pneumonia and hypoxia are observed. **Reye's syndrome** is a poorly understood illness of children recently infected with influenza or varicella. There is progressive metabolic **encephalopathy** and, frequently, death. Its pathogenesis is not understood, nor is the dominant role of aspirin use as a risk factor.

DIAGNOSIS

The clinical manifestations of infection with influenza virus readily suggest the diagnosis. When flu is widespread throughout a community in the winter months, the diagnosis is likely to be correct. Definitive laboratory diagnoses are usually made for purposes of research or for epidemiologic surveillance. The virus can readily be grown from nasopharyngeal swabs or washes by inoculation into cell cultures. Virus replication is detected by a simple assay for the expression of the viral hemagglutinin. Guinea pig red blood cells are added to the cultures and adhere to the surface of cells in which the virus is replicating.

A variety of **serologic techniques** are available for diagnosing past influenza A infection. **Hemagglutination inhibition** (as used in Table 36.4) and neutralization are most often utilized. Their major value is in defining the serologic character of new virus strains and for seroepidemiologic surveillance.

PREVENTION AND TREATMENT

The major treatments for influenza infections are the time-proven ones involving hydration, rest, and antipyretics, especially acetaminophen rather than aspirin (to decrease the likelihood of aspirin-associated postinfluenza Reye's syndrome). For most people these conservative measures are adequate. Influenza A is the first virus for which successful systemic antiviral chemotherapy was developed. In the early 1960s, it was recognized that **amantadine** (Fig. 43.2), a compound now more widely used for the treatment of Parkinsonism, effectively diminishes the duration and severity of influenza A infection. It is most effective when given prophylactically, before an individual is exposed to the virus, leading to a 70–80% reduction in the development of symptoms. Amantadine is, therefore, used for elderly institutionalized individuals and patients with cardiopulmonary compromise for the weeks influenza seems to be in the local community.

A related compound, **rimantadine**, appears equally effective and has improved pharmacokinetics, so that there is a lower incidence of the mild confusion and discomfort that attend amantadine use, particularly in the elderly individual. Unfortunately, both agents are active only against the influenza A strains of virus. Details of the uses of these drugs can be found in Chapter 43, "Strategies to Combat Viral Infections."

Both amantadine and rimantadine block influenza virus replication by interfering with the ion channel of the viral M2 protein, through which the inner core of the particle is acidified. At low pH, the viral ribonucleoprotein complex dissociates, allowing influenza RNA transport to the nucleus, where its replication and transcription takes place. Only influenza A strains have an M2 protein susceptible to these drugs. Mutations in M2 arise readily, and resistance to these drugs has already limited their value in preventing spread of the infection in households.

A different class of agent, represented by the nucleoside analog **ribavirin** (Fig. 43.2), is active against both influenza A and B viruses. In early trials of ribavirin in which the agent was inhaled as a fine-particle aerosol, there was evidence of rapid clearance of virus and resolution of symptoms. The complexity of aerosol administration of ribavirin and modest benefits has limited its use to compassionate treatment of rare hospitalized patients with suspected primary influenza pneumonia.

In reality, none of the medications for influenza are used widely enough to affect our public health. However, the control of influenza is a major international effort. Under the auspices of the World Health Organization, **sentinel clinics** monitor and track the emergence and spread of influenza in both animals and humans. When influenza becomes evident in a country, local public health authorities announce cautionary warnings that the elderly or chronically impaired patients should avoid contact with individuals with upper respiratory infections.

The most powerful thrust of the influenza control program focuses on **vaccination**. The current vaccines contain viral hemagglutinin and neuraminidase proteins from killed virus. These vaccines reduce the incidence and morbidity of influenza by about 75%. The major problem with these vaccines is that they do not provide permanent immunity to the disease. The fault is not with the vaccines themselves, which provide relatively durable immunity, but with the antigenic variations of the virus. Authorities in the United States convene each year to review data on worldwide influenza patterns and attempt to predict the strains that are likely to emerge in the coming season. There is then a frantic effort to prepare adequate vaccine for those strains in time for the onset of the next influenza season. The vaccine formula is altered yearly, and vaccination must be performed annually to afford maximal protection.

Unfortunately, the experts can guess wrong regarding the strains of virus that will circulate in the coming seasons. However, the major problem with influenza vaccination is that most Americans, including those who would benefit the most, are not vaccinated. Many are either apathetic or fear side effects of the vaccine, which in reality are quite minimal.

Newer classes of vaccines are being studied. More effective than the killed virus vaccines are live, attenuated cold-adapted vaccines, which can be rapidly prepared for each season. The viruses in these vaccines grow largely in the cooler parts of the upper respiratory tract of the recipient yet still induce potent cell-mediated as well as humoral immune responses. Thus, they are likely to induce greater and more durable immunity than the current influenza vaccines.

CONCLUSION

We can now answer all of Ms. I.'s concerns about influenza. Although her seronegative children might experience severe influenza, it is unlikely that Ms. I. will come down with severe influenza at this time since substantially altered strains enter the community only infrequently. These new strains develop by mutation and genetic reassortment. It is the antigenic differences in these strains that permit them to infect individuals who have had prior influenza infection. Because Ms. I.'s parents are elderly, they should seek medical consultation for annual vaccination, and, if the influenza season has already begun, possibly receive amantadine prophylaxis along with vaccination. If any of the family members became infected, amantadine treatment should be considered on a case-by-case basis.

SELF-ASSESSMENT QUESTIONS

1. Describe the structure of influenza viruses and their replication cycle. What is peculiar about them?
2. Why do influenza epidemics recur? What causes influenza pandemics?
3. What role do hemagglutinin and neuraminidase play in the pathogenesis of influenza?
4. Compare antigenic drifts and shifts in influenza with antigenic variation in the pill of the gonococcus (Chapter 14, "*Neisseria*") and with the generation of immunological diversity (Chapter 7, "Induced Defenses").
5. Discuss the mechanism of action of amantadine.

SUGGESTED READINGS

Crosby AW Jr. Epidemic and peace, 1918. Westport, CT: Greenwood Press, 1976.

Hay A. The action of adamantanamines against influenza A viruses: inhibition of the M2 ion channel protein. Semin Virol 1992;3:21–30.

Hayden FG, Belshe RB, Clover RD, et al. Emergence and apparent transmission of rimantadine-resistant influenza A virus in families. N Engl J Med 1989;321:1696–1702.

Murphy BR, Webster RG. Orthomyxoviruses. In: Fields BN, Knipe DM, Howley PM, eds. Field's virology. 3rd ed. New York: Lippincott-Raven,1996;1397–1446.

Rotaviruses and Other Viral Agents of Gastroenteritis

CODY MEISSNER

Key Concepts

Rotaviruses:
- Are wheel-shaped, double-stranded RNA viruses
- Are the most common cause of gastroenteritis in children
- Cause a disease with seasonal distribution in the U.S., with peak incidence in the winter months
- Are transmitted by the fecal–oral route
- Cause changes in the small intestine mucosa which lead to diarrhea
- Induce long-term immunity

Other enteric viruses that cause gastroenteritis include:
- Norwalk virus, which is the leading cause of diarrhea in adults
- Two strains of adenovirus, which cause diarrhea especially in children under the age of 2
- Caliciviruses, which cause institutional outbreaks of diarrhea
- Astroviruses, which cause enteric disease mainly in children

---

Worldwide, 410 million children die each year from the complications of **infectious gastroenteritis**. In the U.S., while fewer than 500 children per year die from infectious diarrhea, more than 200,000 children under age 5 are hospitalized for diarrhea-induced dehydration. Before the 1970s, the etiologic agents for diarrhea that could be diagnosed were bacteria or protozoa. Although viruses were often suspected, most cases of viral gastroenteritis went undiagnosed.

Before 1970, viral agents of diarrhea were difficult to identify because they do not grow well in cultured cells. In the 1970s, electron microscopy allowed viral detection in stool specimens, and in 1972, the Norwalk virus was the first viral diarrhea agent identified by electron microscopic examination of stool specimens. When a convalescent serum specimen was mixed with an acute stool specimen, clumped virions were observed. This agent is now recognized as the most common cause of clusters of viral diarrhea in adults. In 1978, **rotavirus** was identified by electron microscopic examination of stool specimens. This agent is now known to be the most commonly recognized agent of gastroenteritis in children. Three additional viral agents of gastroenteritis have been recognized: (a) **enteric adenoviruses**, (b) **caliciviruses**, and (c) **astroviruses** (Table 37.1). It is likely that additional viral agents will be identified as causes of gastroenteritis as 40–50% of diarrhea cases are still of uncertain etiology.

■ CASE

M.A., a 7-month-old girl living in Washington, D.C., was recently switched from breast feeding to bottle feeding. Usu-

Table 37.1. Viral Causes of Gastroenteritis in Humans

Type	Genome	Medical significance
Rotavirus		
Group A	ds-segmented RNA	Major cause of diarrhea in children 6–24 months
Group B, C (atypical rotaviruses)	ds-segmented RNA	Rare in U.S.
Norwalk virus Small, round structured viruses (SRSV)	?RNA	Major cause of diarrhea epidemics in adults
Enteric adenovirus	ds, linear DNA	Second to rotavirus as cause of diarrhea in children, less important in adults
Calicivirus	?RNA	Infects adults and children
Astrovirus	(+)ssRNA	Infects mainly children and elderly

ally a satisfied and happy child, on March 29 she became irritable, began to vomit, and had a low-grade fever. She also had mild upper respiratory symptoms, with cough, nasal discharge, and pharyngitis. After 2 days, she was brought to the pediatrician who diagnosed rotavirus gastroenteritis by detecting viral antigen in the stool with enzyme-linked immunosorbent assay (ELISA) (see Chapter 55, "Diagnostic Principles"). Oral rehydration solution was given at home, and M.A. made an uneventful recovery by the sixth day.

The following questions arise:

1. How did M.A. acquire the virus?
2. Is it significant that M.A.'s disease occurred in springtime?
3. Will M.A. ever have the same disease?
4. Why did the pediatrician suspect this etiological agent?

ENCOUNTER

The peak incidence of rotavirus infection in the U.S. occurs between 6 months and 2 years of age. Most individuals have experienced infection and are immune to severe disease due to rotavirus by age 4. Seropositive older children or adults who are reexposed to a high inoculum of virus or who become immunocompromised may experience mild illness. Parents of young children experiencing a primary rotavirus infection may have mild symptoms. Certain individuals known to be at in-

creased risk for complications of dehydration due to viral gastroenteritis include malnourished children and adults, particularly in developing countries, and the elderly, who may experience waning immunity with age.

Rotavirus-induced disease has a **seasonal distribution** in the U.S., peaking in the winter and becoming rare in the warmer months. In tropical countries, endemic rotavirus infection occurs throughout the year. Recent studies have shown that rotaviruses cause a unique annual epidemic that moves sequentially from west to east. The epidemic first peaks in October and November in Mexico and the Southwestern states, progressing across the country during winter months and peaking in the Northeast and the Canadian Maritime Provinces in March and April (Fig. 37.1). Other viruses, such as influenza virus and respiratory syncytial virus, also have a characteristic seasonal appearance, but this **predictable wave of spread** is unique to rotavirus. It has been suggested that weather conditions, such as low temperature and low relative humidity, facilitate viral survival on fomites, thereby enhancing transmission. However, the epidemic begins in the warm climate of Mexico, but peak activity occurs simultaneously in northern and southern cities with different temperatures and levels of humidity. Therefore, this theory does not fully explain this unusual form of spread.

As with other viral illnesses, it is well recognized that some children will develop rotavirus gastroenteritis without having had contact with symptomatic individuals. Acquisition may result from an encounter with an individual who is asymptomatically shedding virus. Such asymptomatic excretion of rotavirus can occur for weeks before the onset of diarrhea and for days following resolution of symptoms. Other children may shed rotavirus and never experience symptoms.

ENTRY

Endemic rotavirus disease is caused primarily by **person-to-person transmission**. The principal means of transmission is by the **fecal–oral route**. Rotavirus is excreted in stool at high levels that reach 10^9 infectious particles/milliliter stool. Transmission of as few as 10 infectious particles can result in infection. Outbreaks due to contamination of municipal water supplies and foodborne transmission have been reported but appear to be rare. Speculation exists that rotavirus may spread by the **respiratory route** via infectious aerosol. This possibility is based on well-described epidemics in which fecal–oral transmission cannot be documented and on the observation that respiratory symptoms may precede the development of gastroenteritis by a day or two. Most outbreaks of viral gastroenteritis due to the Norwalk agent can be traced to contamination of a common source, such as shellfish, or contamination of municipal or well water.

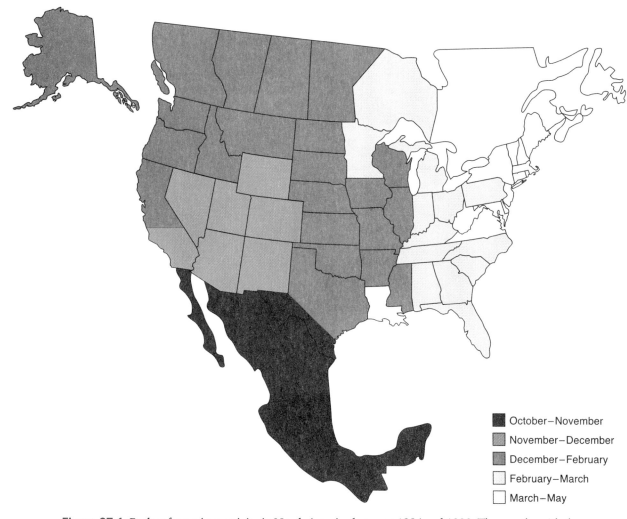

Figure 37.1. Peaks of rotavirus activity in North America between 1984 and 1988. The months with the highest activity are capitalized.

October–November
November–December
December–February
February–March
March–May

SPREAD AND MULTIPLICATION

Rotaviruses are among the few human viruses with a **double-stranded RNA genome**, which resembles double-stranded DNA in structure. Another distinguishing property (shared by the orthomyxoviruses) is that the genome of rotaviruses is **segmented**. Rotavirus particles are shaped like wheels with short spokes and an outer rim (*rota* means *wheel* in Latin) (Fig. 37.2). The particle possesses an icosahedral structure with an inner and an outer capsid. Infectivity requires an intact outer membrane that is necessary for **acid stability**, a critical characteristic for microorganisms that gain entry through the gastrointestinal tract. Two outer capsid proteins, a hemagglutinin (VP4) and a glycoprotein (VP7), induce formation of neutralizing antibodies.

The capsid contains 11 segments of double-stranded RNA as well as a viral **RNA-dependent RNA polymerase (transcriptase)** for transcription of individual RNA segments into mRNA. This enzyme is absent in animal cells and must be introduced from the virion during

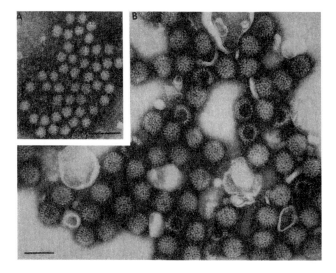

Figure 37.2. Electron micrograph of negatively stained viral particles. A. Norwalk virus. B. rotavirus.

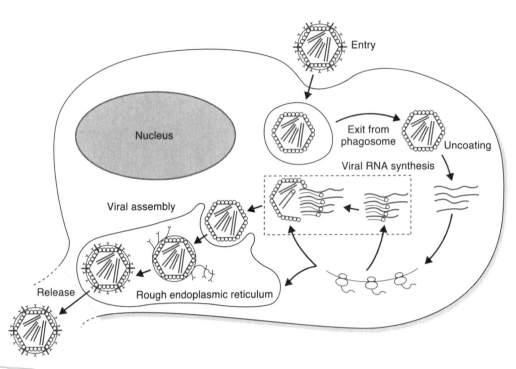

Figure 37.3. The rotavirus replication cycle.

infection. Using in vitro translation and the analysis of viruses that have undergone genomic reassortment, the gene product (structural and nonstructural proteins) of each of the 11 segments has been defined.

Most rotavirus strains require treatment with a protease to become infective. Viral penetration into cells is enhanced by proteolysis of an outer capsid protein. Viral replication then proceeds in the cytoplasm, resulting in the formation of both positive- and negative-strand RNA (Fig. 37.3). The positive-strand RNA functions as mRNA and associates with negative-strand RNA. Viral particles are assembled in the cytoplasm and, after becoming coated with surface proteins, mature by budding through the endoplasmic reticulum. Mature viral particles are then released into the extracellular environment with lysis of the infected cell.

Six groups of rotaviruses have been identified based on antigenic characteristics (A through F). **Group A rotaviruses** share a common antigen and are the only rotaviruses recognized to cause frequent infections in the U.S. **Group B rotaviruses** are best known as a cause of diarrhea in swine, but have caused outbreaks in adults and children in China. The other groups are either infrequent or their role in human disease is not clear.

DAMAGE

Rotaviruses produce a spectrum of disease ranging from asymptomatic infection to mild diarrhea, to severe diarrhea with potentially fatal dehydration. Severe gastroenteritis generally occurs in children between 6 and 24 months, as in the case of M.A. Rotavirus infections typi-

cally have a 2-day incubation period. Vomiting often precedes the onset of gastroenteritis by 2 or 3 days. Watery diarrhea may last 38 days in infants who become symptomatic. Fever and abdominal cramps are common. Red blood cells or leukocytes are generally not found in the stool of patients with rotavirus gastroenteritis.

Morphological changes have been identified from biopsies of the mucosa of the proximal small intestine of infants and children with rotavirus gastroenteritis; these include shortening and atrophy of the villi, denuded villi, and mononuclear cell infiltration of the lamina propria. Viral invasion of the epithelial cells of the small intestine results in destruction of the mature absorptive cells which are then replaced with young, virus-free cells. This process results in diarrhea for at least two reasons. First, immature replacement cells have a reduced ability to absorb salt and water. Second, immature cells have a reduced ability to produce disaccharidases, which results in malabsorption of carbohydrates. The severity of rotavirus-induced diarrhea is proportional to the extent of mucosal damage in the small intestine.

In infants who are under 6 months of age, rotavirus infection is less common, except for premature neonates who may acquire the infection during outbreaks in neonatal units. Normal, term infants often remain asymptomatic even while shedding rotavirus in the stool, for reasons that are not well understood. It may be that maternal antibody transferred during the third trimester protects term infants, and that premature infants are born before they can acquire maternal antirotavirus antibody. In children older than 6 months of age, rotavirus is a major nosocomial pathogen.

Adults generally experience a mild or even asymptomatic infection due to rotavirus because long-term immunity generally follows a primary infection. Symptoms become apparent when the inoculum size is large enough to overcome preexisting immunity. In some instances, rotaviruses may be a cause of travelers' diarrhea in children and adults, although it is less common than other pathogens in this setting.

Chronic diarrhea and prolonged shedding have been associated with rotavirus infection in children with **T-cell immunodeficiencies**. Patients undergoing immunosuppression for bone marrow transplantation are also at increased risk.

DIAGNOSIS

Because most of the viral agents that cause gastroenteritis grow poorly in cell culture, assays that detect viral antigen in stool specimens have become the most widely used method of diagnosis. **Antigen detection** assays, as used in M.A.'s case, are widely available for rotavirus and adenovirus detection. For other viral causes of gastroenteritis, the electron microscope can be used to study an individual stool specimen for characteristic viral morphology. However, a relatively high viral titer must be present in the stool specimen for the virus to be seen by this method. **Immune electron microscopy** increases the sensitivity by adding virus-specific antibody that aggregates viral particles in the field. Serology is feasible but not generally useful, and cultivation is not an option for most intestinal viruses because these agents cannot be easily propagated.

TREATMENT AND PREVENTION

At present, there are no established therapies for the management of viral gastroenteritis. Adherence to universal precautions for infection control, such as hand washing and barrier methods (gloves, gowns) are important for minimizing disease spread. Patient care is directed at supportive measures with particular attention to the prevention of dehydration by the use of intravenous hydration or oral rehydration therapy.

Several potential new approaches to prevention and treatment of viral gastroenteritis are being considered. Since mucosal surfaces may contain only small concentrations of secretory IgA antibodies, oral administration of γ-globulin preparations containing high titers of antibody against enteric viruses may increase antiviral activity. A second approach involves the use of **protease inhibitors** because rotaviruses require proteolytic activity to efficiently penetrate host cells. Other enteric viruses may require a similar activity. By preventing such cleavage with a protease inhibitor, it may be possible to attenuate an infection. Numerous questions need to be considered such as the impact of protease activity on digestion. A third approach involves oral immunization with a **live,** **attenuated rotavirus vaccine**. Rotaviruses of rhesus or bovine origin have been evaluated as candidate vaccines which may induce a protective immune response without inducing disease. Another approach involves the generation of recombinant rotavirus strains which contain genes from both human and animal strains. Two important concerns include (1) the ability of high-risk neonates to mount an effective immune response against a vaccine strain, and (2) ensuring that an attenuated virus cannot cause disease in susceptible contacts.

OTHER ENTERIC VIRUSES

Whereas rotaviruses are the most widely recognized cause of viral enteric infections, other agents are clearly important. The **Norwalk virus** is the prototype of a group referred to as Norwalk-like viruses or small, round structured viruses (SRSV) (see Fig. 37.2). Members of this group are named after the geographic area where an outbreak was described (e.g., Hawaii agent, Montgomery County agent). While these viruses cause sporadic, endemic disease, they usually come to attention through the development of **explosive outbreaks**. These viruses are transmitted by contaminated food or water, or person-to-person contact. **Adenoviruses** are best known as a cause of upper respiratory tract disease (Chapter 39, "Adenoviruses"). However, two serotypes (numbers 40 and 41) in particular are now recognized to cause diarrhea, especially in children who are less than 2 years of age. Outbreaks due to **caliciviruses** have been described mainly in institutions. Based on the prevalence of specific antibodies, most individuals have been infected with these viruses by 12 years of age. **Astroviruses** are another group of incompletely understood viruses that cause enteric disease, primarily in children.

SELF-ASSESSMENT QUESTIONS

1. Discuss the epidemiological features of rotavirus infections in small children
2. What is the season appearance of rotaviruses in North America?
3. Does rotavirus infection protect against further infections with the same strains of virus?
4. What are the most commonly employed diagnostic tools in rotavirus infections?

SUGGESTED READINGS

Dolin R, Treanor JJ, Madore HP. Novel agents of viral enteritis in humans. J Infect Dis 1987;155:365–376.

Ward RL, Bernstein DI, Young EC, Sherwood JR, Knowlton DR, Schiff GM. Human rotavirus studies in volunteers: determination of infectious dose and serological response to infection. J Infect Dis 1986;154:871–880.

Yolken RH, Maldonado Y, Rinney J, Vonderfecht S. Epidemiology and potential methods for prevention of neonatal intestinal viral infections. Rev Infect Dis 1990;12 (Suppl 4):S421–S427.

CHAPTER 38

The Human Retroviruses: AIDS and Other Diseases

CODY MEISSNER

JOHN M. COFFIN

Key Concepts

Retroviruses:

- Are RNA viruses that contain the enzyme reverse transcriptase, which allows them to use RNA as a template to make DNA.
- Are capable of causing chronic disease long after initial infection because the viral DNA integrates with the host cell genome.
- Include human immunodeficiency virus (HIV), the virus that causes acquired immune deficiency syndrome (AIDS); human T-cell lymphoma/leukemia virus-I (HTLV-I), which is associated with leukemia and lymphoma; and HTLV-II.

Human Immunodeficiency Virus (HIV):

- Preferentially binds to the CD4 receptor found on helper T cells and monocytes; the destruction of these cells ultimately disables the immune system and makes the infected individual vulnerable to opportunistic infections.
- Is transmitted through sexual contact, intravenous drug use, and vertically (mother to child)
- Displays antigenic variation.
- Has a long latency period (average of 10 years).
- Can currently be managed with antiviral drugs but is otherwise nearly 100% fatal.

Since five previously healthy homosexual men were diagnosed with pneumocystis pneumonia in May 1981, AIDS has become a major public health concern. During the 8 years between May 1981 and August 1989, the first 100,000 cases of AIDS were reported in the United States. The next 100,000 cases were reported over the subsequent 26 months, and the numbers of new cases continued to increase exponentially until the mid 1990s. After 1994, the epidemic of new cases reached a plateau (Fig. 38.1). More recently, reports of death due to AIDS have actually begun to decrease, an effect most likely attributable to the new and potent combinations of antiretroviral agents that are now in general use. However, by the end of 1996, there had been a total of 581,429 AIDS cases with 362,004 deaths in the United States. Worldwide, 22.6 million people are estimated to be living with HIV/AIDS. By any standards, the impact of AIDS on the U.S. health care system and support services is enormous, and in many parts of the developing world, the impact of the disease has been nothing short of a disaster.

Two attributes make AIDS unique among infectious diseases: It is uniformly fatal, and most of its devastating

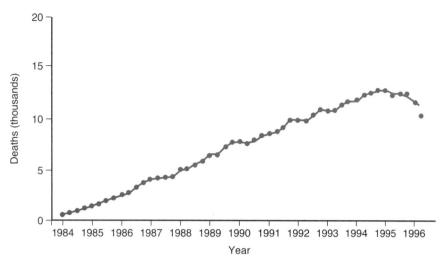

Figure 38.1. Quarterly incidence of AIDS and AIDS-related deaths in the United States, 1984–1996.

symptoms are not caused directly by the causative agent. With suppression of the host's immune response by the AIDS virus (human immunodeficiency virus or HIV), opportunistic organisms are able to cause disease. Most symptoms seen in a person with AIDS result from secondary infections.

AIDS first appeared in the United States in 1978. In 1981, the syndrome was described among gay men with multiple sexual partners. Some evidence suggests that unrecognized cases occurred earlier. By late 1981, the disease was reported in heterosexual intravenous drug abusers. The first cases among individuals with hemophilia receiving transfusions of human factor VIII were described in 1982. Soon, transmission of the presumed infectious agent to heterosexual partners of infected intravenous drug abusers and bisexual men was documented.

The clinical manifestations of AIDS are described in detail in Chapter 68, "AIDS".

CASE

Baby boy G. was born by cesarean section after a 36-week gestation to a 19-year-old prostitute with terminal AIDS. The mother had developed a second episode of *Pneumocystis carinii* pneumonia (PCP) two weeks prior to delivery. Despite intensive therapy, including intubation and mechanical ventilation, the mother died two hours following delivery because of respiratory failure.

IgG antibodies to HIV were detected in the infant by both an ELISA test and by western blot analysis (see "Diagnosis"). The infant received no blood or blood products. By four months of age he experienced poor weight gain, extensive thrush (oral candidiasis), diffuse lymphadenopathy (enlargement of lymph nodes), and persistent diarrhea. He developed a rapidly progressive pneumonia and died of

PCP. Cytomegalovirus was cultured from lung tissue obtained at autopsy.

The diagnosis of AIDS in this infant was based on his birth from a known HIV-infected mother and on the absence of findings to suggest another cause for the neonatal immunodeficient state. The infant's positive HIV serology (i.e., antibodies to HIV), however, may have been due to maternal antibodies transmitted transplacentally. Passively acquired maternal antibodies to HIV may persist until 15 months of age, thus positive serology in young children alone does not mean that they are infected with the virus. Because the child was born by cesarean section, had no contact with his mother after delivery, and had received no blood products, it is most likely that his infection was acquired by transplacental passage *in utero*.

THE RETROVIRUSES

Retrovirus Structure and Life Cycle

Structure

Retroviruses have a small spherical virion surrounded by a lipid envelope (Fig. 38.2). The genome contains two identical RNA molecules linked in a dimeric structure. These molecules resemble eukaryotic mRNA because they contain a **cap structure** at the 5′ end and **poly A sequence** at the 3′ end. Four viral genes are necessary for the replication of retroviruses (Fig. 38.3). The *gag* gene codes for three or four core proteins. The *pol gene* codes for **reverse transcriptase** or **DNA polymerase**, the enzyme responsible for replication of the genome, as well as **integrase**, the enzyme necessary for integration of viral DNA into the host cell genome. The *env* gene codes for the two **env**elope glycoproteins. Noncoding sequences include terminally redundant regions and unique regions near the ends of the genome. The *pro* gene encodes a protease necessary for cleaving the Gag and Pol proteins to their active form. Reverse transcrip-

Humans, Health and History

The History of Retroviruses

Understanding the role of retroviruses as the etiologic agent of AIDS requires a historical detour through the puzzling connection between viruses and cancer. This history includes a challenge to a traditional tenet of molecular biology, that genetic information flows from DNA through RNA intermediates to protein. In the late 1960s, researchers identified an unusual class of viruses that carried genetic information in molecules of RNA. While RNA-containing viruses were not a novelty, these viruses were unique because they contained the formerly unrecognized enzyme, **reverse transcriptase**. Using RNA as a template, this enzyme reverses the conventional flow of genetic information by synthesizing a copy of complementary DNA that ultimately integrates into the genome of the host cell. This DNA, called the **provirus**, serves as an intermediate stage in the replicative cycle.

Some of these viruses (now called **retroviruses** in recognition of their reverse or "retro" mode of replication) are capable of causing tumors. A virus of this type was first isolated in 1911, when Peyton Rous reported that tumors in chickens could be caused by a virus readily transmissible by filtered extracts (later known as **RSV**, for Rous Sarcoma Virus). Since then, hundreds of retroviruses have been isolated from many groups of vertebrates. In the early 1960s, a cancer-inducing cat virus was discovered, now called the **feline leukemia virus**. This virus proved to be important in understanding the biology of retroviruses for two reasons. First, it induces in cats an immunodeficiency similar to the one later observed in humans with AIDS. Second, feline leukemia virus is transmitted among cats in a household setting, providing a valuable model for epidemiological analysis of retrovirus infection.

Until the late 1960s, there was considerable skepticism that a virus could mediate the transmission of cancer. Because cancer appeared to be a genetic alteration, it was difficult to conceive how an RNA-containing virus could interact with the DNA of the host cell to produce oncogenic changes. The discovery of reverse transcriptase suggested a mechanism for the induction of permanent genetic change.

Since 1980, two groups of retroviruses capable of causing disease in humans have been isolated and characterized (Table 38.1). For several years before 1980, researchers suspected that retroviruses may be agents of human disease, but the point could not be proved because these viruses did not grow in cultured cells. Several advances in cell culture technology overcame this obstacle. One of the most important was the discovery of **T-cell growth factor** (or interleukin-2, IL-2), which stimulates the growth of T-lymphocytes in vitro. These lymphocytes could then be used for the isolation of human T-cell lymphotropic viruses (HTLVs). The first of these viruses, **HTLV-I**, was isolated from the cells of two patients with adult T-cell lymphoma. Subsequent HTLV-I isolates from other leukemia patients were shown to be closely related, as determined by serology and nucleic acid hybridization. Epidemiological studies suggested a causal relationship between a childhood infection with HTLV-I and the development of lymphoma in a few percent of infected individuals as many as 40 years later. A similar virus, **HTLV-II**, was later isolated from a patient with hairy cell leukemia, but its role in human disease is less clear at the present time.

The malignant diseases caused by HTLV-I, adult cell leukemia and lymphoma, are uniformly fatal but are relatively rare (even in infected individuals) and have been limited to certain specific populations. More recently, HTLV-I infection has been associated with certain progressive spinal cord diseases, such as tropical spastic paraparesis and HTLV-I-associated myelopathy. HTLV-I has been implicated in these diseases because of the presence of specific antibodies and the isolation of the virus from cerebrospinal fluid (CSF) and serum of such patients.

HTLV-I attracted considerable attention, both because it was the first known human retrovirus and because of the novel features of its biology. Although uncommon in the United States at the present time, the spread of this virus through the blood supply is a major concern. Routine screening of donated blood for the presence of this virus is currently being instituted. Fortuitously, studies of this virus provided the technology needed for the isolation of the AIDS agent several years later. Thus, AIDS was shown to be caused by a retrovirus within three years after it was first described in 1981. When first isolated, this virus had several names, but it is now known as **human immunodeficiency virus** (HIV). The remainder of this chapter focuses on this virus.

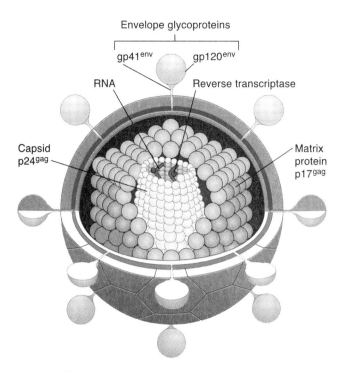

Figure 38.2. Retrovirus structure. A schematic drawing showing the virion proteins and other structures.

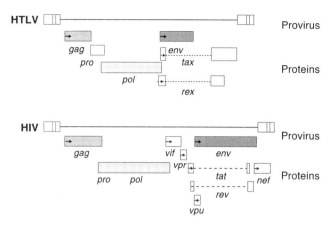

Figure 38.3. The genetic organization of human retroviruses. The top line in each case shows the provirus with control sequences shown as boxes at the ends. The lower boxes indicate the location of the viral genes, with dotted boxes showing genes whose function is uncertain. Note that both these viruses have genes in addition to those that code for virion proteins (*gag*, *pol*, and *env*).

PARADIGM ■ ■ ■

New Epidemics of Infectious Diseases

How do new epidemics of infectious diseases arise? In some cases, such as influenza, the virus is already present in the human or animal population and undergoes antigenic rearrangement to produce new, more virulent strains. In other instances, the agent is present as a relatively innocuous commensal in animals, and by a genetic change becomes virulent in humans.

In the case of the AIDS epidemic, considerable genetic evidence suggests that viruses related to HIV have existed in nonhuman primate populations for a long time. Two possibilities may explain the emergence of the AIDS epidemic in humans. One explanation is that the non human primate viruses have mutated to a more virulent form. The second is that virulent strains have existed all along. In either case, the important variables are changes in human behavior that facilitated the spread of the virus among human. It is likely that sporadic cases of AIDS existed among people in contact with infected monkeys or apes, but that the virus did not spread much beyond the affected individuals. What set off the AIDS epidemic were changes in human behavior, such as the urbanization of certain regions of Africa, changes in sexual habits, and the contamination of intravenous needles used by consumers of drugs. All of these changes led to a dramatic increase in transmission of HIV among people.

Will the Aids epidemic ever come to an end? The AIDS epidemic of today has a vivid historical parallel. At the end of the 15th century, an apparently new disease, **syphilis**, swept through Europe in epidemic proportions. For the first 60 years of its history, syphilis was a very different illness from that we now know: instead of progressing (if untreated) to the chronic manifestations of the tertiary stage, 15th and 16th century syphilis was an acute disease with a high mortality rate. We do not know what caused the abrupt change in the pathological picture of syphilis, but we can speculate as follows: for any disease that is spread directly among people, an agent that causes the death of the hosts eliminates infected contacts. As a result, the transmission of the agent is greatly reduced. Eventually, the deadly strain of the agent will be supplanted by a milder one that causes a chronic illness and thus has a greater chance of being transmitted to a new host. This scenario may in fact have occurred for HIV or HIV-like viruses in monkeys and apes. AIDS in humans, on the other hand, is unlikely to result in such a balanced situation. An HIV-infected person can be the source of transmission of the virus over a long period of time. Thus, the biological basis for the abatement of the AIDS epidemic is not at all obvious. Interrupting the AIDS epidemic cannot depend on evolutionary changes in either the host or the virus but will require effective antiviral vaccination or chemotherapy.

N. CARY ENGLEBERG

Table 38.1. The Pathogenic Human Retroviruses	
A HTLV Group	
HTLV-I	Causative agent of certain cutaneous T-cell lymphoma; as well as HTLV-I myelopathy (also called tropical spastic papaparesis)
HTLV-II	Not conclusively linked to a specific disease; found in cases of T-cell hairy-cell leukemia
B Lentiviruses	
HIV-1	Causative agent of AIDS
HIV-2	Related to, but distinct from HIV-1; described as a cause of AIDS, particularly in West Africa

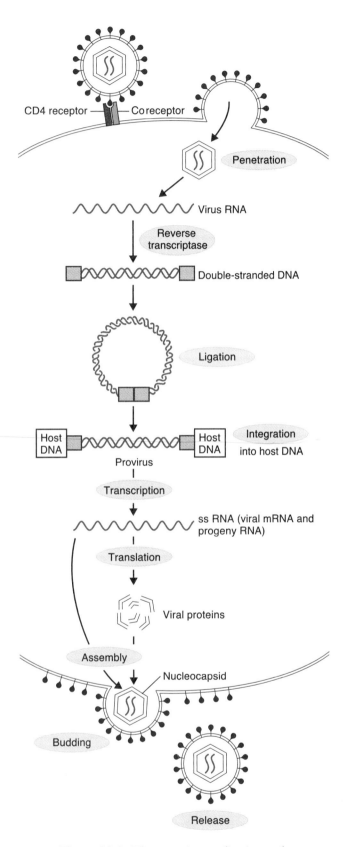

Figure 38.4. The retrovirus replication cycle.

tase (RNA dependent DNA polymerase) molecules are associated with the genome and are carried within the virion.

In addition to the genes common to all retroviruses, *gag, pro, pol,* and *env,* the HIV genome contains at least six other genes (see below). These encode functions that seem to be important in regulating the complex replication cycle of this virus, which may exist in a latent state in the infected cell and then undergo rapid replication at the appropriate time.

The virus life cycle

The replication cycle of HIV (Fig. 38.4) includes the following steps:

- **Binding**. Once in close proximity to a **helper T-lymphocyte**, HIV recognizes and binds to the **CD4 receptor** molecule via its envelope glycoprotein. Antibodies to either the viral envelope protein or the cell receptor block this interaction and prevent infection. The presence of the CD4 molecule on the cell surface, which plays an important role in immunological function (see Chapter 7, "Induced Defenses"), determines the primary target cells for infection.
- **Fusion** of the virus envelope with the cell membrane. This step requires interaction of the envelope protein with a second cell surface molecule, or co-receptor. Co-receptors are receptors for important signaling proteins, called chemokines. As a result, the virion loses its integrity and characteristic morphology. Genomic RNA is released into the cytoplasm within the virus core, which includes molecules of reverse transcriptase.
- **Synthesis of DNA**. Reverse transcriptase now synthesizes a complementary DNA molecule corresponding to the viral RNA genome. The enzyme then synthesizes the second DNA strand (complementary to the first), generating a double-stranded DNA molecule. In the process of making the DNA, portions of ends

of the genomic RNA are copied twice, resulting in a structure at each end of the DNA called the **long terminal repeat (LTR).**

- **Integration.** The double-stranded DNA molecule is transported to the nucleus and integrated into host cell chromosomes. The virus-coded enzyme, **integrase,** is responsible for this reaction, which involves joining the ends of each LTR to cellular DNA. The retrovirus integration process resembles the mechanism of motion of some transposable elements of bacteria (see Chapter 4, "Genetics".) In the integrated state, viral genetic material is called the **provirus.** The provirus behaves like a cellular gene in that it is passed to daughter cells at division and contains signals that control its transcription into RNA.

- **Synthesis of progeny virus.** In the "productive phase", viral DNA is transcribed into messenger RNA by host cell RNA polymerase. Signals that direct the cell's RNA synthetic machinery are found in the LTR and resemble signals used by the cell for making its own RNAs. After transcription, some of these viral RNA molecules are used as messengers for the synthesis of viral proteins. Others become incorporated as genomes into progeny viral particles. Assembly of virions takes place at the cell surface. The structural proteins assemble with genomes and acquire their envelope by passage through the host cell membrane (see Fig. 38.5). Morphological changes in the virion after they bud through the membrane are caused by cleavage of the protein precursors.

- **Latency and trans-activation.** In general the replication cycle described so far is common to all retroviruses. HIV and some related viruses have yet other features. First, infection can also involve a **latent** phase in which infected cells contain a provirus but do not express viral RNA or proteins. Second, expression of HIV macromolecules is subject to regulation by viral gene products that operate as soluble elements (in "trans"). This phenomenon is known as **transactivation.** At least two HIV genes (called *tat* and *rev*) function as **transactivating factors,** which greatly increase the expression of viral RNAs and proteins. *Tat* causes a greater level of RNA to be made by RNA polymerase, and *rev* affects the way that the RNA are processed and translated into protein. Third, HIV proviruses contain signals that can turn on expression when HIV-infected cells are stimulated by antigen or infected by some other viruses (such as a herpesvirus). These features appear to be related in an important way: after infection of lymphocytes and integration of the provirus, the infection process may be halted, to be reinitiated much later in an explosive way by unknown stimuli. The outcome is a high level of trans-activation, resulting in a burst of virus production and rapid death of the cell. While only a small fraction of infected cells enter this latent state, these cells can defeat attempts to

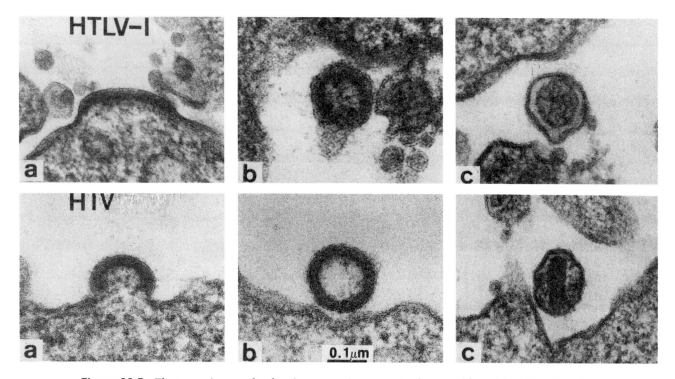

Figure 38.5. Electron micrographs showing successive stages in the assembly and budding of the human retroviruses HTLV-I (top row) and HIV (bottom row). Note the difference in structure of the core in the two types of mature virions (c).

eradicate infection by antiviral therapy even for extended periods.

Antigenic variation

A unique characteristic of infection by HIV is that the immune response of the host is unable to completely curtail viral replication (although it may be important in suppressing it during the latent phase of the disease). This characteristic is a paradox, since for most other viral infections the presence of antibody indicates immunity, protection from infection, and a favorable prognosis. How is HIV able to survive despite the host's immune response? Two mechanisms may be at work here: virus gene products may be relatively invisible to the immune response, and the virus may be able to mask or change its antigenic specificity.

Which HIV gene products are important in directing the immune response of the host? A clue comes from studies of the genetic diversity of the virus genes. HIV genes that code for internal viral proteins *(gag* and *pol)* show relative stability from one isolate to the next, but the *env* gene displays frequent mutations that lead to variations of its product, the surface glycoprotein. Although antibodies to *gag* and *pol* proteins are found in infected individuals, these antibodies do not seem to be important in the infection. Some antibodies to the envelope proteins, on the other hand, can neutralize the virus, although their titers are very low compared to other virus infections. HIV envelope glycoproteins have two unusual features. First, they are extensively coated with polysaccharide side-chains which, because they are added by host enzymes, are antigenically invisible to the host. Second, they contain **hypervariable regions** that permit the virus to present new antigenic configurations to the host. In contrast, the segments of the surface glycoprotein that are involved in the interaction of cellular receptors must be genetically conserved. Conserved segments may then be hidden and protected from neutralizing antibodies by the carbohydrates and the hypervariable regions. As a result, HIV can constantly vary its surface antigenic composition, which may allow it to avoid inactivation. In this regard, HIV resembles influenza viruses and trypanosomes of sleeping sickness in its ability to withstand the immune response by changing major surface antigens. Such a mechanism hinders the development of an effective vaccine containing the surface glycoprotein.

More recently, a new retrovirus has been isolated from patients with AIDS living in West Africa. This new isolate, called **HIV-2**, has an envelope glycoprotein that is more closely related to a monkey virus (simian immunodeficiency virus, SIV) than to HIV-1. (HIV-1 is likely to be closely related to a monkey virus as well; however, no natural host has been definitively identified.) Throughout 1991, seventeen individuals in the United States have been found to be infected with HIV-2. Epidemiological features

Table 38.2. AIDS cases by exposure category reported June 1996 through July 1997 and cumulative totals through July 1997, United States

Adult/adolescent exposure category	June '96–July '97		Cumulative Totals	
	Cases	Percent of total	Cases	Percent of total
Men who have sex with men (MSM)	24,146	38%	298,699	49%
Injecting drug users	16,150	25%	154,664	26%
MSM and injecting drug users	2,684	4%	38,923	6%
Hemophilia/coagulation disorder	265	0%	4,567	1%
Heterosexual contact	8,816	14%	54,571	9%
Receipt of blood, blood products, or tissues	489	1%	8,075	1%
Other/not identified	11,807	18%	44,677	7%
TOTAL ADULT	64,357	100%	604,176	100%

Pediatric (<13 years old) exposure category	Cases	Percent of total	Cases	Percent of total
Mother with/at risk for HIV infection	552	91%	7,157	91%
Hemophilia/coagulation disorder	4	1%	232	3%
Receipt of blood, blood products, or tissues	5	1%	375	5%
Other/not identified	48	8%	138	2%
TOTAL PEDIATRIC	609	100%	7,902	100%

of this virus appear similar to those of HIV-1. Major sequence differences exist between the two HIV types. Antibodies against the surface glycoprotein of HIV type 1 only partially cross react with HIV type 2. Antibodies directed against core proteins of HIV-1 and HIV-2 show some cross reactivity. Thus, AIDS can be caused by at least two distinct but related viruses.

Encounter

The distribution of HIV infection in the population is consistent with an agent that is extremely labile in a free state and that cannot readily enter through intact body surfaces. In this respect, HIV resembles (but is less contagious than) hepatitis B virus, which has a similar epidemiological pattern in the United States. HIV has been detected in a number of body fluids including peripheral blood, semen, cervical secretions, breast milk, urine, CSF, saliva, and tears. It is unlikely that the last four fluids represent an important means of transmission. With few exceptions, HIV transmission in the United States at the present time occurs by one of three routes: sexual contact, intravenous drug abuse, and vertical passage from infected mothers to offspring. At present, heterosexual transmission and congenital transmission from infected mother to child are becoming more important in the spread of AIDS in the United States. The incidence of AIDS associated with various exposure categories in shown in Table 38.2.

In 1991, homosexual and bisexual men accounted for approximately 70% of AIDS cases in the United States (including 8% who were also intravenous drug abusers). Although men who have sex with men are still the most prominent exposure category in 1996-97, they represent a smaller proportion of the total cases than during the earlier stages of the epidemic (Table 38.2). The most prominent risk factors for acquisition of infection are a high number of sexual partners and participation in sexual practices that increase the risk of transmission due to damage of the anorectal mucosa (mainly receptive anal intercourse, which allows the virus to enter the bloodstream through tears in the rectal mucosa or direct infection of the epithelial cells of the rectum).

As the AIDS epidemic has continued, intravenous drug abusers have become the second largest group with HIV infection in the United States, about 25–30% of total cases. Importantly, this group acts as a bridge for the spread of HIV infection to nonhomosexual contacts. Seventy-five percent of AIDS transmission due to heterosexual activity involves at least one partner who uses IV drugs. Transmission among drug abusers occurs due to sharing of contaminated needles and syringes that contain a residue of blood (including infected white blood cells) from previous users.

Although HIV transmission by blood transfusion has been exceedingly rare since March 1985, there are an estimated 12,000 living infected transfusion recipients.

Hemophiliacs have long been identified as a group at risk for blood-borne viruses such as hepatitis B and C because they receive preparations of factor VIII and factor IX obtained from plasma pooled from thousands of donors. Since 1984, factor VIII concentrates have been unlikely to contain HIV because blood donors are screened for HIV antibodies. In addition, since 1984 plasma products have been treated with heat and chemicals to inactivate contaminating viruses. Approximately 80% of recipients of factor VIII prior to 1984 are now infected with HIV or deceased.

Vaginal intercourse can result in HIV transmission to partners of either gender, although the risk is higher for the female. Heterosexual transmission is the most common form of spread of HIV in most countries other than the United States and northern Europe. Transmission rates to long-term heterosexual partners of AIDS patients vary widely, from less than 10% to 70%. In some instances, transmission may occur after one or two sexual contacts only. The low transmission rate seen in spouses of HIV-positive hemophiliacs suggests that, in many instances, the virus is not easily transmitted even over a period of several years. Partners of HIV-infected hemophiliacs appear to have lower rates of infection than partners of infected intravenous drug users. The disparity in transmission rates may be due to differences in the frequency of high-risk sexual practices, unreported drug injection by one of the partners, genetic factors influencing susceptibility, increased virulence of certain strains of HIV, or variable communicability in different stages of the infection. The lower rate of transmission of HIV from females to males versus males to females is not fully understood. Vaginal transmission from females to males may occur less frequently due to unfavorable factors for HIV survival in the vagina, and because such transmission may require penile ulcerations or damage to the male urethral mucosa.

Variation in the rate of HIV transfer from an infected to uninfected partner implies that genetic factors may influence susceptibility to infection. One such factor has been identified as the gene for CCR5, a chemokine receptor that serves as a co-receptor for HIV infection. The defective form of this gene is found in about 10% of individuals of European descent, but it is not found at all in other populations. In the 1% of this group who are homozygous, it confers a very high (though not absolute) level of resistance to HIV infection. Heterozygous individuals are not protected from infection but seem to have a slower rate of progression to AIDS.

Heterosexual transfer of HIV is more common in certain countries. For example, the overall ratio of male to female AIDS cases in Zaire is approximately 1 : 1 as opposed to 13 : 1 in the United States. One study showed that heterosexual African males with AIDS had a markedly higher number of sexual partners than did matched controls without AIDS. Possible other factors include lowered resistance due to coexistent sexually transmitted diseases. Regardless of differences in rates of transmission in the various groups, the prevention of major heterosexual epidemics must focus on all young, sexually active individuals. In some areas of Africa, AIDS is now the leading cause of death among adult males.

Congenital transmission, as in the case of baby G., is the most important route of transmission of pediatric AIDS. The Center for Disease Control estimates that between 1978 and 1993, 15,000 newborns acquired their HIV infection by vertical transmission. Because HIV screening of blood products has been in place since 1985, vertical transmission accounts for more than 90% of all new pediatric HIV infections. The highest seroprevalence rates in women are found among intravenous drug users or women who are sex partners of HIV infected men. Transmission of HIV from mother to infant is considerably more efficient than transmission by sexual contact. In some high-risk areas, such as New York City, more than one in 20 newborns has antibodies to HIV. Between 15% and 30% of children born to untreated HIV-infected mothers are HIV infected. Recent studies have shown that this rate can be reduced to ~5% when HIV-infected pregnant women receive antiviral drugs.

HIV transmission among health care workers is an area of particular concern. Extensive studies have confirmed that HIV transmission in a medical setting is exceedingly rare. The risk of infection following accidental sticking with needles used to draw blood from HIV infected patients is less than 0.5%. The risk from exposure to mucous membranes or by contamination of apparently intact skin is considerably less. With the general adoption of "universal precautions", which assume that blood or other fluids from all patients is potentially infectious, HIV spread to health care workers should remain a rare event. Its rate can be reduced still further by immediate post-exposure treatment with a combination of antiviral drugs. The spread of HIV from health care workers to patients is also exceedingly rare. Only one well-documented case, that of a Florida dentist has been found. At this writing, recommendations for dealing with this important issue are still pending.

It is important to emphasize that spread of HIV among nonsexual household contacts is exceedingly rare. More than 12 studies involving over 700 family members or boarding school contacts of AIDS patients failed to detect a single instance of transmission.

Arthropod vectors have been proposed as a route of transmission, but no evidence exists for this mode of transmission. If arthropods, such as mosquitoes or ticks, were important, children in third world countries would be frequently infected, as they are often victims of bites. In fact, the occurrence of AIDS in children outside recognized risk groups is highly unusual, making vectors an unlikely mechanism of transmission.

Entry, Spread, and Multiplication

The mechanism by which HIV establishes an infection in the host is poorly understood because of the variable course of the disease and the scarcity of infected cells, especially during the long, latent phase of infection. Most likely, HIV enters the host contained within infected cells, e.g., macrophages, lymphocytes, or spermatozoa, although infection with free virus also occurs. HIV enters the body either through micro-abrasions on the surface of mucous membranes or through penetration of intact skin with a needle.

While HIV can infect an expanding list of cell types, two major groups of cells in the body serve as preferred targets for infection by HIV: helper T-lymphocytes and monocytes. The surface of these cells contain the specific CD4 (or T4) protein, which serves as the receptor necessary for viral entry, as well as appropriate co-receptors (Fig. 38.6). Most of our knowledge of HIV replication comes from studies using cells derived from human T-cell tumors, which can be grown in the laboratory.

Damage

Our knowledge of the molecular events that modulate lymphocyte damage in HIV infected patients is still rudimentary. However, on the basis of known abnormalities of humoral and cellular immunity, it is possible to outline a sequence of events that follow HIV infection:

HIV preferentially infects helper T-cells, i.e., lymphocytes that express the CD4 surface protein. The CD4 protein defines this subset of T-cells and serves as the receptor for attachment of HIV. Many of these cells are

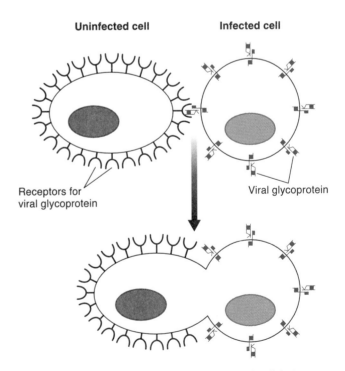

Figure 38.6. Mechanism of HIV-mediated cell fusion.

killed by replication of the virus. Cell death can be direct (i.e., due to either some effect of virus replication) or indirect, [i.e., due to recognition of infected cells by HIV-specific cytotoxic T lymphocytes (CTL)]. Even cells that survive can participate in killing, since such cells express viral envelope protein molecules and, in turn can bind to CD4 receptors on other cells. The result is cell-to-cell aggregation and eventual fusion, resulting in the formation of large multinucleated syncytia.

After the initial primary phase of HIV infection, virus replication is confined largely to the lymphoid organs where CD4 lymphocytes are the primary target. Loss of this cell population results in progressive immunodeficiency that leads to severe opportunistic infections and malignancies. Studies have shown a strong correlation between the absolute number of CD4 lymphocytes and life-threatening opportunistic infections. Although a great individual variation exists, the duration of the symptom-free period before the appearance of AIDS-defining infections is approximately 10 years. During this interval, CD4 counts drop from the normal level of about 1000 to less than 500 cells/mm^3. Patients with advanced HIV disease typically have CD4 counts less than 200 cells/mm^3. The risk of opportunistic infections is greatest in the late stage AIDS, when the CD4 count drops to fewer than 50 cells/mm^3. Serial measurements of CD4 cell counts serve as indicators for the risk of such infections, as well as a guide for the management of anti-retroviral therapy.

The rate of progression to AIDS is related to the extent of virus replication, and it varies considerably from individual to individual. Recent technical advances, based on detection of viral genomes in the blood by sensitive polymerase chain reaction (PCR) or hybridization techniques, make possible the accurate measurement of the amount of virus in blood (the "virus load") at any one time. Individuals with high virus loads (10^5 copies/ml or more) are at high risk for progression within a few years; infected individuals with low loads (less than 10^4 copies/ml) may not progress to AIDS for 10 years or more.

Damage to and depletion of helper T-cells during HIV replication results in a characteristic change in the ratio of helper/suppressor-cytotoxic cells. Depletion of helper T-cells results in a reduction in total circulating lymphocytes (lymphopenia) and a relative increase in the number of suppressor-cytotoxic lymphocytes.

In addition to quantitative T-cell deficits, HIV induces abnormalities in T-cell function. Normally, T cells modulate the function of other cells in the immune system, including B cells, monocytes, and natural killer cells. These interactions require the function of the CD4 protein (see Chapter 7, "Induced Defenses"). Infection with HIV results in loss of the CD4 receptor from the cell surface and can thus derange these functions even if the infected cells survive.

An important unresolved question is how HIV replication results in dysfunction and death of infected helper T-lymphocytes, a small percentage of which are infected. Various mechanisms that interfere with cell metabolism have been proposed. For example, does the formation of large syncytia of T-lymphocytes sequester a sufficient number to explain their depletion? Is there a toxic protein made by HIV but not by other retroviruses? Does unintegrated HIV DNA build up, with possibly disruption of cellular biosynthetic activities? Do the infected lymphocytes undergo premature differentiation and "senility?" Do T-helper cells become inactivated by loss of CD4 from the cell surface? All these phenomena can be observed in cell cultures, but their importance in natural infections is not clear.

The specific CD4 marker characteristic of helper T-lymphocytes is also found in membranes of other cell types, including circulating monocytes and macrophages; natural killer cells; certain B lymphocytes, and cells of the CNS, such as glial cells. These cells may also become infected and damaged by viral replication or, in addition, may serve as a reservoir for virus latency. Defects in killing secondary invading microorganisms may be attributes of HIV infection of macrophages and monocytes, as well as by the loss of helper T-cells. Furthermore, macrophage-related cells called Langerhans cells, which form part of epithelial surfaces, have been found to be highly sensitive to HIV and may be an important entry point for sexually-transmitted infection.

Although many patients with AIDS have elevated immunoglobulin levels in their serum, their ability to produce antibodies against specific antigens may be impaired. For example, children with HIV infections cannot make antibodies against the specific capsular polysaccharide antigens of pneumococcus and *Haemophilus influenzae* type b. This defect may be due to direct impairment of B lymphocytes as well as to the loss of helper T-lymphocytes.

Some Clinical Consequences

AIDS represents the terminal stage of infection by HIV. Clinical syndromes vary with different stages of infection:

Primary HIV infection may be associated with a mononucleosis-like syndrome approximately a few weeks following exposure. This syndrome may include fever, a skin rash, muscle aches, lymphadenopathy, and meningitis. Most of the time, these symptoms are not sufficient to cause the patient to seek medical attention. A few weeks after infection, a strong peak in virus load occurs. With the appearance of an antiviral immune response (particularly the CTL response), the virus load rapidly declines to its steady state value. This pattern implies that the initial immune response effectively eliminates the vast majority of virus and infected cells, but a small surviving population remains. The infected individual often becomes asymptomatic, but HIV antibodies can still be detected in serum and viral replication continues at a low level.

Primary infection is followed by an extended period of clinical latency. Recent studies have shown that this period is not one of latent viral infection, as is true for many viruses (like herpesviruses). Rather, large numbers of CD4 cells are being constantly infected and killed, with an average turnover time of about 2 days. This dynamic situation can be revealed by treatment of infected individuals with antiviral therapy, which leads to a rapid decline in virus load indicative of the rapid death of infected cells. AIDS is now recognized as the cumulative end point of damage acquired during this period.

Once infected, an individual may become completely asymptomatic or develop persistent generalized lymphadenopathy (Table 38.3). Lymphadenopathy may persist or resolve before progressing over months to years to pre-AIDS conditions characterized by diarrhea, oral candidiasis, weight loss, and fever.

HIV-infected individuals will eventually progress to AIDS with opportunistic infections, Kaposi's sarcoma, and/or B cell lymphomas (Table 38.3, categories B and C). In the case described above, both mother and child eventually died of PCP (*Pneumocystis carinii* pneumonia). For information on *P.carinii*, see Chapter 50, "Blood and tissue protozoa", and for details on infections of the compromised patient, see Chapter 67, "Infections of the Compromised host". The majority of adult AIDS patients also develop neurologic symptoms. Neurologic manifestations of AIDS may be due to a secondary infection by opportunistic organisms such as the protozoan *Toxoplasma gondii* or the fungus *Cryptococcus neoformans*, or to the development of malignancies of the central nervous system (CNS). HIV is also known to invade the CNS directly and replicate in glial cells. Presumably, the virus is carried to the CNS by circulating monocytes. It is not known if damage to brain cells is due to the release of toxic substances from the monocytes or to direct damage to brain tissue by replicating virus.

The most important single factor in the development of AIDS in HIV-infected individuals is time. Most, if not all HIV infected individuals will ultimately develop AIDS. Over 95% of HIV-infected individuals progress to AIDS within 15 years of infection. The remaining small fraction of long term—nonprogressors have very low virus loads and may survive for very long times—perhaps indefinitely. Several factors affect survival rates, including age, gender, type of initial diagnosis, and immune status. For example, patients who develop Kaposi's sarcoma have significantly longer survival than patients who present with other opportunistic infections, perhaps because the former are diagnosed at an earlier stage of altered cellular immunity. Overall, the 5-year survival rate of untreated patients with AIDS ranges from 3% to 15%. These figures indicate not only the seriousness of HIV in-

Table 38.3. Clinical Categories of HIV Infection in Persons > 13 Years of Age

Category A (excludes patients with conditions in categories B and C):
- Asymptomatic
- Persistent generalized adenopathy
- Symptomatic, acute (primary) HIV infection

Category B (excludes patients with condition in category C):
If the following conditions are attributable to HIV, follow a course complicated by HIV, or require special management because of HIV:
- Bacillary angiomatosis (disseminated bartonellosis)
- Oropharyngeal candidiasis
- Persistent, recurrent, or poorly responsive vulvovaginal candidiasis
- Cervical dysplasia or cervical carcinoma *in situ*
- Constitutional symptoms, e.g., fever > 38.5°C or diarrhea > 1 month
- Oral hairy leukoplakia
- Recurrent or multidermatomal herpes zoster
- Idiopathic thrombocytopenic purpura
- Listeriosis
- Pelvic inflammatory disease, particularly with tuboovarian abscess
- Peripheral neuropathy

Category C
If any of the following conditions are diagnosed:
- Candidiasis of the trachea, bronchi or lungs
- Esophageal candidiasis
- Disseminated coccidioidomycosis
- Extrapulmonary cryptococcosis
- Chronic cryptosporidiosis, with diarrhea for more than one month
- Cytomegalovirus infection (other than liver, spleen, or nodes)
- Cytomegalovirus retinitis (with vision loss)
- HIV encephalopathy
- Herpes simplex: chronic ulcers for more than one month, or bronchitis, pneumonia or esophagitis
- Disseminated or extrapulmonary histoplasmosis
- Isosporiasis, with diarrhea for over 1 month
- Kaposi's sarcoma
- Non-Hodgkin's lymphoma of B cell or unknown phenotype, including Burkitt's lymphoma
- Primary lymphoma of the brain
- Disseminated *Mycobacterium avium* complex or *M. kansasi*
- Mycobacterium tuberculosis, either pulmonary or extrapulmonary
- Other disseminated or extrapulmonary mycobacterial infections
- *Pneumocystis carini* pneumonia
- Recurrent pneumonia
- Progressive multifocal leucoencephalopathy
- Recurrent *Salmonella* septicemia
- Toxoplasmosis of the brain
- Wasting syndrome due to HIV
- Invasive cervical cancer

fection, but also the magnitude of the health problem in years to come. Even if no one becomes infected with HIV from now on, the incidence of the disease will continue to increase into the next century. It is not known if the probability of progression to AIDS is increased by "co-factors" (e.g., diseases often seen in some risk groups, such as hepatitis, cytomegalovirus, and herpes infections) or by genetic determinants. Before the availability of zidovudine (AZT, azidothymidine), the median survival time among AIDS patients was about 12 months. Recent studies have shown that this figure can be substantially increased among patients who receive antiretroviral and other antimicrobial therapy.

Diagnosis

Before the viral etiologic agent was identified, diagnosis of AIDS was based solely on clinical findings. The presence of specific opportunistic infections or certain tumors such as Kaposi's sarcoma in high-risk groups was necessary before the disease could be suspected. Patients in the early stages of infection could not be identified. In 1993, the CDC issued revised criteria for a **case definition of AIDS** based on the presence or absence of laboratory evidence of HIV infection, the level of CD4 lymphocytes, and the presence of opportunistic illnesses (Table 38.4). Evidence of infection is generally based on the presence of antibodies to HIV. The presence of virus in blood or tissues can be documented by growth of the virus in cell culture or by molecular methods, such as the PCR assay that detects viral genetic material. Remember also that in the early stages of HIV infection only a small percentage of lymphocytes are infected and that such cells may be hard to find. Therefore, laboratory evidence is generally based on serologic or molecular findings.

Serologic tests for HIV infection detect and characterize specific anti-HIV antibodies in serum. The ability to grow HIV in culture provided the antigens that made such tests possible. It is now clear that close to 100% of HIV-infected individuals have measurable antibodies in their serum. The exceptions are a small group of individuals either in the earliest stages of the disease (before seroconversion) or in the terminal stages (when their B

cells are unable to synthesize antibodies). On very rare occasions, certain individuals may "serorevert" (lose detectable antibodies while still carrying the virus). Antibodies may not be detected in an HIV-infected person due to technical problems (false negatives). It is important to remember, therefore, that in a very limited number of instances, the absence of antibodies does not completely rule out an HIV infection. The persistence of detectable antibodies to HIV is generally accepted as an indication of infection and the ability to transmit the virus.

Initial tests for HIV serology generally are performed by an ELISA test (enzyme-linked immuno sorbent assay). This test is carried out by adding a sample of the patient's serum to small plastic cups to which HIV antigen is bound (kits for such assays are commercially available). If antibodies are present, they will bind to HIV antigen. After washing away unreacted components, anti-human immunoglobulin antiserum linked to a readily assayable enzyme, such as a peroxidase, is added. Anti-HIV antibodies in the clinical sample can then be detected by adding a chromogenic enzyme substrate; a positive test is indicated by a suitable color change (see Chapter 55, "Diagnostic Principles", for details). If the serum is found to be positive to HIV antibodies, the test is usually repeated. Results are confirmed by immunofluorescence or "Western blot" analysis. The Western blot detects antibodies against individual viral proteins that have been separated by electrophoresis and transferred ("blotted") onto a thin membrane filter. (See Chapter 55, "Diagnostic Principles", for a full discussion of Western blots, ELISAs and diagnostic principles in HIV infection.)

The ELISA test has a false-positive rate of around 0.4%. With confirmatory Western blot tests, the joint false-positive rate approaches a remarkable 0.005%. However, even these low numbers become worrisome when a population with low prevalence of HIV infection is tested. Thus, it has been estimated that among non-high risk female blood donors in the United States (whose rate of HIV infection is approximately 1 in 10,000), the likelihood that infection is actually present in a woman with a confirmed positive-test is only around 70%. The additional use of PCR or hybridization tests for viral RNA in blood is now standard both for confirmatory and prognostic purposes.

Before the use of viral load tests and the advent of at least partially effective therapy, it was necessary to carefully weigh whether low-risk individuals should be tested. The impact of a positive test result on a person's state of mind, social interactions, marriage, insurance eligibility, and employment opportunities is enormous. It is now recognized that the beneficial effects of initiating anti-HIV therapy prior to the onset of AIDS clearly justifies testing of individuals at risk for HIV infection.

Table 38.4. CDC Definition of AIDS

	Clinical Category*	
CD4+ T-cells	AB	C
>500/μL	A1B1	C1
200–499/μL	A2B2	C2
<200/μL	A3B3	C3

AIDS is diagnosed if the patient meets criteria for category A3, B3, C1, C2, or C3.
* See Table 38.3.

Prevention

Control of the spread of AIDS has proved to be difficult because a vaccine is not yet available. The most effective control of this disease requires a change in the lifestyle for many individuals. Education appears to be the most important means of reducing the spread of AIDS at the present time. The most important measures include curtailing high-risk practices, such as multiple sexual contacts for both the homosexual and heterosexual population; the use of condoms; and awareness of the danger of anal intercourse and the use of uncontaminated needles for intravenous drug abusers. Evidence that education has an impact on sexual practices comes from experience in the gay community in San Francisco, where transmission of other sexually transmitted diseases, especially gonorrhea, is markedly reduced. While it is not yet known if this reduction has also led to a reduction in AIDS cases, it has reduced the spread of HIV in this community.

What problems are encountered in designing an AIDS vaccine? The ability of HIV to change its antigenicity complicates conventional approaches to vaccine development. Early results with viral envelope antigens prepared by genetic engineering techniques have not been encouraging. It should be emphasized that so far researchers have only a limited understanding of the nature of the immune response to HIV infection. Antibody titers in infected individuals are low compared to other viral infections, but the reduction of the initial viremia suggests that the cellular immune response may be partially effective in controlling the infection for many years and raises hope that a similar immune response induced in uninfected individuals may be sufficient to ward off a primary infection.

It is not known whether a vaccine-induced human immune response would confer protection against primary HIV infection. One problem with an HIV vaccine is that the virus is probably transmitted from person to person mainly within infected cells (lymphocytes or macrophages) and, therefore, the virus may not be accessible to the immune system. HIV may be transmitted directly from cell to cell, without going through an extracellular phase. Protection may require a more complex immune response, probably of the cell-mediated type. Another approach to vaccine development involves live recombinant vaccines consisting of bacterial or viral vector genomes that contain and express HIV genes such as *gag*, *pol*, or *nef*. An HIV specific immune response might be induced by replication of the recombinant vector. Conceivably, both humoral and cellular responses, as well as mucosal immunity, might be stimulated by such a vaccine. Experimental recombinant vaccines have been created using vectors such as vaccinia virus, mycobacteria, and adenoviruses.

A number of problems are associated with HIV vaccine development, and testing of an HIV vaccine presents special problems. The chimpanzee is the only animal known to be susceptible to HIV infection (although the infection usually does not progress to AIDS). Vaccine candidates currently being tested include killed whole virus, purified envelope protein, peptides from envelope proteins, and vaccinia virus genetically engineered to produce HIV proteins after infection. The best model system may be the closely related virus (SIVs) found in some monkey species and capable of causing AIDS in other species. In this model, a live, attenuated virus vaccine confers an immune response adequate to protect against challenge with the same virus. These results are grounds for optimism that an effective human vaccine can be developed. However, potential safety concerns may preclude the development of live virus vaccines for human use. Even when a potential HIV vaccine has been developed, human clinical trials will be difficult to accomplish. First, volunteers will have the stigma of becoming HIV antibody positive. Second, criteria need to be established for the volunteers' sexual preference. Third, it is still not known how researchers will determine if a response is protective. Fourth, to provide a statistically significant answer (in view of the low incidence of infection in the population) a huge number of people will have to be vaccinated. Finally, the ability of HIV to establish a latent infection will also complicate vaccine trials. If a vaccinated person becomes infected but remains asymptomatic, is that a vaccine failure or a vaccine success? How long should such a person be followed before results can be meaningfully interpreted? None of these questions have easy answers.

Therapy

Recent progress has been made in the development of anti-retroviral therapy. The life cycle of retroviruses is intimately connected with the replication of mammalian cells, so that only a limited number of metabolic reactions can be singled out for targets of specific chemotherapy. Reverse transcriptase is an attractive target because inhibition of this enzyme should have no effect on the host cell. Several FDA-approved anti-HIV drugs inhibit this unique viral function. Zidovudine (azidothymidine, or AZT) was the first of several dideoxynucleotides to be tested in clinical trials. Other approved drugs in this category include didanosine (ddI), zalcitibine (ddC), stavudine (d4T), and lamivudine (3TC). These drugs inhibit reverse transcriptase after being phosphorylated intracellularly. Inhibition takes place by premature termination of growing strands off DNA into which the drugs has been incorporated. Mammalian DNA polymerases are more resistant to these drugs than viral reverse transcriptase.

A second class of reverse transcriptase inhibitors, the nonnucleoside inhibitors (OR NNRTI's) act by binding directly to the enzyme at a site away from the active site. This class includes the drugs nevirapine and delavirdine.

The third class of antiviral drugs approved for use against HIV comprises inhibitors of the viral protease, such as ritonavir, indinavir, saquinavir, and nelfinavir. These drugs do not affect early stages of virus replication, but rather prevent cleavage of viral proteins into their mature, active form.

The use of all antiviral agents is complicated and limited by the development of genetic resistance of the virus. Any of the antivirals individually is capable of rapidly and effectively halting most or all virus replication in the body. However, in virtually all cases of such monotherapy, virus replication rapidly rebounds and remains resistant to further treatment with the same or related compounds. Much more durable results, strong suppression of virus replication combined with marked clinical improvement, can be achieved in most HIV-infected individuals by using certain combinations of agents. The success and durability of such therapy is dependent on a number of factors, such as lack of prior exposure to any of the compounds and good compliance with rather complex and costly regimens, among others.

Additional improvement in the condition of many people with AIDS has been achieved by therapy directed at opportunistic infections, most notably aerosolized pentamidine for the treatment of *P. carinii* infection (see Chapter 68, "AIDS").

CONCLUSION

AIDS is a uniquely devastating disease: it kills all those that exhibit symptoms. It is a chronic illness, often manifested years after the virus is acquired and after the individual has had the opportunity to transmit it. In the United States, the number of new AIDS cases has stabilized in recent years, and the number of AIDS deaths is declining due to the use of potent antiretroviral drug combinations (Fig. 38.1).

By inactivating a central cellular component of the immune system, the helper T-lymphocyte, HIV produces severe impairment of both humoral and cellular immunity. The disease is lethal because the defense mechanism against opportunistic pathogens is eradicated. Diseases that were practically unseen before AIDS (e.g., encephalitis due to *T. gondii*), or under reasonable control (e.g., mycobacterial infections), have become common and highly dangerous among people with AIDS (see Chapter 68, "AIDS").

AIDS runs counter to the tenet that a successful parasite does not cause lethal injury to its host, suggesting that HIV may be a relative newcomer among human infectious agents. The disease appeared suddenly in the United States and its etiology was established with remarkable speed. We have acquired a great deal of knowledge about HIV and other retroviruses but are still unable to explain many of the features of the disease. We do not understand how helper lymphocytes are killed or impaired, or why the infection of a small proportion of them has such devastating effects. Lack of this knowledge hinders the design of drugs and vaccines. The virus is particularly elusive to immunotherapeutic approaches because of variability in surface antigens and other features of its structure and lifestyle.

Prolonging life among those that have acquired the virus presents a major medical problem. In the absence of an effective vaccine or treatment, prevention of HIV transmission among uninfected members of the population depends on public education.

SELF-ASSESSMENT QUESTIONS

1. Discuss the structure and mode of replication of retroviruses.
2. How does HIV differ from the other known retroviruses?
3. Imagine having to address a community group regarding AIDS. What would you say about its history, transmissibility in the community, and prospects for prevention and therapy?
4. What important aspects of HIV infection have yet to be elucidated? How could understanding their mechanism help prevent or treat AIDS?
5. What problems are associated with designing an effective AIDS vaccine?
6. If you were asked, what specific areas of research and education about AIDS would you target for the award of research funds?
7. What is your guess about the status of AIDS ten years from now? Twenty years from now?

SUGGESTED READINGS

Bloom BR. A perspective on AIDS vaccines. Science 272:1888-1890, 1996.

Centers for Disease Control. HIV/AIDS Surveillance Report. vol. 9, no. 1, 1997.

Graham BS, Wright PF. Drug Therapy: Candidate AIDS Vaccines. N Engl J Med 333:1311-1339, 1995.

Greene WC. The molecular biology of human immunodeficiency virus type I infection. N Engl J Med 324:308-317, 1991.

Haynes BF, Pantaleo G, Fauci AS. Toward an understanding of the correlates of protective immunity to HIV infection Science 271:324-328, 1996.

Henrard DR, Phillips LR, Muenz WA, et al. Natural history of HIV cell free viremia. JAMA 274:554-558, 1995.

Ho DD. Perspectives series: host/pathogen interactions. Dynamics of HIV-1 replication in vivo. J Clin Invest 99:2565-2567, 1997.

Ho DD. Time to hit HIV, early and hard. N Engl J Med 333:450-451, 1995.

Richman DD. Clinical significance of drug resistance in human immunodeficiency virus. Clin Infect Dis 21 (Suppl 2):S166-S169, 1995.

Richman DD. HIV therapeutics. Science 272:1886-1888, 1996.

Adenoviruses

GARY KETNER

Key Concepts

Adenoviruses:

- Most often cause mild infections of the respiratory and gastrointestinal systems; more severe infections caused by adenoviruses include epidemic keratoconjunctivitis and an acute, severe form of pneumonia.
- Are nonenveloped, large DNA viruses.
- Attach to host cells by means of fiber proteins that protrude from the capsid.
- Express their genes following penetration into the host cell in three phases: the pre-early phase, early phase, and late phase.
- Employ both virally encoded and host proteins in the replication process.
- Can evade the cell-mediated immune response by preventing the host cells from expressing MHC proteins, resisting TNF, and preventing protein synthesis in the host cell.
- Have oncogenic potential.

Adenoviruses are among the most common viruses found in healthy people and are often isolated from the tonsils, adenoids, and stool. They frequently cause acute respiratory diseases which range in severity from a sore throat to serious pneumonia. Adenoviruses are also responsible for conjunctivitis and diarrhea. These viruses have a large number of serotypes that are associated with different disease manifestations (Table 39.1). Healthy persons can harbor adenoviruses for long periods of time. Individuals with these persistent infections shed the viruses over periods of months or years.

CASE

Over a period of 3 months, 83 patients who had visited an ophthalmologist's office in Erie, Pennsylvania, reported redness of the eyes, eyelid swelling with discharge, photophobia, and change in vision. Only two of these patients

had fever or diarrhea. The patients ranged in age from 18 to 89 years and all had visited the office between 3 and 29 days before the onset of symptoms. Eventually, all of the patients recovered spontaneously. No further outbreaks were reported after preventive measures were instituted, including reducing the use of procedures that required instruments.

Epidemiologists from the Centers for Disease Control in Atlanta studied this outbreak of **epidemic keratoconjunctivitis (EK)** and documented the presence of adenovirus serotype 37 in 20 of the 22 patients from whom specimens were obtained. The procedures used were immunofluorescence microscopy of eye specimens and culture in cultured human kidney cells. The virus was also found to be present in the ophthalmologist's office. Virus was isolated from instruments used to measure visual acuity, work surfaces, eye drops, and the air-conditioning filter. Neither the ophthalmologist nor members of the staff tested positive for the virus or for specific antibodies.

A number of questions arise:

1. What was the source of the virus that caused this disease?
2. What caused the symptoms in the eyes of patients?
3. Why did the disease resolve spontaneously?
4. What measures helped prevent the further spread of the disease?
5. Why was the medical personnel in the ophthalmologist's office not affected?

Most adenoviruses cause **mild infections of the respiratory and digestive systems**. These infections resemble those caused by other agents and usually remain undiagnosed. Much of our knowledge of adenovirus infection stems from **outbreaks** such as the one described in the above case. Outbreaks leading to eye infections by this virus are frequently reported, indicating that transmission from a contaminated

environment (instruments, surfaces, etc.) readily occurs. Other outbreaks of eye infections (**"pink eye"**) can be caused by contaminated swimming pools. The most serious outbreaks of adenoviral infections are seen among military recruits in the form of serious acute pneumonia. Crowding and physical stress appear to contribute to the occurrence of such outbreaks.

For all their sporadic importance, adenoviruses are common human commensals and relatively mild human pathogens. Although their pathogenic mechanisms are not well known, a great deal is known about their structure and mode of replication. **Emphasis in this chapter is on basic aspects of the replicative strategy of adenoviruses, which serves as a well-studied example of replication among the large DNA viruses.**

Table 39.1. Association of Adenovirus Infections with Specific Phenotypes

Disease	Common adenovirus serotypes
Respiratory infections	1, 2, 5, 6
Pharyngoconjunctivitis	3, 7, 14
Acute respiratory disease (ARD) or recruits	4, 7
Gastrointestinal infection	40, 41
Associated with celiac disease	12
Conjunctivitis	2, 3, 5, 7, 8, 19, 21
Epidemic keratoconjunctivitis	8, 19, 37

THE ADENOVIRUSES

Adenovirus virions are **nonenveloped icosahedral particles** (Fig. 39.1). The shell of the virion is made up of two kinds of capsomeres, **hexons** and **pentons**. Hexons have six neighbors, and pentons, located at the vertices of the icosahedron, have five neighbors. The **pentons** have projecting knobbed **fibers** that give these virions a characteristic "sputnik" appearance. Inside the virion, the viral DNA is associated with several basic proteins in a structure called the **core**. The predominant component of the viral core is an arginine-rich basic protein that presumably aids in the spatial organization of the viral DNA and neutralizes the negative charges of the DNA. This protein serves to package the adenoviral DNA in a manner similar to that of histones in the packaging of cellular chromatin.

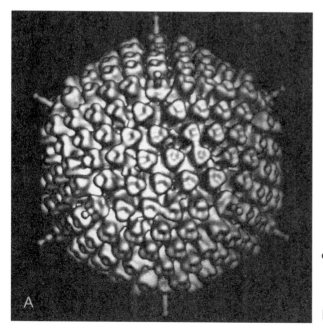
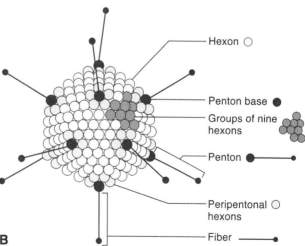

Figure 39.1. The adenovirus particle. A. Three-dimensional image of the adenovirus capsid reconstructed by computer from electron micrographs. **B.** Schematic view of the adenovirus particle with the names of individual capsid proteins indicated.

The genome of the human adenoviruses is a **linear double-stranded DNA** molecule and its sequence has been determined for several serotypes. The adenoviral genome has two unusual structural features. First, it possesses **inverted terminal repetitions**: approximately 100 base pairs are repeated in an inverted orientation at each end of the genome. Second, each strand of the genome is covalently attached at its 5'end to a protein molecule (the **terminal protein; TP**). Both the terminal redundancy and the terminal protein play key roles in the replication of adenovirus DNA.

Adenovirus genes with related functions tend to be clustered on the genome and are expressed from a common promoter. This arrangement, which is more characteristic of prokaryotes than eukaryotes, is also found among other DNA viruses, such as the papovaviruses. Clustering provides an economical mechanism for coordinating expression of genes whose functions are required at similar times during the infection. Thus, clustered genes have related functions. Examples of clustered adenoviral genes are those whose products (a) interact with the host immune system, (b) participate in post-transcriptional events in gene expression, (c) are essential for viral DNA replication, and (d) are components of the virions or involved in its assembly.

ENTRY, SPREAD, AND MULTIPLICATION

Attachment and Penetration

Adenoviruses attach to receptors on the host cell surface via fiber proteins. Most human and many other vertebrate cell types possess surface receptors that bind adenovirus at up to 10^5 copies per cell. The identity and normal functions of these receptors are not known. Following attachment, the virus–receptor complex migrates to clathrin-coated pits, which form endosomes that carry the virus particles into the cell. This internalization is dependent on the interaction of a second virion protein (penton base) with another cell-surface protein, a member of the integrin family of membrane proteins. The pH of the endosome falls, inducing the virions to shed their penton capsomeres and attached fibers. A conformational change in the virions causes the endosome to rupture and releases the partially disassembled virions into the cell cytoplasm. The nucleoprotein complex then enters the nucleus, leaving behind most of the rest of its capsid proteins. The core proteins are replaced with cellular histones to form a chromatin-like complex. The stage is now set for viral gene expression.

Adenovirus Gene Expression

Most DNA viruses display **temporal regulation** of gene expression. That is, viral gene expression takes place in two or more fairly distinct phases, and each phase is characterized by the synthesis of a specific set of viral proteins. Temporal regulation of gene expression contributes to the efficiency of the viral life cycle. Many of the common properties of viral regulatory systems are consistent with this notion. For example, in most cases, the proteins required for viral DNA replication are synthesized before the synthesis of proteins that make up the virus particle. This sequence assures that a large pool of viral DNA has accumulated before the packaging of viral DNA into capsids begins.

Temporal regulation of adenovirus gene expression is accomplished by a cascade of events: each phase of gene expression depends on the expression of specific genes in the previous phase. This mechanism is also employed by other large DNA viruses, including papovaviruses, herpesviruses, and many bacteriophages. In adenoviruses, gene expression occurs in three phases termed pre-early, early, and late (Fig. 39.2). Most regulatory events in ade-

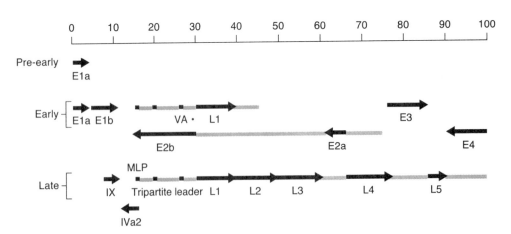

Figure 39.2. Temporal regulation of the adenovirus transcription. The portions of the adenoviral genome transcribed during the pre-early, early, and late phases of viral infection are indicated by arrows under a scale that show their position on the viral DNA molecule. The regions denoted by solid lines encode mRNAs that appear in the cytoplasm. The regions indicated by stippled lines are transcribed but are removed by splicing events from the RNA molecules that enter the cytoplasm. *MLP* indicates the major late promoter. The early regions are numbered E1a–E4; the late regions are L1–L5.

novirus gene expression occur at transcriptional or post-transcriptional steps in cytoplasmic mRNA production. These events take place in the following order:

1.   During the **pre-early phase,** only the portion of the genome called **E1a** is transcribed. Because viral proteins have not yet been synthesized, expression of E1a genes depends on host enzymes. The E1a transcript is spliced (as are essentially all adenoviral mRNAs) to yield two stable cytoplasmic E1a mRNAs. From these transcripts, two proteins are produced. One of these proteins is a **transcriptional activator,** which induces transcription from five viral promoters that are inactive during the pre-early phase. This protein stimulates transcription indirectly by increasing the activity of endogenous host cell transcription factors.

2.   The E1a-dependent activation of the five viral early promoters marks the beginning of the **early phase** of gene expression. During this phase, the newly activated viral promoters direct the transcription of four early regions (**E1b, E2, E3, E4**) and one (questionably named) late region (**L1**). Most of these regions contain several genes and encode several proteins. The RNA transcripts are then spliced to yield the individual mRNAs. Protein products of at least six early genes participate in events necessary for progression to the late phase of gene expression. Three encode the viral proteins necessary for viral DNA replication, and three are required for post-transcriptional events in mRNA synthesis during the late phase.

3.   Under the influence of three of the early proteins, viral DNA replication begins. Coincident with onset of viral DNA synthesis is the transition from the early phase to the **late phase.** The most dramatic events of this transition affect RNA synthesis, which is directed by the so-called **major late promoter.** Transcription from this promoter greatly increases until it makes up the majority of new RNA synthesized in the infected cell. This transcript is a large RNA molecule that when spliced produces about 20 distinct late viral mRNAs. Those mRNAs are then transported to the cytoplasm for translation. Early-phase gene products are required for both the splicing and transport steps in late mRNA production. Because of the efficiency with which late RNA is transcribed and processed and the large number of viral genomes present in the infected cell (due to DNA replication), late mRNAs and proteins are abundantly produced.

Viral DNA replication is a prerequisite for late gene expression. Why? We do not really know, although some evidence suggests that the physical act of replication is in some way necessary for an individual DNA molecule to serve as a template for late gene expression.

As the expression of the viral late genes increases during the early–late transition, the expression of cellular genes decreases. Adenoviral infection interferes with host gene expression in two ways. First, the accumulation of cellular mRNAs in the cytoplasm is prevented. Because the rate of synthesis of host RNAs is not reduced in virus-infected cells, it has been suggested that adenovirus specifically **inhibits the transport of host mRNAs** from the nucleus to the cytoplasm. Apparently, the early proteins are responsible for the inhibition. Second, a virally encoded late protein **appears to inhibit the utilization of existing host mRNAs** in the cytoplasm. The consequence of these two actions is that the **synthesis of host proteins essentially ceases.**

DNA Replication

DNA-containing animal viruses rely to different extents on host cell proteins for the replication of their genomes. The papovaviruses (Chapter 40, "Warts") make a single viral protein that redirects host replication enzymes to replicate the viral genome, whereas herpesviruses (Chapter 41) encode a large number of the enzymes involved in DNA replication. The adenoviruses fall between these extremes, employing both virally encoded and host proteins in replication.

Replication is initiated within the inverted repetitions at one or the other end of the adenoviral DNA molecule (see Fig. 39.3). The two ends of the DNA molecule have identical sequences and initiation of **DNA replication can take place at either end** with about equal frequency. After initiation, DNA synthesis proceeds along the template DNA. One parental strand is copied, while the other is displaced. The completion of the synthesis of the first daughter strand produces a duplex molecule consisting of one parental strand and one daughter strand, plus a displaced parental single strand. Because of the inverted terminal repetition, the displaced single strand assumes a "panhandle" configuration containing a short double-stranded region identical in sequence to the ends of the normal double-stranded genome. DNA synthesis is initiated on this panhandle, and the displaced single strand then serves as the template for the synthesis of the second daughter strand.

The synthesis of viral DNA differs from that of host DNA in three respects. First, a single DNA strand is copied at each viral replication fork, whereas in host cell replication, both strands are copied concurrently. Second, the synthesis of all new viral DNA is continuous; that is, it occurs by the uninterrupted elongation of the growing chain across the entire genome. In host cell DNA replication, one strand at each replication fork is produced continuously, but the other is synthesized discontinuously, as short pieces (Okazaki fragments) that must be joined to produce the finished strand. Finally, host chromosomes replicate by a well-regulated process that occurs once in a division cycle, while viral replication is uncoordinated and takes place continuously over a period of time. The latter strategy is presumably a re-

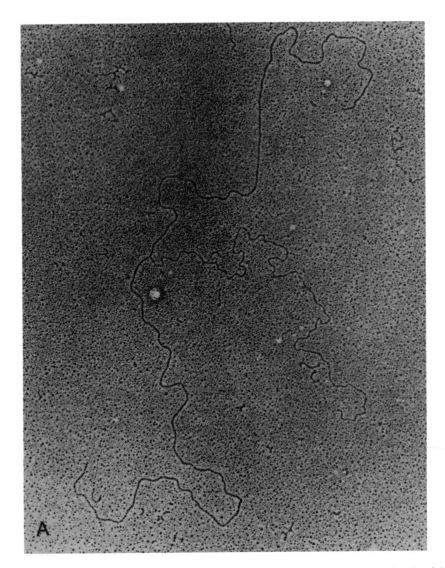

Figure 39.3. Adenovirus DNA replication. A. An electron micrograph of a DNA molecule of the type diagrammed in the second line of Fig. 39.3, panel B, i.e., a duplex with one single-stranded branch.

sponse to the need to produce as many viral DNA molecules as possible over the short course of a viral infectious cycle.

Adenovirus DNA replication can be carried out in vitro in a system composed of purified proteins, which has led to a fairly detailed biochemical understanding of the events in viral DNA replication. Six proteins are required for optimal viral DNA replication in vitro (and, presumably, in vivo). Three of these proteins are virally encoded—a **DNA polymerase**, a **DNA-binding protein (DBP)**, and the **preterminal protein (pTP)**, which is the precursor of the terminal protein found in virions. All three of these proteins are products of early region 2. The remaining three replication proteins are cellular products. Two are DNA-binding proteins that normally function in the transcription of cellular genes in uninfected cells; the third is a topoisomerase.

In the most likely sequence of events, initiation begins with **binding of the host factors** to three adjacent blocks of nucleotides in the terminal repeats. The host proteins probably unwind the end of the DNA molecule, exposing single-stranded DNA that serves as the template for the actual initiation event. This event is the formation of a phosphodiester linkage between deoxycytosine monophosphate (dCMP, the first residue at the 5′ end of the new DNA strand) and a serine residue in the pTP molecule. In this way, **pTP serves as the primer for adenoviral DNA replication** (Fig. 39.3). Protein priming of DNA replication is most unusual; in most systems, primers for DNA replication are short RNA molecules.

After formation of the initial **pTP–dCMP linkage**, elongation of the new daughter strand proceeds conventionally. Viral DNA polymerase sequentially adds nucleotides to the 3′-OH group of the pTP-bound growing

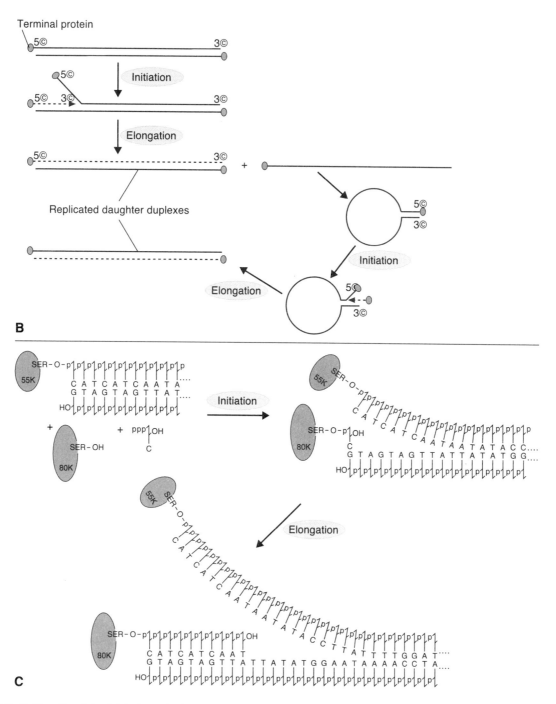

Figure 39.3. B. Details of the initiation of adenovirus DNA replication showing the priming of DNA synthesis by the preterminal protein (pTP is labeled 80K; TP is labeled 55K).

C. Schematic representation of the events in adenovirus replication.

chain. Host proteins do not seem to be necessary for elongation. As DNA is packaged, proteolytic processing cleaves the pTP molecule bound to each DNA strand to generate the form found in mature virions.

Virion Assembly

Particle assembly begins when sufficient amounts of capsid proteins have accumulated. The first step is the assembly of free polypeptide chains into hexon and penton capsomeres. Pentons are assembled spontaneously, but hexon assembly requires the participation of a protein that does not appear in the mature particle. Such proteins that assist in assembly but that do not appear in virions are common and are referred to as **scaffold proteins**. Hexons, as well as several minor virion components, are next assembled into an intermediate structure

DNA Virus Replication and Control of the Cell Cycle

The study of DNA virus-infected cell can teach us a great deal about the complicated workings of normal cells. Because DNA viruses either make use of host cell machinery (sometimes modified by viral proteins) or employ general strategies similar to those of their host cells, understanding the events that occur in a virus-infected cell often reveals much about the events that take place in uninfected cells. Adenoviruses have been particularly useful in this regard. For example, **mRNA splicing** was first detected in studies of the synthesis of adenoviral late mRNAs, and only later was it shown that this process also occurs in normal eukaryotic cells. Similarly, the first in vitro eukaryotic DNA replication system was constructed for adenovirus DNA. The adenovirus system and a system derived from papovavirus-infected cells that more closely simulates host cell replication, have been extremely useful in understanding the biochemistry of cellular DNA replication.

Different DNA viruses exploit the machinery of host cell DNA replication to different degrees. Very large DNA viruses (e.g., the poxviruses) replicate in the host cell cytoplasm independently of host cell DNA replication machinery. The other DNA viruses (e.g., adenoviruses, papillomaviruses, and herpesviruses) exploit the cellular machinery that replicates the host cell DNA. This exploitation is economical for the virus, but it also creates a timing problem, since these shared cellular factors are normally expressed only during the DNA synthetic (S) phase of the cell cycle. Indeed, **very small DNA viruses (i.e., parvoviruses) that have no replicative machinery of their own replicate only during the cellular**

S phase. For most other viruses, however, it is not advantageous to wait for the cell to begin its division cycle, since many of the cells targeted by these viruses are differentiated and do not divide (e.g., superficial epithelial cells).

To overcome this difficulty, adenoviruses and most other DNA maintain a continuous high level of replication and a large supply of the necessary host cell proteins by forcing the infected cells into the division cycle. As one might expect, the identification of the viral factors responsible for this effect and the cellular proteins with which they interact has yielded important insights into the mechanisms controlling the normal cell cycle. For example, an early adenoviral protein **E1b** (as well as proteins from papillomaviruses and herpesviruses) binds to a cellular protein, **p53**, which prevents the cell from advancing into S phase. Binding of the viral protein inactivates this function and permits the cell to express factors necessary for DNA replication. Similarly, other viral proteins bind to the cellular **protein RB**, releasing a transcription factor that enhances the expression of various other required proteins.

By disrupting the normal regulation of the cell cycle, these DNA viruses all pose some **oncogenic potential**. Indeed, the two cellular factors, p53 and pRB, are known as **tumor suppressors**, since mutations in their respective genes are associated with a wide range of human cancers. Both of these factors were originally cloned on the basis of their interactions with DNA virus proteins.

GARY KETNER

that is later filled with DNA. It is not clear how the DNA enters this empty shell, although it has been suggested that it may pass through one of the open vertices. Perhaps surprisingly, the viral core proteins are added to the particles after the DNA enters. Finally, the pentons and fibers become associated with the capsid, and a series of proteolytic events converts precursor proteins within the virion into their mature forms. After assembly, adenovirus particles remain associated with the dying cell and are slowly released as the cells autolyse or are destroyed by the immune system.

INTERACTIONS WITH HOST DEFENSE SYSTEMS

Adenoviruses carry several genes whose functions seem to be to stop host antiviral defenses. The main immunological defense against viral infection, cell-mediated immunity, acts by destroying infected cells. Cytotoxic T lymphocytes (CTLs) have receptors for specific complexes of viral antigens bound to a host protein

found on the surface of almost all cells, the **major histocompatibility complex type I (MHC I)** antigen. These receptors enable CTLs to recognize infected cells. Cells that do not possess MHC I molecules on their surface do not become targets for destruction by CTLs. Adenoviruses evade cell-mediated immune response via two separate mechanisms that interfere with MHC I expression. The first of these mechanisms is mediated by an early viral protein that **blocks the production of MHC I mRNA** in infected cells. The second mechanism is mediated by a glycoprotein that **prevents the transport of newly synthesized MHC I protein** molecules to the cell surface. In an animal model system (cotton rats), infections of the lung with viral mutants that do not express these viral proteins induce a striking pulmonary infiltration of neutrophils, suggesting that this protein in fact influences the course of disease in vivo.

Another way by which adenoviruses protect themselves from cellular immunity is through their resistance to **tumor necrosis factor (TNF)**. TNF is a host protein produced by monocytes exposed to viruses, and it lyses many types of virally infected cells. Once again, a viral protein is required for the induction of this resistance.

A third line of defense against viral infection is the antiviral state that is induced in cells by α and β interferons. Among other effects, the interferons prevent protein synthesis in virus-infected cells by initiating a chain of events that culminates in the inactivation of the cell's translation apparatus. Adenoviruses break the chain and prevent the inhibition of protein synthesis through the action of two small RNA molecules (**VA RNAs**) encoded by viral genes. These VA RNAs closely mimic the structure of double-stranded RNA (dsRNA). The infected-cell dsRNA activates host proteins (DAI) necessary for the inhibition of protein synthesis by interference. dsRNA is produced in the course of infection by most viruses, including adenoviruses. The VA RNAs fold into partially double-stranded structures and bind to DAI, preventing its activation by authentic dsRNA.

As mentioned previously, many DNA viruses have oncogenic potential. Adenovirus type 12 was the first DNA-containing virus shown to cause cancer in animals. This discovery sparked a massive search for evidence that adenoviruses (and other DNA animal viruses) were etiological agents of human cancer and an equally massive effort to determine the mechanism of tumorigenesis by DNA animal viruses. These studies revealed no convincing association between adenoviruses and cancer, but they have contributed considerably to knowledge about the molecular basis of tumorigenesis.

All adenovirus serotypes tested induce permanent morphological changes in cultured cells that resemble those that occur during natural carcinogenesis. This process is referred to as **transformation**. Transformation by adenoviruses requires the products of two viral genes. The role of one of these genes seems to be to "**immortalize**" cells, i.e., confer on them the ability to grow indefinitely in culture. The second gene confers the fully transformed phenotype on immortalized cells. The genome of all cells transformed by adenoviruses contains both of these genes. Researchers have demonstrated that the genes are able to induce transformation if introduced into cells as recombinant DNA molecules. The adenovirus-transforming gene products act by interaction with cellular antioncogene products (see Chapter 40, "Warts"). One of the adenoviral-transforming proteins is the positive transcriptional regulator produced by E1a. Transcriptional stimulation by this protein depends in part on the same interactions involved in transformation. Tumorigenesis by adenoviruses, therefore, seems to be an incidental consequence of the action of mechanisms that regulate viral gene expression.

DAMAGE

Adenovirus infections are widespread in human populations, accounting for between 5% and 10% of all vi-

ral infections. Most of these infections occur in childhood; 75% occur before 14 years of age, and over half occur before 5 years of age. Most adenoviral infections affect either the **respiratory tract** or the **gastrointestinal tract**, in about equal numbers. Although most patients with adenoviral respiratory diseases recover, some mortality has been associated with pneumonia.

The usual symptoms of adenoviral respiratory infections resemble those of the **common cold**, including nasal congestion, inflammation of the upper respiratory tract, and cough. Systemic symptoms such as chills, headache, muscle aches, and fever are common, and **conjunctivitis** sometimes accompanies the other symptoms (**pharyngoconjunctival fever**). In severe cases, **pneumonia** can develop. Different serotypes are associated with respiratory disease and pharyngoconjunctival fever. Serotypes 1, 2, 5, and 6 are endemic in most populations, and 80% of all young adults have neutralizing antibodies to these types. Other serotypes (4 and 7) are associated with outbreaks of a fairly severe febrile respiratory infection (**acute respiratory disease; ARD**) that affects primarily military recruits during basic training. As many as 80% of some groups of recruits are affected, with one-fourth to one-half of them requiring hospitalization. Crowded conditions and fatigue presumably favor the spread of the disease and increase its severity. College freshmen, who are of similar age, do not, however, appear to suffer from ARD. A live virus vaccine is given as an enteric-coated capsule to newly inducted military personnel.

Adenoviruses are also an important cause of acute gastrointestinal disease in children and may be responsible for up to 15% of juvenile intestinal infections. Many serotypes of adenoviruses are present, not only in the stool of patients, but in normal stools as well, in contrast to a number of serotypes that are associated solely with disease. Adenovirus type 12 (Ad12) has been implicated in the development of celiac disease. The development of these diseases from Ad12 appears to depend upon protein sequence homology between an Ad12 early protein and A-gliadin, a component of the cereal grains that activate the disease. It has been suggested that exposure to Ad12 induces an antibody response to A-gliadin, which predisposes to celiac disease.

Less common than respiratory and gastrointestinal disease are adenovirus-induced conjunctivitis without other symptoms. Mild "**swimming pool conjunctivitis**" is probably most often due to adenoviral infection, as is the more serious, highly contagious **epidemic keratoconjunctivitis (EKC)**.

Latent adenovirus infections are very common; adenoviruses can be recovered from as many as 80% of the tonsils or adenoids removed from children and young adults. The mechanism of persistence in these cases is not known. It has been reported that viral DNA can persist in tonsillar tissue free of infectious virus, but it is also possible that persistence may be due to a low-level active infection imperfectly controlled by the immune system.

ADENOVIRUSES AS VECTORS FOR GENE DELIVERY

Virus particles have evolved the ability to efficiently introduce foreign nucleic acid (the viral genome) into living cells. Recently, interest has developed in exploiting this property of viruses to introduce nonviral genes into animals or animal cells. Because adenoviruses have been studied extensively and much is known about their biology and genetics, adenoviruses are considered to be particularly promising vectors for foreign gene delivery.

The use of recombinant adenoviruses to immunize against pathogens other than adenovirus itself is an attractive idea. Several candidate **adenovirus-based vaccine strains** have been constructed. In these strains, a segment of DNA encoding an antigen derived from a pathogen of interest, along with regulatory signals to direct expression of the antigen, replaces a dispensable segment of the adenoviral genome. Such genetically engineered adenoviruses direct the production of the foreign antigen in infected cells, and several (such as a strain that produces the rabies virus surface glycoprotein) have been shown to protect against the target pathogen in animal model systems.

A second potential application for adenovirus is as a vector for **gene therapy**; that is, for the introduction of an exogenous gene into an individual for therapeutic purposes. Gene therapy is usually envisioned as a therapeutic approach to inherited disease. For example, cystic fibrosis (CF) results from the inheritance of nonfunctional alleles of a particular gene (the CFTR gene) from both of an individual's parents. The physiological defect in patients with CF is known, and introduction of a cloned normal CF gene into CF patient cells in tissue culture corrects the defect. Therefore, delivery of the normal gene to a large number of a patient's lung cells (most pathology occurs in the lung) might restore enough CFTR function to relieve the symptoms of the disease. Accordingly, genetically engineered adenoviruses carrying the CFTR gene in place of E1a (such viruses cannot conduct a lytic growth cycle in normal human cells) have been constructed and are being considered for introduction into the lungs of CF patients. Clinical trials to assess safety are now underway, and therapeutic trials may proceed if the results of safety studies are satisfactory.

The development of successful adenovirus-based vaccines and adenovirus-based gene therapy still awaits solutions for a daunting array of technical, medical, and even social problems. Nevertheless, the promise of these technologies is great, and they are well worth careful study.

In fact, a majority of healthy adults examined have very small numbers of peripheral lymphocytes apparently undergoing a typical adenoviral lytic cycle. Early gene products that interact with the host's immune mechanisms may play a role in persistence.

Adenoviruses can be recovered from immunocompromised individuals and have been implicated in mortality in several cases. Recently, numerous isolations from patients with immunodeficiency resulting from HIV infection have been reported, and infection has been associated in some cases with mortality.

CONCLUSION

Adenoviruses are commonly found among healthy persons but also cause a series of infections that range in severity. The eye, the upper and lower respiratory tracts, and the gastrointestinal tract are often involved. In addition, there is evidence that they are linked to oncogenesis in humans, although definitive proof is still lacking.

Adenoviruses are double-stranded DNA viruses whose life cycle has served as a model for the study of mammalian DNA replication. The expression of viral genes follows a defined time table, some genes being expressed early, others late.

Modified adenoviruses strains that are often found in humans without causing overt disease may be suitable candidates for recombinant vaccines to be used in immunizing against a variety of antigens.

SELF-ASSESSMENT QUESTIONS

1. Draw a sketch of the structure of an adenovirus virion and point out the function of the major components.
2. What are the stages in the expression of adenovirus genes? Why is this series of steps necessary?
3. In what ways does adenovirus DNA replication differ from that of host DNA?
4. How do adenoviruses inhibit protein synthesis of infected cells?
5. How do adenoviruses interfere with the action of interferon?
6. Describe briefly the main diseases caused by adenoviruses. Which tend to occur in outbreaks?

SUGGESTED READINGS

Bridge E, Pettersson U. Nuclear organization of adenovirus RNA biogenesis. Exp Cell Res 1996;229:233–239.

Ginsberg HS. The ups and downs of adenovirus vectors. Bull N Y Acad Med 1996;73:53–58.

Jones N. Transcriptional modulation by the adenovirus E1A gene. Curr Top Microbiol Immunol 1995;199:59–80.

Van der Vliet PC. Adenovirus DNA replication. Curr Top Microbiol Immunol 1995;199:1–30.

Wold WS, Hermiston TW, Tollefson AE. Adenovirus proteins that subvert host defenses. Trends Microbiol 1994;2:437–443.

Warts

ELLIOTT J. ANDROPHY

Key Concepts

Human papillomaviruses (HPV):
- Cause warts (papillomas) at various sites, including the hands, feet, and genital regions.
- Are of several types, some of which are associated with malignancy.
- Can be spread by sexual transmission, direct skin-to-skin contact, or through contact with contaminated inanimate objects.
- Replicate within differentiated keratinocytes of the basal skin layer or in other basal epithelial cells.
- Infections are diagnosed usually through clinical signs and symptoms: treatment includes surgical, chemical, or laser removal.

arts usually appear as **slow-growing bumps** of the skin and mucous membranes. They result from infection by human papillomaviruses (HPVs), a large group of related nonenveloped DNA viruses. Clinical manifestations of warts can range from inapparent to large bulky growths. The majority of patients with warts seek medical help because of physical discomfort or concern about the appearance of a new skin lesion. While most papillomavirus-induced warts are biologically benign, some warts become malignant. It is now recognized that **cervical cancer,** one of the most common neoplasms of women, develops from lesions caused by certain types of these viruses.

■ CASE

As a healthy 26-year-old man, M. was almost in a panic. Four months ago he noticed a small bump on the shaft of his penis, but he decided to ignore it with the hope that it would go away on its own. Now however, two new growths had appeared, and he and his wife worried that he had genital warts. The dermatologist he saw immediately confirmed this diagnosis without performing any tests and

applied liquid nitrogen to destroy the warts. He told Mr. M. that genital warts are transmissible and that his wife needed to be examined too. Having been married for 2 years, Mr. M. was anxious about spreading a virus that may cause cervical cancer. The doctor discussed HPV infection and reassured him that with routine gynecological care his wife would be fine.

Several questions arise:
1. What caused M.'s warts?
2. How and when did M. acquire his warts?
3. If Mrs. M. is also infected, what noncancerous manifestations might she have?
4. If she also has warts, how can they eventually result in cancer?
5. How can M. and his wife get rid of their warts?

In this chapter we discuss the biology of human papillomaviruses and address the clinical issues raised by M.'s case. Much of our present understanding of these viruses comes from the application of recombinant DNA technology to medical microbiology and epidemiology. Because papillomaviruses are small infectious agents with the ability to cause human cancers, they provide important insights into the underlying processes that control cell growth.

Table 40.1. Biological Features of Various Papovaviruses

	Papillomaviruses	Polyomaviruses
Human viruses	Human papillomavirus types 1-~60	Human BK virus, human JC virus, human AS virus
Animal viruses	Shope rabbit papillomavirus, bovine papillomavirus, many others	Mouse polyomavirus, simian vacuolating virus 40, and others
Target tissues	Skin, mucous membranes	Brain, kidneys, other organs
Strands transcribed	One	Both
Transforming ability	Yes	Yes
Genome in transformed cells	Usually not integrated	Usually integrated

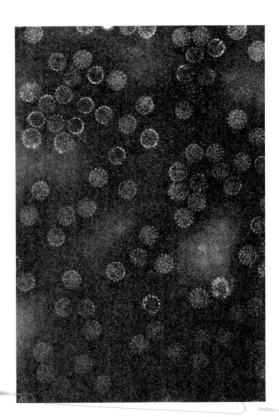

Figure 40.1. Electron micrograph of purified wart viruses.

PAPILLOMAVIRUSES

Papillomaviruses belong to a family known as the Papovaviruses. *Papova* is an acronym for the major members of the group: *papi*llomaviruses, *poly*oma viruses, and *va*cuolating viruses (Table 40.1). All papovaviruses have double-stranded circular DNA genomes which range from about 5000 nucleotide base pairs in SV40 (a well-studied monkey virus) and polyoma to 8000 in papillomaviruses. Papovaviruses also have nonenveloped viral particles. Because papovaviruses are small, about 1/20 the size of herpes viruses, their genetic information is limited and they can encode only a few proteins. For instance, they do not encode a DNA polymerase to replicate their genome and thus must rely on host cell DNA replication proteins to reproduce. Antiviral nucleoside analogs directed against viral polymerase and used in the treatment of herpesvirus infections (or even HIV) are not effective against warts.

Papillomaviruses are actually a large group of related viruses that include pathogens of humans, monkeys, cattle, birds, fish, and most other species. Papillomaviruses are specific; only human HPVs, for instance, can cause human warts. HPVs are classified into types on the basis of **their DNA sequences.** If the nucleotide sequence of a short, highly conserved region found in all papillomaviruses varies by more that 10% from all other known HPV sequences, the isolate is defined as a new type, or more accurately, new genotype. According to this scheme, there are presently over 90 known human papillomavirus types which are divided into several subtypes (Table 40.2).

Table 40.2. Lesions Associated with Human Papillomavirus (HPV) Types

Plantar warts	HPV-1, 4
Common warts	HPV-2
Flat juvenile warts	HPV-3
Anogenital warts[a]	HPV-6
Common warts in meat handlers	HPV-7
Flat warts	HPV-10
Laryngeal and anogenital warts	HPV-11
Macular lesions in EV[b]	HPV-5, 8, 9, 12, 14, 15, 17, 19 to 29
Focal epithelial hyperplasia	HPV-13
Bowenoid papulosis; cervical carcinoma	HPV-16
Cervical carcinoma	HPV-18
Cervical dysplasia	HPV-31
Laryngeal carcinoma	HPV-30
Not described	HPV-32 to 63

[a] Condyloma acuminata.
[b] EV, epidermodysplasia verruciformis, associated with malignant degeneration.

HPV types 1–4 were the first to be discovered because they are found in the majority of **cutaneous warts**. The HPVs in **genital warts** are usually types 6, 11, 16, 18, 31, 33, and 35. These HPV types cause warts of the penis, vulva, and anus, and are able to infect the mucosal epithelium of the vagina, cervix, and oropharynx. The genital-associated HPV types were identified later because the amount of viral DNA present in genital lesions is very low, and thus their identification awaited the advent of recombinant DNA technology. The low content of viral DNA and viral particles in genital warts is sufficient to propagate the infection, since transmission of the virus during sexual contact occurs with high efficiency. In general, each HPV type is usually associated with infection of a specific anatomic region or epithelial environment. For instance, HPV-1 is most frequently found in plantar warts. HPV-2 causes common cutaneous warts but has been isolated from genital warts. HPV-6 and 16, which typically cause genital lesions, have also been infrequently isolated from cutaneous warts.

ENCOUNTER AND ENTRY

HPV particles are present on the surface of warts and the associated keratotic scale. These particles can be spread by direct skin-to-skin contact with other people or from one's own warts, for example, from the side of one finger to the adjacent finger. However, normal skin is highly resistant to entry. These viruses are not highly contagious and epidemics are rare, even within a family. Breaks in the skin barrier promote spread, and scratching a wart can spread the virus to uninvolved areas. Infection also takes place more readily when the virus comes in contact with mucous membranes or with macerated skin. As is discussed later, papillomaviruses are quite stable and remain infectious after exfoliation. Thus it is likely that papillomaviruses present on inanimate objects can be a source of infection. Warts of the soles of the feet probably result from implantation of virus present on microabrasions of the feet caused by contact with rough surfaces, e.g., the concrete surfaces of swimming pools.

The site of viral entry determines the location of the lesions, and it may also be influenced by the HPV type involved. The most frequent sites of warts are commonly traumatized skin surfaces such as the fingers, hands, soles, knees, and elbows. Numerous warts in the hands and fingers of butchers are caused by the inoculation of virus into cuts they sustain at these sites. Microabrasions that occur with vaginal, anal, or oral sex and the moist, mucosal epithelia promote efficient viral spread to the penis, anus, vulva, vagina, cervix, and less frequently, the oropharynx and larynx. Rarely, transmission from mother to child occurs during birth with aspiration of HPV. Infection by this route can cause the devastating disease **respiratory papillomatosis** in the infant. There is no evidence of hematogenous spread of papillomavirus.

It is estimated that 20–30 million people are infected with HPV in the U.S., with about 3 million new individuals infected each year. Over the past three decades, the incidence of genital warts has risen faster than that of genital herpes. Genital warts are now the single most common sexually transmitted infection that leads people to seek medical attention, and are second only to chlamydial infections as the most common sexually transmitted disease. The more rare types of HPVs—those that are usually found in immunocompromised patients—may be maintained as subclinical infections in the population or arise in a susceptible individual from an environmental reservoir.

Many people become infected with wart viruses during their lifetime without exhibiting symptoms. HPVs may lie dormant in the deeper epithelial layers of the skin. Alterations in the epithelium may be so slight that the infection is not recognized. Compelling evidence of frequent asymptomatic infection derives from polymerase chain reaction (PCR) studies of cervical–vaginal cells obtained from healthy college women presenting for routine gynecological care. Prospective studies of college women found 40–50% were HPV DNA positive, although the majority of the cervical cells showed normal histology. Many of these HPV-DNA women subsequently became negative in repeat examination conducted several months later. These findings have led to the belief that many cervical HPV infections are transient. Why some warts persist in the skin or cervix is unknown. Individuals with defective cell-mediated immunity can have numerous warts which are highly resistant to treatment. Women with acquired immune deficiency syndrome (AIDS) are at high risk for development of cervical cancer and HPV-associated anal carcinomas.

MULTIPLICATION AND SPREAD

Papillomaviruses probably establish infection in the **basal cell layer** of the epithelium. This layer represents the replicative area of the skin, where cells continuously divide to replenish the desquamating surface and to heal wounds. The viral genome is present as a single, covalently closed, circular molecule of DNA and constitutes an extrachromosomal **episome** that does not integrate into the cell's genome. Papillomaviruses are not **lytic**: they do not lyse the initial target cell, and basal cells are not packed with virus (which would lead to their death). Because they are not lytic, no blisters or vesicles are observed, as occurs with herpesvirus infection. Instead, the viral episome is duplicated in synchrony with cellular chromosomes; one viral genome is thought to segregate into each daughter cell. As these cells mature and migrate toward the skin surface, the viral episome is transported to upper levels of the epithelium. There, viral genes are expressed and viral DNA replication begins. The late proteins that form the viral capsid (L1 and L2) are synthesized only in the differentiated layers of epithelium.

Like all viruses, HPVs have a genetic content that is minuscule compared to the human genome. To synthesize their macromolecules, viruses must make partial use of the host cell machinery. To orchestrate these activities, viral proteins directly or indirectly coordinate the viral life cycle in concert with the cells they infect. A papillomavirus protein called **E1** maintains the viral DNA as a small closed circle in the infected cell. In this form, the viral genome replicates to high numbers at the proper time, independent of cellular DNA. E1 protein is a **helicase** that unwinds double-stranded DNA to permit replication, and it may also attract cellular DNA replication proteins. A second viral protein, **E2**, binds to a specific sequence of the viral DNA. E2 also binds to E1 protein, which itself is a low-affinity DNA binding factor. The E2 protein is a **transcription factor** that regulates expression of the viral genes by directing the local assembly of cellular transcription factors, including RNA polymerase. The E1/E2 complex can induce the replication of the circular DNA template.

Viral reproduction occurs in concert with the normal differentiation program of **keratinocytes**. These cells are destined to form a nonreplicating, physical barrier that preserves the integrity of the subcutaneous organs and protects the body from exogenous insults. As an epithelium differentiates, upper-level epithelial cells lose their nucleus and are filled with stable, insoluble, structural proteins. These flattened cells are shed as scales into the environment, with fresh cells continually replacing them from below. The papillomaviruses exploit this process for their replication and transmission. After passage to the outer skin layers, the virus somehow senses the differentiated status of the keratinocyte and directs transcription of the late mRNAs that encode its major viral capsid proteins called L1 and L2. These proteins are transported into the nucleus of the differentiated keratinocytes where they assemble with newly replicated DNA to form progeny virions. The nuclear remnant is packed with viral particles and sheds at the surface of the skin.

Viruses such as herpes simplex or HIV-1 incorporate part of the cell membrane into their viral particle as they bud out from a cell. Because of their lipid bilayer, these virions are readily inactivated by heat, drying, or detergents. In contrast, papillomaviruses do not bud from a cell membrane, and their protein capsids are thus resistant to these conditions. For example, nonoxynal-9, a detergent commonly found in condoms as a spermicide, greatly reduces the infectivity of HIV-1. It has no effect, however, on papillomaviruses. Their lack of a lipid envelope and their stable protein capsid allows papillomaviruses to remain infectious after long periods in the environment. These features explain how wart viruses shed from an infected individual onto inanimate objects such as floors may remain infectious and be transmitted to new hosts.

DAMAGE

The hallmark of papillomavirus infection is that the alterations it induces in the host epithelium develop slowly and are often clinically inapparent. As warts enlarge, dermal capillaries proliferate. When these capillaries become thrombosed, usually because of trauma, they create black dots or "seeds" which can be useful in diagnosing warts. Warts often show plates of thin scale and keratotic debris which may be due to altered differentiation induced by viral proteins. Another diagnostic clue to the identification of HPV infection is the absence of normal skin lines in a wart. These changes may not be visible for many months after infection has begun. There is no routine clinical method for determining whether HPV is present in a lesion. Determining the presence of HPV is possible in a research setting, where the tissue is reacted with HPV-specific nucleic acid probes or by polymerase chain reaction (PCR).

Warts look different at different sites. Common warts of the hands and other cutaneous surfaces are elevated, firm, fleshy lesions with a sharp border (Fig. 40.2). On the face, knees, or arms, warts tend to be flat and are more likely to be clustered (Fig.40.3). On the soles of the feet, they tend to be more deeply embedded and more keratotic than those on the hands. Anogenital warts (**condyloma acuminata**) may be either flat or elevated. One or several cauliflower-like lesions may surround the anus, the labia, or the shaft of the penis (Fig. 40.4). Warts of the uterine cervix are usually flat and tend to be missed during visual speculum examinations.

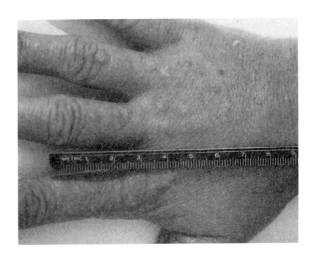

Figure 40.2. Common warts.

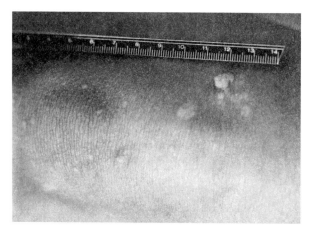

Figure 40.3. Multiple flat warts on knee.

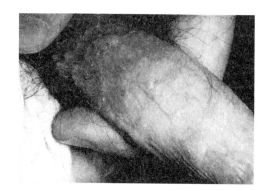

Figure 40.4. Penile warts.

PARADIGM ■ ■ ■

Viral Oncogenesis

The recognized human oncogenic viruses include papillomaviruses, Epstein-Barr virus (associated with Burkitt's lymphoma and nasopharyngeal carcinoma), and hepatitis B virus (associated with primary hepatocellular carcinoma). In the laboratory, some oncogenic viruses can transform cultured cells. Transformed cells can be recognized by their altered morphology, loss of contact-inhibited growth, and decreased nutritional requirements. In many cases, transformed cells are malignant, i.e., they cause tumors when injected into susceptible animals. The oncogenes derived from some oncogenic viruses can induce cell immortalization, i.e., the cells do not undergo the senescence and death characteristic of normal diploid cells in culture. Establishment of the immortal phenotype may be an early step in progression to cancer. Most human cell lines in continuous culture are derived from cancers, whereas normal human cells placed in culture do not become immortal.

Why and how do viruses transform cells? Papillomavirus DNA replication is paradoxical because it occurs in the nondividing upper cell layers. Because papillomaviruses do not encode DNA replication enzymes, they must both prevent the exit of epithelial cells from the cell cycle and activate the cellular pathways that replicate DNA. Many different mechanisms of transformation are used by different viruses, but two recurring themes are inhibition of normal growth regulatory processes and stimulation of cell division.

The process of tumor induction by HPVs is complex because it depends on interactions between virus gene products and selected host cell proteins. Among the eight or nine proteins encoded by high-risk HPVs, only two, **E6 and E7**, are always expressed in cervical cancer cells. Using in vitro cell culture assays, these genes have been shown to immortalize human keratinocytes and to increase their growth rate. E6 and E7 also induce malignant transformation in established mouse cell lines. These findings implicate that these proteins target fundamental growth regulatory mechanisms.

The molecular details of how high-risk E6 and E7 cause these changes are incomplete but are becoming clearer. E7 has amino acid similarities to other viral oncogenes, namely **SV40 Large T** and **adenovirus E1a**. This class of proteins can form complexes with a normal cellular protein called **p105-RB**. The name reflects its size (105 kD) and its association with the human cancer retinoblastoma. The development of retinoblastoma is associated with the absence of p105-RB. Thus, this protein is considered to be a natural suppressor of cell proliferation. By complexing with p105-RB, viral oncoproteins may be able to prevent the cell from exerting the normal check on its inherent potential to proliferate. Binding to p105-RB also releases a **transcription factor** called E2F, which in turn has been shown to activate a series of genes expression necessary for DNA synthesis.

The high-risk E6 proteins inactivate another cellular tumor suppressor protein, p53, by taking advantage of the cell's normal mechanism to **degrade** unwanted proteins. High-risk E6 binds to a cellular factor called E6-AP, which is a component of the **ubiquitination proteolysis pathway**. Ubiquitin is a short peptide which is covalently linked to other proteins to mark them for proteolytic degradation. The E6/E6-AP complex associates with p53 and induces its ubiquitination and subsequent proteolysis. As a result, levels of p53 are very low, and its effects as a tumor suppressor are inactivated. Interestingly, the E6 proteins from HPV types with low cancer risk do not bind p53.

Because papillomaviruses require a differentiated state to complete their replication, virus particles are not found in HPV-induced cancers. In fact, the rapid induction of malignancy would be an evolutionary dead end for papillomaviruses, and cancer should be considered a side effect of some HPVs on cell growth.

ELLIOTT J. ANDROPHY

Cervical papillomas are of special concern because of the association with progression to cervical cancer. More than 90% of all cervical carcinomas contain a subset of HPV genotypes, (e.g., types 16, 18, 31, 35), often called the **high-risk types**. Other HPVs found in genital and cervical warts (e.g., types 6 and 11) are rarely found in cancers and are therefore called **low-risk types**.

Warts of the **oropharynx** occur in two age groups: infants and sexually active adults. In some cases, these warts lead to progressive impairment of laryngeal function and can involve any region of the oropharynx and compromise the airway. Hoarseness is the usual presenting symptom. Respiratory distress and secondary bacterial pneumonias occur in children and signify the presence of obstructing lesions in the bronchial tree. The virus types associated with **respiratory papillomatosis** are the same as those that cause anogenital warts, an observation that, as indicated above, suggests perinatal transmission. Oral-genital transmission is responsible for this clinical syndrome in adults.

How does the host respond to infection by these viruses? Both humoral and cellular immunity probably participate, but their respective roles have not been elucidated. The infection is primarily controlled by cell-mediated immunity. People who are deficient in cellular immunity (transplant recipients, patients with AIDS or lymphoma) are more likely to have multiple chronic warts.

DIAGNOSIS

Papillomaviruses cannot be routinely cultivated in vitro, so a skin specimen cannot be tested for virus by inoculating cultured cells. Viral DNA can be specifically amplified using PCR to determine whether HPV is present. While this test is exquisitely sensitive, it is also fraught with the problems of sample contamination. Thus, it is currently limited to research laboratories. Because the presence of a specific HPV type has implications for the level of risk of progression to cervical cancer, it may be important to confirm the presence and specific type of HPV in these specimens. Technologies such as in situ hybridization, which use highly specific probes to test for the presence of specific HPVs in cervical cell smears, are available but are not routinely used at present. The advent of HPV serology using recombinant L1/L2 complexes may be useful in determining exposure to and persistence of cancer-associated HPV genotypes.

TREATMENT

About 50% of cutaneous warts regress spontaneously within 2 years, although new warts may also appear during this time. It is not possible to predict which warts will regress and whether new warts will develop. Anogenital warts may be obstructive and raise the concern of sexual transmission (as in M.'s case). In the uncommon disease respiratory papillomatosis, significant and life-threatening impairment of laryngeal function may be present. Unfortunately, no specific treatments exist for warts. Nearly all modes of treatment are ablative, e.g., **surgical excision**; destruction with **laser** beams; **liquid nitrogen**; or application of **caustic, keratolytic, or cytotoxic chemicals**. These and other approaches have been used with variable long-term success. A promising new antiwart drug called **imiquimod** is currently awaiting release in the U.S. In a case like M.'s, the treatment may have to be repeated several times. Not only does destruction of the host cell impair wart virus replication, but physical destruction of virally infected cells may expose the viruses to the immune system.

It is not known whether successful treatment of M.'s penile warts actually results in viral cure, i.e., whether HPV DNA is completely gone. However, it is likely that the risk of spread is reduced, since most patients who have complete remission do not develop new warts. An important factor that theoretically limits some forms of therapy is that the viruses often persist in apparently normal tissue adjacent to the warts. Ablation of the lesion may remove one focus of infection but may leave a residual inoculum nearby that may later result in local recurrence.

PREVENTION

The intact skin is an effective barrier to wart virus transmission. Complete avoidance is not practical because papillomavirus can be transmitted by inanimate objects. Latex condoms may act as a physical barrier and reduce the risk of transmission of HPV. In the case study patient M., his wife has likely been infected and therefore she should have regular examination of the external genitalia, vagina, and cervix, including Papanicolaou (Pap) testing. "Painting" the cervix or other suspected mucosal lesions with 3–5% acetic acid whitens them, making the papillomas easier to visualize with magnification (colposcopy). Biopsies of suspicious lesions can then be done to detect precancerous changes in time to permit effective treatment. As discussed previously, HPV are slow viruses, often clinically inapparent, and M. and his wife should be told that when infection occurred cannot be determined.

Laryngeal warts in the neonate may be prevented if an infected woman is aggressively treated prior to pregnancy. Some have suggested cesarean sections for pregnant women with genital warts; however, the risks of surgery are probably greater than the likelihood of developing respiratory papillomatosis.

CONCLUSION

Warts are caused by a large group of related DNA viruses, the papillomaviruses. Papillomavirus cause a wide variety of clinical manifestations ranging from common cutaneous warts to more serious, proliferative lesions. Fortunately, the benign manifestations are by far the most common. Wart viruses have been associated with a variety of epithelial cancers, especially of the cervix.

SELF-ASSESSMENT QUESTIONS

1. Describe the basic properties of wart viruses.
2. Contrast the replication cycle of papillomaviruses in warts with that in virus-associated cancers.
3. Why are warts more than a bothersome clinical problem?

4. Discuss the problems in the treatment of warts.
5. Why are warts difficult to prevent?

SUGGESTED READINGS

Lacey CJ, Fairley I. Medical therapy of genital human papillomavirus-related disease. Int J STD AIDS 1995;6:399–407.

Mansur CP, Androphy EJ. Cellular transformation by papillomavirus oncoproteins. Biochim Biophys Acta Rev Cancer 1993;1155:323–345.

Schiffman MH, Brinton LA. The epidemiology of cervical carcinogenesis. Cancer 1995;76:1888–1901.

Turek LP. The structure, function, and regulation of papillomaviral genes in infection and cervical cancer. Adv Virus Res 1994;44:305–356.

Zur Hausen H. Papillomavirus infections—a major cause of human cancers. Biochim Biophys Acta Rev Cancer 1996;1288:F55–78.

Herpes Simplex Virus and Its Relatives

STEPHEN E. STRAUS

Key Concepts

Herpesviruses:

- Include herpes simplex virus (HSV) types 1 and 2 (genital and oral herpes); cytomegalovirus (infection or immunocompromised individuals); Epstein-Barr virus (mononucleosis); varicella-zoster virus (chicken pox and shingles); human herpesvirus type 6 (roseola in infants); human herpesvirus type 7 and Kaposi's sarcoma virus (Kaposi sarcoma).
- Are characterized by a latent infection that follows the primary infection. Latency leads to recurrent outbreaks of symptoms that persist throughout the infected individual's life.
- Are ubiquitous in humans; for example, almost all individuals have been infected with HSV type 1. Most infections, however, are asymptomatic.
- Are diagnosed in humans through viral isolation in cell culture.
- Can be treated with antiviral therapy such as acyclovir. However, antiviral therapy cannot prevent recurrences. Currently, a varicella vaccine is available to prevent chicken pox.

The term *herpesvirus* refers to several human and animal viruses, the most widely known of which are the **herpes simplex viruses**. These viruses are the causative agents of fever blisters and a sexually transmitted genital infection. Other herpesviruses cause infectious mononucleosis, cytomegalovirus infection, and chickenpox. Because herpes viruses persist for life in cells of the host, they produce a latent infection that can be later reactivated.

CASE

Mr. H., a 26-year-old graduate student, returned home from his first real vacation in years. While on vacation, Mr. H. had engaged in both vaginal and oral sex with Ms. C., who was staying at the same resort. Several days after his last sexual contact with Ms. C. he notices painful, itchy sores on the shaft of his penis and a sore throat. During a difficult telephone call, Ms. C. admits to past episodes of genital herpes. Could he have herpes, he wonders? Mr. H. has heard about herpes infections and knows that there are several types and that some recur.

There are some things you need to know to help Mr. H. with his many questions:

- Many microorganisms can cause genital lesions.
- Genital lesions can be caused by two types of herpes simplex viruses.
- Herpesviruses that cause genital lesions are both fun-

damentally similar to and yet different from other herpesviruses.

- Herpes infections are unique in their ability to recur many times.
- Treatment is still limited and it is not yet known how to prevent the infections.

Despite recent public awareness, herpesviruses are not new causes of human disease. Oral infections similar to those now recognized as associated with herpes simplex virus were described in ancient Greek medical texts. These oral infections are probably what Shakespeare had in mind in *Romeo and Juliet* (Act I, scene iv):

O'er ladies' lips, who straight on kisses dream
Which oft the angry Mab with blisters plagues

Today we know that most humans become infected with herpesviruses during their lifetime. The herpesviruses that cause common oral and genital infections are called herpes simplex viruses (HSV). They are the best understood of all herpesviruses and are the major focus of this chapter, but other herpesviruses also exist. In fact, dozens of different herpesviruses are capable of infecting almost every animal, causing a varied repertoire of diseases (Table 41.1). Two HSV types cause common infections of the skin and mucous membranes: HSV type 1, which is acquired predominantly through the oral route, and HSV type 2, which is acquired through the genital route. Other herpesviruses include the **varicella-zoster virus,** which causes chickenpox and shingles, and **cytomegalovirus,** which causes hepatitis, pneumonia, blinding retinal infections in immunocompromised patients, and serious congenital infections. The **Epstein-Barr virus** is best known as a cause of infectious mononucleosis, but it is also involved in some human cancers. A sixth herpesvirus, called **human herpesvirus type 6**, was discovered in 1986 and causes common illnesses with fever and rash in infants (**roseola**). **Human herpesvirus type 7** was identified in 1990. As yet, no disease has been linked definitively to it. In 1995, DNA segments of a previously unrecognized herpesvirus were found in **Kaposi's sarcoma** biopsies and specimens of an unusual lymphoma.

Herpesviruses are among the most frequent and constant viral companions of humans. It is not surprising that they are also among the most interesting and that "new" herpesviruses are still being discovered.

THE HERPESVIRUSES

Herpesviruses are relatively large, complex viruses with a double-stranded DNA molecule that codes for 70 to 140 proteins (Fig. 41.1, Table 41.1). These viruses replicate and assemble in the nuclei of cells; they then bud through and become enveloped in portions of the nuclear and cytoplasmic host cell membranes. Different herpesviruses cannot readily be distinguished by electron microscopy—they all look very much alike (see Fig. 41.1). They may be distinguished, however, by serological and DNA hybridization tests. Most herpesviruses are relatively unrelated and do not exhibit antigenic or DNA homology. Exceptions include the two types of HSV, which are quite similar. Anti-

Table 41.1. Human Herpesviruses

Herpes simplex virus 1 (HSV-1)
Herpes simplex virus 2 (HSV-2)
Varicella-zoster virus (VZV)
Cytomegalovirus (CMV)
Epstein-Barr Virus (EBV)
Human herpesvirus type 6 (HHV-6)
Human herpesvirus type 7 (HHV-7)
Kaposi's sarcoma–associated herpesvirus (HHV-8)?

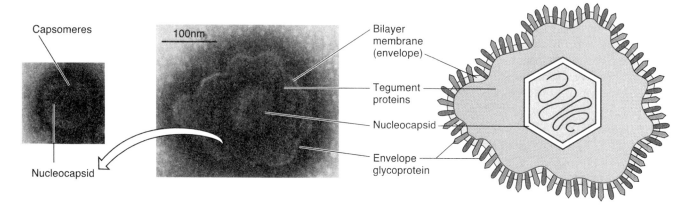

Figure 41.1. Schematic drawing and electron micrograph of a herpesvirus.

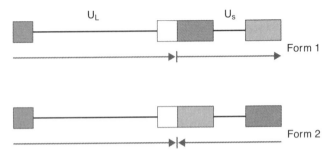

Figure 41.2. Formation of isomers of the herpesvirus DNA. Herpesvirus DNAs can exist in multiple isomeric forms in which the long and/or short genome segments invert. In this example, two isomeric forms are produced by inversion of the short segment. This type of molecular rearrangement is characteristic of varicella-zoster virus (VZV) DNA. HSV DNAs also can independently invert the long segment permitting four possible molecular forms.

bodies made against proteins of HSV type 1 react with many of the proteins of HSV type 2, but proteins that are totally unique to each type have recently been identified. The DNA of one HSV type hybridizes to DNA of the other type with about half the avidity that it hybridizes to itself. The issue of the relatedness of HSV types 1 and 2 is not merely academic. The two viruses cause nearly identical diseases, but the reason for their different yet overlapping clinical manifestations is still a mystery, despite our knowledge of much of their genetic make-up.

The genome of the seven well-defined human herpesviruses has a unique organization: it consists of long, double-stranded linear molecules with several repeated and inverted sequences. The DNA has two stretches of unique sequences, one long (**unique long sequence,** U_L) and one that is much shorter (**unique short sequence,** U_s). Each of these long sequences is bracketed by shorter, identical DNA repeats. For example, at the left-hand end of the HSV U_L is a terminal repeat. An exact copy of this sequence is repeated backwards at the right-hand end of the U_L segment. In addition, in some herpesviruses, each long segment (U_L or U_s) and its terminal repeats can be rearranged in the DNA either in the forward or the backward direction (Fig. 41.2). In HSVs, for example, the various arrangements of the major sequences result in four isomeric forms of the genome. All of the sequences are present, whatever the isomeric form of each herpesvirus. It is not known why this type of genetic organization has evolved, but the rearrangements of DNA during viral replication may provide greater opportunity for the introduction of mutations and evolution of the genome.

ENCOUNTER

Infection with one or more herpesviruses is inevitable in virtually every human. **HSV type 1** is often spread by

kissing or exchange of saliva very early in life. Most children acquire the virus; if they avoid doing so during childhood, they have another opportunity to acquire it when they become sexually active, either through oral–oral or oral–genital contact. Nearly two-thirds of adults possess antibodies to HSV type 1, indicating prior infection. **HSV type 2** is also acquired by oral–oral and oral–genital contact, but it is primarily spread by genital–genital contact. It is uncommon before adolescence, but the prevalence of infection rises rapidly with sexual activity. About one-fifth of all adults are infected with this virus, depending on the nature and number of their sexual encounters.

Most infections with herpes simplex viruses are **asymptomatic.** Perhaps only a third of the individuals who harbor the virus recognize symptoms from it. Clinically evident infection with HSV type 2 is increasing, however. Rough estimates suggest about a 10-fold increase from about 1965 to 1985.

ENTRY

Herpesviruses are very fragile and susceptible to drying and inactivation by heat, mild detergent, and solvents. This susceptibility is imposed by their membrane envelope. Because the viruses do not survive well on environmental surfaces, infection with the herpesviruses requires direct inoculation of virus into areas where they can replicate. Herpesviruses can infect humans by a variety of different routes (Table 41.2). Mucous membranes of the mouth, eye, genitals, respiratory tract, and anus are the sites most readily infected by HSVs. The first line of defense against HSV is the skin, which under normal conditions is not readily penetrated or infected by these viruses. It is likely that the thick, horny keratin layer of the superficial epidermis prevents access of these viruses to their receptors. The mucous membranes do not represent such a formidable barrier, and hence are more readily infected. Thus, our patient, Mr. H., probably acquired genital herpes during sexual contact with the infected tissues of Ms. C.

Cytomegalovirus and Epstein-Barr virus can be transmitted by infected leukocytes during transfusion with blood products, or through saliva and probably semen as well. It is believed that saliva is the most common vehicle for transmitting Epstein-Barr virus, which is why the major disease associated with this virus, infectious mononucleosis, is occasionally called the "kissing disease." Inhalation of viruses borne in **aerosols** is the main way individuals contract chickenpox (varicella). However, direct inoculation is possible. Thus, the mucous membranes provide the primary line of defense against several of the herpesviruses. Nothing is known about the means by which human herpesviruses 6 and 7 are transmitted, but they are acquired early in childhood, so exchange of saliva or contact with some other nongenital mucous membrane surface must be involved. This notion is supported by the demonstration that herpesvirus 7 is frequently shed in the saliva of healthy adults.

MULTIPLICATION AND SPREAD

The life cycle of herpesviruses resembles that of other large DNA viruses that encode many of the enzymes required for its replication. Although these viruses are capable of making many of the enzymes necessary for replication, they are still dependent on cellular enzymes, energy, and metabolite sources. The **lytic** or productive cycle of infection begins with the attachment of virus particles to susceptible cells (Fig. 41.3). The virions interact with specific receptors via glycoproteins that project from the viral envelope. As with most viruses, not much is known about these host cell receptors. Epstein-Barr virus attaches primarily to receptors on B lymphocytes; these receptors also bind complement proteins.

Following binding of the virus to the cell surface, the viral core is released and transported to the cell nucleus where virus-specific synthetic processes are orchestrated. As with all other viruses, the HSV genes are transcribed and translated into proteins in an orderly program. Ultimately, new progeny virions are produced.

DNA Replication

Initially, five HSV **immediate-early genes** are transcribed with the assistance of an **activating protein** carried in the virion tegument, the space between the core and the envelope. In turn, some of these five genes then activate expression of about another dozen early genes

Table 41.2. Transmission of Human Herpesvirus[a]

Virus	Means of transmission	Portal of entry	Initial target cells
HSV-1	Direct contact	Mucous membranes, skin	Epithelial
HSV-2	Direct contact	Mucous membranes, skin	Epithelial
VZV	Inhalation, direct contact	Respiratory tract, mucous membranes?	Epithelial
CMV	Saliva, blood, urine ?, semen ?	Bloodstream, mucous membranes	Neutrophils, monocytes, others
EBV	Saliva, blood	Mucous membranes, bloodstream	B lymphocytes, salivary glands
HHV-6	?	?	T lymphocytes
HHV-7	?	?	T lymphocytes

[a] Means by which HHV-6 and -7 and the putative Kaposi's sarcoma–associated virus spread are not known, but their presence in saliva, blood, and semen is probably relevant.

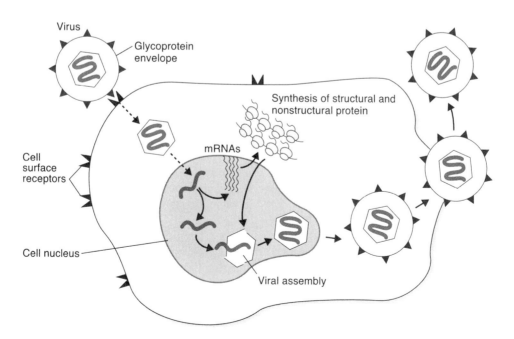

Figure 41.3. Productive infection of a cell by a herpesvirus. The virions are not drawn to scale. In reality they are much smaller in proportion to the cell.

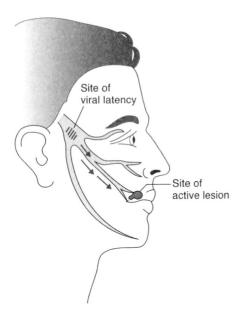

Figure 41.4. The sites of active and latent facial herpes simplex infections.

whose protein products are needed to replicate the viral DNA. Following DNA synthesis, about another five dozen genes are activated. These late genes encode proteins that assemble and comprise the progeny virions. Included among these late proteins are glycoproteins that are inserted into the cell's nuclear and cytoplasmic membranes. As the new viral cores are constructed, they bud through the host cell nuclear and cytoplasmic membranes, becoming enveloped in the process. Some of the host glycoproteins are captured during the process and end up on the outer surface of the virion.

Unlike many other viruses, newly formed herpesvirus particles are not efficiently released into the extracellular space. Rather, as they bud from the host cell, they immediately attach to and penetrate adjacent cells, a process reminiscent of that used by some bacteria, e.g., *Shigella* and *Rickettsia*. This process of cell-to-cell spread has several important implications for the pathogenesis of disease associated with each herpesvirus and the host responses to infection by them. Diseases induced by HSV, for example, are characterized by local spread and progression of lesions. These diseases do not cause systemic illnesses. HSV infection at multiple distant sites is rare and probably requires the circulation of infected cells rather than free virus. Chickenpox, cytomegalovirus, and Epstein-Barr viruses induce multisystem diseases—a feature that may be due in part to their ability to infect and be transported in circulating leukocytes.

HOST DEFENSES

The immune response to herpesvirus infections is multifaceted. Host defenses are adequate to limit the du-

ration and severity of infection and, in some people, are capable of preventing symptomatic recurrences. Within several days of the onset of a herpesvirus infection, antibodies to some of the viral proteins appear in the circulation. However, the development of these antibodies occurs too late to modify the infection, and they have no role in its recurrence. In fact, persons who are unable to make antibodies, have no particular problems with herpesviruses. The likely reason is that these viruses spread from cell to cell, and this mode of spread provides little opportunity for antibodies to come in contact with the virus. The only phase in the herpesvirus infection cycle when infectious extracellular virus circulates is during the initial encounter. If antibodies are present at that time, they can prevent infection. For this reason, antisera to some herpesviruses are administered prophylactically to persons who are at risk of severe infection. Overall, cellular immune mechanisms are the predominant determinants of the severity of the infection and of the likelihood of recurrence.

How do the **lymphocytes** involved in cell-mediated immunity lyse cells in which herpesviruses are replicating? They do so by detecting the "foreign" viral antigens (mostly glycoproteins) that are displayed on the surfaces of the infected cells. Between infections, herpesviruses remain hidden from immune recognition and establish a latent infection. HSV, for example, persists in cells of neural ganglia (Fig. 41.4). Infected neurons avoid immune recognition and killing by lymphocytes via several mechanisms. Part of each neuron is protected by the **blood–brain barrier,** and most of each axon is sheathed in myelin layers, which further protects the neuron from immune recognition. In addition, neurons do not routinely express class I or II major histocompatibility complex (MHC) antigens required for T-cell recognition. Herpesviruses have additional ways by which they avoid immune detection. Some herpesviruses express proteins that block production of MHC antigens. Other herpesvirus proteins block the release or activity of **cytokines** that would normally aid lymphocytes in clearing virus-infected cells.

The ability to mount an adequate cellular immune response to herpesviruses changes with age. The relevant immune effector cells gradually mature during the first month of an infant's life. Until this maturation is complete, herpesvirus infections may be devastating. In fact, neonatal HSV infection is often fatal. By 1 month of age, however, the infant tolerates the virus well. Some herpesviruses become problematic at the other end of the age spectrum. Reactivation of varicella virus that leads to the so-called **zoster** infection (shingles) occurs with increasing frequency as people age, perhaps providing an indication of the senescence of immune responses. The likelihood of having zoster disease is about 10 times greater at age 80 than at age 8.

No better proof of the primacy of lymphocyte-mediated responses in the control of herpesvirus infections can be found than in the response of severely compromised patients to herpes infections. About two-thirds of all bone-marrow transplant recipients experience reactivation HSV infections within the first month after transplantation. Some of these infections may be quite severe and destructive. Similarly, leukemic children and AIDS patients experience frequent and prolonged HSV infections.

DAMAGE

HSVs can be destructive. Epithelial cells in which the virions replicate undergo premature **apoptosis**, or programmed cell death. Under the microscope, changes can be observed in such productively infected cells: their nuclei become enlarged and distorted by viral cores and aggregates of nucleoproteins (Fig. 41.5). Gradually, the nuclear membrane dissolves and the cell swells and ruptures, but not before virus spreads to infect contiguous cells. Thus, a major component of the symptoms and signs of an HSV infection is the destruction of superficial epithelial cells in skin and mucous membranes. The spreading viruses quickly affect regional nerve cells as well, and some of the symptoms of herpes infections may result from damage to these nerves or from the inflammation that surrounds them. The symptoms include itching, tingling, burning, and pain. The host defenses mounted to limit the infection may also contribute to the severity of symptoms and lesions. Degranulation of

---

PARADIGM   ■ ■ ■

Viral Persistence and Latency

Persistent infections and **latent infections** are strategies that some viruses have evolved to maintain themselves in the host for long periods of time and to enhance their spread to other hosts. Both of these types of infection require that the viruses be able to deter or avoid host responses. In persistent infections, the viruses continue to replicate, whereas in latent infections viral genomes are incorporated within infected cells and viral replication does not occur. Periodically, latent viruses shift to a state of viral synthesis, with production of infectious viral particles and possible clinical consequences.

Viral latency is an integral part of the life cycle of retroviruses, adenoviruses, herpesviruses, and papillomaviruses. The processes involved in establishing and maintaining latency are only partly understood. However, it is apparent that different viruses utilize different mechanisms to achieve it. Two well-studied herpesviruses, **Epstein-Barr virus** (EBV) and **herpes simplex virus type 1** (HSV-1), illustrate this diversity.

Latency of EBV requires the expression of a complex array of viral gene products. In latently-infected B-lymphocytes, at least 11 EBV genes are expressed from widely separated regions of the viral genome. The function of only some of these proteins is known, thus we still do not understand how they participate in viral latency. Interestingly, some of these genes participate in the transformation of primary B-cells in culture (i.e., to a malignant-like, immortalized state) and may be play a role in the development of some human malignancies. In particular, **LMP-1** (latent infection membrane protein) has been found to enhance cell growth by interaction with the receptor for tumor necrosis factor (TNF-α). This interaction prevents TNFα—mediated apoptosis, which ensures cell survival. Cells that express LMP-1 form tumors in immunodeficient mice ("nude mice").

Latency of HSV-1 does not appear to depend on the synthesis of virus-encoded proteins. There are suggestions that RNA transcripts, in lieu of proteins, may be involved in HSV-1 latency. Such RNA molecules may inhibit the replication pathway, thus favoring the establishment of latency. Virus-derived mRNA transcripts are found in latently-infected sensory neurons. These **latency-associated transcripts** (LATs) consist of both a primary HSV-1 mRNA and more abundant stable introns derived from the primary transcript. A possible, but unproven, function for LATs is suggested by the overlap of the LAT region with a viral gene known to be expressed during viral replication, the HSV ICPO (infected cell protein αO) gene. Perhaps the LATs act to suppress ICPO by acting as an antisense molecule that hybridizes with its mRNA and thereby inhibit infection.

In latent infections with another herpesvirus, the **cytomegalovirus** (CMV), latently infected cells show no evidence of any viral protein or RNA synthesis. Consequently, the mechanism of latency with CMV is unknown at present, but it is likely to be novel and different from that of EBV and HSV-1.

These three herpesviruses utilize highly diverse mechanisms to achieve latency. Some of the diversity may reflect the different requirements for latency within non-replicative cells (neurons for HSV-1) and replicative cells (lymphocytes or other cells for EBV). A better understanding of these processes in all latent virus infections is of major importance for future antiviral interventions. Although the available antiviral drugs can limit the replication of many of these viruses, truly curative therapy cannot be contemplated without a more complete understanding of the complex interactions with specific host cells that ensure long-term survival of the virus.

AUTHOR: DANIEL BRAUN

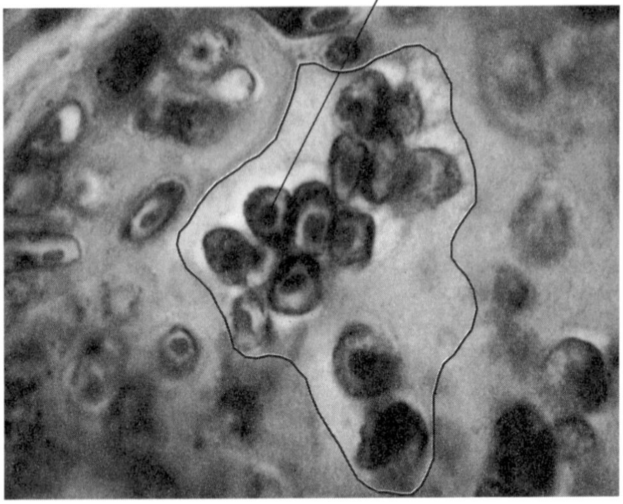

Eosinophilic inclusions

Figure 41.5. Photomicrograph of a biopsy of a skin lesion from a patient with herpes simplex infection. Numerous multinucleated cells containing eosinophilic intranuclear inclusions are apparent.

leukocytes and release of mediators in response to local viral infection augment the tissue swelling and inflammation.

HSV Infections

Now to return to our patient presented in the case of Mr. H. Because immune responses take time to evolve, it can be predicted that healing of all his lesions will require 2 to 3 weeks. Although the outward manifestations of infection disappear completely, Mr. H. will still carry the virus in the sacral sensory nerve ganglia, and he may experience a recurrence of symptoms on an average of 3 to 4 times per year for many years (Table 41.3). Because antibody- and cellular-mediated immune responses are activated during the primary infection, these later recurrences are typically briefer and milder, lasting

an average of 7 to 10 days in all. The immune responses, however, are not adequate to prevent recurrent infection in all individuals.

Mr. H. has a typical adult genital herpes infection. HSV may induce somewhat different conditions depending upon the body site, age, and general host immune capacity (Table 41.4). HSVs may infect nearly any area of the skin. A common site of infection, particularly in health care workers, is the finger tip, acquired by touching active herpetic lesions in patients with an ungloved hand.

HSV can also infect the **conjunctiva** and **cornea** of the eye, a condition known as **herpetic keratoconjunctivitis**. This infection causes inflammation and swelling in the superficial tissues of the anterior eye, with potential scarring and loss of vision.

As mentioned previously, HSV can cause severe and life-threatening infections. Like the newborn, patients with lymphomas, leukemias, or AIDS have inadequate cellular immune defenses. In these individuals, the infection can spread widely across the skin to vital viscera, especially the lungs, esophagus, liver, and brain. A rare form of HSV disease involves reactivation of virus, presumably from the trigeminal ganglion, and its ascent into the brain, rather than the usual descent to the mouth. **Encephalitis** ensues, characterized by an unusually progressive and destructive inflammation of a unilateral and focal nature. This condition is usually fatal if untreated.

Table 41.3. Stages in Herpes Simplex Infection

1. Acute mucocutaneous infection
2. Spread to local sensory nerve endings
3. Establishment and maintenance of neuronal latency
4. Reactivation of virus and distal spread
5. Recurrent cutaneous infection

Table 41.4. Infections Associated with Herpes Simplex Viruses

Infection	Predominant virus type	Frequency	Age group	Usual outcome	Recurrence
Ocular herpes	1	Common	All	Resolution, visual impairment	Yes
Oral herpes	1 > 2	Very common	All	Resolution	Yes
Genital herpes	2 > 1	Common	Adolescents, adults	Resolution	Yes
Neonatal herpes	2 > 1	Very rare	0–4 weeks	Developmental impairment	No
Meningoencephalitis	2	Uncommon	Adolescents, adults	Resolution	No
Encephalitis	1	Very rare	All	Severe neurologic impairment, death	No
Disseminated herpes	1 > 2	Rare	All	Resolution or death	No

INFECTIONS CAUSED BY OTHER HERPESVIRUSES

Each of the other herpesviruses causes important and unique clinical syndromes, which here are reviewed briefly (Table 41.5). Varicella-zoster virus, as its name implies, is associated with only two diseases, chickenpox (varicella) and shingles (zoster). Chickenpox is a familiar, annoying disease of childhood which causes the vesicles to form in the skin. It can be serious in immunodeficient patients. In the United States, 80 to 90% of all adults have had chickenpox. The infection is rarely asymptomatic. Shingles is caused by the reactivation of latent varicella-zoster virus. It occurs in less than 10% of infected people. The rash of shingles is extremely painful and is restricted to the skin area served by a single sensory nerve root in which the virus had lain dormant. The risk of this disease rises sharply with age. In the immunocompromised host, zoster infection can disseminate to cause severe infections.

Most cytomegalovirus infections result in few if any symptoms. However, a series of well-defined syndromes are associated with this virus in individuals of different age and risk category. About 1% of infections occur *in utero*, due to transplacental transmission of virus from a mother experiencing primary or reactivation cytomegalovirus infection. The newborn may suffer from hemolytic anemias, thrombocytopenia, hepatitis, splenomegaly, rash, and developmental disorders. Infection is common in early childhood, particularly in day care settings. In the population as a whole, about 60% of all individuals have been infected by age 40.

Severe visceral infections (lung, eye, brain, liver, colon, etc.) with cytomegalovirus also occur in transplant recipients, leukemia and lymphoma patients, and AIDS patients. Adolescents and young adults with cy-

Table 41.5. Infections Associated with Other Herpesviruses

Virus	Syndrome	Frequency	Age group	Tissues involved	Usual outcome
Cytomegalovirus	Congenital infection	Common	Newborn	Brain, eye, liver, spleen, other	Developmental problems, death
	Mononucleosis	Common	Adolescent, adult	Lymph nodes, liver	Resolution
	Hepatitis	Uncommon	Adolescent, adult	Liver	Resolution
	Pneumonia	Common in immunosuppressed patients	All	Lung	Death
	Retinitis	Common in immunosuppressed patients	All	Eye	Blindness
Epstein-Barr virus	Mononucleosis	Very common	All	Lymph nodes, liver, spleen	Resolution
	Lymphomas	Very rare	All	Lymph nodes, liver, spleen, brain	Death
Varicella zoster	Chickenpox	Very common	All	Skin, others uncommon	Resolution, rarely death
	Shingles (zoster)	Common	Older adults	Skin, nerves, others uncommon	Resolution, chronic pain, rarely death
Herpesvirus type 6	Roseola	Very common	Infants	Skin	Resolution
	Febrile convulsions	Common	Infants	Brain	Resolution, developmental problems ?
Herpesvirus type 7	Roseola	Common	Infants	Skin	Resolution
Kaposi's sarcoma associated virus (HHV8) ?	Kaposi's sarcoma?	Common in immunosuppressed patients	Adults	Skin, "metastatic"	Death
	Lymphoma ?	Uncommon in immunosuppressed patients	Adults	Body cavities	Death

tomegalovirus infection develop hepatitis or a mononucleosis-like illness with fever, sore throat, enlarged lymph nodes, and an increase in the number of circulating lymphocytes, some of which have an atypical appearance. These disorders are particularly prevalent in young gay men, nearly all of whom eventually acquire the virus.

Epstein-Barr virus is also very common. Nearly all children in developing nations are infected before age 5. In industrialized countries the infection is delayed, occurring in only one-half of people by college age, but in over 90% by age 40. Epstein-Barr virus infection in early childhood tends to be mild or asymptomatic. However, if the first exposure to this virus is delayed until adolescence or early adult age, the expression of the infection is dramatically different and infectious mononucleosis often ensues. This syndrome is similar to that caused by cytomegalovirus, with sore throat, fever, and swollen glands. Atypical lymphocytes (reactive T cells) circulate in high number, as do "heterophile" antibodies. As their name implies, these antibodies have broad reactivities and are not specific for Epstein-Barr virus antigens. The appearance of heterophile antibodies reflects the general (polyclonal) stimulation of B lymphocytes. Stimulation of B lymphocytes leads to synthesis of immunoglobulins of diverse specificity, including antibodies to the red blood cells of several different animals. These antibodies serve as the basis for simple and rapid diagnostic tests that involve hemagglutination.

Two recently discovered human **herpesviruses, 6 and 7,** infect T lymphocytes. Little is known about the diseases associated with these viruses, but herpesvirus 6 may be associated with lymphoproliferative disorders. Herpesvirus 6 is known to cause a common, mild, rash-producing infection of early childhood known as roseola, or exanthem subitum. Portions of the genome of another putative herpesvirus have been associated with Kaposi's sarcoma, a multifocal, proliferative disease of skin and viscera. It is epidemic in gay men with AIDS and endemic in Southern Europe and East Africa. The virus has been tentatively called Kaposi's sarcoma–associated herpesvirus (KSHV) or herpesvirus 8. Its DNA sequence shows it to be most similar to Epstein-Barr virus, suggesting that its primary target may be lymphocytes.

In summary, the herpesviruses have many features in common. They are ubiquitous, generally cause mild diseases that may recur, and are especially problematic for patients with cellular immune deficiencies.

WHY DO HERPES INFECTIONS RECUR?

Perhaps the most remarkable aspect of infection with any herpesvirus is the ability of the virus to persist in humans for life. HSV persists because it initiates a latent type of infectious cycle in the sensory nerve cells to which it spreads early in the course of the initial mucocutaneous infection (see Table 41.3, Fig. 41.4). As hosts for HSV, nerve cells are very different than epithelial cells. Rather than permitting a full replicative cycle culminating in the release of progeny virions, the infection of a nerve cell is **abortive** or **latent.** The process is not well-defined, but it appears that only one gene is expressed. The role of this gene may be to facilitate virus reactivation when conditions are optimal, but these conditions are as yet unknown. Viral DNA is not synthesized in latency, nor are progeny virions produced. The viral DNA remains in the neuronal nucleus as a plasmid-like element, replicating rarely if at all in these nondividing cells.

Similar types of latent infections occur in each of the other human herpesviruses. Varicella-zoster viruses also reside in sensory nerve ganglia, whereas cytomegaloviruses reside in neutrophils and monocytes. The Epstein-Barr viruses are harbored in B lymphocytes and salivary gland cells. Herpesviruses 6 and 7 appear to persist in T cells. These latent infections persist for life and—using molecular techniques such as polymerase chain reaction—it is possible to detect the latent viral genomes in appropriate tissues. For example, autopsy studies reveal that nearly all individuals who have been infected with HSV harbor the viral DNA in selected nerve ganglia. The **trigeminal (V) ganglia** are the most commonly affected sites (see Fig. 41.4), followed by certain **sacral root ganglia.** These nerves serve the sites of most common herpes simplex infections. Under certain circumstances, such as when breaks in the skin occur or in open wounds, HSV can penetrate and infect any body site. The virus will establish a latent infection in the sensory nerves serving any such area.

Occasionally, latency is interrupted, and the virus reactivates. Certain factors trigger the reactivation of latent HSV and produce symptoms. These stimuli include sunburn, systemic infections, immune impairment, emotional stress, and menstruation. We do not know how these seemingly unrelated factors induce viral reactivation. Reactivated HSV travel down the axonal processes and bud off from the nerve endings to spread to and infect contiguous mucocutaneous epithelial cells.

The ability of HSV to establish a lifelong latent infection and to undergo episodic reactivation is one of the most fundamental facts that must be imparted to patients. They must know that they are likely to experience repeated episodes of genital herpes, and that during these periods of recurrence they are able to spread the virus to others.

Herpesviruses and Cancer

As we have seen, herpesviruses can cause two types of infection, namely, productive and latent infection. In vitro, most herpesviruses may also initiate an additional and important type of infectious cycle known as a **transforming infection.** Herpesviruses (especially the Epstein-

Barr virus) transform cells in culture. These cells then take on features of malignant tissues. The cells are morphologically altered and have different nutritional requirements. One Epstein-Barr virus protein is known to block lymphocyte apoptosis, thereby immortalizing the cell. Herpesviruses, or at least their proteins or genes, have been found in human cancer cells, but we are not certain whether they induce cancer themselves, participate in cancer induction, or are merely not-so-innocent bystanders. Herpesvirus 8 has been found in nearly all cases of Kaposi's sarcoma. Herpes simplex 2 infection was initially linked to cervical carcinoma, but it is clear that papillomaviruses and perhaps other factors are more important in the pathogenesis of this cancer. The Epstein-Barr virus has been found in the cancerous cells of nasopharyngeal carcinoma, Burkitt's lymphoma, and in other B-cell lymphomas. Burkitt's lymphoma is a common tumor of children in central Africa. In fact, the nearly universal association of African Burkitt's lymphoma with the Epstein-Barr virus is the strongest proof that a human cancer may be caused by a herpesvirus.

DIAGNOSIS

The astute clinician who understands the biology and pathophysiology of HSV infection will have little difficulty diagnosing genital herpes. In the case of Mr. H., the history and physical examination were all that was required to suggest genital herpes. To establish the diagnosis, the presence of virus or its components in active lesions must be demonstrated. Scrapings or a biopsy of lesions can be examined microscopically for multinucleated giant cells whose nuclei contain **eosinophilic inclusions** (Fig. 41.5), the hallmark of herpes replication in tissues. Scrapings may also be stained with specific fluorescein-labeled antisera which will bind to viral proteins and fluoresce when examined with a microscope with an ultraviolet light source.

The definitive diagnostic tool is virus isolation in cell culture (Fig. 41.6). HSV grows well in a wide variety of fibroblastic and epithelial cell lines from animals or humans. Replicating viruses induce the type of deformity and cell destruction described earlier. The appearance of these cytopathic changes characteristic of HSV allows definitive diagnosis (Fig. 41.6).

PREVENTION

Herpesviruses are ubiquitous, and it is not practical to avoid contact with all individuals with herpes infections. It is appropriate, however, to avoid sexual contact during active genital herpes infections. Unfortunately, safe and effective vaccines have not been developed for HSV. Even if an effective vaccine were available, it would probably not help those with existing infection. It is unlikely that a vaccine could induce a better immune

response than a natural infection, which does not suffice to prevent recurrence.

Other herpesvirus infections can be prevented in selected situations. Severe chickenpox in immunodeficient children may be partially prevented by administration of specific human immune globulin promptly after exposure. An approved live, attenuated varicella vaccine prevents chickenpox in normal and some immunologically impaired (leukemic) children. Recombinant DNA–based and live attenuated vaccines for HSV and cytomegalovirus are currently being studied.

TREATMENT

Antiviral therapy is still an evolving science. The first antiviral drugs developed were those for the treatment of HSV infections. Nucleoside analogs (see Chapter 43, "Strategies to Combat Viral Infections") have been developed that are preferentially used by viral synthetic

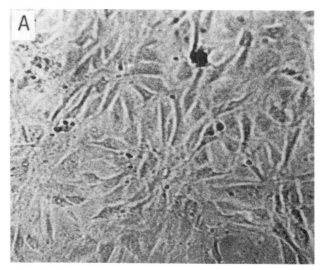

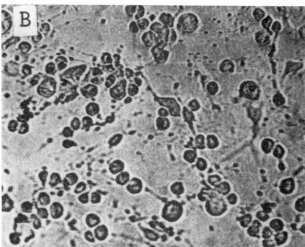

Figure 41.6. Human diploid fibroblasts before (*A*) and 48 hours after (*B*) inoculation with HSV type 2.

pathways. The most useful antiviral drug to be studied extensively in humans is **acyclovir**.

Mr. H. should be given acyclovir because treatment significantly decreases the duration and severity of first episodes of genital herpes. Acyclovir, however, is not a cure because it does not prevent entry of virus into nerve ganglia, nor does it remove virus once there. Therefore, patients treated with acyclovir remain susceptible to later recurrences. Long-term treatment with acyclovir pills will suppress most recurrences, and this regimen would be useful for Mr. H. if his recurrences were very frequent.

Varicella and zoster infections can also be ameliorated by acyclovir or a closely related nucleoside analog, **famciclovir**. Epstein-Barr virus infections do not respond well to the available agents. Two drugs, **ganciclovir** and **foscarnet**, afford effective treatments for sight-threatening cytomegalovirus infections in patients with AIDS. Unfortunately, these drugs are too toxic for use in milder infections by cytomegalovirus. Now that successful antiviral treatment has become routine, so too has the emergence of drug-resistant viruses. For more on this subject, (see Chapter 43, "Strategies to Combat Viral Infections"). Resistance is currently a concern only in selected patients with severe immune deficiencies.

CONCLUSION

Mr. H. has genital herpes, a common sexually transmitted disease most often caused by herpesvirus 2. His symptoms may become ameliorated with acyclovir but recurrence of the disease at a later time is likely. His sexual partners should avoid contact with sites of active infection.

Herpesviruses display a wide range of biological and medical manifestations. They illustrate an important correlation between the life cycle of the viruses and the clinical manifestations of the diseases they cause. This is a fertile area for the study of viral pathogenesis and oncological transformation.

SELF-ASSESSMENT QUESTIONS

1. What are the main types of herpesviruses?
2. Describe the reproductive cycle of a typical herpesvirus, including the latency stage.
3. What is the role of the host defenses in herpesvirus infections? Are there generalizations that apply to most of these infections?
4. What are the main problems in therapy of HSV?
5. If you became involved in work on prevention of HSV infections, what issues would you focus on?
6. How would you counsel a young person with genital herpes?

SUGGESTED READINGS

Fields BN, Knipe DM, Howley PM, Chanock RM, Melnick JL, Monath TP, Roizman B, Straus SE. Field's virology. 3rd ed. New York: Lippincott-Raven, 1996;2221–2342.

Mandell GL, Bennett JE, Dolin R. Principles and practice of infectious disease. 4th ed. New York: John Wiley & Sons, 1995;1330–1382.

Oxman MN. In: Gorbach SL, Bartlett JG, Blacklow NR. Infectious diseases, 2nd ed. Philadelphia: Saunders 1998; 2022–2062.

DAVID W. LAZINSKI

Key Concepts

Hepatitis viruses:
- Display marked tropism for liver cells.
- Use either a "hit and run" infectious strategy (hepatitis A and hepatitis E viruses) that results in acute infection that is cleared by the immune system, or a "hide and infiltrate" strategy (hepatitis B, hepatitis C, hepatitis delta, and hepatitis G viruses) that can lead to chronic infection.
- Cause similar symptoms during the acute stage of infection that are the result of liver damage.
- Can be identified by testing for the presence of specific viral proteins, specific antibodies against these proteins, or viral nucleic acid.
- Can be treated with agents such as interferon; however, treatment for chronic carriers of hepatitis B, C, and D is generally ineffective.
- Cannot be prevented except for hepatitis B and A, for which vaccines exist.

Many viruses can infect the liver and cause disease. These viruses include the yellow fever virus, Lassa virus, herpes simplex virus, varicella zoster virus, adenovirus, Epstein-Barr virus, and cytomegalovirus. However, all of these viruses also cause diseases in other organs or tissues in addition to the liver. In contrast, the viruses discussed in this chapter have a specific tropism for the liver and restrict their replication to the **hepatocyte**, the predominant cell type of this organ. As a result, these viruses are associated with liver disease only.

Some hepatitis virus infections may be asymptomatic, while others can cause debilitating disease and even death. These viruses are a diverse group that includes members from five different taxonomic families (Table 42.1). Of these viruses, hepatitis B virus is the most clinically important and the best understood. For this reason, hepatitis B is the focus of this chapter. The other hepatitis viruses are then briefly discussed.

THE LIVER AS A SITE FOR VIRAL REPLICATION

As the largest organ of the body, the liver represents a potentially fertile site for viral replication. This organ has an extraordinary capacity for regeneration, and it is possible to remove more than two-thirds of it without short- or long-term consequences. Within a few weeks of extensive hepatectomy, the liver and its complex architecture have completely regenerated. Not surprisingly, both properties of excess capacity and rapid regeneration profoundly affect the course of viral infection and disease. For example, diseases caused by hepatitis viruses usually do not become clinically apparent until most or all of the liver is infected. Furthermore, as hepatocytes are killed, either as a direct or indirect consequence of viral infection, new cells are created to take their place. These new cells provide a potentially endless reservoir for additional cycles of viral infection.

Table 42.1. Properties of Human Hepatitis Viruses

Agent	Size (nM)	Nucleic acid composition	Virus family
Hepatitis A	27	Linear (+) single-stranded RNA	Picornaviridae
Hepatitis B	45	Nicked, circular, mostly double-stranded DNA	Hepadnaviridae
Hepatitis C	?	Linear (+) single-stranded RNA	Flaviviridae
		Circular (−) single-stranded RNA	Deltaviridae
Hepatitis E	27	Linear (+) single-stranded RNA	Caliciviridae
Hepatitis G	?	Linear (+) single-stranded RNA	Flaviviridae

Table 42.2. Transmission of Hepatitis Viruses

	A	B	C	D	E	G
Fecal/Oral	Yes	No	No	No	Yes	No
Sexual	Yes[a]	Yes	Yes	Yes	Yes[a]	Probable
Vertical	No	Yes	Yes	Yes	No	Probable
Parenteral	Yes[b]	Yes	Yes	Yes	Yes[b]	Yes

[a] From the combined practices of anal and oral sex.
[b] There is a brief window of viremia in which parenteral transmission occurs.

The liver is armed with potent defenses that ward off unwanted intruders. It is extensively wired with circulatory and lymphatic networks that provide excellent access to the immune system. Thus, a virus that infects the liver is confronted with the complete arsenal of immune responses. Extracellular viruses are neutralized by antibodies, while infected liver cells are promptly killed by cytotoxic T lymphocytes. Liver-specific macrophages, known as Kupffer cells, induce inflammatory responses that also aid in the clearance of virus from the liver. The power of these defenses is illustrated by the relatively low incidence of bacterial infections of this organ.

INFECTIONS STRATEGIES USED BY HEPATITIS VIRUSES

Confronted by such potent immune defenses, hepatitis viruses have evolved two distinct strategies in order to mount infections of the liver. A "hit and run" strategy is employed by **hepatitis A virus** (HAV) and **hepatitis E virus** (HEV). These viruses do not attempt to combat the immune system. Rather, they initiate a rapid acute infection prior to the establishment of the immune response, producing large amounts of infectious virions that can be transmitted to other individuals. Replication by both of these viruses is believed to directly injure hepatocytes. Neither of these two viruses is enveloped, which enables them to survive following introduction into the bile ducts, as fat-dissolving bile salts would de-

stroy a viral envelope. From the bile ducts, these viruses make their way to the intestine and are ultimately excreted in the feces. Thus, the fecal/oral route is the predominant means of transmission for these viruses (Table 42.2). The disease they cause is called **infectious hepatitis**. Provided that the patient survives the initial acute infection by HAV or HEV, which is quite likely, the eventual outcome is not in doubt: the immune response will clear the virus, and the patient will be protected from future infection.

In contrast, **hepatitis B virus** (HBV), **hepatitis C virus** (HCV), **hepatitis delta virus** (HDV), and **hepatitis G virus** (HGV) use "hide and infiltrate" guerrilla-like tactics in an effort to combat the immune response. Each of these viruses is transmitted by the exchange of blood or sexual fluids (see Table 42.2), hence the disease they cause is termed **serum hepatitis**. They first initiate an acute infection which does not injure the infected hepatocyte directly. The immune response that follows is only partly effective. By a number of different mechanisms, most of which are not well understood, these viruses successfully evade certain components of the immune response and are therefore never fully cleared. The resulting chronic infection often lasts for decades and may have severe consequences for the patient (Table 42.3).

Since "hide and infiltrate" viruses do not harm the infected cell, one might wonder why they cause disease at all. However, these diseases are largely a result of the futile attempt of the host to clear the viral infection. When the immune system kills infected hepatocytes, enzymes are that normally exist only within these cells, such as aminotransferases (also known as transaminases) are liberated into plasma. If hepatocyte death is extensive and liver function impaired, bilirubin, an intermediate of heme metabolism that is normally detoxified in the liver, accumulates in the blood causing the patient's skin and eyes to become yellow (jaundice). Although regeneration can replace lost hepatocytes, the process is imperfect and localized scarring occurs. Following one or more decades of continuous scarring throughout the organ, liver function can become permanently impaired in a process known as **cirrhosis**. If the disease progresses, a liver transplant may be necessary to save the patient. In addition, decades of hepatocyte death and replenishment may lead to liver cancer, possibly in connection with viral factors. Chronic infections by HBV and HCV account for more than half of the cases of hepatocellular carcinoma (HCC) worldwide.

■ CASE

Mr. P., a 23-year-old grocery clerk, came to the emergency room of a City Hospital because of jaundice. For several days, he had felt increasingly weak, nauseated, and feverish and had pain on the right side of his abdomen and joints. He had no appetite. Mr. P. thought that he had picked up a bad case of the "stomach flu" until, while shaving, he noted that his eyes were yellow. He reported that he had experimented with a variety of oral and injectable drugs but denied being addicted. He had a stable job and a girl friend with whom he was sexually active.

The emergency room physician suspected that Mr. P. had contracted hepatitis B virus. The laboratory reported elevation of several indicators of liver injury, namely, increased levels of serum aminotransferases, bilirubin, and alkaline phosphatase. Antibodies to hepatitis A and C viruses were absent. A surface antigen associated with hepatitis B, called HBsAg, was detected in his serum, although antibodies directed against this antigen were not found. These findings confirmed the diagnosis of hepatitis B virus infection. The medical personnel who had come in contact with Mr. P. or his blood samples were not particularly concerned about becoming infected because all had received the hepatitis B vaccine.

Consider the following questions:

1. By what route or routes may Mr. P have become infected?
2. What caused Mr. P.'s symptoms?
3. What was the significance of finding viral surface antigen but not anti-surface antibodies?
4. What follow-up tests will be needed to determine his long-term prognosis?
5. What treatment could be instituted?
6. What advice can Mr. P. be given to avoid further transmission?

HEPATITIS B VIRUS

Hepatitis B virus (HBV) belongs to the **hepadnavirus** family, a group of viruses with unusual properties, including a partially double-stranded circular DNA and replication via **reverse transcription**. In addition, HBV exhibits a marked tropism for human and chimpanzee liver cells (hepatocyctes) and cannot be grown in cells in culture. One reason for this tropism is that hepadnaviruses only infect cells that express an appropriate receptor on their surface. Immortalized liver cell lines that have been established in the laboratory do not express such receptors and therefore cannot be used to study infection by these viruses. The lack of these receptors on liver cell lines has greatly hampered research on viral replication. Much of the information about HBV comes from studies of animals infected by other hepadnaviruses. The advent of molecular techniques has made it possible to artificially introduce cloned viral DNA into cells in culture, so that the details of genome replication can be investigated.

Genome and Virion Structure

A map of the HBV genome is shown in Figure 42.1. With less than 3200 nucleotides, HBV has the smallest genome of any human virus (the HDV genome is

Table 42.3. Clinical Comparison of Disease Associated with Hepatitis Viruses

	A	B	C	D	E	G
Incubation period (days)	15–40	60–180	60–120	60–180	21–42	?
Asymptomatic infection	Often	Often[a]	Often[a]	Unusual	Often	Often
Chronicity	No	Yes (10%)	Yes (80%)	Yes	No	Yes
Long-term sequelae	No	Yes[b]	Yes[b]	Exacerbation of HBV	No	?

[a] Asymptomic infections are common only during the acute phase.
[b] Includes cirrhosis and hepatocelluar carcinoma.

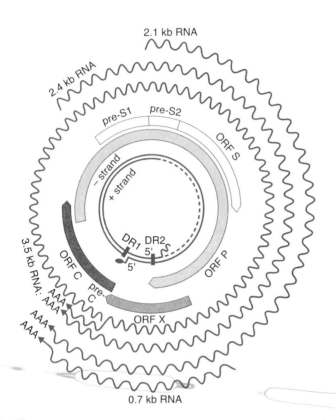

Figure 42.1. Hepatitis B virus (HBV) genome structure and mRNA transcripts.

smaller, but as we will see, this is not a true virus). HBV uses its genome economically by encoding different proteins within the same region of DNA in different reading frames. About half of the genome's nucleotides are used to code simultaneously for two different proteins, and all code for at least one protein. The regulatory signals of this virus are not contained in separate regions as in most genomes; instead, they overlap with coding sequences. These cis acting signals are needed for transcription (promoters and enhancers), polyadenylation, and replication (packaging and reverse transcription). Such unprecedented genome compression limits the degree to which the virus can naturally mutate as well as mutagenic studies by investigators.

The structure of HBV DNA is unique: it is a partly double-stranded circular molecule. The minus strand (i.e., noncoding) is nicked and a polymerase molecule is attached to its 5′ end. The plus strand contains a short RNA oligonucleotide at its 5′ end and is shortened at its 3′ end. Thus, the circular DNA genome has a single-stranded gap (see Fig. 42.1).

The HBV infectious virions (known as "Dane particles") are surrounded by an **envelope** and contain only five proteins. These proteins are called "HB" followed by other letters. The **envelope** layer contains three surface antigens, **HBsAg-S**, **HBsAg-M**, and **HBsAg-L** (for small, middle, and large), embedded in a lipid bilayer.

Each of these proteins is translated from a different initiator methionine codon on their mRNAs, but they share much of their carboxy-terminal sequence. HBsAg-M contains an additional sequence called pre-S2. HBsAg-L has extra sequences called pre-S1 and pre-S2. HBsAg-S is the main constituent of the envelope and is important for virion assembly.

The HBV capsid is icosahedral and composed entirely of **core proteins** (HBcAg) that surround the viral DNA and the reverse transcriptase, which is known as the **pol** protein. A processed form of the core protein, called **e antigen** (HBeAg) is made when translation of the precore message begins upstream from the usual start site. The e antigen is secreted from the cell and is found free in the blood (i.e., not within virions). Although it has the same primary sequence as a portion of the core protein, the e antigen adopts a unique conformation that exposes different epitopes, which makes it a useful diagnostic marker of HBV infection.

The HBV **reverse transcriptase** has some properties in common with those of the retroviruses. Both kinds of enzymes can copy RNA into DNA and DNA into DNA. Furthermore, both enzymes have RNase H domains that digest the RNA template soon after it is copied. However, the HBV pol gene has a unique amino-terminal region, called the **terminal domain**, that is covalently attached to virion DNA. The significance of this covalent linkage is explained below.

In addition to infectious virions, the blood of HBV-infected individuals contains a large amount of empty enveloped particles (i.e., lacking the core and genome). The titer of these so-called **Australia antigen particles** in the blood can reach 10^{13}/ml. Most of the empty particles are spherical and composed mainly of HBsAg-S. Filaments enriched for HBsAg-L are found in smaller amounts (Fig. 42.2). The role of these empty particles in viral replication and disease is still uncertain.

HBV Replication

The HBV replication cycle involves several steps:

- Following its introduction into the bloodstream, HBV travels to the liver and attaches to the surface of hepatocytes. Attachment involves the interaction of the large surface antigen with an unidentified receptor(s).
- After uptake and uncoating, the viral genome is delivered to the nucleus where the partially double-stranded nicked viral DNA is converted into a fully double-stranded, covalently closed, circular species (cccDNA). In this process, the RNA on the plus strand and the pol protein on the minus strand are removed, the gapped single-stranded region is filled in, and the resulting termini are ligated.
- cccDNA serves as the template for transcription of viral RNA, which is synthesized by a **host RNA polymerase**.

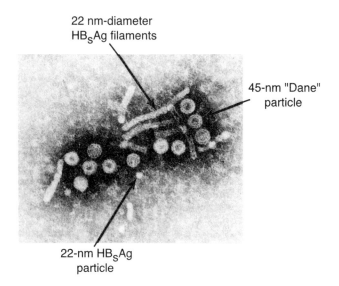

22 nm-diameter
HB_sAg filaments

45-nm "Dane"
particle

22-nm HB_sAg
particle

Figure 42.2. Electron micrograph of 22-nm small, spherical aggregates of hepatitis B surface antigen (HBsAg) particles, 22-nm-wide filamentous aggregates of the antigen, and 42- to 45-nm hepatitis B virus ("Dane") particles.

- Viral RNA is used as a template for reverse transcription, resulting in the formation of viral DNA.
- The viral particles are now assembled and the virions released from infected cells.

Several of these steps have characteristics exclusive to HBV. For example, HBV transcription has properties that help explain its tropism for liver cells. HBV encodes two enhancer elements that have binding sites for host transcription factors uniquely enriched in liver cells. In addition to expressing five mRNA molecules (for making sAg-S, sAg-M, sAg-L, e antigen, and a protein called X), HBV makes a sixth, longer transcript called the **pregenomic RNA** (pgRNA). Following its synthesis, pgRNA is transported to the cytoplasm where it performs two functions: it serves both as the mRNA for translation of the remaining viral proteins (core and pol) and as the template for viral genome synthesis.

The next step in replication is **reverse transcription,** which in HBV is a particularly complex process consisting of the following steps.

- The polymerase binds to a unique stem-loop structure located at the 5′ end of pgRNA (Fig. 42.3, step 1). No other viral or host RNA is known to have such a structure at its 5′ end. This step ensures that only the appropriate RNA is reverse-transcribed.
- Reverse transcription now begins, using a mechanism unique to hepadnaviruses. Instead of using a host tRNA molecule to prime synthesis (as is done by retroviruses), the hepadnaviral polymerase uses one of its own amino acids for this purpose. As a result, the first deoxynucleotide synthesized is covalently

joined to a specific tyrosine residue within the terminal domain of the polymerase.

- Reverse transcriptase now makes a short stretch of 3–4 deoxynucleotides covalently bound to the polymerase, using as a template a single-stranded bulge region within that RNA (Fig. 42.3, step 2).
- The polymerase then translocates to a direct repeat on the 3′ end (DR1) that includes nucleotides complementary to those attached to the polymerase. The deoxynucleotides base-pair with DR1 and the polymerase elongates to make a DNA copy (Fig. 42.3, step 3). As the front end of the polymerase copies RNA into DNA, its trailing portion concomitantly destroys the portion of the template that has already been copied (Fig. 42.3, step 4). When the polymerase reaches the 5′ end of the pregenomic RNA, minus strand synthesis is complete, and a short RNA oligonucleotide at the 5′ end remains undigested.
- The RNA oligonucleotide that remains after minus strand synthesis is used as a primer to initiate plus strand synthesis. After a complex series of synthetic events that include two additional strand translocations (Fig. 42.3, steps 5–6), DNA synthesis stops. For reasons that are not understood, the polymerase pauses before completing the plus strand and a single-stranded gap remains in the final product.

Following reverse transcription, most of the "mature" cores become enveloped by insertion into surface antigen particles that bud from the endoplasmic reticulum. These particles are then transported to the Golgi apparatus, where their envelope proteins become glycosylated. They are then secreted from the cell as infectious virus. However, a small percentage of mature core particles are not enveloped. These particles travel to the nucleus, and following gap repair, replenish the pool of cccDNA.

Readers who find hepadnaviral replication complex and puzzling are not alone. Researchers who have spent much of their scientific careers studying these mechanisms continue to be amazed. The molecular gymnastics that occur during HBV replication are even more remarkable when one considers that the acrobatic polymerase is conducting its maneuvers within the restrictive confines of the capsid, all the while tethered to the 5′ end of the minus DNA strand.

Encounter and Entry

Hepatitis B virus is one of the most clinically important viral pathogens of humans. It is estimated that nearly one-third of the world's population has been infected by HBV, and more than one-quarter of a billion people are chronically infected. Since most of these individuals continue to produce infectious virus for many years to come, they represent an enormous viral reservoir.

Figure 42.3. HBV genome replication. *Step 1.* Reverse transcription begins with the polymerase binding to a unique stem-loop structure, ϵ, located at the 5′ end of pregenomic RNA. *Step 2.* The polymerase uses one of its own amino acids to prime synthesis and copies 3–4 nucleotides derived from a bulged region of ϵ. The polymerase then translocates to the 3′ copy of direct repeat 1 (DR1) which includes nucleotides that are complementary to those attached to the polymerase. *Step 3.* Reverse transcription is then extended from that point. As the leading front of the polymerase copies RNA into DNA, its trailing portion destroys that part of the template which has already been copied. *Step 4.* When the polymerase reaches the 5′ end of the pregenomic RNA, minus strand synthesis is complete. The short pregenomic RNA oligonucleotide that remains undigested is then used to prime plus strand DNA synthesis. That RNA includes the 5′ copy of DR1 and is translocated to a new and complementary region near the 5′ end of the minus DNA strand termed direct repeat 2 (DR2). *Step 5.* Once this second translocation has occurred, positive strand synthesis begins. During plus strand synthesis, when the polymerase reaches the end of the minus strand template, a third and final translocation event occurs. The minus strand DNA has two small terminal redundancies, termed "r". *Step 6.* The 5′ copy of r is dissociated from the plus DNA strand and replaced with the 3′ copy. This dissociation results in the circularization of the DNA molecule and enables further extension of the plus strand.

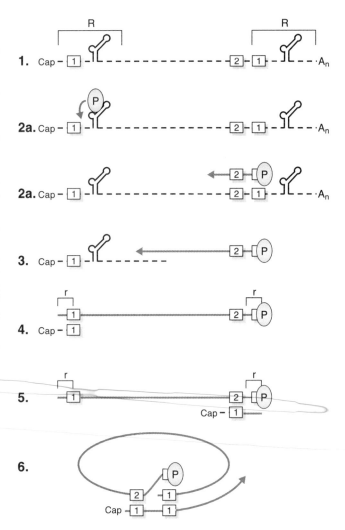

Patterns of HBV infection are not uniform throughout the world. In the United States, Canada, and Northern Europe, HBV infections are only common within high-risk groups such as intravenous drug users. In most of Asia, parts of Southern Europe, Africa, and South America, HBV infection is far more prevalent in the general population. HBV transmission occurs through the exchange of body fluids such as blood, semen, and vaginal secretions. Prior to effective screening for HBV in donated blood supplies, transfusions were a common route of transmission. Today, this route continues to be a problem only in developing countries that lack the resources necessary for proper blood screening.

In addition to parenteral and sexual transmission, HBV is transmitted vertically from mother to baby, probably as a consequence of the newborn's exposure to maternal blood during birth. Returning to our example of Mr. P., it is likely that he became infected by sharing needles with an HBV chronic carrier; however, it is also possible that he may have contracted the virus sexually from his girlfriend.

Diagnosis and Damage

The clinical pattern of HBV infection is complex and may follow several paths. The events can be monitored by determining the presence of viral products and specific antibodies in the patient's blood. Following infection, many patients do not exhibit symptoms for a month or so (Fig. 42.4). Some remain asymptomatic and learn only later from serological testing that they had a prior HBV exposure. After about a month, viral products such as HBsAg may be detected, but no immune response is observed. Soon thereafter, antibodies (IgM class) directed against the viral core protein appear, and the patient may exhibit symptoms similar to those experienced by Mr. P. At this point, the immune system has begun to challenge the infection, infected hepatocytes are destroyed, and associated symptoms occur.

From this point on, three different outcomes are possible. In about 90% of otherwise healthy adults, the immune response will be sufficiently robust to clear the infection. About 10% will progress to a chronic infection, and less than 1% will develop acute liver failure or **ful-**

minant hepatitis that often results in death. In the majority of cases, viral gene products in the blood decline precipitously and anti-HBs IgG antibodies appear (see Fig. 42.4). These antibodies probably play a role in viral clearance and provide protective immunity against future infection. In contrast, chronic patients typically have little or no freely circulating anti-HBs IgG. However, viral products such as HBsAg and HBeAg may be found for decades (Fig. 42.5). Since Mr. P had HBsAg but not anti-HBs antibodies, he may be entering the chronic phase of infection (Table 42.4). The persistence of HBsAg in the blood for 6 months or more confirms the diagnosis of a chronic infection.

We know little about the differences between the immune systems of persons who clear the infection and those who progress to a chronic state. Prior to infection, most chronic carriers display "normal" immune function. Likewise, it is not known if genetic factors of the host have an impact on the outcome of infection, although men are more likely to progress to a chronic infection than women. In addition, chronicity rates are much higher for individuals whose immune responses are immature or suppressed. For instance, in the absence of treatment, the rate of progression to chronic infection among exposed newborns is about 90%. How the virus evades the immune response during a chronic infection

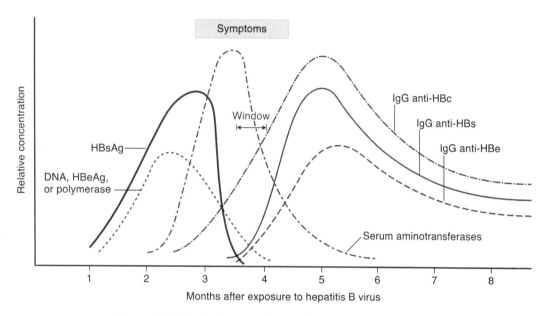

Figure 42.4. Typical course of acute hepatitis B virus infection.

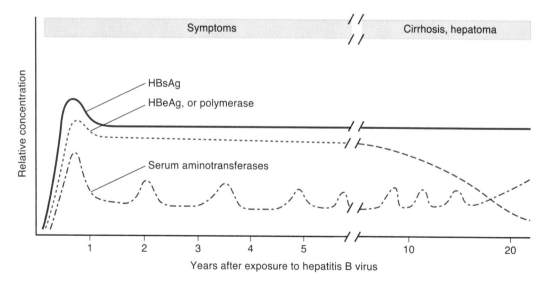

Figure 42.5. Typical course of chronic hepatitis B virus infection. After years of undulating symptoms and aminotransferase levels, the circulating Dane particle activity, as reflected in levels of viral DNA, HBeAg or polymerase, may fall or even disappear. However, cirrhosis and, ultimately, hepatoma may still evolve.

Table 42.4. Interpretation of Serologic Assays for Hepatitis B Virus

HBsAg	α-HBsAg	α-HBcAg	α-HBeAg	HBeAg	Interpretation
Neg	Neg	Neg	Neg	Neg	No prior exposure
Neg	Pos	Neg	Neg	Neg	Prior vaccination
Neg	Pos	Pos	Pos	Neg	Prior acute infection
Pos	Neg	Neg	Neg	Neg	Incubation period
Pos	Neg	Pos	Neg	Pos	Acute or chronic infection
Pos	Neg	Pos	Pos	Neg	Later stage in chronic infection

is also poorly understood. Both the low level of anti-HBs IgG and the underrepresentation of anti-HBV cytotoxic lymphocytes in chronic carriers may contribute to the establishment of a persistent infection.

Once chronicity is established, the patient is likely to suffer from sporadic episodes of active hepatitis associated with liver cell death, which is readily demonstrated by high serum aminotransferase levels (Fig. 42.5). After many years of persistent infection and associated scarring of the liver, some patients progress to cirrhosis, a potentially fatal condition. In addition, after two to four decades of chronic infection, the risk of developing **hepatocellular carcinoma** (HCC) is increased 200-fold. A number of diverse factors may participate in the induction of liver cancer during a persistent infection. In contrast, in healthy adults, with chronic type B hepatitis, hepatocytes are constantly dying and being replenished as the immune system attempts to clear the infection. The net result of HBV infection is to greatly increase the total number of cell divisions in the liver. Since each cell division introduces the chance for mutations that may lead to cancer, perhaps the enhanced rate of liver cell turnover accounts for HBV-induced tumorigenesis. Compounding this effect is the fact that immune-mediated necrosis is accompanied by the production of peroxides and other mutagenic free radicals.

In addition to mechanisms related to the immune response, viral factors might contribute to tumorigenesis directly. HBV has a gene called **X**, whose product is not only able to transactivate viral promoters but also some from the host. Thus, protein X may potentially induce overexpression of host factors involved in cell cycle progression. In animal model systems, X protein induces tumors when expressed at high levels. Integration of HBV DNA into the host genome may also contribute to tumorigenesis. As mentioned above, hepadnaviruses, unlike retroviruses, have no obligatory integration step in their life cycle. The hepadnaviral analog to the retroviral provirus is the cccDNA, which exists as an episomal **plasmid**. Despite the existence of this plasmid, following many years of chronic infection, portions of the HBV genome can be found integrated at apparently random sites in the hot genome.

Prevention and Treatment

An effective vaccine against HBV is available. It consists of HBsAg particles obtained from yeast that harbor recombinant DNA. The HBV vaccine was the first recombinant vaccine approved for use in humans. Currently, HBV vaccination is recommended for all infants in the United States and many other countries. In addition, infants delivered from HBV chronic carriers should receive both the vaccine and HBsAg IgG. Although vaccination programs have reduced the rate of HBV transmission, we are still very far from eradicating this disease. The vaccine requires multiple boosters and is expensive to produce, which is why extensive vaccination in many developing countries has not been achieved. Furthermore, the vaccine is of no benefit to the world's 250 million chronic carriers who continue to represent a major reservoir for both horizontal and vertical transmission.

Unfortunately, the treatment options for HBV chronic carriers are limited. Following administration of α-interferon, a natural antiviral cytokine, many chronic patients respond favorably and their blood level of virus decreases. However, for approximately 70% of the patients, the benefit is transient and viral levels rebound following cessation of treatment. No drugs are yet approved for the treatment of HBV hepatitis, but several nucleoside analogs are being evaluated in clinical trials. One is lamivudine (3TC), a drug also used to treat human immunodeficiency virus (HIV) infection. Thus far, 3TC has proven to be both safe and effective in inhibiting HBV replication. However, in some 3TC trials of longer duration, a rebound in viral levels was observed. The virus that was isolated after rebound contained a mutation located near the active site of the polymerase. Thus, the emergence of drug-resistant mutants may hamper the effectiveness of HBV antiviral therapies.

Regarding Mr. P., the physician could not know with certainty whether his immune response would be ineffective in clearing the viral infection. If Mr. P. does become chronically infected, the exact treatment will depend on a number of factors, including the ongoing severity of his symptoms. In the interim, Mr. P. should be made aware that he can and will infect others unless he uses condoms during sex and does not share needles. In addition, of course, he can no longer donate blood. His friend should be tested for the presence of the virus, and provided that her tests are negative, should be immediately vaccinated to prevent a future infection.

HEPATITIS DELTA VIRUS

Hepatitis delta virus (HDV) is not a true virus but rather a subviral agent incapable of replicating alone. HDV requires the presence of hepatitis B virus as a helper to provide the envelope proteins needed for HDV assembly. As a result of this requirement, HDV only infects people who are simultaneously infected (coinfection) with HBV or who are HBV chronic carriers (superinfection). The requirement for a helper virus is a rare property. Only one other helper-dependent infectious agent of humans is known (the adeno-associated virus).

HDV is associated with an increased risk of death from fulminant hepatitis during the acute phase and higher incidence rates for active hepatitis, liver cirrhosis, and hepatocellular carcinoma during the chronic phase (Fig. 42.6). Currently, approximately 10% of all HBV chronic carriers (25 million people) are coinfected with HDV. Not surprisingly, HDV is acquired by the same routes as HBV, and the geographical prevalence of the two viruses is similar. Furthermore, since the delta virus envelope contains HBsAg, the HBV vaccine also protects against HDV infection. The presence of antibodies directed against HDAg in HBV carriers is diagnostic of delta virus infection. As yet, no effective treatments exist for patients with type D hepatitis. Returning to our example with Mr. P., it is possible that he was coinfected with the delta virus. He should be tested for the presence of anti-HDAg IgG and warned that even if he is not currently infected with HDV, as long as he is an HBV carrier he will continue to be susceptible to HDV superinfection.

HEPATITIS C VIRUS

Hepatitis C virus (HCV) is responsible for the vast majority of non-A, non-B, hepatitis cases. It is estimated that nearly 200 million people are chronically infected with HCV worldwide. In the United States, roughly 15 of every 1000 people have chronic HCV infections. HCV, like HBV, is spread by the exchange of body fluids. Prior to the elimination of HCV from donated blood supplies, transfusions were the most common route of infection. HCV is also transmitted sexually, parentally, and vertically, although, for all three routes, transmission rates appear to be lower than for HBV. HCV infections are diagnosed by the appearance of antibodies directed against viral proteins and by the indirect detection of viral RNA using a variation of the polymerase chain reaction (PCR).

The liver diseases caused by HCV are similar to those caused by HBV, although they are usually somewhat milder and commonly accompanied by fewer overt symptoms. However, the long-term consequences of a chronic infection with HCV can be as devastating as with HBV. This fact is particularly ominous because the rate at which acute infections progress to chronicity in otherwise healthy adults is much higher for HCV than for HBV (80% vs. 10%). Following one or multiple decades of chronic HCV infection, the incidence of liver cirrhosis and hepatocellular carcinoma is very high.

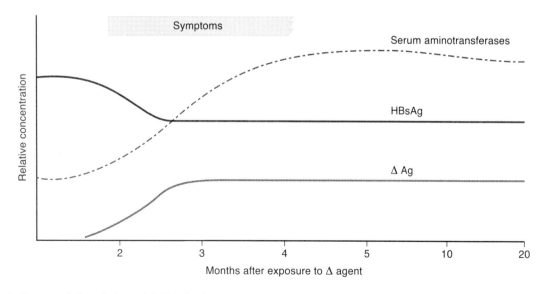

Figure 42.6. Course of chronic hepatitis B infection exacerbated by infection with the hepatitis D or Δ (delta) agent. The levels of aminotransferases may increase and the liver histology may shift from that of a chronic persistent to chronic active hepatitis.

PARADIGM ■ ■ ■

Insights Afforded By Unique Viruses

Viruses that replicate by novel mechanisms can provide us with an enhanced understanding of basic biological processes, reveal new properties of the host cell that were previously unrecognized, and even enable us to formulate hypotheses about the origins of life. Hepatitis delta virus (HDV) is such an example. The HDV replicates like no other mammalian pathogen. At less than 1700 nucleotides, HDV has the smallest genome of any infectious agent of humans or animals. The HDV genome is a single-stranded circular RNA molecule that folds into a characteristic unbranched linear structure. More than 70% of its nucleotides are paired. HDV expresses small and large forms of a single protein, the **delta antigen**. The antigens are identical, except for an additional 19 amino acids at the carboxy-terminus of the large form. These proteins specifically bind to viral RNA to form a ribonucleoprotein (RNP) structure. Upon entry into the cell nucleus, the genomic RNP recruits a host RNA polymerase to copy the genomic RNA directly into an RNA of opposite polarity termed the **antigenome**. This process is surprising because, prior to the discovery of the delta virus, mammalian cells were not thought to possess RNA-dependent RNA polymerase activity. Some evidence suggests that the host RNA polymerase II enzyme transcribes HDV RNA. If this is the case, then HDV has evolved a mechanism by which it induces a DNA-dependent RNA polymerase to accept RNA as its template.

Following the initiation of transcription, replication proceeds by a so-called rolling circle mechanism. Transcription continues many times around the circular genome to generate an antigenomic multimeric precursor. Within this precursor, RNA domains exist which fold in a way that promotes their enzymatic activity. Currently, very few other examples of catalytic RNAs (ribozymes) have been found. Because it functions in both genetic and enzymatic capacities, RNA is believed to have been the first biomolecule to evolve on earth. Thus, it is likely that RNA catalysis was a common feature of prebiotic times and that these ribozymes represent "molecular fossils" that remain from an earlier RNA world.

During replication, the HDV ribozymes within the multimeric precursor self-cleave at unique sites, thereby generating linear monomeric fragments. The resulting termini of the monomers are then joined to create circular antigenomes. These antigenomes serve as the templates for genome amplification. Concomitant with replication, antigenomic RNA is specifically edited (posttranscriptionally modified) by a host enzyme so that the UAG stop codon for the small delta antigen is changed to UGG. As a result, the large delta antigen is synthesized. This protein is required for interaction of the viral RNP with the HBV envelope proteins. Furthermore, it inhibits genome replication and such regulation may be important for the establishment and/or maintenance of a chronic infection. Thus, by ultimately promoting virion assembly and modulating genome replication, editing serves as a pivotal control point in the viral life cycle. In mammalian cells, the editing of host messages is a rare phenomenon and only a handful of examples have been discovered. Therefore, in addition to helper dependence, host-mediated RNA-directed transcription and RNA catalysis, RNA editing is a unique and distinguishing characteristic of HDV replication.

DAVID W. LAZINSKI

HCV infection is also associated with extrahepatic diseases, the most notable of which is **mixed cryoglobulinemia**, an autoimmune lymphoproliferative disorder of the kidneys and other sites. Some evidence shows that HCV can replicate in peripheral blood lymphocytes; this replication may also contribute to the disease.

HCV is an enveloped positive-strand RNA virus (family Flaviviridae). As with HBV, HCV cannot be grown in cultured cells. The only susceptible laboratory animal is the chimpanzee. What little is known about HCV replication has been inferred from its sequence and homology to other viruses or from the expression of viral proteins in the absence of replication.

Like other positive-strand RNA viruses, HCV RNA must be translated upon entry into the cell. At this stage, however, HCV RNA is not capped yet and most ribosomes usually first recognize the presence of a cap structure at the 5' end of an RNA molecule before initiating translation. HCV has circumvented the cap requirement by evolving an *i*nternal *r*ibosome *e*ntry *s*ite (IRES) at its 5' end that binds ribosomes and directs them to initiate RNA translation internally. One long polyprotein is first synthesized. Within this protein precursor are two protease domains where the polyprotein is cleaved into a number of functional proteins. The x-ray crystallographic structure of one of these proteases has recently been determined, giving information that is likely to be useful for the design of specific antiviral protease inhibitors. Once the HCV polyprotein is processed, nonstructural proteins participate in genome replication. One of these, the viral RNA replicase, first copies the (+)RNA into (−)RNA and then the (−)RNA into more (+)RNA.

Currently, no vaccine is available to prevent HCV infection. Vaccine development has been hampered by at least two properties of HCV. First, there are at least nine different genotypes of this virus, each with numerous subtypes. Second, during HCV replication, hypervariable regions within the envelope genes are constantly undergoing mutation. Thus, an infected individual carries not one unique virus but rather a whole population of related quasi-species (reminiscent of HIV). Such properties may allow these viruses to escape immune-mediated clearance. Consistent with this notion is the fact that patients who appear to have cleared an HCV acute infection have no protective immunity to future infection. Few treatment options exist. α-Interferon has been used with some success, but it is effective in no more than 25% of patients. HCV may continue to pose an important threat to worldwide health for decades to come.

HEPATITIS G VIRUS

Hepatitis G virus (HGV) is related to HCV and is an enveloped, positive-strand virus. It causes both acute and chronic infections and may be transmitted by transfusion. The worldwide prevalence of HGV infection is quite high, possibly as high as that of HCV. Little is known about HGV replication and its associated disease; thus, we understand little of the long-term health consequences of HGV chronic infections.

HEPATITIS A VIRUS

Hepatitis A virus (HAV) is responsible for the majority of cases of **infectious hepatitis**. HAV is a nonenveloped, positive-strand virus of the Picornavirus family. This virus is fairly closely related to other picornaviruses, such as poliovirus, and is thought to replicate similarly. Unlike other hepatitis viruses, HAV can replicate in primates such as marmosets, as well as in liver

cells cultured from these animals. This ability to replicate in cell cultures has facilitated study and vaccine development.

HAV is spread primarily through the ingestion of fecally contaminated water or food. Once HAV reaches the intestine, it is thought to be absorbed into the bloodstream and to reach the liver via the portal system. The virus initiates a rapid acute infection prior to the onset of the immune response (Fig. 42.7). Newly synthesized viral particles are shed into the bile ducts and from there are eventually excreted with feces. To a lesser extent, virus is also released into the bloodstream, causing a transient viremia and a brief period during which HAV can be transmitted parentally or by transfusion. Symptoms usually appear coincident with the initiation of an immune response, as gauged by the appearance of IgM class molecules directed against viral structural proteins. The extent of illness during this period varies among individuals; however, in general, symptoms are more severe in adults than in children. In highly endemic regions where sanitation is generally poor, nearly all children become infected in their first few years of life. The majority of these patients remain asymptomatic. In contrast, adults from nonendemic regions who become infected generally display symptoms and can become quite sick. Death associated with HAV fulminant infection is rare. Following the immune response, the virus is rapidly cleared and the patient is no longer infectious and is protected from future HAV infections. HAV does cause chronic infections.

An inactivated HAV vaccine has proven to be both safe and effective; however, boosters are required for long-term protection. Vaccination is recommended for

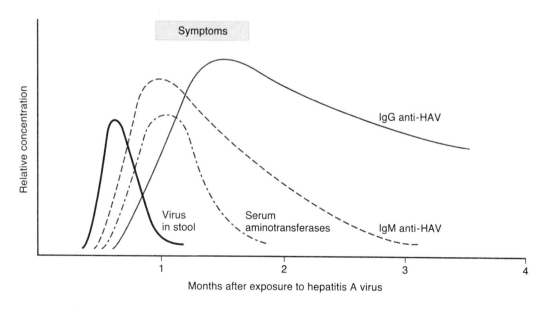

Figure 42.7. Typical course of acute hepatitis A virus (HAV) infection.

members of high-risk groups such as military personnel and others who frequent endemic regions, day-care and institutional staff, and homosexuals. When a patient is diagnosed with an HAV acute infection, the administration of serum globulin can reduce symptoms and expedite recovery.

HEPATITIS E VIRUS

Hepatitis E virus (HEV) is also a major cause of water- and foodborne hepatitis. It resembles HAV in geographical prevalence, routes of transmission, and associated diseases. Therefore, HEV and HAV infections can only be distinguished serologically. Symptoms associated with acute HEV infections may be more severe than those induced by HAV. This is particularly true for pregnant women, in whom an HEV infection can be life-threatening. Like HAV, HEV is a nonenveloped, positive strand RNA virus that only causes acute disease. Efforts to develop an HEV vaccine are currently under way.

CONCLUSION

The hepatitis viruses are a diverse group with representatives that replicate by a variety of different mechanisms. The one attribute these viruses share is a common tissue tropism; each targets the hepatocyte as its focal point for infection. From the standpoint of disease, the hepatitis virus can be grouped into two categories. Hepatitis A and E are "hit and run" viruses which are transmitted by the fecal–oral route and replicate prior to the development of an immune response. Ultimately, these viruses are cleared from the liver and thus only cause acute infections. In contrast, the remaining viruses are transmitted through body fluids and are able to "hide and infiltrate" in the liver even in the presence of an immune response. After one or more decades, the resulting chronic infection can have profound consequences, including the induction of liver cirrhosis and hepatocellular carcinoma. Effective vaccines exist only to prevent

the spread of hepatitis A and B; however, in neither case has wide-scale global immunization been achieved.

During the acute phase of infection, the symptoms induced by all hepatitis viruses are fairly similar and arise as a consequence of liver damage. Elevated serum levels of liver enzymes such as aminotransferases and alkaline phosphatase as well as jaundice (elevated bilirubin) are indicators of liver damage. Determination of the particular virus responsible for the associated damage depends on the use of serological and molecular methods that assay for the presence of specific viral proteins, antibodies directed against these proteins, or viral nucleic acid. Obtaining such a diagnosis is critical for determining the long-term prognosis of the patient. Currently, there are no effective treatments for the majority of patients who suffer from chronic infection with hepatitis B, C, or D.

SELF-ASSESSMENT QUESTIONS

1. Describe the different strategies used by hepatitis viruses for causing disease. Emphasize the different role of the immune response in each.
2. Outline the replication strategies of HEB and HDV.
3. Why do hepatitis viruses show such a marked tropism for liver cells?
4. What are the epidemiological differences and similarities between the major viral hepatitis viruses?
5. Discuss the role of vaccination in the prevention of the major viral hepatitis virus.

SUGGESTED READINGS

Brechot C. Hepatitis C virus: molecular biology and genetic variability. Dig Dis Sci 1996;41(12 Suppl):6S–21S.

Casey JL. Hepatitis delta virus. Genetics and pathogenesis. Clin Lab Med 1996;16(2):451–464.

Ganem, D. Hepadnaviridae and their replication. In: Fields BN, Knipe DM, Howley PM, eds. Fundamental virology. 3rd ed. Philadelphia: Lippincott-Raven, 1996.

Levinthal G, Ray M. Hepatitis A: from epidemic jaundice to a vaccine-preventable disease. Gastroenterologist 1996; 4(2):107–117.

CHAPTER 43

Strategies to Combat Viral Infections

STEPHEN E. STRAUS

"There is always some little thing that is too big for us."

DON MARQUIS (IN *ARCHY AND MEHITABEL*)

The key to successful prevention and treatment of viral diseases is antiviral specificity. An effective antiviral agent must impair the ability of a virus to replicate and spread while sparing the host cells themselves. This chapter deals with some strategies that have shown promise for combating viral infections in people. The emphasis is on antiviral drugs, with some initial discussion of immunoglobulins and interferons as ways of passively augmenting immune responses. Vaccines are historically the most effective and important means of controlling viral infections; vaccines are reviewed elsewhere in the context of specific infections and in a general way in Chapter 44 ("Vaccines and Antisera in the Prevention and Treatment of Infection").

Over the past 50 years, achievements with drugs effective against bacteria, and to a lesser extent against fungi and animal parasites, led to the optimistic assumption that similar chemotherapeutic strategies could be successfully exploited against viruses as well. A key question is, do the facts meet these expectations?

Antiviral drugs have been sought since the early days of animal virology. Thousands of compounds were screened against viruses in many taxonomic groups. Many substances inhibited virus replication but were also toxic to the host cells themselves. It became increasingly clear that virus growth is inextricably tied to host cell processes. The emerging science of animal virology revealed only a few points at which one could safely sever the Gordian knots that link viruses and their hosts. Skepticism initially replaced optimism about the

likelihood of obtaining safe and effective antiviral agents.

During the past 15 years, however, enthusiasm has been restored. Researchers have elucidated biochemical targets at which viral replication may be impaired, and more directly, some drugs have been found to be safe and effective, at least against a few viruses. There are no truly "broad-spectrum" antiviral drugs, as there are for bacteria. The diversity of strategies that viruses evolved to replicate in eukaryotic cells suggests that there never will be a "penicillin" for viruses.

This chapter addresses a variety of strategies by which virus replication can be inhibited and summarizes a series of successful applications to human viral disease.

PHYSICAL AND CHEMICAL APPROACHES

The most obvious approach to treating viral infections is to block the infectivity of the offending agent. Blocking infectivity in the laboratory is easy because many viruses are fragile and easily disrupted. Temperature of 50°C, mild detergent, solvents, chelating agents and numerous other chemical and physical processes all destroy viral infectivity. This results in disinfection, but obviously not in therapeutic options. Nevertheless, such measures can be useful to prevent acquisition of infection. Studies have proven that, for instance, transmission of the common cold viruses by direct contact can be diminished by washing hands or by using iodine-impregnated facial tissues.

Table 43.1. Use of Human Immune Serum Globulins for Postexposure Prophylaxis of Virus Infections

Infection	Preparation	Indication
Measles	Pooled human globulin	Susceptible immunodeficient patients
Poliovirus	Pooled human globulin	Susceptibles
Varicella	Varicella-zoster human globulin	Susceptible immunodeficient pregnant patients
Rabies	Rabies human immune globulin	All cases
Smallpox	Vaccinia human immune globulin	Susceptibles
Hepatitis B virus	Pooled human globulin Hepatitis B human immune globulin	All susceptibles, high-risk susceptibles
Cytomegalovirus	CMV human immune globulin	Susceptible transplant patients
Vaccinia	Vaccinia human immune globulin	Progressive infection
Echoviruses	Pooled human globulin	Chronic myositis or meningoencephalitis
Arenaviruses	Lassa human immune plasma Junin human immune plasma Machupo human immune plasma	Lassa fever Argentinean hemorrhagic fever Bolivian hemorrhagic fever
Hantaan virus	Hantaan human immune plasma	Korean hemorrhagic fever
Respiratory syncytial virus	Pooled human globulin	Bronchiolitis, pneumonia

IMMUNOGLOBULINS

Immunologic approaches to blocking viral infectivity are more practical and some are appropriate and effective in humans. Specific antisera can be raised in animals that, when mixed with viruses, neutralize viral infectivity. Immunoglobulins pooled from human sera are commercially available for prophylaxis and therapeutic management of several infections (Table 43.1).

There are, however, both real and theoretical limitations to the use of immune globulins for managing human viral diseases. First, many sera are not readily available in large amounts or with adequate antiviral antibody titers. Second, sera may be contaminated with viruses or other infectious agents. The methods by which serum immunoglobulins are purified and stabilized kill many known agents, but unknown or nonconventional viruses may resist the process. A classic example of this type of problem occurred during World War II. Several thousand soldiers in the U.S. Army developed infectious hepatitis after receiving a yellow fever vaccine that had been stabilized by the addition of contaminated human serum. Third, the successful prophylactic use of these sera depends on early recognition of exposure. Administration of specific antisera is generally useless once symptoms of an infection appear. Chickenpox represents a practical situation in which the timing of immunoglobulin prophylaxis is critical. Human immunoglobulin pooled from patients recovering from zoster (shingles) infection is effective in preventing severe varicella (chickenpox). But antisera can prevent infection chickenpox reliably only if administered within

the first 3 to 4 days after exposure, which is at least a week before the rash would be expected to appear.

Other immunoglobulin-based approaches to management of viral infections are currently being considered, some of which avoid the limitations of classical serum injections. These approaches primarily involve monoclonal antibodies that can be prepared in large amounts, with high specificity, and without contaminating pathogens.

Antibodies of animal origin cannot be given repeatedly to people without eliciting allergic or other immune reactions to them, so the best antibodies for study are derived from human B cells or by molecularly replacing all but the antigen binding regions of a mouse immunoglobulin with human sequences—a process termed *humanization*. Human and humanized monoclonal antibodies are currently being tested for cytomegalovirus (CMV), hepatitis B virus, and respiratory syncytial virus infections.

Theoretically, monoclonal antibodies directed at the cellular receptor for a virus could sterically hinder virus binding. Unfortunately, the nature of the receptor is not known for many viruses. One virus whose receptor is well characterized is HIV, which binds to the lymphocyte CD4 antigen. Treatment with anti-CD4 was considered but rejected, for fear that binding of an antibody to CD4 would activate T cells and induce further HIV replication within those cells. An alternate strategy was to give patients soluble, recombinant CD4 protein itself. In the laboratory, the soluble CD4 bound to cell-free HIV, preventing its ability to bind to and infect cells. The approach did not work clinically.

Immunoglobulins can only act during the extracellular phase of virus infection. Indeed, most viral infections are initiated by extracellular attachment of free virus. Once the infection is established, though, the therapeutic effects of immunoglobulins are limited to those viruses that infect neighboring or distant cells by freely traversing the extracellular space. The enteroviruses are clear examples of viruses that move between cells (Chapter 32, "Picornavirus"). Immunoglobulins provide effective therapy for some enterovirus infections, such as a serious but rare form of enteroviral encephalitis that develops in patients with agammaglobulinemia. In contrast, infections with herpesviruses, which typically spread directly from cell to cell, cannot be ameliorated by specific immunoglobulins.

A particular limitation of immunoglobulins is in their ability to achieve adequate concentration at mucosal surfaces. A creative means of bypassing this problem is to deliver immunoglobulins in an aerosol for pulmonary infections, such as the bronchiolitis and pneumonia caused by respiratory syncytial virus. Studies in experimentally infected animals showed that similar results can be achieved in treatment of respiratory syncytial virus infection with large quantities of immunoglobulin given parenterally or very small quantities delivered by aerosol. Recent trials in infants are similarly encouraging.

INHIBITION OF VIRUS REPLICATION

Antiviral Drugs

For most viral infections, exposure cannot be determined soon enough to permit effective immunoprophy-laxis. Thus, a more practical and flexible approach is treatment of infected individuals with substances that inhibit the viruses at a specific point in the viral replicative cycle (See Chapter 31, "Biology of Viruses").

Each step and biochemical reaction involved in virus replication is conceivably a target for intervention. But inhibition of these viral processes that depend on host metabolic pools, energy sources, and enzymes is likely to result in unacceptable cell toxicity. Fortunately, some steps in virus replication differ sufficiently from the cellular processes—they can be inhibited with little or no impact on the host cell. Examples of such specific processes include viral penetration, uncoating, nucleic acid synthesis, and protein processing by virally encoded enzymes; the assembly of viral particles; and release of the virus from the cell. Figure 43.1 shows the steps in an idealized virus growth cycle where various agents act.

Two points must be kept in mind when considering the current state of antiviral drug development. First, as indicated earlier, most available compounds have very narrow spectra of activity. Few useful substances inhibit more than one family of viruses. The reason for this may lie in the enormous diversity of viral structures and replicative strategies. In contrast, it is not surprising that antibacterial drugs can have broad activity spectra. Except for differences in the cell envelopes, most bacteria use much the same replicative strategies, often different than those of eukaryotic cells. Thus, bacteria share many potential targets.

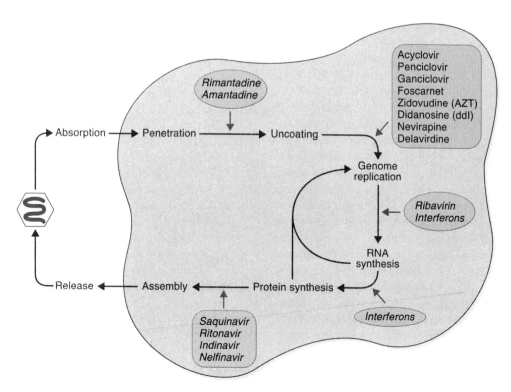

Figure 43.1. Schematic life cycle of viruses showing the steps at which replication can be inhibited by representative drugs. The pink area shows the intracellular space.

Table 43.2. Human Interferons

Current name	Produced by	Typical inducers
α-IFN	Leukocytes	Viruses
β-IFN	Fibroblasts	Viruses
γ-IFN	T cells	Antigens Mitogens

Second, few useful substances impair the earliest and latest stages in virus replication. These phases are most dependent on the proper association of viral structural elements with cellular element rather than on *de novo* synthetic events. To date, nearly all of the potentially useful antiviral substances inhibit nucleic acid synthesis. The following is a survey of some of the major compounds being investigated or in clinical use for viral infections.

Interferons

Interferons were the first extensively studied antiviral substances. They are not synthetic drugs, but rather natural proteins made by the body itself. The discovery of interferon by Isaacs and Lindenmann in 1957 involved a brilliant and fortuitous observation, somewhat analogous to Fleming's recognition of penicillin in moldy cultures. Isaacs was interested in studying viral interference, a poorly understood phenomenon in which infection by one virus renders a cell resistant to subsequent infection with a different virus. This property of virus-infected cells allowed, for example, the first laboratory detection of rubella virus; although this virus does not produce visible damage to cells in culture, it does render them refractory to secondary infection with other viruses that can produce cytopathic damage.

In studying viral interference, Isaacs and Lindenmann noted that resistance to viral infection could be transferred to uninfected cultures by the addition of media from infected cell cultures. The cell-free factors that mediated the transferable resistance to virus infection were found to be proteins, which they termed interferons. Two properties of interferons were quickly appreciated and led to the hope that at last broad-spectrum antiviral therapy may become available. First, interferons released from cells in response to infection by one virus provide resistance to infection by many other viruses; thus, interferons are not virus-specific. Second, the proteins are present in extremely small amounts, indicating that they are very potent molecules. It was reasoned that if interferons could be purified in sufficient quantities, they would be potent therapeutic agents with a broad spectrum of activity. As natural substances, it seemed likely that they would be relatively nontoxic, although

one might wonder why large amounts are not mobilized spontaneously during infections!

Today, we know that many of these earlier assumptions were naive and only partially correct. Large amounts of interferons can now be generated by sophisticated purification methods or by recombinant DNA technology, and their mechanisms of action, biological properties, and therapeutic potencies are relatively well defined. It is now known that there are three classes of interferons, including nearly two dozen different proteins (Table 43.2). Antiviral activity varies with each type and class of interferon. In cell culture interferons exert their antiviral effects by inducing cells to synthesize a number of enzymes that regulate transcription and translation of viral proteins. In both animals and humans, the effect of treatment with interferons is more complex than in cell cultures because these compounds not only inhibit viral replication but also modulate host immune responses to the infection.

Numerous clinical trials have shown that interferons in therapeutic doses, despite their natural origin, cause fatigue, fever, and myalgias, and occasionally bone marrow suppression and neurologic problems. In fact, the recipients of interferons complain so frequently of flu-like symptoms that it can be reasonably argued that many of the constitutional complaints that accompany common viral infections may result from host responses mediated by interferon.

Although interferon treatment ameliorates some severe herpesvirus infections, these actions are not impressive enough to make this the treatment of choice. Nucleotide analogs are much more effective (see below).

In contrast to their lack of useful activity against herpesviruses, interferons are effective for anogenital warts caused by papillomavirus when injected directly into the lesions. Hepatitis B virus and hepatitis C virus infections also respond to recombinant interferon, making it the treatment of choice in the absence of established alternative drugs (see Chapter 42, "Viral Hepatitis"). Most patients with chronic hepatitis B virus infection respond to 4 to 6 months of recombinant α-interferon with marked reductions in circulating virus levels; however, infection persists after completion of treatment in 40 to 75% of cases. Sustained clearance of virus results in histologic improvement in chronic hepatitis. Hepatitis C virus responds to interferon with significant improvements in hepatic function, but sustained virus clearance is uncommon.

Why do interferons not show more dramatic clinical activity for all viruses? Inadequate dosage cannot explain their limitations since circulating levels of the newer recombinant interferon preparations can exceed those observed in untreated infections. Here are some possible reasons why interferons may not be the hoped-for wonder drugs. First, the production of different interferons may vary in response to different viruses. In a given infection the antiviral activity achieved may depend on the relative amount of each interferon expressed at a particular site. This may not be precisely duplicated by exogenous administration. Second, interferons exhibit their most potent activity against a number of RNA viruses that do not cause serious human disease. They are not very active against most DNA viruses and retroviruses.

Even with these limitations, it should be recognized that interferons play other therapeutic roles, with some effectiveness against certain animal parasites and particular types of cancer.

Amantadine

Amantadine and its analog **rimantadine** are primary symmetrical amines (Fig. 43.2). Their chemical structures give no clues about the basis of their antiviral activities. Both compounds are potent inhibitors of influenza A virus replication. (See Chapter 36, "Influenza Virus.")

The anti-influenzal activity of amantadine was first reported in 1961, but enthusiasm for its clinical activity was low. The compound was nearly abandoned but for the fortuitous observation that it is extremely effective in controlling the disordered motor activity in Parkinsonism. This activity may be only a therapeutic coincidence

and does not necessarily suggest an association between Parkinsonism and viral infections.

Controlled studies of laboratory-induced or naturally occurring influenza A infections demonstrate that amantadine and rimantadine exert significant prophylactic and therapeutic effects. Optimal use of these drugs is when the encounter with influenza A can be predicted, such as during epidemics. When treatment is initiated prior to exposure to the virus, these drugs prevent clinical disease in over three-fourths of cases. For patients who begin treatment shortly after the first signs of influenza A infection appear, the reduction in severity of symptoms drops to about 50%.

Both amantadine and rimantadine are fairly well tolerated at the therapeutic dose level. About 3–5% of amantadine recipients (but fewer rimantadine recipients) report mild central nervous system reactions, including jitteriness, insomnia, and difficulty in concentrating. Recent work has shown both agents to be fundamentally similar in therapeutic and toxic potential, but rimantadine achieves lower peak blood levels.

Amantadine is recommended for prophylaxis in individuals who are at increased risk of severe infection during suspected influenza A epidemics. These include the elderly and patients with chronic cardiopulmonary disease. It is also recommended that treatment be initiated in these groups at the first sign of influenza. Even given

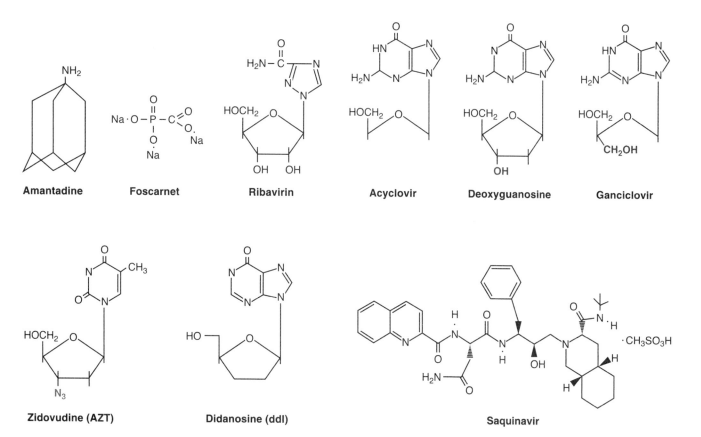

Figure 43.2. Structures of some clinically useful antiviral chemotherapeutic agents.

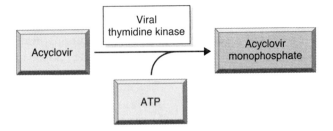

Figure 43.3. Phosphorylation of acyclovir by thymidine kinase.

the limited therapeutic value of amantadine and rimantadine, the medical community has been slow to use these drugs for the prevention and treatment of influenza.

Ribavirin

Ribavirin is purine nucleoside analog with a relatively broad antiviral spectrum (see Fig. 43.2) meaning that in cell culture it inhibits some DNA viruses, including herpes simplex, and many RNA viruses, including influenza A and B, respiratory syncytial virus, parainfluenza virus, measles virus, and several arenaviruses. Ribavirin seems to inhibit viruses by several different mechanisms, perhaps explaining its range of activity. The triphosphate form of ribavirin inhibits virally encoded, DNA-dependent polymerases and, possibly, RNA-dependent polymerases as well. Ribavirin monophosphate inhibits inosine monophosphate dehydrogenase, leading to an overall reduction in cellular pools of GTP (guanosine triphosphate). This, in turn, restricts viral (as well as cellular) nucleic acid synthesis. In addition, as a more circumscribed mechanism, ribavirin has been found to impair capping of virus-specific messenger RNA (the addition of especially methylated guanine nucleotides to the 5′ end of RNA molecules).

The relatively broad spectrum of ribavirin is accompanied by a concomitant lack of potency at nontoxic doses, probably because the mechanisms by which it inhibits viruses are so nonspecific. This translates into poor clinical activity for most virus infections. Oral and intravenous ribavirin seem useful in dramatic hemorrhagic fevers caused by Lassa virus. Ribavirin is being tried for the hantavirus pulmonary syndrome recently described in the American Southwest.

A novel method of administering ribavirin avoids its systemic toxicity and yet enhances its antiviral activity. It involves delivery of the drug in high concentrations directly to the critical site of influenza infection, namely the lung. Inhalation of an aerosol of ribavirin was shown to significantly limit the severity and duration of influenza A and B infection. Studies have proven the efficacy of this delivery system for severe infections with respiratory syncytial virus, which are associated with severe bronchiolitis and pneumonia in infants.

Acyclovir

Acyclovir is the standard against which all other antiviral drugs are compared (see Fig. 43.2). It was the first agent approved for clinical use that resulted from a rational and directed search for antiviral compounds. This strategy is being increasingly exploited. Once we know that a compound has some activity, it can be further modified and its derivatives tested for increased activity and better pharmacologic properties such as stability, solubility, or gastrointestinal absorption.

Acyclovir is an inhibitor of some herpesvirus DNA polymerases. When its activity against cellular and viral polymerases is compared, acyclovir exhibits a therapeutic ratio that substantially exceeds that of older drugs, namely, about 1000. The reason is interesting: in order for acyclovir to inhibit DNA polymerase, it must be phosphorylated in vitro by thymidine kinase (Fig. 43.3). It turns out that the herpes simplex virus encodes a thymidine kinase that has the unique property of phosphorylating acyclovir far better than does the cells' own kinase. The resulting monophosphate is then further phosphorylated by cellular enzymes to generate acyclovir triphosphate. This moiety inhibits the DNA polymerases of some herpesviruses because its incorporation into nascent strands of DNA blocks further replication. Viral DNA polymerase is unable to attach bases beyond the point of addition of acyclovir because the drug lacks the 3 carbon of the sugar ring at which phosphodiester bonds link nucleosides together.

How do these biochemical mechanisms translate into acyclovir's in vitro potency for each herpesvirus? Herpes simplex virus types 1 and 2 are effectively inhibited with submicrogram concentrations of acyclovir (Table 43.3). Epstein-Barr virus and varicella-zoster virus are less sensitive to the drug, whereas cytomegalovirus is not well inhibited.

The clinical response to acyclovir therapy seen in patients is similar to these in vitro results. The most significant benefits accrue in patients with herpes simplex virus infections. Clinical responses to acyclovir therapy are also seen in patients with varicella and zoster infec-

Table 43.3. Typical Concentrations of Acyclovir Required for 50% Inhibition of Herpesvirus Replication in Cell Culture

Virus	μg/ml
Herpes simplex 1	0.1
Herpes simplex 2	0.3
Varicella-zoster virus	3
Epstein-Barr virus	3
Cytomegalovirus	>40

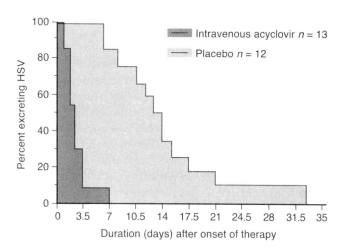

Figure 43.4. Comparison of intravenous acyclovir and placebo treatment on the duration of virus shedding in normal patients with first episode genital herpes.

tions. Acyclovir has not reproducibly helped alleviate cytomegalovirus infections.

The greatest benefit from acyclovir comes in treatment of prolonged or severe mucocutaneous herpes simplex virus infections. These include the first infections of normal patients or any infection of immune deficient hosts. Topical, oral, and intravenous formulations of acyclovir speed the clearing of virus, hasten the resolution of symptoms, and shorten the healing time (Fig. 43.4). Herpes infections in normal patients, which are inherently milder, are not helped by topical acyclovir treatment; these infections do not warrant intravenous therapy. A modest reduction in the severity of the milder forms of herpes infections can be achieved with prompt administration of oral acyclovir.

Acyclovir does not prevent or terminate latency of herpesviruses. In other words, the infection is as likely to recur whether or not acyclovir treatment is instituted promptly. Nevertheless, there is an effective way of circumventing this limitation. Long-term treatment with oral acyclovir suppresses most expected herpetic recurrences (Fig. 43.5). The suppressive effect of the drug is limited to the period of treatment. Even after years of continuous treatment, recurrences may develop promptly after its termination. This leads to an unusual dilemma for practitioners. Should patients take prolonged treatments for a nonprogressive illness like recurrent genital herpes? An additional source of concern is that the virus may develop resistance to the drug (see below). Thus, one needs to exercise restraint and judgment in instituting long-term acyclovir treatment in young patients.

Ganciclovir

The most serious gap in acyclovir's antiviral spectrum is its lack of activity against cytomegalovirus. A major

cause of morbidity and mortality in transplant recipients and AIDS patients, cytomegalovirus has long been a major target for antiviral chemotherapy. The drugs mentioned above, alone or in various combinations, all fall short of ameliorating cytomegalovirus disease.

In studying modifications of the acyclovir molecule, one compound, ganciclovir was found to have greatly improved activity against cytomegalovirus (Fig. 43.2). Its mechanism of action is similar to that of acyclovir, with preferential phosphorylation by viral enzymes and inhibition of the viral DNA polymerase. However, it is more toxic than acyclovir, very possibly because cellular polymerases can utilize ganciclovir triphosphate better than acyclovir triphosphate. Furthermore, its free 3' hydroxyl permits chain elongation beyond the points of its incorporation, thus making the compound a potential mutagen.

Ganciclovir proved to be the first agent to reduce the amount of cytomegalovirus in an infected patient. Cytomegalovirus-induced retinitis and gastroenteritis in AIDS patients are stabilized by this drug, but reactivation and progressive infections are seen in many patients once the treatment is stopped. Thus, essentially lifelong suppressive therapy is required. In some AIDS patients with CMV disease, treatment has to be changed because of the bone marrow toxicity of ganciclovir or the emergence of resistant strains.

Organ and bone marrow recipients are also at risk for serious CMV infections, especially pneumonia. Ganciclovir treatment is not effective in these cases, because the disease causes too much lung injury before it can be correctly diagnosed. A good strategy is to observe transplant recipients closely, taking frequent blood cultures for CMV. When ganciclovir is started as soon as there is

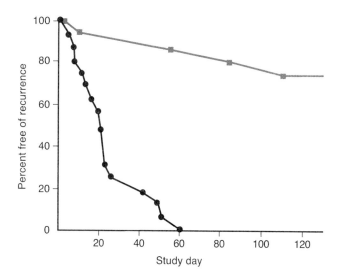

Figure 43.5. Patients with frequently recurring genital herpes were treated chronically with placebo (black) or acyclovir capsules (red). The likelihood of remaining free of recurrence is shown by study day.

evidence of an evolving CMV infection, the likelihood that pneumonia will develop is greatly diminished.

Newer Acyclovir-like Antiviral Drugs

Acyclovir and ganciclovir have established the standards for therapy of a spectrum of herpesvirus infections ranging from simple and recurrent to rare or life-threatening. Their successes have spawned a competitive industry trying to improve on these drugs. Two compounds are worth mentioning as examples of antiviral drug development. The limitations of acyclovir are addressed in each of these new compounds. The first is the poor solubility and absorption of acyclovir from the gastrointestinal tract, meaning that the maximum serum levels that can be achieved with oral acyclovir are relatively low. An analog known as valacyclovir (see Fig. 43.2) is very well absorbed. It has a valine side chain that is enzymatically clipped off as the drug traverses liver cells, yielding higher, and clinically more effective, acyclovir blood levels. Valacyclovir, then, is considered a "prodrug" that is turned in the body into an active antiviral drug.

Another limitation of acyclovir is its relatively short half-life. That is, its levels disappear so quickly from the blood and cells that it must be given 5 times per day to be most effective. Of the many antiherpesvirus synthetic compounds, one, penciclovir—similar in activity to acyclovir but persisting longer—was chosen for clinical development. Unfortunately, penciclovir is also poorly absorbed, so a prodrug of it was designed by adding two acetyl groups that are cleaved off after it gets into the bloodstream. The end result is famciclovir, a drug that is effective when given orally 2 to 3 times daily (see Fig. 43.2).

Foscarnet

All of the above antiherpes drugs are nucleoside analogs that must be phosphorylated before they can inhibit herpesvirus DNA polymerase. Another drug, foscarnet, is a phosphonate rather than a nucleoside. It directly inhibits herpesvirus DNA polymerases. It is poorly soluble, relatively weak, and moderately toxic. Why use it? Because it is the only good drug for treatment of herpesviruses that are resistant to acyclovir (see below).

Zidovudine and Other AIDS Drugs

The strategies that led to the development of effective anti-herpes agents are now being widely exploited. The synthesis of nucleoside analogs that can inhibit RNA and DNA polymerases, as well as other known viral enzymes, is leading to drugs with many additional therapeutic indications. Nowhere is the need more urgent than for agents that inhibit reverse transcriptases or other retrovirus-specific enzymes. Screening compounds for their ability to inhibit the growth of HIV has identified many candidates for clinical testing. Some of these have already proven too toxic, but a few of them work!

The first AIDS drug was zidovudine (see Fig. 43.2). It inhibits HIV virus replication at concentrations of 0.1 to 0.5 μg/ml, readily achieved via oral or parenteral routes but below the cytotoxic level. Zidovudine has proven to benefit patients with HIV disease. Treatment improves the immune status, weight, and feeling of well-being, and prevents opportunistic infections. Most importantly, zidovudine-treated patients live longer, and when used in asymptomatic patients with only moderately reduced $CD4^+$ counts, the drug slows the relentless progression to AIDS-related complex (ARC) and AIDS. Unfortunately, this drug is toxic for the bone marrow, and its use over months and years often necessitates repeated blood transfusions.

The strategies that led to zidovudine have resulted in a series of related nucleosides that comprise an "alphabet soup" of drug options for HIV-infected patients—ddI, ddC, d4T, 3TC (see Fig. 43.2), and more. It is not important at this point that you know them all, but rather that you appreciate their merits and limitations as a group.

Each has its own toxicity profile, dose schedule, and evolving role in AIDS therapy. All are taken orally, as is needed for virtually lifelong, daily care. It has become clear that combinations of AIDS drugs are better than single drugs, an observation that comes as no surprise when considering the best management of other difficult, chronic infections such as tuberculosis. Current studies are exploring the "ideal" mix of 2 or 3 of these HIV-targeted nucleoside analogs.

An obvious benefit of combination therapy is avoidance of drug resistance (see below). Combination therapy also allows the use of drugs against different virus targets. All of the above nucleoside analogs, though, act by inhibiting the retroviral reverse transcriptase. Other drugs under study target the HIV protease that cleaves larger viral proteins into smaller ones. There are many candidate HIV protease inhibitors (see Fig. 43.2). Protease inhibitors like saquinavir (Fig. 43.2) are chemical mimics of the peptide sequences recognized by the active site of the enzyme. They were designed rationally, based on the known crystal structure of the protease enzyme and the specific sequence that it cleaves. It is already clear that their use together with one or more nucleoside reverse transcriptase inhibitors yields a more potent regimen that may yet prove to benefit patients more and for a longer time.

DRUG RESISTANCE

The early days of antibacterial chemotherapy were marked by blissful naiveté about the impact of drug resistance. Those who study antiviral compounds are now forearmed with this knowledge and are careful to screen virus isolates from treated patients for evidence of drug resistance. Not surprisingly, resistant mutants can be readily obtained in the laboratory by growing viruses at subinhibitory drug concentrations. Resistant strains have been recovered from patients as well. The good news is that, in the normal host, resistance has not proven to be especially troublesome. There may be two major reasons for this:

- Most viral infections resolve spontaneously as a result of the successful efforts of the cellular immune defenses. The goal of antiviral therapy in most such instances is to speed resolution. Emergence of drug resistance may lead to delay in virus clearing, but in general the resistant viruses would present a problem mainly for individuals with impaired immune defenses.
- Development of drug resistance may actually reduce the inherent virulence of some viruses. Herpes simplex strains become resistant to acyclovir predominantly because of mutations in the gene for thymidine kinase. But thymidine kinase deficiency renders strains less virulent in animals and less likely to establish latent neural infection. In fact, patients with strains resistant to acyclovir do not suffer severe infections. Moreover, recurrences are associated with reactivation of the original drug-sensitive strains that remained unaltered in the nerve ganglia.

Unfortunately, antiviral resistance is a problem in severely immunocompromised patients. The best-studied examples are acyclovir- or ganciclovir-resistant herpesvirus infections in AIDS patients. Foscarnet, with its completely distinct mechanism of action, is the current answer to the treatment of these difficult, resistant infections.

Resistance of HIV is a major issue in AIDS. Chronic administration of single drugs such as zidovudine leads to selection of resistant virus clones. After several months of treatment, the benefit of the drug begins to fade, leaving patients the choice of alternative or additional drugs. Intense, multinational efforts are being made to determine which "cocktail" of several drugs with distinct actions would be useful. Theoretically, they could be given to patients whose immune systems have not been too badly damaged by HIV (high CD4$^+$ counts), could be safely given over many years, and could retain their potency throughout. The goal is to make the emergence of resistant virus an exceedingly rare event.

SUGGESTED READINGS

Galasso GJ, et al, eds. Antiviral agents and viral diseases of man. 3rd ed. New York: Raven Press, 1990.

Hirsch MS, Kaplan JC, d'Aquila RT. Antiviral agents. In: Fields BN, et al, eds. Field's virology. 3rd ed. New York: Lippincott-Raven, 1996;431–466.

CHAPTER 44

Vaccines and Antisera in the Prevention and Treatment of Infection

SHERWOOD L. GORBACH

Key Concepts

Vaccines:

- Induce either active immunization (the induction of an antibody and other immune response to prevent infectious diseases) or passive immunization (the administration of exogenously produced antibodies to provide temporary treatment or prevention of infectious diseases).
- Consist of live, attenuated microorganisms; live, unattenuated microorganisms; killed microorganisms; or toxoids. In general, live vaccines provide longer immunity than those composed of killed organisms or toxoids.
- Can, in some instances, produce B-cell type–specific protective antibody without contribution of helper T-cells.
- Can induce secretory immunity at critical steps of microorganism replication or penetration; examples of these vaccines include those against polio, rubella, influenza, and cholera.
- Should be administered to infants, the elderly, and other people at risk of contracting diseases that are particularly severe in these groups.
- Are being developed by cloning genes encoding foreign antigens from a pathogen and inserting them into suitable vectors.

The dramatic decrease in the incidence of infectious diseases since the middle of the 19th century is due largely to two factors, improved sanitation and development of vaccines. The availability of potable water supplies and sewage disposal, along with improvements in housing, have reduced the incidence of diseases transmitted by food and water and those associated with close living quarters, e.g., typhoid fever, cholera, tuberculosis, typhus, and plague. Immunization with vaccines has eradicated smallpox and reduced the incidence of polio, measles, rubella (German measles), diphtheria, pertussis, and tetanus. Despite these advances, infectious diseases still cause havoc in developing countries because of inadequate sanitation or the unavailability of vaccines. These often represent failures of economics and politics rather than deficiencies in scientific knowledge or public health awareness.

Infectious diseases also cause serious morbidity and

mortality in industrialized countries. Vaccines have not been developed for many pathogens, and institutional public health control measures have proven difficult for some diseases, for example, sexually transmitted diseases. Unconquered infections include most viral diseases, particularly those of the respiratory and gastrointestinal tracts; sexually transmitted diseases (syphilis, gonorrhea, and chlamydia); and AIDS. While rejoicing in the triumphs over many infectious diseases, we should not be complacent about the tremendous tasks ahead in dealing with those insidious microbes that continue to attack the human population.

APPROACHES TO IMMUNIZATION

Several immunization strategies are available to prevent or to treat infectious diseases; the choice depends on the type of microorganism, the age of the host, and the time frame of contact between the host and the pathogen (Box 44.1). **Active immunization** with vac-

---

BOX 44.1. DEFINITIONS

Active immunization: The induction of antibody and other immune mechanisms to prevent infectious diseases.

Vaccine: An immunizing agent derived from microorganisms (or parasites), consisting either of:

Live, attenuated microorganisms (Sabin polio vaccine, measles vaccine)

Live, not attenuated microorganisms (adenovirus vaccine, given by the oral/GI route to induce immunity in the respiratory tract)

Killed microorganisms or fractions

Killed whole agents (Salk polio vaccine)

Extracts of microorganisms, such as soluble capsular polysaccharide (pneumococcal vaccine) or immunologically active fractions (hepatitis B vaccine)

Toxoid: An inactivated bacterial toxin that has lost its damaging ("toxic") properties but is able to induce protective antibody; diphtheria and tetanus toxins are adsorbed with aluminum salts to produce their respective toxoids.

Passive Immunization: Administration of exogenously produced antibodies to provide temporary treatment or prevention of infectious diseases

Immune globulin: A mixture of antibodies produced by fractionating large pools of blood plasma

Specific immune globulin: Antibody produced by fractionating donor blood pools selected for high antibody titer to a specific microorganism.

---

cines or toxoids leads to prolonged immunity and is generally preferred over **passive immunization** (administering immune globulins) for prevention of infection. Vaccines currently licensed for use in the U.S. are listed in Table 44.1. Vaccination alone may not ensure protection from disease. As a rule, antibody response to a live vaccine takes at least 13 weeks to develop; to a killed vaccine or toxoid, antibody response can take several weeks, and often requires two or three doses at 3-week intervals. Because most infectious diseases have a short incubation period, usually less than 2 weeks, it is often a futile gesture to use active immunization for postexposure control. If available, passive immunization with specific globulins or antitoxins should be used after contact (Table 44.2). Certain diseases have a long incubation period (e.g., the incubation period for hepatitis B is 6–24 weeks) or a variable incubation period (e.g., rabies, tetanus); combined active and passive immunization are used for postexposure control in these settings.

Live vs. Killed Vaccines

Vaccines are made with either live, attenuated microorganisms; killed microorganisms; or microbial extracts. Polio and typhoid vaccines are each available in live or killed versions. Killed vaccines have traditionally been used because they are easier to manufacture and pose no risk of vaccine-associated infection. The advantages and disadvantages of the two types of polio vaccines are discussed in detail in Chapter 32 ("Picornavirus") and are listed in Table 32.2.

Currently, the favored approach in vaccine development is to attempt to define the active virulence factors of the pathogen. A vaccine can then be manufactured using extracts of the critical virulence factor, e.g., the capsular polysaccharides of the pneumococcus vaccine, the surface antigen of the hepatitis B vaccine, and the hemagglutinin and neuraminidase antigens of the "split" influenza vaccine. But immunity to a killed vaccine is not as effective or long-lasting as immunity to a live, attenuated vaccine, which more closely mimics the natural disease. However, attenuation of the virulent pathogen to a tame vaccine strain can be technically difficult to achieve. Even when successful, a small but finite danger that the vaccine strain will revert to a pathogen in a susceptible host exists. Vaccine-associated poliomyelitis, for example, occurs approximately once with every one to three million doses of live polio vaccine.

TYPE OF IMMUNE RESPONSE

Immunizing agents can produce immunity through B-cell proliferation leading to antibody production, with or without helper T cells. Pneumococcal polysaccharide induces B-cell type–specific protective antibody (Chap-

Table 44.1. Vaccines Licensed for Use in Humans in the U.S.

		Live	Killed	Fractions
Viral		Adenovirus Measles Mumps Polio (Sabin) Rubella Varicella Yellow fever	Hepatitis A Influenza (whole virus) Polio (Salk) Rabies (human diploid)	Hepatitis B (inactivated surface antigen) Influenza ("split" vaccine)
Bacterial		BCG (tuberculosis) Typhoid (oral)	Cholera Pertussis Plague Typhoid	Diphtheria (toxoid) *Haemophilus* B polysaccharide PRP (polyribosylribitol phosphate) Meningococcal (polysaccharide) Pneumococcal (polysaccharide-23 valent) Tetanus (toxoid) Typhoid (Vi capsular polysaccharide)

ter 13, "Pneumococcus B"). Similarly, the polysaccharide of *Haemophilus influenzae* type B induces B-cell production of antibody without a contribution of helper T cells. These **T-cell-independent antigens** are characterized by low antibody titers, particularly in children less than 18 months of age. Thus, a conventional *H. influenzae* polysaccharide vaccine does not provide protection for the age group (3 to 18 months) in which infection with this organism is most deadly. By conjugating (covalent linkage) the *Haemophilus* polysaccharide known as **polyribosylribitol phosphate** (PRP) to a protein antigen such as diphtheria protein or the outer membrane protein from *Neisseria*, *Haemophilus* vaccines have been developed that produce a T-cell-dependent antibody response. In contrast to the PRP-only vaccines used in the past, the conjugate vaccines induce antibody in infants at 3 months of age. These vaccines produce higher levels of serum antibody and a higher proportion of the immunoglobulin M (IgM) class antibodies. In addition, a strong booster response is produced with revaccina-

tion. Surveys carried out since widespread use of the new conjugate vaccines have demonstrated significant protection of infants against serious infections caused by *H. influenzae* type B, particularly meningitis.

Many pathogenic microorganisms use mucosal surfaces either for replication and/or penetration. Secretory IgA antibodies produced at the mucosal surface offer protection against organisms such as polio, rubella, influenza, gonorrhea, and cholera. The optimal strategy against these pathogens is a vaccine that induces secretory immunity at the critical site. Only a few such vaccines have been developed, but they are notably effective, e.g., polio, adenovirus, and the oral typhoid vaccine. Other mucosal invaders have eluded the vaccine researchers.

The live adenovirus vaccine represents a novel approach to vaccination. In this case, the live vaccine virus strains are not attenuated, and are administered by the oral route (via ingestion of an enteric-coated tablet). This administration results in an asymptomatic intestinal infection that stimulates a systemic immune response against subsequent adenovirus-induced respiratory infections.

Table 44.2. Specific Immune Globulins and Antitoxins

Human Immune Globulins
   Hepatitis B
   Cytomegalovirus
   Rabies
   Tetanus (antitoxin)
   Vaccinia
   Varicella zoster
Equine Antitoxins
   Botulism (types A, B, E)
   Diphtheria

Age of Immunization

Newborns receive a supply of serum IgG antibody from their mothers, which gives them substantial protection for 36 months against those diseases to which the mother was immune. Maternal milk also contains secretory antibodies that provide some protection against intestinal and respiratory tract infections. The infant's antibody-producing capacity develops slowly during the first year of life. Although immunization is not yet fully efficient because the immune system is not fully developed, it is desirable to begin immunization at 2 months of age because diseases are common in this age group and can be particularly severe (e.g., whooping cough, *H. influenzae* meningitis). As with infants, the **elderly** have a reduced antibody response to vaccines. For this group, a larger dose of influenza vaccine is needed to achieve adequate protection. Pneumococcal infections are particularly severe in the elderly, and they should be protected by the pneumococcal polyvalent polysaccharide vaccine.

Duration of Immunity

As a rule, live vaccines give longer, even lifelong, immunity, whereas vaccines composed of killed organisms, extracts, or toxoid have shorter term immunity lasting months to years. However, the immunity to live, attenuated vaccines may also wane, leaving the host susceptible to natural disease that can occur with atypical features later in life.

The best example of faltering immunity with a live virus vaccine is that of measles vaccination. Before 1956, when initial trials of measles vaccines were undertaken, virtually every adult in the U.S. had contact with measles, as indicated by the high prevalence of serum antibody to this virus (Chapter 34, "Paramyxoviruses"). The immunization campaign in the 1960s and 1970s reduced measles cases to less than 1% of previous numbers. In recent years, however, dramatic increases in measles cases have occurred, principally in two age groups: preschool children, in whom the disease has been traditionally most common, and older children and young adults. The increase in measles cases in the preschool group can be explained by the low vaccination rates in parts of the U.S. In older children and young adults, most of whom have been vaccinated appropriately, the presentation of an atypical form of measles is related to failure of vaccination to continue to provide immunity. As a result of these trends, current recommendations for vaccination against measles include two doses, the first one given at 15 months of age (vaccine efficacy in younger children under 11 months of age is low), and the second dose at entrance to middle school (11 to 12 years of age). Whether this schedule will produce lifelong immunity can only be resolved by future observations.

Selection of Antigens

Infective agents possess tens, hundreds, or even thousands of antigens. Such diversity is reflected in their number of genes, which can vary from as few as six in polyoma virus to several thousand in protozoa such as malaria. The principal immune response that establishes protection in the host is usually related to a small number of antigens, often located on the surface of the microorganism. In some instances, a vaccine protects against all strains of the organism, as with the hepatitis B vaccine, which is composed of surface antigen. With other agents, such as the pneumococcus, protective antibody is produced against a specific capsular polysaccharide, of which

more than 80 distinct types have been discovered. Immunity to one polysaccharide type does not convey immunity to any other type. For this reason, the pneumococcal vaccine is composed of 23 different polysaccharides, comprising the most common types causing disease. In the case of rhinovirus infections, the most common cause of the common cold, at least 100 types of the virus are known, and it has proven impractical to develop a vaccine that confers protection to a sufficient number of these antigenic types. Influenza virus vaccines change each year to counter the different antigens of the influenza A and B virus strains in circulation. Minor antigenic "drifts" occur annually in both influenza A and B virus strains, whereas major antigenic changes, known as antigenic "shifts," occur about every 10 years. Vaccines must be modified to accommodate both antigenic drifts and shifts (Chapter 36, "Influenza").

Immunization of Special Populations

Individuals with underlying illnesses are at high risk of certain infections for which efficient immunizing agents are available (Table 44.3). Such individuals should receive active immunization, even though they may mount a less complete immune response and have reduced benefits of such intervention. Patients with sickle cell disease may acquire a fatal pneumococcal infection, which progresses with astounding rapidity and leads to death by septicemia and disseminated intravascular coagulation (DIC). The pneumococcal vaccine, while not fully effective in these patients, nevertheless provides some protection. Similarly, persons who are either born without a spleen or who have had their spleen removed surgically are also at high risk for overwhelming infections with encapsulated organisms such as pneumococci, meningococci, and *H. influenzae*; these persons should receive the respective vaccines.

Other special groups that should be targeted for vaccination are the elderly, for influenza and pneumococcal vaccines; children with leukemia who have been exposed to chickenpox; health care workers, who may be exposed to hepatitis B and rubella; and travelers, depending on local health conditions at their destination.

Live, attenuated vaccines should be avoided in immunocompromised hosts because the organism may be sufficiently pathogenic to cause progressive disease in such individuals. The only exception, based on experience, is the use of the live measles, mumps, and rubella (MMR) vaccine in HIV-positive children to avoid the potentially severe effects of the natural diseases, particularly measles.

DPT (DIPHTHERIA, PERTUSSIS, TETANUS) VACCINE

DPT vaccine is the oldest and most successful combination vaccine used in childhood. It consists of a combi-

Table 44.3. Immunization in Special Populations

Population	Immunization	Comment
Sickle cell disease; splenectomized patient	Pneumococcal, meningococcal, and *H. influenzae* vaccines	Infections are often fatal
Elderly	Influenza, pneumococcal tetanus–diphtheria vaccines	High risk (immunity has waned)
Children with leukemia	Varicella zoster immune globulin (postexposure)	Chickenpox causes severe, often fatal disease in leukemics
Health care workers	Hepatitis B, mumps, rubella, and measles vaccine; influenza vaccine	If not immune, annually
Travelers	Hepatitis A and B, yellow fever, rabies, Japanese encephalitis, measles, meningococcal, polio vaccines	Depends on local conditions
Pregnancy	Hepatitis B	Prenatal screening for HbsAg; newborns of carriers receive HBIG and vaccine
	Tetanus toxoid	Particularly in developing countries to prevent neonatal tetanus

nation of two toxoids (**diphtheria** and **tetanus**) and a killed, whole-cell vaccine (pertussis). Administration of the vaccine is legally mandated for all children in the U.S. The preferred schedule is initial vaccination at 2 months of age, followed by three injections given up to 15 months of age. A booster is given at entry to primary school. Thereafter, a booster of tetanus toxoid (full dose) and diphtheria toxoid (reduced dose) is given every 10 years. A booster dose of pertussis vaccine is not recommended after school age because the disease is less common and less severe in older children and adults. To emphasize the efficacy of these vaccines, two of these classic infections are reviewed below. The third, tetanus, is covered in Chapter 20, "Clostridia."

Diphtheria

Before widespread introduction to immunization, diphtheria was a major and, in some areas, the leading cause of death in young children. Epidemics of diphtheria in colonial America killed up to one-third of the children in a community. The organism is spread mainly by airborne respiratory droplets. Occasionally, direct contact with persons with diphtheria of the skin is responsible for epidemic spread. Communicability is fostered by close living quarters, especially in the fall and winter months.

Widespread vaccination in childhood has had an extraordinary effect on the occurrence of this disease in the U.S.; hundreds of thousands of cases were reported annually in the 1920s, compared to only five cases per year at present. While immunized and partially immunized persons can develop diphtheria, the disease occurs more frequently and is more lethal in unvaccinated individuals.

The clinical picture of diphtheria consists of local infection of the nasopharynx, which can lead to obstruction of the airway, and the later complications associated with elaboration of toxin. While *Corynebacterium diphtheriae* does not invade the mucosal surface, it does produce a thick, mucoid, gray membrane that coats the entire oral cavity, extending upward into the nasal passages, and downward to the respiratory tract and even into the bronchial tree. Obstruction of the airway can lead to death in the early phases of the disease. Most of the serious complications, however, are associated with the exotoxin (Chapter 9, "Damage by Microbial Agents"). Although all cells of the body are sensitive to the toxin, the major clinical effects occur in the heart and nervous system. Up to 25% of patients with diphtheria experience cardiac complications, consisting initially of irregular heart beat and progressing to myocarditis and congestive heart failure. The effects on the cardiac conduction system are severe, and many patients have permanent arrhythmias and abnormal electrocardiograms. Neuropathy is also common, especially in patients with severe diphtheria. The initial manifestations are local paralysis of the palate and swallowing mechanisms, followed by cranial nerve abnormalities and peripheral neuritis.

Antibiotic therapy is used to kill the organism at the local site of infection, but it has no effect on the liberated toxin nor on the obstructive problems in the respiratory tract. Diphtheria antitoxin is an immune serum produced in horses. It can neutralize circulating toxin, but does not bind to toxin that has entered the cell; hence, it should be given early. Horse serum may cause serum sickness, a serious complication of passive immunization with diphtheria antitoxin.

Pertussis

Whooping cough is not a single toxin disease, as is tetanus and diphtheria. *Bordetella pertussis* produces an array of proteins, toxins, and biologically active substances, many of which play a role in the complex evolution of the clinical disease (Chapter 19, "*Bordetella pertussis*"). The organism initially attaches, but does not penetrate, the ciliated respiratory epithelial cells. The various toxins are then released, which cause local damage to the mucosa and suppress mobilization of mucus, leading to accumulation of thick secretions. The pertussis toxin also produces systemic signs and complications.

Worldwide, more than 50 million cases of whooping cough are reported annually, and over half a million deaths are attributed to pertussis. Most of these cases occur in developing countries, although relaxation of immunization schedules in certain developed countries has led to epidemics in recent years. The disease is remarkably contagious, with attack rates as high as 90% among those susceptible. Nearly half of reported cases occur in children under 1 year of age, and infants also experience the highest mortality. Inexplicably, females are infected more often than males. In older children and adults, in whom the disease has occurred with increased frequency in recent years because of waning immunity following vaccination or lack of primary vaccination altogether, pertussis may cause a mild illness with a prolonged, hacking cough.

Antibiotic treatment for whooping cough is only marginally effective. Because of the high incidence of complications and the considerable mortality seen in infants, prevention by vaccine is clearly preferred to treatment with antibiotics.

The standard pertussis vaccine is a killed suspension of the whole organism ("**whole-cell vaccine**"). In communities in which the vaccine is widely employed, pertussis has become a rare disease in childhood. Conversely, when pertussis vaccination was allowed to decline as a result of concerns about vaccine safety, as in England and Japan during the 1970s, sharp epidemics of pertussis occurred which required reinstitution of a vaccine program.

Adverse reactions are common after DPT vaccination and are related mostly to the pertussis component. More than 60% of recipients experience reactions at the injection site and fever. About 1 in 2000 recipients have seizures; these seizures are related to the fever rather than to the vaccine itself. Serious neurological reactions leading to permanent brain damage or death have been ascribed to whole-cell pertussis vaccine. Because of these safety concerns, new **acellular pertussis vaccines** have been developed. These vaccines consist of inactivated bacterial components such as filamentous hemagglutinin, pertactin, and pertussis toxin. Field trials have shown higher protection rates and fewer side effects with the acellular vaccines compared to the standard whole-cell vaccine. It is expected that an acellular vaccine will replace the current pertussis component in the DPT vaccine by 1997.

USE OF BACILLE CALMETTE-GUERIN (BCG) AND VACCINIA VIRUS AS RECOMBINANT VACCINE VECTORS

Recent technological developments have enabled the introduction of **recombinant DNA** into avirulent but persistent agents, such as BCG (Bacille Calmette-Guerin) (Chapter 23, "Mycobacteria") and vaccinia virus. The feasibility of introducing foreign genes may lead to development of these agents into recombinant multiple vaccine vehicles. A multivaccine could be made by cloning a gene encoding a foreign antigen from another pathogen and inserting this gene into BCG or vaccinia virus. When the live, genetically engineered carrier agents are administered to an animal or human, protective immune responses would be elicited not only to these agents but also to the pathogenic agent from which the antigen was cloned.

BCG has numerous attractive advantages as a vaccine vector. First, BCG itself is a safe vaccine. Since 1948, it has been administered to over 2 billion people and the number of side effects is minimal. Second, BCG is the only live vaccine other than oral polio that can be administered soon after birth. This feature could increase the number of children that receive the vaccine and also allow for immunization against agents active early in life, such as measles. Third, BCG is a potent adjuvant and confers protection for a period of 5–50 years. Fourth, since BCG lives within macrophages, it provides the possibility of generating T-cell-mediated immunity to the cloned foreign antigen. A drawback of BCG is that it will only "take" if the person has no immunity to tuberculosis. BCG will not establish itself in people who have been colonized by *M. tuberculosis* or some other cross-reacting mycobacteria. For this reason, BCG can only be given once and more research is needed to formulate a BCG-recombinant vaccine that can be used on a wide scale. Similar considerations apply to a recombinant vaccinia virus multivaccine.

SUGGESTED READINGS

Guide for adult immunization. 3rd ed. Philadelphia: American College of Physicians, 1994;1–218.

Klein JO. Immunization of children and adults. 2nd ed. In: Gorbach SL, Bartlett JG, Blacklow N, eds. Infectious diseases. Philadelphia: WB Saunders, 1998.

Plotkin SA, Mortimer EA Jr, eds. Vaccines. Philadelphia: WB Saunders, 1988.

Recommendations of the Advisory Committee on Immunization Practices (ACIP). General recommendations on immunization. Morbid Mortal Weekly Rep (CDC) 1994;43(No. RR-1):1–38.

Review of the Main Pathogenic Viruses

This chart is intended to review the main human viruses. Included are the agents of greatest medical relevance. Many of the viruses that cause relatively uncommon diseases are not included. This chart may be completed to review material you have covered under this topic.

Virus	Group or Family	Nucleic Acid, Cellular Site of Replication State if Enveloped	Other Important Attributes	Disease(s) and Systems Involved	Relevant Chapters
Poliovirus					32
Coxsackie and other enteroviruses					32
Rhinoviruses					32
Arbovirus encephalitis					33
Rubella					33, 49
Measles					34
Respiratory syncytial virus					34
Rabies					35
Influenza					36
Rotavirus					37
HIV					38
Adenovirus					39
Papillomavirus					40
Herpes simplex					41
Epstein-Barr virus (EBV), cytomegalovirus (CMV, varicella-zoster)					41
Hepatitis A					32, 42
Hepatitis B					32
Smallpox					<?>

Fungi

CHAPTER 45

Introduction to the Fungi and the Mycoses

GEORGE S. KOBAYASHI

GERALD MEDOFF

Key Concepts

Pathogenic fungi:
- Are eukaryotes and belong to the kingdom Eumycota.
- Can be filamentous (molds) or unicellular (yeasts). Some species are dimorphic, i.e., can exist as both forms under different environmental conditions.
- Cause superficial, cutaneous, subcutaneous, or systemic infections.
- With some exceptions, are free-living in nature and are acquired from environmental sources.
- Cause damage by eliciting the inflammatory response or through direct invasion or destruction of tissues.

WHAT ARE THE PATHOGENIC FUNGI?

In many people's minds, the word "fungi" conjures up the image of mildew and old shoes, moldy bread, or skin infections with graphic names like "athlete's foot" or "jock itch." In fact, fungi have a major influence on the health and livelihood of people throughout the world. They cause a wide spectrum of clinical disease, from simple cosmetic problems to potentially lethal systemic infections. They also play an important role in degrading organic waste material in nature but are also economically destructive and cause widespread damage to food and fabrics. Finally, fungi are used commercially in many fermentations, and produce steroid hormone derivatives and antibiotics, such as penicillin.

Fungi are **eukaryotes**, with a defined nucleus enclosed by a nuclear membrane, a cell membrane that contains lipids, glycoproteins, and sterols, mitochondria, Golgi apparatus, ribosomes bound to endoplasmic reticulum, and a cytoskeleton with microtubules, microfilaments, and inter-mediate filaments (Chapter 3, "Biology of Infectious Agents"). Of course, this description applies to animal cells as well, a fact that constitutes a major problem when treating fungal infections. The infecting organisms are so similar to their host cells that it is difficult to devise therapeutic strategies specific for the parasite and nontoxic to the host.

SHAPES AND STRUCTURES

Pathogenic fungi have two forms, **filamentous**, the **molds**, and **unicellular**, the **yeasts**. Molds grow as microscopic, branching, threadlike filaments. These filaments are called **hyphae** and are collectively referred to as the **mycelium**. A mycelium is what you see when you look at the white mat on moldy fruit. The hyphae are either septate (divided by partitions) or coenocytic (multinucleate without cross walls), features that are used in laboratory diagnosis (Fig. 45.1). On agar, hyphae grow outward from the point of inoculation by extension of the tips of filaments and then branch repeatedly.

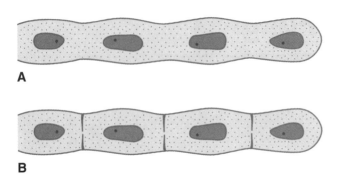

Figure 45.1. Somatic hyphae. A. Apical portion of non-septate (coenocytic) hypha; the protoplasm is continuous and multinucleated. **B.** Apical portion of septate hyphae; protoplasm is interrupted by cross walls.

Yeasts are single cells, ovoid or spherical, with a rigid cell wall and the same cellular complexity as the hyphae. Most yeasts divide by budding, although some species divide by binary fission like bacteria (Fig. 45.2). On agar, they form colonies that are similar to those of bacteria but usually become considerably larger. Some also produce a polysaccharide capsule, an important characteristic of the yeast that causes the disease cryptococcosis, *Cryptococcus neoformans.*

DIMORPHISM AND GROWTH

Many important pathogenic fungi display both growth forms and can exist either as molds or as yeasts. For example, the agent of histoplasmosis, *Histoplasma capsulatum* grows as yeast in some conditions and as mycelium in others (Fig. 45.3). This phenomenon is called **dimorphism**. In the laboratory, the transition between these two phases can be reversibly induced by changes in temperature; the yeast phase is more typical at human body temperature.

The yeast–mycelium or mycelium–yeast shift frequently occurs when a free-living organism becomes a parasite. With most fungi that cause systemic infections, e.g., the agents of histoplasmosis and blastomycosis, the yeast is the parasitic form, while the mold form is found in the environment (soil). In a few unusual instances, such as in *Candida*, this rule is reversed and the mycelial form is usually found in host tissues.

Not all pathogenic fungi are dimorphic and undergo morphological changes when they infect a host. Aspergilli, among the most common molds in the environment, are always filamentous, whereas *C. neoformans* is always a yeast. Certain yeasts, particularly species of *Candida*, carry out a modified form of budding in which newly budded cells remain attached to the parental cells and become elongated like links of sausages. These aggregates are called pseudohyphae or, in the aggregate, pseudomycelium (Fig. 45.4).

Most of the molecular biology and genetics of fungi has been studied using the common baker's or brewer's yeast, *Saccharomyces cerevisiae,* and to a lesser extent, the molds *Aspergillus nidulans* and *Neurospora crassa.* Less is known about pathogenic fungi, although active studies are being carried out on their virulence factors and dimorphic transitions. In the laboratory, most fungi are grown in media similar to those used for bacteria, although usually at a lower pH. All fungi are basically aerobic, but baker's yeast can grow for short periods without oxygen. In general, fungi prefer 25–30°C, although some of the organisms that cause deep mycoses grow well at 37°C and one thermophilic pathogen, *Aspergillus fumigatus,* grows well up to 50°C.

Fungi belong to a discrete kingdom, the **Eumycota,** and are classified on the basis of their mode of sexual and asexual reproduction, morphology, life cycles, and to some extent, physiology. Until recently, the mode of sexual reproduction of most human fungal pathogens was unknown. For this reason, they were dumped into a catch-all category, the **Fungi imperfecti.** Since the 1960s, researchers have elucidated the sexual reproductive states of an increasing number of skin pathogenic fungi. Although the rules of nomenclature give preference to names of the "perfect" or sexual state (if known), the longer-established and more familiar names of the imperfect state are still used because the asexual phase is routinely isolated on primary culture. Thus, the diagnostic laboratory will report the isolation of *C. neoformans* or *H. capsulatum* rather than the less familiar names of the sexual states.

MYCOSES

Fungal infections can be classified by areas of the body that are primarily affected.

- **Superficial mycoses** are infections limited to the outermost layers of skin and hair. These are generally mild infections with minimal or no inflammatory response. They are mainly cosmetic problems that are readily diagnosed and respond well to therapy. Four infections comprise this group. Two involve hairs of the scalp (black and white piedra), and two involve

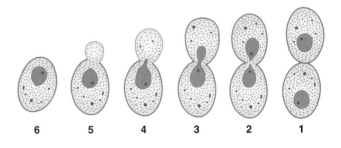

Figure 45.2. Vegetative reproduction of yeast. Cell reproducing by budding (blastospores formation).

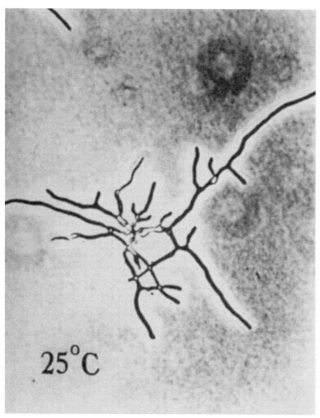

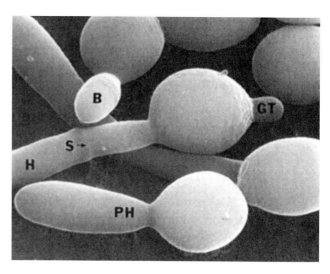

Figure 45.4. Electron photomicrograph of *Candida albicans*. The following cellular morphological characters are illustrated: pseudohypha (*PH*); hypha (*H*) with septum (*S*); germtube (*GT*); blastospore (*B*).

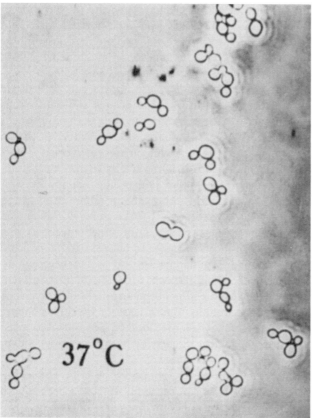

Figure 45.3. Temperature-induced morphogenesis in *Histoplasma capsulatum*. Cultures grow in the mycelial phase at 25°C and as yeasts at 37°C.

the glabrous (hairless) skin (tinea nigra and tinea versicolor).

- Slightly deeper in the epidermis are found the sites of the **cutaneous mycoses**, like **athlete's foot** or **ringworm**. These conditions are caused by fungi called the **dermatophytes**. The diseases they cause may be acute or chronic, depending on the etiological agent and immunological status of the patient. In general, these conditions are more difficult to treat than the superficial fungal infections. The etiological agents belong to three genera, *Microsporum*, *Trichophyton*, and *Epidermophyton*. The clinical diseases are called the **tineas** and are described according to the area of the body involved (e.g., tinea capitis involves the head, tinea pedis the feet, tinea corporis the body, etc.)

- The **subcutaneous mycoses** are a distinctive group of fungal diseases that involve the dermis and the subcutaneous tissue. They are caused by fungi that are commonly isolated from the environment and produce disease only under circumstances that are associated with trauma. Many of these infections mimic those caused by bacteria. With two exceptions (lymphangitic sporotrichosis and chromoblastomycosis), subcutaneous mycoses do not respond well to antifungal chemotherapy. Excision of the lesion or amputation is sometimes necessary to manage these infections. Examples are subcutaneous phycomycosis, eumycotic mycetoma, phaeohyphomycosis, chromoblastomycosis, and lymphangitic sporotrichosis.

- **Systemic mycoses** are infections that invade the internal organs of the body. Systemic mycoses are caused by **primary pathogens**, such as *H. capsulatum* or

Coccidioides immitis, which affect healthy individuals, or they may be caused by **opportunistic fungi,** such as *Candida albicans*, which are only marginally pathogenic and generally require a debilitated host for progressive infection to take place. In the primary systemic mycoses, most healthy people affected usually have mild signs or subclinical manifestations. In contrast, opportunistic fungal infections in the debilitated host almost always produce significant disease.

ENCOUNTER

With a handful of important exceptions, fungi implicated in human diseases are **free-living** in nature. Most mycoses are acquired as a result of accidental encounters by inhalation or traumatic implantation from an exogenous source. For example, *H. capsulatum* is found in soil contaminated by the excreta of bats, chickens, and starlings. *C. neoformans* is associated with pigeon roosts and soils contaminated by pigeon droppings.

Some fungi have distinct **geographic preferences.** Thus, *Coccidioides immitis* is found in the bioclimatic area known as the Lower Sonoran life zone of the southwestern U.S. and similar geographic sites in Central and South America. This region has arid or semiarid climates, hot summers, few winter freezes, and alkaline soils. *C. immitis* has been found only in the New World (North, Central, and South America). Thus, paracoccidioidomycosis, a disease caused by *Paracoccidioides brasiliensis*, is geographically limited to South and Central America. *Blastomyces dermatitidis*, once thought to exist only in the North American continent, has been found to have endemic foci in Africa. *Sporothrix schenckii*, an agent of subcutaneous mycoses, has been isolated frequently from rose and barberry thorns and decaying vegetation.

In contrast to these environmental habitats, many of us carry *C. albicans* in the mouth, gastrointestinal tract, and other mucous membrane linings as part of our normal flora. *Malassezia furfur* (*Pityrosporum ovale*) are yeasts found on the healthy human skin, particularly in the upper trunk, face, and scalp, the areas that are rich in sebaceous glands, which produce lipids used by these organisms. Finally, dermatophytes that cause ringworm and athlete's foot are occasionally found on the skin and scalp of individuals in the absence of symptoms; they are thought to represent transient colonization or a carrier state.

ENTRY

The level of innate immunity to pathogenic fungi is high in most humans, as witnessed by the fact that fungal infections are usually mild and self-limiting. The intact skin or mucosal surfaces are the primary barriers to infection. Desiccation, epithelial cell turnover, fatty acids, and the low pH of the skin are believed to be important factors in host resistance. In addition, the bacterial flora of the skin and mucous membranes compete with fungi and hinder their unrestricted growth. Alterations in the balance of the normal flora by use of antibiotics or changes in nutrition allow fungi such as *C. albicans* to proliferate, thus increasing the likelihood of entry and infection. Violation of the natural barriers by trauma or foreign bodies allows entry of fungi into sterile areas of the body. As in all infections, the outcome is determined by the virulence of the infecting organism, the size of the inoculum, and the adequacy of the host defenses.

SPREAD AND MULTIPLICATION

Within host tissues, fungi are restrained by a variety of nonspecific mechanisms. Using *C. albicans* as an example, the fungistatic effect of serum has been shown to be due, in part, to transferrins, the human iron-binding proteins that deprive microbes of the iron they need for making respiratory enzymes. In addition, β-globulins found in serum cause a nonimmunological clumping of *Candida* and facilitate their elimination by inflammatory cells.

Tissue reaction to the presence of fungi varies with the species, the site of proliferation, and the duration of infection. Some mycoses are characterized by a low-grade inflammatory response, which does not eliminate the fungi. Fungal cells can sometimes persist within macrophages or giant cells without being killed. For example, yeast cells of *H. capsulatum* can proliferate within the cytoplasm of macrophages and neutrophils and spread to other organs of the body within those cells (Fig. 45.5). Why they are able to survive within macrophages is not known, but recent work suggests that they may neutralize the acidity of the phagolysosome. In general, however, nonspecific inflammatory reactions are critically important in eliminating fungi. Phagocytosis by neutrophils is the primary mechanism that prevents the establishment of fungal infections, and is usually the most effective. In fact, the frequency and virulence of disseminated *Candida* and *Aspergillus* infections is greater in patients with low numbers of neutrophils or with disorders of neutrophil functions, such as chronic granulomatous disease or myeloperoxidase deficiency. In the case of *Candida*, phagocytized yeast cells are killed intracellularly by both oxygen-dependent and -independent mechanisms.

Sometimes, however, phagocytosis fails. For example, *C. neoformans* can cause meningitis in people with normal phagocytic function. Just as with the encapsulated bacteria, these organisms escape phagocytosis because they are surrounded by a thick viscous **capsule.**

Fungi that are too big to be ingested can, nevertheless, be killed by immunological mechanisms. Fungal cells

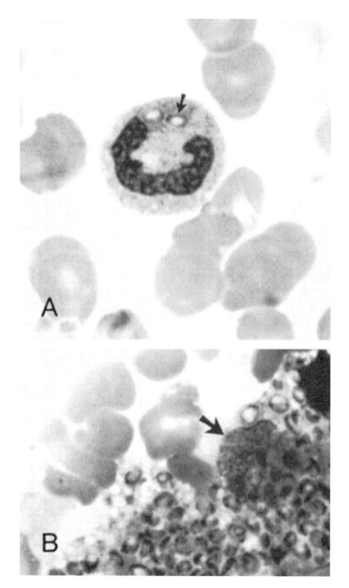

Figure 45.5. A. Peripheral blood smear showing neutrophil with phagocytized yeast cells (*arrow*) of *Histoplasma capsulatum*. **B.** Bone marrow aspirate showing histiocytes (*arrow*) filled with phagocytized yeast cells of *H. capsulatum*.

and their extracellular products are highly antigenic and evoke both cellular and humoral responses. Evidence exists that antibodies play a role in the elimination of fungi from the body. Along with complement, antibodies participate in the extracellular killing of *A. fumigatus* and pseudohyphae of *C. albicans* by lymphocytes and phagocytic cells (Fig. 45.6). Instead of "ingesting" and "digesting" the fungi, phagocytic cells appear to secrete lethal lysosomal enzymes.

Resistance to fungal disease is due mainly to cellular- or T-lymphocyte-mediated immunity. This can be inferred from animal experiments and from the clinical observation that patients with depressed cellular immunity are especially prone to invasive and serious systemic fungal disease. For example, patients with AIDS commonly have mucocutaneous candidiasis and serious systemic infections with *C. neoformans*. As can be expected, patients with AIDS who live in endemic areas have an increased propensity to acquire or to activate the fungi that cause disseminated histoplasmosis or coccidioidomycosis.

DAMAGE

Fungi that cause invasive disease are not known to secrete toxins that harm the host. Tissue damage most probably results from direct invasion with displacement, destruction of vital structures, and toxic effects of the inflammatory response. Fungi may also grow as masses of cells (fungus balls) that can occlude bronchi in the lung or tubules or even ureters in kidneys, leading to obstruction of outflow of biological fluids (sputum, urine) and

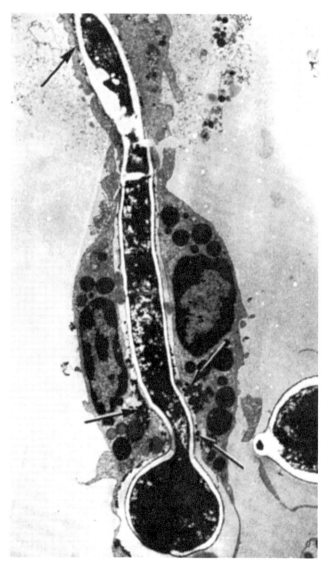

Figure 45.6. Electron photomicrograph of phagocytic cell ingesting a hypha of *Candida albicans* (*arrows*).

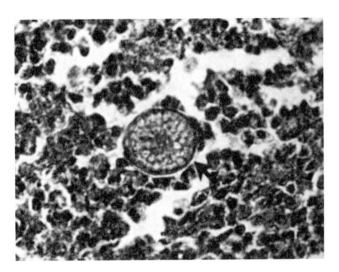

Figure 45.7. Surgical specimen of lung showing mature spherule of *Coccidioides immitis*–containing endospores.

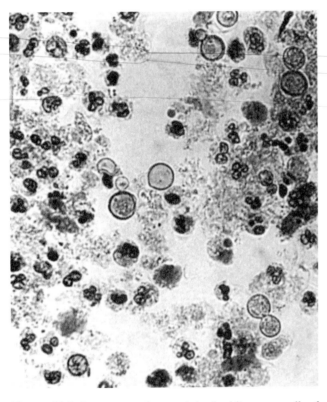

Figure 45.8. Sputum sample containing budding yeast cells of *Blastomyces dermatitidis*.

secondary infection and tissue damage. *Aspergillus* and *Mucor* species have a propensity for growth in the walls of arteries or veins, leading to occlusion and ischemic tissue necrosis. Mats of fungi are formed as vegetations on heart valves in fungal endocarditis. Pieces of these fungal mats can break off and travel through the blood to any organ in the body and cause arterial occlusion with resultant tissue necrosis.

DIAGNOSIS

Fungal infections are diagnosed in the laboratory by **direct microscopy, culture,** and **serology.** Morphological characteristics of the organisms aid in the identification of all fungi, both in tissues and in culture. These are particularly useful in the diagnosis of serious systemic infections. Among the distinctive characteristics are the spherules of *C. immitis* in tissue (Fig. 45.7), the typical large budding yeasts of *B. dermatitidis* in pus (Fig. 45.8), the coenocytic hyphae of mucormycosis (Fig. 45.9), and the encapsulated yeast cells of *C. neoformans* in cerebrospinal fluid or brain tissue (Fig. 47.3). Their detection provides an immediate and reliable diagnosis in systemic infections. For opportunistic pathogens such as *Mucor, Candida, and Aspergillus*, microscopic examination of clinical specimens is particularly useful because culture alone may not be helpful (inasmuch as these organisms are in the environment and can be part of the normal flora of the body). Here, histological evidence of infection in tissue is usually the single most valuable diagnostic procedure, although a negative finding does not rule out infection.

Pathogenic fungi may also be recovered from infected tissues using **culture procedures.** When the organism isolated is a primary pathogen, such as *H. capsulatum*, the diagnosis is unequivocal. Isolation of opportunistic or-

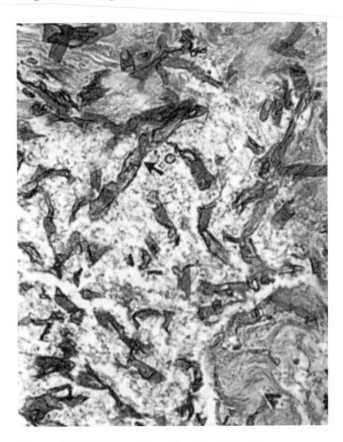

Figure 45.9. Section of lung showing ribbonlike nonseptate hyphae (*arrows*) characteristic of agents such as *Mucor* spp. that cause zygomycosis.

Table 45.1. Antifungal Antibiotics

Class	Compounds	Mechanism	Uses
Polyene	Amphotericin B Nystatin	Binds to sterols causing perturbations in cell membrane	Systemic disease Topical disease
Azole	Clotrimazole Miconazole Ketoconazole Fluconazole Itraconazole	Inhibits ergosterol biosynthesis	Topical disease; systemic disease
Pyrimidine	5-fluorocytosine (5FC)	Inhibits DNA and RNA synthesis	Systemic disease
Grisans	Griseofulvin	Inhibits microtubule assembly	Topical disease

ganisms like *Candida* from superficial locations may have little clinical significance because it could represent colonization, but culturing these organisms from blood is always significant.

Culturing clinical specimens does not always result in growth of the organism. For example, invasive *Aspergillus* infections yield positive blood cultures in less than 10% of cases. We do not know why. Perhaps only a small portion of the mycelium is actively growing and capable of producing a positive culture, or possibly, a large inoculum of these fungi is required for growth in vitro.

Because fungi grow slowly, there is often considerable delay between the time the specimen is obtained and a positive culture. Relying on the results of the cultures may, therefore, cause a significant delay in starting therapy. Despite these limitations, cultures should always be performed because when they work, they work well.

Detection of antibodies specific for fungal antigens is sometimes helpful in diagnosis, particularly for the deep-seated mycoses. Many serological and skin tests are available, but the results provide only presumptive evidence for infection and must be interpreted in light of clinical findings. It is particularly difficult to interpret the significance of positive skin tests to *H. capsulatum* in parts of the world where the disease is endemic. Almost everyone living in these areas has been exposed to this fungus and has developed a **positive skin test** indicative of delayed-type hypersensitivity. The tests are further limited in usefulness because the antigens available are not sufficiently specific. False-positive tests may also be due to symptomless colonization, previous subclinical infections, or anamnestic response owing to previous skin tests. Delayed or false-negative responses, particularly in the immunosuppressed host, may also be a problem.

Recently, procedures for detecting circulating fungal antigens in body fluids have been developed. The most successful one detects soluble capsular polysaccharides of *C. neoformans* in cerebrospinal fluid. It is highly specific and sensitive. Similar tests for other fungi are not available but are currently under development.

TREATMENT

It is extremely important to realize that not all fungal infections require treatment. As stated previously, humans have a high innate resistance to most of these agents. Most infections with *H. capsulatum* or *C. immitis* are subclinical, self-limiting, and do not result in disease. Some candidal infections respond to supportive measures, such as improving the nutritional status of the host or eliminating predisposing factors, e.g., intravenous lines, catheters, and the administration of broad-spectrum antibiotics. These fungal infections are easily managed when predisposing factors are recognized and corrected.

Most antifungal agents in common use target fungi more than host cells, but not by much (Chapter 5, "Biological Basis for Antibacterial Action"). Toxicity is a problem in the treatment of these diseases. In addition, many antifungal compounds have limited therapeutic value because of problems with solubility, stability, and absorption. Compared to antibacterial agents, the number of effective antifungal agents is quite small. With the increase in frequency of fungal infections, the search for additional effective agents has expanded.

Most useful antifungal antibiotics fall into one of two categories: those that affect fungal cell membranes, and those that are taken up by the cell and interrupt cellular processes (Chapter 5, "Biological Basis for Antibacterial Action"). Table 45.1 lists some of the useful antifungal agents and their most likely mechanisms of action.

SUGGESTED READINGS

Chandler FW, Kaplan W, Ajello L. Histopathology of mycotic infections. Chicago: Year Book, 1980.

Kwon-Chung KJ, Bennett JE. Medical mycology. Philadelphia: Lea and Febiger, 1992.

Medoff G, Brajtburg J, Kobayashi GS, Bolard J. Antifungal agents useful in therapy of systemic fungal infections. Ann Rev Pharmacol 1983;23:303–330.

Sutcliffe J, Georgopapakakou NH: Emerging targets in antibacterial and antifungal chemotherapy. New York: Chapman and Hall, 1992.

CHAPTER 46

Systemic Mycoses Caused by Primary Pathogens

GERALD MEDOFF

GEORGE S. KOBAYASHI

Key Concepts

A paradigm of systemic mycoses caused by primary pathogens, *Histoplasma capsulatum*:

- Is a soil organism whose growth is enhanced by bird or bat excreta.
- Causes histoplasmosis in an area of the midwestern United Stated called the "histo belt."
- Transforms into a yeast when exposed to internal body temperatures.
- Enters macrophages and resists phagocytosis if the size of inoculum is large or the macrophages are not activated.
- Histoplasmosis resembles tuberculosis. The organisms may remain viable within calcified lesions and thus can be reactivated.
- Causes progressive histoplasmosis in immunodeficient patients.

INTRODUCTION

In this chapter we discuss the systemic fungal infections caused by primary pathogens. The distinguishing features of these infections are that they may affect healthy people, whereas another group of fungi are usually seen in immunodeficient patients only. The mycotic infections caused by primary pathogens are caused by fungi that often have a geographic predilection, such as the San Joaquin Valley of California for coccidioidomycosis, or the midwestern United States for histoplasmosis. The diseases they cause are generally chronic and have a clinical picture resembling that of tuberculosis. To illustrate this kind of diseases, we will use histoplasmosis as an example.

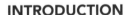 CASES

An Outbreak

Thirty-five members of several families from the Midwest camped on a farm in northwestern Tennessee for 2 weeks. In return for the use of the site, they helped the farmer clean out an old barn on the property. The barn had not been used for about 20 years and had become a gathering place for starlings. The walls and ground were caked with bird droppings and, inasmuch as the weather had been dry, considerable dust was stirred up when the campers raked the ground. The cleaning took several hours. Everyone then went home.

Over the next 6–12 days, 18 members of the group got sick with chills, fever, cough, and headache (Table 46.1). Several had substernal discomfort and others had painful red bumps on the front of their legs below the knee. Two patients had severe joint pains that shifted from the knees to the ankles and wrists.

In approximately 2 weeks, 14 of the campers got well without treatment. Several of these patients had seen their physician and had chest x-rays. These x-rays showed infiltrates that disappeared after several weeks. Repeat chest x-rays on these patients 1 year later showed calcified hilar lymph nodes and calcified nodules in the periphery of the lungs (Fig. 46.1). Over the next year, one of these patients

Table 46.1. Outcome of Infection with *H. capsulatum* in 35 Patients

Number of patients	Clinical course	Physical findings	Chest X-rays	Laboratory results
17	Asymptomatic	None	Lung infiltrates or mild increase in lymph node size, calcifications	Positive antibody reaction to antigens of *H. capsulatum*; positive skin tests with histoplasmin
18	Symptoms	Enlarged lymph nodes, rales on auscultation, skin lesions	Patchy infiltrates, enlarged hilar lymph nodes, calcified lymph nodes with calcified granulomas in the lung	Most developed; positive antibody tests; most developed positive skin tests with histoplasmin antigen; cultures of sputum of the 14 patients were positive for *H. capsulatum*

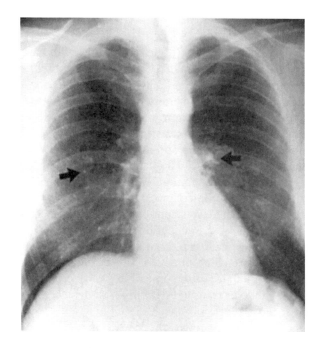

Figure 46.1. Chest x-ray showing calcifications of the lung and mediastinal lymph nodes consistent with healed histoplasmosis.

developed shortness of breath and progressive swelling of the lower extremities and the face. Subsequent x-rays showed a mass in his mediastinum, which compressed several bronchi. A venogram showed compression of the superior and inferior vena cava as well. Four of the other campers developed progressive histoplasmosis.

This is a description of a typical outbreak of histoplasmosis, the disease caused by *Histoplasma capsulatum*. Analysis of the case histories (Table 46.1) will reveal the most important points about the pathophysiology of the disease.

ENCOUNTER

The outbreak occurred in Tennessee, which is located in the so-called **"histo belt,"** a geographic area in the southeastern United States bordering the Mississippi and Ohio River valleys. The outbreak described is typical because cases often occur in clusters after a common exposure. The endemic zone extends through many of the tropical countries of the world. A clinically distinct form of histoplasmosis occurs in Africa (caused by a variety known as *Histoplasma capsulatum* var. *duboisii*) and affects subcutaneous tissue, the skin, and bones, with little or no evidence of pulmonary disease.

H. capsulatum is a soil organism whose growth is enhanced by bird or bat excreta. Common sources of infection are spores present in old barns used as roosting sites by starlings, grackles, or chickens. Bat-roosting sites, such as trees or caves, are also important sources of the organism, particularly in the tropics. In the outbreak described, the dry weather, coupled with the vigorous activities of the group, led to the aerosolization of spores and fragments of hyphae. The particles were inhaled, and their small size allowed them to evade the anatomic defense mechanisms of the respiratory tract and reach the alveoli of the lung (Chapter 59, "Respiratory System").

ENTRY

The events following entry of *H. capsulatum* into the alveoli are unknown, but based on the physiology of the organism and the relevant factors in host defense, we can construct the following scheme: when spores or mycelial fragments of *H. capsulatum* are exposed to human body temperatures of 37°C, they transform into the yeast phase. Experiments with animals indicate that this transformation is required for pathogenicity. Also, only yeast cells are seen in tissues of infected hosts. The virulence of different strains of *H. capsulatum* is related to their level of tolerance to the elevated temperature; low levels of virulence and tolerance to elevated temperatures are associated with a delayed transformation to the yeast phase and slower growth of the yeast.

SPREAD AND MULTIPLICATION

In tissue, yeast cells of *H. capsulatum* are found within macrophages only. However, phagocytosis does not always lead to killing, and the intracellular habitat paradoxically results in protection of the fungus from other defenses of the host. What determines whether or not the macrophages will kill the yeast phase? Here again, we lack information but the following factors are probably important:

- If the inoculum of organisms is very large, macrophages are simply overwhelmed by the sheer numbers of organisms.
- Macrophages have to be activated to kill the fungi efficiently. Activation of macrophages, which occurs rapidly in a host sensitized by previous infection, limits the infection.
- After ingestion, the organisms avoid being killed, perhaps by preventing the oxygen burst, or phagosome–lysosome fusion, or by resisting or neutralizing the degradative effects of lysosomes.

The outcome of the initial interaction between the host cells and the fungi is either death of the organisms or inhibition of their multiplication and spread to local lymphatics and from there to other organs. After 1–2 weeks, cellular immunity is stimulated and host reticuloendothelial cells become more efficient in limiting growth and multiplication of the fungus. The infection is thus curtailed and eventually resolves. However, yeast cells may remain viable within calcified lesions for years and may be a source for reactivation of infection when immunity wanes. This sequence of events is the same as in tuberculosis, and, in fact, the granulomas formed in response to *H. capsulatum* are very similar to those seen in tuberculosis (and, for that matter, all primary systemic mycoses).

Seventeen of the people exposed to *H. capsulatum* in the barn were asymptomatic. Perhaps they only inhaled a small number of organisms or had been sensitized by prior infection to deal efficiently with renewed exposure. About 80–90% of adults who have lived in the "histo belt" have positive skin tests to antigens of *H. capsulatum*, evidence of their cellular immunity. This test is analogous to the tuberculin test or to the one used to determine exposure to *Coccidioides immitis*, the fungus that causes coccidioidomycosis.

DAMAGE

Fourteen of the people presented here experienced a self-limited disease that disappeared, presumably as cel-

lular immunity developed. These people were left with the scars of the disease, seen on chest x-rays as calcified granulomas (Fig. 46.1). It is not known why calcifications occur, but macrophages in granulomas make a factor that elevates calcium levels in the blood. All of these people had elevated antibody titers to fungal antigens. One person in this group developed a particularly intense immune response, which resulted in a proliferative tissue reaction (mediastinal granulomatosis). Eventually, the advanced fibrosis impinged on vital structures in the chest (sclerosing mediastinitis). This process was not due to active infection but to the immune response gone awry. This rare complication of infection with *H. capsulatum* can only be treated by surgical removal of the fibrotic tissue.

Each of the four people who developed progressive disease after the initial infection illustrates the failure of an important component of host defenses to limit infection.

- Patient A had severe chronic obstructive pulmonary disease and emphysema. Because of the anatomic abnormalities and scarring in his lung, he could not clear the infection. An effective systemic response and the use of potent antifungal therapy limited the infection to the lung. Increasing damage to the lung by continued infection and local spread resulted in further destruction and a relentless downhill course until he died from pulmonary insufficiency 5 years after the onset of infection.
- In Patient B, there was continued disease in the lungs and, ultimately, dissemination of the infection to other organs. Failure to limit and to contain the infection may have resulted from a particularly large inoculum inhaled at the time of exposure or from some subtle or transient defect in host defenses. In disseminated histoplasmosis, T-cell function is defective but it is not known whether this is the cause or the result of the disease. One of the manifestations of the disease is ulcerations of the oral mucosa. It is not unusual to find mucosal lesions as the sole sign of disease. We do not understand why *H. capsulatum* has this unusual tropism for mucous membranes. It is not unique to this disease, but does help in the diagnosis. The fungus also spreads to many other organs, including the bone marrow and the adrenal glands, where it causes insufficiency of adrenal function (Addison's disease), a complication also seen in disseminated tuberculosis. This patient was treated with ketoconazole and eventually recovered. In general, when disseminated disease is diagnosed early in an otherwise apparently normal host, the prognosis is good.
- Patient C suffered an acute overwhelming pulmonary infection, probably because she had been previously sensitized and, on this occasion, may have inhaled a

Table 46.2. Systemic Mycoses Caused by Primary Pathogens

Disease	Etiologic agent	Epidemiology	Clinical disease	Histopathology	Therapy
Histo-plasmosis	*Histoplasma capsulatum:* dimorphic; mycelial in the environment; in tissue, a budding yeast found within phagocytes	Endemic in the U.S. in the Ohio and Mississippi River valleys; also worldwide; Soil organism whose growth is enhanced in locations contaminated by bird or bat excreta	About 90% of all primary cases are not clinically significant; In the endemic area, many individuals have x-ray signs consistent with past disease (i.e., calcification) but cannot give a history of relevant infections; they will require treatment; here there may be underlying conditions that makes these individuals prone to progressive disease	Yeasts are usually found within histiocytes; there are epithelioid granulomas	Ketoconazole is the drug of choice; amphotericin B is used in treatment of failures or rapidly progressive disease
Blasto-mycosis	*Blastomyces dermatitidis:* dimorphic; in tissue, a yeast with buds attached to parent cell by broad base usually found in microabscesses	Isolated cases occur all over North America	Pulmonary infection with chronic skin and bone disease; other forms are urogenital disseminated disease involving multiple organs; like the fungi causing the other primary systemic infections, the organism is inhaled and invades via the lungs; however, in disseminated disease the lung fields are frequently clear and free of disease	Large budding yeasts with broad bases are characteristic and seen in microabscesses and granulomas	Same drugs as in histoplasmosis
Coccidioi-domycosis	*Coccidioides immitis:* dimorphic; in tissues, the organism develops into a sporangium ("spherule") 10 to 70 μm in diameter, filled with endospores	Southwestern U.S. and parts of Central and South America; epidemics may be associated with dust storms	Approximatedly 60% of these infections are asymptomatic; 40% are symptomatic with the spectrum of disease ranging from mild influenzae-like complaints to frank pneumonia and spread to other areas of the body, including the central nervous system; dark-skinned patients (African-Americans and Orientals) appear to be more prone to develop progressive disseminated disease	Pyogenic, granulomatous, and mixed cellular reactions are present; spherules and endospores are seen	Ketoconazole is effective in nonmeningeal disease; parental amphotericin B and direct instillation of the drug into the CNS is required to treat meningitis; oral fluconazole may be effective in CNS
Paracoccidi-oidomycosis	*Paracoccidioides brasiliensis:* dimorphic; in tissues, a yeast with several budding cells attached to its surface	Most countries of South America and parts of Central America. The infection is strikingly more common in males than in females	Pulmonary disease is often inapparent, as in blastomycosis; ulcerative granulomas of buccal, nasal, and occasionally the gastrointestinal mucosa indicate dissemination	Very similar to that seen in blastomycosis	Itraconazole or fluconazole is effective; amphotericin B is used in treatment failures

very large inoculum. The damage to her lungs probably resulted from direct tissue damage by the fungi and from the inflammatory reaction made more severe by the previous sensitization. This patient was critically ill because her pulmonary function was severely compromised. After treatment with amphotericin B, the patient improved and the pulmonary infiltrates cleared rapidly.

- Patient D had AIDS. Because he lacked a normal T-cell response, he succumbed to an overwhelming infection, which spread to every organ. He was unresponsive to intensive therapy with amphotericin B. This patient's clinical course underlines the importance of the cooperation between host defenses and chemotherapy for a successful outcome. Disseminated histoplasmosis occurs in patients with AIDS either as the result of newly acquired infection or by reactivation of old disease. Like the tubercle bacillus, *H. capsulatum* may persist in a dormant state in cells of the reticuloendothelial system for many years after primary infection and may reactivate when host resistance becomes severely impaired.

OTHER SYSTEMIC MYCOSES

The pathophysiology and clinical manifestations of histoplasmosis are very similar to those of the other primary systemic mycoses listed in Table 46.2 and all can be categorized along with tuberculosis as granulomatous infections.

SUGGESTED READINGS

Bradsher DA. Blastomycosis. Inf Dis Clin North Am 1988; 2:877–898.

Stevens DA. Coccidioidomycosis, a text. New York: Plenum, 1983.

Wheat JL. Histoplasma. In: Gorbach SL, Bartlett JG, Blacklow NR. Infectious Diseases. 2nd ed. Philadelphia: WB Saunders, 1998, 2335.2346.

Derensk: SC, Kemper CA. *Coccidioides immitis*. In: Gorbach SL, Bartlett J.G., Blacklow NR. Infectious Diseases. 2nd ed. Philadelphia: WB Saunders, 1998, 2344–2361.

Systemic Mycoses Caused by Opportunistic Fungi

GERALD MEDOFF

GEORGE S. KOBAYASHI

Key Concepts

Opportunistic fungi:
- Are not very pathogenic and therefore only infect individuals with impaired defenses, particularly a decreased number of functioning neutrophils.
- Include *Candida albicans*, which is part of the normal flora.
- Also include *Aspergillus fumigatus*, an environmental pathogen that causes invasive disease in profoundly immunocompromised patients.
- Include *Cryptococcus neoformans*, a common cause of meningitis in AIDS patients, and other species.

The more pathogenic the infecting microorganism, the less host susceptibility it needs to cause disease. The fungi we describe in this chapter are not very pathogenic. Therefore, these fungi only cause disease when host resistance is decreased. Understanding the underlying host defects in opportunistic fungal infections may allow us to identify persons with predisposing factors and to take steps to reverse or reduce the conditions that predispose these individuals to these infections. If we cannot accomplish this, the prognosis is often serious.

Patients at high risk for opportunistic fungal infections include individuals with malignancies, organ or bone marrow transplants, AIDS, burns, trauma, or illnesses that require long-term use of intravenous or intra-arterial catheters. Patients who have undergone bone or organ transplants and other surgical procedures are also at risk. In addition, opportunistic fungal infections occur in patients who have received broad-spectrum antibacterial therapy and whose normal intestinal bacterial flora has markedly decreased. In such cases, fungi like

Candida albicans proliferate unchecked and can replace the bacteria of the normal flora.

On the basis of clinical experience, a decrease in the number of functioning neutrophils is the most important host defect that affects the response to fungal infection. These infections are difficult to treat in a normal host, but cure is almost impossible when there are few functioning white cells. Premature babies and the elderly also tend to do poorly when infected with fungi.

The weakly pathogenic fungi that cause opportunistic systemic mycoses are nearly ubiquitous. They may be part of our flora or they may be inhaled or ingested from the environment.

A CASE OF ENDOGENOUS INFECTION

A 19-year-old woman, Ms. J., was involved in a bicycle accident and sustained severe cervical spinal cord trauma resulting in quadriplegia. She required an indwelling urinary catheter, which led to multiple urinary tract infections. These infections were treated with a variety of broad-spectrum antibiotics. She has also had several episodes of *Candida* infections of her mouth, perineal area, and vagina.

At the time of the present admission to the hospital, Ms. J. again had signs and symptoms of urinary tract infection, including cloudy urine and fever. On the tenth hospital day, urography revealed an enlarged left kidney with delayed function and poor urine concentration.

Microscopic examination of sediment obtained by centrifuging urine samples and specimens of tissue obtained surgically showed budding yeast cells, pseudohyphae, and hyphal elements; this evidence permitted a rapid presumptive diagnosis of *Candida* infection. Further laboratory tests identified the organism as *C. albicans*. Blood cultures taken after a febrile episode grew the same organism.

C. albicans is the most frequent species that causes this type of infection, although infection may also be due to other species. Careful examination of the retina with an ophthalmoscope revealed a "fluffy" cottony growth caused by the organism. Ms. J.'s heart valve became infected and she developed a heart murmur. In addition, she developed weakness on the right side of her face.

Candida are present in the posterior pharynx and the bowel of many healthy individuals. In the case of Ms. J., overgrowth of this organism occurred because the normal flora was suppressed by the multiple courses of antibiotics. This yeast then contaminated the bladder and the infection spread into the urinary system. *Candida* appears to have a particular tropism for the kidney. From the kidney, the yeast probably spread through the blood to the several different organs described above. This spread was probably a result of an organism-laden clot that traveled to her brain from her infected heart valve. Disseminated candidiasis often follows such a series of devastating events. Systemic infection is usually preceded by other superficial infections, such as those involving the mouth, pharynx, esophagus or other parts of the gastrointestinal tract or the vagina.

All forms of systemic *Candida* infections are potentially life-threatening and require therapy. Consideration should always be given to the primary predisposing factors, and these should be minimized or reversed. In the case of Ms. J., the catheter and intravenous lines were probably infected at the time of the candidemia and had to be replaced. Ms. J. received carefully monitored doses of amphotericin B and 5-fluorocytosine. Had the response not been adequate, Ms. J.'s infected heart valve would have had to be removed and replaced by a prosthesis.

This case is an example of an opportunistic infection resulting from anatomic defects in the host. The white blood count and the immune responses were normal, yet successful management with antifungal drugs required repair of the anatomic defects. The prognosis is guarded.

■ CASE

Exogenous Infection

Mr. S., a 25-year-old man, was hospitalized for treatment of acute lymphocytic leukemia. The initial diagnosis was made 20 months earlier when he complained of general malaise and weakness. At that time, his white blood cell count was greater than 100,000/mm^3 with 93% lymphocytes and lymphoblasts, all values much greater than normal. A bone marrow aspiration established the diagnosis of leukemia. He was treated with anticancer drugs, which produced a complete remission.

One year later he had a relapse of leukemia. He was treated with large doses of the anticancer agents cyclophosphamide and cytarabine, which resulted in leukopenia and thrombocytopenia. A chest x-ray showed nodular lesions in both lungs. Blood cultures were negative. Microscopic examination of sputum specimens and a skin biopsy of a purpuric lesion revealed septate branching hyphae 7–10 μm in diameter and several hundred micrometers in length (Fig. 47.1). Cultures resulted in colonies of a white mold that quickly developed a smoky gray color. This, and the shape and arrangement of the asexual spores identified the organism as *Aspergillus fumigatus*.

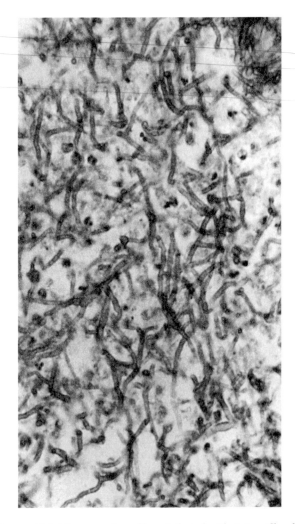

Figure 47.1. Tissue section of lung infected with *Aspergillus fumigatus*. Septate hyphae and dichotomous branching are characteristic features of organisms belonging to this group of fungi.

Serological tests yielded an antibody titer of 1:4 to *Aspergillus* antigens, which is not diagnostic for *A. fumigatus* infection. Nevertheless, based on the clinical findings and the microscopic and culture results, a diagnosis of invasive aspergillosis was made. Therapy with amphotericin B was immediately initiated on Mr. S. Treatment for fungal infections in this kind of host is often initiated on the basis of clinical suspicion because diagnosis by culture of blood or other body fluids is inconclusive.

Aspergilli are a group of molds so ubiquitous that they may be easily cultured from the air, soil, or moldy vegetation. The major pathogenic species is *A. fumigatus*, but others may also cause disease. They are not part of the normal flora of humans and do not grow in normal tissue. They cause invasive disease only in profoundly immunocompromised subjects, particularly those with neutropenia, like Mr. S. The initial site of invasion is usually the lung or the paranasal sinuses, which was probably the case in this patient. The lesions seen in x-rays include focal consolidation, lobar pneumonia, and lung cavities that contain "fungus balls" of the mold (Fig. 47.2). Patients with such invasive infections also have intracerebral abscesses, necrotic ulcers of skin, and lesions of bone, liver, and the breast.

Aspergillus may also cause noninfectious disease, such as allergy or asthma following inhalation and growth of the fungus in the bronchial tree (**allergic bronchopulmonary aspergillosis**. They also elaborate toxic metabolic products, the **aflatoxins**, which are hepatotoxic or carcinogenic, although their role in cancers of humans has not been established.

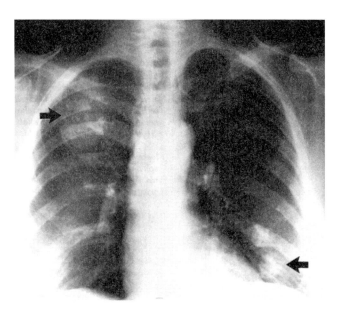

Figure 47.2. A chest x-ray of primary *Aspergillus* pneumonia *with "fungus balls"* (arrows).

OTHER MYCOSES CAUSED BY OPPORTUNISTIC FUNGI

Severely immunocompromised hosts suffer from a large number of other opportunistic systemic fungal infections as well. The etiology of the most frequent of these infections is listed in Table 47.1. The so-called **zygomycoses** have two principal clinical presentations. The **rhinocerebral form** is unique to diabetics, particularly those with diabetic ketoacidosis. These patients often have sinus infections, periorbital cellulitis (infection of the connective tissue around the eye), and tissue necrosis that may extend to the central nervous system. It is not known why diabetes predisposes to this infection, but it has been postulated, on the basis of laboratory data, that the acidotic state of the diabetic patient stimulates growth of this fungus.

The second type of opportunistic systemic fungal infections, **disseminated zygomycosis**, has a clinical presentation almost identical to that of disseminated aspergillosis. In contrast to the hyphae of *Aspergillus* and *Candida*, the fungal elements seen in pathologic specimens of mucormycosis are nonseptate, branch irregularly and produce bizarre balloon-shaped cells.

Table 47.1. Mycoses Caused by Opportunistic Fungi

Disease	Fungus	Predisposing factors	Involvement	Therapy
Cryptococcosis	*Cryptococcus neoformans*	Immunosuppression, none	Lung, most prominent in CNS, kidney, bone	Amphotericin B + 5-FC, fluconazole
Candidiasis	*Candida albicans*	Immunosuppression, broad-spectrum antibiotics, foreign bodies	Mucosal areas, GI tract, blood, kidney, other organs	Amphotericin B + 5-FC, fluconazole
Aspergillosis	*Aspergillus fumigatus* and other species	Immunosuppression	Lungs, other organs	Amphotericin B
Zygomycosis	Several genera and species of *Zygomyces*	Diabetes, burn, immunosuppression	Blood vessels, eye, CNS, nose, sinuses, lungs	Amphotericin B
Other	Many other genera and species (each one infrequent)	Immunosuppression, trauma, or not known	Lungs, CNS, soft tissue, joints, eye, disseminated infection	Amphotericin B, miconazole

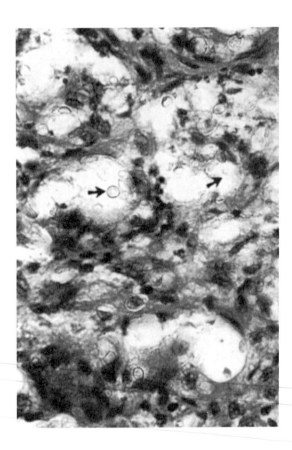

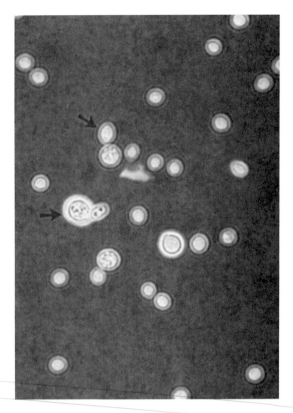

Figure 47.4. India ink preparation of spinal fluid containing encapsulated yeast cells of *Cryptococcus neoformans.*

Figure 47.3. Tissue section of brain of patient with crypto-coccosis. Note yeast cells *(arrows)* typical of *Cryptococcus neoformans* within spaces occupied by capsular material and general absence of cellular response

Cryptococcosis is usually listed among the opportunistic fungal infection, although it also occurs in immunocompe-tent persons. In recent years cryptococcal infection, partic-ularly meningitis, has occurred most prominently in pa-tients with AIDS (see Chapter 68, "AIDS"). In fact, 90% of patients with cryptococcal meningitis in the United States have AIDS, and it is estimated that this form of meningitis will eventually develop in 5–10 percent of all AIDS patients.

The etiologic agent of cryptococcosis is an encapsulated yeast, *Cryptococcus neoformans*, which is found in the excreta of birds, particularly pigeons. The organism is also found on rotted fruits and vegetables. The organism is in-haled into the lungs where it can cause pneumonia. How-ever, the most frequent clinical presentation is meningitis. No explanation currently exists for the striking tropism of this organism for the central nervous system. Brain ab-scesses caused by *C. neoformans* have a particularly inter-esting feature: they usually elicit little or no tissue response (Fig. 47.3). Thus, damage is caused by displacement and pressure on brain tissue rather than by inflammation. The mechanism for the lack of immune response is also not known, but may be related to the properties of the capsule.

The diagnosis of cryptococcal meningitis is made by ex-amining samples of cerebrospinal fluid for budding yeast cells with capsules outlined by India ink particles (Fig. 47.4). A serologic test can detect soluble capsular polysaccharide in the cerebrospinal fluid of over 90% of patients with this disease. Both microscopic and serologic tests can be per-formed right after lumbar puncture and the diagnosis can be made before obtaining results from a culture, which takes several days. The accuracy of microscopic and serological tests in establishing the diagnosis allows early therapy with a combination of amphotericin B and 5-fluorocytosine. More recently, fluconazole has also been used successfully.

Prognosis depends on the overall clinical status of the patient. A good prognostic sign is a falling antigen titer followed by the detection of circulating antibodies to the cryptococcal polysaccharide. If there is no underlying dis-ease, 80–90% of patients respond to therapy. If patients are severely immune-compromised, less than 50% will survive. Patients with AIDS respond to therapy but will relapse after treatment is stopped. For this reason, lifelong antifungal therapy is required to suppress the infection.

SUGGESTED READINGS

Levitz SM. Aspergillosis. Inf Dis Clinics North Am 1988;3:1–18.
Macher AM, DeVinatea ML, Tuur M, Anzritt P. AIDS and the mycoses. Inf Dis Clinics North Am 1988;2:827–840.
Odds FC. Candida and candidiosis. 2nd ed. Philadelphia: WB Saunders, 1988.

Subcutaneous, Cutaneous, and Superficial Mycoses

GERALD MEDOFF

GEORGE S. KOBAYASHI

A distinctive group of fungal diseases involve the subcutaneous tissue, dermis, and epidermis. These infections originate in the deeper tissue layers and eventually extend out through the dermis and the epidermis. Spread through the bloodstream is unusual but the lymphatics may be involved as far as the draining lymph nodes. Most of these mycoses, along with other "jungle rots," are confined to tropical climates. Sporotrichosis is the only relatively common infection in temperate climates.

Subcutaneous infections are called **mycoses of implantation** because the organisms enter the skin via thorns or splinters. Consequently, sporotrichosis is considered to be an **occupational risk** for gardeners, florists, and plant hobbyists. In addition to involving the subcutaneous tissue, the diseases of this group have several other features in common:

- Encounter: The etiologic agents are ubiquitous and usually found in soil or decaying vegetation.
- Entry: Infections occur on the parts of the body that are most prone to be traumatized, e.g., feet, legs, hands, buttocks. The patient usually gives a history of trauma preceding the appearance of lesions.
- Spread: These infections progress slowly and lesions evolve over many months. This persistence may be due to the noninvasive properties of this group of organisms and may also be fostered by tissue damage and foreign material in the wounds. Malnutrition, which is common in the populations most frequently infected, may also be a factor.
- Diagnosis: Some of these organisms are commonly encountered in the laboratory, and single isolations must therefore be confirmed by repeated cultures. The presence of fungi with a characteristic morphology in tissue specimens is helpful in diagnosis.

- Treatment: With few exceptions (sporotrichosis, chromoblastomycosis), the subcutaneous mycoses are difficult to treat and often require surgical intervention. The reason for the lack of response to drug therapy is unknown. It is possible that the organisms are only marginally sensitive to antifungal agents; a more likely explanation is that the chronic inflammatory reaction they cause makes these fungi inaccessible both to drugs and to host defense mechanisms.

Subcutaneous sporotrichosis responds to potassium iodide, which is puzzling since this compound has no in vitro effect against the fungus. The reason for its therapeutic effect is not known, although some researchers think that the compound may affect the host response to infection. It is interesting to note that only the subcutaneous form of sporotrichosis responds well to this compound.

Several bacterial infections, such as those caused by *Staphylococcus*, *Nocardia*, or *Actinomyces* or by atypical mycobacteria may mimic clinical and pathological manifestations of the subcutaneous fungal infections. Since most of these can be treated with antibacterial antibiotics, it is extremely important to determine the etiology of the infection. This is most effectively done by surgical biopsy. In the case of sporotrichosis, culture is more useful than histology, since the yeastlike organisms are difficult to find on histopathological examination. Table 48.1 summarizes the important features of the principal subcutaneous mycoses.

CUTANEOUS MYCOSES OR DERMATOMYCOSES

The dermatomycoses of humans include a wide spectrum of infections of the **skin** and its **appendages** (hair

Table 48.1. Fungi—Subcutaneous Mycoses

Disease	Etiologic agent(s)	Clinical disease	Therapy
Sporotrichosis	*Sporothrix schenkii*	Lymphocutaneous sporotrichosis is the disease most commonly associated with this fungus The organism gains access to the deep layers of skin by traumatic implantation: a small hard plainess nodule appears at the site of injury and it enlarges into a fluctuant mass that eventually breaks down and ulcerates; as the primary lesion enlarges, several other nodules begin to develop along lymphatics that drain that site; they also become fluctuant and ulcerate; the infection rarely extends beyond regional lymphatics	Saturated solution of potassium iodide given orally is the drug of choice; amphotericin B is used for diseases involving the lung and other organs
Chromoblastomycosis	*Fonsecaea pedrosoi*; many species	The most common form of chromoblastomycosis; surgical excision and cryosurgery; consists of warty, vegetative lesions that look like a cauliflower	5-fluorocytosine has been used successfully, but response depends on the organism
Others, e.g., rhinosporlidiosis lobomycosis, etc.	Many species	Many manifestations: deep subcutaneous masses, wart-like lesions, polyps, etc.	Surgical excision, antifungal drugs

and nails) by fungi known as dermatophytes. In the asexual state these fungi are classified in the genera *Microsporum, Trichophyton,* and *Epidermophyton* on the basis of sporulation patterns and morphologic features of development. Some species are found worldwide, while others are geographically restricted to certain parts of the world. These patterns are becoming disrupted by the increasing mobility of the world's population.

■ CASE

Two adult teaching volunteers in a school for mentally handicapped children were seen by their physicians because each had developed well-demarcated, scaly, itchy lesions on their skin (Fig. 48. 1). Clinical history revealed that the volunteers had developed these lesions over a period of several weeks since they started their work. Both were childless and had no contact with domestic or wild animals. Microscopic examination of skin scales taken from the lesions showed the presence of fungal elements (Fig. 48.2), and cultures grew *Trichophyton tonsurans*.

An epidemiologic inquiry and clinical survey of seven students in the school revealed that two had patchy hair loss (alopecia). One of these students had typical ringworm of the scalp and the other had highly inflammatory lesions

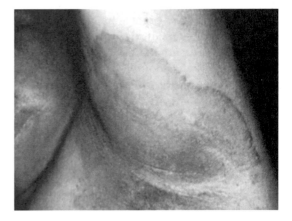

Figure 48.1. Clinical appearance of tinea corporis. Note the well-demarcated border of the lesions, which suggest that a worm or larva is at the margin, hence the terms *ringworm* or *tinea* (worm) to describe the lesions.

associated with ringworm called **kerion** (Fig. 48.3). The five other students appeared asymptomatic except for mild dandruff. Cultures of scalp scrapings of two of these were positive for *T. tonsurans*.

The parents of the children were notified of these findings and asked to have their family physician examine the

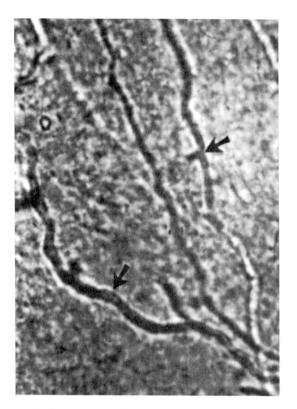

Figure 48.2. Specimen taken from skin of patient with tinea corporis, treated with 10% potassium hydroxide. A positive preparation is indicated by presence of hyphae (*arrows*).

siblings of each student. The brother of one of the asymptomatic students who had a positive culture for *T. tonsurans* was found to have ringworm of the scalp. All of the children and the two adults were treated with griseofulvin, and all responded well.

This example of an outbreak of dermatophytosis illustrates several points:

- In occupations where adults come into close contact with children, such as nursing and teaching of the handicapped, it is not uncommon to find ringworm of the body in adults during outbreaks of ringworm of the scalp in the children: both conditions are caused by the same organism.
- The clinical manifestations of these infections are variable. Of the five students who had what appeared to be dandruff, two grew the fungus from the scalp. The two others had hair loss and distinct clinical diseases, regular ringworm and kerion.
- Ringworm of the scalp is a frequent problem in the pediatric population. At puberty it spontaneously disappears, treated or untreated. In the adult population ringworm of the scalp is rare. The patient usually has close association with infected children or animals with clinical disease.

Encounter

Different species of dermatophytes have different ecological niches. Some species are most frequently isolated from the soil and are called **geophilic.** Other species, found most often in association with domestic and wild animals, are called **zoophilic.** A third group, the **anthropophilic** dermatophytes, are found almost exclusively in association with humans and their habitat.

It is important to identify the species in order to determine the possible source of infection. Identification even has some prognostic value. The anthropophilic dermatophytes tend to cause chronic infections and may be difficult to treat. The zoophilic and geophilic dermatophytes tend to cause inflammatory lesions that may heal spontaneously.

Dermatophytes are not members of the normal skin flora. Although they are occasionally found in people's toe clefts, these fungi almost always cause some minor pathology once they become established. The disease caused by these fungi is called **ringworm** or **tinea.** The term *tinea* comes from the Latin word for worm and refers to the serpentine lesions that characterize these infections and which look as if a worm is burrowing at the margin. This term is used in conjunction with the part of the body that is affected to describe the disease, e.g., **tinea capitis** (head), **tinea pedis** (feet), **tinea corporis** (body), **tinea cruris** (crotch). Other terms often used by the layperson to describe these diseases include athlete's foot, jock itch, jungle rot, etc.

Entry

Experimental studies on dermatophyte infections have been useful for understanding their clinical mani-

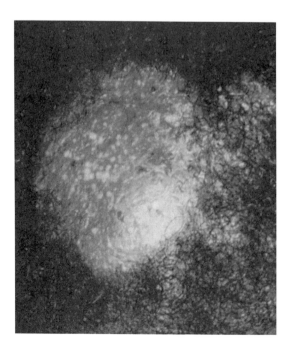

Figure 48.3. Clinical photograph of tinea capitis showing the inflammatory lesion called "kerion."

festations. Volunteers who immersed their feet in water teeming with viable spores of the causative fungi did not get athlete's foot unless the skin was first traumatized. Continuous moist conditions were also important, and infections took place when the skin was occluded with nonporous materials. This occlusion increases hydration and temperature of the skin and interferes with the natural barrier function of the superficial layer, the **stratum corneum**. Such conditions are caused by wearing nonporous shoes or covering the skin with occlusive bandages.

Spread and Multiplication

A classical ringworm lesion is characterized by the presence of fungal mycelium in the stratum corneum. Growth of the fungus sometimes results in minimal clinical signs of infection. In active disease, there is an inflammatory reaction in the underlying epidermis and dermis. Scaling often occurs, indicating increased epidermal turnover. Toe nails and finger nails as well as hair follicles and hair shaft may be invaded. The fungi particularly prefer keratinized tissues and do not invade living cells or the incompletely keratinized zone of the hair bulb. Although keratinases have been found in some dermatophytes, their role in the disease is unknown.

Damage

The clinical features of this disease are all related to the **inflammation** of the epidermis, dermis, and the hair follicles. What sets this off is an immunologically mediated reaction to the fungal antigens that diffuse from the infected epidermis. This process could be called a **biological contact dermatitis**. The extent of the inflammatory response and cellular infiltration correlate well with the degree of delayed hypersensitivity of the skin to extracts of the dermatophyte ("trichophitin"). The term **kerion** is used to describe the highly inflammatory pustular form of infection in the scalp and beard areas. The pus results from secondary bacterial infections.

The ring shape characteristic of dermatophyte lesions is the result of the organism growing outwardly in a centrifugal pattern. The area of the lesion that yields viable fungal elements is located at the inflamed margin. The central area generally has few or no viable fungi, and the healing tissue is refractory to infection. This pattern simulates the centrifugal growth of "fairy ring" mushrooms in a grassy field.

Systemic infections by dermatophytes are extremely rare, no matter how impaired the host. The most likely reasons are inability of dermatophytes to grow at human body temperature and the presence of nonspecific serum factors (e.g., transferrin).

Environmental and cultural habits associated with types of clothing and shoes contribute to the incidence of dermatophytosis. Studies performed on institutionalized populations and families show that close and crowded living conditions are important factors in the spreading of the infections. Immunologic factors also contribute to their incidence and evidence suggests that natural cell-mediated resistance to these infections is important.

Because these diseases do not have to be reported to the U.S. Public Health Service, the prevalence of dermatophytes and the incidence of disease are both difficult to determine. Fragmentary surveys from epidemiologic studies and case reports indicate that dermatophytes are among the most common of human diseases. They are among the most common skin disorders in children under the age of 12, and the second most common skin disorder in older populations.

Different age groups manifest these diseases at different anatomic sites. In the pediatric population the most prevalent problem is **ringworm of the scalp**, which is most common in the 5- to 10-year old. After puberty, this disease ceases to be a problem. On the other hand, **athlete's foot**, which rarely occurs in childhood, gradually becomes the predominant infection and remains so throughout life. The reason for this shift is not well understood, but may be due to changes in the composition of sebum that occur at puberty, particularly in the even-numbered saturated fatty acids that have natural fungistatic activity. The fact that humans are generally shod is perhaps the major factor that leads to the high incidence of athlete's foot in adults.

In the United States there is a disproportionate incidence of ringworm of the scalp in black children. We don't know why. Natives of India have higher incidence of this disease than resident Europeans. Studies from the Vietnam War revealed that athlete's foot in U.S. servicemen was mainly caused by *Trichophyton mentagrophytes*, whereas the native Vietnamese were more susceptible to *T. rubrum*.

The incidence of dermatophytosis is higher in males than females, with ratios of 3:1 for ringworm of the scalp and 6:1 for athlete's foot. **Jock itch** (Tinea cruris) is also common in males and rare in females. Infection of the nails of the hands is more common in females, but nails of the feet are more often involved in males.

Diagnosis

When examined microscopically in scrapings of the skin surface in infected areas, dermatophytes all look alike. In culture, however, dermatophyte colonies have complex morphological characteristics that distinguish genus and species. Under the microscope, they differ in the morphology of specialized large multicelled spores, the macroconidia.

Treatment

The dermatophytoses are treated topically or systemically. Systemic treatment is necessary when hair or nails are infected because locally applied fungicides do not penetrate the tissue matrix where the fungus resides.

Various local applications, creams, ointments, lotions, and paints are available that, when used regularly for 3 weeks or more, will clear many of the localized ringworm infections. Controlled trials have not demonstrated a clear leader among antiringworm drugs. In most cases, regular application is more important than the choice of agent.

Two antiringworm agents are given systemically by oral administration: the antibiotic griseofulvin and the imidazole derivative ketoconazole.

SUGGESTED READINGS

Hay RJ. Dermato phytosis and other superficial mycoses. ln: Principles and Practices of Infectious Diseases. 4th ed. Maudell GL, Bennett JE, Dolin R, eds. New York: Churchill Livingstone. 1995;2375.

SUPERFICIAL MYCOSES

Many of us harbor fungi on our skin and hairs without signs of disease. Sometimes, these fungal members of our normal flora cause superficial infections that go no deeper than the stratum corneum. They are frequently mild, do not stimulate an inflammatory response, and may go unnoticed. These conditions are often seen in warm and moist climates, but one, **tinea versicolor**, is frequently found in temperate areas. Superficial mycoses are usually easy to treat with topical keratolytic agents.

Rosenthal JR. Fungal Infections of the Skin. ln: Gorbach SL, Bartlett JG, Blacklow NR. Infectious Diseases. 2nd ed. 1998; 1276-1295.

Review of the Medically Important Fungi

This chart may be completed to review material covered under this topic.

	Name of Disease or Fungus	Epidemiology	Main Symptoms
Systemic "true pathogens" 1.			
2.			
3.			
Systemic opportunistic 1.			
2.			
3.			
Subcutaneous 1.			
2.			
Superficial 1.			
2.			

Animal Parasites

Introduction to Parasitology

DONALD J. KROGSTAD

N. CARY ENGLEBERG

Key Concepts

- Knowledge of the parasites' life cycles is essential to understanding the rationale for preventive interventions.
- Local ecology (e.g., climate, arthropods) and socioecoconomic factors (e.g., sanitation, housing) determine whether a particular parasitic life cycle can be completed and thereby govern the geographic distribution of the disease.
- Parasites that have evolved within human hosts usually cause asymptomatic infections, in which case the host response does not usually hinder the completion of the parasitic life cycle. Symptoms typically results when the parasite burden is high or when the duration of infection is prolonged. There are notable exceptions to this generalization (e.g., malaria).
- Many parasites survive in the human host by evading or subverting the immune response. Damage induced by these pathogens is usually a direct consequence of host hypersensitivity.
- For many parasitic infections, the capacity to occupy certain tissues (tropism) is an essential feature of the life cycle.
- Diagnosis often depends on direct identification of parasitic forms in human samples. Therefore, knowledge of the tissue tropisms and modes of transmission determines which samples should be collected and examined.

In developed countries, parasitology suggests the strange and exotic—"worms, wheezes, and weird diseases." Although **parasitic infections** are among the most prevalent diseases in developing countries, they are also common in developed countries. Often, these infections cause no clinical symptoms (Table 49.1). In North America and Europe, parasitic infections are being recognized with increasing frequency, particularly among patients with immunosuppression caused by AIDS or malignancies.

INFECTION VERSUS DISEASE

As with other agents, parasitic infection must be distinguished from parasitic disease. For example, a large number of adults in the United States are infected with the protozoan *Toxoplasma gondii*, as demonstrated by the prevalence of antitoxoplasma antibodies in the population. However, few normal humans become ill from this infection. Another example is hookworm infection. Hookworms consume small amounts of blood to survive, mate, and release eggs in the human intestine. Because the amount of blood consumed by each worm is small (0.03–0.15 ml/day), infections with only a few worms are clinically insignificant. However, infections with large numbers of hookworms may produce a life-threatening anemia.

Like other infectious agents described in this textbook, parasites have evolved to exploit their hosts in order to grow and procreate. Since they depend on the host for their survival and to complete their life cycle, killing or disabling the host is not to the parasites' advantage.

Toxoplasmosis	1–2 billion
Ascariasis	1 billion
Hookworm disease	800–900 million
Amebiasis	200–400 million
Schistosomiasis	200–300 million
Malaria	200–300 million
Filariasis	250 million
Giardiasis	200 million
Pinworm infection	60–100 million
Strongyloidiasis	50–80 million
Guinea worm infection	20–40 million
Trypanosomiasis	15–20 million
Leishmaniasis	1–2 million

Parasitic diseases are often the consequence of prolonged or repeated infection. These diseases are usually subacute or chronic and, even if untreated, are rarely fatal over short periods of time. There are, however, important exceptions, such as malaria caused by *Plasmodium falciparum*, which may be rapidly fatal (within 3–5 days). Other parasites that normally produce quiescent, asymptomatic infections in immunocompetent hosts can cause disseminated and potentially lethal diseases in immunocompromised persons (e.g., toxoplasmosis).

PARASITIC INFECTIONS AS ZOONOSES

Several parasitic infections of humans are zoonoses, that is, are caused by agents that infect animals such as birds, reptiles, and other mammals (see Chapter 70, "Zoonoses" and the paradigm in Chapter 28, "Rickettsiae"). Many human parasites require both human and nonhuman hosts to complete their life cycles. For example, humans may carry an adult beef tapeworm in the intestinal lumen, but an infected human cannot transmit the parasite to another human. To complete its life cycle, this parasite must undergo larval development in the muscles of cattle (cysticercosis). Humans may become infected with the tapeworm by eating undercooked beef. Both stages (adult and larval) and both hosts (cattle and humans) are required to complete this life cycle. Other animal parasites do not require a developmental stage in humans but can nevertheless infect humans and cause disease. In these cases, humans are **dead-end hosts**. For example, the blood fluke (schistosome) of birds alternates between birds and snails. Humans are sometimes "substitute" for a bird as a vertebrate host, however, the life cycle of the parasite is not completed in humans. The infecting larvae cannot penetrate beyond the skin. They die there and cause an irritating dermatitis, called "swimmer's itch," which resolves spontaneously.

TYPES OF PARASITES AND MODES OF TRANSMISSION
Protozoa

Protozoa are one-celled eukaryotes. Protozoan parasites of medical importance include the agents of malaria (*Plasmodium*), as well as *Giardia*, *Cryptosporidium*, *Leishmania*, and trypanosomes. Infections with any of these pathogens may be initiated by relatively small inocula. Disease is generally a consequence of the replication of the parasites in large numbers within the host. This replication may be intracellular (e.g., *Plasmodium*, which grows within red blood cells, and *Leishmania*, which grows within macrophages), or it may occur extracellularly, such as in the lumen of the gastrointestinal tract (e.g., of amebae and *Giardia*).

Intracellular protozoa are typically unable to withstand dessication (drying) in the external environment. Consequently, their life cycles usually do not include free environmental stages. They are most commonly transmitted from one host to another by vectors, such as arthropods. For example, *Plasmodium* is transmitted by mosquitoes. In contrast, extracellular protozoa are often transmitted by the fecal–oral route. Extracellular intestinal protozoa typically alternate between two distinct forms: an active **trophozoite** form that grows and replicates by binary fission, and a dormant **cyst** form that is transmitted between humans. Cysts are relatively impermeable because of their double membranes and can thus resist dessication in the external environment.

Helminths

Helminths (worms) are multicellular animals (metazoa) considerably larger than protozoa. Those of medical importance include both roundworms and flatworms. One human intestinal roundworm (*Ascaris lumbricoides*) bears a remarkable resemblance to an earthworm. Many different helminths cause human disease, including tapeworms, roundworms, and flatworms (flukes). Because of their large size, helminths are typically extracellular. However, the larvae of some helminths, such as the roundworm that causes trichinosis (*Trichinella spiralis*) and most tapeworms, develop into dormant cysts.

Helminthic infections may be transmitted by oral ingestion (ascariasis), by the direct penetration of unbroken skin (hookworm) infection, or by the bites of arthropod vectors (filariasis). Although many of these helminths live in the gastrointestinal tract, several infect the internal organs or skin, and a few cause disease in both the intestine and deeper tissues. Because helminths are protected from the environment by a cuticle, they often have complex life cycles involving environmental or animal reservoirs. With rare exceptions, helminthic parasites do not complete their life cycle within a single human host. Therefore, disease is not normally a consequence of parasites growing in number within the host, as it is with protozoa. Instead, the parasitic burden (and the likelihood of pathologic consequences) is directly related to the number of parasites that the host acquires from the environment.

Vectors

Vectors are living transmitters of disease. Most vectors are **arthropods**. Perhaps the best-known example of a vector is the female *Anopheles* mosquito, which transmits malaria. Other important vectors include tsetse flies, which transmit sleeping sickness; black flies, which transmit river blindness; kissing bugs, which transmit Chagas' disease; and ticks, which transmit babesiosis. Arthropods may transmit not only parasites but also bacteria (e.g., the agents of Lyme disease and Rocky Mountain spotted fever) and viruses (e.g., yellow fever, dengue, and encephalitis viruses).

Arthropods are not simply passive agents that transfer parasites from one mammalian host to another. They are also involved in essential steps of the parasitic life cycle. To a large extent, the prevalence of a parasitic disease in a given geographical location may depend on whether the local conditions are favorable to arthropod breeding, e.g., stagnant water for mosquito breeding or foliage, moisture and suitable animal hosts for the propagation of ticks. Because of the obligatory role that arthropods play in the development of some protozoal and helminthic pathogens, their elimination from the environment can theoretically eradicate the respective diseases they cause in humans.

Reservoirs

Reservoirs are sources of parasites in the environment that do not participate directly in transmission to humans. Reservoirs of human parasites include other humans (malaria parasites, amebae), other animals (pigs for trichinosis and pork tapeworm, cattle for beef tapeworm and cryptosporidiosis) and the environment (soil contaminated with parasitized human feces).

ENTRY

One intriguing aspect of human parasites is the number of different strategies they have evolved to enter the host. The most common modes of entry are oral ingestion (ascariasis) or penetration of the skin (hookworm, schistosomes). Thus, the transmission of parasites is frequently due to the ingestion of contaminated food or water or to inadequate control of human wastes in soil or water.

Most arthropod-borne infections are transmitted through bite wounds. Arthropod-borne transmission may be extraordinarily efficient. In fact, malaria may be acquired from the bite of a single infected mosquito during a stop at an airport in an endemic area. In addition, some arthropod-borne infections may also be transmitted by the transfusion of blood from asymptomatic infected humans.

SPREAD AND MULTIPLICATION

Inoculum Size

The effective inoculum size has been determined for a few parasites by experimental infections in human volunteers and animals, usually in conjunction with quantitative epidemiologic studies. For example, large inocula are required to cause amebiasis in humans, whereas symptomatic cryptosporidiosis can be produced by the ingestion of only relatively few cysts. In most helminthic infections, the severity of the infection is proportional to the inoculum size (or the cumulative inoculum).

Parasite Survival Mechanisms in Immunologically Normal Hosts

Parasites, like other microorganisms, elicit both antibody and cell-mediated responses. However, they are adept at circumventing those host defenses. For example, adult schistosomes (blood flukes) coat themselves with host plasma proteins and are thus not recognized as foreign by the host's immune system. As a result, they are able to persist within the bloodstream for decades without immune-mediated destruction. Trypanosomes elude their hosts' immune systems by varying their surface antigens. In contrast, intracellular parasites are protected by special adaptations. For example, *Leishmania*, which live in the phagolysosomes of macrophages, secrete a superoxide dismutase that protects them from the toxic superoxide produced in the phagolysosome.

Species and Tissue Tropisms

The life cycles of parasites are determined by species and tissue **tropisms**, which define the hosts that parasites can infect and the organs and tissues in which they can survive. As yet, very little is known about the biologic basis of these tropisms. Thus, it is not clear why the larvae of *Strongyloides* invade the intestinal wall, whereas those of hookworms remain in the intestinal lumen. Nor is it clear why the pork tapeworm can cause cysticercosis (infection of the deep tissues) in humans, whereas the beef tapeworm cannot. Recent studies have shown that some tropisms depend on specific receptors. For example, the presence of the Duffy factor antigen on the surface of the red blood cell is necessary for the entry of *Plasmodium vivax* malaria parasites (merozoites) into human red blood cells. Thus, subjects whose red blood cells lack the Duffy factor (black Africans) are resistant to *P. vivax* infection.

Temperature also plays an important role in the ability of parasites to infect humans and cause disease. For example, *Leishmania donovani* replicates well at 37°C and causes visceral leishmaniasis (kala-azar), a disease of the bone marrow, liver, and spleen. (Note that the temperature of these tissues is, of course, 37°C). In contrast, *Leishmania tropica* grows well at 25–30°C but poorly at 37°C and causes infections of the skin (where temperatures are 25–30°C). Temperature changes also induce stage-specific transitions in many parasites. For example, *Leishmania* transform from the promastigote to amastigote form, when they move from a cooler insect vector to a warmer human host (from 25°C to 37°C). They also synthesize heat-shock protein.

DAMAGE

As with other infectious agents, the clinical manifestations of parasitic disease may reflect tissue damage by the parasite, the effects of the host immune response, or both. The pathogenic amebas are examples of pathogens that cause most of their tissue damage by a direct cytolytic effect (see below). Characteristic colonic ulcers and amebic liver abscesses are produced by direct destruction of host cells, whereas the host response contributes little or nothing to this pathology of amebiasis. In contrast, many other parasitic infections that involve deep tissues elicit an inflammatory response that may be exclusively responsible for the histopathology. Chronic **inflammation** is the hallmark of diseases such as schistosomiasis and cutaneous filariasis. In these helminthic infections, the adult parasites are innocuous, but their progeny (i.e., schistosoma eggs and microfilaria) induce intense inflammatory responses when they degenerate in host tissues. In some parasitic diseases, the host inflammatory response may cause persistent disease even after the parasites have died (trichinosis). In cysticercosis, the infected individual may remain asymptomatic for long periods of time until the parasite dies. Then, the leakage of parasite antigens into the tissues may trigger a hypersensitivity reaction and produce symptoms in the host.

Eosinophilia

Eosinophils are leukocytes that participate in neutralizing infections with parasitic worms. In helminthic infections, eosinophils appear in the blood in large numbers. This eosinophilicism occurs in response to the parasites' surface glycoproteins and polysaccharides, particularly when the parasites invade or migrate through tissues. Eosinophilia is typically accompanied by increased levels of IgE and is driven by elevated levels of IL-5. Together, eosinophils and IgE play a critical role in killing multicellular parasites. Because these responses (eosinophilia and increased levels of IgE) occur with helminthic infections and are most striking with helminths that invade the deep tissues, they are useful in diagnosis. Note that neither eosinophilia nor elevated IgE levels are characteristics of protozoan infections.

Timing of Clinical Complications

The most important complications of many parasitic diseases occur years after the initial infection. For instance, persons with schistosomiasis typically have bleeding from either the gastrointestinal tract (*Schistosoma mansoni*) or the urinary tract (*Schistosoma haematobium*), which continues for years. Years or decades later, persons with heavy, chronic infections may develop complications such as portal hypertension with esophageal varices (*S. mansoni*), obstructions, or cancer of the urinary tract (*S. haematobium*).

Important complications may also occur at distant sites. For example, pork tapeworm (*Taenia solium*) infections are asymptomatic as long as the adult parasite remains in the intestine. Late complications result if larval forms of the parasite hatch from the egg, cross the intestinal epithelium to enter the bloodstream, and encyst in the deep tissues as cysticerci. These cysts are small (0.5–1.5 cm) and produce no signs or symptoms if they lodge in skeletal muscle. However, when they lodge in the central nervous system, they may produce seizures (similar to those caused by a mass lesion in the brain) or hydrocephalus by blocking the flow of cerebrospinal fluid.

A chronic protozoan infection, Chagas' disease (American trypanosomiasis), typically produces a relatively trivial skin lesion at the time of the initial infection. Although in rare cases the initial infection may progress rapidly to death in young children, it is usually asymptomatic or minimally symptomatic. Years later, older persons with chronic infection may develop heart block from damage to the cardiac conducting system, or impaired swallowing or defecation from damage to the nerves responsible for the motility of the esophagus or colon. Although the majority of infected persons do not develop these complications, there are no predictors to identify the persons at greatest risk of these late complications.

DIAGNOSIS

Diagnostic Strategies Based on the Parasite Life Cycle

Most parasitic infections are diagnosed by identifying the parasites or their characteristic progeny (cysts,

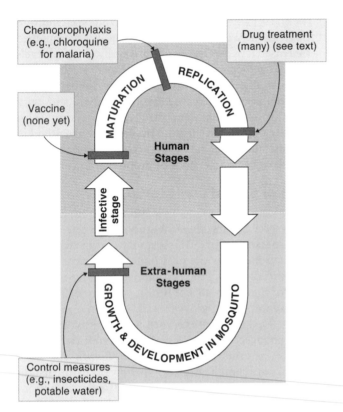

Figure 49.1. Idealized (model) parasite life cycle and points of intervention. The human stages of the life cycle are located in the top half of the diagram. The extrahuman stages (in animate or inanimate reservoirs) are in the lower half. When the parasite reaches the infective stage, it invades the human host, matures, replicates, and ultimately completes the life cycle by producing infective forms. These infective forms are taken up by a vector or released into the environment. Control measures interfere with the replication or the survival of the extrahuman stages of the parasite. They reduce the incidence of infection by reducing the number of infective stages to which humans are exposed. Immunization (vaccination) prevents symptomatic infection by inhibiting or killing the parasite as it enters (or replicates within) the human host. Chemoprophylaxis is used to inhibit parasite replication in order to prevent symptomatic infection. Neither immunization nor chemoprophylaxis prevents the initial entry of the parasite. Drug treatment is used to prevent death or severe morbidity in persons with established infections.

eggs, or larvae) in clinical specimens. In order to pursue the most effective diagnostic strategies, it is important to understand the parasite's life cycle (Fig. 49.1). For instance, in the life cycle of hookworms, the adult female lives in the lumen of the human intestine, suggesting that the adult female will release her eggs into the stool. As a result, examination of the stool for hookworm eggs is an effective and sensitive method for the diagnosis of hookworm infection. In contrast, in the life cycle of *Strongyloides*, the adult female invades the intestinal wall in order to release

her eggs. Intact eggs are rarely seen in the stool. However, the larvae that emerge from eggs in the intestinal wall can be found in the stool of persons with *Strongyloides* infection, and their presence is diagnostic for this infection.

One species of filarial helminths (*Wuchereria bancrofti*) is transmitted to humans by mosquitos that bite only at night. To maximize their transmission to mosquitos, these parasites release their microfilaria into the human bloodstream during the later hours of the evening. Consequently, in order to examine blood for these particular microfilaria, blood samples must be typically drawn at midnight!

Environmental Constraints on Transmission

Examination of the parasite life cycle often also explains why a given parasitic disease is found in one area of the world and not another (Table 49.2). For example, the transmission of schistosomiasis depends on the intermediate snail host, which is not present in North America or Europe. Thus, viable eggs in the stool or urine of infected persons cannot produce the forms infective for humans (cercariae) because there are no intermediate snail hosts in which the parasite can mature. For this reason, schistosomiasis is not endemic in the United States and will not be, unless an intermediate snail host becomes established. For this disease, it does not matter how many infected persons enter the U.S. and contaminate the environment with infective eggs. In contrast, *Anopheles* mosquitoes capable of transmitting malaria are found in the United States. Therefore, recent immigrants or travelers who acquired malaria in endemic areas may infect the indigenous mosquito pool. Local transmission of malaria by this mechanism occurs a few times each year in the United States (recent cases have occurred in California, New Jersey, and Michigan). These rare events often present a diagnostic dilemma, since the infected individual typically has no history of foreign travel. For this reason, ongoing malaria surveillance is particularly important when large numbers of people from malaria-endemic areas enter the U.S. and settle in parts of the country where substantial numbers of anopheline mosquitoes are present.

TREATMENT AND PREVENTION

Antiparasite strategies fall into three general categories: (1) drugs for prevention (chemoprophylaxis) and treatment, (2) immunization, and (3) control measures in the field. Eradication programs have generally been effective only when more than one of these strategies were used simultaneously.

The parasite life cycle also provides important clues

Table 49.2. Geographic Context of Parasitic Infection	
Currently or historically indigenous to the U.S. mainland	Imported
Intestinal Helminths	
Ascaris lumbricoides (roundworm)	*Ancylostoma braziliensis* (hookworm)
Enterobius vermicularis (pinworm)	*Schistosoma mansoni* (schistosomiasis)
Trichuris trichiura (whipworm)	*Schistosoma hematobium*
Strongyloides stercoralis (threadworm)	*Schistosoma japonicum*
Necator americanus (hookworm)	
Taenia saginata (beef tapeworm)	
Taenia solium (pork tapeworm)	
Diphyllobothrium latum (fish tapeworm)	
Hymenolepis nana (dwarf tapeworm)	
Toxocara canis, T. cati (visceral larva migrans)	
Trichinella spiralis (trichina)	
Echinococcus	
Echinococcus granulosus	*Echinococcus multilocularis*
Filaria	
Dirofilaria immitis (canine filariasis)	*Wuchereria bancrofti*
	Brugia malayi
	Onchocerca volvulus
	Loa loa
	Dracunculus medinensis
Flukes	
	Paragonimus westermani (lung fluke)
	Clonorchis sinensis (liver fluke)
Protozoa	
Entamoeba histolytica (amebiasis)	*Plasmodium vivax, falciparum, ovale, malariae*
Giardia lamblia (giardiasis)	*Leishmania donovani, tropica*
Toxoplasma gondii (toxoplasmosis)	*Balantidium coli* (balantidiasis)
Babesia microti (babesiosis)	*Trypanosoma cruzi* (Chagas' disease)
Pneumocystis carinii (pneumocystosis)	*Trypanosoma brucei* (African sleeping sickness)
Trichomonas vaginalis (trichomoniasis)	
Naegleria fowleri (meningoencephalitis)	
Cryptosporidium (cryptosporidiosis)	

for treatment and control strategies (see Fig. 49.1, Table 49.3). For example, hookworm larvae from eggs in human stool mature to the filariform stage in the environment; they then cause infection by penetrating unprotected human skin. Therefore, sanitation (appropriate disposal of human waste) and wearing shoes can reduce the transmission of hookworms and thus decrease the number of people infected. Hookworm infection and disease were very common in the southern United States until these preventive measures were instituted on a large scale by the Rockefeller Commission in the 1930s. Sanitation is particularly effective in reducing infection rates with parasites transmitted through contaminated stool or urine, such as ascariasis, strongyloidiasis, and hookworm infection.

An understanding of the parasite life cycle is also helpful in selecting antiparasitic drugs. For example, dif-

ferent drugs are necessary for the intestinal and tissue stages of the pork tapeworm (*T. solium*): one drug, niclosamide, is effective against taeniasis (intestinal infection); another drug, praziquantel, is used to treat the tissue stage of the infection (cysticercosis).

Drugs

Chemoprophylaxis

Drugs used for chemoprophylaxis must meet more stringent requirements than drugs used only for treatment. Minor drug side effects acceptable for short periods of time in sick persons (e.g., headache, nausea, or gastrointestinal disturbances) are unacceptable for prolonged periods of time in persons who are healthy.

One example of successful chemoprophylaxis is the use of chloroquine to prevent malaria. Chloroquine is effective against all four species of *Plasmodium* that cause

Table 49.3. Modes of Spread of Some Parasitic Diseases

Route of transmission			
Mode of exit	Mode of entry	Human-to-human	Animal-to-human
Feces	Mouth	Cryptosporidiosis Amebiasis Giardiasis Strongyloidiasis[a] Ascariasis[b] Trichuris infection[b] Pork tapeworm	Cryptosporidiosis Toxoplasmosis Visceral larva migrans Echinococcosis
Feces	Skin	Strongyloidiasis Hookworm	Creeping eruption (dog or cat hookworm) Schistosomiasis[c]
Arthropod bite	Arthropod bite	Lymphatic filariasis Onchocerciasis Malaria Leishmaniasis	Trypanosomiasis (sleeping sickness, Chagas' disease) Leishmaniasis

None (parasite encysts
  in muscle)
	Ingestion (inadequately-cooked
	  meat)
			Trichinosis
			Toxoplasmosis
			Beef tapeworm
			Pork tapeworm
			Fish tapeworm

[a] Usually transmitted by fecal-cutaneous contact but may also be transmitted by the fecal-oral route.
[b] May require a period of time outside the human host in order to be infectious.
[c] Mode of exit may also be urine.

malaria in humans. Oral administration once a week produces effective plasma levels of the drug because chloroquine is well-absorbed and has a plasma half-life greater than 4 days. The main disadvantage of chloroquine is that many strains of *P. falciparum* have become resistant to it. Another example of successful chemoprophylaxis is the use of trimethoprim–sulfamethoxazole to prevent *Pneumocystis carinii* infection in persons with AIDS. Before this prophylaxis was implemented, pneumonia due to *P. carinii* was the most common cause of illness and death among persons with AIDS in the U.S.

Treatment

When does treatment influence the transmission of parasites? Mass treatment may be an effective control strategy for diseases that depend on humans as a reservoir. In contrast, treatment of those with zoonotic and "dead-end" infections will not influence the occurrence of these diseases. In general, treatment of symptomatic infections is usually an inefficient strategy for controlling transmission because a long delay often occurs between the initial infection and the onset of symptoms (e.g., 10–20 years or more for schistosomiasis). During this long asymtomatic interval, infected humans are able to transmit the infection. If treatment is to be effective in reducing transmission, it must be given to patients who are all infectious persons, both symptomatic and asymptomatic.

The goal of many treatment regimens for parasitic infection has been to prevent the long-term complications of infection (such as portal hypertension in schistosomiasis or seizures in cysticercosis). In the last 10 years, several new drugs have appeared which represent significant advances in the treatment of parasitic diseases, such as praziquantel for cysticercosis and schistosomiasis; ivermectin for onchocerciasis (see Chapter 53, "Tissue and Blood Helminths"); and difluoromethylornithine (DFMO) for African trypanosomiasis (see Chapter 50, "Blood and Tissue Protozoa"). In each of these diseases, the previously available drugs were toxic and often ineffective. Prior to praziquantel, no medical treatment existed for cysticercosis (the tissue-invasive form of pork tapeworm infection). Now, researchers expect that widespread use of these drugs will significantly decrease seizures and hydrocephalus from cysticercosis, cirrhosis from schistosomiasis, and blindness due to onchocerciasis.

Immunity and Immunization
Major problem in designing vaccines—evasion of the host immune response

Many important parasites survive to produce disease because they are able to evade the host immune response. Schistosomes masquerade as "self" by covering themselves with host antigens. Because of this protection, circulating antibodies against schistosomal antigens (produced spontaneously or by immunization) are unlikely to bind to the relevant schistosomal antigens and are thus unlikely to be effective against these parasites. Trypanosomes use another strategy to evade the host immune response: they alter their surface antigens (see Chapter 50, "Blood and Tissue Protozoa" and the paradigm, Chapter 14, "Neisseriae"). When the host develops an effective immune response to one antigen, clones of the trypanosomes emerge that express different antigens on their surfaces, leading to successive bouts of high-grade parasitemia. An effective vaccine against all these antigenic types seems extremely unlikely.

Other problems in designing vaccines—stage-specific antigens and antigenic variation

Parasites typically have different proteins or polysaccharides on their surfaces at different stages of their life cycles. Many of these surface components are antigenic, imparting different immunological characteristics to each stage of the parasite life cycle. For example, the form of the malaria parasite that is injected into humans by the mosquito is antigenically distinct from the form that infects red blood cells. Consequently, a person immunized with the mosquito stage (the sporozoite) is susceptible to infection by the red blood cell stage of the parasite (the merozoite). Thus, an effective malaria vaccine will likely need to contain major antigens derived from each of the several different stages of the parasite's life cycle. Efforts to develop vaccines are under way for several important parasitic diseases in addition to malaria, including schistosomiasis, onchocerciasis, lymphatic filariasis, and toxoplasmosis.

Control Measures

Effective control measures are potentially available for all parasitic diseases. The most effective measures are those based on the mode of transmission as defined by the parasite's life cycle (see Fig. 49.1). For example, mosquitoes that transmit malaria often bite at night, when people are sleeping. Because many of these mosquitoes rest under the eaves of houses after biting humans, insecticides such as DDT have reduced malaria transmission substantially when sprayed at these sites. Unfortunately, this strategy is limited because many mosquitoes have developed resistance to DDT and because this strategy selects for mosquitoes that bite outside the house during daylight hours.

In developed areas such as North America and Europe, transmission of parasitic disease is typically low because sanitation interrupts the parasite's life cycle. However, in developing countries—where the major parasitic diseases are endemic—even simple sanitary methods of interrupting transmission are difficult to implement. Potable water, for example, is unavailable or too expensive in many parts of the world. During the dry season, the transmission of infection by waterborne and fecal–oral routes increases in these regions because the small amounts of water available are used for both washing and drinking.

CONCLUSION

The most striking differences between parasites and other infectious agents are their variety of hosts, vectors, and stages in their life cycles. These life cycles of parasites provide important clues to understanding the parasitic diseases and help in diagnosis and in the development of public health strategies. In most cases, we still do not know the biological basis for the ability of different stages of parasites to invade different hosts and different types of tissues.

Although parasitic diseases are more prevalent in areas with inadequate sanitation, they are also found in regions with apparently high sanitary standards, such as Europe and North America. The presence of parasitic diseases in these areas is frequently due to the susceptibility of immunocompromised patients to these infections. For example, toxoplasmosis and pneumocystis are quite prevalent in developed countries, but do not produce disease in immunologically normal individuals. In immunocompromised patients, some parasites escape their normal constraints and may multiply to high and dangerous numbers.

SUGGESTED READINGS

Beaty BJ, Marquardt WC. The biology of disease vectors, Niwot, CO: University of Colorado, 1996.

Boothroyd JC, Komuniecki R, eds. Molecular approaches to parasitology. MBL lectures in biology; Vol 12. New York: Wiley-Liss, 1995.

Cohen S, Warren KS. Immunology of parasitic infections. 2nd ed. London and Boston: Blackwell, 1986.

Desowitz RS. New Guinea tapeworms and Jewish grandmothers: tales of parasites and people. New York: Norton, 1981.

Harries JR, Harries AD, Cook GC. One hundred clinical problems in tropical medicine. London: Bailliere Tindall, 1987.

Kean BH, KE Mott, AJ Russel. Tropical medicine and parasitology: classical investigations. Ithaca, NY: Cornell University Press, 1978.

Liu LX, Weller PF. Antiparasitic drugs. N Engl J Med 1996; 334:1178–1184.

Orihel TC. Parasites in human tissues. Chicago: ASCP Press, 1995.

Peters W, Gilles HM. Color atlas of tropical medicine and parasitology. 4th ed. London: Mosby-Wolfe, 1995.

Rose ME, McLaren JD, eds. Pathophysiological responses to parasites. London: British Society for Parasitology, 1986.

Strickland GT. Hunter's tropical medicine. 7th ed. Philadelphia: WB Saunders, 1991.

Trager W. Living together: the biology of animal parasitism. New York: Plenum Press, 1986.

Wyler DJ. Modern parasite biology. New York: WH Freeman, 1990.

Blood and Tissue Protozoa

DONALD J. KROGSTAD

N. CARY ENGLEBERG

Key Concepts

- Most tissue invasive protozoa have intracellular stages during their life cycle.
- Fever is a cardinal symptom of disseminated protozoal infections. Some species become dormant in tissues and cause prolonged, asymptomatic infection.
- Malaria is transmitted between humans by *Anopheles* mosquitoes. Its propagation depends on the presence of a reservoir of partially-immune, asymptomatic human carriers. Non-immune persons (e.g., young children in endemic areas and adult travelers from non-endemic areas) may experience severe, or even fatal illness. *Plasmodium falciparum* must be distinguished from other plasmodia and treated promptly, because this species is more virulent and more likely to be resistant to antimalarial drugs.
- Like malaria, babesiosis is a protozoal infection of erythrocytes, but it is more geographically-localized and less prevalent partly because it is transmitted by ticks rather than mosquitoes.
- Cats are the definitive (intestinal) host for *Toxoplasma gondi*; all other animals develop dormant toxoplasmal cysts in their muscles and viscera. Humans acquire infection by ingesting oocysts from cat feces or muscles cysts in undercooked meat. Manifestations in humans include a mononucleosis-like primary infection, chorioretinitis, congenital infection, or mass lesions in the brain (in person with AIDS)
- *Pneumocystis carinii* causes a potential fatal pneumonia in AIDS and other forms of severe immunodeficiency. The epidemiology of this infection is still not well understood. Nucleic acid analysis suggests that this agent is more closely related to the fungi than the protozoa.
- Virulence attributes of different *Leishmania* species determine whether infection results in a chronic skin ulcer at the site of the sandfly bite or a disseminated chronic febrile illness involving the liver, spleen and lymph nodes.
- Long-standing infection with the agent of Chagas' disease, *Trypanosoma cruzi* may result in immunopathologic damage to the heart and the gastrointestinal tract.
- The agent of African sleeping sickness, *Trypanosoma brucei*, evades the host immune response by a genetically-determined mechanism of antigenic variation.

Protozoa that produce bloodstream infection typically cause anemia by destroying red blood cells. Diseases caused by such protozoa include malaria and babesia. Protozoa that infect tissues may cause significant damage to the eyes, the brain, or the heart (toxoplasmosis), to the brain (African sleeping sickness), or to the heart and the gastrointestinal tract (Chagas' disease).

The major blood and tissue protozoa are presented in Table 50.1.

PARASITES OF RED BLOOD CELLS
Plasmodium

Malaria is the most important of all protozoan diseases and is said to have caused "the greatest harm to

Table 50.1. Comparison of Major Blood and Tissue Protozoa

Organism	Reservoir	Mode of transmission	Clinical manifestations
Blood Protozoa			
Plasmodia (malaria)	Infected humans	Vector-borne by the female *Anopheles* mosquito	Fever and chills with red blood cell lysis
Babesia (babesiosis)	Rodents—voles, deer, mice	Vector-borne by the hard-bodied *Ixodes* tick	Fever and chills with red blood cell lysis
Tissue Protozoa			
Toxoplasma gondii (toxoplasmosis)	Sheep, pigs, cattle, cats	Food-borne by the ingestion of inadequately cooked beef or lamb / Fecal-oral by the ingestion of infectious oocysts in cat feces	Intrauterine (congenital) infection may produce severe retardation / Mononucleosis-like illness most common / Infection of the brain (encephalitis) or heart (myocarditis) in severely immunocompromised patients
Leishmania (leishmaniasis)	Infected humans, dogs, jackals, foxes, rats, ground squirrels, gerbils	Vector-borne by infected *Phlebotomus* sandflies	Trivial or mild (self-healing) skin lesions / Disfiguring mucocutaneous lesions / Systemic illness with involvement of liver, spleen, and bone marrow
Pneumocystis carinii[a] (pneumocystosis)	Probably in infected humans and animals	Probably air-borne for initial infection / Disease typically represents activation of previously quiescent infection with natural or iatrogenic	Pneumonia
Trypanosoma cruzi (Chagas' disease, American trypanosomiasis)	Wildlife and domestic animals (zoonosis)	Vector-borne by reduviid bugs followed by rubbing infected feces in the bite wound	GI tract dysfunction from autonomic nerve damage (megacolon, megaesophagus) / Cardiac dysfunction from damage to the conducting system (right bundle branch block)
Trypanosoma brucei gambiense or *rhodesiense* (African trypanosomiasis, sleeping sickness)	Infected humans / Wildlife and cattle	Vector-borne by the tsetse fly	Systemic illness with fever, headache, muscle, and joint pains / Progresses to CNS involvement with altered speech, gait, and reflexes (encephalitis)

[a] Recent evidence suggests that this organism is a fungus.

the greatest number" of all infectious diseases. It occurs in many tropical and semitropical regions of the world (see Table 49.1), with approximately 200–300 million cases annually. An estimated 2–3 million people die of malaria each year, especially malnourished African children. Malaria in humans is caused by four different species of the *Plasmodium* protozoa: *Plasmodium falciparium*, *Plasmodium vivax*, *Plasmodium ovale*, and *Plasmodium malariae*. Infected humans are the only reservoir for the plasmodia that infect humans; transmission occurs via the bite of infected female anopheline mosquitoes.

CASE

Mr. M. is a 54-year-old businessman from Liverpool who traveled to East Africa (Kenya and Tanzania) on a business trip and then went on a photographic safari. After 1 week in Nairobi, he embarked on a 10-day trip through the wildlife preserves of Serengeti and Ngorogoro, with a final visit to Mombassa on the Indian Ocean. During his flight home, 9 days after leaving the game parks, he developed a flulike syndrome with headache, muscle aches, and a temperature of 38°C. After he returned home, he saw a physician who diagnosed influenza (which can also cause headache, muscle aches, and fever). He had returned to England in February during an outbreak of influenza A.

Mr. M. was given acetaminophen, which initially reduced his fever and muscle aches. However, he felt worse the next day. He suddenly developed an intense chill that lasted for about 30 minutes, followed by a fever to 40.2°C which lasted for 6 hours. As the fever abated, Mr. M. became drenched in sweat and felt exhausted and drained. These symptoms continued to worsen and he was brought to the hospital unconscious 2 days later. On examination, he had edema of the lungs. He showed no signs of endocarditis and a lumbar puncture was negative for bacterial meningitis.

The attending physician, drawing on his experience while serving in the armed services abroad, recognized that the clinical manifestations of Mr. M. were typical of a **malarial paroxysm**. The recent history of travel to endemic areas helped sharpen his suspicion of the disease, and the diagnosis was confirmed when a Giemsa-stained smear of the patient's blood revealed large numbers of parasites within red blood cells. The parasites were identified as *P. falciparum* by their characteristic ring shape. Mr. M's hematocrit (packed red cell volume) was 18% (normal is 40–45%). Urinalysis revealed dark urine, suggesting extensive hemolysis. His serum creatinine (a measure of renal function) was 5.4 mg per 100 ml (normal is 1 mg or less per 100 ml).

Because Mr. M had traveled in Kenya, a country in which drug-resistant malaria is endemic, treatment was begun with intravenous quinidine, which is effective against *P. falciparum* strains resistant to other antimalarial drugs. Mr. M. was also given intravenous glucose as a precaution against hypoglycemia (which may produce coma in patients with severe *P. falciparum* malaria). Hypoglycemia may result both from consumption of glucose by large numbers of parasites and from the direct release of insulin from the pancreas caused by quinidine or quinine. For his pulmonary edema, Mr. M. required artificial ventilation with a respirator. He was given multiple transfusions for his anemia and was put on a dialysis machine because of his kidney failure. He recovered and was discharged after spending 10 days in the intensive care unit.

Encounter and entry

Malaria is transmitted to humans by the mosquito vector 9 to 17 days after a female *Anopheles* mosquito ingests blood from a person infected with a species of *Plasmodium* that infect humans. Infected persons typically develop malaria symptoms 8 to 30 days later. Most cases of malaria that occur in Europe and North America are acquired in endemic areas and then imported into the nonendemic areas during the incubation period (**imported malaria**). However, mosquitoes that can serve as vectors (*Anopheles*) exist in the United States. When these mosquitoes bite returning travelers infected with plasmodia, malaria may be introduced into the United States, i.e., it may be transmitted to persons who have never traveled abroad. Introductions of malaria have oc-

curred with the return of large numbers of infected veterans after war or in regions that receive large numbers of recent immigrants. Malaria may also be transmitted by blood transfusion or by the sharing of needles among intravenous drug users (**induced** malaria).

Spread and multiplication

The life cycle of the malaria parasite is complex and rich in morphological detail (Fig. 50.1). In the infected mosquito, plasmodia inhabit the salivary glands as **sporozoites**, a stage of the parasite that is infectious for humans. The organisms are injected into the human bloodstream when infected mosquitoes bite and feed. The sporozoites travel through the bloodstream and enter liver cells within 30 minutes of injection. Over the next 8–14 days, they multiply and mature inside liver cells to very large numbers. At the end of this period (**the hepatocellular cycle**), they are released once again into the bloodstream in a form that can invade red blood cells (**merozoites**). Once inside these cells, the organisms divide and mature. After 2 or 3 days, the red blood cells burst, liberating a new generation of infective merozoites which infect previously unparasitized red blood cells (the **erythrocytic cycle**). In the liver and red blood cells, the parasites multiply asexually (i.e., by fission). Some of the plasmodia in the blood may also develop into forms capable of sexual reproduction called **gametocytes**. Male and female gametocytes are taken up by biting mosquitoes. In the mosquito gut, the male and female gameocytes participate in the portion of the reproductive cycle. The parasites undergo further changes in the mosquito before migrating to the salivary glands and once again becoming infective sporozoites. In each of these stages, the plasmodial cells are morphologically distinguishable (see Fig. 50.1).

The four species of plasmodia that cause human malaria vary in their virulence. A major reason for this difference is that the various plasmodial species prefer red blood cells of different ages: *P. falciparum* invades erythrocytes of all ages, producing the highest parasitemias and the greatest risk of mortality. *P. vivax* prefers reticulocytes and young red blood cells; *P. malariae*, older red blood cells. Both *P. vivax* and *P. malariae* infect only 1–2% or less of red blood cells, thus producing less severe disease. The fourth species, *P. ovale,* is virtually identical to *P. vivax* clinically and morphologically. *P. vivax* and *P. ovale* are also notable for the fact that some infected hepatocytes may harbor these parasites for a long period of time before they are released into the bloodstream. Thus, infection with these species may cause a series of relapses that may occur months, or even years, after the initial episode. Recurrent malaria is prevented by treatment with an antimalarial agent that targets the dormant parasites (hypnozoites) within liver cells.

The intracellular location of the malaria parasite

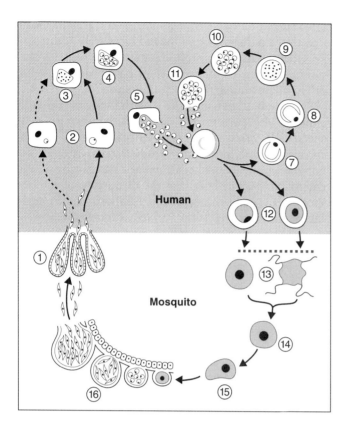

Figure 50.1. Malaria life cycle. Sporozoites released from the salivary gland of the female *Anopheles* mosquito are injected under the skin when the mosquito bites a human (*1*). They then travel through the bloodstream and enter the liver (*2*). Within liver cells, the parasites mature to tissue schizonts (*4*). They are then released into the bloodstream as merozoites (*5*) and produce symptomatic infection as they invade and destroy red blood cells (RBCs). However, some parasites remain dormant in the liver as hypnozoites (*2, dashed lines from 1–3*). These parasites (in *P. vivax, P. ovale*) cause relapsing malaria. Once within the bloodstream, merozoites (*5*) invade RBCs (*6*), and mature to the ring (*7,8*), trophozoite (*9*), and schizont (*10*) asexual stages. Schizonts lyse their host RBCs as they complete their maturation and release the next generation of merozoites (*11*), which invades previously uninfected RBCs.

Within RBCs, some parasites differentiate to sexual forms (male and female gametocytes, *12*). When gametocytes are taken up by a female *Anopheles* mosquito, the male gametocyte loses its flagellum, producing male gametes. These male gametes fertilize the female gamete (*13*) to produce a zygote (*14*). The zygote invades the gut of the mosquito (*15*) and develops into an oocyst (*16*). Mature oocysts produce sporozoites, which migrate to the salivary gland of the mosquito (*1*) and repeat the cycle. The *dashed line* between stages *12* and *13* indicates that absence of the mosquito vector precludes natural transmission via this cycle. Note that infection by the injection of infected blood bypasses this constraint and permits transmission of malaria among intravenous drug addicts and to persons who receive blood transfusions from infected donors.

within the red blood cell has two important consequences:

- Red blood cells infected with *P. falciparum* develop special "knobs" on their surfaces as a result of parasite-induced changes in the red blood cell membrane. Surface molecules associated with these knobs bind to receptors on the endothelial cells of venules and capillaries (e.g., intercellular adhesion molecule-1 [ICAM-1], thrombospondin). Parasitized red blood cells adhere to these cells, accumulate, and impede blood flow through the deep vascular beds. This process may have dire pathological consequences.
- The presence of plasmodia within red blood cells makes the cells less deformable. The spleen recognizes and removes older and less deformable red blood cells from the circulation, thus removing parasitized red blood cells from the circulation. Not surprisingly, splenectomized people have higher degrees of parasitemia and more severe infections.

Damage

The main manifestations of malaria are fever, chills, and anemia. The typical malarial paroxysm (as in Mr. M.'s case) coincides with the simultaneous lysis of many red blood cells and the release of large numbers of merozoites. Parasite replication can be synchronous and may produce a regular fever pattern—every 2 days with *P. vivax* or *P. ovale*, every 3 days with *P. malariae*. In contrast, the fever pattern is often irregular with *P. falciparum*. Other frequent clinical presentations include an influenza-like syndrome (fever, muscle aches, and malaise) and gastroenteritis (nausea, diarrhea, vomiting). Patients with these signs and symptoms are often misdiagnosed, especially if the physician is not acquainted with malaria or fails to obtain a history of recent travel to endemic areas.

Although the cause of these manifestations and the mechanism that maintains synchronous parasite development in vivo are still not clear, researchers believe that an immune-mediated mechanism may be involved. Malaria parasites may release a substance that induces the release of the cytokines tumor necrosis factor (TNF) and/or interleukin-1 from macrophages. TNF may be responsible for the paroxysmal fever and many malaria complications, such as edema of the lungs and shock, as seen in the case of Mr. M. (see also Chapter 63, "Sepsis"). The anemia that occurs in malaria is usually more severe than can be accounted for by the degree of parasitemia. Thus, uninfected red blood cells may also be destroyed prematurely, presumably by an immunologically mediated mechanism.

Human Genetics and Malaria

Genetic polymorphism of several human genes affects the entry, multiplication, and survival of malarial parasites. Genes are also important in determining the outcome of the infection. For example, parasite invasion of red blood cells depends on the presence of specific surface molecules. For *P. falciparum* and *P. vivax*, these surface molecules are glycophorin A and the Duffy blood group antigen, respectively. The variable susceptibility of black Americans to *P. vivax* infection is consistent with the distribution of Duffy antigen. Black Africans are Duffy-negative and are thus resistant to *P. vivax* infection.

Because falciparum malaria is such a devastating disease, it has probably been a powerful selective force in human evolution. Many epidemiological studies have shown that sickle cell disease—a recessive genetic disorder that causes red blood cells to become sickle-shaped—is common in areas of Africa with a high incidence of *P. falciparum*. A defective form of hemoglobin, called sickle cell hemoglobin (HbS) causes this disease. Malaria is seldom found in heterozygous carriers of HbS (sickle cell trait), which suggests that this genetic determinant imparts a selective advantage to people living in areas where the parasite is common. Furthermore, in vitro studies have shown that at oxygen tensions similar to those in tissue, the parasites grow poorly in red blood cells from persons with sickle cell disease or the sickle cell trait (Fig. 50.2). Thus, in the black African population, a trade-off exists between the risk of a fatal disease—sickle cell disease in those who are homozygous for HbS—and the protection of a larger group of the population, the heterozygous HbS carriers. This is an example of a balanced genetic polymorphism.

How does the sickle cell trait protect from malaria? *P. falciparum*–infected red blood cells adhere to the walls of blood vessels via knobs that form as the parasites mature. This adherence to the peripheral microcirculation sequesters the parasitized red blood cells in an area of reduced oxygen tension, which facilitates sickling, potassium loss, and the killing of the parasites.

Other genetic abnormalities that restrict the growth of malarial parasites within red blood cells are glucose-6-phosphate dehydrogenase deficiency (G6PD) and thalassemia. In the case of G6PD, it is thought that the reduced ability of the red blood cells to produce NADPH via the pentose phosphate shunt results in an oxidative stress that inhibits parasite growth.

Diagnosis

Malaria is diagnosed in the laboratory by microscopic examination of a Giemsa-stained smear of peripheral blood using the oil immersion objective (Fig. 50.3). Wright's stain, which is used more often in the clinical hematology laboratory, stains the parasites less well. If the degree of parasitemia is low, a "thick smear" may be used to increase sensitivity. Because red blood cells are lysed in the preparation of thick smears, this procedure provides no information about the size of the

infected red blood cells or about the intracellular location of the parasite within the red blood cells (central or peripheral). These morphological characteristics that can be seen on a "thin smear" of blood can be used to differentiate among the species of plasmodia.

In acutely ill patients, the malarial species is usually either *P. falciparum* or *P. vivax*. In contrast to these species, *P. malariae* most often causes subacute or chronic infections (but may produce acute infections in nonimmune people). *P. ovale* malaria is clinically so similar to *P. vivax* malaria that the distinction of the two species is usually of no practical importance. *P. vivax* can be differentiated from *P. falciparum* on the basis of morphological characteristics. For example, *P. vivax* causes infected red blood cells to progressively enlarge as the parasite matures and produces eosinophilic "stippling" in the red blood cells (Schüffner's dots). Neither red cell enlargement nor Schüffner's dots occur with *P. falciparum*. This distinction is important because *P. falciparum* infection poses a greater risk of death and may be resistant to treatment with chloroquine, whereas *P. vivax* may cause post-treatment relapses due to slowly growing or dormant parasites in the liver.

Serologic testing is of little value for the diagnosis of malaria in the acutely ill patient. The reason is that treatment must begin within 1–2 days of the onset of symptoms, and patients do not develop species-specific antibodies to the parasites for 3–5 weeks. Hybridization with DNA probes and polymerase chain reaction (PCR)

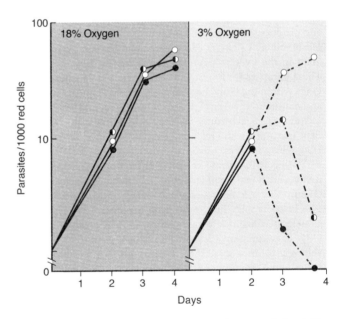

Figure 50.2. Effect of hypoxia on parasite growth in sickle hemoglobin red blood cells. In 18% oxygen, *P. falciparum* grow as well in sickle hemoglobin (*SS*) red blood cells (*filled circles*) as in either heterozygous (*SA*) red blood cells (*half-filled circles*) or normal (*AA*) RBCs (*open circles, left panel*). In contrast, at 3% oxygen, *P. falciparum* parasites grow less well in SS cells than in SS or SA cells (*right panel*).

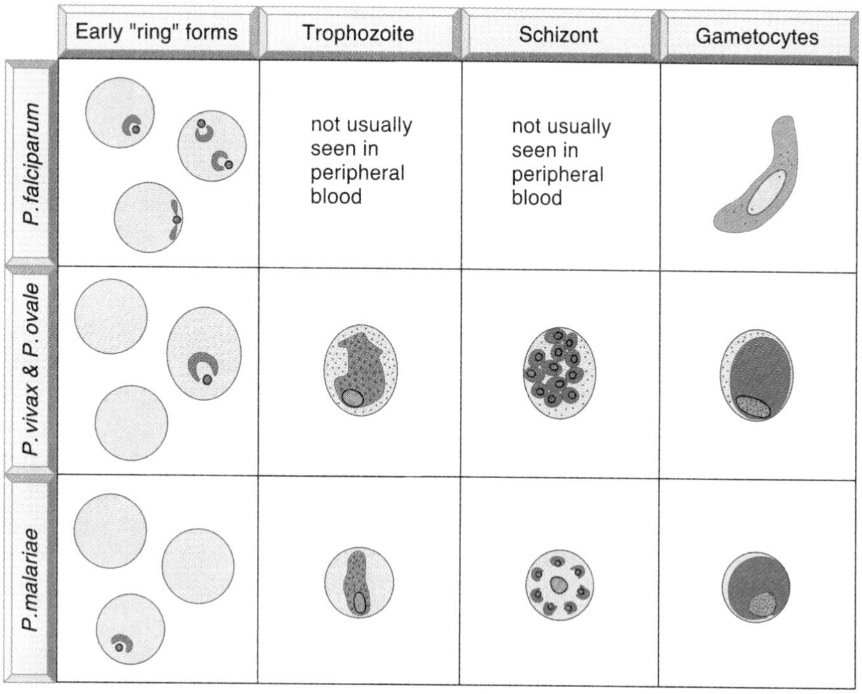

	Early "ring" forms	Trophozoite	Schizont	Gametocytes
P. falciparum		not usually seen in peripheral blood	not usually seen in peripheral blood	
P. vivax & P. ovale				
P. malariae				

Figure 50.3. Malarial parasites in blood cells. This schematic drawing illustrates the most prominent morphological features that distinguish human malarial species in blood smears. The nuclear chromatid bodies of all of the malarial parasites are shaded in dark gray in this diagram but actually appear red in Giemsa-stained preparations.

P. falciparum usually appears as small, fine, ring forms, sometimes more than one per red blood cell. More mature forms of this species are not usually seen in the peripheral blood. The gametocyte is characteristically banana-shaped.

P. vivax and *P. ovale* are distinguished by details not illustrated here. Infected cells and ring forms are larger than those of *P. falciparum*. At the trophozoite stage, red Schüffner's dots are seen. The schizont contains more than a dozen merozoites before it ruptures.

P. malariae infects smaller, senescent cells. Schüffner's dots are not present. At the schizont stage, 8–12 merozoites are arranged peripherally around the brown-colored, central malarial pigment.

may be useful in the diagnosis of malaria (see Chapter 55, "Diagnostic Principles"). Several technical modifications of PCR will have to be made before this test can be used in the field in developing countries.

Prevention and treatment

Natural immunity to malaria is imperfect. Persons who have lived in malarious areas all their lives and who have evidence of humoral and cellular responses to parasite antigens are nevertheless infected on a regular basis. However, their infections tend to be less severe than those of nonimmune persons, suggesting that the immune response plays a significant role in controlling infection. Some researchers have shown that antibodies directed against sporozoites, the form introduced by the insect (see Fig. 50.1), are not sufficient to protect against infection. Effective protective immunity may involve cell-mediated cytotoxicity of infected liver cells or antibodies against certain surface proteins of the merozoite stage. An effective future vaccine will probably stimulate cell-mediated immunity and include antigens derived from the various stages of the parasite. Unfortunately, studies of cell-mediated immunity

are not as advanced as those of humoral immunity. The future will tell if such a "combined" vaccine is possible.

Chloroquine is the most widely used drug for antimalarial chemoprophylaxis and treatment. It is effective against all strains of *Plasmodium*, except for resistant strains of *P. falciparum*. Such strains are now widespread in most of Southeast Asia, South America, and Africa. Chloroquine resistance complicates the prophylaxis and treatment of malaria acquired in these geographic areas. Thus, Mr. M. might well have acquired *P. falciparum* infection in East Africa even if he had been on chloroquine chemoprophylaxis. In contrast, he would have been protected in Haiti, where there is no chloroquine resistance. Updates on the prevalence of chloroquine-resistant *P. falciparum* and recommendations for antimalarial prophylaxis are published annually by the Centers for Disease Control and the World Health Organization.

Patients infected with chloroquine-resistant *P. falciparum* can be treated with other agents, such as mefloquine, quinine, quinidine, or Fansidar (a fixed combination of sulfadoxine and pyrimethamine). Although Fansidar was once considered an effective alternative to chloroquine for chloroquine-resistant *P. falciparum*, resistance to this agent has recently emerged in the same geographic areas where chloroquine resistance is prevalent. In addition, Fansidar has been associated with rare but potentially fatal skin reactions. At present, *P. falciparum* cases acquired in areas where drug resistance is prevalent are usually treated with a combination of doxycycline and quinine or quinidine. Mefloquine is a quinine derivative that is also active against chloroquine-resistant strains, but it is often toxic at treatment doses. However, it is a mainstay for chemoprophylaxis in travelers to most areas with chloroquine-resistant malaria. Unfortunately, resistance to mefloquine has also been detected in parts of Southeast Asia, and travelers to these areas are now being advised to take daily doxycycline to prevent infection.

Although chloroquine is effective in controlling acute infection caused by *P. vivax* or *P. ovale*, it is not effective against the liver (hypnozoite) stages of these species. Primaquine, a derivative of quinine, is effective against these stages. It is used with chloroquine to prevent late relapses associated with maturation of the hypnozoite to the tissue schizont stage and the subsequent release of infectious merozoites. However, primaquine is more toxic than chloroquine and causes nausea, vomiting, and diarrhea. In patients with glucose-6-phosphate dehydrogenase (G6PD) deficiency, this drug induces hemolysis. Primaquine is not indicated for either *P. falciparum* or *P. malariae* infections because these parasites do not produce a dormant (hypnozoite) stage in the liver.

Mosquito control with insecticides and drainage of aquatic breeding sites have been used to control malaria in many countries, and these measures have resulted in a dramatic decline in the incidence of the disease. Unfortunately, these measures have some drawbacks: they are expensive and are not always effective because mosquitoes may become resistant to some of the insecticides. In endemic areas, individuals should protect themselves with mosquito netting, house screening, and insect repellents. The best hope for controlling malaria is the development of improved antimalarials and/or an effective vaccine.

Babesia

Like the plasmodia of malaria, *Babesia* are protozoal parasites that cause illness by destroying the red blood cells they infect. Unlike malaria, babesiosis is endemic in the United States. *Babesia microti* is the most recognized cause of human babesiosis in the United States. Interestingly, it is concentrated geographically in the same areas as endemic Lyme disease because *B. microti* and *Borrelia burgdorferi* (the bacterial cause of Lyme disease) infect the same animal reservoir—the white-footed mouse—and are transmitted to humans by the same deer tick, *Ixodes scapularis* (see Chapter 25, "Lyme Disease"). Cases of babesiosis outside this geographic area (e.g, from the Midwest and Pacific Coast) appear to be due to other babesial species which are more closely related to the principal European species, *Babesia divergens*, than to *B. microti*.

Clinical and parasitological features

Babesiosis is difficult to recognize clinically, because the illness it causes is nonspecific. Infected persons experience a flulike illness with fever, chills, sweats, muscle aches, and fatigue. Since the illness usually occurs in the summer months, when ticks are feeding, babesiosis has been likened to a "summer flu." Illness is usually mild, but as in malaria, more severe disease occurs in splenectomized patients. In persons with an intact spleen the percentage of infected red blood cells is usually 0.2% or less; it can rise to over 10% in splenectomized patients. In fact, the disease was first detected in postmortem studies of splenectomized patients. As in malaria, the spleen is thought to remove the less deformable babesia-infected red blood cells from the circulation.

The life cycle of *Babesia* is shown in Fig. 50.4. The

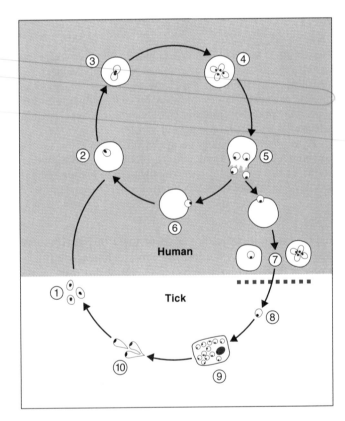

Figure 50.4. *Babesia* life cycle. Infectious merozoites are injected under the skin by the hard-bodied tick (*Ixodes*) vector (*1*) and they invade red blood cells directly (*2*). There is no intermediate liver stage in babesiosis as there is in malaria. Once within the red blood cells, parasites replicate asexually by binary fission (*3*). *Babesia* characteristically form tetrads (*4*), lyse their host red blood cells as they mature (*5*), and complete the cycle when parasitized red blood cells are ingested by the tick vector (*6*). The *dashed line* between *7* and *8* indicates that natural transmission does not occur in areas lacking the hard-bodied tick.

epidemiology of the disease is restricted by the presence of a suitable tick vector and wildlife reservoir, as well as by human contact with them. Humans are infected accidentally in endemic areas and are not thought to contribute to the maintenance of the parasite's life cycle.

Diagnosis and treatment

The laboratory diagnosis of babesiosis depends on finding the parasites in Giemsa-stained blood films using the oil immersion objective. The parasites are seen as small rings, often in tetrads. These are the only forms found in peripheral blood and may be easily missed when parasitemia is low. Their ring shape makes them easy to confuse with a similar form of *Plasmodium falciparum*. The distinction between the two parasites is important because *Babesia* infections are treated with different chemotherapeutic agents than malaria: clindamycin plus quinine for babesiosis, versus a variety of different drugs for malaria (see above).

Antibodies to *Babesia* can be detected in most infected persons. However, they often appear too late (3–4 weeks after the onset of infection) to be helpful in the diagnosis and treatment of acute babesiosis.

TISSUE PROTOZOA

Toxoplasma

Infection with the agent of toxoplasmosis, *Toxoplasma gondii*, is common in humans. Tests for antitoxoplasma antibodies have revealed that infection with toxoplasma is common among adults in the United States. However, less than 1% are ever diagnosed with toxoplasmosis. In the few persons with signs and symptoms of active infection, the clinical presentation of the disease varies (see below). Toxoplasmosis is particularly damaging for immunocompromised patients, such as those with AIDS, and for the developing fetus. *T. gondii* can cause three distinct syndromes:

- A "mononucleosis"-like syndrome in which tests for the common viral agents of mononucleosis—Epstein-Barr virus and cytomegalovirus—are negative.
- A congenital infection that may have severe consequences if acquired in the first trimester of pregnancy. A more detailed discussion of the effects of *T. gondii* on the developing fetus is presented in Chapter 69, "Congenital Infections."
- Infections in immunocompromised hosts (especially those with AIDS), often involving the brain or the heart.

Encounter

People acquire toxoplasma infection by eating inadequately cooked meat or by ingesting food contaminated with infected cat feces (Fig. 50.5). The more common mode of transmission appears to be via the ingestion of inadequately cooked meat (lamb, mutton, and possibly beef) that contains parasitic tissue cysts (produced by asexual reproduction, see Fig. 50.6). Less frequently, humans become infected by accidentally ingesting minute amounts of cat feces containing fertile cysts called oocysts. The frequency with which this type of transmission occurs is in dispute and is difficult to determine for two reasons. First, only a small percentage of toxoplasma-infected cats excrete oocysts in their stools, and second, we do not know how frequently humans accidentally ingest cat feces.

The evidence that cats are important in the transmission of *T. gondii* to humans comes from the observation that toxoplasmosis is absent from areas that do not have cats, such as isolated Pacific atolls. Once cats are introduced into an area, humans become infected. Cats harbor the sexual cycle of the organisms and produce environmentally resistant infective cysts in their stool, thus making them necessary to maintain the life cycle of the parasite.

After ingestion, the parasites are released from tissue cysts (oocysts) in the small intestine and penetrate the gut wall, invading the bloodstream and disseminating throughout the body, including the brain and the heart. In the first 4–6 weeks after the parasites enter the body, normal hosts mount an immune response that controls the infection. The parasites are not eliminated but form dormant tissue cysts in different parts of the body. Unless the person becomes immunosuppressed at some time in the future, the infection remains inactive.

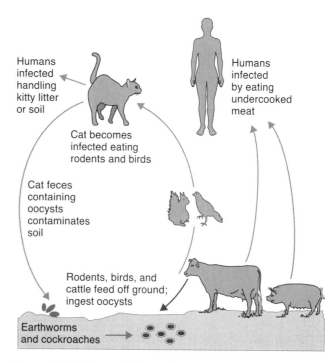

Humans infected handling kitty litter or soil

Humans infected by eating undercooked meat

Cat becomes infected eating rodents and birds

Cat feces containing oocysts contaminates soil

Rodents, birds, and cattle feed off ground; ingest oocysts

Earthworms and cockroaches

Figure 50.5. Transmission and spread of *Toxoplasma gondii*.

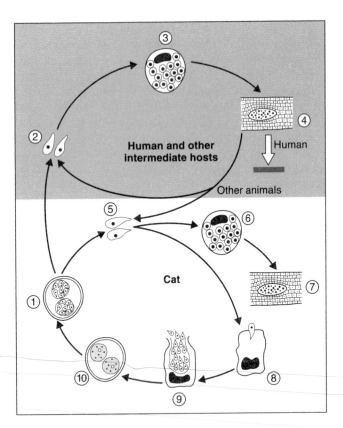

Figure 50.6. *Toxoplasma* life cycle. Humans and other mammals become infected with *Toxoplasma* by ingesting inadequately cooked meat containing tissue cysts or by ingesting infectious oocysts excreted in the feces of infected cats (*1*). Once in the human host, the oocysts mature to tachyzoites (*2*). Tachyzoites enter the bloodstream and disseminate throughout the body (*3*). After the initial acute infection, most people mount a successful immune response that eliminates the active infectious (tachyzoite) form of the parasite and leaves only tissue cysts with dormant organisms (*4*). A similar progression is observed within the cat (steps l–4), where the parasite also invades intestinal epithelial cells (*6*). In addition, the organism establishes a sexual cycle (*8,9*) in the cat, in which infectious oocysts are formed (*10*) and released (*11*). The *solid line* below step 4 in the *upper half* of the diagram indicates that human tissue infection is a dead end. Unless an animal or human consumes infected human flesh, human tissue cysts disintegrate after the death of the host.

Pathogenesis, diagnosis, and treatment

In the active phase of infection, toxoplasma are found within macrophages and can be observed under the microscope with the high dry or oil immersion objectives. The parasites survive intracellularly in part by preventing acidification of phagosomes and/or their fusion with lysosomes. However, activated macrophages are able to kill *T. gondii*.

In the immunologically competent host, the diagnosis of acute toxoplasmosis is made by an elevated antibody titer, especially of IgM antibodies. Most previously healthy persons do not need treatment for self-limited, acute toxoplamosis.

Serologic diagnosis is often insensitive in the immunocompromised patient, such as those with AIDS, who may be unable to produce a diagnostic rise in antibody titer. Other methods must be used to diagnose toxoplasmosis in immunocompromised patients. The appearance of any new neurologic symptom or symptoms and the presence of multiple, ring-enhancing lesions on a CT or MRI scan of the brain should raise suspicion of nervous system toxoplasmosis. On biopsy, the trophozoites associated with acute infection may be difficult to detect morphologically. Staining brain biopsy material with fluorescent or peroxidase-labeled antitoxoplasma antibodies increases the sensitivity of detection. In the absence of an adequate immune response, toxoplasma will cause local inflammation that may result in severe necrosis, tissue damage, and death. Since biopsy of the brain is a complicated and potential hazardous procedure, most AIDS patients with a suggestive history, positive brain scan, and serological evidence of prior toxoplasma exposure (e.g., specific IgG antibody) are treated presumptively for cerebral toxoplasmosis. Lifesaving treatment is usually initiated with pyrimethamine plus either sulfadoxine or clindamycin.

T. gondii may be transmitted to a developing fetus if the mother acquires infection during pregnancy. Because most of the potential damage occurs in utero, treatment for congenital infections after the baby is born is usually too late. For this reason, most physicians screen women for antitoxoplasma antibody at the time of marriage or when pregnancy is first detected. Women with preexisting antibodies at the time of pregnancy (indicating prior infection) have virtually no risk of producing a congenitally infected child. Women who are seronegative can be given preventative advice, and those who seroconvert during pregnancy can be counseled, offered therapeutic abortion (if early in pregnancy), or given treatment with experimental drugs, such as spiramycin. The risk of severe complications in the fetus is greatest for women who seroconvert in the first trimester of pregnancy. The frequency of congenital infection is greatest in the third trimester, but most of the children infected late in gestation have no detectable disease at the time of birth. Chorioretinitis, which many develop early or many years after birth, is sometimes the only manifestation of congenital infection. Unfortunately, a variety of developmental problems may also be seen among these initially "asymptomatic" children later in childhood.

Pneumocystis

As with *Toxoplasma*, *Pneumocystis* infection is common, but overt disease is rare in healthy individuals. The widespread distribution of *Pneumocystis* is demonstrated by the large percentage (70%) of people over the age of 4 who have antibodies to this in the United States. In fact, *Pneumocystis* qualifies as a member of the normal human flora.

In contrast to toxoplasma, this organism typically causes only one disease—pneumonia. It has become a sentinel infection in persons with AIDS, for whom it is highly virulent (see Chapter 68, "Acquired Immunodeficiency Syndrome"). It also causes serious disease among malnourished children and other immunosuppressed persons, and may produce disease at other sites (such as the spleen and bone marrow).

■ CASE

Ms. F., a 45-year-old woman, had been generally healthy before admission to the hospital. In the preceding 4 months her weight decreased from 128 to 103 lbs. and she reported night sweats and fatigue. Her history included the usual childhood diseases, two uneventful pregnancies, and two blood transfusions in Haiti 3 years ago, which she received for injuries sustained during an automobile accident.

On admission she had a fever of 38.4°C, a nonproductive cough, bilateral pulmonary infiltrates on chest film, and moderate hypoxia. On the basis of her history of blood transfusion in Haiti, she was tested for HIV antibodies and was found to be positive. Because examination of an induced sputum specimen revealed no pathogens, the patient underwent bronchoscopy with bronchoalveolar lavage. The fluid collected by this procedure was examined using a fluorescent monoclonal antibody against *Pneumocystis carinii* and revealed multiple characteristic, glowing cysts by fluorescence microscopy. She was treated with trimethoprim–sulfamethoxazole (an antibacterial combination that has been shown to be effective against this protozoan), and a tapering course of corticosteroids. However, her white blood count decreased with this treatment, and she was switched to pen-

tamidine. Over the next 10 days, her white blood cell count increased, and she recovered from the illness despite some renal insufficiency caused by pentamidine.

Pathogenesis, diagnosis, and treatment

The full life cycle of this organism is not known. Until recently, *P. carinii* was classified as an animal parasite; newer studies based on the homology of its ribosomal RNA indicate that it is probably a fungus. The organism is frequently found during careful examination of sections of lungs of people who have died from other causes. The epidemiological evidence for person-to-person or animal-to-human transmission is confusing and controversial. Active *P. carinii* infection may be elicited by giving steroids to normal rats, suggesting that they normally carry these organisms. In rats and infected humans, the alveoli of the lungs are typically filled with proteinaceous material and cysts. *P. carinii* is an extracellular parasite and does not readily invade tissues; thus, it is usually confined to the pulmonary air spaces. It is not clear why *P. carinii* produces only pneumonia (perhaps it requires an increased oxygen tension). Rarely, the organism is seen at other sites, such as the spleen, lymph nodes, or bone marrow.

The diagnosis of *P. carinii* infection requires microscopic demonstration of the organism in body fluids or tissues (Fig. 50.7). Often, the organisms can be identified in sputum samples induced by inhalation of nebulized saline, but it is sometimes necessary to perform an invasive procedure, such as bronchoalveolar lavage, transbronchial biopsy, or even open lung biopsy to obtain adequate mate-

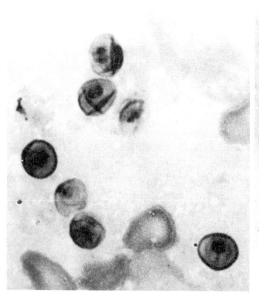
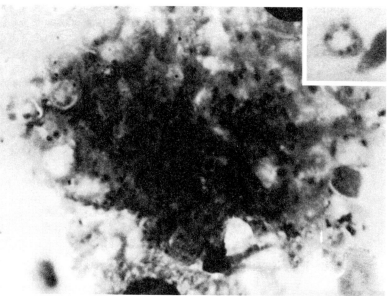

Figure 50.7. *Pneumocystis carinii. Left:* P. carinii is usually identified by the staining of cysts with Gomori methenamine silver nitrate (as in this figure). The cysts contain dark bodies which, in some instances, look like parentheses (see the two upper organisms). The cyst wall often appears folded. *Right:* A

Giemsa-stained preparation showing *P. carinii* trophozoites, but not cysts. The large clump of cells is typical of that seen in AIDS patients. Giemsa does not stain the cysts, which appear as round, clear areas. The *inset* shows a *P. carinii* cyst in which nuclei of the intracystic organism are arranged in clockface fashion.

rial for examination. Rapid microscopic staining techniques must be used because of the need for timely diagnosis. Serologic tests are of limited value because a diagnostic rise in antibody titer often takes 2–3 weeks after the onset of symptoms and may not occur in severely immunocompromised patients. Antigen detection tests are being developed but are not yet sufficiently sensitive or specific. The two treatment regimens used in the case of Ms. F. are thought to be equally effective. Other antimicrobials that have been used successfully for treatment include dapsone–trimethoprim, the antiparasitic agent atovaquone, the antifolate drug trimetrexate, and the combination of clindamycin plus primaquine. Corticosteroid therapy has been shown to improve survival in pneumocystosis associated with moderate or severe hypoxia and may be used concurrently with any of these antimicrobial agents. Severely immunocompromised patients, such as those with AIDS, bone marrow transplants, and malignancies requiring intensive cancer chemotherapy may be given intermittent doses of trimethoprim–sulfamethoxasole, dapsone, or inhaled aerosolized pentamidine to prevent the occurrence of pneumocystis pneumonia.

Leishmania

Leishmania species produce a spectrum of clinical syndromes, from superficial ulcers to severe lesions of the liver, spleen, and bone marrow accompanied by systemic signs such as fever, weight loss, and anemia. Several species are pathogenic for humans. The reason for the wide diversity in clinical disease is not well understood, but it is probably due in part to the temperature preferences of the different species. Superficial lesions are produced by *Leishmania* species that grow better at lower temperatures (25–30°C), whereas those that invade the viscera grow better at 37°C.

■ CASE

Mr. Q., a 26-year-old graduate student in anthropology, returned from a 6-month expedition to Peru with a non-healing 2 × 5 cm lesion on his right shin. A smear taken from the edge of the lesion stained with Giemsa revealed *Leishmania*-containing macrophages. Mr. Q. was given the antimony-containing, antiprotozoal drug pentostam for 4 weeks. The lesion began to heal slowly and he eventually recovered completely.

Transmission

Leishmania are small protozoa that belong to the flagellates because they possess a prominent flagellum during part of their life cycle. The flagellum is connected to an organelle called the kinetoplast which, like the mitochondria, has its own DNA.

Leishmania are transmitted by the bite of sandflies—small, short-lived insects that feed on many mammals. The phlebotomine sandflies that transmit leishmaniasis are generally found in tropical or subtropical parts of the world, which explains why this disease is rare in North America and Europe. However, phlebotomine sandflies are occasionally found in more temperate regions, and indigenous cases have been reported in the United States. Like malaria, leishmaniasis in the United States is seen mainly among travelers returning from tropical countries and has been observed in military personnel returning from the 1991 Gulf War. Reservoirs of *Leishmania* include rodents, dogs, other animals, and infected humans.

Pathogenesis, diagnosis, and treatment

There are several species of *Leishmania*, each with different tissue tropisms and clinical manifestations. The diseases they cause include localized skin ulcers, such as "chiclero disease" (after the harvesters of chewing gum, "chicle"), mucocutaneous lesions ("espundia"), disseminated cutaneous leishmaniasis, and disseminated visceral leishmaniasis ("kala azar"). Mr. Q. had a form of cutaneous leishmaniasis that usually heals poorly and requires treatment.

The life cycle of *Leishmania* is shown in Fig. 50.8. A protein on the parasites' surface binds to one of the complement receptors on macrophages. Phagocytosis then takes place with a minimal degree of oxidative burst. *Leishmania* also produce superoxide dismutase, which protects them from superoxide produced by the macrophages. After they are taken up into phagosomes, the parasites differentiate into a nonflagellate form, called the amastigote. Although the parasite-containing phagosomes fuse with lysosomes, the amastigotes are resistant to killing by lysosomal enzymes. In addition, the amastigotes depend on the low pH of the phagolysosomes for the uptake of nutrients such as glucose and proline.

Immunity against leishmaniasis involves cell-mediated mechanisms and the induction of γ-interferon (a Th1 response, see Chapter 7, "Induced Defenses"). It is thought that the parasite may facilitate it own survival by possessing immunodominant antigens that preferentially induce a Th2 response, which is not protective. Patients with AIDS, who lack coordinated cell-mediated immunity altogether, may develop severe *Leishmania* infections. In fact, leishmaniasis is one of the most common causes of fevers in persons with AIDS who live in the Mediterranean region.

Leishmaniasis is best diagnosed by histologic examination of biopsy material using the high dry objective. However, the different species look alike and cannot be distinguished morphologically. *Leishmania* species can be distinguished by culture or by analyzing patterns of isoenzymes or DNA restriction endonuclease fragments. A DNA hybridization technique allows the differentiation of parasite species in biopsy material without the need for culture. The increased sensitivity of this method takes advantage of the presence of repetitive DNA sequences ("minicircles") in the kinetoplast.

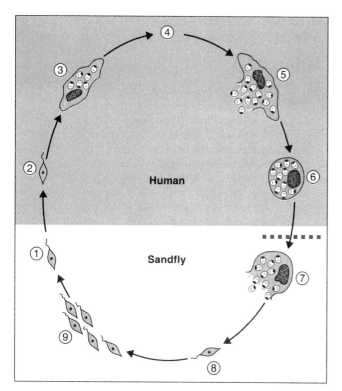

Figure 50.8. *Leishmania* life cycle. The flagellated (promastigote) insect form of the parasite (*1*) is injected under the skin by the sandfly (*Phlebotomus*) vector (*2*). Once within the human host, the parasite transforms into a nonflagellated (amastigote) form that is more capable of evading the host immune response than the promastigote form (it stimulates less release of H_2O_2 from mononuclear cells than the promastigote and produces its own superoxide dismutase). The parasite then invades lymphoreticular cells (*3*), replicates (*4*), lyses the cells (*5*), and repeats the same sequence in other reticuloendothelial cells (*6*).

In endemic areas, the cycle is completed when previously uninfected sandflies acquire infectious leishmanial amastigotes by biting infected humans (*7*). The amastigotes then transform into flagellated promastigotes (*8*) and replicate in the sandfly GI tract (*9*). Infective promastigotes are injected under the skin of another human when the parasitized sandfly takes a blood meal (*1* and *2*). The *dashed line* between 6 and 7 indicates that transmission is blocked at this point in nonendemic areas such as the United States because the sandfly vector is not present.

A variety of drugs are used to treat leishmaniasis, especially the invasive forms of the disease. Antimony-containing compounds are modestly successful. However, disease of deep organs, such as the bone marrow, may produce fatal anemia and granulocytopenia, despite treatment.

Trypanosoma cruzi

Chagas' disease, caused by *Trypanosoma cruzi*, occurs throughout Latin America. Overt disease is much less common than infection, but the reasons for this difference are poorly understood.

CASE

Senhor R., a 58-year-old Brazilian businessman, was admitted to a hospital in Sao Paolo for the evaluation of chronic constipation. Radiologic examination of his gastrointestinal tract revealed a large dilated colon (megacolon) and a somewhat less dilated esophagus (megaesophagus). A blood sample revealed antibodies to *T. cruzi*. Because no drugs are effective after the onset of complications, Senhor R. was not given antiparasitic treatment. His chronic constipation was treated symptomatically with a high-fiber diet. A few years later, Senhor R. was hospitalized for treatment of cardiomyopathy with congestive heart failure. Although this complication was adequately compensated with medical therapy, Senhor R. expired suddenly at home 1 year later.

Pathogenesis

The life cycle of *T. cruzi* is shown in Fig. 50.9. In the

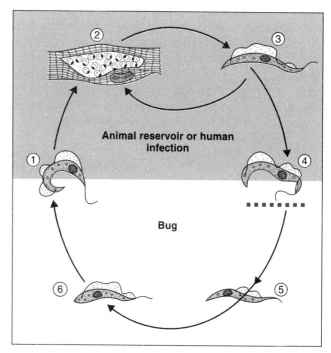

Figure 50.9. Chagas' disease (American trypanosomiasis). The reduviid bug vector deposits feces containing infectious trypomastigotes on the skin (*1*). The human host rubs the itching bite wound, allowing the parasites to enter the bloodstream. In the human host, the trypomastigote transforms into an amastigote (analogous to the leishmanial amastigote) as it invades tissue such as muscle (*2*). Cells containing large numbers of amastigotes often rupture, liberating large numbers of trypomastigotes (*3*). Trypomastigotes invade other host cells (*arrow* from 3 back to 2) or may be taken up by the vector to complete the cycle.

In the vector (*5*), the parasite replicates as an epimastigote and produces additional infectious trypomastigotes (*1*). The *dashed line* below 4 indicates that natural transmission does not occur in areas lacking the reduviid bug vector. Although reduviid bugs are present in the southern United States, indigenous cases are rare.

endemic areas of South and Central America, most persons are infected by *T. cruzi* in childhood by the bite of an infected reduviid bug (or "kissing bug"). A chancre or tissue and lymph node swelling may develop at the bite site. Although some persons develop serious (even fatal) illness, most develop a relatively mild disease with fever, recover spontaneously, and remain asymptomatic. A small proportion of individuals infected with *T. cruzi* develop complications 10–20 years later. The complications of Chagas' disease result from damage to nerves in the gastrointestinal tract (megaesophagus, megacolon), the conducting tissue in the heart (right bundle branch block), or the heart muscle (cardiomyopathy). Sudden death due to cardiac arrhythmia is common. Infected reduviid bugs are present in the southern United States and are presumably responsible for the sporadic cases of Chagas' disease observed among lifelong residents of Florida, Louisiana, Mississippi, and California.

It is not clear why infection with *T. cruzi* produces autonomic nerve damage in the gastrointestinal tract or why it damages the cardiac conduction system. Usually, few organisms and a number of lymphocytes are seen in damaged tissue. Fibrosis is the hallmark of the pathology. Consequently, several investigators have postulated that autoimmune mechanisms may play a significant role in the pathogenesis of these complications.

Diagnosis and treatment

The diagnosis of early infection is usually based on the appearance of the patient. Organisms may often be found in the blood if it is cultured in an appropriate medium. Early infection can also be diagnosed by detecting infection in reduviid bugs that have purposely been allowed to feed upon the patient. Antibodies appear within several weeks. Antibody titers usually remain positive for years. The diagnosis of chronic infection with complications is based on a positive antibody titer or history of exposure plus a known complication.

Patients with early acute Chagas' disease may respond to treatment with either of two drugs, nifurtimox or benznidazole. However, there is no effective treatment for patients with late complications, perhaps because the critical damage has already occurred and is no longer reversible.

Trypanosoma brucei

African sleeping sickness is caused by *Trypanosoma brucei* (Fig. 50.10). This disease is endemic in Africa and is transmitted by the bite of infected tsetse flies. A remarkable feature of these parasites is their ability to change their predominant surface antigens as the host develops immunity to the previous surface antigen. *T. brucei* and its vectors differ in several biological characteristics from *T. cruzi* (the agent of Chagas' disease) and its vectors. For example, *T. brucei* resides in the salivary glands of tsetse flies, and is transmitted directly by bites. *T. cruzi*, on the other hand, grows in the intestine of re-

duviid bugs and is transmitted when feces deposited by the biting insect are introduced into the bite by scratching.

CASE

Mr. S., a 32-year-old student from Kenya living in Canada, had fevers to 38°C and swollen lymph nodes at the back of his neck for 8 months. Two weeks ago, he developed a severe headache, stiff neck, and an aversion to light (photophobia). Trypanosomes were seen on Giemsa-stained specimens of blood and cerebrospinal fluid under the oil immersion objective. Mr. S was treated with two drugs: suramin for hemolymphatic infection and an arsenical (tryparsamide) for central nervous system infection. He recovered after 4 weeks of treatment.

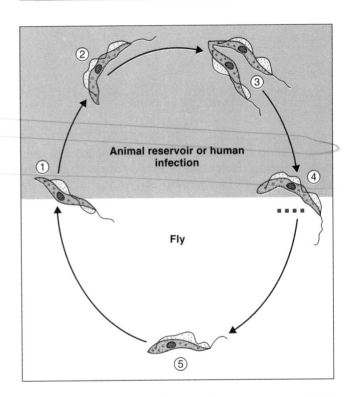

Figure 50.10. Sleeping sickness (African trypanosomiasis). The tsetse fly vector inoculates infectious trypomastigotes under the skin (*1*) when it bites humans or other mammals. Once inside the new host (*2*), the parasite replicates in the bloodstream by binary fission as a trypomastigote (*3*). Unlike *Leishmania* and the trypanosome that causes Chagas' disease, the trypanosomes that cause African sleeping sickness do not have promastigote or amastigote forms. The rate of movement of trypomastigotes from the bloodstream and lymph nodes to the central nervous system defines the point at which the illness changes from a systemic (hemolymphatic) infection to an encephalitis. Circulating trypomastigotes (*4*) taken up anew by tsetse flies complete the cycle.

Within the tsetse fly, the parasites replicate in the GI tract and transform into epimastigotes (*5*). The *dashed line below 4* indicates that natural transmission does not occur in countries such as the United States where the tsetse fly vector is not present.

Pathogenesis and diagnosis

The spread of African trypanosomiasis is restricted by the distribution of its tsetse fly vector (*Glossina*) and of its animal reservoirs. In East Africa, the main reservoirs are wild game animals (such as impalas); in West Africa, infected humans and domestic animals, such as cattle. Several weeks to months after the initial infection, patients develop a systemic illness with fever and swollen lymph nodes, and trypanosomes are present in the bloodstream. After several months (the East African form) or years (the West African form), the parasites invade the central nervous system and infect the brain and spinal fluid.

During months or years of chronic bloodstream infection, patients undergo bouts of parasitemia (Fig. 50.11). During each bout the parasite changes its dominant surface antigen (variable surface glycoprotein), thus avoiding immune destruction by the host. As with bacterial pathogens that undergo similar antigenic variation, the basis for this variability is genetic rearrangement. Each parasite expresses only one glycoprotein gene from an "expression locus," but it also carries a repertoire of numerous, alternative versions of the gene that are not expressed. When one of these "silent copies" recombines into the expression locus, the parasite expresses an immunologically distinct surface glycoprotein. For a full discussion of antigenic variation, review the paradigm in Chapter 14, "Neisseriae."

Treatment

Several drugs, including pentamidine and suramin, are useful in the systemic stage of the infection. However, treatment is much more difficult after the central nervous system has become involved.

Free-living Amebae

In this section, we discuss only those amebas that do not have human or animal reservoirs. Amebas with a human animal reservoir, such as *Entamoeba histolytica* (see Chapter 51, "Intestinal and Vaginal Protozoa"), are discussed in other chapters. A number of protozoa, principally *Naegleria*, *Acanthamoeba*, and *Hartmanella*, have no known animal reservoir but may cause rare but serious systemic diseases, such as meningoencephalitis (inflammation of the meninges and the brain). These organisms may also infect the eye, especially among persons wearing contact lenses.

▌ CASE

E., a 6-year-old girl living in rural Virginia, swam in a lake in the month of August. Although she was well previously, 2 days later she developed a severe headache, neck stiffness, and eye pain on exposure to light (photophobia). Spinal fluid obtained a day later had 300 mononucleated cells per mm³ and a few neutrophils. Many of these cells

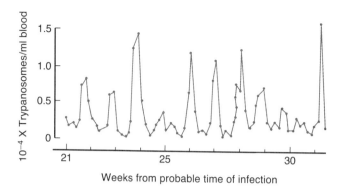

Figure 50.11. Periodic fluctuation in the number of *Trypanosoma brucei* in the blood of a patient with African trypanosomiasis.

---

were actively motile in a wet mount, suggesting that they were not leukocytes but amebae. Despite treatment with antimicrobial drugs, the patient died 3 days later. Several other children who swam in the same lake also had headaches and mild neck stiffness, but recovered spontaneously.

Pathogenesis

There are two types of amebic meningoencephalitis. The first is a usually fatal disease caused by *Naegleria fowleri* which, as in this case, typically occurs in young, previously healthy people. This form of amebic meningoencephalitis is associated with exposure to warm, freshwater lakes that harbor these amebae. The second form is a disease caused by *Acanthamoeba* or *Hartmanella*, and is typically seen in older patients who are immunocompromised (such as those with lymphoma or diabetes). Both types of disease, once clinically apparent, tend to progress despite treatment. Although there are reports of recovery using multiple drugs (amphotericin B, miconazole, and rifampin), these regimens have not proven to be reproducibly effective.

In the meningoencephalitis caused by *Naegleria*, the parasite is thought to enter the central nervous system via the cribriform plate along the olfactory nerve tracts. Note that this site is the area in which the nervous system is in nearest proximity to the exterior; it can thus serve as a unique portal of entry into the central nervous system. Trauma or increased pressure, as may occur when diving into water, are believed to facilitate the entry of the organisms. *Acanthamoeba* or *Hartmanella*, on the other hand, are thought to spread to the central nervous system via the bloodstream, as suggested by the postmortem finding of foci of infection at distant sites, such as the lung.

Infection of the cornea (keratitis) is produced by some free-living amebae and is an increasingly important (often undiagnosed) cause of visual loss among contact lens wearers or persons with other ocular trauma. It is important to recognize this infection (by morphologic examination of Giemsa-stained material using the high dry or oil immersion objectives), because treatment with topical or systemic imidazoles may save the patient's sight. These parasites may gain access to the eye from contaminated fluids used to clean contact lenses.

CONCLUSION

The global morbidity and mortality associated with tissue-invasive protozoal infections is staggering. Malaria is a leading cause of death in young children in endemic regions. Toxoplasmosis is estimated to affect over a billion people and is cosmopolitan in its distribution. Although public health measures to control vectors, mass treatment programs, and chemoprophylaxis (for malaria and toxoplasmosis) has dramatically reduced the impact of some diseases in countries that can economically support such measures, the best hope for worldwide eradication rests on the development of effective vaccines.

SUGGESTED READINGS

Hopewell PC, Masur H. Pneumocystic carinii pneumonia: current concepts. In: Sande MA, Volberding PA. The medical management of AIDS. 4th ed. Philadelphia: WB Saunders, 1995.

Jones TR, Hoffman SL. Malaria vaccine development. Clin Microbiol Rev 1994;7:303–310.

Magill AJ, Grogl M, Johnson SC, Gasser RA, Jr. Visceral infection due to *Leishmania tropica* in a veteran of Operation Desert Storm who presented 2 years after leaving Saudi Arabia. Clin Infect Dis 1994;19:805–806.

Masinde GL, Krogstad DJ. Biologic and geographic factors in prevention and treatment of malaria. Curr Clin Topics Infect Dis 1994;14:80–102.

Miller LH, Good MF, Milon G. Malaria pathogenesis. Science 1994;264:1878–1883.

Nussenzweig RS, Long CA. Malaria vaccines: multiple targets. Science 1994;265:1381–1383.

Pearson RD, Sousa AQ. Clinical spectrum of leishmaniasis. Clin Infect Dis 1996;22:1–13.

Persing DH, Herwaldt BL, Glaser C, Lane RS, Thomford JW, Mathiesen D, Krause PJ, Phillip DF Conrad PA. Infection with a babesia-like organism in northern California. N Engl J Med 1995;332:298–303.

Sibley LD. Interactions between *Toxoplasma gondii* and its mammalian host cells. Semin Cell Biol 1993;4:335–344.

Simonds RJ, Hughes WT Feinberg J, Navin TR. Preventing Pneumocystis carinii pneumonia in persons infected with human immunodeficiency virus. Clin Infect Dis 1995; 21(Suppl 1):S44–S48.

Su TH, Martin WJ Jr. Pathogenesis and host response in Pneumocystis carinii pneumonia. Annu Rev Med 1994;45: 261–272.

Vickerman K. Trypanosome sociology and antigenic variation. Parasitology 1989;99(Suppl):S37–S47.

Intestinal and Vaginal Protozoa

DONALD J. KROGSTAD

N. CARY ENGLEBERG

Key Concepts

- Intestinal protozoa are acquired by ingestion of cysts by the fecal-oral route of transmission, usually involving contaminated food or water.
- *Entamoeba histolytica* lyses cells in the colon and feeds on their contents, resulting in colonic ulcerations and dysentery (diarrhea with blood and mucus). Asymptomatic human carriers are the reservoir of infection; occasionally the parasite enters the portal circulation and produces abscesses in the liver or other distant organs.
- *Giardia lamblia, Cryptosporidium, Cyclospora,* and *Microsporidia* are zoonotic and therefore cannot be prevented by control of human sanitation alone. They infect the small intestine and cause non-inflammatory, watery diarrhea that may last for days or weeks.
- A chronic inflammatory response to persistent giardiasis may result in the loss of intestinal villi, malabsorption syndrome, and weight loss.
- Patients with AIDS and other immunodeficiencies may experience intractable diarrhea due to these agents. *Cryptosporidium* infection is particularly serious since there is no specific antimicrobial treatment for this parasite.
- Trichomoniasis is a common form of sexually-transmitted vaginitis and urethritis that requires treatment of all contacts to ensure that reinfection will not occur.

The protozoa are classified according to their motility and their replicative cycles. The intestinal and vaginal organisms discussed in this chapter are a varied group: an ameba (*Entamoeba histolytica*), two flagellates (*Giardia lamblia* and *Trichomonas vaginalis*), three coccidia (*Cryptosporidium, Cyclospora,* and *Isospora*), and microsporidia (a group of organisms that are not true protozoa, but occupy a phylum of their own) [see Table 51.1]. The coccidian protozoa are nonmotile and reproduce by alternating sexual and asexual cycles (as do *Toxoplasma gondii* and malaria parasites; see Chapter 50, "Blood Protozoa").

Between 5% and 10% of all people in developing countries harbor the ameba *Entamoeba histolytica* in their stool. In the United States, the figure is less than 1%.

Giardia and *Cryptosporidium* are more frequent in the U.S. Both have caused large waterborne outbreaks, but their prevalence varies considerably in different regions. *Cyclospora* was recognized only recently as a human pathogen when it was implicated in a series of foodborne outbreaks. *Isospora* and the microsporidia are agents that are most serious when they affect persons with AIDS. Other protozoa also live in tissues other than the intestine. For example, *Trichomonas vaginalis* is a common agent of vaginitis. It is usually transmitted sexually.

ENTAMOEBA HISTOLYTICA

Entamoeba histolytica causes a disease called amebiasis. As its species name indicates, *E. histolytica* may

Table 51.1. Comparison of Major Intestinal and Vaginal Protozoa

Organism	Reservoir	Modes of transmission	Clinical manifestations
Entamoeba histolytica (amebiasis)	Infected humans	Fecal-oral transmission by the ingestion of feces containing infectious cysts	Bloody diarrhea (dysentery) Distant abscesses (especially liver) Asymptomatic intestinal infection
Giardia lamblia (giardiasis)	Infected humans, and other mammals	Fecal-oral transmission by ingestion of feces containing infectious cysts	Watery diarrhea; may also cause steatorrhea and malabsorption
Cryptosporidium parvum (cryptosporidiosis)	Infected humans and a wide variety of other animal hosts (zoonosis)	Fecal-oral transmission by the ingestion of feces containing infectious cysts	Watery diarrhea; intractable diarrhea in people with AIDS
Cyclospora cayetanensis	Unknown	Food and waterborne; person-to-person spread unlikely	Watery diarrhea
Isospora belli	Infected humans	Food and waterborne	Watery diarrhea; intractable diarrhea in AIDS
Microsporidia	Unknown	Unknown	Watery diarrhea, biliary tract infection, etc.

cause destruction of host tissue, especially in the colon. The lesions start as small ulcerations of the intestinal epithelium. Amebae within the lesions spread laterally as they encounter the deeper layers of the colon, sometimes producing flask-shaped ulcers that undermine the mucosal epithelium. The organisms may also spread through the bloodstream to produce abscesses in the liver, and less commonly in the brain or other organs. Despite their pathogenic potential, these organisms cause few or no symptoms in the majority of infected individuals. In addition, many humans carry non-pathogenic amebas that are morphologically indistinguishable from *E. histolytica*. The species name *Entamoeba dispar* is used to designate these avirulent strains, which can be identified only by biochemical or nucleic acid–based techniques.

■ CASE

Mr. A. is 26 years old and was discharged from the U.S. Army 2 years previously. He spent three of his six military years abroad, including tours of duty in Korea, Panama, and Germany. During the last 2 years he developed intermittent diarrhea, with blood and mucus visible in the stool (i.e., dysentery). Sigmoidoscopy (endoscopic examination of the colon) and an x-ray study of the intestine following a barium enema revealed pseudopolyps, consistent with inflammatory bowel disease. He was diagnosed with ulcerative colitis, an inflammatory bowel disease of unknown cause, and was treated with steroids.

At the time of admission to the hospital, 4 months after beginning steroid therapy, Mr. A. reported the loss of about 24 lbs. of weight (down to 147 lbs.) and a recent increase in bloody stools and abdominal pain. He had no fever (probably because he was medicated with large doses of steroids). Examination of his stool under the microscope showed many white and red blood cells but no amebae. However, a serological test for *E. histolytica* antibodies in serum (indirect hemagglutination) revealed a high titer (1:2000). A CT scan showed abscesses in the liver, lungs, and brain.

He had a stormy hospital stay with several episodes of bacteremia (secondary to disruption of the intestinal mucosa by the parasite). He finally recovered after the steroids were tapered and he was treated with the antiamebic agent metronidazole.

Encounter

E. histolytica is transmitted from person to person via the fecal–oral route. It has a simple life cycle, with two forms: the actively growing, vegetative **trophozoite** and the dormant but highly resistant **cyst** (Fig. 51.1). The critical factors responsible for the transformation from trophozoites to cysts and vice versa are not understood. The transmission of *Entamoeba* and *Giardia* has a paradoxical aspect. Patients with diarrhea pose only a minor threat of transmission because they excrete the actively growing, yet labile trophozoites—they are destroyed by drying in the environment or acid in the stomach. Conversely, asymptomatic carriers excrete the tough, cyst form of the parasite. Asymptomatic carriers thus represent a greater danger of transmission because the cysts are resistant to drying and to gastric acid. This paradox illustrates the biological principle that successful parasites generally do not harm the host: when amebae are in balance with their host (when they do not cause symptoms), they are excreted as cysts, which ensures their transmissibility.

Because the parasite is infectious in the cyst stage and does not require a period of maturation in the environment, transmission of amebiasis is not restricted to warm climates. In fact, *E. histolytica* can even be transmitted in polar regions. The only requirement for transmission is that contaminated feces of the carrier be ingested with food or water. Sexual transmission (anal–oral or oral–genital) is also important, particularly among homosexual men.

Spread, Multiplication, and Damage

E. histolytica is frequently found in the human colon in persons without symptoms of disease. The amebae must adhere to specific receptors containing galactose on host cells. In experimental models, attachment to cells and subsequent cytotoxicity is inhibited by adding galactose. This attachment is also inhibited by intestinal mucus, which suggests that disruption of the mucus layer may be a critical event in the pathogenesis of amebiasis. Damage to host cells requires intimate cell-to-cell contact and takes place in three distinct steps: receptor-mediated attachment to the mammalian target cell, contact-dependent killing (probably by insertion of pore-forming proteins into the host cell membrane), and ingestion of the killed host cell by the ameba. Although certain strains of *E. histolytica* produce an enterotoxin, it is not yet clear whether enterotoxin production correlates with virulence.

White blood cells do not control amebic infection in nonimmune hosts: pathogenic strains of amebae actually kill neutrophils and nonactivated macrophages (note the reversal of the usual "phagocyte ingests invader" theme). The situation is different in immune hosts, in whom the most important line of defense appears to be cell-mediated immunity (which was suggested by the finding that amebae can be killed in vitro by activated macrophages). Also, persons given steroids (which suppress cell-mediated immunity) tend to have disseminated infection despite high titers of antibodies, as is the case with Mr. A. Thus, circulating antibodies may not play a critical role in protection against amebic infection.

Diagnosis

E. histolytica trophozoites can be identified in freshly passed dysenteric stool or in scrapings from colonic ulcers obtained through a sigmoidoscope. On a warm microscopic slide, the parasite can be observed to move and may contain ingested red blood cells. The identification of this pathogen in stools by microscopic examination is one of the most challenging diagnostic procedures in microbiology. Nonpathogenic amebae or even white blood cells in stool can be mistaken for amebae,

resulting in false-positive laboratory reports. Reliable results require examination by an experienced technologist using a high dry or oil immersion objectives. False-negative results are frequently due to the insensitivity of microscopic examination or to interfering substances, such as barium given for x-rays. Thus, although a positive stool examination is helpful, a negative stool examination does not prove that amebiasis is absent. For this reason, serological diagnosis is often attempted and is of considerable value. Serology is positive in over 80% of people with invasion of the intestinal mucosa and in 96–100% of persons with systemic (metastatic) disease. In the United States, 1% or less of the general population has antibodies to *E. histolytica*. Among asymptomatic carriers the prevalence of antibodies is approximately 10–15%. Thus, although circulating antibodies to *E. histolytica* are of little protective value, they are an excellent marker for disease.

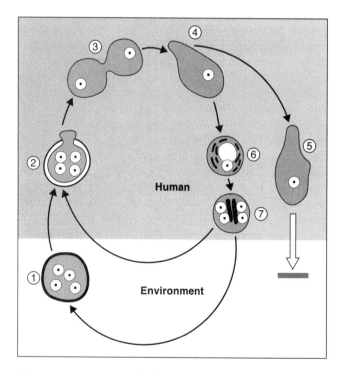

Figure 51.1. *Entamoeba histolytica* **life cycle.** Humans acquire amebic infection by oral ingestion of the cyst form of the parasite (*1*). Viable cysts may be ingested from the external environment (where they remain stable and infectious for prolonged periods after excretion), from the stool of other infected persons, or from the stools of the patients themselves (the *arrow* from 7 to 2). In the upper GI tract, the parasite excysts after passing through the stomach (*2*), replicates asexually by binary fission (*3*) and transforms to the potentially pathogenic trophozoite form (*4*), which is typically found in the large intestine. Trophozoites die rapidly when they are shed into the external environment (*5*) (*solid line below 5* on the diagram). When conditions in the GI tract are unfavorable, trophozoites transform into cysts (*6* and *7*) which can remain dormant for long periods of time in the host and the environment.

Treatment

The drug of choice for active amebic infection is **metronidazole**, the same antimicrobial used to treat infections caused by anaerobic bacteria. Pathogenic amebae carry out anaerobic metabolism and convert metronidazole to its active form in the same way as *Bacteroides* (see Chapter 3, "Biology of Infectious Agents" and Chapter 15, "Bacteroides"). This drug is particularly effective for invasive infections because it penetrates well into most tissues, including the brain. Since metronidazole is less efficient at killing amebae within the intestinal lumen, a second drug is given to eradicate the luminal forms. Drugs such as diloxanide, paromomycin, and diiodohydroxyquin are used for this purpose and may also be used to treat asymptomatic carriers of pathogenic strains.

GIARDIA LAMBLIA

Giardia lamblia is the intestinal protozoan that causes giardiasis. *G. lamblia* is distributed all over the world. Giardiasis is a zoonosis, an animal disease that affects humans only accidentally. It is commonly acquired by ingestion of water contaminated by feces from animal carriers. Since giardial cysts are resistant to chlorine, waterborne outbreaks associated with municipal water systems have occurred in the United States and around the world. In the United States, giardiasis is commonly found in areas of poor sanitation such as in daycare centers, where there is frequent opportunity for direct fecal–oral transmission. Giardiasis is also an important infection among homosexual males. *Giardia* typically produces a mild but persistent diarrheal disease, often localized to the duodenum and jejunum. Occasionally, chronic infection causes intestinal malabsorption.

▮ CASE

Ms. R. is a 36-year-old woman. She visited Colorado for 10 days of backpacking 2 months before seeing her physician. One week after returning she developed abdominal bloating, belching, and diarrhea with 3–5 watery stools per day. The stool contained no pus or blood, and she had no fever or chills. A stool examination was positive for *G. lamblia*. She was treated with metronidazole and improved markedly over a 7-day period. Subsequently, symptoms recurred and the organisms were again found in her stool.

Entry, Spread, Multiplication, and Damage

As with *E. histolytica*, giardiasis is acquired by ingestion of the cyst form of the parasite (Fig. 51.2). Giardial cysts are highly resistant in the environment and are found in ostensibly "pure" mountain streams contaminated by the feces of infected animals or humans. When asked, Ms. R. admitted drinking water drawn directly from a mountain stream. Like pathogenic amebae, these organisms may be transmitted in cold as well as in warm climates.

Stomach acid does not kill giardial cysts. Moreover, stomach acid actually stimulates the cysts to transform into the vegetative trophozoite form in the duodenum. *Giardia* trophozoites attach to the epithelium of the duodenum and jejunum using a ventral sucking disk. The vegetative forms have the characteristic appearance of a face adorned with mustache-like flagella (see Fig. 51.2).

Signs of malnutrition due to malabsorption may occur as a result of extensive, prolonged infection. In these cases, the organisms may literally cover the mucosal surface of the small intestine (Fig. 51.3). Unlike *E. histolyt-*

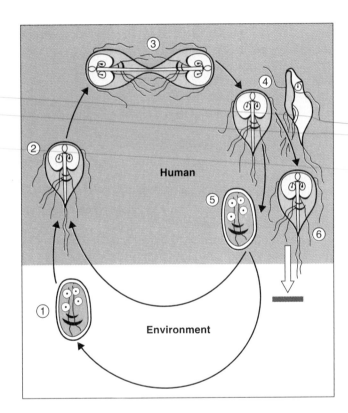

Figure 51.2. *Giardia lamblia* life cycle. Humans acquire giardiasis by ingesting the cyst form of the parasite (*1*). After contact with the gastric contents, the parasite excysts and transforms to a trophozoite in the upper gastrointestinal tract (*2*), where it replicates asexually by binary fission (*3*). Trophozoites cause disease by attaching to the epithelium of the small intestine via a ventral sucking disk (*4*). As indicated by the *solid line* and *open arrow below 6*, trophozoites are not infectious for others because they are readily killed by drying in the external environment. As in amebiasis, humans acquire infection by ingesting cysts from the external environment (*1*), from the stools of other patients, or from their own stool (*arrow from 5 to 2*).

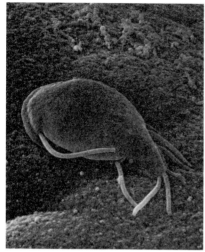

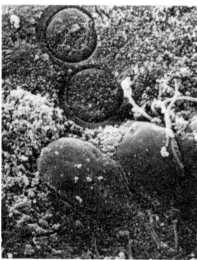

Figure 51.3. Scanning electron micrograph of *Giardia lamblia*. Top. Scanning electron micrograph of *G. lamblia* adhering to the gastrointestinal epithelium via its ventral sucking disk. Patients with giardiasis may have a significant reduction in the amount of absorptive surface available because of the large number of adhering parasites. **Bottom.** Upon detaching from the intestinal epithelium, the organisms often leave a clear impression on the microvillous surface (*upper circles*).

ica, Giardia is not invasive and does not produce bloody diarrhea or metastatic infection. However, the host responds to chronic giardial infection with a submucosal infiltrate of inflammatory cells and an effacement of the normal intestinal villi. With the loss of villi, the total absorptive area of the intestine is significantly diminished. In particular, malabsorption of fats can lead to greasy, foul-smelling stools; diarrhea associated with unabsorbed fatty acids in the lumen; deficiencies of fat-soluble vitamins (i.e., A, K, D, and E); and weight loss.

Diagnosis and Treatment

The standard approach to diagnosis of giardiasis is by direct examination of stool or duodenal aspirates.

Trophozoites are actively motile in fresh specimens. Alternatively, giardial antigens can be detected in stool samples by an ELISA test or by a direct fluorescent antibody test (see Chapter 55, "Diagnostic Principles").

In the United States, giardiasis is usually treated with metronidazole. Hikers and campers may prevent unpleasant episodes of diarrhea by boiling or filtering their drinking water or by treating it with adequate amounts of iodine or chlorine.

CRYPTOSPORIDIUM

Cryptosporidia cause a zoonosis that was first discovered among veterinary students and animal handlers who acquired it from calves they were treating for diarrhea. It is now clear that cryptosporidiosis is an important diarrheal disease in both developed and developing countries.

■ CASE

Mr. H. is a 40-year-old gay male with HIV infection who lives on a farm in rural Michigan. Despite a low CD4 count and periodic episodes of oral candidiasis, he had been well. Six weeks ago he began to have watery stools 3 to 8 times a day. He reported no fever, nor did he see blood or pus in the stools. A microscopic examination of his stool (with the oil immersion objective) using an acid-fast stain revealed the presence of cryptosporidia (these organisms have the property, unusual for protozoa, of being acid-fast). Although the patient was treated with oral rehydration and a synthetic hormone that reduces intestinal secretion, he continued to have persistent but manageable diarrhea.

Encounter

Cryptosporidiosis is often acquired in rural areas because of greater contact with animals. However, it may also spread from person to person in crowded urban environments such as day care centers. It is now recognized as a frequent cause of diarrhea in Great Britain and the United States, and it has been identified as a potential cause of diarrhea in travelers to developing countries. It is particularly troublesome in patients with AIDS.

Recent attention has focused on outbreaks associated with public water systems. Cryptosporidium oocysts can be found in most surface waters in this country, and most public utilities draw on these sources to provide public water service. Several outbreaks of cryptosporidiosis have involved drinking water or swimming pools. The largest single waterborne outbreak in the history of the United States (Milwaukee, Wisconsin, 1993) was due to *Cryptosporidium*. Over 400,000 persons were affected, and more than 4,000 people were hospitalized after contamination of the municipal water supply.

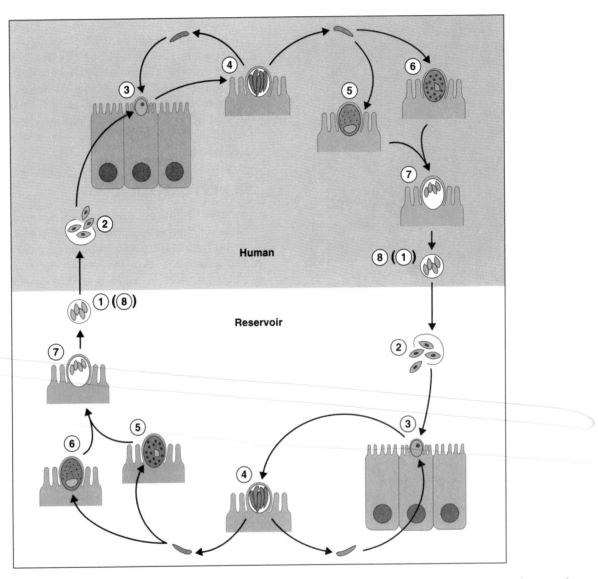

Figure 51.4. Cryptosporidium life cycle. Humans acquire infection by ingesting infectious oocysts (*1*) after direct contact with infected animals or humans, or by ingesting water or food contaminated with human or animal feces. Autoinfection can also occur. Once inside the human host (*2*), sporozoites are released from the oocyst, enter the epithelial cells of the GI tract, and develop into trophozoites (*3*). Trophozoites develop into structures containing individual merozoites (*4*). These trophozoites can either recapitulate the asexual cycle (*3*) or evolve into one of two sexual gametes (*5,6*). The gametes join and form oocysts (*7*). When mature and released, oocysts are the infectious form of the parasite that is excreted in the feces (*8*). The identical events take place in the reservoir.

Spread and Multiplication

Cryptosporidium resembles *Toxoplasma* in that infectious oocyst forms are produced in the intestine and spread to other animals. However, unlike *Toxoplasma*, cryptosporidia do not invade the intestinal epithelial cells, nor do they disseminate to produce systemic infection. They carry out their entire life cycle among the microvilli of the small intestine (Fig. 51.4). In immunocompetent individuals, the life cycle takes place only once or twice, resulting in a single episode of diarrhea that usually lasts 2 weeks or less. In immunocompromised patients, the life cycle of the organism is repeated many times and is associated with persistent and often intractable watery diarrhea.

Diagnosis and Treatment

The diagnosis of cryptosporidiosis is made by identifying characteristic, acid-fast cysts in the stool. Because the cysts have few distinguishing features, a direct fluorescent antibody test has also been used to find and identify these structures in specimens. There is currently no effective antimicrobial therapy for cryptosporidiosis. Treatment is supportive only.

CYCLOSPORA CAYETANENSIS

Cyclospora cayetanensis is a protozoal parasite that resembles *Cryptosporidium* in producing acid-fast cysts in stools, although these are roughly twice the size of those of cryptosporidium (Fig. 51.5). In the late 1980s and early 1990s, *Cyclospora* was increasingly recognized as a cause of epidemic diarrhea in the United States and chronic diarrhea in developing countries around the world. In 1996, over 40 separate outbreaks of cyclosporiasis occurred in several states. Most of these outbreaks were linked to ingestion of raspberries imported from Central America. In Lima, Peru, *Cyclospora* was found in the stools of 6% to 18% of young children, often associated with diarrhea. The species *C. cayetanensis* is named for the Peruvian University ("Cayetano Heredia") where these observations were made.

Spread and Multiplication

Unlike *Entamoeba and Giardia* cysts, *Cyclospora* oocysts are not infectious when excreted in human feces. The parasites become infectious (sporulate) only after days to weeks of incubation in environmental sites with warm temperatures and high humidity. Therefore, most new infections are acquired by ingestion of contaminated food or water. Person-to-person spread, if it occurs at all, is probably very rare.

Diagnosis and Treatment

Infection with *Cyclospora* causes watery diarrhea which may be associated with loss of appetite, bloating, cramps, nausea and vomiting, fatigue, muscle aches, and low-grade fever. The illness may last for only a few days, or it may persist for a month or longer. Relapses are common.

Diagnosis depends on the identification of the large acid-fast oocyst in the stool. Treatment with trimethoprim–sulfamethoxazole appears to relieve symptoms and to shorten the course of infection.

OTHER INTESTINAL PARASITES

Isospora

Isospora belli is a coccidian protozoa that causes transient watery diarrhea in healthy individuals. This infection tends to occur more frequently in tropical areas. Cases recognized in the United States occur mostly in AIDS patients. In people with AIDS, *I. belli* can cause a persistent watery diarrhea, like that associated with *Cryptosporidium.*

The diagnosis is made by examination of stool for characteristic oocysts. Fortunately, trimethoprim–sulfamethoxazole appears to be effective in controlling this infection in immunocompromised patients.

Microsporidia

Microsporidia belong to a phylum containing almost 1000 species that are ubiquitous among vertebrate and invertebrate animals and in the environment. They have been studied for decades as causes of insect and fish diseases; only recently have they been associated with human disease. These obligate intracellular parasites are very small relative to the other pathogens discussed in this chapter (see Fig. 51.5). They lack mitochondria and possess small ribosomal RNA, suggesting a procaryotic origin. These features distinguish them from other protozoa and have caused taxonomists to place these parasites into their own phyllum, Microsporidia.

A few of these species have been associated with human diseases, particularly but not exclusively in immunocompromised patients. Various species have been associated with infections of the GI tract, respiratory tract, urinary tract, liver, brain, and eye. The modes of transmission have not been clearly elucidated. Symptomatic intestinal infection is primarily associated with the species *Enterocytozoon bieneusi.*

E. bieneusi is believed to cause transient diarrhea in healthy hosts but a protracted watery diarrhea in AIDS patients. The organism infects the mucosal epithelial cells and, in AIDS patients, may also disseminate to distant sites. Thus, *E. bieneusi* may ascend into the biliary tree and cause symptoms of cholangitis. The diagnosis can be made by microscopic examination of stool or in-

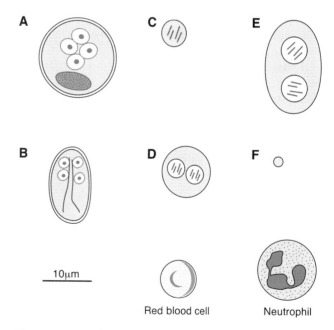

Figure 51.5. Schematic representation and relative sizes of protozoal cysts and oocysts found in human feces. (*A*) Round *Entamoeba histolytica* cyst with four nuclei. (*B*) Oval *Giardia lamblia* cyst with four nuclei and a central axostyle (encysted flagellae). (*C*) *Cryptosporidium parvum* oocyst with four internal sporozoites. (*D*) *Cyclospora cayetanensis* oocyst with two sporocysts, each containing four sporozoites. (*E*) Oval *Isospora belli* oocyst containing two sporocysts. (*F*) A tiny microsporidial organism with few distinguishing features by light microscopy.

testinal biopsy material after special staining procedures. Optimal treatment has not yet been found, as common antibacterial and antiprotozoal drugs are not very effective. Oddly, the best responses are seen with an antihelminthic drug, albendazole.

TRICHOMONAS VAGINALIS

Trichomonas vaginalis is a common inhabitant of the vagina and is found in 15% or more of women, where it occasionally causes vaginitis. Less common and less pathogenic are species of *Trichomonas* found in the GI tract (*Trichomonas hominis*) or the mouth (*Trichomonas tenax*).

Spread, Multiplication, and Diagnosis

T. vaginalis infection is transmitted by sexual intercourse. Vaginitis is typically associated with a frothy creamy discharge. Symptomatic *T. vaginalis* infection is uncommon among men, although most partners of symptomatic woman become infected. On occasion, men develop symptomatic *T. vaginalis* infection of the urethra, epididymis, or prostate.

CONCLUSION

Most intestinal protozoa produce self-limited illness with watery diarrhea, abdominal cramps, and characteristic protozoal forms in the stool. Amebiasis is unique among these diseases since it involves direct destruction of tissues and occasionally disseminates to vital organs. Accordingly, the clinical features of amebiasis may include bloody stools (dysentery), fever, or abscess formation in the liver and elsewhere. Amebiasis is also distinct from the other protozoa in that the transmission depends on a reservoir of asymptomatic human carriers, rather than non-human source. Thus, infection always results from a failure to dispose of human feces safely in contrast to giardiasis and other intestinal protozoa, which may result from contamination of food and water at its source. Understanding of the pathophysiologic differences among these parasites aids in the diagnosis of diarrheal illness, and an appreciation for their epidemiology may direct attention to the circumstances and source of infection.

Treatment

Single-dose metronidazole treatment is recommended by most investigators. In pregnant women (in whom there is particular concern about the potential carcinogenic effects of metronidazole), douching with vinegar may suppress symptomatic infection by lowering vaginal pH. Male sexual partners must also be treated to prevent "ping-pong" relapse, a common feature of sexually transmitted diseases.

SUGGESTED READINGS

Amebiasis

Allason-Jones E, Mindel A, Sargeaunt P, Williams P. *Entamoeba histolytica* as a common intestinal parasite in homosexual men. N Engl J Med 1986;315:353–356.

Martinez-Palomo A, ed. Amebiasis. Amsterdam: Elsevier, 1986.

Petri WA Jr, Mann BJ. Molecular mechanisms of invasion by *Entamoeba histolytica*. Semin Cell Biol 1993;4:305–313.

Reed SL. New concepts regarding the pathogenesis of amebiasis. Clin Infect Dis 1995;21(Suppl 2):S182–S185.

Giardiasis

Erlandsen SL, Meyer EA, eds. Giardia and giardiasis: biology, pathogenesis and epidermiology. New York: Plenum, 1984.

Wright SG. Giardiasis. In: Strickland GT, ed. Hunter's tropical medicine. 7th ed. Philadelphia: WB Saunders, 1991.

Cryptosporidiosis, Cyclospora, Isospora, and Microsporidia

Goodgame RW. Understanding intestinal spore-forming protozoa: cryptosporidia, microsporidia, isospora, and cyclospora. Ann Intern 1996;124:429–441.

Guerrant RL. Cryptosporidiosis: an emerging, highly infectious threat. Emerg Infect Dis 1997;3:51–57.

Herwaldt BL, Ackers ML. An outbreak in 1996 of cyclosporiasis associated with imported raspberries. The Cyclospora Working Group. N Engl J Med 1997;336:1548–1556.

Madico G, McDonald J, Gilman RH, Cabrera L, Sterling CR. Epidemiology and treatment of *Cyclospora cayetanensis* infection in Peruvian children. Clin Infect Dis 1997;24:977–981.

Marshall MM, Naumovitz D, Ortega Y, Sterling CR. Waterborne protozoan pathogens. Clin Microbiol Rev 1997;10:67–85.

Soave R. Cyclospora: an overview. Clin Infect Dis 1996;23:429–435.

Intestinal Helminths

DONALD J. KROGSTAD

N. CARY ENGLEBERG

Key Concepts

- The common intestinal helminthic infection are caused by nematodes (roundworms) and cestodes (tapeworms). The life cycles of these infections require indiscriminate handling of human wastes leading to fecal helminth eggs contamination of soil, foodstuffs, animal feeds, etc.
- Nematode infections are acquired by ingestion of eggs (e.g., *Ascaris, Trichiuris, Enterobius*) or by direct penetration of soil larvae through the skin (e.g., *Strongyloides*, hookworm).
- These infections are often asymptomatic unless the worm burden is very large. Then, pathologic features may include intestinal obstruction (*Ascaris*), rectal prolapse (*Trichiuris*), anal itching (*Enterobius*), and iron-deficiency anemia (*hookworm*).
- Sustained autoinfection is a unique feature of strongyloidiasis. Immunosuppressed individuals may develop a syndrome of *Strongyloides* hyperinfection with diarrhea, pneumonitis, rash, and eosinophilia.
- Three species of tapeworm infections are acquired by ingesting encysted worm larvae in undercooked tissues of beef, pork, or fish. Fish tapeworms may successfully compete for vitamin B_{12} and cause anemia in the host. The presence of beef or pork tapeworms in the intestines rarely produces systemic signs or symptoms.
- Diagnosis of intestinal helminths relies on identifying the characteristic eggs, larvae, or adult worms (or segments) in feces.

Tapeworm infections are usually asymptomatic. The tissue invasive form of the pork tapeworm (cysticercosis) can cause severe central nervous system manifestations, but this disorder occurs in only a minority of tapeworm carriers and often occurs in persons without intestinal tapeworms (see Chapter 53 "Tissue and Blood Helminths").

The helminths or worms are multicellular animals. They include many free-living, harmless species as well as some pathogenic species which infect a high proportion of all people on earth (Table 49.1). Helminthic diseases are sometimes mistakenly thought to be a problem only for people living in the tropics. In fact, some of these infections are common in temperate zones; others are relatively rare but have major consequences when they go unrecognized, especially in immunocompromised persons.

Helminths are the largest parasites that affect humans, ranging in size from 10-yard-long tapeworms to barely visible pinworms. Helminths fall into three large groups: **roundworms** *(Nematodes)*, **tapeworms** *(Cestodes)*, and **flukes** *(Trematodes)*. The three groups are generally distinguishable by their shape. Examples of each type of worm are discussed in the next two chapters. However, the number and range of all helminthic parasites is beyond the scope of this text, and specialized parasitology textbooks should be consulted for details. From the point of view of human disease, helminths can be divided into the **intestinal helminths** (this chapter) and the **blood and tissue helminths** (Chapter 53). The generalities about helminths mentioned below apply to both intestinal and tissue-invasive helminths.

In small numbers, helminths often cause chronic infec-

Table 52.1. Pathophysiologic Mechanisms in Helminthic Diseases

Mechanism	Example
Mechanical obstruction or mass effect	
Intestinal obstruction	*Ascaris* "worm ball"
Lymphatic obstruction	Lymphatic filariasis (elephantiasis)
Displacement of normal tissue	Echinococcosis ("hydatid disease")
	Cysticercosis
Facilitating bacterial invasion into normally sterile spaces	
	Strongyloidiasis
Production of anemia (nutritional)	
Due to sucking blood	Hookworms
Due to vitamin B_{12} depletion	Fish tapeworm
Chronic inflammation	
	Schistosomiasis
	Onchocerciasis

tions that are well tolerated by their human host. Helminths reproduce sexually. Therefore, humans must harbor both a male and female worm for the infection to produce fertilized eggs or larvae. A few species (tapeworms) are hermaphroditic, and thus a single parasite can produce eggs. In massive numbers, intestinal parasites may cause disease by contributing to the malnutrition of their host, occluding the intestinal lumen, or triggering a symptomatic immune response (Table 52.1). Tissue-invasive helminths in large numbers cause disease by immunopathologic mechanisms or by creating an obstructing mass in vessels or organs (see Table 52.2, p. 477).

The developmental stages of some helminths (e.g., hookworms) take place outside the human body, sometimes involving insect vectors and/or animal reservoirs. In these complex life cycles, the hosts that harbor the adult, sexual form of the parasites are called the **definitive host**. The other animal hosts that harbor developmental stages are called **intermediate hosts**. Since multiple steps are required for infectivity, direct transmission from human to human does not occur with these species. In some infections (e.g., *Enterobius*), an infected patient may pass feces containing eggs or larvae that are immediately infectious for other humans. Person-to-person transmission or **autoinfection** is then possible. In all of these species, however, the total number of parasites does not increase during the course of infection since the life cycle cannot be completed entirely within the human body. As a result, the intensity of infection (i.e., the **worm burden**) is determined by the size of single or repeated inocula (i.e., the number of eggs or larvae acquired from the external environment).

A few helminthic species (e.g., *Strongyloides*) can carry out their entire life cycle within the human body. Here, a continuous reinfection cycle prolongs the duration of the infection long beyond the life span of a single worm. In such infections, the immune system may provide a check on the continuous propagation of worms, while an immunocompromised individual may experience uncontrolled growth of the worm burden.

In general, established adult worm infections are not eliminated by the host immune response. Most helminth infections resolve spontaneously when the adult parasites reach senescence (after a few months or years, they die of old age). Longevity differs by species. In some infections, immunity to developing stages of the parasite may develop to keep continuous acquisition in check. Unfortunately, in most helminthic infections, the major contribution of the host immune response is to cause the pathophysiologic features of the disease. Most of the pathologic features of these infections are not due to the direct action of the parasite on tissues but rather on the host's response to the products of parasites (eggs, larvae, and soluble antigens).

Eosinophilia is often regarded as a characteristic host response to parasitic infection. Indeed, specific antibodies together with eosinophils may adversely affect some parasites. However, a significant systemic eosinophilia occurs only when parasites are invading or migrating through host tissues. Although some intestinal parasites have stages of migration through the tissues and lungs which may provoke eosinophilia, worm infections confined to the intestinal lumen do not cause this systemic response.

INTESTINAL NEMATODES (ROUNDWORMS)

The comparative life cycles of the intestinal nematodes (roundworms) are summarized in Fig. 52.1. Some of these parasites enter the body through the mouth by the ingestion of eggs. Others develop into larvae that penetrate through the intact skin. The species discussed below infect large numbers of people and cause infections that range from asymptomatic to severe.

Nematode Infections Acquired by Ingestion—*Ascaris*

Ascaris is one of the largest of the human parasites, up to 30 cm in length, and one of the most frequently encountered worldwide. It affects perhaps one quarter of the human population, including a substantial number of people in the southern United States. A few *Ascaris* are generally well tolerated, but a large worm load may cause serious illness.

■ CASE

A 4-year-old-boy living in the southern United States had been well until 3 weeks before a visit to the doctor, al-

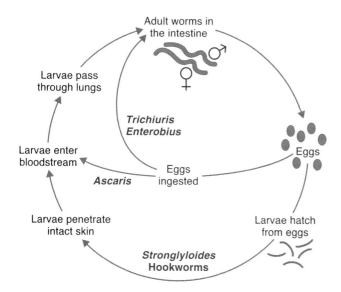

Figure 52.1. Comparative life cycles of intestinal nematodes.

Large numbers of larvae (from a large number of ingested eggs) may produce pneumonia as they cross from the bloodstream into the lungs. This reaction may be particularly severe if the patient has been sensitized by a previous ascaris infection. Later, if adult worms are present in large numbers in the intestine, they may form a large mass (worm ball) and produce intestinal obstruction, as in the case presented. Occasionally, indi-

though he had always been small for his age (height and weight at the l0th percentile). His parents reported that he passed "earthworms" with his stool. For the previous 2 to 3 weeks he had vague abdominal pain with nausea. He had been unable to eat, his abdomen was distended, and he had had no bowel movements for 5 days. X-rays of his abdomen were consistent with intestinal obstruction. Stool examination revealed large numbers of *Ascaris* eggs. He was given mebendazole and placed on intravenous fluids. One day after beginning treatment, he passed large numbers of *Ascaris*. Three days later, his abdomen was no longer distended, he was able to eat and drink, and he had a normal bowel movement

Encounter and pathobiology

After excretion in the stool, *Ascaris* eggs require several weeks in a warm environment to mature to the infective stage (Fig. 52.2). For this reason, ascariasis, like hookworm disease, is restricted to warm climates and to areas where the soil is contaminated by untreated human feces. The eggs must be ingested to complete the cycle. Ingestion may occur by placing soiled hands in the mouth or by eating food contaminated with soil-containing eggs. Fruits and vegetables growing near to the ground become contaminated by direct contact with fecally contaminated soil, either inadvertently or deliberately (as when human feces are used as fertilizer).

Once ingested, the eggs hatch in the small intestine and release larvae, which penetrate the mucosa and submucosa and enter venules or lymphatics. The parasites travel to the lung and migrate up the trachea to the pharynx, where they are swallowed, regaining access to the gastrointestinal tract. The worms mature in the intestinal lumen and the females release their eggs into the stool.

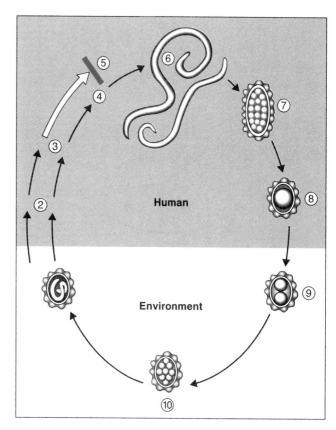

Figure 52.2. *Ascaris* life cycle. *Ascaris lumbricoides* (human roundworm) and dog or cat roundworm (visceral larva migrans). Humans acquire these infections by ingesting embryonated roundworm eggs from the environment (*1*). After ingestion, the parasites hatch in the upper intestine (*2*), cross the bowel wall (*3*), and enter the bloodstream. The human *Ascaris* (innermost set of *arrows* in the *top half* of the diagram) enters the lung by crossing into the alveolus (*4*). It then travels up the trachea, is swallowed, and reenters the GI tract to develop to a mature adult (*6*). The *open arrow* and *solid line* on the diagram indicate that neither dog nor cat *Ascaris* are able to enter the lung from the bloodstream. As a result, these parasites wander aimlessly through deep tissues and are unable to return to the gastrointestinal tract (*5*). Thus, stool examinations are negative in patients with visceral larva migrans and positive in patients with human *Ascaris* infection (*7*).

In the environment, fertilized *Ascaris* eggs (*8*) germinate and divide (*9,10*) and produce embryonated eggs (*11*) which are infectious on oral ingestion. This process takes several weeks and requires a warm, moist climate. In visceral larva migrans, the infectious eggs are shed by infected dogs or cats, rather than humans.

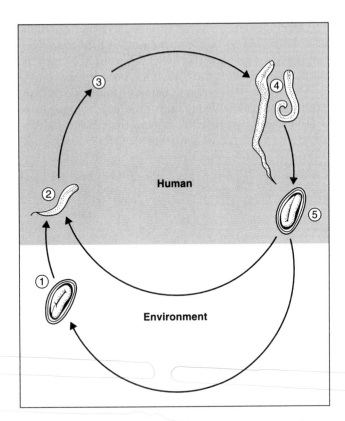

Figure 52.3. Pinworm life cycle (*Enterobius vermicularis*). Humans acquire pinworm infection by the ingestion of embryonated eggs (*1*). After ingestion, these eggs hatch in the small intestine (*2*), mature to adults in the large intestine (*3,4*) and produce eggs (*5*). Because the gravid female lays her eggs in the perianal area, the eggs may be shed into the environment (*lower half* of diagram) or inadvertently ingested by patients or their close contacts when fingers used to scratch the perianal area are licked or used to prepare food.

vidual worms may produce biliary obstruction (by migrating up the bile duct and occluding it) or peritonitis (by perforating the intestinal wall). Moderate intestinal worm burdens, on the other hand, may be totally asymptomatic.

Humans may also be infected by ingesting ascarid worms native to dogs, cats, or raccoons. Transmission is also by the fecal–oral route. The resulting infection is known as **visceral larva migrans**. Animals are the definitive hosts for these worms, which are unable to complete their cycle in humans. After leaving the intestine, dog or cat ascaris wander randomly through the tissues rather than crossing the lung to the trachea. Enlargement of the liver and spleen (hepatosplenomegaly) may result from the inflammatory response to the worms. Eosinophilia is usually marked because the worms invade the deep tissues. Because the worms cannot complete their life cycle in humans, they are considered **dead-end hosts** for these animal infections. The aborted nature of human infection by parasites of other primary hosts (dog or cat *As-*

caris in visceral larva migrans; dog or cat hookworms in creeping eruption) is a vivid reminder of the specificity of host–parasite interactions.

Diagnosis and treatment

Ascariasis is usually readily diagnosed by stool examination using low power (×100) magnification, since each adult female worm releases approximately 200,000 eggs per day into the intestinal lumen. One can estimate the number of worms present by the numbers of eggs in the stool.

Mebendazole, pyrantel pamoate, piperazine, and a number of other agents are effective in treating *Ascaris* infection of the gastrointestinal tract. Medical treatment with these agents typically relieves intestinal obstruction without surgical intervention.

Nematode Infections Acquired by Ingestion—*Enterobius* (Pinworm)

Pinworm infection is common in both temperate and tropical regions, affecting at least 200 million people worldwide. It is most prevalent among small children, who typically infect their siblings and parents, and among institutionalized persons. Pinworms seldom produce serious disease but may cause considerable discomfort. A typical case would be that of a healthy 3-year-old girl who is brought to the pediatrician because she has developed what the mother considers "unacceptable behavior"—she frequently scratches herself in the anal and vulval areas.

Encounter and pathobiology

Pinworms do not require an extrinsic incubation period, thus the infection is transmitted readily in areas with fecal–oral contamination (Fig. 52.3). The eggs resist drying and may be transmitted from an infected person to other members of the household from bed clothes or dust. After oral ingestion, the eggs hatch in the duodenum and jejunum. After maturation and fertilization, the larvae mature in the ileum and large intestine. Gravid females migrate out of the rectum to the perianal skin to lay eggs. This results in the most typical presentation, perianal itching, which may be caused by dermal sensitivity to parasite antigens. Scratching facilitates the spread of the infection because infective eggs may be spread to the same person (autoinfection) or to others by putting the infected fingers into the mouth. Other moist areas, such as the vagina, may also be affected. On occasion, the parasite may be found in the lumen of the appendix, although it is thought to rarely produce appendicitis.

Diagnosis and treatment

Pinworm infection is easy to diagnose using the microscope. The buttocks are gently separated and a microscope slide covered with Scotch tape (adhesive side out) or its commercially prepared paddle version is placed between them before the patient arises in the morning. Pinworm eggs are large enough to be identified under the microscope using low-power (×100) magnification.

A number of anthelminthics, including mebendazole, pyrantel pamoate, and other drugs, are effective in the treatment of pinworm infection. Because one untreated person may easily infect others, the entire family must be treated (including relatives who live with or visit the infected child, babysitters, and other children at the day care center).

Intestinal Roundworms That Penetrate the Skin—*Strongyloides*

Strongyloidiasis is prevalent in tropical areas of the globe but may also be found elsewhere. In large numbers, these worms may cause intestinal malfunction. They may perforate the intestinal wall, resulting in serious bacterial septicemias. In addition, they may reinfect the same host, especially if immunocompromised, to produce a lethal systemic disease.

■ CASE

A 57-year-woman was hospitalized for her fourth episode of unexplained Gram-negative bacteremia. The only other pertinent medical history was that the patient had recently begun treatment with corticosteroids for asthmatic bronchitis. Paradoxically, her cough worsened with this therapy, and she began to experience abdominal pain and diarrhea. Likewise, the other episodes of bacteremia also followed the initiation of steroid therapy.

The patient was a resident of Michigan who had lived in rural Eastern Kentucky as a child and teenager. She was treated with antibiotics for the organism causing her bacteremia. Because a CAT scan of the patient's abdomen showed a thickened intestinal wall, the patient underwent a small intestinal biopsy that revealed the presence of helminthic parasites attached to the mucosa. Subsequently, examination of the patient's stool revealed numerous immature larvae of *Strongyloides stercoralis*. More developed larvae were also identified in the patient's sputum.

Encounter and entry

Strongyloides penetrate human skin as filariform larvae (perhaps best remembered by thinking of them as "filing" their way through the skin). Thus, transmission of these parasites does not require the ingestion of contaminated feces; transmission is typically via the fecal–cutaneous route, not the fecal–oral route. People become infected with *Strongyloides* by contact with infected human stool or with soil that has been contaminated by human stool containing filariform larvae. After they penetrate the skin, the larvae enter the bloodstream and lymphatics and become trapped in the lungs. Here, they break through the alveolar wall into the alveolar lumen, are coughed up, and are then swallowed into the

GI tract where they continue their life cycle (Fig. 52.4), primarily in the duodenum and jejunum.

The life cycle of *Strongyloides* does not require an external soil phase (see Fig. 52.4). In areas of poor sanita-

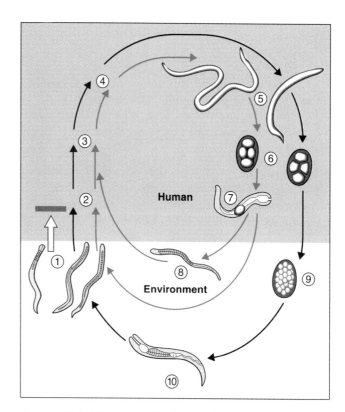

Figure 52.4. The *Strongyloides* and human hookworm life cycle. The invasive filariform larvae of these parasites penetrate unbroken human skin (*1*). Once inside the host, *Strongyloides* and human hookworm larvae migrate through the subcutaneous tissues to the bloodstream (*2*), enter the lung by crossing into the alveoli (*3*), travel up the trachea, and are coughed up and swallowed into the gastrointestinal tract (*4*). In contrast to *Strongyloides* and hookworm, the filariform larvae that cause creeping eruption (the larvae of dog or cat hookworms) are unable to enter the bloodstream and migrate to the lung. Instead, they wander through the subcutaneous tissues causing cutaneous larva migrans. The *solid line* and *open arrow* (above and to the left of *1*) indicate that the larvae of this parasite are unable to complete their normal life cycle in a human host. The larvae of *Strongyloides* and hookworm mature (*5*) within the upper gastrointestinal tract. As shown on the *right side* of the diagram, female hookworm larvae remain within the lumen of the gastrointestinal tract, releasing their eggs into the stool (*6*), which then pass into the environment (*9*). Because the female *Strongyloides* larvae enter the bowel wall, their eggs do not appear in the stool (*left side of 6*) and only the larvae (*7*) are normally found in the stool. On occasion, these larvae mature to the filariform stage in the gastrointestinal tract (*8*) to produce endogenous reinfection (autoinfection). Because hookworm larvae require maturation in the environment to become infectious (*bottom half* of the diagram), autoinfection cannot occur in this disease.

tion, this worm is transmitted via human feces, regardless of climate. Thus, outbreaks of strongyloidiasis have been reported from institutions for the mentally retarded in temperate zones, from Eskimo settlements north of the Arctic circle, and from the tropics. In past decades, strongyloidiasis was a common infection in the Appalachian region of the United States.

Damage

Many people infected with *Strongyloides* carry only a small number of the worms in the intestine, and few have clinical manifestations. Like other intestinal roundworms, *Strongyloides* has three opportunities to cause damage during its life cycle:

- While passing through the skin—*Strongyloides* does not usually cause damage at this step, but other worms (e.g., hookworms) may produce itching and a rash, neither of which tend to be severe.
- During passage through the lungs—*Strongyloides* may elicit a transient response characterized by cough, wheezing, and fever.
- In the intestine—Although *Strongyloides* infection is usually asymptomatic, it may cause pain, vomiting, and diarrhea when the number of worms becomes large.

Unlike the other intestinal roundworms, female *Strongyloides* have the unusual ability to invade the bowel wall to lay their eggs. This invasion may cause severe disease because the so-called rhabditiform larvae hatching from the eggs can cross the intestinal wall into the peritoneum and cause intestinal perforations, permitting intestinal bacteria to follow and produce peritonitis. As a result, strongyloidiasis may produce acute clinical syndromes (such as peritonitis) or may mimic chronic abdominal problems such as peptic ulcer or gallbladder disease.

Because the female *Strongyloides* lay their eggs in the bowel wall instead of the intestinal lumen, the larvae may hatch and mature while still in the body. Reinfection may then occur from larval invasion of the perianal skin even if the patient has not been exposed to new external sources of infection. Strongyloides reinfection produces a characteristic snakelike (serpiginous) urticarial rash ("larva currens"), typically located near the anus. As in the case, the process of endogenous reinfection may produce a fatal hyperinfection syndrome that is sometimes fatal. In the case described above, the patient may have acquired the infection as a youth in rural Kentucky. She apparently maintained an asymptomatic *Strongyloides* infection by the mechanism of autoinfection described above. With the administration of corticosteroids later in life, the infection was no longer controlled and she experienced respiratory and abdominal symptoms. She later died.

Immunosuppression and strongyloidiasis

Patients immunosuppressed by malnutrition or drugs have a much greater risk of dissemination and progression to hyperinfection syndrome. In fact, strongyloidiasis is a major cause of death in kidney transplant recipients in the tropics. Presumably, these patients can control the infection before transplantation. However, they become unable to control the infection when their cell-mediated immunity is compromised by the immunosuppressive drugs used to prevent rejection of the transplanted kidney.

Because the hyperinfection syndrome is often seen in patients with impaired cell-mediated immunity, it seems likely that this kind of immunity is the critical factor in the control of strongyloidiasis. The relative role of mononuclear cells and eosinophils has not been elucidated, nor is it known if these worms coat themselves with host proteins.

Strongyloides infections may become chronic and produce symptoms for decades. Persistent infections lasting over 35–40 years have been described among former prisoners of war (from World War II). These persons often have chronic syndromes that are misdiagnosed as peptic ulcer or gallbladder disease and fail to respond to medical or surgical treatments for those conditions. Patients in whom autoinfection has been controlled may develop urticarial skin lesions from the migration of larvae at the surface of the skin.

Diagnosis and treatment

Strongyloidiasis is often difficult to diagnose because the worms lay their eggs in the bowel wall, and thus the eggs are rarely found in the stool. In addition, *Strongyloides* larvae are easily confused with hookworm larvae.

Patients with strongyloidiasis typically have a marked eosinophilia (10–20% of white blood cells, over 10–20,000 eosinophils per μl of blood). However, lack of eosinophilia does not exclude the disease. The magnitude of the eosinophilia in persons with the hyperinfection syndrome may be limited by the basic T-cell defect(s) predisposing to the syndrome, the outpouring of neutrophils resulting from secondary bacterial infection, and corticosteroid therapy. Note the difference between determining the percentage of eosinophils among all white blood cells and their absolute number per microliter. Patients thought to have strongyloidiasis should be studied first by stool examination. Even if three or more stool examinations reveal no larvae, examination of the duodenal contents or duodenal biopsy may be positive.

Thiabendazole has been the drug of choice for strongyloidiasis although it may produce vomiting and has other side effects. Thiabendazole is thought to act by binding to β-tubulin of the parasite. Recent studies suggest that ivermectin may also be effective.

Table 52.2. The Main Intestinal Helminths

Example	Reservoir	Clinical manifestations
Acquired by passage through the skin		
Roundworms		
Strongyloides stercoralis	Infected humans	GI manifestations that may mimic peptic ulcer or gallbladder disease; disseminated infection ("hyperinfection syndrome")
Hookworms	Infected humans	Iron-deficiency anemia from chronic GI blood loss
Necator americanus		
Ancylostoma duodenale		
Acquired by ingestion		
Roundworms		
Ascaris lumbricoides	Infected humans	Often asymptomatic except for passage of 25- to 30-cm worms; may produce GI or biliary obstruction, or peritonitis from intestinal perforation
Pinworm	Infected humans, especially children	Itching of the perianal or genital region
Enterobius vermicularis		
Whipworm	Infected humans	Often asymptomatic.
Trichuris trichiura		Damage to intestinal mucosa; malnutrition and anemia if severe.
Tapeworms		
Taenia solium	Pigs	Intestinal infection (teniasis) is typically asymptomatic; for cysticercosis, see Table 53.1
T. saginata	Cattle	Intestinal infection (teniasis) is typically asymptomatic
Diphyllobothrium latum	Fish	Intestinal infection is typically asymptomatic, but may lead to vitamin B_{12} deficiency

INTESTINAL NEMATODES THAT PENETRATE THE SKIN—HOOKWORMS

Hookworm disease is caused by two species of roundworms: *Necator americanus* and *Ancylostoma duodenale*. Human hookworms have a life cycle similar to that of *Strongyloides*, but with the following differences:

- After being shed in the stool, hookworm eggs require a period of maturation in a warm environment to produce infective filariform larvae (unlike *Strongyloides*). Consequently, hookworm infection is restricted to warm climates. Transmission of hookworms requires contamination of the soil with untreated human feces and subsequent exposure of unprotected human skin to the infected feces. Hookworm infection may be prevented by sanitation (using indoor or outdoor toilets or treating feces used for fertilizer), or by wearing shoes. Hookworm infection was common in the Southern United States up until the early part of this century.

- Hookworms cannot complete their life cycle in the human host (unlike *Strongyloides*). Thus, hookworm infection cannot produce a hyperinfection syndrome.

- Unlike *Strongyloides*, hookworms do not invade the bowel wall and thus do not produce severe bacterial superinfections.

- Hookworms produce chronic anemia by hanging onto the intestinal mucosa with their teeth, secreting an anticoagulant, and sucking the patient's blood. This mode of attachment results in a slow, steady blood loss (0.03 ml per worm per day for *Necator americanus*, 0.15 ml for *Ancylostoma duodenale*). Hookworms affect some 800–900 million people throughout the globe; it has been estimated that the total loss of human blood to hookworms is at least 1 million liters daily. The severity of the anemia is proportional to the worm burden. Severe infections in children may produce chronic anemia which may lead to developmental retardation.

- As they penetrate the skin at the time of initial infection, hookworm larvae may also cause local manifestations, namely itching and irritation ("ground itch"). People may also become infected with cat and dog hookworms; this condition is known as creeping eruption (or cutaneous larva migrans). Unlike *Strongyloides* or human hookworm, the filariform larvae of dog or cat hookworms cannot make their way from the skin into the circulation. As a result, filariform larvae crawl randomly in the skin and die after several days to a week.

Diagnosis and treatment

The adult female hookworm releases 10,000–20,000 eggs per day into the bowel lumen, which makes it easy to diagnose significant hookworm infections by stool

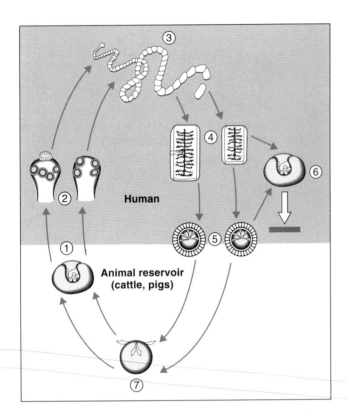

Figure 52.5. Intestinal tapeworm life cycle—*Taenia solium* (pork tapeworm) and *Taenia saginata* (beef tapeworm). Humans acquire these infections by ingesting the tissue stage of the parasite (cysticercus) in inadequately cooked meat (*1*). The parasite then hatches in the intestine (*2*) and matures to an intestinal tapeworm 10 meters or more in length (*3*). The pork tapeworm (*outside* of diagram) has a crown of spines on its head and fewer pairs of lateral uterine branches in its proglottids (segments) than the beef tapeworm (*4*). The eggs of these two parasites (*5*) are identical morphologically. As shown in the diagram, only the pork tapeworm (*T. solium*) produces human cysticercosis (*6*). When human feces containing viable eggs are ingested by either pigs or cattle, the eggs hatch (*7*) and produce the tissue (cysticercal) stage of the infection in those animals (*1*) to complete the cycle.

examination using low power (×100) magnification. In fact, it is possible to estimate the number of worms present and the average daily blood loss by quantitating the number of eggs in the stool.

Mebendazole, pyrantel pamoate, and several other drugs can be effectively used to treat hookworm infection. Emergency treatment is not required because hookworms produce chronic, but not acute or invasive disease. Patients with hookworm disease may require dietary supplementation with iron and folic acid to produce sufficient numbers of red blood cells to correct their anemia.

INTESTINAL TAPEWORMS

As the name suggests, tapeworms are long and ribbonlike and are composed of chains of rectangular seg-

ments. An individual tapeworm is actually an animal colony, since each segment (known as a proglottid) is a self-contained unit capable of reproduction, metabolism, and food uptake (tapeworms have no gut). Tapeworms attach to the intestinal wall by a head (scolex) which has sucking discs or grooves (Fig. 52.5). In their intermediate animal host, these worms penetrate deep tissues and develop into infective larval forms.

The most common human tapeworms are acquired by eating uncooked or inadequately cooked beef (*Taenia saginata*), pork (*Taenia solium*), or fish (*Diphyllobothrium latum*). Tapeworms cause two types of disease:

- Intestinal infection (teniasis) is caused by ingestion of larval cysts in pork, beef, or fish. The clinical picture of intestinal infection is generally mild and is essentially the same for all tapeworms.
- Deep tissue infection is caused by ingestion of eggs from the pork tapeworm (cysticercosis) or the carnivores' tapeworm (echinococcosis or hydatid disease). See Chapter 53, "Tissue and Blood Helminths."

These two types of diseases are very different and must be distinguished. Unfortunately, confusion is possible because one tapeworm (pork tapeworm) may produce both teniasis and deep tissue infection in the same patient.

■ CASE

The wife of a high-ranking government official accompanied her husband on a trip to the Near East. During a diplomatic reception they were served steak tartare (raw beef), a traditional dish in that region. Three months later she noticed thin, white, rectangular segments in her stool (approximately 1 × 2 × 0.2 cm). She experienced nausea, apparently brought about by seeing the worms in her stool. Laboratory studies revealed that the segments were proglottids of *T. saginata*. Her stool also contained eggs of this worm.

She was reassured by her physician, who told her that this infection is unlikely to have clinical consequences in a healthy person. On the other hand, he could understand her revulsion at seeing the worm segments in her stool and visualizing the rest of the worm inside her. The physician prescribed niclosamide, which eliminated the rest of the tapeworm.

Encounter

The life cycle of beef tapeworm requires both humans (definitive host) and cattle (intermediate host) (see Fig. 52.5). Cattle become infected by ingesting human feces containing the parasite's eggs; humans become infected by eating beef that contains larvae (cysticerci). The eggs hatch in the intestine of cattle and enter the bloodstream to lodge in peripheral tissues, where they develop into cysticerci (Chapter 53, "Tissue and Blood Helminths"). Beef tapeworm infection only exists in areas where infected humans defecate near cattle. These areas, however, are found in most countries of the world.

All human intestinal tapeworm infections correlate with gastronomic preferences: they are found mainly among people who consume their meat undercooked or raw (as in the case described). Transmission also clearly depends on lack of sanitation. These diseases are common in many parts of the world, but are infrequent in Western Europe and the United States. Cooking effectively destroys the larvae, but cooks have been known to become infected by tasting raw food during preparation: fish tapeworm infection is said to be an occupational hazard of Jewish or Scandinavian grandmothers making "gefilte fish" or "lutefisk."

Damage

The infectious tissue larvae from the intermediate host (beef, pork, fish) hatch in the human small intestine and mature into adult tapeworms. The worms may live in the human intestine for several decades and attain lengths of up to 10 meters, which has given rise to the popular but mistaken notion that they increase a person's appetite by consuming a significant amount of their food intake.

Most patients are asymptomatic, but some have nausea, diarrhea, and weight loss. The infection is usually noted only because of the presence of proglottids in the stool. Almost half of those infected with fish tapeworm have low levels of vitamin B_{12}, leading to serious so-called megaloblastic anemia. This deficiency appears to be due to competition between the host and the parasite for this vitamin in the diet. Note that the intestinal disease caused by tapeworm is very different from that in the tissues (see Chapter 53, "Tissue and Blood Helminths").

Diagnosis and treatment

Most tapeworm infections are readily diagnosed by stool examination. The proglottids are macroscopic and can be seen by the naked eye. The eggs are large enough (3l to 43 μm in diameter) to be seen using low-power magnification ($\times$100). Although the eggs of pork and beef tapeworms are identical, their proglottids may be distinguished by the experienced observer (those of *T. solium* have uteri with fewer pairs of lateral branches).

Most patients (>90%) are cured with a single dose of niclosamide. Those who are not cured often have nausea or vomiting with their first treatment and typically respond to a second treatment with the drug.

CONCLUSION

Intestinal helminthic infections are usually benign, but can cause significant illness if the worm burden in very large. With the exception of *Strongyloides*, these parasites have no capacity to increase their numbers in the infected host. Therefore, the worm burden in infections other than by *Strongyloides* is directly related to the size of the ingested inoculum (or the accumulation of repeated inocula). Since *Strongyloides* infection can be asymptomatic and sustained, the hyperinfection syndrome can occur during immunosuppression decades after the initial exposure.

SUGGESTED READINGS

Genta RM, Weesner R, Douce RW, Huitger-O'Connor T, Walzer PD. Strongyloidiasis in U.S. veterans of the Vietnam and other wars. JAMA 1987;258:49–52.

Liu LX, Weller PF. Strongyloidiasis and other intestinal nematode infections. Infect Dis Clin North Am 1993;7:655–682.

Mahmoud AA. Strongyloidiasis. Clin Infect Dis 1996;23: 949–952.

Phillis JA, Harrold AJ, Whiteman GV, et al. Pulmonary infiltrates, asthma and eosinophilia due to *Ascaris suum* infestation in man. N Engl J Med 1972;286:965–970. (An account of a fraternity stunt in which unsuspecting students were given pig ascaris.)

Weber M. Pinworms. N Engl J Med 1993;328:927.

Fuessl H. *Ascaris lumbricoides*. N Engl J Med 1994;331:303.

Brennick J, Mattia A. *Strongyloides stercoralis* infestation. N Engl J Med 1996;334:1173.

Tissue and Blood Helminths

DONALD J. KROGSTAD
N. CARY ENGLEBERG

Key Concepts

- Tissue invasive helminths enter humans by ingestion (*Trichinella*, invasive cestodes), penetration through the skin (*Schistosoma*), or arthopod bites (various filariae).
- Trichinosis is maintained by a "cycle of carnivorism" in which predators and scavengers feed on each other and acquire larvae encysted in muscles. Humans usually acquire infection from undercooked meat from pigs or carnivorous game animals. Fever, severe muscle pain, and intense eosinophilia occur when larvae disseminate to human skeletal muscles.
- Invasive cestode infections occur when humans ingest tapeworm eggs (pork tapeworm eggs from human feces or *Echinococcus* eggs from canine feces). Larvae that emerge from ingested eggs migrate to and encyst within the brain (*Taenia solium*, pork tapeworm) or in the liver or lungs (*Echinococcus granulosum*). Symptoms develop after prolonged infection because of pressure effects of the enlarging cysts or hypersensitivity to released parasite antigens.
- Schistosomiasis is prevalent in geographic areas where: 1) fresh, surface waters are used for bathing or washing, 2) the waters are contaminated with human feces or urine, and 3) certain types of snails are present to host the intermediate stages of the parasite. In humans, adult worms localize to the mesenteric or pelvic veins. The manifestations of disease are caused by the granulomatous reaction to helminth eggs that are trapped in tissues (e.g., intestine, bladder, liver).
- Lymphatic filariasis results from chronic obstruction of lymph channels by adult worms and progressive swelling of extremities or genitals (e.g, elephantiasis). Adult worms are often inapparent in cutaneous filariasis, but their microfilaria (larvae) disseminate subcutaneously and produce chronic hypersensitivity reactions which may lead to chronic dermatitis or blindness (e.g., onchocerciasis, or "river blindness").

Helminths cause a variety of diseases by establishing residence in deep tissues. As with the intestinal helminths, some are acquired by ingestion and others by penetration of the skin—either by direct entry of the parasites or by insect bites. The diseases they produce almost invariably involve chronic inflammation and thus are caused in part to the host immune response to the parasite. As with the intestinal helminths, when the worm burden is low, infections are rarely symptomatic. Since many worms are long-lived in humans, they may gradually accumulate in large numbers as the consequence of repeated encounters. When present in sensitive target organs, helminths may produce severe disease and even death. Helminths that cause deep tissue infections include members of all three helminth groups: roundworms, tapeworms, and flukes (Table 53.1).

TISSUE HELMINTHS ACQUIRED BY INGESTION

The main helminths in this group are the roundworm *Trichinella* and the deep tissue-invading tapeworms.

Table 53.1. The Main Tissue and Blood Helminths

Examples	Reservoir	Mode of transmission	Clinical manifestations
Acquired by ingestion			
Tapeworms			
Hydatid disease: *Echinococcus granulosus*	Sheep, cattle, horses	Fecal-oral (eggs)	Tissue-displacing and invasive lesions, most common in liver but seen in lung, CNS, and elsewhere
Cysticercosis: *Taenia solium* (cysticerci)	Pigs	Foodborne	Tissue-displacing lesions, most critical in CNS
Roundworms			
Visceral larva migrans:			
Toxocara canis	Dogs	Fecal-oral (eggs)	Systemic illness with malaise, eosinophilia, often enlarged liver and spleen
T. catis	Cats		
Trichinosis: *Trichinella spiralis*	Pigs (also bears) (larvae)	Foodborne	Mild infection produces malaise, mild diarrhea and periorbital edema; severe infection may be life-threatening with CNS and heart involvement
Guinea worm: *Dracunculus medinensis*	Infected humans (larvae)	Waterborne-oral	Malaise, fever, other systemic symptoms when the adult worm emerges 1 year after initial infection
Flukes			
Lung fluke: *Paragonimus westermani*	Animals, humans?	Foodborne (metacercariae in crabs)	Cysts rupture in lung, leading to secondary bacterial infection, chronic bronchitis, and a tuberculosis-like picture
Liver fluke: *Chlonorchis sinensis*	Fish, animals, humans	Foodborne (metacercariae in fresh-water fish)	Often asymptomatic; if worm load is high, can lead to biliary stones, chronic inflammation, liver cancer
Acquired by passage through the skin			
Blood flukes			
Schistosomes *S. mansoni, S. haematobium, S. japonicum*	Infected humans	Water-cutaneous (cercariae)	Symptoms vary with the intensity of infection, from asymptomatic to hematuria and bladder cancer (*S. haematobium*), and blood in stool and portal hypertension (*S. mansoni* and *S. japonicum*)
Roundworms			
Cutaneous larva migrans (dog, cat hookworms)	Dogs, cats	Fecal-cutaneous (filariform larvae)	Superficial skin lesions progressing at a rate of 2 cm/day
Filaria			
Lymphatic filariasis *Wuchereria bancrofti, Brugia malayi*	Infected humans (larvae)	Mosquito bite	Vary from asymptomatic to massive enlargement of the legs, scrotum, and breasts with recurrent filarial fevers
River blindness: *Onchocerca volvulus*	Infected humans (larvae)	Black fly bite	Multiple subcutaneous nodules; blindness from reaction to microfilariae crossing the eye

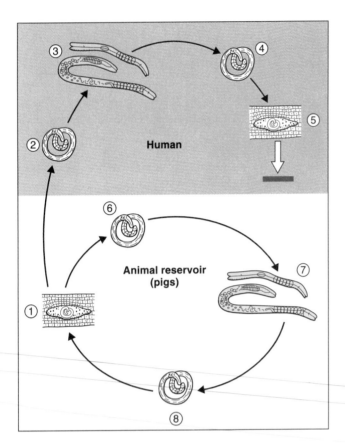

Figure 53.1. Trichinella life cycle (*Trichinella spiralis*). Humans acquire trichinosis by eating undercooked pork containing viable encysted *Trichinella* larvae (*1*). After ingestion, these larvae hatch in the intestine (*2*), mature to adults (*3*), and release larvae that invade the intestinal wall and enter the bloodstream (*4*). The larvae then encyst in striated or cardiac muscle (*5*). As indicated by the *open arrow* and *solid line below 5* on the diagram, human infection is normally a dead end in the natural transmission of trichinosis. Similar phenomena are observed in the pig reservoir, and in other carnivores that may also harbor *Trichinella* larvae (*6–8* on the *lower half* of the diagram).

Trichinella spiralis

The presence of *Trichinella spiralis* larvae in the heart, skeletal muscle, brain, or GI tract causes trichinosis. Most infected people are asymptomatic and are not seriously ill. Paradoxically, trichinosis is more common in the United States than in many developing countries. The reason for this higher prevalence is that many other countries ensure that pigs are not fed uncooked garbage contaminated with viable *Trichinella* larvae. Fortunately, only a few hundred clinically significant cases occur in the U.S. each year.

▮ CASE

A 45-year-old immigrant from Laos living in Iowa had been well until a few days after a family celebration that featured a highly seasoned but undercooked pork dish. Two days after the celebration, he developed diarrhea and abdominal pain. About a week after the onset of diarrhea, he developed severe muscle pain, swelling around the eyes, and headache. Physical examination revealed "splinter" hemorrhages in his fingernails. Laboratory studies demonstrated a marked eosinophilia (12,000/μl). Biopsies of his tender muscles and of the splinter hemorrhages revealed *Trichinella* larvae.

Encounter and pathobiology

The life cycle of *Trichinella* is illustrated in Figure 53.1. After the ingestion of meat containing viable encysted *Trichinella* (usually in undercooked pork), the infective larvae hatch and mature in the small intestine of pigs or humans. After a few days, the adult worms release larvae which cross the mucosa to enter the intestinal lymphatics and the bloodstream (producing diarrhea and pain in the process). These larvae are then carried to all parts of the body via the bloodstream. The larvae **encyst** in striated and cardiac muscle fibers and produce a marked initial inflammatory response. The cysts usually calcify, although the worms may remain viable for up to 30 years. The life cycle of the parasite is completed in non-human vertebrates when their muscle (meat) containing viable larvae is eaten by another carnivore. Thus, the propagation of this disease depends on a "cycle of carnivores" (Fig. 53.2).

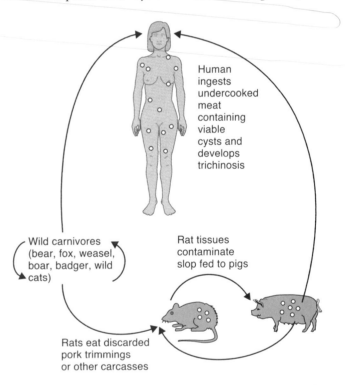

Figure 53.2. The epidemiology of trichinosis. In temperate climates, the infection is maintained in the food chain of wild carnivores by a "cycle of carnivorism." Carnivorous rodents may contaminate garbage that is fed to domestic pigs, and humans can become infected by eating undercooked pork or game meats. In arctic climates, indigenous peoples are commonly infected by eating undercooked bear, walrus, or seal meat. In the tropics, bushpigs and warthogs are potential sources.

Recently, the incidence of trichinosis has diminished, as judged by the prevalence of *Trichinella* cysts at autopsy. The figure has decreased from 16% to less than 1% over the last 30–40 years, partly because of legislation prohibiting the use of uncooked garbage for feeding pigs, and partly because of increased public awareness about the danger of eating undercooked pork. *Trichinella* is also found in other carnivorous animals such as wild pigs and bears, including polar bears, and has caused several outbreaks among hunters and in Eskimo communities.

The manifestations of this disease correlate with the load of worms in tissues and range from asymptomatic to fatal. Several studies suggest that larger inocula (ingestion of many viable larvae) result in more severe disease with a shorter incubation period (2–3 days versus 10 days or more). Patients with 1,000–5,000 larvae per gram of tissue may die from involvement of the heart or central nervous system. Studies in experimental animals suggest that cell-mediated immunity is important in the control of *Trichinella* infection.

Diagnosis and treatment

A rise in antibody titer is diagnostic. However, this increase typically occurs 3–4 weeks or more after the initial infection and is thus useless for the management of severely ill patients (in whom the incubation period may be as short as 2–3 days). In severely ill patients (as in the case presented), muscle biopsy often reveals *Trichinella* larvae under low power magnification ($\times100$) and permits a definitive diagnosis long before serologic testing.

Treatment of trichinosis is problematic. In the early stages of infection, antihelminthic drugs (thiabendazole, albendazole, mebendazole) are useful because they kill adult parasites in the intestine and may prevent ongoing production of invasive larvae. In contrast, antihelminthic agents are of uncertain therapeutic value against the encysted larval forms and may actually provoke symptoms. Bed rest and anti-inflammatory agents (such as aspirin) are most useful for controlling symptoms. Corticosteroids have been used for their anti-inflammatory effects in severely ill patients with myocarditis and/or encephalitis.

Infections by Tissue Forms of Tapeworms

The larvae of a few species of tapeworms infect deep tissues of humans and cause diseases that may have severe manifestations. Illness caused by the tissue form of the pork tapeworm is known as **cysticercosis**; that due to tapeworms of carnivores is known as **echinococcosis**. The life cycle of echinococcos is illustrated in Figure 53.3.

■ **CASES**

Case 1—Cysticercosis

A 33-year-old nurse had been a Peace Corps volunteer in Thailand 10 years earlier. While in Thailand, she had occasionally passed tapeworm segments (proglottids) in her stool, but she was never treated. Eight years after her return to the U.S., she developed multiple subcutaneous nodules across her chest and arms and began having headaches. After two generalized seizures, she was brought to the emergency room. A CT scan of her brain revealed numerous lesions consistent with cysticerci. After treatment with praziquantel, her headaches worsened. Corticosteroids were given to reduce brain swelling and antiepileptic drugs were given to control her seizures, and she was able to complete the praziquantel treatment. She was withdrawn from the antiepileptics 1 year later and has had no additional seizures.

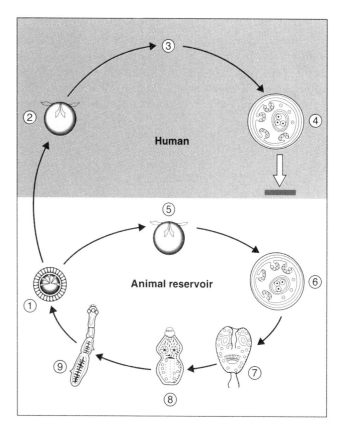

Figure 53.3. Echinococcal life cycle. Humans acquire infection by ingesting eggs in the feces of infected carnivores (*1*), such as dogs or wolves. After ingestion, the eggs hatch in the intestine (*2*). The larvae cross from the GI tract to the tissues (*3*), where they develop into cysts containing daughter cysts and scolices (heads) from which tapeworms can develop under the appropriate circumstance (*4*). As indicated by the *open arrow* and *solid line below 4*, this infection is a dead-end in humans. However, domestic animals (e.g., sheep and goats) may acquire infection by grazing in fecally contaminated pastures (see Figure 53.4). The tissue cysts that develop in these animals are identical to those in humans (*5,6*), but when the animals eventually die in the pasture (often from unrelated causes), dogs or wolves may eat their remains and ingest the tissue cysts. In the canine intestine, the ingested heads (scolices) may develop into adult tapeworms (*7–9*), which eventually produce eggs (*1*) to complete the cycle.

Case 2—Echinococcosis

A 39-year-old Navajo woman was examined for abdominal pain. Two years previously she had first noticed a sensation of fullness in the right upper quadrant of her abdomen. Since that time, this sensation has increased and she now has an obvious swelling (8 × 10 cm) in the area of the liver. Stool examination revealed no tapeworm eggs. A CT scan of the liver revealed a large (12-cm diameter) encapsulated lesion consistent with an hydatid cyst. Serologic testing revealed antibodies against *Echinococcus*. Because of the size of the liver lesion, the mass was removed surgically, using liquid nitrogen to freeze it and prevent spillage of its contents into the peritoneum.

Encounter

Human **cysticercosis** is acquired by ingesting *T. solium* eggs from the feces of humans who harbor an adult tapeworm. The egg hatches into an invasive larva after passage through the acidic stomach. Occasionally, cysticercosis may also develop endogenously in a person who carries a tapeworm (by autoinfection with their own feces or by regurgitation of intestinal tapeworm eggs into the stomach). Endogenous infection may have occurred in the case of the Peace Corps volunteer described above.

The life cycle of *T. solium* requires that pigs become infected by ingesting the eggs of this parasite and that humans eat inadequately cooked pork (analogous to the beef tapeworm life cycle) (Fig. 53.4). These conditions exist in many areas of the developing world. In Mexico, as many as 10–15% of persons hospitalized for neurologic problems have evidence of central nervous system cysticercosis at autopsy.

Echinococcosis or **hydatid disease** is found in most areas of the world, including the United States. *Echinococcus* infections are acquired by ingesting infectious eggs, rather than tissue cysticerci. The usual source of *Echinococcus granulosus* is the feces of dogs or other carnivores (wolves, coyotes). Thus, transmission is by the fecal–oral route, not by eating contaminated meat. The eggs hatch in the small intestine but do not reside

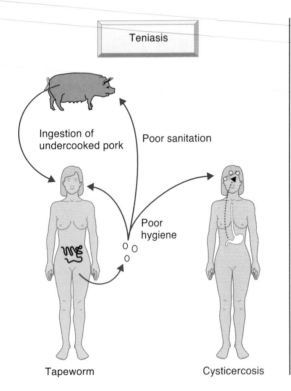

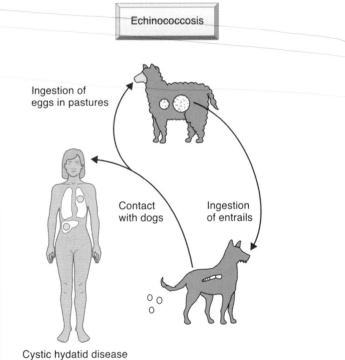

Figure 53.4. Comparative epidemiology of two tissue-invasive tapeworm infections—cysticercosis (due to pork tapeworm, *Taenia solium*) and cystic hydatid disease (due to *Echinococcus granulosus*). Left panel: In "pork tapeworm," the definitive host is the human, not the pig, since only humans harbor the adult tapeworms. Pigs are an intermediate host, since they develop only the tissue invasive form of infection (cysticercosis) after ingestion of eggs from feces of infected humans. Humans also develop the tissue-invasive stage of infection after ingesting eggs from human feces. Although tapeworm carriers can infect themselves with eggs from their own

feces, many humans acquire cysticercosis directly by ingestion of fecally contaminated food and never actually harbored a tapeworm themselves. *Right panel:* In echinococcosis, the definitive host for the tapeworm is the canine (dog, wolf, or fox). Intermediate hosts that harbor the invasive tissue forms become infected by ingesting eggs from canine feces. In humans, tissue-invasive disease with either tapeworm is considered a "dead-end" infection, since humans are rarely cannibalized (to complete the Taenia life cycle), and human remains are buried or incinerated in most cultures (making completion of the echinococcal life cycle improbable).

there. Rather, they penetrate the intestinal wall and form so-called **hydatid cysts** in many organs.

The cycle of *Echinococcus* is maintained between sheep and sheep dogs in the southwestern United States (see Fig. 53.4). Native Americans who keep sheep in that region are sometimes victims of the disease. A "sylvatic" cycle is also present in the northern United States and Alaska, with wolves as the carnivores and elk and other large game as the herbivores. *Echinococcus multilocularis* is an analogous parasite in colder climates, for which foxes and cats are the carnivore hosts and mice and voles are the herbivores.

Pathobiology

The sequence of events in echinococcosis and cysticercosis is generally similar. The parasites lodge under the skin or within internal organs, such as the brain or liver, and develop a cyst wall surrounded by a fibrous capsule of host origin. In echinococcosis, the hydatid cysts are lined internally by a germinal membrane that generates numerous embryonic tapeworm heads (each of which has the potential to develop into a tapeworm in the canine intestine). Most hydatid cysts occur in the liver or the lung. They usually produce few symptoms until they reach 8–10 cm or more in diameter, which may take years or even decades. The growing mass may produce symptoms by compression of vital structures, or the cysts may leak or rupture and pose a significant risk of death from anaphylactic reactions.

Tapeworm larvae (or cysticerci) each contain only one potential tapeworm head. The cysts are generally more numerous than hydatid cysts, but rarely grow larger than 1–2 cm. When a cyst dies, its contents leak into the surrounding tissues and induce a host inflammatory response. Cysts outside the central nervous system rarely produce symptoms. However, even small cysticerci in the brain may cause cerebral dysfunction, including seizures, increased intracranial pressure, and blindness. Cysticerci thus provide a good example of the correlation between the location and the severity of a disease. Cysticerci may cause symptoms when the parasites die and displacement of normal tissue is magnified by the host's inflammatory response. This typically occurs 5–10 years after infection, but may occur as much as 50 years later.

Diagnosis and treatment

Because cysticerci may be present in patients without evidence of intestinal infection, *T. solium* cysticercosis is usually diagnosed by its deep tissue manifestations (including lesions visible by CT scan or by "soft" x-ray technique in the long axes of skeletal muscles). A positive serologic test for antibodies to *T. solium* is helpful, especially among persons who live in Europe, the U. S., or other areas of low incidence. This test is typically negative in persons with intestinal *T. solium* infection only.

Praziquantel and albendazole are both effective in the treatment of cysticercosis. Drug treatment kills the organism and decreases the size of the lesions. The fluid-filled cysts collapse and the parasite is ultimately resorbed by the host or calcified. During treatment, central nervous system symptoms may transiently worsen because of the inflammatory response to dying cysticerci. As in the case presentation, the concomitant use of steroids typically alleviates the headaches and seizures that may be caused by this treatment.

The antihelminthic drug albendazole administered over a period of weeks may kill growing echinococcal cysts as well. Alternatively, surgical removal of a large cyst can also cure the infection, although great care must be taken to avoid spillage and dissemination of the infection. For the same reason, it is unwise to attempt blind needle aspiration of a cystic structure that may be an hydatid cyst. Nevertheless, and despite the potential hazard of needle puncture, procedures for aspiration of cysts have been developed that are safe and effective. Quite often, patients with echinococcosis are discovered after their cyst(s) have died. In these cases, the cysts appear calcified in x-rays or CT scans, and no treatment is needed (Fig. 53.5).

TISSUE HELMINTHS THAT PENETRATE THROUGH THE SKIN

This group includes worms that can cross the skin directly (the schistosomes or blood flukes), and those that penetrate via insect bites, the filariae (members of the roundworms).

Schistosomes

Schistosomiasis is an important and common disease in tropical regions. It is estimated that about 200–300 million people are infected worldwide. Schistosomiasis produces a variety of clinical syndromes, depending on the anatomic location of the adult worms and the eggs they release. There are three main pathogenic species with different geographic distributions, found largely in warm climates: *Schistosoma haematobium*, *S. mansoni*, and *S. japonicum*. Their geographic distribution depends on the presence of the snail intermediate host (Fig. 53.6). The schistosomal life cycle is illustrated in Figure 53.7.

■ CASES

Case 1—Intestinal Schistosomiasis

A 48-year-old woman from Egypt had noticed for many years that she had dark stools. During the past year, she also had two episodes of vomiting blood. Examination of her esophagus and stomach with a fiberoptic gastroscope revealed dilated veins in the esophagus which were oozing large amounts of blood. Because viable eggs of *S. mansoni* were found in her stool, she was treated with praziquantel.

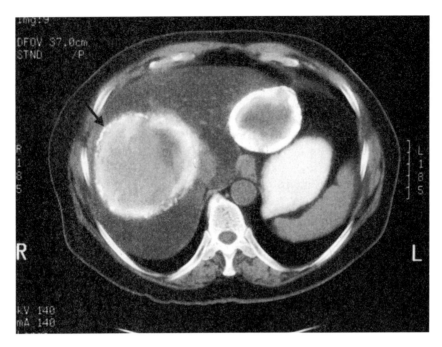

Figure 53.5. Abdominal CT scan of an asymptomatic 55-year-old Lebanese woman. The patient was scheduled to have surgery for an unrelated problem. A routine, preoperative chest x-ray showed a large calcified mass. The CT scan shows two large calcified structures in the liver which represent dead hydatid cysts (*white arrows*).

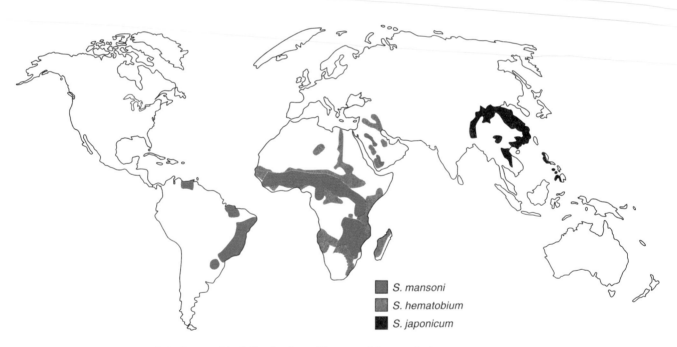

Figure 53.6. Geographical distribution of human schistosomiasis.

Case 2—Schistosomiasis of the bladder

A 38-year-old European man had worked in West Africa for 10 years on a rice-growing irrigation scheme. During the past year, he noticed blood in his urine. Under the microscope, his urine showed the presence of *S. hematobium* eggs. At cystoscopy, his bladder had a cobblestone pattern, consistent with the granulomatous changes seen in schistosomiasis. Typical eggs were seen in the bladder biopsies taken during cystoscopy. He was treated with a single dose of praziquantel (40 mg/kg).

Encounter and pathobiology

The life cycle of schistosomes requires development in certain species of fresh water snails which are their intermediate hosts. The infective stage of the parasite

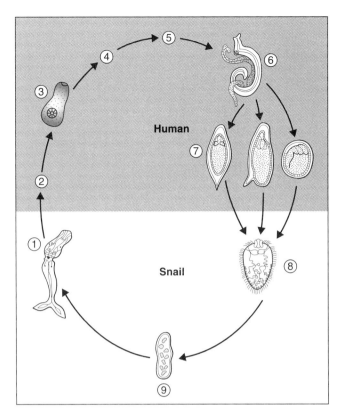

Figure 53.7. Schistosomal life cycle. Humans acquire schistosomiasis by exposure of unprotected skin to water containing infectious cercariae (*1*). The cercariae penetrate unbroken skin (*2*), lose their tails, and become schistosomulae (*3*). They then travel throughout the bloodstream, cross the lungs (*4*) and mature (*5*) in the venous system of the liver to adult worms (*6*). After a period of 6–8 weeks, pairs of adult worms travel to the venous plexuses of the bladder (*S. haematobium*) the large intestine (*S. mansoni*), or the small intestine (*S. japonicum*), where they remain for decades releasing their characteristic eggs (*7*, left to right, *S. hematobium*, *S. mansoni*, and *S. japonicum*). Eggs released into fresh water hatch to miracidia (*8*), which invade the snail intermediate host where they mature to sporocysts (*9*). They then release cercariae (*1*) to complete the cycle.

emerges from the snails and swims in water until it finds a suitable host. Because these snails are not present in the United States, schistosomiasis cannot be transmitted in the U.S., despite the migration of infected persons from Africa and the Middle East. Suitable snails are present in parts of the Caribbean.

The infective forms released from the snails are called cercariae. They are capable of burrowing through the skin of people standing, swimming, or walking through infected water, as in rice paddies (Case 2). In the body, the cercariae lose their tails and change into forms called schistosomulae, which can enter the bloodstream. The parasites then pass through the pulmonary circulation to the portal venous system, where they mature. After sev-

eral weeks, pairs of male and female adults move to the venous plexuses of the large intestine (*S. mansoni*), small intestine (*S. japonicum*), or bladder (*S. hematobium*). The mating worms remain locked together, copulating in the venous system for 10 years or more. The eggs they release may be excreted via the stool (*S. mansoni, S. japonicum*) or the urine (*S. hematobium*). The life cycle is completed when the eggs are released into fresh water, where they hatch and penetrate the appropriate snail intermediate host.

S. mansoni and *S. japonicum* adult worms reside in the venous plexuses of the intestine. There, they release eggs which travel to the intestine and the liver. Eggs that are trapped in host tissues induce the formation of granulomas. The granulomas eventually undergo fibrosis. Over many years of infection, this process results in the pathological changes of schistosomiasis, such as periportal fibrosis in the liver, which may lead to portal hypertension and thus to dilated collateral veins in the esophagus (esophageal varices, as in Case 1). *S. hematobium* adults live in the venous plexus of the urinary bladder and produce blood in the urine (hematuria), granulomatous inflammatory changes in the bladder, and sometimes bladder carcinoma. Fibrotic changes in the bladder and ureters may cause ureterovesical obstruction and recurrent secondary bacterial infections of the bladder, leading occasionally to Gram-negative septicemia.

As in other helminthic infections that invade the tissues, eosinophilia and elevated IgE levels are common in persons with schistosomiasis. Two important anomalous host–parasite interactions are central to the pathogenesis of schistosomiasis:

- Profound fibrotic reactions to schistosome eggs, probably mediated by cytokines. These reactions account for the important pathology of the disease and its long-term complications.
- Lack of an effective immune response to the male and female adult worms, which can reside in the vascular system for decades without being eliminated by the host. Studies have shown that adult worms adsorb host proteins (including serum albumin and HLA antigens) on their surfaces. Essentially, the parasite camouflages itself with these host proteins in order to evade the host's immune response.

Cercariae often produce itching as they penetrate the skin. The cercariae of nonhuman schistosomes (of birds and fish) also cause itching as they penetrate the skin (swimmers' itch, clam diggers' itch), but do not enter the bloodstream or mature within the human body.

Diagnosis and treatment

Most schistosome infections are diagnosed readily by microscopic examination of stool (*S. mansoni, S. japonicum*) or urine (*S. hematobium*) or by biopsy of a rectal

Table 53.2. Control of Human Schistosomiasis	
Rationale	Methods of Control
Reduce carriers	Mass treatment program
Eliminate snail hosts	Molluscicides Destroy snail habitats Snail-eating fish
Prevent contamination of water	Provide latrines, sewage systems Public health education
Prevent human exposure	Provide clean water systems for washing, bathing, drinking, and recreation

valve (*S. mansoni*). Schistosome eggs (150 × 60 μm) are large enough to be identified easily under the microscope with low-power (×100) magnification. Unfortunately, it can be difficult to find schistosome eggs in the stool or urine of patients who are chronically infected and at risk of developing long-term complications. In such patients, serologic testing for antischistosome antibodies may be valuable. However, a positive serologic test does not distinguish between recent versus old or light versus severe infections. Serologic testing is most useful in people who have had single defined exposures in endemic areas. It is of little use for lifelong residents of endemic areas, since most are seropositive but may or may not experience complications.

Praziquantel is the treatment of choice for schistosomiasis. This drug exerts its lethal action by increasing the calcium permeability of the parasite. Drug treatment eliminates the production of eggs by killing the adult worms, but the fibrosis associated with chronic infection is not reversible.

Schistosomiasis can be prevented by disrupting any point in the parasitic life cycle. Potentially effective public health measures and their rationales are shown in Table 53.2.

Filaria

The main filarial infections in humans are onchocerciasis (river blindness) and lymphatic filariasis (elephantiasis). In onchocerciasis, the adult filarial worms live in subcutaneous tissue; in lymphatic filariasis, the adult larvae live in lymphatic tissue. Their offspring, known as microfilariae, travel through the subcutaneous tissue or circulate in the blood. Some 50 million persons in Africa, Asia, and tropical Latin America have onchocerciasis. About 10% of them will become blind from the disease and approximately 30% will have visual impairments unless they are treated. There are West African villages where most people become blind from this disease by the time they reach adulthood. None of these diseases are endemic in the United States.

Lymphatic filariasis affects approximately 200 million people in tropical regions, especially in Asia. This disease leads to tissue swelling, sometimes to elephantine proportions (hence the name elephantiasis). The life cycle of filariae is illustrated in Figure 53.8.

■ CASES

Case 1—Onchocerciasis

A 32-year-old man from Nigeria was seen for an evaluation in a hospital of a nearby town. His village was situated near a rapidly running stream where the men fish and hunt. Like many of his neighbors, he began to lose vision in his late twenties. Three nodules (2 × 3 × 2 cm) are present on his trunk. Skin snips reveal microfilariae of *Onchocerca volvulus*. He was treated with a single oral dose of ivermectin.

Case 2—Elephantiasis

A 48-year-old native of a Philippine island lived in a village where many men and women had elephantiasis. He

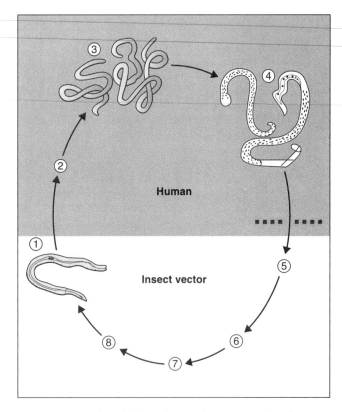

Figure 53.8. Filarial life cycle (*Onchocerciasis*, lymphatic filariasis). Humans acquire infection with the filariae that cause onchocerciasis or elephantiasis by the bite of black flies or mosquitoes, respectively. After third-stage larvae (*1*) are injected under the skin by the vector, the larvae mature (*2*) to adult worms (*3*) that release microfilariae in the subcutaneous tissue (onchocerciasis) or in lymphatics (lymphatic filariasis) (*4*). Microfilariae ingested by the insect vector during feeding mature through a series of stages (*5–8*) to infectious third-stage larvae (*1*) within approximately 2 weeks.

first noticed swelling of his right leg when he was 20 years old. Since that time he has had intermittent fevers to 38.5–39.0°C associated with red streaks from his groin to the foot on both legs. Both feet and his scrotum are now chronically swollen. Typical microfilariae consistent with *Wuchereria bancrofti* were seen in a Giemsa-stained blood smear taken at 2 AM. His recurrent episodes of lymphangitis were treated with an antimicrobial effective against streptococci. The antifilarial drug diethylcarbamazine was given but discontinued when it produced shock and hypotension.

Encounter and pathobiology

The distribution of the diseases is limited primarily by that of their vectors and of infected persons. Onchocerciasis is transmitted by *Simulium* black flies. In contrast, lymphatic filiariasis is transmitted by mosquitoes. Neither infection is transmitted within the United States; there is no reservoir of infected humans to serve as a source of infection for susceptible insect vectors. In the case of onchocerciasis, there are also no *Simulium* flies to become infected. With both diseases, filarial larvae enter the host during a bite by an infected insect.

The typical manifestations of lymphatic filariasis are low-grade fever and inflammation of lymphatics and lymph nodes, induced by the adult worms (usually in the inguinal or pelvic nodes). With repeated episodes, the lymphatics become occluded and fluids leak into tissues, producing severe swelling. After many years, the lower limbs and the scrotum may swell to gigantic size. The diurnal cycle observed in lymphatic filariasis facilitates transmission because the microfilariae are more prevalent in the bloodstream at night, when mosquitoes bite more frequently.

In contrast, the microfilariae of onchocerciasis and other skin-dwelling filariae invade the subcutaneous tissues, where they can be acquired by a biting fly. The adult *Onchocerca* worms congregate in a subcutaneous nodule and, like adult schistosomes, are invisible to the host immune system. Females released by the adult female worms are disseminated under the skin in all directions from a mature nodule. The pathology of the disease is caused by a type III hypersensitivity reaction to antigens released from dying microfilariae (Chapter 7, "Induced Defenses"). Thus, the clinical manifestations include chronic dermatitis and loss of eyesight (due to nodules on the head with migration of microfilariae into the anterior chamber of the eye).

Diagnosis and treatment

Infections that release microfilariae into the bloodstream (lymphatic filariasis) may be diagnosed by examining smears of peripheral blood. The microfilariae may be scarce and difficult to find. The sensitivity of the method can be increased by lysing red blood cells and concentrating the remainder of the specimen and by sampling blood at night for microfilariae with nocturnal periodicity (e.g., with *W. bancrofti*). Onchocerciasis is diagnosed by examining for microfilariae in a superficial "skin snip." In all of these specimens, microfilariae are identified with Giemsa stain under the high dry or oil immersion objectives. Recent studies suggest that antigen detection using antifilarial antibodies may be a more sensitive and convenient method.

The treatment for lymphatic filariasis is less than ideal. The drugs diethylcarbamazine and ivermectin reduce the number of circulating microfilariae but do not eliminate the adult worms. In any form of filariasis, diethylcarbamazine may produce systemic reactions, presumably due to the sudden release of filaria antigens from damaged microfilariae (as in the case presented above). In heavy infections with *Onchocerca*, diethylcarbamazine can cause severe reactions, including sudden blindness, vascular collapse, or even death. Ivermectin is less likely to produce these effects and is the preferred treatment for this form of disease. This drug has been used in preemptive mass treatment campaigns in parts of the world where there is significant morbidity and blindness. Surgical resection of subcutaneous nodules in onchocerciasis removes the source of microfilariae and may thus decrease the risk of blindness. However, it is impossible to be sure that all nodules have been removed because they are often in deep tissue and are not palpable.

Prevention of these diseases relies mainly on vector control. Unfortunately, the flies that transmit onchocerciasis breed in clean, fast-running streams and rivers. Although they can be controlled readily with insecticides, effective spraying may be difficult in these areas.

CONCLUSION

Tissue invasive helminthic infections are a diverse group of pathogens with distinct and complex life cycles. To diagnose and treat these infections, it is essential to know where the parasites reside within the human host and which tissues, body fluids, or excreta harbor the characteristic eggs or larvae. Antihelminthic drugs are active against these parasites; however, infections of long duration with high worm burdens can produce chronic, fibrotic changes that are irreversible with treatment. To control these infections in endemic regions, it is necessary to understand the parasitic life cycles and to know what environmental conditions, vectors, or intermediate hosts enable the parasites to deliver their progeny from one human to the next.

SUGGESTED READINGS

Carpio A, Santillan F, Leon P, Flores C, Hauser WA. Is the course of neurocysticercosis modified by treatment with antihelminthic agents? Arch Intern Med 1995;155:1982–1988.

Clausen MR, Meyer CN, Krantz T, Moser C, Gomme G, Kayser L, Albrectsen J, Kapel CM, Bygbjerg IC. Trichinella infection and clinical disease. Quarterly J Med 1996;89: 631–636.

Khuroo MS, Dar MY, Yattoo GN, Zargar SA, Javaid G, Khan BA, Boda MI. Percutaneous drainage versus albendazole therapy in hepatic hydatidosis: a prospective, randomized study. Gastroenterology 1993;104:1452–1459.

Ottesen EA. Immune responsiveness and the pathogenesis of human onchocerciasis. J Infect Dis 1995;171:659–671.

Ottesen EA. Filarial infections. Infect Dis Clin North Am 1993;7:619–633.

Public health impact of schistosomiasis: disease and mortality. WHO Expert Committee on the Control of Schistosomiasis. Bull WHO 1993;71:657–662.

Taylor MG. Schistosomiasis vaccines: farewell to the God of Plague? J Trop Med Hyg 1994;97:257–268.

White AC Jr. Neurocysticercosis: a major cause of neurological disease worldwide. Clin Infect Dis 1997;Feb 24(2): 101–113; quiz 114–115.

Addressing Emerging Infectious Diseases

JAMES M. HUGHES

INTRODUCTION

In 1969, the Surgeon General of the United States said optimistically: "It is time to close the book on infectious diseases." Considerable progress has indeed been made in eliminating some infectious diseases. The most dramatic example is the global eradication of **smallpox,** with the last case occurring in 1977. More recently, **polio** was eradicated from the Western Hemisphere, and substantial progress is being made toward its global elimination (Fig. 54.1). These achievements took years of effort that involved global leadership and a major commitment of human and financial resources. In the United States, substantial progress has been made in reducing the incidence of several preventable diseases with vaccines. The incidence of **measles** was at a record low level in 1995. Recent progress in reducing the incidence of Haemophilus influenzae type B invasive disease following the introduction of the conjugate vaccine is particularly impressive (Fig. 54.2).

These achievements illustrate the progress that can be made when the commitment exists and resources are mobilized. However, despite the impact of improvements in sanitation and the availability of antibiotics and vaccines, the Surgeon General's 1969 statement has not been realized. Infectious diseases remain the leading cause of death worldwide (Table 54.1) and an important cause of death in the United States (Tables 54.2 and 54.3). **Acquired immunodeficiency syndrome** (AIDS) is now the leading cause of death among persons 25 to 44 years of age in the United States.

EMERGING INFECTIOUS DISEASE CONCEPTS

In 1992, a National Academy of Science's Institute of Medicine (IOM) Committee issued a report entitled "Emerging Infections: Microbial Threats to Health in the United States." In this report, **emerging infections** were defined as those that have increased in incidence in the past 20 years or threaten to increase in the near future. The report documents the complacency concerning infectious diseases, describes the threats posed by microbial agents, identifies the factors that contribute to disease emergence and reemergence, and stresses the need to heighten vigilance and strengthen response capacity.

The report also cites a number of important examples of emerging infections, the most dramatic of which is the global epidemic of **human immunodeficiency virus** (HIV) infection resulting in AIDS, which was first recognized in New York and Los Angeles in 1981. More recent examples cited by the committee include the resurgence of measles in 1989–91, the resurgence of **tuberculosis** beginning in the late 1980s, and the emergence of **multidrug-resistant tuberculosis** in the early 1990s.

The IOM Committee report identifies six factors that contribute to the emergence of infections that are listed in Table 54.4 along with concrete examples of their impact. Most emerging infectious diseases are caused by existing pathogens that have been given a chance to grow and spread because of natural or induced changes in their environment. In some cases, specific infections have increased in frequency because an environmental change has made transmission more efficient. Certain other infections have flourished because of an increase in the population of susceptible hosts. In yet other situations, changes or manipulations of the microenvironment have permitted variants of existing agents to emerge selectively. A preeminent example is the upsurge of drug-resistant microorganisms, which is clearly attributable to the use and overuse of antimicrobials.

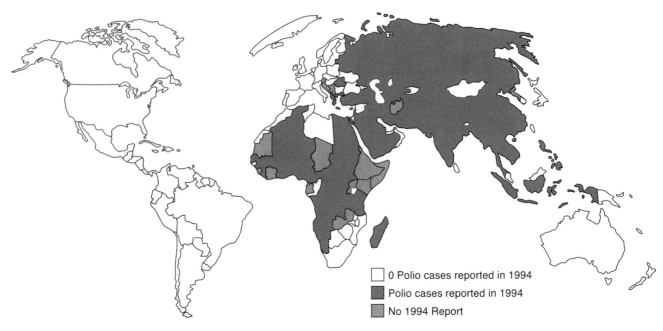

Figure 54.1. Global status of polio, 1994.

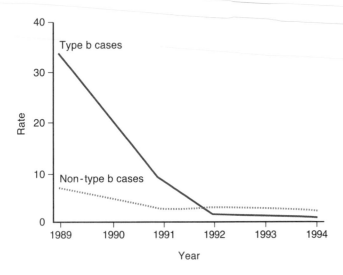

Figure 54.2. Race-adjusted incidence rate of *Haemophilus influenzae* type b and non-type b disease detected through laboratory-based surveillance among children <5 years, United States, 1989–1994.

Table 54.1. Leading Infectious Causes of Death Worldwide, 1993

Acute respiratory infection	4.1 million
Diarrhea	3.0 million
Tuberculosis	2.7 million
Malaria	2.0 million
Measles	1.2 million

Table 54.2. Actual Causes of Death in United States,[a] 1990

Cause	No. deaths	% of total
Tobacco	400,000	19
Diet/activity	300,000	14
Alcohol	100,000	5
Microbial agents	90,000	4
Toxic agents	60,000	3
Firearms	35,000	2
Sexual behavior	30,000	1
Motor vehicles	25,000	1
Illicit drug use	20,000	< 1
Total	1,060,000	50

[a] Composite approximation of external (nongenetic) factors leading to death, drawn from studies that use different approaches to derive estimates, ranging from actual counts (e.g., firearms) to population attributable risk calculations (e.g., tobacco).

EXAMPLES OF EMERGING INFECTIONS

Within a few months of publication of the IOM Report, clinicians, microbiologists, and public health officials in the United States were confronted with an interstate foodborne disease outbreak of **hemorrhagic colitis** and **hemolytic-uremic syndrome** caused by Escherichia coli 0157:H7, which was linked to undercooked hamburger served by a fast food restaurant chain. This organism was first recognized as a cause of disease only in 1982. A few months after this foodborne outbreak, the largest waterborne disease outbreak in U.S. history resulted in more than 400,000 cases of **cryptosporidiosis** in Milwaukee, Wisconsin. *Cryptosporidium parvum*, the organism responsible for this outbreak, was first recognized as a cause of human disease in 1976.

In May 1993, an outbreak of adult respiratory distress syndrome, now known as **hantavirus pulmonary syndrome** (HPS), was recognized in the southwestern U.S. Healthy young adults were primarily affected by this disease. Early signs and symptoms included fever accompanied by muscle aches. Sudden onset of interstitial pulmonary edema rapidly progressed to respiratory failure and, in most cases, death. In early June 1993, sero-

logic tests provided the first clue to a hantavirus etiology. Primers were designed for polymerase chain reaction (PCR) to amplify hantavirus-specific RNA from tissues. Subsequent studies implicated the deer mouse as the virus reservoir. Identification of hantaviral antigens in capillary endothelium of the lung using immunohistochemical techniques provided an important link to the pulmonary edema observed in patients. A previously unrecognized hantavirus was finally identified as a cause of HPS, which is totally different from illnesses caused by hantaviruses in other parts of the world. This identification permitted the development of prevention strategies that were implemented a few months before the virus was finally isolated in cell culture. Large parts of the genome of the new virus obtained from infected human tissues were cloned, the nucleotide sequence determined, and viral proteins expressed and used as diagnostic antigens in an improved serologic technique. This diagnostic technique plays a critical role in ongoing national surveillance of HPS (Figs. 54.3 and 54.4).

In the past 20 years, several "new" infectious agents have been identified (Table 54.5). In reality, the evolution of a truly new human pathogen is an uncommon event. HIV is such a pathogen, since it is believed to have evolved to cause human disease only in recent history. Most other newly described pathogens have actually been present in the human population for numerous past generations, but came to attention either because a large

---

Table 54.3. Leading Underlying Causes of Death in United States,[a] 1992

1. Heart diseases
2. Malignant neoplasms
3. Infectious diseases
4. Cerebrovascular diseases
5. Chronic obstructive pulmonary disease
6. Accidents

[a] "Underlying cause of death" is defined as the disease or injury that initiated the train of events leading directly to death.

Table 54.4. Factors Contributing to the Emergence of Infectious Diseases

Factor	Specific circumstances	Examples
Ecological/environmental changes	Reforestation leading to increased tick populations	Lyme disease
	Construction of dams	Schistosomiasis
	Weather anomalies	Hantavirus pulmonary syndrome
Human demographics and behavior	Sexual behavior and IV drug use	AIDS
	Urbanization and increased population density	Dengue and dengue hemorrhagic fever
International travel and trade	International shipping	Spread of cholera to South America
	Air transport of mosquitoes	"Airport" malaria in nonendemic countries
	Globalization of food supply	Numerous foodborne outbreak related to imported foods
Technology and industry	Mass food processing technology	Enterohemorrhagic *E. coli*
	Blood and tissue products for medical use (blood, serum)	Hepatitis B and C
	Feeding scrap meat to cattle	"Mad cow" disease
	Superabsorbent tampons	Toxic shock syndrome
Microbial adaptation	Overuse of antimicrobials	Antibiotic-resistant organisms
	Lack of cross-reactive immunity from prior infection	Emergence of new influenza strains
Breakdown in public health systems	Relaxation of public health services	Multidrug-resistant tuberculosis
	Inadequate water treatment	Spread of cholera in South America; *Cryptosporidium* outbreaks

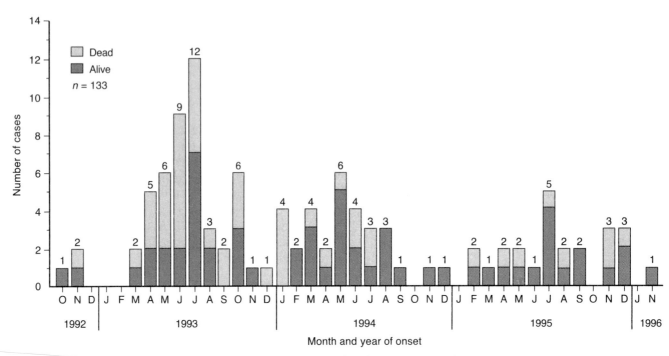

* Twenty-six additional cases (sixteen deceased) with onset before October 1992 not shown.

Figure 54.3. Hantavirus pulmonary syndrome cases by outcome, United States, as of April 17, 1996.

concentration of cases was identified (e.g., Legionnaires' disease, Lyme disease) or because advances in technology permitted the isolation and identification of the microbe (e.g., hantavirus).

EMERGING DRUG-RESISTANT INFECTIONS

The incidence of **nosocomial infections** caused by **vancomycin-resistant enterococci** has increased in hospitalized patients. Such drug resistance causes untreatable infections and raises concerns that genes mediating vancomycin resistance might be transferred to *Staphylococcus aureus*. Because surveillance of drug resistance in community-acquired infections in the United States has been limited to infections caused by *Mycobacterium tuberculosis*, *Neisseria gonorrhoeae*, and *Streptococcus pneumoniae*, new surveillance methods are needed to detect and control these emerging resistant pathogens. The frequency of high-level penicillin resistance in *Streptococcus pneumoniae* can be assessed by monitoring the sensitivity of pneumococcal isolates from normally sterile body sites, e.g., blood, cerebrospinal fluid. Sterile site isolates of pneumococcus from patients in 13 hospitals in 12 states increased more than 60-fold from 0.02% in 1987 to 1.3% in 1991 and to 3.1% in 1993. The frequency of high-level resistance is even greater in some geographic areas (e.g., 7.1% in metropolitan Atlanta in 1994). It is therefore important that clinicians have

available data on drug resistance for their own geographic area.

Combating drug resistance requires a coordinated effort among clinicians, microbiologists, and public health personnel. Programs to improve antimicrobial use must be implemented to help preserve the effectiveness of these valuable drugs as few new antimicrobial agents are being introduced. For example, not a single new drug for the treatment of bacterial infections was approved for use in the United States in 1994.

INTERNATIONAL PERSPECTIVE

Reminders of the challenges posed by infectious diseases are numerous in other parts of the world. Examples include the emergence of epidemic cholera in Latin America in 1991, the identification of a new epidemic strain of Vibrio cholerae (*V. cholerae* 0139) in India in 1992; and the recent introduction of the fourth serotype of **dengue virus** into the Western Hemisphere, which increases the risk for outbreaks of dengue hemorrhagic fever. Diseases emerging around the world have direct implications for clinicians, microbiologists, and public health officials in the United States.

ADDRESSING EMERGING INFECTIOUS DISEASES IN THE UNITED STATES

In 1994, the Centers for Disease Control and Prevention (CDC), in consultation with outside experts in clin-

Table 54.5. Selected Infectious Agents Identified Since 1975

Year	Etiologic agent	Disease	See chapter
1975	Parvovirus B19	Fifth disease	69
1976	*Cryptosporidium paroum*	Acute enterocolitis	51
1977	Ebola virus	Ebola hemorrhagic fever	54
1977	*Legionella pneumophila*	Legionnaires' disease	21
1981	Staphylococcal TSST-1	Toxic shock syndrome	11
1982	*E. coli* O157:H7	Enterohemorrhagic *E. coli*	17
1982	*Borrelia burgdorferi*	Lyme disease	25
1983	HIV	AIDS	38
1983	*Helicobacter pylori*	Peptic ulcer disease	22
1989	*Ehrlichia chaffeensis*	Human ehrlichiosis	28
1989	Hepatitis C	Non-A, non-B hepatitis	42
1992	*Vibrio cholerae* O139	Epidemic cholera	16
1992	*Bartonella henselae*	Cat scratch disease, bacillary angiomatosis	26
1993	Hantavirus isolates	Hantavirus pulmonary syndrome	54
1994	*Cyclospora cayetenensis*	Acute and chronic enteritis	51
1996	New variant Creutzfeld-Jacob disease agent	"Mad cow" disease	31

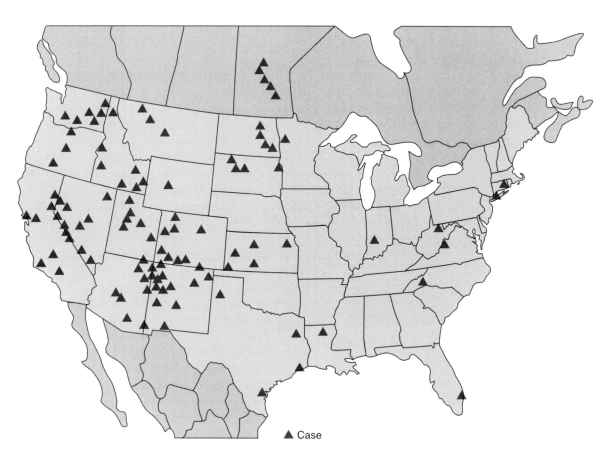

▲ Case

Figure 54.4. Location of Hantavirus cases, as of April 17, 1996.

ical infectious diseases, microbiology, and public health, developed a strategy for addressing emerging infectious diseases. The strategy contains four goals:

- strengthening surveillance and response capability
- addressing research priorities
- improving prevention and control strategies
- strengthening the public health infrastructure at the local, state, and federal levels.

Implementation of the CDC plan requires effective partnerships with other federal, state, and local public health agencies, clinicians, clinical microbiologists, academic institutions, industry, the World Health Organization (WHO), and other international organizations and agencies. CDC has begun implementing this strategy by establishing **Emerging Infections Programs** (EIPs) based in four state health departments, initiating publication of the journal *Emerging Infectious Diseases*, and organizing a laboratory training fellowship program in collaboration with State Public Health Laboratories.

Strengthening surveillance is critical to the successful implementation of this strategy. The use of uniform case definitions, including laboratory components, is essential. Also critical in an infectious disease surveillance system is the flow of information (Fig. 54.5). One of the approaches to strengthening surveillance and response capacity has involved establishment of EIPs in several states. These programs establish partnerships between state and local health departments, academic institutions, and health maintenance organizations. Each program is conducting two core projects that focus on invasive bacterial diseases and the etiology of unexplained deaths in persons between the ages of 1 and 49 years.

For example, under this program, Minnesota identified an outbreak caused by Salmonella serotype *enteriditis* in the fall of 1994 when the state laboratory noted an increase in the expected number of isolates submitted to the state public health laboratory. Prompt epidemiologic investigation identified the vehicle as a contaminated ice cream product produced in Minnesota and dis-

tributed to 48 states. The product was removed from distribution; follow-up investigation identified culture-confirmed cases in 41 states and approximately 250,000 cases of illness nationwide.

Oregon identified an increase in the incidence of **meningococcal disease** in the state between 1992 and 1994 associated with the emergence of a clone of group B meningococci (called ET-5), which has caused epidemic disease in other countries. Recently, cases have been identified in the adjacent state of Washington, raising concerns about epidemic disease.

ADDRESSING EMERGING INFECTIOUS DISEASES AROUND THE WORLD

Repeatedly, outbreaks of infectious diseases in different parts of the world illustrate the global implications of a local problem and provide evidence of the disruption of commerce and industry that such outbreaks can cause. For example, cases of illness associated with two contaminated, widely distributed foods have recently been detected and reported by state laboratories to the Centers for Disease Control (CDC). The first outbreak involved cases of *Salmonella* serotype agona infection associated with a contaminated infant snack food imported from Israel. The cases were identified in the United States following notification of an outbreak in England. The second outbreak involved cases of *Salmonella* serotype Stanley infection in a number of different states. Epidemiologic investigation implicated contaminated alfalfa sprouts from a single U.S. distributor. Cases were also identified in Canada and England.

Local diseases of especially high severity underscore the importance of surveillance, prompt epidemiologic investigation, and availability of adequate diagnostic laboratory capacity. The **Ebola virus** infection outbreak in Zaire in 1995 served as a reminder that only six "maximum containment laboratories" are operational in the world. Personnel from three of these six laboratories participated in the investigation. Other recent examples that have required international coordinated efforts are **plague** in India in the fall of 1994 and **leptospirosis** in Nicaragua in the fall of 1995.

Responding to such threats will require strengthened surveillance and the formation of multidisciplinary response teams at the local, national, and international levels with expertise in epidemiology, laboratory science, behavioral science, and disease control. The National Science and Technology Council recently established a working group on emerging infectious diseases. This working group, which includes members of 17 U.S. government agencies and organizations, considers ways in which these agencies could collaborate more effectively to address emerging infectious diseases domestically and to

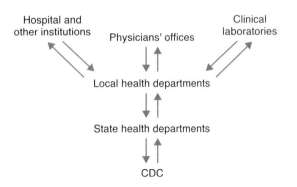

Figure 54.5. National surveillance of infectious diseases: the vision.

> **Table 54.6.** Emerging Infections United States, 1995

Salmonella Hartford, several states

Salmonella Stanley, several states

Human granulocytic ehrlichiosis, New York and Connecticut

Cyclospora cayetanensis, Florida

Malaria, Michigan

Dengue, Texas

Fluoroquinolone-resistant *Neisseria gonorrhoeae*, Colorado and Washington

> **Table 54.7.** Emerging Infections, International, 1995

Ebola hemorrhagic fever, Zaire

Dengue hemorrhagic fever, Western Hemisphere

Venezuelan equine encephalitis, Venezuela and Colombia

Cholera, Cape Verde Islands

Leptospirosis, Nicaragua

> **Table 54.8.** Global Population and Distribution Estimates, United Nations Population Fund Report, 1993

	1980	1990	2025
Industrialized nations	33%	23%	16%
Developing world	67%	77%	84%
Total population (billions)	2.5	5.3	8.5

support WHO efforts internationally. Recommendations focus on the need for (1) a global infectious disease surveillance and response system, (2) enhanced domestic infectious disease surveillance, (3) improved response capacity through collaboration with the private sector, (4) assistance to other countries to strengthen their national infectious disease surveillance systems, (5) enhanced authority of U.S. agencies to make the most effective use of their expertise in addressing emerging infections, and (6) establishment of an Interagency Task Force to facilitate implementation of the report's recommendations.

CONCLUSION

Infectious diseases are important, evolving, complex public health problems. Their prevention and control will increasingly require sophisticated epidemiologic, molecular, biologic, statistical, and behavioral approaches and technologies and the integration of epidemiologic and laboratory sciences.

Ensuring information exchange and technology transfer through intercountry networks is critical if future emerging infectious disease threats are to be recognized in time to implement cost-effective control measures. As the authors of the IOM Report noted, "Pathogenic microbes can be resistant, dangerous foes. Although it is impossible to predict their individual emergence in time and place, we can be confident that new microbial diseases will emerge."

While it is difficult to predict specific future challenges posed by infectious agents, the experience in the United States and globally in 1995 (Tables 54.6 and 54.7) indicates that we will continue to be confronted by national and international outbreaks, new syndromes caused by recognized microbial agents, and increasing problems posed by drug-resistant organisms. The likelihood of future challenges seems even higher when population projections are considered (Table 54.8). These statistics are particularly sobering when the potential impact of these diseases on the population of large urban areas, sometimes referred to as "megacities," in the developing world is considered.

SELF-ASSESSMENT QUESTIONS

1. Describe the factors involved in emergence of infectious diseases.
2. Identify and describe factors contributing to the recent emergence of hantavirus pulmonary syndrome.
3. Identify the leading infectious causes of death worldwide.
4. Identify two important antibiotic-resistant organisms and discuss strategies required to address threats posed by these organisms.
5. Describe some of the critical elements in identifying and responding to emerging infectious diseases domestically and internationally.

SUGGESTED READINGS

Berkelman RL, Bryan RT, Osterholm MT, et al. Infectious disease surveillance: a crumbling foundation. Science 1994; 264:368–370.

Berkelman RL, Hughes JM. The conquest of infectious diseases: who are we kidding? Ann Intern Med 1993;119:426–428.

Centers for Disease Control and Prevention. Addressing emerging infectious disease threats: a prevention strategy for the United States. Atlanta, Georgia: U.S. Department of Health and Human Services, Public Health Service, 1994.

Centers for Disease Control and Prevention. Progress toward elimination of *Haemophilus influenzae* type b disease among infants and children—United States, 1993–1994. MMWR 1995;44:545–550.

Cohen ML. Epidemiology of drug resistance: implications for a post-antimicrobial era. Science 1992;257:1050–1055.

Garrett L. The coming plague: newly emerging diseases in a world out of balance. New York: Farrar, Straus and Giroux, 1994.

Gubler DJ, Clark GG. Dengue/dengue hemorrhagic fever: the emergence of a global health problem. Emerg Inf Dis 1995; 1:55–57.

Lederberg J, Shope RE, Oaks SC. Emerging infections: microbial threats to health in the United States. Washington, DC: Institute of Medicine, National Academy Press, 1992.

Pinner RW, Teutsch SM, Simonsen L, et al. Trends in infectious diseases mortality in the United States. JAMA 1996; 272:189–193.

Robbins FC. Eradication of polio in the Americas. JAMA 1993;270:1857–1859.

Satcher D. Emerging infections: getting ahead of the curve. Emerg Inf Dis 1995;1:1–6.

Tauxe RV, Mintz ED, Quick RE. Epidemic cholera in the new world: translating field epidemiology into new prevention strategies. Emerg Inf Dis 1995;1:141–146.

Review of the Main Pathogenic Animal Parasites

These charts are intended to help you review the main animal parasites only. Included are the parasites of greatest medical relevance.

Many of the animal parasites that cause relatively uncommon diseases are not included. These charts may be completed to review material covered under this topic.

PROTOZOA

	Reservoir	Mode of Transmission	Location in Body	Disease and Main Attributes	Relevant Chapters
Blood					50, 63
Malaria (*Plasmodium vivax, malariae, falciparum*)					50
Babesia					50
Deep tissue					50, 63
Toxoplasma					60, 69
Pneumocystis					50, 67
Leishmania					50
Trypanosomes (Sleeping sickness and Chagas' disease)					50
Intestinal					51
Entamoeba histolytica					51
Giardia lamblia					51
Cryptosporidium					51
Cyclospora					51

HELMINTHS (WORMS)
(Try to *recognize* Latin names. You need not memorize them.)

	Reservoir	Mode of Transmission	Location in Body	Disease and Main Attributes	Relevant Chapters
Intestinal					51
Tapeworms (*Taenia*, several)					52
Hookworms (*Ancylostoma*, *Necator*)					52
Ascaris (*A. lumbricoides*) (+ visceral larva migrans)					52
Pinworms (*Enterobius vermicularis*)					52
Whipworms (*Trichuris, trichiura*)					52
Blood and deep tissue					50, 63
Cysticercus (*Taenia solium*) and Echinococcus					53
Trichina (*Trichinella spiralis*)					53
Schistosomes (*S. haematobium*, *S. mansoni*, *S. japonicum*)					53
Filaria (*Wuchereria*, *Brugia*, *Onchocerca*)					53

Pathophysiology of Infectious Diseases

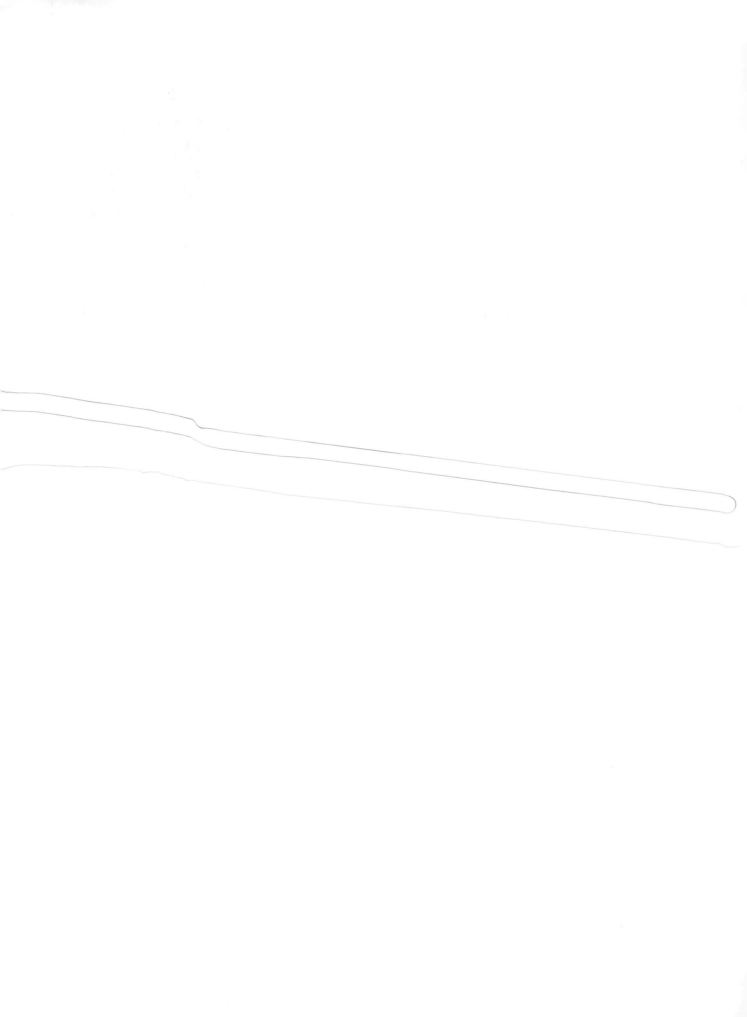

CHAPTER 55

Diagnostic Principles

N. CARY ENGLEBERG

The role of the clinical microbiology laboratory is to determine whether potential pathogens are present in tissues, body fluids, or secretions of patients, and if present, to identify them. This service is indispensable to the modern clinician, since information about the pathogen's identity is of critical importance in predicting the course of the infection and in guiding the selection of appropriate therapy. This information can be generated in four ways:

- Microscopic examination of patient samples
- Cultivation and identification of microorganisms from patient samples
- Measurement of a pathogen-specific immune response in the patient
- Detection of pathogen-specific macromolecules in patient samples

The extent and reliability of the information that the laboratory can provide varies depending on the nature of the pathogen. Some pathogens (e.g., *Staphylococcus aureus*) are easily detected, cultivated, identified and characterized; others (e.g., *Toxoplasma gondii*) require extraordinary measures merely to establish their presence. However, thanks to the technological advances in molecular biology, the capabilities of the modern clinical microbiology laboratory are expanding and improving rapidly. New diagnostic procedures are being introduced into clinical practice at an ever-increasing pace. Clinicians need to understand the principles underlying both the new and old methods to make an informed and critical assessment of their value and reliability and to use them wisely.

ASSESSING THE PERFORMANCE OF LABORATORY TESTS

No laboratory test is perfect. Therefore, to interpret the results of tests, clinicians must have a sense of how reliable they are. When a microbiologic test correctly predicts the presence of a pathogen, the result is referred to as a **true-positive**. Similarly, a negative test obtained in the absence of the pathogen is a **true-negative**. Inac-

curacies occur either because the laboratory test is negative in the presence of the pathogen (**false-negative**) or positive in the absence of the pathogen (**false-positives**).

The terms sensitivity and specificity defined in Fig. 55.1 are commonly used to describe the performance and value of all diagnostic tests. The **sensitivity** of the test is the likelihood that it will be positive when the pathogen is present. The **specificity** of the test measures the likelihood that it will be negative if the pathogen is not present.

In clinical practice, diagnostic tests with 100% sensitivity and 100% specificity do not exist. If available, a combination of tests may often yield a higher level of diagnostic certainty. In addition, clinicians may make use of less than perfect tests to advantage. Thus, a test that is very sensitive but not particularly specific may be useful in screening for the presence of an infection. For example, the so-called RPR (rapid plasma reagin) or VDRL (Venereal Diseases Reference Laboratory) tests are commonly used to screen patients for syphilis, even though several other infectious and noninfectious conditions can cause these tests to be falsely positive. However, nearly all patients who have syphilis have positive RPR or VDRL tests after the primary (chancre) stage. Therefore, the test has few false-negatives and is useful to "rule out" the diagnosis of syphilis. If the RPR or VDRL is positive, then a second, confirmatory test must be employed in order to determine whether syphilis is actually present. In contrast to a screening test, a confirmatory test used to "rule in" a suspected diagnosis must be highly specific. Take as an example a patient found to have a positive enzyme-linked immunosorbent assay (ELISA) screening test for human immunodeficiency virus (HIV) after a blood donation. A more specific (and costly) confirmatory test, the Western blot assay, is used to determine whether the patient actually has HIV infection or whether the screening test result was falsely positive.

The predictive value of a diagnostic test is influenced by the frequency of the infection in the population being tested. Because the specificity of the HIV-ELISA is 99.8%, it will register a false-positive in one of every

Test results

	Positive	Negative
Organism present	true-positives	false-negatives
Organism absent	false-positives	true-negatives

$$\text{Sensitivity} = \frac{\text{true-positives}}{\text{true-positives} + \text{false-negatives}} \times 100\%$$

$$\text{Specificity} = \frac{\text{true-negatives}}{\text{true-negatives} + \text{false-positives}} \times 100\%$$

Figure 55.1. Definitions of terms used in evaluating diagnostic tests.

500 negative individuals tested. If less than one person in 500 in a given population is infected with HIV, then there will be more false-positive tests than true-positive tests, and the positive predictive value will be poor. For example, HIV infection is extremely rare among elderly women with no apparent risk factors, and a positive result in such a patient is most likely to be a false-positive. In contrast, in populations with a high prevalence of HIV infection, e.g., among intravenous drug users, there will be a higher proportion of true-positive tests. The lesson is this: the interpretation of a laboratory result depends not only on the technical accuracy of the method used but also on the prevalence of the infection in the population to which the patient belongs.

DIAGNOSIS OF INFECTIONS BY MICROSCOPY

Because they possess characteristic morphologic features, staining properties, or movement, some pathogens can be accurately identified by direct microscopic examination of clinical material. For certain infections, microscopic diagnosis is highly sensitive and specific. It is also a rapid technique that permits the physician to initiate treatment without waiting for the results of a culture.

Nearly all helminthic and most protozoal infections are routinely diagnosed by microscopy. Many fungal pathogens also have characteristic morphologic features. Notably, *Cryptococcus neoformans* meningitis is diagnosed most rapidly by finding encapsulated yeast in the spinal fluid. By staining the fluid background with India ink, the transparent capsule of the yeast is visualized (Fig. 55.2). In contrast, the morphology of most bacteria is too simple to permit microscopic identification; however, few exceptions exist. Syphilis can easily

be diagnosed by observing the characteristic helical form and bending motions of spirochetes in fresh scrapings of primary or secondary lesions. Although viruses cannot be seen in the light microscope, virus-induced changes in host cell morphology may be diagnostic. Examples include the multinucleated giant cells in scrapings from herpes simplex or varicella-zoster virus lesions (the "Tzanck smear") and the specific intracellular inclusion bodies in tissues that are actively infected with cytomegalovirus.

Stains

Although a species identification is rarely possible, bacterial pathogens may be visualized and assigned to morphologic and functional groups using special stains. The basic principles of the **Gram stain** and the **acid-fast stains** were described in Chapter 3, "Biology of Infectious Agents." The Gram stain is both rapid and simple to perform and can be carried out on virtually any body fluid or tissue sample. It may yield clinically useful information of three kinds.

- The presence of bacteria in a normally sterile body fluid (e.g., cerebrospinal fluid [CSF], pleural fluid, urine).

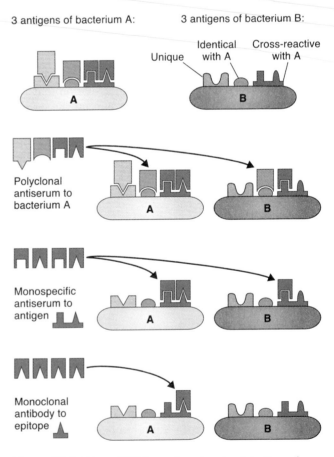

Figure 55.2. Direct ELISA serology for the detection of specific antibodies in patient serum.

- Staining properties and morphology of the organisms in a sample or culture that can direct further efforts at species identification and the empirical selection of antibiotics for the patient.
- For certain clinical specimens, a diagnosis. For example, the presence of Gram-negative diplococci inside the leukocytes of urethral pus is highly specific for gonococci. The same morphologic type seen in samples of CSF is nearly always the meningococcus.

The Gram stain is much less useful when samples are obtained from nonsterile body sites, owing to the presence of normal flora. Considerable experience and skill are required to interpret Gram stains of coughed sputum specimens, since they are typically contaminated with oropharyngeal bacteria which are indistinguishable from respiratory pathogens. In contrast, acid-fast bacteria (i.e., mycobacteria) are not normally found in the respiratory tract, and seeing them in a coughed sputum suggests pulmonary tuberculosis. In general, acid-fast bacteria in smears of sputum or normally sterile tissues are assumed to be tubercle bacilli until proven otherwise.

A variety of other stains are used to visualize pathogens. Among the most commonly used stains are the **Giemsa stain** for systemic protozoal infections (e.g., malaria), iodine stains for intestinal helminths, and silver stains for systemic fungal pathogens. Special stains may be used to visualize the characteristic cysts of *Pneumocystis carinii* in a sample of bronchial fluid from an AIDS patient.

Antibody-based Identification

The accuracy of microscopic identification of bacterial and viral pathogens is enhanced when **specific antibodies** are used in conjunction with direct microscopy. A classic example is the identification of pneumococci by the addition of anticapsular antiserum to a wet preparation of bacteria. Visible swelling of the capsule in the presence of antiserum identifies the organism as the pneumococcus and establishes its serotype. Modern approaches to antibody-directed diagnosis involve the attachment (or conjugation) of a detectable substance to the antibody molecules so that the microscopist can actually see where the antibodies bind. For example, in the **direct fluorescent antibody (DFA) test** for *P. carinii*, a monoclonal antibody has been conjugated to a fluorescent compound. To diagnose the infection, a deep respiratory specimen is fixed to a slide and then treated with the conjugated antibodies. After washing, the slide is examined using a **fluorescence microscope.** *P. carinii* cysts appear as bright yellow-green, glowing spheres when illuminated with ultraviolet light. Since the organisms are so distinct against the dark background, they are easy to pick out when scanning the slide. The DFA technique can be used to identify any pathogen to which specific antibodies can be produced.

Clearly, the specificity of antibody-based identification of pathogens depends on the specificity of the antibodies used. Most antisera are polyclonal mixtures of antibodies that bind to different domains of a variety of different antigenic molecules (Fig. 55.3). When polyclonal antiserum is used in a diagnostic test, therefore, there is a high likelihood of unwanted cross-reactions with other microorganisms. The specificity of the test may be enhanced with the use of monoclonal (monospecific) antibodies, as suggested in Figure 55.3. The principles illustrated in this figure apply to all antibody-based methods of diagnosis,

Agglutination

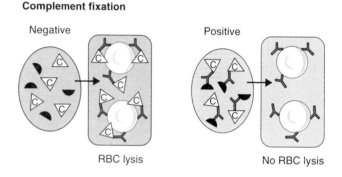

Complement fixation

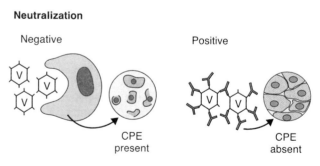

Neutralization

Figure 55.3. The cross-reactivity of three types of immunoglobulin preparations. Antibodies raised to react with bacterium A may cross-react with bacterium B. Polyclonal antisera are cross-reactive because bacteria A and B have protein antigens in common. Additionally, in this case, monospecific antiserum raised against a single antigen of bacterium A is also cross-reactive, because one of the antibody binding sites (epitopes) on this antigen is shared by an antigen of bacterium B. However, a monoclonal antibody against an epitope on this antigen was found to be unique to bacterium A and to have no cross-reactivity.

including the serologic antigen detection tests described in the next few sections of this chapter.

DIAGNOSIS OF INFECTIONS BY CULTURE

Culturing is usually the most specific way to establish the presence of a particular pathogen in a patient sample. However, in many situations, culturing may not be sensitive or clinically practical. Culture is routine for most bacterial and fungal infections but is virtually never performed for helminthic and protozoal pathogens. Some microorganisms cannot be cultured at all in clinical microbiology laboratories (e.g., hepatitis viruses, *Treponema pallidum, Mycobacterium leprae, Pneumocystis carinii*), either because the necessary conditions for their cultivation in vitro are not yet known or because the available culture systems are inefficient and impractical. Since chlamydiae and viruses are obligate intracellular pathogens, they can be propagated and identified only in appropriate cell cultures. Cultivation of some other pathogens, such as rickettsiae, is shunned by most clinical laboratories because of the hazards involved in handling these microorganisms.

General Principles

In general, the choice of culture methods and media is tailored to the nature and source of the specimen and the question that the culture is meant to address. For example, when a specimen of pus from a brain abscess is cultured, the implied question is: What microorganism(s) is (are) present in the abscess? The assumption is that any organisms present are causative and that chemotherapy directed against them will be beneficial. To look for the etiologic agents, the sample is cultured on a variety of agar-based media and in broth medium under both aerobic and anaerobic conditions. In this situation, the culture strategy is to recover any and all microorganisms that might inhabit such an abscess.

In contrast to this open-ended approach, other cultures are performed primarily to determine whether a particular pathogen is present or not. An example is the throat culture for *Streptococcus pyogenes* in cases of exudative pharyngitis, since this is the only culturable bacterial agent for which treatment is indicated. Throat swab specimens are inoculated only onto nutrient sheep's blood agar plates, which not only support the growth of streptococci but also show the characteristic β-hemolysis of *S. pyogenes*.

Cultures from nonsterile body sites present yet another problem, namely the inhibition or obscuring of the pathogen's growth by an abundant normal flora. For this reason, **selective media** are needed. An example of a selective medium is that used to culture gonococci, the so-called Thayer-Martin medium or chocolate agar (made with boiled blood, not chocolate) containing antibiotics that inhibit the growth of members of the normal flora in the genitourinary tract but not gonococci. Selective and semiselective media are also used to cultivate enteric pathogens from the bacteria-rich stool specimens or respiratory pathogens from sputum. One disadvantage of selective media is that they may inhibit the growth of some strains of the pathogen of interest. Therefore, selective media should be used only for specimens that are likely to contain contaminating normal organisms.

As with all diagnostic methods, culture results require interpretation by the physician. In some situations (e.g., meningitis, urinary tract infection), a negative culture is quite reassuring that the etiology of the patient's problem is not a bacterial or fungal infection. In other situations, the sensitivity of culture diagnosis is relatively poor. For example, a negative culture for pneumococci does not rule out this agent as the cause of a bacterial pneumonia, since the sensitivity of sputum culture for this fastidious pathogen may be 50% or lower in some clinical settings.

When cultures are positive, one must always question whether the isolate is the actual cause of the patient's illness. In cultures from nonsterile body sites, the problem is whether the isolate represents normal flora (colonization) or an etiologic agent (infection). In cultures from normally sterile body sites, contamination may occur when patient samples are obtained using faulty sterile technique. Typically, specimens obtained by needle puncture are contaminated with normal skin flora (e.g., *Staphylococcus epidermidis*, diphtheroids, streptococci). Since these bacteria may occasionally cause true infections, the physician must consider the clinical circumstances of the individual patient to judge whether the isolate is a contaminant. In many cases, it is necessary to reisolate the same organism by repeated cultures to be convinced of its significance. As another example, almost all voided urine collections have some degree of contamination; true infection is associated with a relatively high concentration of bacteria in the specimen. But a urine sample that sits for hours will soon be grossly contaminated as the microorganisms in the specimen start growing.

Blood Culture

The simplest blood culture involves the direct inoculation of a blood sample into nutrient broth, followed by incubation at 37°C and periodic checks for turbidity as an indicator of microbial growth. Microorganisms from broth cultures are eventually transferred to agar plates, or **subcultured**, to permit species identification. In recent years, newer methods have gained popularity for their increased sensitivity and rapidity. In one method, the **lysis–centrifugation technique**, blood is collected directly into a tube containing a solution that lyses blood cells. The remaining dense material, which includes any microorganism, is pelleted by centrifugation to the bottom of the tube, where it is removed and inoculated directly onto an appropriate agar-based media. In addition to its increased sensitivity for some pathogens, this technique has the advantage of bypassing the usual subculture step, since the isolates grow directly as colonies on agar plates. Blood cultures can also be automated by periodically assaying for a byproduct of microbial growth (e.g., CO_2). Using such sensitive techniques, growth of organisms can be detected long before visible growth develops.

Culture Identification

Classically, bacteria cultured from clinical specimens are identified by determining **phenotypic properties**, such as motility, utilization of various nutrient substrates, production of enzymes, toxins or byproducts of metabolism. Since regrowth is required for many of these tests, definitive identification typically requires an extra day or more.

Microorganisms in culture are sometimes identified more rapidly using **antibody-based techniques** that are discussed in more detail in the next section. Viruses are frequently identified in culture by their reaction with specific antiviral antibodies or by the ability of a specific antiserum to neutralize them when inoculated into fresh tissue culture. Another recent development in culture identification involves the use of nucleic acid probes, as discussed in the final section of this chapter.

Antimicrobial Sensitivity Testing

Perhaps the most important advantage of culturing is that the isolate can be tested for susceptibility to antimicrobial agents, often the most important piece of therapeutically related information to be obtained. A discussion of antibiotic sensitivity testing of bacteria is found in Chapter 30, "Strategies to Combat Bacterial Infections." Fungal and viral pathogens can also be tested for drug susceptibility, but these tests are beyond the scope of most clinical microbiology laboratories.

MEASUREMENT OF THE ANTIBODY RESPONSE TO INFECTION

Serologic tests measure the patient's humoral immune response to an infection. Since human serum contains many different antibodies, these tests are designed to measure only those that are directed at specific microbial antigens. Older serologic methods measure these specific antibodies by detecting their activity in the presence of antigen. For example, the addition of patient serum to a sample of killed organisms may result in visible **agglutination** (clumping), if agglutinating antibodies are present. In more specific agglutination tests, purified microbial antigens are used to coat inert particles, such as latex beads (**latex agglutination**) or red blood cells (**hemagglutination**). The **complement fixation test** measures the depletion ("fixation") of a limited amount of serum complement by the patient's antibodies when the cascade is triggered by adding antigen, and **neutralizing antibody tests** measure the capacity of serum to inhibit growth in culture (Fig. 55.4). Neutralization assays are rarely used clinically, but are used frequently in research

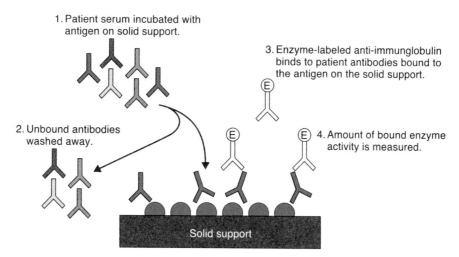

1. Patient serum incubated with antigen on solid support.

2. Unbound antibodies washed away.

3. Enzyme-labeled anti-immunglobulin binds to patient antibodies bound to the antigen on the solid support.

4. Amount of bound enzyme activity is measured.

Solid support

Figure 55.4. Functional methods for detection of specific antibodies. Agglutination: When specific antibodies (*Y-shaped structures*) are present in the patient's serum, they bind to the particle coated with microbial antigen (*black semicircles*). The bivalent antibody forms bridges between particles and causes visible clumping. When there is much more antibody than antigen in the mixture, a false-negative, or **prozone** phenomenon, may occur. Paradoxically, a serum sample that is negative because of a prozone, becomes positive when it is diluted. **Complement fixation:** Patient serum is incubated with antigen and complement (the numerous individual complement components are contained in each *triangle*). Sheep red blood cells (RBCs) coated with anti-RBC antibodies (*gray Y-shaped struc-*

tures) are then added. If specific antibodies are absent in the serum, complement is free to be "fixed" by the anti-RBC antibodies, and the RBCs are lysed by the complement attack complex. If specific antibodies are present in the serum, they will have bound to antigen during the first incubation step and fixed all available complement, so that none is available to lyse antibody-coated RBCs in the second step. **Neutralization:** In the absence of specific neutralizing antibody, virus added to tissue culture results in infection and cytopathic effect (CPE). When specific antibodies are present, they block viral structures critical for binding and uptake into host cells; no infection or CPE is observed.

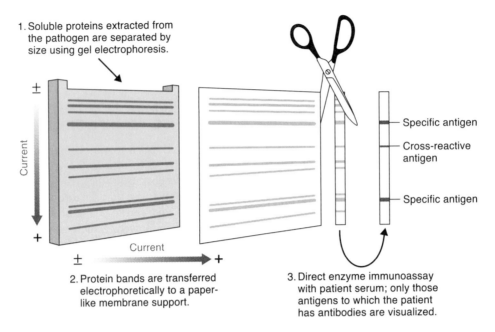

1. Soluble proteins extracted from the pathogen are separated by size using gel electrophoresis.

Current

Current

± +

2. Protein bands are transferred electrophoretically to a paper-like membrane support.

Specific antigen

Cross-reactive antigen

Specific antigen

3. Direct enzyme immunoassay with patient serum; only those antigens to which the patient has antibodies are visualized.

Figure 55.5. Western blot. By noting the antigens ("bands") with which the patient serum reacts, it is possible to determine whether the reactivity is due to specific or cross-reactive antibodies.

to assess protective immunity to viral infections. In all of these tests, the amount of specific antibody present in the patient's serum is quantified by testing dilutions of the serum. The highest dilution of the patient's serum that still can exert the measured function, or **endpoint** (i.e., agglutination, complement fixation, or neutralization) is the positive **titer** for that assay.

Later generations of serologic tests do not measure the activity of specific antibody, but measure their presence directly. Most of these tests are **solid-phase assays**, that is, they use either the pathogen or antigens from the pathogen fixed to a solid support, such as the wells of a multititer plate or inert beads (Fig. 55.2). In these assays, patient serum is added to this system, and specific antibodies are bound and immobilized to the fixed antigen. All nonreacting antibodies and serum components are washed away. The presence of the bound specific antibody is typically detected by adding a labeled antibody directed against human immunoglobulin molecules (raised in animals by immunization with human antibodies). A popular format for these tests is the **ELISA**. In ELISAs, the "second antibody" is conjugated to an enzyme, such as peroxidase or alkaline phosphatase, that catalyzes the production of visibly colored compounds from colorless precursors and makes the detection far more sensitive. A microscopic method, the **indirect fluorescent antibody (IFA) test,** uses a second antibody labeled with fluorescein, and the fixed antigen is usually an intact microorganism. In a positive test, the fixed microorganisms glow when illuminated with ultraviolet light. In both of these direct assays, the anti-immunoglobulin may also be made specific for IgG or IgM; these tests recognize only antibodies of a certain class.

The specificity of a serologic test is determined largely by the antigen used to capture the antibody in the direct test formats. An **immunoblot** (or **"Western blot"**) is one of the most specific serologic methods available. In this test, the antigenic molecules from a pathogen are first separated according to their size using electrophoresis. The whole series of antigens is then "blotted" onto a solid support and incubated with the patient's serum (Fig. 55.5). It is then possible to determine whether the patient's antibodies are directed against pathogen-specific or cross-reactive antigens. This additional level of analysis allows the discrimination of specific and nonspecific reactions. Western blotting has become a mainstay for confirming the diagnosis of HIV infection by ELISAs (Fig. 55.6).

Serological tests for particular infectious diseases may be both sensitive and specific, but their utility in clinical management is often limited. Since these tests depend upon the immune response to infection, they have limited use in the early diagnosis of acute infections, before the patient develops specific antibodies. Serology is typically more useful in determining whether infection with a particular pathogen has occurred in the past. The physician must decide whether the positive serology is due to the patient's current illness or to an infection that took place months or years earlier. There are two ways to make this determination. One way is to measure the patient's specific antibody titer at two points in time, usually several weeks apart (**acute and convalescent titers**). A significant increase in the amount of antibody indicates a recent or ongoing infection with the pathogen. Another way to diagnose a recent infection serologically is to measure specific **IgM antibodies** against the pathogen. In the course of most infections, these antibodies appear first and tend to disappear a few weeks or months after onset.

DIAGNOSIS OF INFECTION BY DETECTING MICROBIAL MACROMOLECULES

In the investigation of a crime, a detective may look for traces left by the perpetrator. Similarly, the microbial culprit associated with an infection can often be identified by recognizing its products or parts, provided that these "parts" are as specific for the pathogen as fingerprints are for an individual criminal. In microbiology, these identifications are made either by detecting an antigen(s) or a nucleic acid sequence that is specific for a particular pathogen. As you know from recent, celebrated criminal cases, prosecutors may also use these laboratory methods when traces of blood or body fluids are the available clues.

Macromolecular detection tests have inherent disadvantages and advantages compared to standard culture diagnosis. Among the disadvantages are the imperfect specificity, the inability to further study the infecting pathogen (e.g., for antimicrobial sensitivity, strain typing), and the need to perform separate tests for each suspected pathogen. Advantages include the capacity to diagnose the infection within hours rather than days and greater sensitivity in certain settings (e.g., the detection of a pathogen after treatment with antimicrobials has rendered the culture negative).

Detection of Microbial Antigens

Antigen detection tests are like serologic tests in reverse; instead of using the microbial antigen to capture antibodies from patient serum, specific antibodies are used to capture microbial antigens from a patient sample. In most of these assays, the "capture" antibody is bound to a solid support. Certain antigens, such as capsular polysaccharides, can be detected by a simple agglutination assay (Fig. 55.6). Several widely performed tests use antibody-coated latex beads (latex agglutination tests) to detect capsular material from meningococcus, pneumococcus, *Haemophilus influenzae, Cryptococcus neoformans,* and others. These tests may be performed as a panel on cerebrospinal fluid samples to make an early diagnosis of meningitis.

For many antigens, the presence of the "captured" molecule is detected using a second antibody (e.g., in the "sandwich ELISA"; Fig. 55.7), analogous to what is done for antibody detection. In this test, the sample is incubated with an antibody-coated solid support, and the unbound material in the sample is washed away. An enzyme-labeled second antibody, which is also directed against the microbial antigen, is then added forming a "sandwich" of the antigen between two layers of anti-

body. This basic format has been used to develop simple tests for several pathogens (e.g., *Chlamydia,* gonococcus, rotavirus) that can be used in office practice.

Another common antigen detection format is the radioimmunoassay (RIA) (see Fig. 55.7). This test is a competitive assay in which measured amounts of radio-labeled antigen specifically compete with antigen in the sample for binding to a fixed amount of specific antibody. These tests are particularly sensitive and are used not only in microbiological diagnosis but to detect hormones and other important molecules as well.

Nucleic Acid–Based Diagnosis of Infection

DNA is composed of two separate strands held together by hydrogen bonding between complementary bases. Because they are bound by relatively weak hydrogen bonds, the two strands of DNA can be separated into single strands by heating. When the temperature is once again lowered, the complementary strands will reconnect (or hybridize), reforming double-stranded DNA. Hybridization will occur only when the two strands are a genuine complementary pair. A short, single-stranded DNA sequence (or probe) can be chosen so that it will hybridize *only* to a perfectly complementary "target" sequence. The precision of this interaction accounts for the high degree of specificity of these tests.

It is always possible to find unique probes from among the sequences that encode structures or functions specific to a particular group of organisms. A commonly used target sequence for probe tests is ribosomal RNA (rRNA) or the genes that encode rRNA (rDNA). These

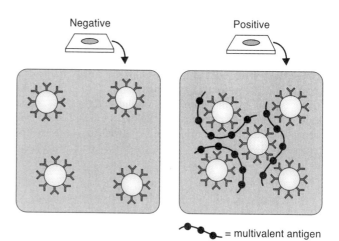

Figure 55.6. Detection of a polyvalent antigen by particle agglutination. Particles are coated with specific antibodies. If a multivalent antigen is present in the patient sample, bridges form between the particles, causing clumping. As with antibody detection by agglutination, false-negative prozones may occur if there is an overabundance of antigen (see Fig. 55.4). In these cases, dilution of sample will give a positive reaction.

A. ELISA for antigen detection
(direct "sandwich" assay)

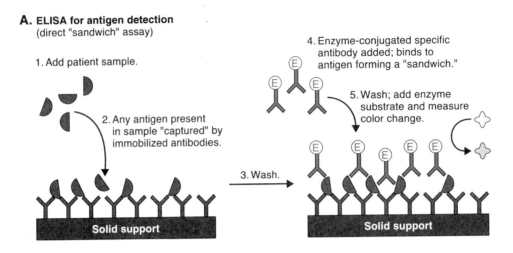

1. Add patient sample.

2. Any antigen present in sample "captured" by immobilized antibodies.

3. Wash.

4. Enzyme-conjugated specific antibody added; binds to antigen forming a "sandwich."

5. Wash; add enzyme substrate and measure color change.

Solid support

B. Radioimmunoassay for antigen detection
(competition assay)

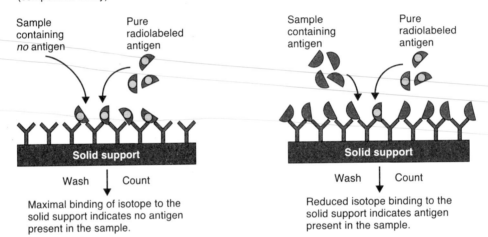

Sample containing *no* antigen

Pure radiolabeled antigen

Sample containing antigen

Pure radiolabeled antigen

Solid support

Wash   Count

Maximal binding of isotope to the solid support indicates no antigen present in the sample.

Solid support

Wash   Count

Reduced isotope binding to the solid support indicates antigen present in the sample.

Figure 55.7. Detection of a microbial antigen by "sandwich" ELISA and radioimmunoassay (RIA). ELISA: A "capture antibody" bound to a solid support binds antigen from the patient sample. Nonspecific contents of the sample are washed away. The presence of the captured antigen is detected using a second, specific antibody conjugated to an enzyme. Lastly, the activity of the enzyme bound to the solid support is measured using a color-producing substrate; color production signals the presence of the antigen which is "sandwiched" between the two antibodies. **RIA:** The patient sample is combined with a measured, small amount of purified, radiolabeled antigen in the presence of a specific antibody. If the patient sample contains no antigen, then all of the labeled antigen will complex with the antibody, and all of the radioactivity will be bound in immune complexes. If the patient sample contains antigen, it will compete with the labeled antigen for binding to the available antibody, and there will be less radioactivity associated with immune complexes. RIAs may be done in solution (with immune complexes precipitated and counted) or as solid-phase assays (with specific antibody bound to a solid support).

sequences are used by taxonomists to classify microorganisms, since organisms that are closely related phylogenetically tend to have similar rRNA sequences. This property makes rRNA a convenient source of probe sequences to detect individual species. In addition, the presence of many copies of rRNA in microorganisms (one for every one of the cell's ribosomes) increases the sensitivity of any assay using this molecule as a target.

Diagnostic nucleic acid probe tests have a similar basis, although the format may differ (see Fig. 55.7). Single-stranded probe DNA are labeled with a radioisotope, an enzyme, or other detectable labels. The patient's sample is treated so that microorganisms are disrupted and DNA and RNA are released and then heat denatured (i.e., converted to single strands). The mixture of labeled probe and sample is incubated and the amount of probe hybridized to nucleic acids measured. Bound and unbound probe are distinguished, which is commonly done by using probes attached to a solid support, just like in the separation steps in antibody and antigen detection tests. On the microscopic level, **in situ hybridization** may be performed on tissue sections (Fig. 55.8).

Most nucleic acid hybridization tests are very sensitive, but patient samples must contain at least several thousand organisms to elicit a positive probe test, as compared to only a few for a positive culture. Therefore, direct diagnosis by these techniques is most suited for infections with pathogens that are difficult to grow in culture or identify by other means, such as viral infections (e.g., HIV, herpesviruses) or sexually transmitted diseases (e.g., chlamydiae, gonococci).

Some nucleic acid probe tests, although not sufficiently sensitive for testing clinical samples directly, may be useful for rapid identification of pathogens that have been cultured. For example, some viruses can be detected in tissue culture using DNA probes well before any cytopathic effects are noticed by microscopy. (DFA and other antigen detection techniques may also be used for this purpose.) Cultures of mycobacteria require 4–6 weeks of incubation before colonies are visible, and then several more days for species identification. Early testing by incubating cultures with DNA probes for *Mycobacterium tuberculosis* or *M. avium-intracellulare* significantly hastens correct diagnosis and treatment.

Nucleic Acid Amplification

In many instances, the amount of specific nucleic acid in a sample is insufficient for direct detection. In such cases, it may be possible to use **nucleic acid amplification methods**, such as the **polymerase chain reaction (PCR)**. To design a PCR test, a specific sequence of microbial nucleic acid must be known. Two short DNA probes (**"primers"** or **"amplimers"**) are then chemically synthesized so that they will hybridize to the opposite strands of the target DNA sequence at a given distance (Fig. 55.9). In the assay, three components are added to DNA extracted from the patient's specimen: the primers, deoxyribonucleotides (deoxynucleotide triphosphates [dNTPs]), and a heat-stable DNA polymerase. The reactants are subjected to repeated cycles of temperature shifts which result in denaturation of DNA (heating), hybridization of the primers, and DNA synthesis (cooling). In each cycle of the reaction, the DNA spanned by the two primers is duplicated. With the synthesis of each new strand of DNA, new primer-binding sites are generated. Consequently, each new strand also becomes a new template for subsequent rounds of primer-initiated synthesis. With every cycle, the number of copies of the DNA segment between the primers doubles, thus doubling the templates for further synthesis. This "chain reaction" results in the geometric increase in the amounts of target DNA. In this respect, PCR is analogous to the biological process of DNA replication that occurs in

populations of dividing cells; however, in PCR, the exponential synthesis is limited to the DNA segment bounded by the two synthetic primers.

Once the reaction is carried out, the amplified sequences (or **"amplicons"**) are detected by gel elec-

A. *In situ* hybridization

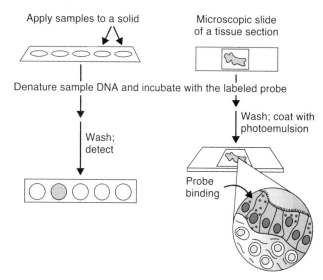

B. Solution hybridization

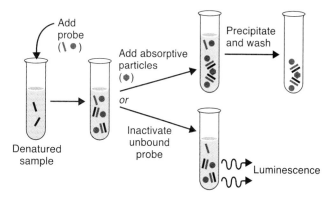

Figure 55.8. Nucleic acid probes—the basic formats. **A. Solid phase** or **in situ hybridization** involves hybridization of the probe with nucleic acids fixed to a solid support. The sample may be a lysate of a patient specimen, purified DNA, or a tissue section. In the latter case, DNA in the tissue is denatured on the microscopic slide. If a radiolabeled probe is used, the slide is overlaid first with the probe; then after washing, with a photographic emulsion that creates opaque, microscopic grains at sites of radioactive emissions. The anatomical structures to which the probe has hybridized can then be seen under the microscope. **B.** In **solution hybridization**, the probe and the denatured patient sample are incubated together in solution. After hybridization, the double-stranded hybrids are precipitated from solution and separated from unbound probe DNA. If the target sequence was present in the sample, then radioactive counts, representing hybridized probe, are detected in the precipitated fraction.

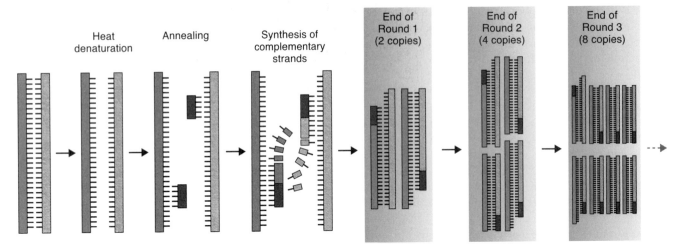

Figure 55.9. Nucleic acid amplification: the polymerase chain reaction. In this assay, the DNA in the patient sample is mixed with specific primers, deoxynucleotide triphosphates (dNTPs), and a thermostable DNA polymerase enzyme. The reaction involves three steps that are repeated in sequence: (1) **Heat denaturation**, which permits complementary strands of the target DNA to separate. (2) **Annealing**, as the primers hybridize to opposite strands of the targeted sequence when the temperature is lowered. (3) **Synthesis**, as the polymerase incorporates the dNTPS into a new complementary strand of DNA, in a sequential and unidirectional manner, beginning at each hybridized primer. Note that synthesis from either primer generates a new site to which the opposite primer can hybridize in the next cycle. Each time this cycle is repeated, the number of double-stranded target DNA sequences available to bind the two primers doubles. One target DNA molecule subjected to 30 repetitions of the PCR would result in 2^{30} copies of the target sequence. The products of the reaction are detected by gel electrophoresis or by a gene probe specific for the sequences between the two primers.

trophoresis as fragments of a predicted size. Some commercial PCR kits detect amplicons by automated methods. One test system uses labeled primers, thus the amplicons produced at the end of the cycling will be labeled. Instead of analyzing the PCR products by electrophoresis, the amplicons are used as probes to hybridize target DNA bound to a solid support. If the labeled amplicons hybridize to the bound DNA (i.e., are captured on the solid support), the microbial nucleic acid of interest was initially present in the patient sample. This method is called the **"reverse capture"** technique.

The great power of PCR is its sensitivity. Theoretically, the chain reaction can be initiated by a single copy of the target sequence. But this exquisite sensitivity is also the major pitfall of the procedure as a clinical diagnostic tool. There is a serious potential for cross-contamination ("microcontamination") in laboratories that process numerous, similar samples every day. The prevention of false-positive PCR results is a matter of great concern to physicians and lawyers, since there may be no equally sensitive, alternate method to verify a positive PCR result. The most celebrated example of this pitfall occurred in the O. J. Simpson trial, in which questions about mishandling of specimens and cross-contamination of evidence may have influenced the verdict. To avoid such problems in clinical diagnostic laboratories, specimen preparation, amplification, and analysis of the reaction products are each performed in separate areas

to avoid cross-contamination. In addition, positive tests are usually retested.

PCR and other methods of nucleic acid amplification are presently being used to detect infectious agents that elude more conventional methods of diagnosis. For many infectious diseases, PCR may be the only method that is sufficiently sensitive to detect a particular pathogen in routine clinical specimens.

CONCLUSION

Many different techniques are available to establish the presence of a pathogenic microorganism in an ill patient. All methods have the potential for inaccuracy, either in failing to detect a pathogen or immune response when present or in signaling their presence when the pathogen or the immune response is absent. Some tests are more sensitive or more specific than others, and these measures of performance determine how and when they are used. But even when a test accurately analyzes a given sample, the simple presence of a microorganism in the specimen or of antibodies against a pathogen in patient serum does not always indicate active infection, nor does it necessarily establish the cause of illness. For these reasons, there is always a need for interpretation with any microbiologic test, regardless of its technical performance characteristics. In the final analysis, there is no substitute for the interpretive skills of the clinician in placing microbiologic test results into the context of the patient's illness.

Principles of Epidemiology

DAVID R. SNYDMAN

Epidemiology is the study of the determinants of disease in a population. Epidemiologists deal with both infectious and noninfectious etiologies. When infectious agents are involved, the aim is to understand their mode of transmission and what predisposes a population to a particular agent. The practical purpose of epidemiology is to control the spread of disease in a population, either by limiting microbial transmission or by altering the susceptibility of a population. Common control measures include removing the source of the agent, controlling its transmission, and immunizing the population.

This chapter considers epidemiological concepts and methods through the examination of an epidemiological "case," the investigation of a new disease. Following the case discussion, the chapter considers general epidemiological issues.

AN EPIDEMIOLOGICAL "CASE"

In October, 1975, the Department of Health of Connecticut received separate calls from two mothers living on rural roads in the towns of Lyme and Old Lyme. They reported that several children in their households and the neighborhood had what appeared to be arthritis. They had voiced their concern to local physicians and were not deterred by being told that arthritis is "not infectious."

Given the unusual nature of these reports, the epidemiologists considered the following questions:

1. Were these cases related?
2. Were there other similar cases?
3. Did the children have an infectious form of arthritis?
4. What forms of arthritis are infectious?

After discussing the cases with the parents and local physicians, the epidemiologists decided that this situation deserved looking into. What steps did they take and what principles did they apply to their study?

EPIDEMIOLOGICAL METHODOLOGY

The Connecticut epidemiologists undertook what is known as an **epidemic investigation**, the study of the extent, characteristics, mode of transmission, and etiology of a cluster of cases. It is perhaps the most self-evident of the methods used in epidemiology, but by no means the only one. Others, including **case-control studies**, **cohort studies**, and **epidemiological interventions**, are discussed below.

An epidemic investigation is undertaken when the number of cases of a disease increases over what is considered to be the norm or standard. In the Connecticut study, it was necessary to determine first if indeed the arthritis cases represented an epidemic. The determination of an epidemic depends solely on the background incidence of the disease in the population and not on an absolute cutoff point. For example, before the advent of the polio vaccine in the 1950s, about 50,000 cases of the disease occurred in the U.S. annually. After the vaccine was put into widespread use, the number of case dropped dramatically to about 10 per year. Therefore, one or two cases of polio is considered to be an epidemic!

In addition to epidemics, there are **endemic** and **pandemic** diseases. An endemic infectious disease is one that is consistently found in the population, such as dental caries, gonorrhea, or athlete's foot. A pandemic is a worldwide epidemic; examples are the current AIDS pandemic, or the Spanish flu pandemic of 1918–1919.

Case Definition

The investigators of the cases of Connecticut arthritis began by asking whether other individuals had the same disease. They first had to establish a set of clinical crite-

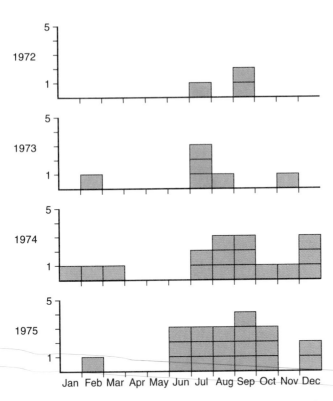

Figure 56.1. Time course of Lyme disease in three towns in Connecticut (Old Lyme, Lyme, and East Haddam) between 1972 and 1975.

ria known as the **case definition**. After all, many people have arthritis. From the mothers, physicians, and school nurses in the area, they obtained a list of other individuals who may have had the same symptoms. After examining the patients and taking careful histories they included, as fitting the case definition, those with the following clinical picture: (a) a sudden onset of swelling and pain in a knee or other large joint lasting a week to several months; (b) those affected had had several attacks that recurred several times at intervals of a few months; (c) nearly one-half of those affected also had fever and fatigue.

Time, Place, and Personal Characteristics of Patients

Armed with a usable case definition, the investigators found other cases in Old Lyme and two adjacent towns. The best source of additional cases were the two determined mothers who had made the original phone calls. From current and past episodes, the investigators collected 51 cases that conformed to the case definition. They could now proceed to determine what epidemiologists call the time, place, and personal characteristics of these cases. The **time characteristics** include the **time of onset** of the disease and its **duration**. As shown in Figure 56.1, many of the Connecticut cases clustered in the summer and early fall. The duration of each bout of the

disease varied from a week to a few months, and 69% of the patients had recurrences of the symptoms. Not knowing at this time the etiology of the disease, they could not determine another important time characteristic, namely the **incubation period**, or the interval from exposure to the first onset of symptoms.

Place characteristics are primarily the site of residence and the area in which the patients lived. For occupation-related illnesses, this can also include the place of work. The cases were concentrated in three adjacent towns on the eastern side of the Connecticut River. Most of the patients lived in wooded areas near streams and lakes.

Personal characteristics include the age and sex of the patients and any possible genetic predisposition to the disease. Of the 51 cases, 39 were children, nearly evenly divided by gender. No familial pattern was discerned. The epidemiologists now listed the cases by the time of onset and constructed what is called an **epidemic curve**. They named this outbreak "Lyme arthritis," which was later modified to Lyme disease, its current eponym.

The epidemiologists now posed other questions. Was the outbreak a surveillance artifact based on the fact that many questions about arthritis were being asked by outsiders? The simplest way to assess this was to go elsewhere and ask the same questions. The answer, from surveying towns across the Connecticut River, was that increased interest did not result in an increase in the number of cases of arthritis reported. The team then asked, is this an infectious disease? The most common arthritic conditions of childhood, such as juvenile rheumatoid arthritis, are collagen vascular problems and are not known to be infectious. Nonetheless, the clustering of cases, the fact that most of the cases began in the summer or early fall, and that most patients lived in wooded areas along lakes or streams suggested an arthropod transmitted disease, possibly viral. If so, the investigators wondered, is the disease new?

Is Lyme Disease Communicable?

Many infectious diseases are **communicable**, e.g., measles, polio, or tuberculosis. Others, such as a ruptured appendix, urinary tract infections, or osteomyelitis, are not. Was Lyme disease communicable, or did it merely affect especially susceptible individuals? To answer this question, the investigators attempted to trace contacts, but even in families with multiple affected members, the onset of illness had usually taken place in different years. Next, they tried to identify a common exposure, but none could be found. However, an intriguing clue surfaced. About one-quarter of the patients had reported that the symptoms of arthritis were preceded by an unusual skin rash. The rash had started as a red spot that spread to form a 6-inch ring. What was the connection? An astute dermatology consultant remembered that similar rashes had been described in 1910 in Sweden and had been attributed to tick bites. This rash went by the impressive name of "erythema chronicum migrans."

The investigators undertook a **case control study** in 1977, in which the cases are matched with a similar group of control or unaffected persons. After matching for age, sex, and any other relevant factors, the epidemiologists looked for any differences between the two groups that could give clues as to possible risk factors. They found that those affected were more likely to live in a household with pets. One consequence is that they were more likely to come in contact with the ticks that dogs and cats pick up in the woods of that region. In a roundabout way, this clue became more credible when the investigators remembered the suggestive clinical finding of the Swedish researchers.

So far, the connection between the rash and Lyme disease depended on **retrospective evidence**. To make the connection stronger, it became appropriate to ask if patients with the signs of erythema chronicum migrans progress to develop Lyme disease? In 1977, the team set up a **prospective study**, looking for patients with the rash and observing them for some time. Indeed, of 32 new cases of erythema chronicum migrans, 19 progressed to Lyme disease. Meanwhile, the "tick connection" became even more plausible after a thorough entomological survey. Insects and ticks were collected from Lyme and surroundings, with the finding that adult ticks were 16 times more abundant on the east side of the Connecticut River than on the west side. This corresponded roughly to the proportion of incidence of cases of Lyme disease in the two areas. In addition, many more tick bites were reported by the arthritis patients than by their neighbors without the disease. Thus, the tick–rash–arthritis connection seemed more and more plausible. We will see that the final proof of this scheme awaited the discovery of the etiological agent and the direct demonstration of its transmission via ticks.

At the same time, a **surveillance network** had been set up in Connecticut and part of the adjacent states to gather information about other cases. A careful study revealed that, contrary to the early reports, the disease was more frequent in adults than in children. It was easier to recognize arthritis as an unusual occurrence in children. Many arthritis patients had serious manifestations, such as neurological dysfunction and myocarditis. Thus, the disease turned out to be considerably more complex than described by the original case definition. This illustrates an important epidemiological point. An early case definition is, by necessity, tentative, and may be modified when the full spectrum of the disease becomes known. As an example of a complex case definition, see the one developed for AIDS (see Table 38.4).

Search for the Etiological Agent

So far, the investigators could conclude with assurance that Lyme disease was an infection, most likely transmitted by ticks. It appeared to be a new clinical entity. However, until this time, the search for the etiological agent had proved unproductive. Despite many attempts, no laboratory had succeeded in isolating a virus, which, at the time, seemed to be a good candidate for being the agent of the disease. On the other hand, the investigators collected anecdotal evidence that tetracycline, erythromycin, and penicillin were clinically effective. With time, more physicians reported the beneficial effect of antibiotics, making a bacterial etiology more likely. At about this time, in 1979–1980, entomologists and microbiologists at the Rocky Mountain Public Health Laboratory in Montana, who were experts on tickborne diseases, examined ticks sent from the affected area and found that the gut of many specimens contained unusual spirochetes. Were these the agents of Lyme disease?

Using a culture medium that supports the growth of tick- or louseborne spirochetes, the microbiologists succeeded in growing a newly recognized spirochete. Soon thereafter, they isolated the spirochete from human cases and the immune responses of patients were linked to this organism. The spirochete was classified among the *Borrelia*, a group that includes the agent of another tickborne disease also found in the U.S., relapsing fever. The agent of Lyme disease was given the name *B. burgdorferi*, in honor of the entomologist who discovered the organism in the ticks.

With a simple diagnostic test at hand, investigators in many parts of the world could carry out serological surveys or serosurveys, that is, they determined the proportion of persons with antibodies to *B. burgdorferi*. In general, serosurveys allow recognition of a wide range of clinical manifestations, from asymptomatic cases to full-blown disease. This recognition is important because, in most infectious diseases, there are many more asymptomatic than clinically overt cases. Using these techniques, Lyme disease has been diagnosed in other parts of the U.S., especially on the East and West Coasts, as well as in Canada, Europe, Asia, and Australia. It is considered a serious disease, mainly because of its important and chronic neurological manifestations.

The original puzzle of "Lyme arthritis" had been solved. A few years after the original phone calls, a new disease was described, its agent and mode of transmission were identified, and preventive and therapeutic measures had been instituted. Note that it took the joint efforts of epidemiologists, clinicians, entomologists, microbiologists, and alert and determined members of the public.

VARIETY OF THE ROUTES OF TRANSMISSION
Humans As Reservoirs

We now turn from a specific example to a more general consideration of epidemiological principles. These

Table 56.1. Examples of Modes of Transmission

Modes of transmission	Example	Factor	Route of entry
Direct contact			
Respiratory aerosol	Influenza	Crowding?	Lung
	Tuberculosis	Household	Lung
Nasal secretions	Respiratory syncytial virus	Household, nosocomial	Upper respiratory tract
Droplets	*Meningococcus*	Crowding	Nasopharynx
Skin	*Streptococcus* (impetigo)	Crowding	Skin
Semen	AIDS	Sexual contact	Mucous membrane
Transplacental	Hepatitis B	Carrier	Mother
Indirect contact			
Blood	Hepatitis B	Transfusion, needlestick	Blood
	AIDS	Transfusion	Blood
Stool	Hepatitis A	Ingestion	GI tract
Animal	*Salmonella*	Ingestion	GI tract
Inanimate	*Legionella*	Water contamination	Respiratory tract
Arthropod vector			
Tick	Lyme disease	Bite	Skin, blood
Mosquito	Malaria	Bite	Blood

principles include the routes of transmission, incubation periods, communicability, and individual susceptibility. The first is the mode of transmission (Table 56.1). **Transmission from human to human** may take place from parent to offspring or between mature individuals. **Vertical transmission** refers to the passage of an agent from an infected mother to her fetus or infant. The most intimate mode is via the **transplacental route**. Examples of such congenitally acquired diseases are syphilis and rubella. Newborns may also pick up chlamydiae, gonococci, cytomegalovirus, or hepatitis B virus during passage through the birth canal. Other organisms may be transmitted via mother's milk.

Horizontal transmission may be between individuals in close proximity or living far away, and includes intimate modes, such as sexual intercourse, or more casual contacts, such as touching another person, breathing of aerosols, etc. The actual path of an organism from one person to another depends on the way the agent exits the body of the donor. Thus, bacteria or viruses that infect the respiratory tract are often expelled as aerosols during coughing and even talking, and may be inhaled by bystanders. If the organism is resistant to drying, as is the case with the tubercle bacillus, the danger of inhalation may persist for a long time. Intestinal pathogens often cause diarrhea, which increases their distribution in the environment and, under conditions of poor sanitation, results in contaminated drinking water and foodstuffs.

Some diseases are acquired by breaching the skin or mucous membranes by trauma, insect bites, blood transfusions, or contaminated hypodermic needles. Agents that are transmitted in this fashion include the AIDS or hepatitis B viruses. Many of the agents that are transmitted by insect **vectors** have different life cycles in the vector and in the host. Note that some of these organisms may be transmitted by more than one of these routes. Thus, HIV infection may be transmitted transplacentally, by sexual intercourse, or by the use of needles.

Nonhuman Reservoirs

Other diseases are acquired from **nonhuman reservoirs**. These include the zoonoses (Chapter 70, "Zoonoses"), in which the reservoir is an animal. Transmission from the animal may be direct, as in the bite from a rabid dog, or via insect vectors, as in the plague or the viral encephalitides. Lyme disease is also a zoonosis in which the natural reservoir are mammals such as deer that share the same ticks with humans. Transmission may be indirect as well from contact with a contaminated environment, such as with rodent excreta in the newly described Haanta virus outbreak in the Southwestern United States.

In other diseases, the reservoir is the **inanimate environment** and the organisms live freely in nature. For example, the clostridia of gas gangrene are commonly found in soils. However, humans or animals may contribute to the frequency with which the agents are found in nature. Thus, cholera bacilli grow naturally in warm estuaries, probably on the surface of shellfish. However, contamination from human feces may help the organisms become established in a previously unaffected area.

Incubation Periods and Communicability

The length of the incubation period differs considerably among infectious diseases, from a few hours to months and years (Table 56.2). It is influenced by many factors. For example, a large infective dose may shorten it and a small one may lengthen it. To the epidemiologists, the incubation period is particularly important because, during this time, some diseases may be transmitted from asymptomatic patients. Control of transmission may therefore rely on special surveillance methods that include infected but asymptomatic persons. The periods of incubation and of communicability are not always the same. For example, the incubation period in hepatitis A most commonly lasts for 34 weeks. However, individuals can communicate the virus for only 1 or 2 weeks before the onset of the disease.

The period of communicability may extend long after the disease symptoms abate, as in the case of **chronic carriers**. For example, hepatitis B carriers can usually transmit the virus for the length of time they carry it. In many of the preceding chapters, the carrier state has been discussed at some length (see Chapter 14, "Neisseriae"; Chapter 17, "Invasive Enterics"; Chapter 27, "Chlamydiae"; Chapter 38, "Human Retroviruses"; Chapter 41, "Herpesvirus"; and Chapter 42, "Viral Hepatitis").

Individual Susceptibility

Human beings differ in their susceptibility to infectious diseases. We have all encountered individuals who seem more prone to respiratory or intestinal infections than the majority. For many of these persons, we do not know the reason for this variability. They may have subtle deficiencies in certain of their defense mechanisms. When these deficiencies become severe and the risks are more evident, the cause is often easier to ascertain.

Table 56.2. Examples of Incubation Periods

Disease	Range of period
Staphylococcal food poisoning	1–6 hours
Clostridial food poisoning	12–24 hours
Hepatitis A	14–42 days
Hepatitis B	30–180 days
Gonorrhea	2–9 days
Salmonellosis	0.5–3 days
Epstein-Barr virus infection	21–49 days
Mycoplasma pneumoniae infection	8–21 days
Varicella	10–21 days
AIDS	21 days to 5 years or more
Leprosy	7 months–5 years

Chapter 68 ("AIDS") discusses the consequences of the major kinds of innate and acquired immune deficiencies.

The epidemiologist must be aware of the different susceptibility of members of the population. Age, sex, nutritional status, previous exposure, and immune competence all influence susceptibility to a particular infectious disease. Thus, children and older persons are frequently more susceptible to bacterial pneumonia or intestinal infections. The incidence of the carrier state of hepatitis B is greater in males than in females. It is also more frequent among individuals with Down syndrome or those receiving hemodialysis.

Genetic factors are also known to play a role in susceptibility, although the data are generally inconclusive. The importance of these factors is often difficult to unravel from a myriad of socioeconomic factors, such as those that contribute to the state of health and nutrition. Nonetheless, the role of genetic factors has been well established in certain diseases. It has been shown, for example, that among identical twins living apart, if one twin contracted tuberculosis, the other had a greater chance than average of getting the disease. Nonidentical twins did not show this pattern. One of the most intensively studied genetic effects is the decreased susceptibility to malaria of persons with the sickle cell trait (Chapter 50, "Blood and Tissue Protozoa"). It is also well established that non-Caucasians are more prone to the disseminated form of coccidioidomycosis than Caucasians.

PRACTICAL ASPECTS OF EPIDEMIOLOGY

In a civilized society, epidemiology is everyone's business. The practicing physician and all members of the health care team must be aware of the public health implications of a given patient's infectious disease. To safeguard both the public interest and individual rights to privacy, a considerable body of local and national laws has been developed in most countries of the world. For instance, in the U.S., certain communicable diseases are notifiable, that is, physicians are obliged to report cases to the U.S. Public Health Service. The information collected is published in a readily available pamphlet, the *Morbidity and Mortality Weekly Reports*, or *MMWR*, which lists all routine information and calls attention to unusual occurrences. In addition, each state has its own surveillance mechanism and reporting requirements for the study of communicable diseases within its borders. Each has a **State Board of Health** and a **Reference Laboratory** equipped to carry out special diagnostic tests that are often outside the scope of hospital laboratories.

CONCLUSION

Epidemiology may appear to be a remote discipline, practiced mainly by public health officials. In fact, it pervades all forms of medical practice and furnishes important clues for the diagnosis of infectious diseases. Thus, inquiry into time and place characteristics should be part of the usual process of taking a clinical history. Epidemiological information may reveal how people encounter disease agents and can help reduce exposure and spread of infectious diseases.

SUGGESTED READINGS

Esdaile JM, Feinstein AR. Lyme disease: a medical detective story. 1985 Medical and Health Annual. Encyclopedia Britannica: 267–271.

Giesecke J. Modern infectious disease epidemiology. Boston: Little, Brown, 1991.

Lederberg J, Shope RE, Oaks SC, eds. Emerging infections: microbial threats to health in the United States. Washington, DC: National Academy Press, 1992.

Sackett DL, Haynes RB, Guyatt GH, Tugwell P. Clinical epidemiology. A basic science for clinical medicine. 2nd ed. Boston: Little, Brown, 1991.

Steere AC, Malawista SE, Snydman DR, et al. Lyme arthritis. An epidemic of oligoarticular arthritis in children and adults in three Connecticut communities. Arthrit Rheum 1977;20: 717.

CHAPTER 57

Digestive System

GERALD T. KEUSCH
DAVID W.K. ACHESON

The digestive system is a microbiologist's paradise. In health or disease, the digestive tract is a microbial garden of unsurpassed variety and complexity, and feces is the seed of its creation. It varies in the level of colonization from the "buggiest" parts of the body, at both ends, to the nearly sterile environment of the mid-small intestine (Fig. 57.1). The alimentary tract is studded with different ecosystems occupied by site-specific microbial populations. The normal stomach is an effective sterilization chamber that limits the entry of microorganisms to the small bowel and beyond, thus providing nonspecific protection against many enteric pathogens.

A community of well over 400 distinct species of bacteria, in addition to a few fungi and protozoa, form the resident flora of the normal gastrointestinal (GI) tract. Bacteria in the colon are present at approximately one-tenth of the theoretical limit of packing cells into a defined space (about 10^{12} bacteria/g) and, amazingly, produce no intestinal dysfunction. On the contrary, they enter into a symbiotic relationship with the host (see Chapter 2, " Normal Microbial Flora"). While we furnish this microbial population with room and board, it provides a number of essential services for us. Among these are accessory digestive functions such as converting unabsorbable carbohydrates to absorbable organic acids, energy for colonic epithelial cells in the form of butyrate, vitamin K needed for synthesis of blood clotting factors, and assistance in the reabsorption and conservation of estrogens and androgens excreted in the bile. In addition, their mere presence helps us resist colonization by invading pathogens.

The frequency of infections of the digestive system varies from the most prevalent human infectious disease, dental caries, to fairly common diarrheas and food poisoning, to unusual opportunistic infections of immunocompromised patients. Worldwide, diarrheal diseases are a far greater cause of morbidity and mortality than are the more familiar diseases of the industrialized nations (heart disease, cancer, and strokes). Unfortunately, infants and small children are disproportionately affected, especially in poor developing countries with poor nutrition and even poorer environmental sanitation. While diarrheal disease is not a frequently fatal disease in the U.S., it remains among the most common complaints of people seen in general medical practice.

Intestinal infections range in severity from asymptomatic (e.g., polio) through mild diarrhea (e.g., most rotavirus infections) to life-threatening loss of fluid and electrolytes (e.g., cholera) or severe mucosal ulceration complicated by intestinal perforation (e.g., bacillary dysentery). This variation in clinical manifestations is not surprising when one considers the striking local differentiation in the alimentary tract and the variation in virulence genes among the pathogens (Fig. 57.2).

ENTRY

Barriers to Infection

Each portion of the alimentary tract has special anatomic, physiological, and biochemical barriers to infection (see Fig. 57.2). The most general impediment to infective agents is an **unbroken mucosal epithelium** covering all parts of this system. Its importance is illustrated when people receive ionizing radiation or cytotoxic cancer chemotherapy, which interferes with the normal replacement of sloughed epithelial cells. Some of the earliest manifestations of damage are nausea, vomiting, and mucositis, superficial ulcerations of the mucosa of the entire GI tract. Members of the normal flora can now reach deep tissues through these ulcerations and may even disseminate through the bloodstream to other organs.

Some defense mechanisms, such as **mucus formation** and **gut motility**, hinder the adherence of microorganisms to the epithelial wall. In the intestine, the mucus

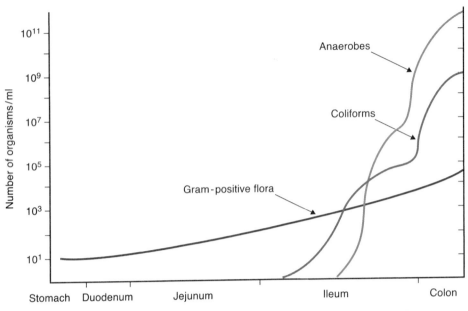

Figure 57.1. The GI tract and typical numbers of bacteria at the main sites.

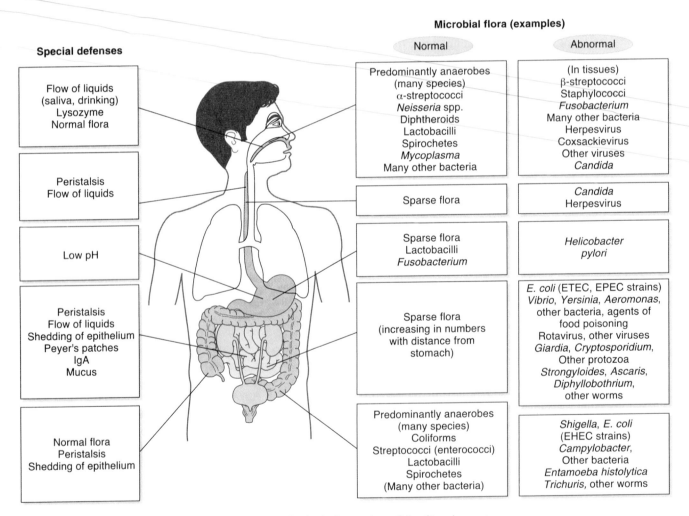

Figure 57.2. A microbiological overview of the digestive system.

layer functions as a mechanical obstacle to protect the epithelium; it also coats bacteria, which makes it easier to pass them along by peristalsis. Glycocalyx, the glycoprotein and polysaccharide layer that covers the surface of cells, has "decoy" binding sites that entrap certain invading organisms and facilitate their excretion in feces. In some instances, however, mucus may promote virulence by triggering the synthesis of virulence factors. **Bile** plays an important role in selecting those bacteria and viruses that are able to colonize the intestines. Organisms that survive in the intestinal lumen, both normal flora and pathogens, are often resistant to the detergent action of bile salts. Most enteric viruses, polio or hepatitis A for example, lack a lipid-containing envelope that would make them sensitive to bile. Certain bacteria, e.g., the Gram-negative typhoid bacillus and Gram-positive enterococci, are so highly bile resistant that they can even grow in the gallbladder.

A number of cellular and soluble factors have less well-understood defensive functions. For instance, **secretory IgA immunoglobulins** and the protein **lactoferrin** in mother's milk may help prevent colonization of the infant by certain bacteria. While it is likely that IgA has a similar function in older children and adults, it has been difficult to prove its role as a host defense mechanism, in part because some individuals with IgA deficiency (the most common immunoglobulin defect) have no evidence of an increase in susceptibility to infections. The intestinal tract is also the major disposal site for senescent white blood cells, especially neutrophils. It is likely, but not proven, that movement of these cells through the mucosa into the lumen of the gut plays a role in controlling pathogens or in maintaining balance with the normal flora. This putative role may explain the frequency of gut-based systemic infections in granulocytopenic patients, especially the enterobacteriaceae.

Establishment of Infectious Disease in the Digestive System

Several circumstances predispose to the establishment of infectious disease in the alimentary tract either by pathogens or members of the normal flora:

- **Anatomic alterations.** Obstructions to the flow of secretions remove one of the most powerful defensive mechanisms of the hollow organs. Thus, stones in the gallbladder or the common bile duct that impede the flow of bile predispose the biliary tree to infections. Surgery may also create intestinal "blind loops" which are isolated from the moving stream of the intestinal contents. Bacterial overgrowth can occur in the blind loop and result in malabsorption.
- **Changes in stomach acidity.** Alteration of the acid barrier of the stomach by disease, surgery, or drugs increases the survival of certain, but not all, pathogens in this organ. Bacterial infection down-

stream can thus result from a smaller inoculum. This scenario is particularly true of cholera and *Salmonella*, but not *Shigella* or *Escherichia coli* O157:H7.
- **Alterations in the normal flora.** In the regions of the digestive tract that are most heavily colonized—the mouth and the colon—changes in the density or composition of the flora may permit pathogens to become established. The most frequent cause of such an alteration is the use of **broad-spectrum antibiotics**.
- **Encounter with specific pathogenic agents.** Certain bacteria, viruses, protozoa, and helminths cause disease even in the absence of predisposing host factors. At each site, pathogens must be able to resist the specific local defenses. Because microorganisms face different survival problems in the mouth, stomach, small intestine, or the colon, they must possess different attributes to survive in each site.

DAMAGE

The signs and symptoms of infections related to the digestive system are caused by several general mechanisms:

- **Pharmacologic action.** Some bacteria produce toxins that alter normal intestinal function without causing lasting damage to their target cells. Typical examples are the **enterotoxins** made by *Vibrio cholerae* or by some strains of *Escherichia coli*, which provoke copious watery diarrhea. Because the small bowel is primarily responsible for absorbing most of the 9–10 liters of fluid that pass through the gut each day, even small reductions in its absorptive capacity cause large amounts of fluid to enter the colon, overwhelming its relatively modest absorptive capacity. The excess unabsorbed fluid results in diarrhea; it may rapidly lead to profound dehydration, electrolyte loss, depletion of the intravascular volume, and shock, as seen in cholera.
- **Local inflammation.** In certain areas of the alimentary tract, an inflammatory reaction may occur as the consequence of microbial invasion. Often, the invasion is limited to the epithelial layer but may spread to contiguous tissue and beyond. In the mouth, usually the gums, infections with anaerobic bacteria cause inflammation in the gingival pocket (periodontitis). In the large intestine, inflammation due to *Shigella* infection of the lamina propria can result in bloody diarrhea or dysentery.
- **Deep tissue invasion.** Some organisms are able to invade deeper and enter the circulation. Examples are the worm *Strongyloides* or the protozoan *Entamoeba*, which are capable of burrowing through the intestinal wall, and *Salmonella*, which penetrates the lamina propria and eventually reaches the blood-

stream. Interestingly, *Strongyloides* itself is often colonized by gut bacteria; as a result, invasion with this worm can result in polymicrobial septicemia.

- **Perforation.** When the mucosal wall is necrotic or perforated, the normal flora can spill into the normally sterile peritoneal cavity and invade the bloodstream, often with serious consequences. Thus, rupture of an inflamed appendix may lead to peritonitis, while traumatic perforation of the esophagus results in mediastinitis.

The variety of infectious agents and the intestinal diseases they can cause is daunting. We organize this chapter by the principal sites of infection: the mouth, stomach, biliary tree, and intestines.

INFECTIONS OF THE MOUTH

Virtually all of the pathogens of the alimentary tract enter through the mouth. Because most of these pathogens come from the stool of an infected person, this route is known as "fecal–oral transmission". The organisms reach the mouth by hitching a ride aboard food, fluids, or fingers.

The specific defenses of the mouth include the following:

- The nonpathogenic resident flora, including bacteria (Table 57.1), fungi (e.g., *Candida*), and protozoa (e.g., the ameba *Entamoeba gingivalis*). These organisms resist the establishment of newcomers by occupying suitable sites and repelling other organisms, presumably by the production of acids and other metabolic inhibitors.
- The mechanical action of **saliva** and the **tongue.** We produce more than a liter of saliva per day. With as-

sistance from the tongue, saliva mechanically dislodges and flushes microorganisms from mucosal surfaces. If salivary flow is reduced, as with dehydration or during fasting, the bacterial content of saliva increases markedly.

- Antimicrobial constituents of saliva, notably **lysozyme** and **secreted antibodies.** As mentioned above, secretory IgA selectively inhibits the adherence of certain bacteria to mucosal cells or to tooth surfaces. Lysozyme is effective mainly against Gram-positive bacteria.

Several properties allow bacteria to evade these host defenses. Some are able to stick to teeth or mucosal surfaces. Attachment to teeth is not direct; rather bacteria adhere to a coating of sticky macromolecules, mainly proteins, called the **dental pellicle.** The bacteria themselves produce polysaccharides that help them adhere. For example, *Streptococcus mutans* transforms sucrose into polysaccharides which are particularly sticky. They are layered on the pellicle to form a matrix that allows adherence of other organisms. The result is dental plaque, one of the densest collections of bacteria in the body. Microbial metabolism in plaque transforms dietary sugar into acids, mainly lactic acid, that are responsible for dental caries (cavities). Other bacteria, especially strict anaerobes, reside in the gingival crevices between the tooth and gum, where they evade the washing effects of the saliva and normal tooth brushing.

The bacteria of the indigenous oral flora are not highly virulent, but when a break occurs in the mucosal barrier, such as with advanced gingivitis (periodontal disease), they may invade surrounding healthy tissue. The mouth is also the likely portal of entry of α-hemolytic streptococci that cause subacute bacterial endocarditis in patients with rheumatic heart disease. A

Table 57.1. Composition of the Intestinal Flora of Adult Humans

Bacterial species	Bacterial concentration (Log$_{10}$/ml or g)			
	Stomach	Jejunum	Ileum	Colon
Total viable count	0–10^3	0–10^5	10^2–10^7	10^{10}–10^{12}
Aerobes or facultative anaerobes				
Enterobacteria	0–10^2	0–10^3	10^2–10^7	10^4–10^{10}
Streptococci	0–10^2	0–10^4	10^2–10^6	10^4–10^9
Staphylococci	0–10^2	0–10^3	10^2–10^5	10^4–10^{10}
Lactobacilli	0–10^3	0–10^4	10^2–10^5	10^4–10^{10}
Fungi	0–10^2	0–10^2	10^2–10^4	10^4–10^6
Anaerobes				
Bacteroides	Rare	0–10^3	10^3–10^7	10^{10}–10^{12}
Bifidobacteria	Rare	0–10^4	10^3–10^9	10^8–10^{12}
Streptococci	Rare	0–10^3	10^2–10^6	10^{10}–10^{12}
Clostridia	Rare	Rare	10^2–10^6	10^6–10^{11}
Eubacteria	Rare	Rare	Rare	10^9–10^{12}

synergistic cooperation between several different types of bacteria, both aerobic and strictly anaerobic, can also lead to a severe and rapidly advancing mixed infection of the soft tissues surrounding the oral cavity. Ludwig's angina, a polymicrobial infection of the sublingual and submandibular spaces that arises from a tooth (often the second and third mandibular molars), is a cellulitis —an inflammation of submucosal or subcutaneous connective tissue—that may progress rapidly, press against the airway, and compromise respiratory airflow and threaten the patient with asphyxiation.

Thrush

▌ CASE 1

C., a 7-month-old girl, was treated by her pediatrician for a middle ear infection. She was prescribed a 7-day course of a penicillin, amoxicillin, which cleared the infection within 4 days. Antibiotics were continued, but on the sixth day of therapy, the mother noticed that the child was irritable and feeding poorly. During a follow-up visit at the clinic, her pediatrician noted several creamy white, curdlike patches on the tongue and buccal mucosa. When scraped, they were clearly painful and left a raw, bleeding surface. Microscopic examination of the exudate scraped from the affected areas revealed yeast. Thrush, or oral **candidiasis** was diagnosed. Antibiotics were stopped, a topical antifungal solution was administered, and the patches disappeared within 2 days.

Pathobiology

In the case, the white patches adhering to the oral mucosa consisted of "pseudomembranes" made up of the yeast *Candida*, mixed with desquamated epithelial cells, leukocytes, oral bacteria, necrotic tissue, and food debris. *Candida albicans* and related species are yeasts found in the environment that establish themselves in the alimentary tract early in life (see Chapter 47, "Systemic Mycoses"). The adult vagina is commonly colonized with these organisms, and they may be acquired by infants during delivery. Small numbers of *Candida* live harmlessly in the alimentary tract until the balance between indigenous bacterial flora and host defenses is upset. In the case of C., antibiotic therapy killed many of the normal oral bacteria and allowed the *Candida* to proliferate.

Candida exploits changes in the normal host flora to multiply locally. If the number or function of neutrophils is decreased, or if defects in cellular immunity are present, they may invade beyond the mucosal surface. Predisposing conditions for oral and other forms of candidiasis include diabetes, malnutrition, malignancy, immunosuppressive drugs or infections, genetic abnor-

malities of the immune system, and HIV infection. Normal individuals are also frequently affected. *Candida* vaginitis is commonly encountered in postpubertal women who are taking broad-spectrum antibiotics, often for a urinary tract infection. The prolonged use of inhaled steroids for asthmatics may also predispose to candidal overgrowth in the mouth. In more severe forms of immunodeficiency, the organism may disseminate through the bloodstream and infect virtually any organ system, but most commonly the liver, lung, and kidney.

Candida may also invade the esophagus, an organ that is rarely prone to infection. Candidal esophagitis is seen in patients with specific T-cell abnormalities, such as chronic mucocutaneous candidiasis or AIDS. The differential diagnosis of esophagitis in immunocompromised patients includes infection by herpes simplex type 1 virus (HSV) and cytomegalovirus (CMV). These infections can cause particularly troublesome mucosal ulcerations, with severe pain and difficulty in taking nourishment.

Diagnosis

Thrush is characteristic in appearance and the diagnosis is usually suspected on oral inspection. It is confirmed by examination of the exudate under a microscope and detection of characteristic yeast forms. Culture is not necessary and often misleading, because *Candida* is a commensal and can be cultured from the mouths of some healthy people.

Prevention and treatment

Because candidal colonization of the GI tract is frequent, prevention and treatment consist primarily of correcting the reversible predisposing factors and avoiding the unnecessary use of antibiotics. Candidiasis of the mouth is usually superficial and responds to oral antifungal agents such as nystatin. If the infection extends more deeply than the mucosa, it may be necessary to use an absorbed oral antifungal agent, such as fluconazole, or intravenous amphotericin B.

STOMACH

Until recently, the stomach received little attention as a locus of infections of the alimentary tract. It was not considered to be susceptible to infection. However, its role in protecting the gut further downstream by its secretion of acid was always appreciated. The majority of oral or foodborne bacteria, washed with saliva into the stomach, are destroyed by stomach acid.

In some individuals, the stomach is indeed sterile, and in most others, the concentration of bacteria is very low, generally less than 10^3 bacteria/ml. The predominant bacteria found in the stomach are acid-resistant Gram-positives, e.g., *Streptococcus*, *Staphylococcus*, *Lactobacillus*, and *Peptostreptococcus*. The normal stomach contains very few enteric Gram-negative rods, *Bacteroides*, or *Clostridium* organisms that are typically associated with the lower GI tract.

It is now known that gastric infections do occur and much more frequently than was previously thought. In particular, *Helicobacter pylori* is able to colonize regions of the stomach and may be involved in the production of gastritis and peptic ulcers. Human and experimental animal studies have demonstrated that *H. pylori* is a real pathogen of major clinical significance (see Chapter 22, "*Helicobacter pylori*"). Gastric ulcers have now entered the ever-expanding ranks of infectious diseases.

Some bacteria, including pathogens, if introduced into the stomach with food, will survive and enter the small intestine alive. Survival depends largely on the buffering effects of food, especially in patients who do not produce normal amounts of gastric hydrochloric acid because of disease, partial or total gastrectomy, drug therapy (e.g., H_2- or proton pump blockers), or antacid consumption. The infective dose of cholera bacilli or salmonellae in human volunteers, for example, was ten thousand-fold lower when the organisms were administered with 2 g of sodium bicarbonate.

Low or absent acid production, known as hypo- or achlorhydria, often leads to colonization of the stomach and upper small intestine by enteric Gram-negative rods. This colonization can have two important consequences:

1. Development of a disease called the bacterial overgrowth syndrome (see below);
2. Regurgitation of the abnormal gastric flora, which becomes a source of nosocomial (hospital-acquired) aspiration Gram-negative pneumonia (see Chapter 59, "Respiratory System").

BILIARY TREE AND THE LIVER

Infections of the **gallbladder** (cholecystitis) are a frequent complication of obstruction to the flow of bile due, for example, to gallstones migrating into the cystic duct or common bile duct. The clinical presentation is often sudden and dramatic, as the obstruction causes increased pressure and distention. Mechanical, chemical, and bacterial inflammation caused by *E. coli, Klebsiella pneumoniae*, group D streptococci, *S. aureus*, or *Clostridium perfringens* can result. The hallmark of cholecystitis is pain in the right upper quadrant of the abdomen, which may build to a crescendo and then subside, only to soon recur. This pattern is called **biliary colic**. Nausea and vomiting usually accompany the pain and may be intractable. The majority of patients with common duct obstruction have shaking chills, high spiking fever, jaundice, and tenderness over the gallbladder. Biliary colic, jaundice, and chills and spiking fever,

known as **Charcot's triad**, are characteristic of acute cholecystitis.

Inflammation and infection can cause ischemia of the gallbladder wall, sometimes progressing to gangrene and perforation. Gangrene and perforation may lead to contamination of the peritoneal cavity with bacteria and abscess formation. The spread of infection up the biliary ducts in the liver, known as **ascending cholangitis**, is common. With complete obstruction, the combination of pus and increased pressure leads to abscess formation, bacteremia, and symptoms of septic shock.

Primary bacterial infections of the **liver parenchyma** itself are not common, and are perhaps prevented by the defensive capacity of the phagocytic Kupffer cells. Liver abscesses can develop from portal vein bacteremia from an infected intra-abdominal site, from systemic bacteremia via the hepatic artery, from ascending cholangitis, and from contiguous infections. Intracellular pathogens that survive in macrophages can cause granulomatous infections. Examples are the agents of typhoid fever, Q fever, brucellosis, and tuberculosis.

Infectious diseases of the liver are not discussed in detail here. The most important diseases are due to hepatitis viruses (see Chapter 42, "Viral Hepatitis"). The liver is also the site of parasitic infections such as amebiasis (see Chapter 51, "Intestinal and Vaginal Protozoa"), schistosomiasis (see Chapter 53, "Tissue and Blood Helminths"), leishmaniasis (see Chapter 50, "Blood and Tissue Protozoa"), and others. An important, although clinically silent, part of the life cycle of the malarial parasites also takes place in the liver.

Cholecystitis

■ CASE 2

Ms. F., an obese 48-year-old mother of eight with a vague history of intermittent "stomach problems," awoke with moderate midepigastric pain. Approximately 2 hours before going to bed, she had eaten a large meal of fried chicken and vegetables. The pain soon shifted to her right upper quadrant and was occasionally felt in the area of the right scapula. She vomited several times and then improved but had residual pain for several days with numerous similar but less intense attacks. By the sixth day, she felt sick again and developed jaundice and a shaking chill. In the emergency room, she was in obvious pain and had a temperature of 40°C. Her skin was slightly yellowish. The right upper quadrant of her abdomen was markedly tender to palpation. An 8-cm tubular mass was felt under the margin of the right ribs. Her white blood cell count was elevated (14,000/μl), suggesting a bacterial infection. Her liver function tests were abnormal; her serum bilirubin and alkaline phosphatase levels were elevated, suggesting biliary obstruction.

Blood was cultured and antibiotic therapy was begun. An ultrasound examination showed that her gallbladder was markedly distended and contained several stones. The diagnosis of acute cholecystitis was made. Within 36 hours of admission, the pain improved and the fever resolved. The blood cultures grew *E. coli* and enterococci. Ms. F. was scheduled for surgery to remove the affected gallbladder and stones.

Pathobiology

Both infections of the gallbladder (**cholecystitis**) and of the bile duct (**cholangitis**) are secondary consequences of obstruction. The process begins with obstruction and distention, resulting in inflammation of the gallbladder wall. The disease may not progress, but the process increases the risk of infection caused by the small number of bacteria normally present in bile. Patients with cholecystitis commonly have a history of recurrent attacks of biliary colic resulting from obstruction of the biliary outlet. It is possible that Ms. F.'s vague "stomach problems" of the past were episodes of mild biliary colic caused by transient and/or partial obstructions of the duct by her gallstones. In the most recent episode, infection developed and the character of her illness changed.

Once bacterial infection becomes established, tissue damage may be accelerated by the resulting inflammatory response. Healing is unlikely to occur without surgical or spontaneous relief of the obstruction and specific antimicrobial therapy.

A particularly rapid and severe form of gallbladder infection occurs in patients with compromised arterial blood supply to the gallbladder wall, such as diabetics or the elderly. If the infecting organisms invade the gallbladder wall, they may produce a condition called **emphysematous cholecystitis**. This condition is distinguished by rapid clinical onset, extensive gangrene, presence of gas in the gallbladder wall (when gas-forming species, such as clostridia or *E. coli* are present), and a high mortality rate. Surgical removal of the gallbladder (cholecystectomy) is required because of the frequent occurrence of gangrene, perforation, and extensive peritonitis.

The typical clinical presentation of cholangitis is similar to cholecystitis, as in Ms. F.'s case, but is typically accompanied by high spiking fever, chills, jaundice, and constant pain. The most common obstructing causes are gallstones and neoplasms, but occasionally, a worm infection, such as *Ascaris lumbricoides*, is responsible. Considerable pressure within the duct seems to be a prerequisite for infection. Experiments in dogs have shown that the normal common duct pressure of 70 mm H_2O must be raised to 250 mm H_2O before *E. coli* injected into the bloodstream produces infection in the gallbladder. It is not known why the resulting distention facilitates bacterial invasion of the duct wall, but microscopic tears or ischemic damage are obvious possibilities.

Organisms that infect the gallbladder and bile duct are usually derived from the GI tract, *E. coli* being the single most frequent organism. Approximately 40% of these infections are caused by a mixed facultative and strictly anaerobic flora that ascends from the duodenum.

Typhoid bacilli have an unusual predilection for the gallbladder (see Chapter 17, "Invasive and Tissue-Damaging Enteric Bacteria"). These organisms may persist for a long period of time within gallstones, where they are protected from the effects of antibiotics. They produce little or no inflammation, and the person may not be aware he or she is a carrier. All carriers, cognizant or not, shed the typhoid bacteria into the environment and may infect other people.

Diagnosis

When the clinical presentation of cholecystitis is typical, as in Ms. F.'s case, a tentative diagnosis of cholecystitis can be made on clinical grounds. Unfortunately, this disease is prone to misdiagnosis, because it often presents in a less typical form. A helpful test is abdominal ultrasound, an imaging technique that can reliably visualize obstruction or distention in the biliary system. Direct culture of the infected bile is rarely performed, because of the difficulty in obtaining a specimen; antibiotics are chosen on the basis of expected flora. The diagnosis is confirmed when blood cultures grow the culprit organisms, but cultures are often negative.

Prevention and treatment

Patients with cholangitis should receive antibiotics appropriate for the expected mixed bacterial species typically present, before the diagnosis is confirmed and bacteria are identified in the blood, but not before blood cultures are obtained. Correct antibiotics are not sufficient, however. To effect a definitive cure, the underlying obstruction must be relieved. Relief of the obstruction may occur spontaneously or with surgery. The timing and need for surgery to remove stones and an inflamed gallbladder is controversial, and the surgeon's decision depends on many factors specific to each patient.

SMALL AND LARGE INTESTINE

We now discuss diseases that illustrate the diversity of infectious problems of the gut, based on host factors and on virulence attributes of the organisms. Examples of other classic infections of the intestines caused by bacteria are discussed in Chapters 16, "Secretory Diarrhea," and 17, "Invasive and Tissue-Damaging Enteric Bacteria," and by animal parasites in Chapters 51, "Intestinal and Vaginal Protozoa," and 52, "Intestinal Helminths".

Bacterial Overgrowth Syndrome

The anatomy and physiology of our alimentary tract ensure that we have first crack at the food we eat (Fig. 57.3). Thanks to the sterilizing power of the stomach

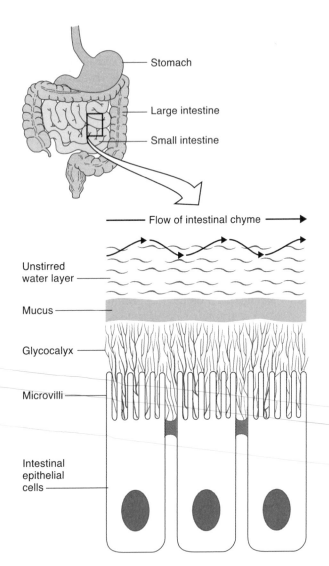

Figure 57.3. Schematic representation of host barriers faced by intestinal pathogens.

and the defenses of the small intestine, we absorb most of our nutrients without microbial competition. The upper intestinal contents, rich in unabsorbed sugars, fats, and other nutrients, do not normally come in contact with large numbers of bacteria.

The presence of a large microbial biomass in the absorptive small intestine leads to competition for certain vitamins and malabsorption of fats and produces a disease known as **bacterial overgrowth syndrome**. The study of bacterial overgrowth in the small intestine has helped us understand the normal relationship of the gut flora to gut function.

■ CASE 3

Two years before his current illness, Mr. O., a 65-year-old man, had an operation for removal of a tumor that ob-

structed his stomach outlet. The surgeon removed part of the stomach and duodenum and connected the remainder of the stomach with the jejunum (gastrojejunostomy), bypassing the unresected duodenum. Mr. O. subsequently developed chronic diarrhea and his weight dropped from 63 to 44 kg. His nutritional history indicated that his food intake was adequate and thus malnutrition could not account for the weight loss. The diarrhea had recently become bulky, smelly, and greasy. He felt fatigued, was short of breath on exertion, and had numbness and tingling in his hands and feet. On examination, he was extremely thin and appeared ill with a pale complexion.

Laboratory tests showed a severe anemia with large red blood cells ("megaloblastic" anemia) and leukopenia with many neutrophils with extra nuclear lobes. The serum level of vitamin A and its precursor, carotene, was depressed and that of vitamin B_{12} was undetectable, although intrinsic factor was present in his gastric juice. Specific tests of intestinal function revealed malabsorption. The diagnosis of bacterial overgrowth syndrome was made. (Although not done in this case, intubation of the small bowel might have revealed approximately 10^9 *Bacteroides fragilis* and 10^6 *E. coli* per ml of bowel content). Fat-soluble vitamins and vitamin B_{12} were replaced and Mr. O. was placed on a course of tetracycline. The diarrhea resolved and the tests of absorptive function improved. He continued on antibiotic therapy and, over the next several months, he returned to his normal weight and felt entirely well.

Pathobiology

Prior surgery left this patient with a loop of small bowel diverted from the main flow of intestinal contents. The result of this "blind loop" was stasis of the intestinal contents due to the lack of the continuous flushing action of the intestinal secretions. Bacterial proliferation occurred, leading to impaired absorption of fats and fat-soluble vitamins (see below).

Bacterial overgrowth in the small intestine may also arise from other causes, such as motor abnormalities that depress peristalsis (diabetic neuropathy, scleroderma, gastric atony), or gastric achlorhydria which permits large bacterial inocula to reach the proximal small bowel. Under these conditions, bacterial overgrowth occurs rapidly. As stagnation progresses, the small number of bacteria normally present increases dramatically. Careful anaerobic sampling of the small intestine in these conditions has revealed counts as high as 10^{10} bacteria/ml, levels comparable to those in the colon. By far, the most numerous bacteria and those most likely to be responsible for the physiological derangement are strict anaerobes, mainly *Bacteroides*.

Damage

Bacterial overgrowth in the small intestine may have the following effects:

- Increased fecal fat, or **steatorrhea** is due primarily to malabsorption of fat as a consequence of depletion of the bile acid pool. Why this depletion? Because bile acids such as cholic acid are normally conjugated with glycine or taurine in the liver, secreted in the bile, and reabsorbed in the terminal ileum in the conjugated form. The bacterial overgrowth flora can deconjugate these compounds, making them unavailable for reabsorption and ultimately depleting bile salts needed to form fat micelles necessary for fat absorption in the proximal gut.

- **Deficiency of vitamin B$_{12}$.** Normally, vitamin B$_{12}$ (or cobalamin) is bound to intrinsic factor from the stomach, and this complex is absorbed from the terminal ileum. With bacterial overgrowth, dietary B$_{12}$ is utilized by bacteria, making it unavailable for uptake by the host. With prolonged B$_{12}$ malabsorption (longer than 1 year), endogenous stores are depleted. Cellular systems with a high rate of turnover and DNA synthesis (bone marrow, central nervous system, gut epithelium) are severely impaired, and megaloblastic anemia and structural gut abnormalities may result. The epithelial villi are shortened due to decreased turnover and atrophy of enterocytes, decreasing the absorptive area. Thus, bacterial overgrowth sets off a cascade of malabsorptive events. Vitamin B$_{12}$ is also required for myelin synthesis, and its deficiency results in degeneration of the spinal cord, producing the classic neurological syndrome of pernicious anemia.

- **Diarrhea,** an increase in fecal water and electrolyte excretion above normal amounts. Diarrhea does occur in all patients with bacterial overgrowth. It usually results from the degradation by the normal flora of malabsorbed oligosaccharides reaching the colon. As a result, the concentration of osmotically active solutes increases. Water then moves across the mucosa to maintain isosmolarity and diarrhea occurs. Deconjugated bile salts in the colon can also cause diarrhea.

- **Malabsorption of vitamins A and D.** Malabsorption of fat-soluble vitamins, particularly A and D, causes severe visual disturbance (night blindness) and softening of the bones (osteomalacia). Interestingly, vitamin K deficiency does not usually occur. The reduced absorption of this fat-soluble vitamin is offset by the markedly increased vitamin production by the plentiful bacteria, ordinarily our main source of vitamin K.

Diagnosis and treatment

Bacterial overgrowth syndrome is usually diagnosed when malabsorption and nutritional deficiencies are present together with predisposing anatomic or physiological conditions, such as intestinal blind loops. Noninvasive breath tests are available to document the presence of the overgrowth flora in the proximal small bowel. Treatment requires correction of the surgical or medical predisposing condition in conjunction with careful nutritional repletion and, most importantly, broad-spectrum antibiotic therapy. Relapse may occur and repeated courses of therapy may be necessary.

Diarrhea and Dysentery

Diarrhea is the final common pathway of intestinal responses to many inciting agents, both infectious and noninfectious. Diarrhea is defined as an increase in the daily amount of stool water, although patients usually refer as much to the frequency of movements as to their consistency (see Chapter 16, "Secretory Diarrhea"). **Dysentery**, in contrast, is a distinctive syndrome involving the colon, in which a brisk inflammatory response results in abdominal pain and small-volume stools consisting of blood, pus, and mucus (see Chapter 17, "Invasive and Tissue-Damaging Enteric Bacteria"). Dysentery is a more severe problem than bloody diarrhea. Not only is its pathophysiology distinctive, but so too are the organisms involved, usually *Shigella* spp. Therapy is directed toward elimination of the pathogen using antibiotics, an issue now complicated by multiple antibiotic resistance.

In contrast, in recent years, foodborne outbreaks of bloody diarrhea have occurred primarily in young children and the elderly, associated with clinical signs due to formation of platelet-fibrin thrombi in the glomeruli or the brain. A group of *E. coli* that produce toxins related to Shiga toxin (from *Shigella dysenteriae* type 1), most notoriously *E. coli* O157:H7, are responsible. This is truly a new and emerging infectious disease.

The cases presented here illustrate distinctive ecological features of the pathogens and their interactions with the host.

■ CASE 4—*VIBRIO CHOLERAE*

Approximately 2 days after returning from Mardi Gras in New Orleans, Mr. V., a 24-year-old student who was the runner-up in the raw oyster eating contest, abruptly started to vomit. Within hours, he was restricted to the bathroom with voluminous and nearly continuous but painless watery diarrhea. Soon thereafter, he became lightheaded, with a rapid pulse and a feeling of marked lethargy and weakness. Later that evening, his roommate brought him to the emergency room, where he was found to be afebrile but profoundly dehydrated, with severely altered levels of serum electrolytes.

In the hospital, his stool was composed of an opaque fluid with small flecks of mucus, giving it a typical "rice water" appearance (so-called because it resembles the starchy water in which rice has been washed), and without a fecal, bloody, or bilious appearance. Although the diagnosis is often missed in the United States, the emergency room physician had worked in the Rwandan refugee camps and recognized the cholera syndrome. Vigorous intravenous rehydration was administered. When the fluid losses were repleted and the diarrhea rate slowed, fluid balance was maintained with an oral rehydration solution until the diarrhea ceased. The physician requested that the laboratory look for *V. cholerae,* and stool was cultured on a special medium called TCBS agar (TCBS = thiosulfate–citrate–bile salt sucrose). *V. cholerae* was isolated in 24 hours. No antibiotics were used, and by the end of the fourth hospital day, he was discharged with all symptoms and abnormalities resolved.

CASE 5—*SHIGELLA FLEXNERI*

Mr. T., a 26-year-old former Peace Corps worker in East Africa, returned from a visit to the village he had lived in with a low-grade temperature and mild watery diarrhea. The next morning his symptoms were worse, with a fever of 40.0°C; abdominal pain, mostly in the left lower quadrant; and the presence of blood in his stool. Mr. T. recognized the problem as *Shigella* infection and went to his local hospital. The infectious diseases clinician looked at the stool under light microscopy and noted the presence of sheets of neutrophils consistent with shigellosis. Mr. T. was given an oral fluoroquinolone agent and sent home with instructions to return if the symptoms worsened. The next day, *Shigella flexneri* was isolated and was found to be resistant to ampicillin and trimethoprim–sulfamethoxazole. The patient steadily improved over the next 48 hours.

CASE 6—*ROTAVIRUS*

M.A., a 7-month-old girl, was recently switched from breast to bottle feeding. Usually a satisfied and happy child, she became irritable, began to vomit, and had a low-grade fever. She also developed mild upper respiratory symptoms, with cough, nasal discharge, and pharyngitis. Watery diarrhea, without blood or leukocytes, developed, and persisted for 2 days. The infant was brought to the pediatrician who made the clinical diagnosis of rotavirus gastroenteritis. Specific laboratory tests, for example, detecting viral antigen in the stool with ELISA (enzyme-linked immunosorbent assay) were not performed because the insurance plan did not pay for such diagnostic tests. Fortunately, the pediatrician was convinced of the diagnosis and did not prescribe antibiotics. Instead, oral rehydration solution was given at home and M.A. made an uneventful recovery by the sixth day.

CASE 7—*YERSINIA ENTEROCOLITICA*

Mr. C. took his family to southern Sweden to visit his parents who were dairy farmers outside Malmö. S., 5 years of age, and I., 12 years of age, enjoyed helping their grand-

parents care for the numerous domestic animals on the farm and loved the home-cured meat and fresh raw milk served to them. Between 7 and 10 days after arrival, all members of the C. family became ill. S. developed watery, mucoid diarrhea with occasional flecks of blood, low-grade fever, and diffuse abdominal pain, all of which resolved spontaneously after 4 days. I.'s episode began similarly, but worsened after 3 days, when her pain localized to the right lower quadrant and became associated with high fever and leukocytosis. She was brought to the local hospital and a tentative diagnosis of acute appendicitis was made. During surgery, her appendix was found to be normal; however, the terminal ileum was inflamed, with many enlarged mesenteric lymph nodes.

Stool cultures done on admission were incubated at 25°C for several days before culturing, and these cultures grew *Y. enterocolitica.* By that time, I. had made a nearly complete recovery. Mr. C., like S., developed an acute mucoid diarrhea, abdominal pain, and fever that remitted by the fourth day. Three weeks later, he developed painful swelling of several joints and a painful raised rash over his shins (erythema nodosum). Despite a lack of gastrointestinal symptoms, his stool tested positive for *Yersinia* and he was treated with trimethoprim–sulfamethoxazole. The rash and arthritis slowly resolved but returned several months later and then spontaneously remitted for good.

CASE 8—*E. COLI O157:H7*

L.J., a 3-year-old girl, became ill 24 hours after eating at a fast-food hamburger restaurant, with cramps, fever, and mild watery diarrhea. Her pediatrician advised giving fluids but no antibiotic. The diarrhea turned bloody on day 3, and the child was hospitalized. Laboratory tests revealed moderate leukocytosis but no other abnormalities.

On day 5, *E. coli* O157:H7 was isolated from the initial stool culture. Laboratory studies the next day revealed a leukocytosis of 27,000 with 85% neutrophils and 5% bands, anemia (hematocrit of 30%), thrombocytopenia (34,000 platelets per μl), and an elevated creatinine of 88 μmol/L). Erythrocyte fragments characteristic of red cell damage secondary to endothelial cell injury (microangiopathic hemolytic anemia) were seen on the blood smear. Over the next 2 days, anemia, thrombocytopenia, and uremia progressed, without evidence of consumptive coagulopathy. These signs established the diagnosis of **hemolytic-uremic syndrome** (HUS). The patient required a week of hemodialysis for oliguria, hypertension, and uremia. She also required red cell and platelet transfusions, but then improved. She was discharged after 3 weeks, and by 3 months, all laboratory tests had returned to normal. She remains well after two additional years of follow-up.

Encounter

The list of intestinal pathogens is expanding as well-known organisms appear in unexpected frequency and in new settings, and as new organisms are recognized (Figs. 57.4 and 57.5, Table 57.2). In other chapters, we discuss some of the more common agents of intestinal infections (see Chapter 16, "Secretory Diarrhea"; Chapter 17," Invasive Enteric Bacteria"; Chapter 51, "Intestinal and Vaginal Protozoa"; Chapter 49, "Introduction to Parasitology"; and Chapter 52, "Intestinal Helminths"; food poisoning is discussed in Chapter 72). To this list we should add a few more. *Campylobacter jejuni*, formerly thought to be a rare cause of diarrhea in the United States, is now emerging as one of the most common, transmitted via poultry which are almost always colonized by this organism. Within the last several years, *Aeromonas hydrophila* and *Pleisomonas* spp. have become established as occasional agents of waterborne or shellfish-associated outbreaks. Other common agents of diarrhea here and abroad include the protozoan *Cryptosporidium* (see Chapter 51, "Intestinal and Vaginal Protozoa"), which was responsible for a massive waterborne outbreak in Milwaukee in 1993 involving almost half a million people and a newly described foodborne coccidian parasite, *Cyclospora cayetanensis* (transmitted in a 1996 U.S. outbreak via contaminated imported raspberries). Another protozoan group, microsporidia (including *Enterocytozoon bienensi* and *Septata intestinalis*), can cause chronic diarrhea in some AIDS patients. Viral diarrhea is common in all age groups. Viral diarrheal agents include rotavirus and others (calicivirus, astrovirus, enteric adenovirus) in normal

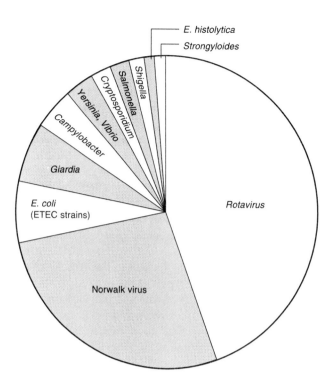

Figure 57.5. Distribution of agents of diarrhea in residents of the U.S.

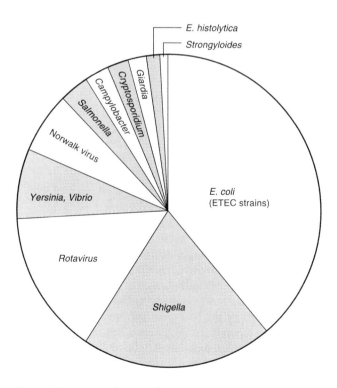

Figure 57.4. Distribution of agents of diarrhea in travelers to the U.S.

Table 57.2. Some Etiologic Agents of Diarrhea	
Organism	Source
Escherichia coli	Human feces–contaminated foods
Salmonella	Contaminated foods, especially poultry products
Shigella	Fecal–oral
Campylobacter	Farm animals, contaminated food (e.g., raw eggs)
Yersinia enterocolitica	Animal products
Vibrio cholerae	Water and shellfish
Vibrio parahemolyticus	Seafood (e.g., sardines, shellfish)
Bacillus cereus	Contaminated foods (e.g., recooked rice)
Clostridium perfringens	Contaminated foods (e.g., reheated meat)
Entamoeba histolytica	Fecal–oral and water
Giardia lamblia	Fecal–oral and water
Cryptosporidium, Cyclospora	Fecal–oral and water

young children, small-round structured viruses such as Norwalk virus in young normal adults, or viruses associated with diarrhea and inflammatory enteritis in immunocompromised patients (cytomegalovirus, herpes simplex virus). As the list of enteric pathogens lengthens and we begin to understand how they produce disease, the practical challenge of diagnosis and treatment increases.

The cases described illustrate the relationship of microbial ecology to the transmission of certain microorganisms. *V. cholerae* serogroup O1, long thought to be a human adapted pathogen, is actually a marine organism inhabiting coastal waters where it lives in association with plankton. In the United States, it is endemic in the Gulf of Mexico near New Orleans and in the Chesapeake Bay near the nation's capital. Because shellfish can concentrate bacteria present in the waters in which they live, Mr. V., the cholera patient, was no doubt infected by eating a large helping of contaminated oysters. He may have been at greater risk due to achlorhydria (which was not evaluated), or his meal may have been flavored by an unfortunately high concentration of the organisms.

In cholera endemic areas, infected persons can transport the organism to other areas and initiate epidemics of cholera where water and food cannot be protected and environmental sanitation is poor. These events occurred in Latin America in early 1993, resulting in over a million cases of cholera over the subsequent 2 years and approximately 5,000–10,000 deaths. It has recently been discovered that the segment of DNA that encodes cholera toxin is actually contained on a filamentous bacteriophage that infects the cholera bacteria. This bacteriophage is named CTX-ϕ. The possibility that a functional set of cholera toxin genes can be acquired by phage transduction raises questions about the safety of cholera vaccines based on deletions of the toxin gene. Attesting to the constant evolution of microbes and emerging diseases, a new epidemic serotype of *V. cholerae*, previously unknown and now designated O139 Bengal, was first detected in India in 1992 and spread in epidemic fashion beginning in 1993 (Fig. 16.1). The new strain resulted from deletion of O1 LPS synthesis genes and insertion of new LPS synthesis genes into the current pandemic serogroup O1 cholera strain. The O139 strain causes severe clinical cholera, and it continues to spread in Asia.

In contrast, *Shigella* is found only in close association with humans. Relatively few organisms are required to cause shigellosis (also known as bacillary dysentery). As a result, the disease readily spreads between persons in close contact. It is also typically a disease of children, and in the United States, the most common species, *Shigella sonnei*, is a common cause of watery diarrhea in infants and children in day-care centers. The species infecting Mr. T., *S. flexneri*, is no longer common in the United States, but remains important in developing countries, where *S. sonnei* is rare. *Y. enterocolitica* has yet another ecological characteristic; it is often zoonotic (acquired from infected animals, see Chapter 69 "Congenital and Neonatal Infections") and may be transmitted by drinking raw milk.

Diarrhea affecting infants who are younger than 2 years of age is most likely of viral etiology, with rotavirus by far the most common. In temperate regions, this diarrhea is seasonal and produces "winter vomiting disease"; in tropical zones, it occurs all year round. Adults may be infected when a child introduces the virus into the household, but they are usually asymptomatic, presumably because of preexisting immunity. In areas of the world where malnutrition is prevalent, severe diarrhea is associated with measles, which is highly contagious and kills large numbers of infants. The use of the measles vaccine in these populations may reduce the incidence of this life-threatening diarrhea.

A distinct group of enteric infections is also seen in male homosexuals. The special conditions of anal intercourse permit infection of the distal bowel with pathogens typically associated with sexually transmitted diseases. Proctocolitis due to *Neisseria gonorrhoeae, Chlamydia trachomatis,* herpes simplex virus, or *Treponema pallidum* has been recognized as the Gay Bowel Syndrome. The modifications of sexual practices among homosexual men initiated by the AIDS epidemic have diminished the frequency of these infections. More usual enteric pathogens, such as *Campylobacter, Shigella,* and *Entamoeba histolytica,* may be transmitted sexually on occasion via analingus.

Damage

The diarrheal disease pathogens have distinctive sets of virulence properties and preferentially attack specific areas of the bowel (Table 57.3). For this reason, we will consider the small and large intestine separately.

Small intestine. The mechanisms involved in diarrhea arising in the small intestine differ according to the type of pathogenic agent:

- Viruses that cause death of intestinal epithelial cells. The main agents are the rotaviruses (Case 6), Norwalk virus, and related viruses (e.g., Snow Mountain agent, and enteroviruses). These viruses cause diarrhea by destroying enterocytes at the villi, but they do not affect those in the crypts. Villus cells are sodium-absorbing cells, whereas crypt cells secrete chloride ions. Damage of villus cells leads to decreased sodium and water absorption, which results in net accumulation ("secretion") of fluid in the lumen and damage to the disaccharidase-containing microvillus membranes, leading to sugar malabsorption. Instead of being hydrolyzed locally and absorbed, these sugars enter the colon where they are metabolized by the bacterial flora to osmotically more active products. As a result fluid is drawn into the lumen, which worsens the diarrhea. It is also partly responsible for a postenteritic syndrome seen in children, in whom mild diarrhea persists for considerable time after the infection is resolved.
- Bacteria that colonize the upper small intestine, e.g.,

Table 57.3. Clinical Features of Diarrheal Disease

	Small bowel	Large bowel
Pathogens	*V. cholerae* *E. coli* (LT/ST strains) Rotavirus Norwalk agent (virus) *Giardia* *Cryptosporidium* *Cyclospora*	*Shigella* *E. coli* (EIEC, or invasive) *Campylobacter* *Entamoeba histolytica*
Location of pain	Midabdomen	Lower abdomen, rectum
Volume of stool	Large	Small
Type of stool	Watery	Mucoid
Blood in stool	Rare	Common
WBCs in stool	Rare	Common (except in amebiasis)
Proctoscopy	Normal	Mucosal ulcers; hemorrhagic friable mucosa

V. cholerae, and enterotoxigenic *E. coli*. In cholera and enterotoxigenic *E. coli* infections, diarrhea is secondary to the production of toxins by these organisms. These toxins activate the enzymes responsible for synthesis of cyclic nucleotide mediators (cAMP, cGTP), which, in turn, stimulate net chloride secretion and/or inhibit sodium uptake resulting in fluid loss. These mechanisms are discussed in detail in Chapter 9, "Damage by Microbial Agents."

■ Protozoa, *Giardia* and *Cryptosporidium*, which infect the small bowel (see Chapter 51, "Intestinal and Vaginal Protozoa"). It is not yet known if a toxin is involved in these infections, nor how these organisms colonize or invade the gut epithelium.

■ Bacteria that cause true food poisoning. This form of diarrhea occurs when toxigenic bacteria (e.g., *S. aureus, Bacillus cereus*) multiply in food some time before it is eaten. As a result toxins accumulate, and they are ingested along with the food. Because the signs and symptoms of food poisoning are not caused by bacterial multiplication in the body, the effects are often felt within a few hours after the tainted meal is eaten. Examples are discussed in Chapter 73, "Foodborne Diseases".

Clearly, not all infections of the small intestine produce a secretory diarrhea. Some organisms such as *Campylobacter jejuni* or *Y. enterocolitica* (as illustrated

by the C. family in Case 7) may infect the terminal ileum, producing a watery, sometimes bloody stool. The varied presentations of illness in the C. family also illustrate the age-related differences in disease caused by a single organism. *Y. enterocolitica* is unique in this respect, and little is known about the reasons for this diversity. *Y. enterocolitica* infects primarily the terminal ileum and colon in all patients, but in infants who are younger than 5 years of age, infection manifests as watery diarrhea. In older children, like S., bacteria from the intestine invade the mesenteric lymph nodes and cause focal inflammatory responses. Interestingly, diarrhea may be minimal or absent, and the mesenteric adenitis can mimic acute appendicitis. Many adults infected with *Y. enterocolitica* develop reactive arthritis within weeks after the onset of diarrhea. The same symptoms occur after *S. flexneri, C. jejuni*, and nontyphoidal *Salmonella* gastroenteritis. Reactive arthritis is probably an immunological phenomenon, as organisms are not found in the joint fluid. Interestingly, individuals affected most severely by arthritis often possess the histocompatibility antigen HLA-B27.

Large intestine. Bacterial pathogens that infect the large intestine tend to produce epithelial damage, mucosal inflammation, and bloody diarrhea or the dysentery syndrome. The major large bowel invasive pathogens causing dysentery are **Shigella** and the amebae *Entamoeba histolytica*. Because inflammation in shigellosis is prominent and is usually located in the distal large bowel, pain often worsens with bowel movements, a symptom known as tenesmus. The mucosa is easily damaged and looks ulcerated when examined by proctoscopy. Initially, the stools may be watery and substantial; later, they decrease in volume and consist of blood, mucus, and pus. White blood cells are typically scarce in amebic dysentery because they are lysed by a contact lysin produced by the amebic trophozoites present in the lesions. Certain bacteria (*Campylobacter, Salmonella*, and *Yersinia*) produce an inflammatory illness in the terminal ileum. This inflammation is associated with bloody diarrhea containing leukocytes. The inflammation occasionally extends to the colon, resulting in dysentery.

E. coli O157:H7 is a normal inhabitant of the intestine of meat and dairy cattle. In about 50% of cases, contaminated beef products, most often ground beef, is the source of infection. This organism, and a number of other serotypes of Shiga-toxin producing *E. coli* (STEC), infect the large bowel. They adhere to the colonic epithelial cell, causing a characteristic lesion in which the brush border is effaced by a dramatic change in cytoskeletal structures beneath the attached organism. This lesion causes diarrhea that appears to be almost pure blood; this characteristic syndrome is known as hemorrhagic colitis. A different disease is caused by *Clostridium difficile* and its toxins. *C. difficile* usually arises in infection after administration of antibiotics, which wipe out or alter the other resident flora. This infection is characterized by an adherent pseudomembrane with considerable mucosal inflammation and damage but without tissue invasion (see Chapter 20, "Clostridia").

Serious complications arise occasionally from infection of the colon by invasive organisms. Shigellosis may be associated with severe malnutrition, leading to a protein deficiency syndrome in children known as kwashiorkor. Shigellosis sometimes results in rectal prolapse or in a frequently fatal distention of the colon known as toxic megacolon, with a complete cessation of colonic peristalsis. Systemic complications may also occur, leading to clinical manifestations known as the hemolytic-uremic syndrome (HUS), leukemoid reactions with high white blood cell counts, encephalopathy, and others. Amebiasis may lead to intestinal perforation or obstruction, or the organisms may spread to produce abscesses in other organs, especially in the liver.

STEC infections are associated with the production of one of two related and potent toxins called Shiga toxin 1 or 2 (STX1 or STX2, but also called "Shiga-like toxins" or "Verotoxins"). These toxins appear to cross the intestinal mucosa and attack the endothelium of the intestinal lamina propria, the glomeruli, and the brain. The toxins cause HUS in children and a more prominent neurological disease in older adults, usually called thrombotic thrombocytopenic purpura, or TTP. HUS is associated with an immediate mortality rate of 5–10% and an unknown frequency of renal failure after many years. In the past TTP was usually fatal, but the mortality rate has dropped to 20% with improved therapy and the use of exchange transfusion.

OTHER GI INFECTIONS

Gut-associated Lymph Tissue

A different type of enteric infection is exemplified by typhoid fever (see Chapter 17, "Invasive and Tissue-Damaging Enteric Bacteria"). It is characterized by invasion of the gut-associated lymph tissue of the small bowel. From there, the organisms disseminate to the liver and spleen where the organism, *Salmonella typhi*, proliferates. When the number of organisms is sufficient, it enters the bloodstream, causing the persistent bacteremia and fever characteristic of enteric fever. Diarrhea may be absent or transient; some patients complain of constipation. Other characteristic findings are a low white blood cell count in relation to fever and enlargement of the liver and spleen. With sustained bacteremia, the organisms invade the lymphatic tissue of Peyer's patches and may cause severe inflammatory lesions, bleeding, and perforation. The mortality rate is high if the disease is untreated. Early use of effective antibiotics curtails the acute illness but predisposes to relapse, presumably by interfering with the protective immune response.

Surgical Complications of Intestinal Infections

Perforation of the wall of either the small or the large intestine may be caused by certain intestinal infections that induce inflammatory responses and tissue damage. Trauma, such as a penetrating knife injury or motor vehicle collision, may also cause perforation of the wall of the gut. Perforation results in spillage of intestinal contents into the normally sterile peritoneal cavity. The severity of the resulting peritonitis is generally related to the volume of the spill, its spread in the abdomen, and the ability of the omentum to wall off (contain) the abscess. A small amount of fecal contents may be handled by the defenses in the peritoneum, but a large inoculum can easily overwhelm them; the presence of blood worsens the response. These infections tend to be severe, and if untreated are often life-threatening. They are caused by a mixture of strict anaerobes, in particular *Bacteroides fragilis*, and facultative Gram-negative enterobacteriaceae. Peritonitis represent a classic therapeutic challenge, as it requires antibiotics for both groups of organisms. The pathogenic mechanisms are discussed in Chapter 15, "*Bacteroides*."

Diagnosis

Most patients with acute diarrhea have a mild and self-limited course and never seek medical attention. It is not practical or cost-effective to search for enteric pathogens in all patients with diarrhea. In a large percentage of cases, it is not warranted to do more than to replenish fluids and electrolytes, usually by oral rehydration and avoid the use of intravenous fluids unless the patient is in hypovolemic shock. A careful history of symptoms is the most important part of the investigation and often narrows the diagnostic possibilities. The clues that suggest disease requiring specific therapy (e.g., antimicrobial drugs) include fever, tenesmus, and persistent or severe abdominal pain (the triad of dysentery); weight loss; blood in the stool; recent antibiotic use; raw seafood meals; male homosexual practices; travel, especially to Mexico or other developing countries; and prolonged duration of symptoms.

Culturing of stool samples for enteric pathogens is primarily intended to isolate species of *Salmonella* and *Shigella*. Isolation or identification of other enteric pathogens requires special culture techniques, evaluation of serotype, or tests for toxin production that are not part of the laboratory routine (see Chapter 55, "Diagnostic Principles"). Animal parasites, protozoa, or helminths are detected by direct microscopy of fresh or appropriately preserved stools, but the specimens may require special concentration or staining procedures. Therefore, it is important to narrow the list of possible organisms that are sought. For example, if cholera is suspected, the laboratory should be instructed to inoculate the sample on to TCBS agar, which is not used in routine stool cultures. Similarly, if *E. coli* O157:H7 is suspected, the laboratory should inoculate a sorbitol-containing MacConkey agar (SMAC), because this serotype of *E. coli* is typically sorbitol nonfermenting, and it stands out from the other sorbitol fermenting *E. coli* of the normal flora. However, this test does not distinguish the non O157:H7 STEC, which are now known to be an important group of organisms that cause a disease similar to that caused by O157:H7. A commercial enzyme immunoassay is available to detect the STX toxins in stool produced by any STEC.

If nonbloody diarrhea persists or remains unexplained, tests for protozoa, especially *Giardia lamblia* and *Cyclospora* are indicated. If the patient is HIV-infected, samples should be examined for *Cryptosporidium parvum, Isospora belli*, or microsporidia species. Immunoassays to detect antigens of *Giardia* and *Cryptosporidium* are also available. *Cryptosporidium, Cyclospora*, or *Isospora* infection can also be readily diagnosed in stool or in biopsy specimens because these organisms are positive when stained by the acid-fast technique used for mycobacteria, an unusual feature among protozoa.

The clinical value of a particular test depends on whether or not the results will meaningfully affect the management of the patient. Sometimes the information is used not for treatment of the individual patient but to determine if special isolation measures are warranted. Thus, the presence of rotavirus in M.A.'s stool (Case 6) did not materially change the treatment plan. However, the positive ELISA test for rotaviruses suggested that if she were hospitalized or near other susceptible infants, she would have to be isolated from them.

Treatment

Most acute infectious diarrheas are mild, self-limited, and best treated with oral fluid replacement and continued feeding. The decision to employ specific antimicrobial or more aggressive intravenous replacement therapy is determined by the severity or duration of diarrhea or the presence of shock or dysenteric symptoms. In general, infections caused by toxigenic and invasive *E. coli, V. cholerae*, and *Shigella* are improved with antibiotics, but these infections often resolve before the diagnosis is made. The disadvantage of treating all infections with antibiotics is that these organisms may develop drug resistance. Also, antibiotic treatment (except for the use of new fluoroquinolones) may not alter the course and may also increase the risk of inducing a carrier state, with the potential of increased spread of the infection, as with *Salmonella*. Other specific antimicrobials are prescribed for *G. lamblia, E. histolytica, Cyclospora*, or *Isospora*. To date, *C. parvum* defies truly effective therapy.

Antidiarrheal agents may reduce the frequency of stools and improve their consistency, but no evidence suggests that these drugs shorten the course of the illness, or (with the exception of loperamide) reduce the volume of fluid lost. In fact, by decreasing gut transit time, antimotility agents may impair the clearance of the pathogens and, thus prolong the infection and enhance severity. In addition, anticholinergics or opiates may produce the life-threatening condition of intestinal stasis known as toxic megalocolon, especially in children and those with inflammatory diarrhea.

An important medical breakthrough has been the development of oral rehydration therapy for mild to moderate diarrhea. Following the discovery that sodium and glucose transport are coupled in the small intestine, it was observed that the oral administration of glucose with essential electrolytes dramatically accelerates absorption of sodium, with water following passively (i.e., without the expenditure of energy) to maintain osmolality. Moderate dehydration associated with cholera or other small bowel diarrheas should now be corrected with oral replacement. Even in severe dehydration, which requires rapid intravenous fluids to correct or prevent shock, oral rehydration may later be used alone for maintenance of adequate hydration. The impact of this simple concept on worldwide mortality from dehydration cannot be overstated, especially in the poorest areas of the world where the problem is prevalent and severe. In these areas, the use of intravenous therapy is too expensive and trained personnel are too scarce to provide it to more than a small proportion of patients. Technically uneducated people can be trained to mix the proper ingredients (sometimes using bottle caps as measuring devices) or to dissolve prepackaged mixtures. The recipe for oral rehydration is remarkably simple.

To one liter of water add:

½ teaspoon salt (3 g)
¼ teaspoon bicarbonate (1.5 g)
¼ teaspoon KCl (1.5 g)
4 tablespoons sugar (20 g)

SUGGESTED READINGS

ESOPHAGITIS
Sutton FM, Graham DY, Goodgame RW. Infectious esophagitis. Gastrointest Clin North Am 1994;4:713–729.
Wilcox CM, Karowe MW. Esophageal infections: etiology, diagnosis and management. Gastroenterologist 1994; 1:188–206.

GASTRITIS
Cave DR. Transmission and epidemiology of *Helicobacter pylori*. Am J Med 1996;100:12S–17S.
McGowan CC, Cover TL, Blaser MJ. *Helicobacter pylori* and gastric acid: biological and therapeutic implications. Gastroenterology 1996;110:926–938.
Mobley HL. Defining *Helicobacter pylori* as a pathogen: strain heterogeneity and virulence. Am J Med 1996;100:2S–9S.

BACTERIAL OVERGROWTH SYNDROME
Berg RD. Bacterial translocation from the gastrointestinal tract. Trends Microbiol 1995;3:149–154.

Riordan SM, McIver CJ, Duncombe VM, Bolin TD, Thomas MC. Factors influencing the 1 gram ^{14}C-D-xylose breath test for bacterial overgrowth. Am J Gastroenterol 1995;90: 1455–1460.

Thorens J, Blum A, Bille J, Gonvers JJ, Gyr K. Duodenal bacterial overgrowth during treatment in outpatients with omeprazole. Gut 1994;35:23–26.

INTESTINAL INFECTIONS

Angulo FJ, Swerdlow DL. Bacterial enteric infections in persons infected with human immunodeficiency virus. Clin Infect Dis 1995;21:S84–S93.

Dellert SF, Cohen MB. Diarrheal disease. Established pathogens, new pathogens, and progress in vaccine development. Gastroenterol Clin North Am 1994;23:637–654.

Echeverria P, Sethabutr O, Serichantalergs O. Modern diagnosis (with molecular tests) of acute infectious diarrhea. Gastroenterol Clin North Am 1993;22:661–682.

Mahon BE, Mintz ED, Greene KD, Wells JG, Tauxe RV. Reported cholera in the United States, 1992–1994: a reflection of global changes in cholera epidemiology. JAMA 1996;276:307–312.

Su C, Brandt LJ. *Escherichia coli* O157:H7 infection in humans. Ann Intern Med 1995;123:698–714.

Central Nervous System

Infections of the central nervous system (CNS) are relatively infrequent but can have extremely serious consequences. Untreated bacterial meningitis, for example, is fatal in over 70% of cases. Antibiotics have reduced mortality in these diseases to less than 10%, but this is still unacceptably high. In addition, some CNS infections in childhood leave serious **neurological sequelae** that impair mental development and produce sensory deficits.

From a microbiological point of view, the brain and the spinal cord have distinctive attributes: They are very well protected and isolated by the skull and the blood–brain barrier, but also highly vulnerable. In a limited space, the effects of infections tend to be magnified; even minor swelling and inflammation cause significant damage. This is especially true in view of the essential functions of the CNS. These two sides of the coin are also apparent on the physiological level; the **blood–brain barrier** inhibits passage of microorganisms and toxic substances into the brain and cerebrospinal fluid (CSF), yet the same barrier impedes the passage of humoral and cellular defensive elements from the blood. It also hinders the passage of many antimicrobial drugs, which sometimes narrows the therapeutic options.

To understand the pathogenesis and outcome of infections in this distinctive part of the body, you will need to recall general aspects of neuroanatomy and neurophysiology. The brain and spinal cord are suspended in the CSF and are surrounded by three layers of meninges: the pia mater and arachnoid, which constitute the leptomeninges, and the dura mater or pachymeninges (Fig. 58.1). Infections of the CNS can be grouped by the anatomic part of the brain affected. For example, infection of the brain parenchyma is **encephalitis**; infection of meninges, **meningitis**; and infection of spinal cord tissue, **myelitis**. This anatomic separation of CNS infections is somewhat artificial, because all of these areas are connected and may be infected at the same time. In many cases, therefore, it is more accurate to speak of meningoencephalitis or even meningomyeloencephalitis

Infections of the CNS may be caused by bacteria, viruses, fungi, or animal parasites that are either encountered in the environment or are members of the normal flora. The main types of infections and the most common etiologies are listed in Table 58.1. In almost all CNS infections, the causative agents were previously introduced into peripheral tissues of the host and traveled to the CNS either via the systemic circulation or via neural pathways. For instance, pathogens may have colonized the respiratory epithelium and penetrated it (e.g., the meningococcus) or entered the bloodstream via the bite of an arthropod (e.g., Eastern equine encephalitis virus), from the bite of a bat (e.g., rabies virus), or through the placenta (e.g., rubella virus). A third way that microorganisms may enter the CNS is by direct inoculation, usually associated with trauma. In certain infections, the organisms are lodged for a period of time within the CNS in a latent state and then manifest active disease some time in the future (e.g., tuberculosis or polyoma viruses).

ENCOUNTER

Infections of the CNS are caused by only a small number of the pathogens that infect humans. Thus, these organisms must possess special characteristics that permit them to localize in the CNS. The most frequent agents and the types of disease they cause fall into distinct categories. Certain bacteria (pneumococci, *Haemophilus influenzae,* meningococci) classically caused meningitis but rarely caused infections of brain parenchyma, whereas others (staphylococci, anaerobic streptococci) cause brain abscesses but seldom cause meningitis. Some viruses cause encephalitis (herpes simplex virus); others cause meningitis (enteroviruses).

Once inside the CNS, viruses sometimes localize in

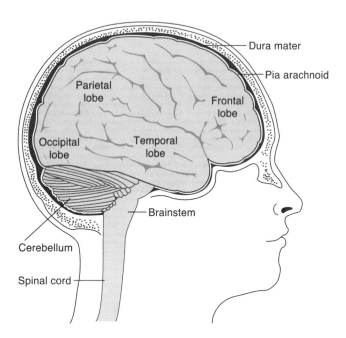

Figure 58.1. Gross anatomy of the cranium. The brain is located within a closed space, surrounded by the meninges (dura mater and pia arachnoid) in close approximation to mucosal surface containing commensal flora (the nasopharynx).

specific regions. Certain viruses show a marked **tropism** for certain neural cell types, e.g., polio for the motor neurons of the spinal cord and medulla, and mumps virus for the cells of the ependyma of the fetus. The basis for such tropism is probably the distribution of viral receptors on specific neural cells. Some clues regarding this point come from experiments with reoviruses. Depending on their type of surface hemagglutinin, reoviruses cause different kinds of severe infections of the CNS when they are injected into laboratory animals. There are two types of reoviral hemagglutinins, which differ in their ability to bind to receptors on distinct neural cells. Viruses with Type 1 hemagglutinin bind to ependymal cells, replicate, and cause inflammation at that site. Damage to the ependymal cells leads to occlusion of the ventricular aqueduct and thus to hydrocephalus (i.e., dilation of the ventricular system due to obstruction of CSF flow). In contrast, Type 3 viruses bind to neurons and cause a fatal encephalitis (without ependymal cell infection). Thus, the anatomic location of these viruses depends, at least in part, on the specificity of their surface proteins for host cell receptors. This, in turn, determines the type of disease produced.

Localization is also believed to be influenced by differences in blood flow. Does this explain why polio virus commonly infects the anterior horn cells of the spinal cord on the side of the dominant hand? Right-handed people are indeed more often affected on their right side, which may have greater blood flow.

Different bacteria cause CNS infections in patients of

different ages (Table 58.2). Thus, in the newborn, bacterial meningitis is most commonly caused by *Escherichia coli* and group B β-hemolytic *Streptococcus agalactiae*. Both are encapsulated strains. Over one-half of all *E. coli* strains have a capsule composed of **K1 antigen,** suggesting that neuropathogenic strains have been specially selected from the many antigenically distinct *E. coli* strains. In contrast to other *E. coli* capsular antigens, K1 is a **polysaccharide rich in sialic acid.** So are capsular polysaccharides of group B streptococci. Why sialic acid? Apparently, polysaccharides containing this compound aid in bacterial adherence (and growth) on the meninges. K1 antigen also has antiphagocytic properties and inhibits the alternative pathway of complement activation.

WHO, WHERE, AND WHEN

The most important epidemiological features of infections of the CNS are age, geographic location of the pa-

---

Table 58.1. Type of Central Nervous System Infection and Frequent Causative Agents

1. Acute meningitis
   Bacteria
   　　N. meningitidis
   　　H. influenzae, type b
   　　S. pneumoniae
   　　Group B streptococci
   　　E. coli
   　Viruses
   　　Mumps virus
   　　Enteroviruses
2. Chronic meningitis
   　M. tuberculosis
   　C. neoformans
   　Other fungi
3. Acute encephalitis
   　Viruses
   　　Arboviruses
   　　Herpesviruses
   　　Enteroviruses
   　　Mumps virus
4. Acute abscesses
   　Bacteria
   　　Staphylococci
   　　Mixed anaerobe/aerobe flora
   　　Group A or D streptococci
5. Chronic abscesses
   　Bacteria
   　　M. tuberculosis
   　Fungi
   　　C. neoformans
   　Animal parasites
   　　Cysticercus (*Taenia*)

Table 58.2. Etiology of Bacterial Meningitis

Age	Underlying disease	Bacterial pathogen	
		Most common	Other
Birth–2 mo	None	*Streptococcus agalactiae* (group B)	Escherichia coli Listeria monocytogenes
2–60 mo	None	*Haemophilus influenzae*	*Neisseria meningitidis* *Streptococcus pneumoniae*
>60 mo	None	*Streptococcus pneumoniae*	*N. meningitidis* *
Any age	Cranial surgery	*Staphylococus aureus*	*Staphylococcus epidermidis*
Any age	Immunosuppression from cancer chemotherapy	Streptococci	*E. coli* *Pseudomonas aeruginosa* Klebsiellae

* Occurs in epidemics.

Table 58.3. Viruses Causing Encephalitis

Virus	Geographic location	Major age group	Predominant season	Notable features
Herpes simplex	All	All	None	Focal symptoms
St. Louis encephalitis	All	Older Adults	Summer–fall	Most cases mild
Eastern equine encephalitis	East coast and Texas	Children	Summer–fall	Disabling sequelae
Western equine encephalitis	West of Mississippi	Infants to children	Summer–fall	
California equine encephalitis	East of Mississippi	Older children	Summer–fall	
Enteroviruses	All	Infants to children	Summer	Severity inverse to age
Rabies	All	All	All	Animal bite
Varicella	All	Children	Winter	Rare
HIV	All	Adults	All	Dementia in AIDS patients

tient, and the time of the year. For example, encephalitis in infants is more likely to be due to enteroviruses, because enteroviruses are spread by the fecal–oral route and children are more likely to come in contact with contaminated feces (Chapter 34, "Picornavirus"). In adults, encephalitis is more likely to be due to arboviruses (Table 58.3). Spread of arboviruses by arthropods also has seasonal variations, which follow the life cycle of the vectors (Chapter 33, "Arthropod-borne Viruses"). Overall, herpes simplex virus is the most common cause of viral encephalitis in adults and it does not have a specific seasonal distribution. The geographic distribution of some of these viruses is well illustrated by the names given to the diseases caused by arboviruses (Eastern, Western, Japanese encephalitis, etc.) This is sometimes misleading. For example, although St. Louis encephalitis was first studied in that city, it is the arbovirus disease most commonly encountered throughout the U.S.

In addition to acute encephalitis, in which the symptoms coincide with viral invasion of the CNS, there is also **postinfectious encephalitis,** and "slow virus" CNS infection. Postinfectious encephalitis appears to come about by two mechanisms— persistent infection of cells of the CNS by viruses in a latent state, or an autoimmune reaction to sequestered CNS-specific antigens. In certain types of postinfectious encephalitides, both mechanisms appear operative. Chronic progressive, uniformly fatal CNS infections are believed to be caused by a group of agents called **prions,** which are not viruses but misfolded proteins (see Chapter 34, "Paramyxovirus"). **Creutzfeldt-Jakob disease** (CJD) and **kuru** are human examples of what are believed to be prion infections and there are similar diseases in animals (e.g., **bovine spongiform encephalopathy** or "mad cow disease" and **scrapie** in sheep). Patients who develop an illness characterized by primary immune deficiency (i.e., Hodgkin's disease), or who become immune deficient secondary to anticancer chemotherapy, can develop a **progressive multifocal**

leukoencephalopathy (PML). PML is caused by activation of a polyomavirus called JCV. JCV is usually acquired early in childhood, when it causes a self-limited disease; the virus then becomes latent within the CNS. Immune suppression subsequently permits renewed viral replication and progressive disease.

ENTRY

Hematogenous Route

Most cases of CNS infection are caused by entry of the organisms from the **circulation** (Fig. 58.2). The precise mechanism by which organisms penetrate the blood–brain barrier is not known. It is presumed that the **choroid plexus**, the site where most of the CSF is formed, provides the most common site of entry. These structures are highly vascular, and inflammation on the blood side may result in the spillage of microorganisms into the CNS side. The likelihood of CNS infection is generally correlated with the microbial load of the blood. Certain viruses (e.g., rubella) can also be delivered to the CNS during the neuroma phase of the illness (see Chapter 34, "Paramyxovirus").

Neural Route

Although most neurotropic viruses also reach the CNS by the circulation, a few utilize special neural path-

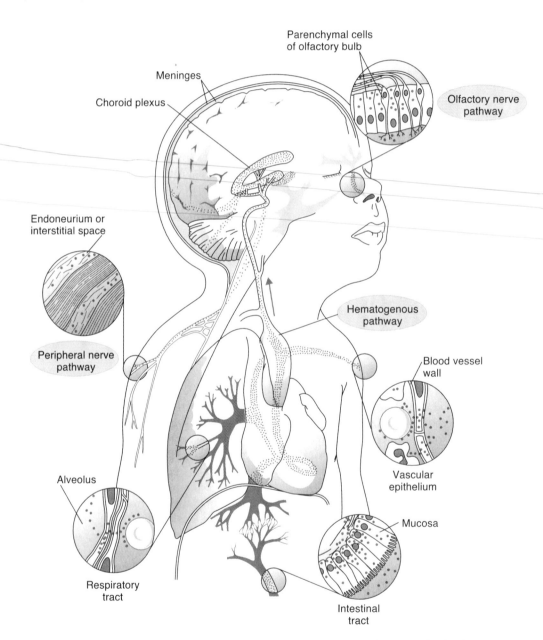

Parenchymal cells of olfactory bulb

Meninges

Choroid plexus

Olfactory nerve pathway

Endoneurium or interstitial space

Hematogenous pathway

Peripheral nerve pathway

Blood vessel wall

Vascular epithelium

Mucosa

Alveolus

Respiratory tract

Intestinal tract

Figure 58.2. Pathways of entry of agents that cause CNS infections. In bloodborne infections, agents from the respiratory tract, gut, or vascular epithelium enter via the choroid plexi. Inside the CNS, they spread either by contiguity or through extracellular spaces. Some neurotropic viruses reach the brain via peripheral nerves or olfactory nerve endings.

ways (Fig. 58.2). The best known case of neural transmission is **rabies**, where the virus travels to the anterior horns of the spinal cord via peripheral nerves. Rabies virus enters the axon of a peripheral nerve and travels to neuronal perikaryon in retrograde fashion, presumably on a microtubular filament. Another well-known example of neural transmission is herpes simplex virus (HSV), where the virus ascends via the trigeminal nerve root (Chapter 41, "Herpesvirus"). As mentioned above, experimental studies with reoviruses showed that the choice of the hematogenous or the neural route depends on genetic differences in the viral hemagglutinin.

A speculative but intriguing notion is that viruses and other infectious agents may penetrate the body via the olfactory nerve endings, which are the only elements of the nervous system in direct contact with the exterior. Experimental studies suggest that herpes viruses may reach the brain by this route. The ameba *Naegleria fowlerii*, which causes a rare but lethal meningoencephalitis, is also thought to penetrate the CNS by trauma to the cribriform plate, as might happen when a person dives into water containing these amebae.

SPREAD AND MULTIPLICATION

Once a pathogen has reached the CNS, it finds itself in a relatively sequestered compartment that does not have as ready a recourse to defense mechanisms as most other regions of the body. For example, complement levels are very low in the CSF, apparently due to poor penetration from the blood, and also because the CSF contains a substance that partially inactivates complement. Therefore, lysis or phagocytosis of bacteria does not readily occur in the brain, the meninges, and the CSF. However, the CNS is not as immunologically restricted as was once supposed. It possesses an intrinsic immunological surveillance mechanism in the **microglia**. Microglia have many surface markers identical to peripheral blood monocytes, suggesting that the latter migrate to the brain to evolve into microglia. In addition, it is now believed that the CNS has a lymphlike system consisting of the Virchow-Robin spaces (the perivascular sheaths surrounding the blood vessels as they enter the brain). These spaces contain macrophages and lymphocytes and are thought to be the site where these cells enter the CSF. Does the existence of these mechanisms suggest that infections of the CNS are more frequent than is believed, but are often kept in check by host defenses?

DAMAGE

Tissue dysfunction in CNS infections is caused in a variety of ways. Death of host cells may be due directly to the action of bacterial toxins, to lytic cycles of viral replication, or as the result of intracellular growth of bacteria and fungi. In most infections, however, cell death and tissue destruction result from the host's own inflammatory response. The multiplication and spread of microorganisms in the CNS elicits an inflammatory response similar to but generally less intense than that seen in other areas of the body. Characteristic of inflammation of the CNS are infiltration of microglia and proliferation of **astrocytes**. As in other parts of the body, the inflammatory response of the CNS has both a humoral and a cellular component. The humoral component develops first and consists of edema caused by increased capillary permeability. Neutrophils and macrophages then infiltrate the area and phagocytize microorganisms as well as dead cells. Neutrophils often lyse in the process, releasing enzymes that digest cells and tissue material in the immediate area.

Swelling of the brain due to inflammation within the closed cranial vault (cerebral edema) may, by itself, produce cerebral cortical symptoms from decreased capillary perfusion. More severe forms of cerebral edema can cause herniation of the temporal lobe through the falx, or of the brainstem into the foramen magnum, producing severe brain damage or death. Thus, neurological symptoms that arise during infection of the CNS may be due to focal tissue lesions, which produce specific functional deficits, or to cerebral edema that leads to a global loss of higher cerebral cortical function.

The functional characteristics of the CNS often help diagnose specific kinds of infections and identify the areas involved. For example, psychosis, impairment of memory, and seizures suggest herpes simplex encephalitis (because of the preferred involvement of the temporal lobe); stiffness of the neck without severe impairment of cerebral function is characteristic of enteroviral meningitis; flaccid paralysis of the lower extremities suggests polio virus infection of the motor neurons of the spinal cord. Figure 58.3 depicts focal symptoms produced by certain CNS infections.

The following case histories and discussion describe characteristic infections of the CNS and their diagnosis. They include cases of meningitis, acute encephalitis, postinfectious or late encephalitis, and brain abscess.

MENINGITIS

The majority of cases of meningitis can be classified in the following ways:

- By clinical presentation: acute, subacute, or chronic;
- By etiology: bacterial, fungal, or viral;
- By epidemiology: sporadic or epidemic.

Acute meningitis is caused by bacteria, chiefly *E. coli* and group B streptococci in young infants, meningococci and pneumococci in children, and pneumococci in adults. *H. influenzae* type b used to be the most common cause of bacterial meningitis. However, the introduction of vaccines in the mid 1980s in which the type b carbo-

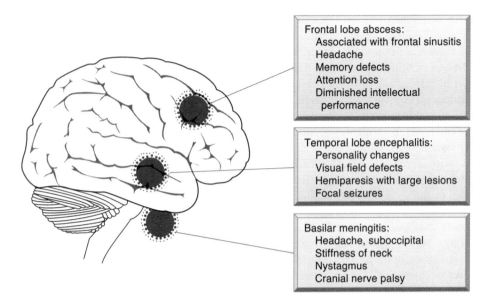

Frontal lobe abscess:
Associated with frontal sinusitis
Headache
Memory defects
Attention loss
Diminished intellectual
performance

Temporal lobe encephalitis:
Personality changes
Visual field defects
Hemiparesis with large lesions
Focal seizures

Basilar meningitis:
Headache, suboccipital
Stiffness of neck
Nystagmus
Cranial nerve palsy

Figure 58.3. Anatomic basis of localization of symptoms in CNS infections. Focal involvement of cerebral cortex produces specific signs and symptoms depending on the primary function of that part of the brain. In contrast, pyogenic meningitis produces global cerebral cortical dysfunction due to diffuse cerebral edema.

hydrate capsule was covalently linked to protein vaccinogens (tetanus or diphtheria toxoids) made them immunogenic in young infants. The presence of antibody directed against the type b capsule confers immunity against *H. influenzae* b infection. Subacute or chronic meningitis is usually caused by fungi (mainly *Cryptococcus)* or by tubercle bacilli (all organisms that cause chronic inflammatory, granulomatous tissue reactions). Below we discuss an outbreak of meningococcal meningitis.

▮ CASE

Outbreak of Acute Meningitis

One week after arriving at the Army recruit camp at Fort Ord (California), Pvt. T.A. had become the first of three cases of meningitis. He had a precipitous onset of fever and headache and felt a pain in his neck when he moved his head. On lumbar puncture, his pressure was slightly elevated, 220 mm H_2O (the normal range is <150 mm H_2O). A smear of the CSF revealed small Gram-negative coccobacilli and numerous leukocytes (Fig. 58.4). A culture grew the meningococcus, *Neisseria meningitidis.* Two weeks after intravenous administration of penicillin G, Pvt. T.A. nearly completely recovered. At this time, Pvt. F.H. developed the same symptoms and was admitted to the hospital. When Pvt. B.W. was diagnosed the next morning with the same illness, the remaining soldiers in the camp became alarmed. Their fears calmed when the medical corps personnel explained that this meningococcal meningitis "epidemic" would be stopped by the prophylactic administration of antibiotics to all.

At about the same time, Pvt. V.L. was assigned to Fort

Leonard Wood (Missouri). When he arrived, he had a fever, slight headache, and some nausea. The next day, when putting on his boots, he noticed that his neck was stiff. When he went to the infirmary, he immediately had a lumbar puncture: the CSF pressure was 90 mm H_2O, in the normal range, and the fluid contained 76 neutrophils/μl, 80 mg/dl of protein (an elevated value), and 66 mg/dl of glucose, also in the normal range. He was observed in the hospital for 3 days and was discharged with a diagnosis of aseptic meningitis when his CSF proved to be sterile and his symptoms resolved.

Why did meningococcal meningitis, the illness of Pvt. B.W., produce alarm and call for preventive measures, whereas aseptic meningitis, that of Pvt. V.L., was just observed? How does the pathobiology of these diseases differ and how can they be differentiated?

Encounter and Entry

Meningococci are acquired by inhalation of aerosol droplets from asymptomatic human carriers. It is likely that, in the outbreak at Ford Ord, most of the recruits were exposed to the organisms from another individual, since meningococci are found in the oropharynx of about 10% of healthy people. The frequency of colonization does not, however, always correlate directly with outbreaks, because individual strains of meningococci vary considerably in virulence. The reason why so many people become colonized but only a few get sick is not truly known. The best clue comes from the observation that susceptible individuals lack antibodies against the meningococcal capsular antigen, whereas carriers have protective antibodies. There is also a striking association between congenital deficiency in the late components of the complement cascade and neisserial infection, particularly with meningococci. These findings suggest that the immunological repertoire of an individual plays a role in determining whether he or she manifests the disease.

Spread, Multiplication, and Damage

Meningococcal meningitis may be a distinct clinical event, such as in the cases of the soldiers at Fort Ord, but it may also follow an overwhelming septicemia caused by these organisms. In such cases, the symptoms of meningitis only add to an already grave clinical picture; the presence of large numbers of organisms in the blood causes severe non-neural manifestations, such as shock and intravascular coagulation. These signs are due to the high blood content of Gram-negative endotoxin. In such cases, it is proper to speak of **meningococcal septicemia**, rather than meningococcal meningitis.

The clinical manifestations of acute meningitis, caused by meningococci or other bacteria, are fever, a stiff neck (nuchal rigidity), headache, and occasionally global focal CNS dysfunctions. These symptoms are caused by the inflammatory response to meningeal invasion. Pus in the subarachnoid spaces may spread over the brain, the cerebellum, and the spinal cord. It tends to be particularly thick in pneumococcal infections and those due to Enterobacteriaceae, which leads to blockage of various foramina and increased CSF pressure. In meningococcal meningitis, the CSF pressure is usually only slightly elevated. Increased intracranial pressure due to cerebral edema invariably makes the patient vomit, as well as have a severe headache. The extent of inflammation varies considerably, with the intrinsic virulence of the strains and the immune state of the patient. Severe signs and symptoms of meningeal irritation, "meningismus," include involuntary extension of the neck and back to prevent stretching of the dura at the point where spinal nerves exit the spinal foramina. Additional symptoms, such as altered vision, may be caused by compression of the nerves that emanate from the base of the brain. Spasm or thrombosis of blood vessels may lead to small or large strokes.

In general, meningitis leaves fewer traces when caused by meningococci than by the other bacteria. *H. influenzae* meningitis is often followed by mental retardation, deafness, or both. Sequelae from pneumococcal meningitis tend to be severe and frequent. Some of these deficits are cortical, presumably because of decrease in cerebral cortical blood flow during the acute stages of the disease.

Diagnosis

An acute infection of the CNS presents a diagnostic problem of grave urgency. Saving the life of a child with meningococcal meningitis sometimes requires instituting proper therapy within minutes. Fortunately, examination of a Gram stain of the CSF obtained by lumbar puncture can rapidly yield a presumptive diagnosis. Examination of the CSF is absolutely necessary when acute meningitis is suspected. Table 58.4 shows the pattern of inflammation in the CSF in various CNS infections.

The elements of inflammatory response in the CSF can also help in determining whether the infection is likely to be bacterial or viral and even in suggesting specific infectious agents. A large number of neutrophils points to a bacterial infection, whereas the predomi-

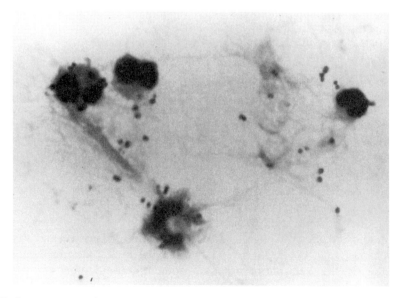

Figure 58.4. Gram stain of CSF from a patient with meningococcal meningitis. Gram-negative coccobacilli and neutrophils are evident.

Table 58.4. Usual Composition of the Cerebrospinal Fluid in Various Infections

	None	Acute bacterial meningitis	Fungal and viral meningitis	Herpes encephalitis	Brain abscess
Leukocytes (no./μl)	0–6	>1000	100–500	10–1000	10–500
% Neutrophils	0	>50	<10	<50	<50
Red blood cells (no./μl)	0–2	0–10	0–2	10–500	10–400
Glucose (mg/dl)[a]	40–80	<30	≤40	>30	>40
Protein (mg/dl)	20–50	>100	50–100	>75	50–100

[a] Diagnostic values are best interpreted as the ratio of glucose levels in blood of those in the CSF.

nance of lymphocytes suggests a viral etiology. Recall that the symptoms of Pvt. B.W. were almost identical to those of Pvt. V.L.; the nature of their illnesses was discerned by CSF examination. Gram stain examination of the spinal fluid should be a routine procedure because it reveals infecting bacteria in about 50% of the cases of meningitis.

Culture of CSF can definitively establish the etiology of meningitis and is also useful for choosing the specific antibiotics. More rapid tests are based on identification of unique microbial constituents in the CSF. Most of these tests involve detecting a specific antigen, such as bacterial or fungal capsular polysaccharides (see Chapter 55, "Diagnostic Principles"). These tests are commonly used, as the reagents (specific antisera and an indicator system) are readily available. It is also possible to identify a specific bacterium by detecting a species-specific gene, but the more technically demanding DNA-based tests have not replaced the easily performed antigen detection.

Prevention and Treatment

Vaccination against meningococci is limited to high-risk groups, such as military recruits. Currently, U.S. military personnel receive a meningococcal vaccine when they arrive in a recruit camp. The vaccine contains capsular polysaccharides of Type A and C meningococci, the most common types to cause meningococcal epidemics, plus two rare types. An effective vaccine against Type B meningococci, which cause the majority of cases of meningococcal meningitis in the U.S., is not available. However, even if it were available, it would probably not be used because most of these cases are sporadic and do not occur often enough to warrant widespread vaccination. Chemoprophylaxis with rifampin or minocycline eradicates nasopharyngeal carriage in 90% of the recipients.

To treat bacterial meningitis effectively, antibiotics to which the bacteria is susceptible must penetrate the CSF in an active form. β-Lactams are usually administered for the common forms of bacterial meningitis. These drugs are highly polar and enter the CSF poorly by diffusion through the blood–brain and blood–CSF barriers. The average drug concentration in CSF normally achieved is 15% that of serum. However, β-lactams also enter the CSF through capillary leaks enhanced by inflammation, thus allowing these drugs to reach therapeutic levels in patients with meningitis. It has been estimated that for the drugs to be effective, it is necessary to achieve a CSF concentration that is eight to ten times that of the minimal bactericidal concentration (MBC) measured in the laboratory. The reason for this requirement is not really known.

Newer β-lactams, such as **cefotaxime** and **ceftriaxone**, are very potent and produce CSF concentrations that exceed the MBC by 20-fold or more. As the inflammation resolves, the β-lactam concentration decreases but is still adequate to sterilize the CSF. Other antibiotics, such as **chloramphenicol** and **tetracycline,** are lipophilic and diffuse readily across blood–brain and blood–CSF barriers. They achieve effective CSF concentrations independent of the presence or magnitude of the meningeal inflammation and are bactericidal against *H. influenzae* and meningococci. Chloramphenicol, however, may produce a serious side effect, and its serum levels should be monitored (a practice that may be prohibitive in economically disadvantaged countries). Tetracycline may cause permanent discoloration of the teeth, mitigating its administration to young children.

An important aspect of the treatment of meningitis is to control the increased intracranial pressure. Cerebral edema may further decrease the already diminished cerebral blood flow and depress oxidative glucose metabolism. Death may ensue from compression of the brainstem into the foramen magnum (i.e., herniation). Supportive measures must ensure that the patient is adequately oxygenated and that blood glucose is in the normal range. Dexamethasone, a glucocorticoid with potent anti-inflammatory activities, has been shown to decrease the incidence of deafness occurring as a sequelae of *H. influenzae* meningitis. Dexamethasone may have the same beneficial effect on meningitis due to the pneumococcus and other bacteria when the disease occurs in children. It is not known if dexamethasone improves the outcome of meningitis in newborns or the aged. Rapid institution of antibiotic therapy is of utmost importance. Antibiotics should be administered intravenously very early and in doses high enough to achieve adequate CNS concentrations. Bacterial meningitis is a true medical emergency.

VIRAL MENINGITIS

Viremia gives viruses the opportunity to invade the CNS and cause so-called **aseptic meningitis.** This traditional term means only that the CSF is sterile on routine bacteriological culture. The term is also used for infections by other agents that do not grow on the usual bacteriological media (e.g., fungi, leptospira, *Treponema pallidum).* Aseptic meningitis may also have noninfectious etiology such as certain cancers or cerebral collagen–vascular disease. In viral meningitis, the brain is usually involved as well, and the illness, therefore, should be described as a meningoencephalitis. However, the meningeal signs (stiff neck and headache) are more prominent than those of cerebral involvement.

Viral meningitis can be distinguished from bacterial meningitis because it produces a milder disease with low to moderate inflammatory reaction in the CSF consisting primarily of lymphocytes. Pvt. V.L. had the clinical disease and CSF findings typical of viral and not fungal meningitis (chiefly, a large number of leukocytes and normal glucose level; see Table 58.4). For this reason, antibiotics were not administered and he was only observed in the hospital. His improvement without antibacterial or antifungal treatment further points to a viral etiology. If Pvt. V.L. had not improved, another cause for his symptoms and the presence of leukocytes in the CSF would have had to be found. Viral meningitis can be proved by isolation of a virus from the CSF. However, viral isolation is seldom accomplished early enough to aid in treatment. Isolating a virus known to cause aseptic meningitis from the throat or stool of a patient with appropriate symptoms suggests, but does not prove it is the etiology of aseptic meningitis.

In infants less than 1 year of age, it is often difficult to distinguish bacterial from aseptic meningitis. The newborn has a limited repertoire of immune responses when the CNS is infected, and the relative immaturity of its reticuloendothelial system may not permit an adult-type inflammatory response. The presence of bacterial polysaccharide in the CSF helps make this distinction. However, the absence of bacterial antigens does not eliminate the diagnosis of bacterial meningitis. As a result, most infants with the symptoms of acute meningitis and leukocytes in the CSF are treated with antibiotics.

CHRONIC MENINGITIS

CASE

Ms. L., a 32-year-old woman, immigrated to the U.S. 1 year ago from the Solomon Islands with her husband and three children. Four weeks later, her oldest child came home from day care with chickenpox. Two weeks later, she and the rest of the family also developed the disease. As her rash faded, she developed a headache and again had fever. Over the next week, she lost her appetite and vomited a few times. These symptoms persisted for an additional week and she became apathetic. When she became stuporous 4 days later, she was taken to a hospital.

The diagnosis of varicella (chickenpox) encephalitis was considered, but because her chickenpox began a month previously, this diagnosis was unlikely. Invasion by this virus would have occurred earlier, during active disease. On physical examination, she was deaf in her right ear and the right side of her face was paralyzed. A chest radiograph showed a right upper lobe pneumonia. A technetium-99 brain scan showed increased uptake at the base of her brain, and a cranial CT indicated increased intracranial pressure. A lumbar puncture revealed a CSF pressure of 310 mm H_2O (highly elevated) and 350 leukocytes/μl, of which 87% were lymphocytes, and a protein concentration of 168 mg/dl (elevated) . A Gram stain and an acid-fast stain did not show any organisms, but the CSF contained a lipid typical of tubercle bacilli, tuberculostearic acid, which allowed the diagnosis of tuberculous meningitis (see Chapter 23, "Mycobacteria"). Subsequently, *Mycobacterium tuberculosis* grew from her CSF and was found to be susceptible to streptomycin, rifampin, and isoniazid. Ms. L. was treated with these agents for 6 weeks and was then discharged, to continue on oral rifampin and isoniazid for an additional 9 months.

Pathobiology

Ms. L. came from a geographic region in which pulmonary tuberculosis is endemic. During primary pulmonary infection, tubercle bacilli were deposited in many organs (including the brain), where they were contained within granulomas. Ms. L.'s chickenpox suppressed her cell-mediated immunity, and the tubercle bacilli were now able to multiply and cause inflammation. In the brain, granulomas located near the ventricles spilled tubercle bacilli into the CSF. The organisms then spread throughout the subarachnoid space, and, for unknown reasons, became most prevalent in the basilar cisterns. As cell-mediated immunity returned, it elicited an intense delayed hypersensitivity-type reaction to the organisms. Granulomas formed around cranial nerves caused them to malfunction. In Ms. L.'s case, the nerves affected were cranial VII and VIII (as indicated by deafness and paralysis of the side of the face, respectively). Inflammation of the meninges compromised her cerebral blood flow, leading to the stupor (which could have progressed to coma). Ms. L.'s CSF findings and indolent course were consistent with chronic meningitis and both fungi and *M. tuberculosis* had to be considered. The presence of a **tubercular lipid** (tuberculostearic acid) in the CSF made the diagnosis of tuberculous meningitis likely, and it was confirmed by the isolation from the CSF of *M. tuberculosis*.

Because the diagnosis of tuberculous meningitis is so important, DNA-based methods have been developed. Using primers specific for certain genes of *M. tuberculosis*, the organism can be rapidly detected in CSF. DNA-based methods, although technically sophisticated, are less cumbersome than the gas chromatographic techniques used to detect tuberculostearic acid.

ENCEPHALITIS

Acute encephalitis is almost invariably caused by a virus, with HSV the most frequent in the U.S., followed by the togaviruses (encephalitis viruses). These viruses are listed in Table 58.3 and described in detail in Chapter 41, "Herpesvirus" and Chapter 33, "Arbovirus." They cause serious illnesses which, if untreated, have mortality rates of 75% or greater. Fortunately, herpes simplex encephalitis can be treated if diagnosed early.

Herpes Simplex Encephalitis

Ms. H., a 19-year-old woman living in the inner city, was brought to the emergency room by her mother because she was "acting funny." Her mother reported that, on arising, she thought "there were devils in the room," and she nearly destroyed her bedroom trying to escape them. On her way to the hospital, Ms. H. hallucinated intermittently, telling her mother that she was smelling roses. Three days previously, she had had some mild nausea and vomiting. In the emergency room, her urine was found to contain "angel dust" (phencyclidine) and she was admitted to the psychiatric ward. There she was noted to have a low-grade fever and received a phenothiazine tranquilizer (haloperidol). After 2 days, she had a generalized seizure and then became comatose.

Because convulsions are not associated with phencyclidine intoxication and are not a side effect of phenothiazines, it was likely that Ms. H. had a CNS infection. Her fever and seizures made this suspicion more probable. CSF obtained by lumbar puncture contained 280 erythrocytes and 350 mononuclear leukocytes/μl. The glucose content was in the normal range (48 mg/dl) and the protein concentration was elevated (126 mg/dl; see Table 58.4 for normal values). A technetium-99 scan showed increased uptake in the left temporal lobe, indicating involvement of brain tissue (see under "Diagnosis"). In light of her recent neurological history, these findings prompted a biopsy of the temporal lobe, a preferred site for HSV. A tissue sample was sectioned and,

upon examination by immunofluorescent microscopy, indicated the presence of herpes simplex antigen. Herpes virus grew in cell cultures inoculated with the biopsy material. Ms. H. was treated with acyclovir for 2 weeks, which halted the progression of her neurological symptoms, but she had many residual signs of neurological impairment, which needed extensive rehabilitation therapy.

Pathobiology

Herpes simplex encephalitis is not a common disease, although it is the most common of the severe encephalitides. It usually follows the chronic latent infection characteristic of this virus. Genital herpes may also produce infection of the lower spinal cord and meninges, but this progression is rare. It is not known why, in some individuals, the virus travels centripetally (up the nerve) from the trigeminal ganglia, instead of following the more usual centrifugal route to the vermilion border of the lip. Fibers emerging from the trigeminal ganglia innervate the dura of the middle and anterior fossae and the meningeal arteries of the area. HSV may use this route to spread to the meninges and meningeal arteries and, from there, to the meningeal nerves and the contiguous cortex. This postulated pattern may explain the frequent localization of herpes virus in the temporal and frontal lobes.

The characteristic manifestation of viral encephalitis is **cerebral dysfunction** (e.g., abnormal behavior, altered consciousness, and seizures). Fever, nausea, and vomiting are also common, possibly because of increased intracranial pressure. Thus, Ms. H. had many of the typical signs and symptoms of the disease. Many of the manifestations of herpes simplex encephalitis are due to necrosis of neurons, especially of the temporal and frontal lobes. Necrosis is accompanied by inflammation with infiltration of mononuclear cells from the perivascular sheaths (Virchow-Robin spaces). Ms. H.'s sites of involvement included the portion of the temporal lobe responsible for the sense of smell; hence her olfactory hallucination (smelling roses). The lesions are usually on one side only, because the viruses ascended only from one (her left) trigeminal ganglion.

Diagnosis

Patients are suspected of having herpetic encephalitis if they have fever and focal cerebral cortical lesions, particularly in the frontal and temporal lobes. Diagnostic tests are necessary to document the clinical impression of inflammation (e.g., CSF pleocytosis, an increase in the number of cells in the CSF) and focal involvement of cerebral tissue. A **radioactive brain scan** with technetium is the most sensitive test to indicate brain tissue involvement. Technetium-99, an artificial radioactive element, is injected in the blood covalently bound to serum albumin. Leakage from cerebral capillaries is detected by radioactive technetium spilling into tissues. If the area of brain that is destroyed by HSV is large enough, damage may sometimes be detected by cranial CT or MR examination.

Herpetic encephalitis is conclusive diagnosed by a brain biopsy, as was done with Ms. H. However, in patients with a history and physical findings of herpes encephalitis, **acyclovir** (a relatively nontoxic drug) is usually administered without further studies. The value of a brain biopsy is demonstrated by the fact that in approximately one-fourth of adults suspected of having herpes encephalitis, pathological examination of biopsy material reveals other diseases, e.g., cancer, bleeding, fungal infections, which require other forms of treatment. If HSV-specific DNA is present in the CSF, a brain biopsy can be avoided.

Many clinical conditions mimic herpetic encephalitis, particularly in adults. These include enterovirus or arbovirus encephalitis, cerebral collagen vascular disease, tumors, and even cryptococcal meningitis. To distinguish HSV encephalitis from these conditions, brain tissue obtained on biopsy is examined by conventional microscopy and is tested for herpes-specific antigens using fluorescent conjugated monoclonal or polyclonal antisera directed against an HSV glycoprotein. Culturing HSV from brain tissue provides unequivocal evidence of encephalitis, but takes more time. Since HSV spreads by contiguous cell-to-cell contact, it can rarely be cultured from the CSF. However, some viral DNA leaks from the lesion (or from a dying phagocyte) and it can be readily detected by polymerase chain reaction (PCR). With widespread availability of the PCR test, the brain biopsy—an invasive and hazardous—procedure will no longer be necessary.

Treatment

As stated above, in patients with encephalitis, it is essential to determine if the disease is due to herpes simplex, because the morbidity and mortality of this disease can be decreased by drug treatment. Two antiviral agents, **acyclovir** and **arabinosyl adenine**, are available for the treatment of herpes encephalitis (Chapter 43, "Antiviral Strategies"). In a randomized chemotherapy trial carried out chiefly with adult herpetic encephalitis patients, the mortality rate and the sequelae were reduced with acyclovir treatment (in one study, the overall mortality rate was reduced from 70% to 20%). With either agent, the outcome is related to the severity of disease at the time antiviral chemotherapy is begun, hence the urgency to begin treatment. As with the bacterial meningitides, supportive care must also be instituted. Sequelae are caused by destruction of cerebral gray matter. Such lesions in the temporal or frontal lobes may result in personality changes, whereas involvement of the white matter may lead to significant paralysis.

LATE ENCEPHALITIS

Inflammation of brain substance can occur some time after the initial invasion of the CNS. This can be the result of an autoimmune reaction, continued unrestricted viral replication, or reactivation of latent virus.

▥ CASE

T. was 13 months old when he was placed in a large day care center in Philadelphia after moving from American Samoa. After 1 month of daily attendance (approximately 6 hours each day), he developed a fever of 101°F, cough, watery eyes, and runny nose. Each day his maximum temperature increased slightly and on the third day of illness, he developed a rash. The rash began as small (3–4 mm diameter) red macules on the face and neck. Within hours it spread down over the chest, became bright red and palpable. T was taken to his physician who, after examining him, told the mother he had measles. Over the next few days, his rash became more extensive, but his fever and respiratory symptoms lessened. T. was well until 8 years of age, when he began having problems in school. His teachers first felt T.'s problems were behavioral, but over a period of a few months they noted that his ability in math (a subject he loved) was regressing. T.'s parents took him to a neurologist who, on additional questioning, found that T's skill in baseball had also been slipping; he appeared more awkward and was stumbling often. The neurologists performed a lumbar puncture and obtained an electroencephalogram. Several weeks later, without any perceptible change in T's clinical condition, the neurologist told the family that T's illness was due to the measles virus. The disease was called subacute sclerosing panencephalitis (SSPE) and was ultimately fatal.

T.'s parents were devastated and doubtful. How could the physician be sure T.'s condition was due to measles? Why did T. develop the illness? Could it have been prevented? Is there a treatment now?

Pathobiology

T. suffered from SSPE, a rare complication of measles virus infection. During the initial infection, the virus invaded virtually all organs in the body. In the majority of measles patients, the virus replication and spread is terminated by host immunity. In rare patients with unrecognized deficiency in cell-mediated immunity, progressive encephalitis with seizures and motor deficits appears after 1 week of disease. This illness is due to unrestricted viral replication and spread and is different from "postinfectious" encephalitis. In this form of measles-associated encephalitis, the patient begins recovering from measles but precipitously develops obtundation or coma, coincident with the reappearance of fever. This complication is relatively common, affecting 1 in every 1000 children with measles. It is one of the major reasons for measles vaccination. Why didn't T. receive the measles vaccine? A modified measles virus, along with mumps and rubella, is given to children at 15 months of age. Before this age, most children still have maternal antibody (received in utero), which prevents an effective immune response. Thus, T. was too young to receive the measles vaccine, when he was exposed to children not living within the continental United States, who are often not immunized.

T.'s symptoms are typical of SSPE, in which mental deterioration is followed by loss of motor skills. The physician made the diagnosis of SSPE from a characteristic pattern on the electroencephalogram and the increased concentrations of antibodies to measles virus–specific proteins in the CSF. Often, patients with SSPE have high serum antibody titers, but measles virus replication in the brain evokes local production of antibodies. This results in the CSF concentration of specific antibodies greater than that in serum. SSPE is an extremely rare complication of measles, occurring in only 1 of 100,000 cases of measles.

It is not clear how the measles virus manages to become latent. Virus is present in neurons and glial cells, but it appears that genes encoding for membrane antigens are deleted. The virus is thus sequestered from the host immune response. Latency also appears to be due to selective inhibition (or mutation) of viral genome expression. One measles virus–specific protein, termed M-protein, is involved in the budding of mature virus from the cell. Failure of the virus to assemble into mature virions would favor its retention in the cell. Because cells of the CNS do not turn over (as liver cell do, for example), the virus can remain latent for a long period of time. Slow replication of the defective virus leads to slow progression of CNS symptoms in SSPE. Unfortunately, no specific treatment exists for SSPE. In addition to measles, rubella and the polyomaviruses can cause latent infection of the CNS, i.e., reactivation of these viruses at a time after the acute infection can produce encephalitis.

ABSCESSES

Brain abscesses typically follow two distinct diseases: congenital heart disease and chronic parameningeal infections. In a patient with endocarditis, a septic embolus from the heart may rarely cause a brain abscess.

▮ CASE

Ms. T., a 29-year-old housewife, complained of earache. She had had many such episodes since childhood, especially of the left ear, but this one was associated with a headache that made her nauseated. She vomited once. After 4 days of these symptoms, she was driven to the hospital because she had developed a large blind spot in her right field of vision. At the hospital, it was noted that she had a low-grade fever of 38.1°C. A CT scan of the head revealed a 4 × 3 cm mass in her left occipital lobe, consistent with an abscess (Fig. 58.5).

A neurosurgeon performed a needle aspiration of the abscess under CT guidance. A smear of the aspirate revealed Gram-positive cocci and some Gram-negative rods, and the material grew only *Staphylococcus aureus* when cultured. Ms. T. was treated with intravenous nafcillin (to cover *S. aureus*) and metronidazole (to cover anaerobic bacteria) for 4 weeks. During this period, serial CT examinations showed the abscess to be shrinking. She recovered completely, but a remaining small blind spot remained in her right visual field.

Pathobiology

The case of Ms. T. may well have started with a chronic infection of the middle ear or mastoid. Her long-term earache points to that scenario. Chronic infections of the middle ear, mastoid, or sinuses often involve the bony structures that surround them, plus their vasculature. Veins that bridge the temporal bone and the cerebral cortex may become infected (septic thrombophlebitis), leading to a decrease in local blood supply and providing a reservoir of bacteria.

Abscesses may appear at many locations of the brain

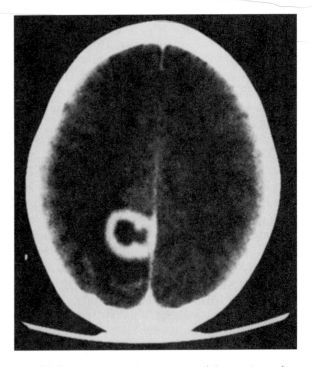

Figure 58.5. Computerized tomogram of the cranium of a patient with an abscess in the left occipital lobe. The liquefied (necrotic) material in the abscess center appears dark. The white rim surrounding the abscess is its wall, which is visualized because of its vascularization and contiguous vasodilation. All of the intracranial vasculature is visualized because contrast material was infused intravenously at the time the radiograph was obtained.

and the subdural or epidural meningeal spaces. Infarction of superficial cerebral cortex during meningitis can produce a subdural abscess that is poorly localized, a condition called **subdural empyema.** If an empyema is not completely drained, it slowly resolves, as do abscesses in other parts of the body. In contrast with intracerebral abscesses, those located on the outside of the dura mater (**epidural abscesses**) are invariably related to contiguous infection of bone, sometimes secondary to infection of the paranasal sinuses or mastoids.

Decrease in the blood supply to an area of the brain leads to a condition called **encephalomalacia,** a softening of the brain tissue that accompanies cell death. Bacteria that are transiently found in the circulation may lodge in these softened and necrotic areas and cause abscess formation. Children with cyanotic congenital heart disease have multiple areas of encephalomalacia throughout their brain and many suffer from brain abscesses. In Ms. T.'s case, septic phlebitis of veins that pass from the temporal bone to the cortex not only produced encephalomalacia and infarction, but also supplied the bacteria causing the abscess. Abscesses may also be a complication of meningitis, if cerebral vasculitis is severe enough to produce infarction of brain substance. Abscesses usually occur in the watershed areas, on the margin between adjacent vascular territories where the vasculature least overlaps.

The symptoms caused by brain abscesses are due to increased intracranial pressure and to destruction of tissue at specific locations. When the frontal lobe is involved, there is diminished intellectual performance, memory deficits, drowsiness, and perhaps some memory loss (Fig. 58.3). Temporal lobe involvement results in visual field defects and, occasionally, in difficulty in speaking. In some patients, mastoiditis leads to cerebellar abscesses, resulting in incoordination, ataxia, and falling toward the affected side.

Acute abscesses in the CNS are frequently caused by a mixed bacterial flora consisting of strict and facultative anaerobes. The mixture of bacteria is similar to that found in the mouth, or a parameningeal focus such as an infected middle ear, mastoid, or sinus. Staphylococci can also infect brain tissue if delivered to that location in a septic embolus from an infected heart valve.

Chronic abscesses may be located in either the meninges or brain tissue. The most common causative agents are tubercle bacilli, *Cryptococcus,* and other fungi. Chronic abscesses are invariably due to metastatic spread from foci elsewhere. Sometimes, however, the CNS manifestations may be the first indication of the presence of the organisms. These abscesses usually follow a course of remission and relapse. They are often associated with a loss of cell-mediated immunity, when the causative agents are no longer kept in check at the primary focus.

Brain abscesses may also develop from head injuries that allow the direct penetration of microorganisms. Some fractures of the temporal bone may never heal completely and thus become a chronic portal of entry for bacteria from the middle ear and the mastoid. Invasion of the CNS may follow neurosurgical or orthopaedic procedures of the brain or spinal column. Brain abscesses that result from trauma or surgical procedures are usually due to *S. aureus* or nosocomial Gram-negative bacilli.

Diagnosis

Diagnosis of brain abscess is aided by several imaging techniques. A brain scan with technetium-99 will reveal an area of increased radioactivity in the wall of the abscess (where the capillaries are inflamed and leaking) and an avascular central portion (the abscess cavity). This area often looks like a "donut" on the scan (Fig. 58.5). Cranial CT may also demonstrate the same structures—a fluid avascular abscess cavity and an overly vascularized (hyperemic) rim surrounding the cavity. Magnetic resonance imaging can also delineate the necrotic center of the abscess, the denser abscess wall, and the adjacent edematous brain tissue. Lumbar puncture is inadvisable in an individual suspected of having a brain abscess, as the increased intracranial pressure may cause brainstem herniation with lumbar "decompression."

Aspiration of the abscess cavity yields material for cytological analysis, Gram stain, and culture. Anaerobes are common in brain abscess and the aspirate should immediately be cultured anaerobically. Often a smear will show the presence of many Gram-positive cocci, Gram-positive rods, and perhaps a few Gram-negative rods, yet only S. *aureus* will grow in culture. In such cases the bacteria that failed to grow can be assumed to be oxygen-sensitive anaerobes.

Treatment

Like abscesses elsewhere, brain abscesses must usually be drained to effect resolution. In addition, aspiration of the contents of an abscess helps lower the increased intracranial pressure and improves the patient's condition. Focal symptoms due to tissue destruction will not be improved, but the lesion can be contained from further increase in size by the administration of antibiotics.

Antibiotic therapy is not always effective in the treatment of brain abscesses. Inflammation of the meninges is usually too slight to enhance penetration of antibiotics into the CSF. In addition, most antibiotics function poorly in an abscess. Ideally, an antibiotic should be chosen based on the susceptibility of organisms isolated from the abscess cavity, but aspiration of material for culture and susceptibility testing is not always practical. Usually a β-lactam and a lipophilic antibiotic active against anaerobes are administered together.

CONCLUSION

The anatomic and physiological protective mechanisms of the CNS effectively limit access of microorganisms. However, if infective agents succeed in penetrating the tissues of the system, these same mechanisms tend to exacerbate the symptoms of disease.

The most frequent infections of the CNS are caused by relatively few agents. Typically, the organisms tend to cause specific disease manifestations; encephalitis is almost exclusively caused by viruses, acute meningitis by bacteria, and chronic meningitis by tubercle bacilli and *Cryptococcus*. Bacterial abscesses, in contrast, are frequently caused by a mixture of bacteria derived from the normal flora of the mouth and oropharynx.

Infections of the CNS are often severe and life-threatening. Many require immediate action based on acute clinical assessment and, when available, rapid diagnostic tests. The most important diagnostic procedure is the examination of the CSF for microorganisms, white blood cells, and the determination of the concentration of glucose and protein. Fortunately, drugs are available that are effective against many of even the most dangerous conditions, such as herpetic encephalitis.

SUGGESTED READINGS

Johnson RT. Acute encephalitis. Clin Infect Dis 1996; 23;219–226.

Mandell GL, Bennett JE, Dolin R. Principles and practice of infectious diseases. 4th ed. New York: Churchill Livingstone, 1995; Section H.

Quagliarello VJ, Sheld WM. Treatment of bacterial meningitis. New Engl J Med 1997;336:708–716.

Rosenblum ML, Hoff JT, Norman D, Edwards MS, Berg BO. Nonoperative treatment of brain abscesses in selected high-risk patients. J Neurosurg 1980;52:217–225.

Weiner LP, Fleming JO. Viral infections of the nervous system. J Neurosurg 1984;61:207–244.

Respiratory System

GREGORY A. STORCH

The respiratory tract is the most common site for infection by pathogenic microorganisms. Perhaps because respiratory infections are so common and are usually mild, they are frequently taken for granted. But in fact, they represent an immense disease burden on our society and thus, have a major economic impact. Upper respiratory infections (URIs) account for more visits to physicians than any other diagnosis. It has been estimated that, in the U.S., influenza-like illnesses are responsible for more than 400 million days of restricted activity each year. In addition, some respiratory infections have severe consequences, especially in individuals compromised by other diseases. Pneumonia, the most severe form of respiratory infection, is frequently life threatening and still accounts for a large number of deaths in the U.S. population.

It is not surprising that the respiratory tract becomes infected frequently. It is in direct contact with the environment and is continuously exposed to microorganisms suspended in the air we breathe. Some of these microorganisms are highly virulent, and only a few of them are needed to infect even a healthy person. However, most of these microorganisms do not cause infection unless other factors interfere with host defenses. The warm, moist environment of the respiratory tract is an ideal place for the growth of microorganisms. One of the questions that this chapter addresses is why these frequent infections are not even more frequent.

Infection may be localized at any level of the respiratory tract, and the location is a major determinant of the clinical manifestations. The clinical syndromes associated with infection at different locations are shown in Figure 59.1. Infections of the conjunctivae, the middle ear, and the paranasal sinuses are included because these areas are continuous with the respiratory tract and are lined by respiratory epithelium. Several important diseases of the respiratory system are discussed in other chapters (pneumococcal pneumonia, Chapter 13; whooping cough, Chapter 19; pulmonary tuberculosis, Chapter 23; chlamydial pneumonitis, Chapter 27; mycoplasma pneumonia, Chapter 29; rhinoviruses, Chap-

ter 32; respiratory syncytial virus, Chapter 34; influenza, Chapter 36; infections of the sinuses and middle ear, Chapter 65).

The clinical manifestations of respiratory tract infection also depend on the causative agent. Thus, viruses are important pathogens in the upper respiratory tract and account for most cases of pharyngitis. Bacteria are the most important causes of otitis media, sinusitis, pharyngitis, epiglottitis, bronchitis, and pneumonia. Fungi and protozoa rarely cause serious respiratory tract infection in healthy individuals but are important causes of pneumonia in the immune compromised host. Some of the common pathogens that produce infection at different locations in this system are listed in Table 59.1. Their relative contribution to respiratory tract disease is shown in Figure 59.2.

To a casual observer it may appear that respiratory tract infections are constant in the population. However, close observation coupled with laboratory studies reveal that specific respiratory infections occur in large and small epidemics. The results of careful viral surveillance carried out in Houston, Texas over a period of several years are shown in Figure 59.3.

Some microorganisms have a strong predilection for certain sites in the respiratory tract, either because of specific tropism or selective survival. The reason that the common cold occurs in the nose and not further down the respiratory tract is that the cold viruses grow best at 33°C. This is the temperature found in the nose but not in the lungs.

This chapter divides the respiratory system into three major anatomic regions:

Nose and throat, airways, and the lungs.

INFECTIONS OF THE NOSE AND THROAT

CASE 1: PHARYNGITIS

F., a 5-year-old child who was in good general health, was brought to the pediatrician because of fever, irritabil-

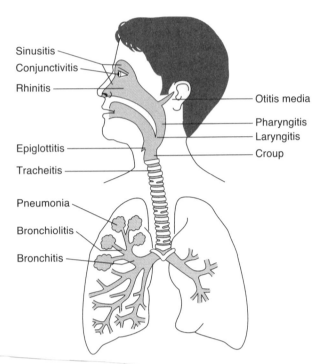

Figure 59.1. Clinical syndromes associated with infection at different locations within the respiratory tract.

Table 59.1. Pathogens Producing Disease at Different Levels of the Respiratory Tract

Location	Common pathogens
Nasopharynx	Rinovirus, *Coronavirus*, other respiratory viruses, *Staphylococcus aureus*
Oropharynx	Group A streptococcus (*Streptococcus pyogenes*), *Corynebacterium diphtheriae*, Epstein-Barr virus, adenovirus, enteroviruses
Conjunctiva	*Streptococcus pneumoniae*, *Haemophilus influenzae*, *Neisseria gonorrhoeae*, *Chlamydia trachomatis*, adenovirus
Middle ear and paranasal sinuses	*S. pneumoniae*, *H. influenzae*, *Moraxella (Branhamella) catarrhalis*, Group A streptococcus (*S. pyogenes*)
Epiglottitis	*Haemophilus influenzae*
Larynx–trachea	Parainfluenza viruses, *S. aureus*
Bronchi	*Streptococcus pneumoniae*, *H. influenzae*, *Mycoplasma pneumoniae*, influenza viruses, measles virus
Bronchioles	Respiratory syncytial virus
Lungs	(See Table 59.4)

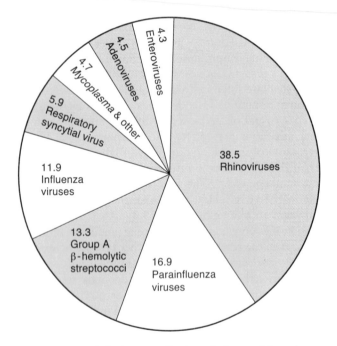

Figure 59.2. Relative contribution of viruses, *Mycoplasma*, and group A streptococci to total respiratory infection of known etiology in Tecumseh, Michigan.

ity, and a sore throat that began 1 day earlier. On examination, F. had a 102°F temperature, and his conjunctivae and oropharynx were erythematous. In addition, his tonsils were enlarged and coated with a patchy white exudate, and his anterior cervical lymph nodes were enlarged and tender.

The remainder of the examination was unremarkable. A throat culture was negative for group A streptococcus. F.'s symptoms worsened slightly over the next day and then resolved without treatment over a 5-day period.

Although the posterior nasopharynx merges with the oropharynx, important differences exist between infections of the nose and throat. Some are illustrated in the above case. Most infections of the nasopharynx are caused by viruses and give rise to the signs and symptoms that are known collectively as the common cold (See Fig. 32.7). Approximately 40–50% of colds are caused by the rhinovirus group (which are discussed in detail in Chapter 31). Coronaviruses are the next most common group of agents, accounting for approximately 10% of colds. The remainder are caused by a variety of respiratory viruses listed in Table 59.2. Although the patient with a cold may experience a "scratchy" throat, nasal symptoms are usually more prominent. Bacterial infection of the nose occurs occasionally, although it is not common.

Infection of the oropharynx, pharyngitis, is associated with discomfort in the throat, especially during swallowing. Nasal symptoms may also present. Viruses and bacteria are the most common etiological agents (Table 59.3). It is difficult to differentiate between viral and bacterial pharyngitis on the basis of clinical findings. Therefore, a throat culture or a rapid diagnostic

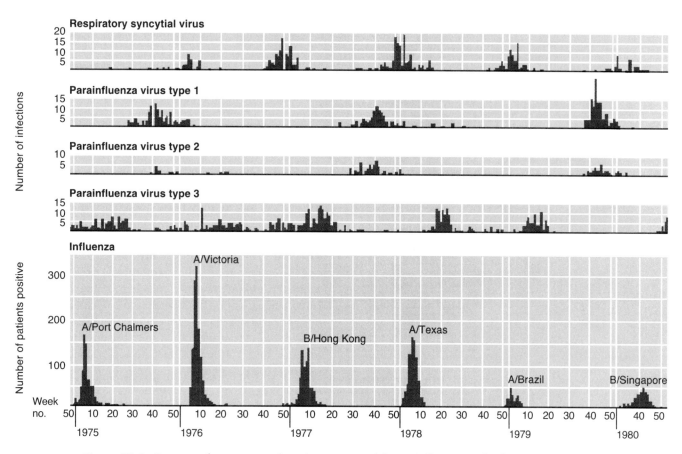

Figure 59.3. Patterns of occurrence of respiratory syncytial, parainfluenza, and influenza virus infections in Houston, Texas.

Table 59.2. Causes of the Common Cold	
Agent	Relative importance
Rhinovirus	+ + + +
Coronavirus	+ +
Parinfluenza virus	+^{a}
Respiratory syncytial virus	+^{a}
Influenza virus	+
Adenovirus	+
Other viruses	+ +
Unknown	+ + + +

^{a} + + or more in children.

Table 59.3. Causes of Pharyngitis	
Agent	Relative importance
Streptococcus pyogenes (Group A β-hemolytic)	+ + + +
Rhinovirus	+ +
Adenovirus	+ +
Coronavirus	+ +
Epstein-Barr virus	+ +
Herpes simplex virus	+
Parainfluenza virus	+
Influenza virus	+
Coxsackie virus	+
Mixed anaerobic bacteria	+
Neisseria gonorrhoeae	+
Corynebacterium diphtheriae	+
C. hemolyticum	+
Mycoplasma pneumoniae	+
Francisella tularensis	+
Unknown	+ + + +

test should be performed to detect group A streptococci, which is the most important bacterial cause of pharyngitis. Other streptococci account for a small proportion of cases, as do gonococci in sexually active individuals. In the past, oropharyngeal diphtheria caused an important form of pharyngitis, but this disease is rarely seen in the U.S. today. Recently, an organism called *Arcanobac-*

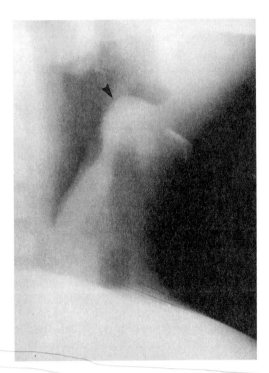

Figure 59.4. X-ray of the neck taken in a lateral projection, reveals marked swelling of the epiglottis *(arrow)*.

terium haemolyticum has been found to cause some cases of pharyngitis in older children and young adults. This organism may be easily overlooked in a routine throat culture. Among the viruses, the adenovirus group is particularly prominent and may be suspected if conjunctivitis is also present (pharyngoconjunctival fever). In adolescents and young adults, Epstein-Barr virus is a common cause of pharyngitis, which is one of the manifestations of infectious mononucleosis. The enteroviruses, especially the group A coxsackie viruses, sometimes produce small vesicles on the mucous membrane of the throat. This clinical picture is known as herpangina.

INFECTIONS OF THE EPIGLOTTIS

■ CASE 2: EPIGLOTTITIS

G., a 3-year-old girl, was put to bed by her parents with a low-grade temperature. In the middle of the night she awoke and her parents found that her fever was higher and that she was having trouble breathing. The family pediatrician told the parents to take G. immediately to the local hospital. On examination, the child was sitting upright and drooling. A presumptive diagnosis of epiglottitis was made and the child was taken to the operating room, where an endotracheal tube was inserted. An x-ray of the lateral neck

was taken en route to the operating room and revealed swelling of the epiglottis (Fig. 59.4). When her throat was examined as she was being intubated, her epiglottis was seen to be very red and swollen. She was treated with antibiotics effective against *Haemophilus influenzae* type b. The next day, the laboratory reported that blood and epiglottis cultures grew H. influenzae. She responded promptly to treatment and completely recovered.

Acute epiglottitis is probably the most serious form of URI. This distinct clinical syndrome can be rapidly fatal because the airway may become completely obstructed from swelling of the epiglottis and surrounding structures. Acute epiglottitis occurs most often in young children, with the cause almost invariably H. influenzae type b. Fortunately, since immunization of infants against *H. influenzae* type b has become universal, this feared clinical entity has become rare. Cases also occur in adults and are more often caused by bacteria other than *H. influenzae* type b. Despite the current rarity of this condition, the practitioner must always be vigilant because early recognition of acute epiglottitis may make the difference between life and death.

Epiglottitis probably becomes established by direct extension of infection from the nasopharynx. Bacteremia is almost always present and is secondary to infection of the epiglottitis. We do not know the factors that determine who among the many individuals colonized with *H. influenzae* type b will develop this disease. Nor do we understand the marked tropism of this organism for the epiglottis nor why other bacteria or viruses rarely cause epiglottitis.

Epiglottitis is an acute inflammation and is accompanied by edema and infiltration with neutrophils. Microabscesses containing *H. influenzae* type b may be present. Metastatic complications are less common in epiglottitis than in *H. influenzae* meningitis, possibly because patients with epiglottitis seek medical attention earlier in the course of their illness. Fortunately, epiglottitis responds readily to treatment with antibiotics, and the outcome is good if early recognition allows for airway intervention, as illustrated in the above case.

INFECTIONS OF THE LARYNX AND TRACHEA

■ CASE 3: CROUP

H., a 19-month-old boy, developed a runny nose, hoarseness, cough, and a low-grade temperature. His pediatrician diagnosed a viral URI and prescribed no specific treatment. That night, H. had a barking cough. His breathing was forced and noisy, especially with inspiration. Alarmed, the parents called the pediatrician, who told them that the child probably had croup. He advised them to take H. into the bathroom and to fill the room with steam by running the hot water in the shower. He also advised them to call back 15 minutes later if the respiratory difficulty worsened. In fact, it subsided and H. fell back to sleep. A similar but milder episode occurred the next night. Over the next few days, all of the symptoms gradually resolved.

Infection of the larynx and upper airway in young children is often associated with the clinical syndrome of croup, as in this case. Croup (the obstruction of the upper airway) is characterized by sudden onset, barking cough, difficult respiration, and often sudden resolution. Almost all cases are caused by viruses, especially the parainfluenza viruses. Infection with parainfluenza virus types 1 to 3 is common in young children, and repeated infections may occur. Rarely, bacteria particularly *Staphylococcus aureus,* cause clinical findings similar to those of viral croup. Typically, mild upper respiratory symptoms such as nasal discharge and dry cough are present 13 days before the signs of airway obstruction become evident. In most cases, the illness is self-limited and resolves after 37 days.

In croup, infection begins at or near the site of original inoculation in the upper airway and spreads downward by direct extension. Viremia and spread to sites outside of the airway are highly unusual. The upper airway obstruction characteristic of croup results from swelling of the tracheal mucous membrane. Because the tracheal wall has nonexpandable rings of cartilage, swelling of the mucous membrane results in narrowing of the tracheal lumen. This narrowing worsens during inspiration and results in inspiratory stridor. Histamine and IgE, antibody specific for parainfluenza virus have been detected in nasopharyngeal secretions of children with croup, suggesting that immunological mechanisms involving inflammatory mediators may be involved in its pathogenesis.

Some children experience recurrent episodes of croup, suggesting that they may have a predisposition to airway hyperreactivity, although the basis for hyperactivity remains unknown. Most children admitted to the hospital with croup have greater reduction in the oxygen content of their blood than can be explained by the degree of obstruction to airflow. This finding suggests that the lungs as well as the airways may be involved in the infectious process. No specific drug treatment for parainfluenza virus infection is currently available. Management of croup consists of providing oxygen, administration of epinephrine by aerosol in some cases, and support of the airway if needed.

In adults, the major clinical manifestation of infec-

tions of the larynx is hoarseness. Most acute laryngeal infection in adults is caused by respiratory viruses. Although annoying, these infections are generally mild and self-limited. Other less common causes of laryngeal infection include tubercle bacilli and yeast such as *Candida albicans*, especially in immunocompromised patients.

INFECTIONS OF THE LARGE BRONCHI

▌ CASE 4: INFLUENZA

J., a 28-year-old physician, developed symptoms of cough, myalgias (aches and pains in the muscles), headache made worse by coughing, substernal chest pain, and high fever. She suspected influenza because an outbreak was in progress and she had recently cared for several patients with similar symptoms. During the next 3 days, she was bedridden because of weakness and a persistent temperature of 103[dg]F. The symptoms gradually resolved over the next few days without specific treatment. After 7–10 days, J. was able to resume her usual activities. A viral throat culture she took on the first day of illness confirmed the diagnosis of influenza.

Many different organisms cause infections of the large bronchi. Among viruses, the prototype is influenza, illustrated here and more fully discussed in Chapter 30 ("Strategies to Combat Bacterial Infections"). Bronchitis is also caused by other viruses, mycoplasmas, chlamydiae, pneumococci, and *H. influenzae.*

INFECTIONS OF THE BRONCHIOLES

Bronchiolitis is a common clinical syndrome in the first two years of life and is usually associated with respiratory syncytial virus. See chapter 34 ("Paramyxoviruses") for a full discussion of this entity.

INFECTIONS OF THE LUNGS

Pneumonia, or infection of the lung parenchyma, may be caused by many different pathogens, sometimes with distinctive clinical manifestations. Thus, pneumonia is not one disease, rather, pneumonia represents a variety of diseases that share a common anatomic location. Pneumonias can be classified in various ways. Here we use a clinical and epidemiological classification (Table 59.4) both of which are based on the perspective of the clinician encountering patients with pneumonia. This classification is important because it can form the basis for managing the patient's illness even before a specific cause has been proven.

In this classification, the first important distinction is between acute pneumonia (fairly sudden onset with progression of symptoms over a very few days), and subacute and chronic pneumonia. Among the acute pneumonias, a second important distinction is made between community-acquired cases and nosocomial cases acquired by patients in hospitals. Nosocomial pneumonias are classified separately because the responsible pathogens are frequently different from those that produce pneumonia in nonhospitalized individuals.

Most of the common forms of acute community-acquired pneumonia are caused by pathogens that are transmitted from person-to-person (for example, pneumococci). A second group, encountered less frequently, includes pneumonias caused by pathogens that have an animal or environmental reservoir. In many cases of animal or environmentally transmitted pneumonias the diagnosis is difficult unless the physician seeks out the circumstances of exposures (for example, exposure to a parrot leading to psittacosis). Pneumonias in infants and young children are placed in a third group because they have a distinctive etiological spectrum.

Because of the frequency of HIV infection, physicians must also be aware that patients presenting with acute community acquired pneumonia may, if they are infected with HIV, be severely immunocompromised. These patients may develop pneumonia caused by the common causes of community acquired pneumonia, but they are also at risk for pneumonia caused by so-called opportunistic pathogens. These pathogens, such as *Pneumocytis carinii*, cause infections only in immunocompromised individuals.

Acute Pneumonias

In contrast to patients with acute pneumonia are those with lung infections that have been present for weeks or months. Several forms of subacute and chronic pneumonias can be distinguished. These forms include tuberculosis, fungal pneumonia, and anaerobic lung abscesses. It is important to realize that although this classification is based on the common clinical patterns of disease, exceptions do occur. For example, patients with tuberculosis, histoplasmosis, or lung abscesses may sometimes experience acute, rapidly progressing disease.

■ CASE 5: COMMUNITY-ACQUIRED PNEUMONIA

P., an 8-month-old Native American boy who had been previously in good health, was brought to a physician because

---

Table 59.4. Classification of Pneumonia Syndromes

I. Acute	
A. Community-acquired	
1. Person-to-person transmission	*Streptococcus pneumoniae, Mycoplasma pneumoniae, Haemophilus influenzae, Staphylococcus aureus, Streptococcus pyogenes, Klebsiella pneumoniae, Neisseria meningitidis, Branhamella catarrhalis, Chlamydia pneumoniae* (?), influenza virus
2. Animal or environmental exposure	*Legionella pneumophila, Francisella tularensis, Coxiella burnetii, Chlamydia psittaci, Yersinia pestis* (plague), *Bacillus anthracis* (anthrax), *Pseudomonas pseudomallei* (melioidosis), *Pasteurella multocida* (pasteurellosis)
3. Pneumonia in the infant and young child	*Chlamydia trachomatis*, respiratory syncytial virus and other respiratory viruses, *S. aureus*, Group B streptococci, cytomegalovirus, *Ureaplasma urealyticum* (?), *Pneumocystis carinii* (?), *S. pneumoniae, H. influenzae* type b.
B. Nosocomial pneumonia	Enterobacteriaceae, *Pseudomonas aeruginosa, Acinetobacter calcoaceticus, S. aureus*
II. Subacute or Chronic	
A. Pulmonary tuberculosis	*Mycobacterium tuberculosis*
B. Fungal	*Histoplasma capsulatum, Blastomyces dermatitidis, Coccidioides immitis, Cryptococcus neoformans*
C. Aspiration pneumonia and lung abscess	Mixed anaerobic and aerobic bacterial organisms
III. Pneumonia in the immunocompromised patient	*P. carinii*, cytomegalovirus, atypical mycobacteria, *Nocardia, Aspergillus, Phycomycetes, Candida*

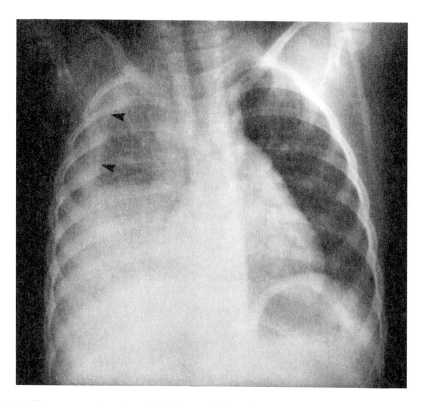

Figure 59.5. Chest x-ray of patient with *Haemophilus influenzae type b pneumonia reveals consolidation of the middle and lower lobes.* A plural effusion is also present *(arrows).*

of fever and rapid breathing. On examination, he was noted to look acutely ill, to have a temperature of 104.4°F, and a respiratory rate of 70/minute. A chest x-ray revealed consolidation of the right middle and lower lobes (Fig. 59.5). His white cell count was 26,000/µl, which is markedly elevated over the normal. Because sputum samples cannot usually be obtained from young children, a rapid latex agglutination test for *H. influenzae* type b antigen was performed on the boy's urine. The result was positive, suggesting that this organism was responsible for the pneumonia. (Antigen detection tests such as latex agglutination are convenient because they give rapid answers. They are especially useful when the patient has been treated with antibiotics which can render cultures negative. In P.'s case, antigen was still detectable). P. was treated with antibiotics effective against H. influenzae type b and recovered uneventfully. Blood cultures drawn before antibiotics were given were positive for H. influenzae type b.

Note that although the causative bacterium in this case was *H. influenzae* type b, the pneumococcus (*Streptococcus pneumoniae*) can produce an identical illness, and most such cases are in fact produced by this organism.

CASE 6: PNEUMONIA IN A CHRONIC ALCOHOLIC

Mr. L., a 52-year old man with severe chronic alcoholism, was brought to an emergency room by a police of-

ficer who had found him lying on a street. Physical examination revealed a lethargic, disheveled, middle-aged man with a temperature of 102.0[dg]F and a respiratory rate of 36/minute. During respiration, the left side of the chest moved much less than the right side (splinting). Auscultation, revealed evidence of consolidation of the lower lobe of the left lung. A sample of bloody sputum was obtained by tracheal suction, and a Gram stain revealed many neutrophils and Gram-negative rods. A chest x-ray confirmed the consolidation of the left lower lobe (Fig. 59.6).

Mr. L. was treated with broad-spectrum antibiotics. The sputum culture was reported to have a heavy growth of *Klebsiella pneumoniae,* one of the Enterobacteriaceae. Mr. L's hospital course was stormy and he required mechanical ventilation for 4 days. Eventually he recovered and was discharged to a chronic care hospital after 3 weeks.

What are the signs and symptoms that lead physicians to make the diagnosis of pneumonia? Most patients with the disease have fever and feel sick. Many also present with clues, often very obvious, that point to the chest as the location of disease. Some clues are chest pain, frequently pleuritic (exacerbated by respiratory motion), and a cough that may or may not be productive of sputum. Patients with extensive involvement of the lungs may have shortness of breath, rapid respiration, and poor color, even cyanosis. If breathing is painful, expan-

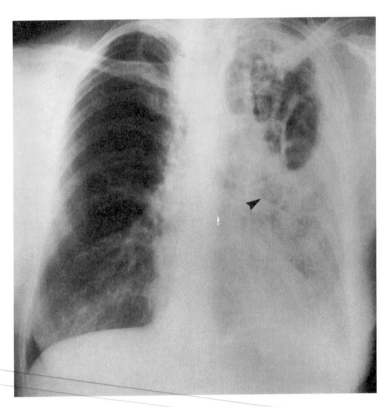

Figure 59.6. Pneumonia caused by *Klebsiella pneumoniae.* Chest x-ray reveals extensive consolidation of the left lower lobe. Cavity formation is apparent within the involved area (*arrow*).

sion on of the chest may be limited (splinting). Auscultation may reveal "rales," which are usually indicative of alveolar disease. The most important diagnostic finding is a chest x-ray that reveals a shadow or "infiltrate," the pattern of which may be a clue to the identity of the pathogen causing pneumonia. Skilled interpretation is important, because other processes, tumors, pulmonary edema, or pulmonary hemorrhage may produce radiographic changes very similar to those of pneumonia.

In general, the most common forms of acute community-acquired pneumonias are those caused by the pneumococcus and *Mycoplasma pneumoniae*, described in Chapters 13 ("The Pneumococcus") and 29 ("Mycoplasma"), respectively. A newly recognized organism, *Chlamydia pneumoniae* (described in Chapter 27 "Chlamydiae"), may also be an important cause of community-acquired pneumonia. In Case 5, P.'s signs and symptoms (his ill appearance, high temperature, elevated white blood cell count, and chest x-ray), all point to an acute bacterial pneumonia. These manifestations are characteristic of pneumococcal pneumonia, which is common in all age groups (see Fig. 13.1 for a chest x-ray of a patient with pneumococcal pneumonia). However, the astute physician may be tipped off to *Haemophilus* as the cause in this case by the age and ethnic background of the child. *H. influenzae* type b accounts for a high proportion of serious systemic bacterial infections

in children in the first year of life. Although it affects children in all socioeconomic groups the incidence is higher in nonwhites and is particularly high among Native Americans and Alaskan Eskimos. It is important to recognize this etiological agent, first because of its tendency to cause meningitis and other forms of invasive infection and second, because it is frequently resistant to antibiotics that may be used to treat pneumococcal pneumonia. However, if the infant had been immunized against *H. influenzae* type b, infection with this organism would be very rare.

A particular aspect of acute pneumonia occurring in children under 2 years of age is that they are more often caused by viruses than by bacteria. Illness caused by RSV, influenza, and parainfluenza, viruses or adenoviruses tends to be milder, and spontaneous recovery is the rule unless the child is compromised in some other way. This situation is unique because viruses are unfrequent causes of community-acquired pneumonia in other age groups. Although influenza virus may lead to pneumonia in adults, pneumonia in this situation is usually caused by bacterial superinfection. Children who develop pneumonia in the first few months of life are often infected with organisms acquired from the mother, including *Chlamydia trachomatis* and cytomegalovirus.

Case 6 illustrates another form of acute community-acquired pneumonia, that caused by aerobic Gram-negative bacilli. The factors that placed Mr. L. at risk for this disease, chronic alcoholism and exposure, also predispose him to pneumonia caused by pneumococcus, Legionella pneumophila, and anaerobic bacteria (aspiration pneumonia). The bloody sputum is characteristic of pneumonia caused by *K. pneumoniae,* which causes necrosis of the lung. Other features of Klebsiella infection are occurrence in the upper lobes and bulging at an interlobar fissure (indicative of the expansive nature of the inflammatory process). However, these characteristics are not unique, and similar illness may be caused by many other bacteria. Laboratory testing is required to make the specific etiological diagnosis. In current medical practice, most cases of pneumonia caused by members of the Enterobacteriaceae occur in hospital patients or residents of nursing homes.

Encounter

The agents that cause pneumonia can be encountered in different ways:

In colonization-infection, the causative organism is transmitted from person-to-person usually without environmental reservoirs. Transmission is typically airborne over short distances, or by contaminated secretions or fomites. In the case of some pathogens such as pneumococcus, *H. influenzae,* and *Staphylococcus aureus,* most individuals who encounter the organism become colonized, but only a few develop disease directly or after a variable period of colonization.

Pneumonias may be caused by organisms associated with the environment or with animals. Most of these organisms are transmitted by the air-borne route, although some have insect vectors. Organisms that follow this pattern are shown in Table 59.5. An example is Legionnaires' disease discussed in detail in Chapter 21("Legionella").

Aspiration pneumonias usually occur when the normal microbial contents of the upper respiratory tract enter the lungs. Typical cases lead to lung abscess and other anaerobic lung infections. The causative agents are part of the normal oral flora, which may cause disease when translocated in large numbers to an abnormal location.

Entry and spread

Pathogens may reach the lungs by one of five routes: (a) direct inhalation, (b) aspiration of upper airway contents, (c) spread along the mucous membrane surface, (d) hematogenous spread, and rarely, (e) direct penetration. Of these, inhalation and aspiration are the most common.

Inhalation and aspiration. Obviously, the respiratory tract is exposed to potential pathogens suspended in the inhaled air. Less obvious is that it is also exposed to potential pathogens by aspiration of oropharyngeal contents. Studies with radioactive tracers have shown that

in normal individuals, aspiration is no uncommon during deep sleep. In addition, intoxication or unconsciousness may cause an individual to aspirate large amounts of oropharyngeal material or even material from the stomach and upper small intestine (see Chapter 57, "Digestive System"). Defenses that protect against aspiration include the epiglottis, which physically protects the airway; the laryngeal spasm reflex, which prevents material from entering the airway; and the cough reflex, which expels material from the airway. Aspiration of oropharyngeal contents is the most important mode of entry for organisms that exhibit the colonization-infection pattern.

Direct spread. Respiratory viruses such as influenza and RSV initiate infection in the upper airway and spread to the lower respiratory tract by spreading directly along the respiratory epithelium, a route possibly facilitated by aspiration.

In hematogenous spread, the lung is a secondary site of infection. This mechanism is unusual but clearly implicated in cases of staphylococcal pneumonia in intravenous drug abusers. In many of these patients, the tricuspid heart valve is infected, and pulmonary infection results when infectious material from the valve embolizes to the lungs. Hematogenous spread has also been implicated in some cases of pneumonia caused by *Escherichia coli* and other Gram-negative rods.

Defense mechanisms of the lungs. The defense of the lungs (Fig. 59.7) begins in the nose, where specialized hairs, known as vibrissae, filter large particles suspended in inhaled air. Large particles (more than 10 [gm]m in

---

Table 59.5. Pneumonia Resulting From Unusual Exposure

Disease	Causative organism	Source
Psittacosis (parrot fever)	*Chlamydia psittaci*	Infected birds
Q fever	*Coxiella burnetii*	Infected animals
Histoplasmosis	*Histoplasma capsulatum*	Infected soil, bats
Coccidioidomycosis	*Coccidioides immitis*	Soil
Cryptococcosis	*Cryptococcus neoformans*	Soil, pigeons
Plague	*Yersinia pestis*	Infected animals, insect vectors
Melioidosis	*Pseudomonas pseudomallei*	Soil
Tularemia	*Francisella tularensis*	Infected animals, ticks

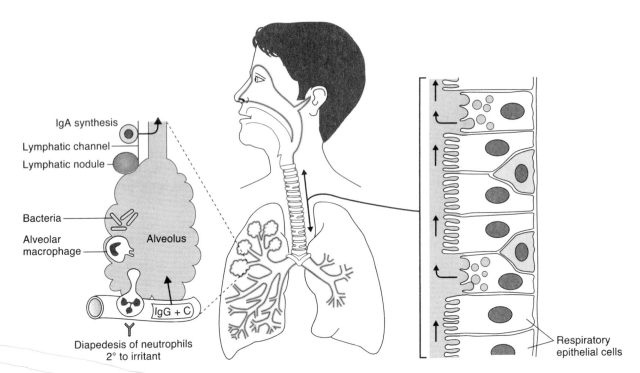

IgA synthesis

Lymphatic channel

Lymphatic nodule

Bacteria

Alveolar macrophage

Alveolus

IgG + C

Diapedesis of neutrophils 2° to irritant

Respiratory epithelial cells

Figure 59.7. The defense mechanisms of the respiratory tract. Aerodynamic factors include the presence of vibrissae in the nasal passage and abrupt changes in the direction of flow of the air column. The epiglottis and cough reflex prevent introduction of particulate matter into the lower airway. The cili- ated respiratory epithelium propels the overlying mucus layer *(red)* upward toward the mouth. In the alveoli, macrophages, humoral factors (including immunoglobulins and comple- ment), and neutrophils (when inflammation is present) all as- sist in preventing or clearing infection.

diameter) tend to settle at points where abrupt changes in the direction of airflow occur, such as the posterior nasopharynx. Smaller particles, (less than 3 [gm]m in diameter) are likely to elude these barriers and reach the terminal bronchioles and alveoli. The importance of the upper airway structures in defending the lungs is illustrated in patients in whom these structures are bypassed. Endotracheal tubes used in anesthesia and mechanical ventilation provide a conduit from the outside environment to the lower airway; patients with these tubes in place are markedly predisposed to pneumonia.

The respiratory epithelium itself has specialized defenses against infection. The tight junctions between cells prevent direct penetration. Epithelial cells from the nose to the terminal bronchioles are covered with cilia that beat coordinately. Overlying these cilia is a covering of mucus containing antimicrobial compounds such as lysozyme, lactoferrin, and secretory IgA antibodies. Each ciliated cell has approximately 200 cilia, which beat at speeds up to 500 times per minute. Cilia serve to move the overlying mucus layer upward toward the larynx at a rate as high as 46 mm/minute. The cilia and mucus are together called the mucociliary escalator. Many patients with impaired ciliary function have frequent respiratory infections. Ciliary dysfunction occurs in Kartagener's syndrome, in which patients have structurally and functionally altered cilia (these patients also exhibit the dramatic condition called dextrocardia, or right-sided heart). Ciliary function may also be impaired by viral or mycoplasma infections and may also be damaged by smoking (Fig. 59.8).

The final lung defenses are found in the alveoli: Alveoli contain IgA antibodies, complement components possibly surfactant itself, and most important, alveolar macrophages. These phagocytic cells function as active scavengers, ingesting and killing invading pathogens. When they cannot contain infection by themselves, they are helped by other phagocytic cells that do not normally reside in the lungs, especially neutrophils. Encapsulated bacteria can effectively evade phagocytosis; others not only survive but can multiply within phagocytic cells. Thus, tubercle bacilli, *Histoplasma capsulatum,* and *Legionella* find a haven within macrophages, resist killing, and multiply in large numbers. If macrophages become activated through nonspecific or specific immune mechanisms, they can limit the multiplication of such intracellular invaders.

In viral infection, the viruses usually invade cells that are not phagocytic and thus lack obvious means to kill the invader. Histopathological studies of the lungs (or other affected tissues) of patients with viral infection show infiltration by large numbers of lymphocytes and plasma cells, suggesting that viral infection stimulates the recruitment of lymphoid cells rather than neutrophils. These lymphocytes contribute to host defense by antibody production and by attacking infected cells via cytotoxic T-lymphocytes, natural killer cells, and antibody-dependent cell-mediated cytotoxicity.

Damage

The deleterious effects of pneumonia on the host fall into two categories: systemic effects and local effects in the lungs.

Systemic effects are those that result from infection any place in the body. These effects include fever, shock (particularly with Gram-negative bacilli), and wasting (for example, in chronic tuberculosis);

Local effects in pneumonia are those that interfere with the ability of the lungs to carry out air exchange. For example, the membrane that separates erythrocytes from inspired air in the alveoli may thicken. In bronchopneumonia, difficulty in gas exchange probably results from regional mismatches in the ventilation and perfusion of the lungs.

The various pneumonias cause markedly different in the amounts of permanent lung damage. It is remarkable that, in severe pneumococcal pneumonia, the lung often heals completely without any scar formation (see Fig. 13.4). The reason for lack of scarring is that although an exuberant inflammatory response occurs within the alveoli, necrosis of the underlying lung parenchyma does not occur. Necrosis provokes scar formation and per-

manent loss of functional lung tissue. In contrast, lung infections caused by Gram-negative rods and anaerobic bacteria frequently result in permanent lung tissue destruction. The fibrotic healing of a necrotizing pneumonia is referred to as healing by organization.

The specific manifestations of pneumonia vary widely and fall into several patterns. The commonly used terminology is confusing because it derives, in part, from gross pathology, microscopic histopathology, and chest x-ray. Adding to the confusion is the custom of using terms differently in different settings. Nevertheless, these terms are in widespread use and here we attempt to define them.

Lobar pneumonia refers to a homogeneous involvement of a distinct region of the lung such as a lobe or a segment of a lobe. Most of the involvement is within the alveoli, and the bronchioles and the interstitium are relatively spared. The infection spreads between alveoli until it is contained by the anatomic barriers that separate one segment from another. Thus, an entire segment or even an entire lobe becomes involved (see Figs. 13.1 and 59.9). The most frequent agents of lobar pneumonia in adults are the pneumococcus, *H. influenzae*, and Legionella.

In bronchopneumonia, the pathological process originates in the small airways and extends to nearby areas of the lung. The process is much more patchy than lobar pneumonia, often occurring in more than one area of the

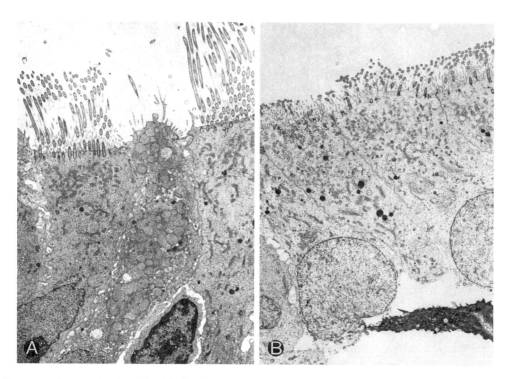

Figure 59.8. Electron micrograph of nasal epithelium from a healthy child (A) *and a child with adenovirus infection* (B). The nasal epithelium in A is characteristic of the pseudostratified ciliated columnar epithelium lining the large conducting airways. Normal ciliated cells are seen on either side of a mucous cell that is filled and distended with secretory material. B shows the altered ultrastructure and loss of ciliated cells that may accompany viral infection.

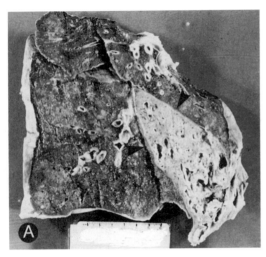

Figure 59.9. Lobar pneumonia. A is an autopsy specimen in which homogeneous consolidation of the right middle lobe is evident *(arrow).* **B** is a microscopic view showing lung alveoli filled with an infiltrate of inflammatory cells including both neutrophils and mononuclear cells. Note the lack of involvement of the interstitium.

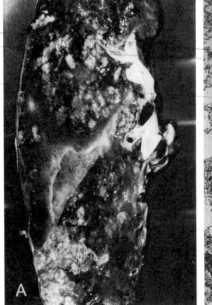
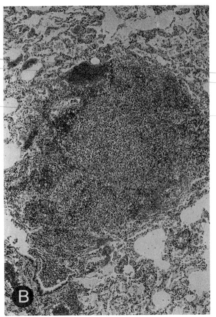

Figure 59.10. Bronchopneumonia. A is an autopsy specimen showing multiple areas of bronchopneumonia. Each area represents inflammation centered around an airway. **B** is a microscopic view showing an area of inflammation in a region distal to a respiratory bronchiole.

lung and not confined by the anatomic barriers (Fig. 59.10). Typical causes of bronchopneumonia include *M. pneumoniae* and respiratory viruses.

Interstitial pneumonia refers to involvement of the lung interstitium. When viral infections such as influenza involve the lung, they tend to produce an interstitial pneumonia (Fig. 59.11). One of the most common causes is cytomegalovirus, which usually infects patients with severe suppression of the immune system. *P. carinii* pneumonia in AIDS patients falls in this category.

A fourth pattern of involvement is the lung abscess. Here, one or more areas of lung parenchyma are replaced by cavities filled with debris generated by the infectious process. Many bacteria and fungi are capable of producing lung abscesses, but currently, a large proportion of cases are caused by anaerobic bacteria.

Infections may spread from the lung beyond the respiratory tract; for example, into the pleural space, creating a condition called **empyema.** More rarely, the process may extend to involve mediastinal structures such

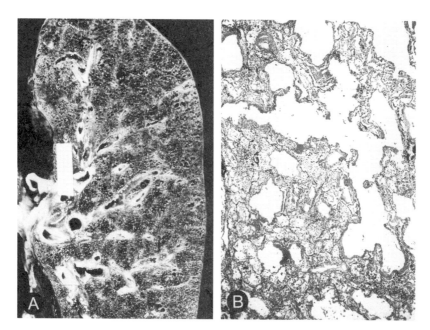

Figure 59.11. Interstitial pneumonia. A An autopsy specimen showing diffuse interstitial involvement of the lung from a patient who died with influenza pneumonia. Characteristic features are the uniform panlobar involvement with no predictable relationship to microscopic air passages and the accentuation of air spaces. **B** A microscopic view of the same

lung revealing involvement of both the interstitium and the alveoli. A uniformly dilated alveolar duct is present lined in areas by hyaline membrane, which would appear eosinophilic and refractile when viewed microscopically. The interstitium is widened and sparsely infiltrated by mononuclear cells.

as the pericardium. Microorganisms may spread outside of the chest via the lymphatic drainage of the lung and reach the bloodstream via the thoracic duct. Brain abscess, pyogenic arthritis, and endocarditis are all unusual but well-known complications of bacterial pneumonia.

Some Examples of Other Pneumonias
Aspiration pneumonias

■ CASE 7: ASPIRATION PNEUMONIA LEADING TO A LUNG ABSCESS

Mr. A., a 46-year-old man with a poorly controlled seizure disorder, was brought to a physician because of cough, fever, and weight loss occurring over a 2-week period. Physical examination revealed an ill-appearing man with a temperature of 101°F and foul-smelling breath. He had "amphoric" breath sounds (resembling those produced by blowing across the mouth of a bottle), suggestive of a lung cavity. A chest x-ray showed a large cavity in the left midlung with extensive surrounding inflammation (Fig. 59.12). He was admitted to the hospital and treated with high-dose intravenous penicillin. He began to feel better almost immediately and his fever disappeared over the course of a week. After 3 months on oral penicillin, he was judged to be cured.

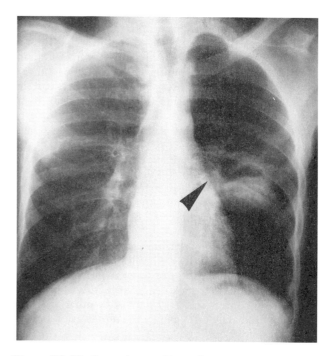

Figure 59.12. Lung abscess. X-ray showing a cavitary lesion *(arrow)* with surrounding infiltrate.

Lung abscesses such as these of Mr. A. (Case 7) are usually a consequence of gross aspiration of oropharyngeal or gastric contents. The resulting infection has a number of distinguishing features.

The clinical course tends to be less acute than that of most other forms of bacterial pneumonia. Mr. A may have been ill for several weeks or even months before seeking medical attention.

The typical lung abscess represents a polymicrobial infection with multiple species of bacteria. The bacteria most commonly involved are anaerobes and microaerophilic organisms from the normal flora of the mouth. Lung abscesses can also result from infection with other organisms that can also destroy lung tissue, including *S. aureus, K. pneumoniae*, mycobacteria, and others.

Although the definitive diagnosis is usually made on the basis of the chest x-ray, there may be clues that may lead the astute physician to suspect a lung abscess. Cough, malaise, and fever of several weeks' duration, sometimes accompanied by unexplained weight loss, should make the physician think of subacute processes in the chest, both infectious and noninfectious. Risk factors, if present, can provide important clues. Finally, as in the case of Mr. A., the patient's breath and sputum may have a putrid odor that is highly suggestive of anaerobic infection. In some cases, this odor is so strong that the diagnosis can be suspected as soon as the physician enters the patient's room.

Lung abscesses typically occur following the aspiration of a larger quantity of oropharyngeal content that can be disposed by the normal defense mechanisms of the lung. Thus, the disease occurs most often in individuals who are prone to aspirate. The most important risk factor is alteration of consciousness for any reason, including anesthesia, sedation, intoxication, drug overdose, injuries, and seizures. Lung abscess may also be caused by fragments of teeth aspirated during dental procedures.

In some cases of severe aspiration, gastric contents may enter the lungs. Probably because of their low pH and proteolytic enzymes, gastric contents induce an intense chemical pneumonitis that is not in itself, an infection; but secondary infection of the injured lung may occur.

If not treated promptly, lung abscess may spread to involve the pleural space, resulting in empyema. An unusual distant complication of lung abscess is brain abscess, which results from spread of the infection via the bloodstream. Infections at distant sites other than the brain are extremely infrequent as a complication of lung abscesses.

Pneumonias in immune compromised patients

Pneumonia is a common occurrence in immunocompromised individuals, including individuals who undergo cancer chemotherapy, with AIDS, and with congenital immunodeficiencies (Chapters 67 "Infections" and 68 "Acquired Immunodeficiency Syndrome"). Most cases are caused by opportunistic pathogens that rarely cause infections in normal individuals. Examples include *P. carinii*, the fungus *Aspergillus fumigatus*, and the virus cytomegalovirus. Many of these infections can be diagnosed only by carrying out invasive procedures such as bronchoscopy or lung biopsy. Some patients, especially those with more severe forms of immunodeficiency, may be infected with more than one pathogen at a time. At the extreme, patients with AIDS may be infected simultaneously with *P. carinii*, cytomegalovirus, and others.

Pneumonias resulting from unusual exposures

A number of pneumonias not commonly result from agents found in animals or in the environment (Table 59.6). These infections occur when peoples' activities bring them into contact with these organisms. For example, *Chlamydia psittaci* is a common cause of disease in birds, and psittacosis or parrot fever may be acquired by inhalation (Chapter 27 "Chlamydiae"). This illness is unlikely to be diagnosed correctly unless the physician obtains the history of contact with birds.

Another example is Q fever, caused by the rickettsia *Coxiella burnetii* and usually acquired from sheep, goats, and cattle. The organism is stable in the environment, and infection can occur after exposure to contaminated material from infected animals. Here too, the diagnosis is difficult unless the physician elicits the history of exposure to animals or their environment. Several fungal infections also affect the lungs (Chapter 46 "Systemic Mycoses") e.g., histoplasmosis, especially in the Mississippi and Ohio river valleys, particularly where the soil has been enriched by bird droppings; coccidioidomycosis in the deserts of the southwestern U.S.; and cryptococcosis in areas frequented by pigeons. The latter is frequently but not exclusively found in individuals who are immunocompromised. A recent example is of an unusually acquired pneumonia outbreak in New Mexico of a deadly disease in which patients' lungs filled with fluid. This outbreak was found to be caused by a virus in the hantavirus group that has since been named the Sin Nombre virus. The hantaviruses infect rodents, and the Sin Nombre virus has been found to cause chronic infection of *Peromycus maniculatis*, the common deer mouse. People apparently became infected when they came in contact with environments contaminated with rodent urine containing Sin Nombre virus.

Diagnosis

Considerable overlap exists in the clinical manifestations of pneumonia, but the astute physician may be able to use some refined clinical and epidemiological indicators to arrive at a specific diagnosis. For instance, although pneumococcal pneumonia may occur at any age, it has a predilection for the very young and the elderly. It usually has a rapid onset and an acute course. *H. influenzae* is suspected in children less than 4 years old and in adults with chronic lung disease. Lobar involvement is less common with staphylococci than with pneumococci; progression is even more rapid. Patients with staphylococcal pneumonia are more likely to belong to several risk groups, such as debilitated nursing home residents, individuals who have recently had influenza, intravenous drug users, or children under 1 year of age. Patients with cystic fibrosis may also suffer from staphylococcal pneumonia, although in these cases, pneumonia is most frequently caused by *Pseudomonas aeruginosa*. Pneumonia caused by *K. pneumoniae* occurs in hospital or nursing home residents, but is also seen in the community, usually in debilitated individuals. Because pneumonia by this organism is also a necrotizing process, the sputum is often bloody, resembling currant jelly.

A markedly elevated neutrophil count is generally indicative of bacterial infection, especially when accompanied by an increased proportion of immature cells. The examination of sputum is often quite revealing. For example, thick yellow or greenish sputum is suggestive of bacterial infection. The presence of squamous epithelial cells in large numbers indicates contamination by oropharyngeal contents, and a culture of such a specimen may yield misleading information. Large numbers of neutrophils indicate bacterial infection. However, the absence of neutrophils should not rule out bacterial infection, especially if the patient is neutropenic. Finding a predominant organism in the Gram stain may point toward the etiological agent. Thus, lancet-shaped, Gram-positive diplococci suggest pneumococci: large, round, Gram-positive cocci in clusters, staphylococci; small, pleomorphic, Gram-negative rods, *H. influenzae*; and larger and thicker Gram-negative rods, enterics such as *K. pneumoniae*. Unfortunately, the microscopic examination of sputum has limitations. Some patients cannot produce sputum, and the agents of Legionnaires' disease and *Mycoplasma pneumonia* are not visible by routine microscopy.

Sputum culture has other limitations. First, mycobacteria, mycoplasma, and viruses require specialized culture methods. Second, many of the bacteria that frequently cause pneumonia are also common colonizers of the upper airway, so that culturing these organisms is not proof that they are causing illness. This particular problem may be circumvented, although with difficulty, by bypassing the contaminated upper airways and obtaining the specimen directly from the site of infection in the lower airways. Several procedures are available. One is transtracheal aspiration, a procedure in which a large-bore needle is inserted through the cricoid membrane of the trachea and is used to aspirate secretions. This procedure is not widely used because of its potential complications. A second method, used only occasionally, is transthoracic needle aspiration, usually under fluoroscopic or computed tomographic guidance. The most widely employed method for obtaining a specimen from the lower airways is by bronchoscopy, or passage of an endoscope into the bronchial tree. This procedure allows visualization of the airway as well as aspiration of material for specimens. In actual practice, bronchoscopy is usually reserved for immunocompromised patients and individuals with severe disease.

Treatment

Making a specific etiological diagnosis in pneumonia is important because treatment differs markedly depending on the causative agent. For example, penicillin is highly effective for pneumococcal pneumonia but would be ineffective in most cases of mycoplasma, staphylococcal, or Haemophilus pneumonia. It would certainly not be effective for tuberculosis or histoplasmosis.

The tremendous diversity of potential etiologies makes it impractical to discuss the coverage for all possible agents. What should be remembered is that careful consideration of clinical and epidemiological factors often allows the physician to institute a rational and effective plan while efforts are underway to establish a specific microbiological diagnosis.

SUGGESTED READING

Bisno AL. Acute pharyngitis: etiology and diagnosis. Pediatrics 1996;97:949–954.

Denny FW, Clyde WA Jr. Acute lower respiratory infections in non-hospitalized children. J Pediatr 1986;108:635.

Dick EC, Jennings LC, Mink KA, Wartgow CD, Inhorn SL. Aerosol transmission of rhinovirus colds. J Infect Dis 1987;156:442–448.

Green GM. In defense of the lung. Am Rev Respir Dis 1970;102s:691–705.

Huxley EJ, Viroslav J, Gray WR, Pierce AK. Pharyngeal aspiration in normal adults and patients with depressed consciousness. Am J Med 1978;64:564–568.

Mandell G, Bennett JF and Dolion. *Principles and Practice of Infectious Diseases.* Chapters 39–46. 4th ed. 1995. New York: Churchill Livingstone.

Marston BJ, Plouffe JF, File TM Jr, Hackman BA, Salstrom SJ, Lipman HB, Kolczak BS, Breiman RF. Incidence of community acquired pneumonia requiring hospitalization. Arch Intern Med 1997;157:1709–1718.

Pennington JE, ed. *Respiratory infections: diagnosis and management.* New York: Raven Press, 1983.

Sande MA, Hudson LD, Root RK, eds. *Respiratory infections.* New York, Edinburgh, London, Melbourne: Churchill Livingstone, 1986.

Urinary Tract

MICHAEL BARZA

INTRODUCTION

From the distal urethra to the calyces of the kidney, the urinary tract is lined with a sheet of epithelium that is continuous with that of the skin. Thus, the epithelial surface represents a potential portal of entry for microorganisms from the outside world. Most urinary tract infections are caused by fecal organisms (especially *Escherichia coli*) which are inadvertently introduced into the periurethral area. Hematogenous infection of the kidney is much rarer. The main defenses against urinary tract infections are the flow of urine and the sloughing of epithelial cells to which bacteria may be attached. Immune defenses (humoral or cellular) play little role here in defending against the infections.

In view of the ready access of bacteria to the urinary tract, it is not surprising that urinary tract infections (**UTIs**) are second in incidence only to infections of the respiratory tract. They are the most common bacterial diseases for which adults seek medical attention. The majority of patients are women, presumably because the female urethra is much shorter than the male urethra. An antibacterial effect of prostatic secretions may also offer some protection to the male. Thus, **bacteriuria** (the presence of bacteria in the urine), whether symptomatic or asymptomatic, is generally more common in women than in men at all ages (Fig. 60.1). As many as 20% of all women have experienced an episode of urinary tract infection by the age of 30. An estimated 3 million office visits for this complaint take place each year in the United States alone. **Recurrent episodes** of urinary tract infections afflict about 1 in 10 of women at some time in their lives.

All areas of the urinary tract may be affected, but the most common UTIs are those of the bladder (**cystitis**) and the kidney (**pyelonephritis**). Infection of the urethra alone, or **urethritis**, is discussed with the sexually transmitted diseases (see Chapter 66, "Sexually Transmitted Diseases"). Prostatic infection is usually considered as

separate from UTI, although chronic bacterial prostatitis may lead to recurrent UTI. **Renal abscesses** may occur as a result of ascending UTI or bacteremia, and pyelonephritis may also result from bacteremia, without other involvement of the urinary tract. As in other infectious diseases, the physician usually suspects urinary tract infection on the basis of characteristic symptoms and signs and confirms the diagnosis by means of culture.

PATHOBIOLOGY OF UTI

As in other sites, host–parasite interactions in the urinary tract include the entry of microorganisms, their spread and multiplication, and the damage they cause (Fig. 60.2). However, in the urinary tract, **mechanical factors**, especially those that obstruct the normal flow of urine, play a particularly important role in disease. Cellular and humoral immunity are not as important in the defense against UTI as the normal flow of urine and other anatomic factors.

Entry

Access of infectious agents to the urinary tract is nearly always by ascent from the urethra. Bloodborne infections are a relatively infrequent cause and are more likely to result in renal abscesses than in ordinary UTI. Renal abscess following bacteremia probably results from the presence of bloodborne organisms in the glomeruli. Most ascending UTIs are caused by enteric or skin bacteria. Chlamydiae, the fungus *Candida albicans,* and rarely, viruses, protozoa, or worms also cause UTIs, but less frequently. The fecal bacteria, the most frequent cause of UTI, are not a random sample but are a selected subset of the intestinal flora. Strict anaerobic species of bacteria rarely cause UTI. Over 80% of acute UTI in patients without anatomic abnormalities (**uncomplicated UTI**) are caused by strains of *E. coli* that possess certain virulence factors. Other members of the enteric bacilli and the group B and D streptococci are also prominent (Table 60.1). Some infections, especially in women, are caused by *Staphylococcus saprophyticus* or by *C. albi-*

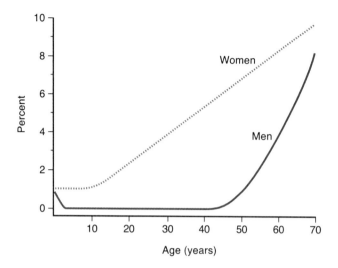

Figure 60.1. Prevalence of bacteriuria according to age and sex.

cans. Adhesion to epithelial cells appears to be the most important single determinant of pathogenicity of those species.

Some prospective studies in women with recurrent urinary tract infections indicate that shortly before the onset of bladder infections, an increasing number of fecal bacteria colonize the epithelium of the vagina and the area around urinary meatus. If the number of bacteria becomes large enough, the organisms may enter the urethra and the bladder and overwhelm the normal defense mechanisms. However, large numbers of bacteria alone may not be enough to cause UTI; mechanical and other factors may contribute to causing infection.

Host factors

The much greater prevalence of UTI among women than men has been attributed to the shorter distance that invading microorganisms have to travel up the female urethra to reach the bladder. Once bacteria have colonized the urethral opening, their entry into the urinary bladder is facilitated by mechanical factors including sexual intercourse, the use of a contraceptive diaphragm, or the presence of a Foley catheter. The preva-

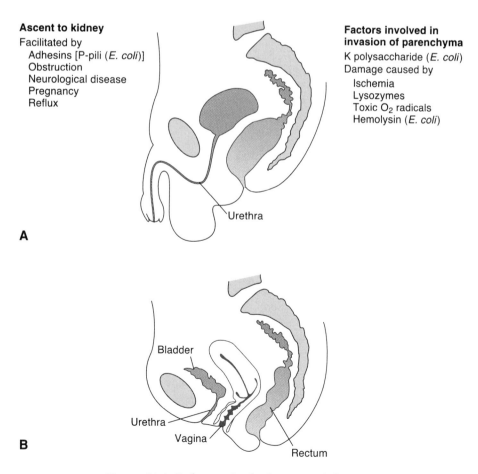

Figure 60.2. Pathogenesis of urinary tract infections.

Table 60.1. Causative Agents of Urinary Tract Infection

Uncomplicated	%	Complicated[a] or nosocomial	%
Escherichia coli	80%	*Escherichia coli*	20%
Proteus mirabilis		*Klebsiella*	
Other Enterobacteriaceae		Other Enterobacteriaceae	
Staphylococcus saprophyticus	20%	*Pseudomonas aeruginosa*	80%
Streptococci (enterococci and group B streptococci)		*Serratia*	
Chlamydiae			

[a] Patients with structural or neurological abnormalities of the urinary tract.

lence of bacteriuria in women rises sharply with sexual activity; celibate women have a smaller frequency of bacteriuria than sexually active women. Sexual intercourse contributes to UTI, perhaps by introducing bacteria upward into the bladder, hence the term "honeymoon cystitis." Knowledge of these issues may allow the physician to help the patient who is subject to recurrent UTI. Voiding after intercourse protects against the development of infection. Contraceptive diaphragms make it more difficult to empty the bladder completely, and the presence of residual urine in the bladder fosters bacteremia. Likewise, neurological disease affecting the bladder muscles impairs emptying of the bladder and also appears to contribute to UTI. Women who are particularly prone to recurrent UTI have been found to possess a greater than normal density of bacterial receptors on their uroepithelial cells; their epithelial cells are particularly "sticky" for bacteria. Individuals with certain blood group antigens are more prone than others to develop recurrent UTI. The hypothesis is that these individuals lack substances on their epithelial cells that obscure receptors for *E. coli*.

Men are less prone to get UTI, possibly because of their longer urethra and the presence of antimicrobial substances in the prostatic fluid. An increased frequency of UTI in older men correlates with the onset of prostatic hypertrophy, which leads to obstruction to voiding. Occasionally, the prostate gland itself may become infected and serve as a source from which bacteria may emerge periodically to cause relapsing infections.

UTIs in patients with structural abnormalities of the urinary tract, including stones, obstructions, or catheters, are known as "**complicated UTIs.**" These infections, especially those associated with urinary catheters, are often caused by species of Gram-negative organisms such as *Klebsiella, Enterobacter, Acinetobacter, Serratia* spp., or *Pseudomonas aeruginosa*, that are relatively resistant to antibiotics (Table 60.1). These species are often selected for by antimicrobial agents given for the treatment of other infections, particularly

in hospitalized patients. The administration of antimicrobial agents to prevent UTI in patients with urinary catheters has little effect except to foster infection by resistant organisms. Patients with urinary stones often have infection caused by urea-splitting microorganisms, especially *Proteus* spp., which raise the pH of the urine and lead to the formation of "struvite" calculi. Complicated UTI is also important medically because of the high likelihood of spread to the kidney (pyelonephritis) and the bloodstream (sepsis), as discussed below.

Bacterial factors

Of the bacterial factors predisposing to UTI, the best studied one is the ability of organisms to stick to the mucosa of the urinary tract. Adhesion to epithelial cells ensures that bacteria are not readily washed out by the flow of urine. Many causative agents of UTI have strong **adhesins**, usually in the form of pili (sometimes called fimbriae, see Chapter 3, "Biology of Infectious Agents"). These protein appendages help overcome the repulsive forces between the surface of bacterial and epithelial cells, as types of cells are hydrophobic and negatively charged. In *E. coli*, the so-called **P pili** appear to play a role in the establishment of infection both in the bladder and in the kidney. These pili stick specifically to galactose-containing receptors on epithelial cells; the receptors are contained in the P group blood antigen, which is present in 99% of the population. In one study of women with recurrent UTI, P pili were present in 29% of random fecal isolates of *E. coli*, in 65% of isolates from patients with cystitis, and in 100% of isolates from patients with pyelonephritis.

Spread to the kidney

The most serious consequence of bladder infection is the ascent of microorganisms to the kidneys to produce pyelonephritis. Any factor that contributes to the retrograde flow of urine may contribute to the establishment of pyelonephritis. The most common examples of such predisposing factors include:

- **Reflux of urine** from the bladder into the ureters. This problem is common in children and is caused by incomplete closing of the ureterovesical valves. It can lead to regurgitation of contaminated urine from the bladder into the ureter and the calyces. Reflux is frequently corrected spontaneously as the child grows.
- **Other physiological malfunctions. Neurological disorders** lead to poor emptying of the bladder. The hormonal and anatomic effects of **pregnancy** cause dilatation and decreased peristalsis of the ureters. Diabetic patients are also prone to pyelonephritis for reasons that are not fully understood.
- **Urethral catheters.** Catheters present at least two risk factors for cystitis and pyelonephritis: they serve as a conduit along which bacteria can spread, and as a source for persistent infection. Most patients who acquire UTI in the hospital become infected as the result of instrumentation of the urinary tract, especially from the use of an indwelling catheter. Scrupulous adherence to good technique, such as maintaining closed drainage and placing the collection bag below the level of the bladder, is helpful but cannot fully prevent these infections. The prevalence of bacteriuria in patients increases by about 5% for each day the catheter is in place. In these patients, many of the infecting strains do not have the usual adhesins: they are able to ascend along the catheter without having to adhere to the mucosa.
- **Urinary tract stones.** Once colonized by bacteria, stones serve as a source for relapsing infections of the bladder and the kidney. Bacteria themselves may also contribute to the formation of such "infection stones." Species of *Proteus* split urea to form ammonium hydroxide, which raises the pH of the urine and facilitates the formation of "struvite" calculi. These calculi consist of ammonium magnesium phosphate, which becomes increasingly insoluble as the pH rises.

Damage

Bacteria do not generally invade the mucosa of the lower urinary tract. The symptoms of cystitis and urethritis are caused mainly by superficial irritation. In contrast, bacteria that reach the parenchyma of the kidney (i.e., the upper urinary tract) produce the systemic manifestations of fever, chills, and leukocytosis, which, together with the localized symptoms of flank pain, are the hallmarks of pyelonephritis. Pyelonephritis is often accompanied by bacteremia, but it need not be present to produce the systemic manifestations. It has been suggested that hyperosmolarity in the renal pelvis diminishes the function of neutrophils and thereby facilitates invasion of the kidneys, but this theory is disputed. Although antibody is produced as the result of tissue invasion, it probably plays little role in host defenses.

Strains of *E. coli* that possess certain capsular polysaccharides appear to be particularly invasive, perhaps because these polysaccharides inhibit phagocytosis. For reasons that are not clear, hemolysin production by some *E. coli* strains also appears to contribute to renal damage; and of course the endotoxin of Gram-negatives may also contribute to inflammation and damage of the renal parenchyma (see Chapter 62, "Bone, Joints, and Muscles"). As stated previously, *Proteus* is associated with stone formation. Stones often cause obstruction, which by itself can significantly damage the kidney. Obstruction with infection is particularly dangerous because it can lead to life-threatening sepsis and rapid kidney destruction.

Diagnosis

Bacteriuria and colony counts— a diagnostic problem

As mentioned in the introduction, laboratory confirmation of the diagnosis of UTI depends upon culture of the urine. However, interpretation of such cultures is difficult because voided urine usually contains contaminating bacteria from the urethral meatus. Normal precautions of cleansing the external genitalia and collecting a "clean catch" midstream specimen reduce the degree of contamination but do not totally prevent the problem. Urine collected by needle aspiration of the bladder or by urethral catheterization contains fewer contaminants than voided urine (Table 60.2), but these procedures are not practical. Certain species that are common members of the skin flora, including coagulase-negative staphylococci and diphtheroids, are more likely to be contaminants than are enteric Gram-negative bacilli; however, this knowledge is not a reliable means to distinguish between true bacteriuria and contaminated urine. Repeated cultures may be obtained to determine the reproducibility of the findings, but such repetition is costly and time-consuming.

For practical purposes, the distinction between signif-

Table 60.2. Definitions of "Significant Bacteriuria" in Selected Groups of Patients

Population	"Significant bacteriuria"
Asymptomatic bacteriuria	$\geq 10^5$ cfu/ml
Acute pyelonephritis	$\geq 10^5$ cfu/ml
Women with acute dysuria	$\geq 10^2$ cfu/ml in women with abnormal pyuria (best shown for coliforms; not clear if same criteria are applicable for staphylococci)
Patients with indwelling urinary catheters	$\geq 10^2$ cfu/ml

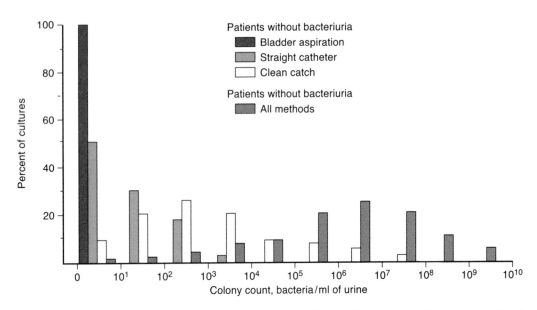

Figure 60.3. Colony counts for women with and without bacteriuria. Results are similar for men except that colony counts from those without bacteriuria are lower using the clean-catch technique for urine collection.

icant bacteriuria and contamination of the urine is based on counting the number of bacteria in the urine. This approach relies on the experimental observation that more bacteria are usually present in the urine of patients with "true bacteriuria" than in the urine of patients in whom the microorganisms are present only as contaminants. The following guidelines have been developed that apply mainly to the Gram-negative bacteria. In the asymptomatic patient, a level of 10^5 colonies per ml of urine or greater is considered indicative of infection (Fig. 60.3, see Table 60.2). In patients with symptoms of cystitis, even 10^2 colonies per ml is considered significant. The reason for the difference in threshold is that the likelihood that low counts represent contamination rather than true bacteriuria is greater in asymptomatic patients.

The reasons why some patients with cystitis have high and others have low bacterial counts in the urine are not known. Indeed, the same patient may have high counts on one occasion and low ones on another. Of course, urine must be cultured as soon as possible after it has been obtained in order to avoid bacterial growth in vitro, which would produce spuriously high counts.

As shown in Figure 60.1 and Table 60.2, asymptomatic bacteriuria is infrequent in both sexes at birth. The incidence of all urinary tract infections begins to rise in young women as they reach the sexually active years. In contrast, the frequency remains low in males until they reach the age when hypertrophy of the prostate becomes common (see Fig. 60.1 and Table 60.2).

Problem in distinguishing upper from lower UTI

Clearly, upper and lower UTI differ in their potential to cause serious disease. As we shall see, they also have different implications for therapy, in that treatment of pyelonephritis is usually more intensive and carried out for a longer time than treatment of lower UTI. Unfortunately, it is not always easy to distinguish between these infections. Upper UTIs are often accompanied by fever and flank pain. These symptoms strongly suggest involvement of the kidney. However, 30% to 50% of women with symptoms of cystitis alone have bacteria in the upper urinary tract, even though they have no symptoms of kidney involvement. These patients have a mild, subclinical pyelonephritis. Radiological studies sometimes help in pinpointing to upper UTI but are costly and not highly sensitive; they also involve some risk.

Presently, the most accurate way to determine the site of involvement in UTI is to catheterize the ureters and obtain a sample directly. To avoid this costly and somewhat risky procedure, a test has been developed based on the assumption that invasion of the kidney leads to the production of specific antibodies that coat the bacteria in the urine. This test is called the **antibody-coated bacteriuria test.** Coating by antibodies can be seen in a smear of urine sediment stained with fluorescein-labeled anti-human γ-globulin antibody. Unfortunately, thus far, the test has proven to be falsely negative in as many as 40% of patients with pyelonephritis and falsely positive in as many as 15% of patients without pyelonephritis. Men with bacterial prostatitis, for example, often have a positive reaction because this infection invades tissues.

On practical grounds, the distinction between upper and lower UTIs may be made empirically, based on the response to the administration of antibiotics (see below). In the absence of symptoms pointing to renal involvement or factors predisposing to renal involvement, physicians will often treat patients for cystitis alone. Relapse of the infection may be the first clue to renal involvement and may lead to more intensive treatment.

Principles of Treatment

The basic tenets in the treatment and prevention of UTI follow the concepts of the pathogenesis of these infections (Table 60.3). The choice of antibacterial drugs should include the following considerations: Is the infecting agent susceptible to the drug or drugs? Can an effective drug concentration be achieved at the site of infection? What is the likely effect of therapy on the recurrence of infection? It is not generally necessary to do a follow-up urine culture in patients with UTI whose symptoms resolve with treatment unless the patient belongs to one of the risk groups in which asymptomatic bacteriuria merits treatment (see below).

SPECIFIC INFECTIONS OF THE URINARY TRACT

Most patients come to medical attention for UTI because they have symptoms. In young children such as baby David (Case 2), the symptoms may not call particular attention to the urinary tract. In adults the symp-

toms of UTI are usually related to the lower portion of the urinary tract (**cystitis**) or to the upper one (**pyelonephritis**).

Cystitis

▇ CASE 1: RECURRENT CYSTITIS

Ms. C., a 23-year-old woman, had five attacks of acute **cystitis** (painful urination, increased frequency, and urgency) in the year since her marriage. The diagnosis was based on the clinical picture and the laboratory finding of bacteriuria. Three attacks were caused by *E. coli*, one by *Staphylococcus saprophyticus*, and one by *Proteus mirabilis*. Urinary colony counts in the various episodes ranged from 10^2 to 10^6 /ml. Each attack responded either to treatment with trimethoprim–sulfamethoxazole or ampicillin for 1 week. Recurrences were noted at 1-week to 3-month intervals after stopping therapy. After long-term antibiotic prophylaxis was instituted, Ms. C. had no further recurrences.

Pathobiology

Patients with cystitis, like Ms. C., have dysuria (painful urination), urgency (the need to urinate without de-

Table 60.3. Principles of Treatment of Urinary Tract Infection

Type of Infection	Treatment	Rationale
Cystitis	Single-dose or short course (e.g., 3 days)	Effective for bacterial cystitis; will not be effective in patients with early pyelonephritis, chlamydial cystitis, or infection caused by resistant bacteria, which will be detected by follow-up culture or by relapse of symptoms
Acute urethral syndrome with "abnormal pyuria"	Single-dose Rx, if no response, 10 days of doxycycline or TMP-SMX	Coliforms or staphylococci respond to many agents, chlamydiae (found in 20%) should respond to doxycycline or possibly TMP-SMX; patients without abnormal pyuria do not respond to antibacterial drugs.
Pyelonephritis	At least 2 weeks (some say 4–8 weeks) of full doses IV or by mouth; tend to prefer bactericidal drug, but one based on susceptibility tests.	Not many data re importance of bactericidal vs. bacteriostatic drug or optimal duration of Rx, but with shorter courses the relapse rate is high (e.g., 10–50% relapse after 7–14 d treatment)
Asymptomatic bacteriuria	Mainly indicated for pregnant women, young children, or patients about to undergo instrumentation of the urinary tract	25–40% of pregnant women with asymptomatic bacteriuria develop pyelonephritis if not treated
Recurrent infection		
Multiple reinfection	Individual attack usually responds well to short-course treatment	Main issue is of prophylaxis: continuous or postintercourse
Relapse	Long-term treatment (e.g., 4–8 weeks)	Usually suggests tissue invasion or structural abnormality and usually merits IVP or other evaluation

lay), and increased frequency of urination. These symptoms result from irritation of the mucosa of the lower urinary tract as a result of the infection.

Vaginitis may produce symptoms that resemble those produced by UTI. Vaginitis may result from infection with *Trichomonas* or *C. albicans*. "Nonspecific vaginitis" appears to be the result of complex interactions among various anaerobic bacteria, including the newly recognized *Mobiluncus* spp., and possibly *Gardnerella vaginalis*, a taxonomic cousin of *Haemophilus*. Although patients with vaginitis may experience pain on urination, they perceive the discomfort as external and they usually do not experience urgency or frequency of urination (in contrast to the symptoms of UTI).

Treatment of cystitis

In about 10–20% of patients with cystitis, the infection is caused by chlamydiae, which are missed by the usual bacteriological culture techniques. Most patients with cystitis have an increased number of white cells in their urine, or **abnormal pyuria**. Most patients with both cystitis and abnormal pyuria respond to treatment with antibacterial drugs, whether their urinary bacteria counts are low ($<10^2$ colonies/ml) or high ($>10^5$ colonies/ml). However, about 30% of patients with cystitis and low bacterial counts do not have abnormal pyuria; these patients do not respond to antibiotics, and the etiology of their disease remains unknown.

Most cases of cystitis are caused by organisms that are relatively susceptible to antibacterial antibiotics. A single large dose of a drug suffices to eradicate most uncomplicated infections, presumably because of the high concentration of the drug in the urine and the lack of tissue invasion by the bacteria. Slightly higher cure rates are obtained if the treatment is given for 3 days. It does not matter if the antibacterial agent is bacteriostatic or bactericidal. Short-course treatment has the advantage of lower drug cost, lower rate of side effects, and lesser chance of selection of resistant strains. (This practice is not always followed. Ms. C. was treated with several week-long courses of drug therapy.)

The most common choice is trimethoprim–sulfamethoxazole (Bactrim, Septra), which is effective against the usual Gram-negative pathogens, is inexpensive, and generally well tolerated. Ampicillin (or amoxicillin) works less well for reasons that are not clear. For infection caused by resistant organisms, a quinolone is a good choice or possibly amoxicillin with the β-lactamase inhibitor, clavulanic acid (Augmentin) or an oral cephalosporin. For patients with suspected chlamydial infection, doxycycline or another tetracycline should be used. About 80–90% of patients with uncomplicated cystitis can be cured with a 3-day course of therapy. Patients in whom failure of treatment of cystitis occurs should be suspected of having occult (subclinical) pyelonephritis or prostatitis and should be retreated, but for a longer period.

Asymptomatic Bacteriuria

Asymptomatic bacteriuria is common, especially in older patients. In the past, it was thought that asymptomatic bacteriuria was an important contributor to chronic nephritis, renal failure, hypertension, and even premature death. Although the issue remains somewhat controversial, it is now believed that asymptomatic bacteriuria generally does not have significant consequences and need not be treated in most patients. Indeed, in the elderly, debilitated patients in whom it is commonly detected, it is difficult to eradicate the infection, and recurrence after treatment is usual.

There are three main groups in whom asymptomatic bacteriuria should be treated. **Pregnant women** should be treated, because without treatment, 25–40% of them will develop pyelonephritis with possible adverse consequences for the pregnancy. **Preschool children** should be treated, because reflux from the bladder to the ureters may lead to ascent of the infection into the kidneys with resultant renal scarring. Finally, patients with structurally **abnormal urinary tracts** and those who are about to undergo **instrumentation** of the urinary tract should also receive treatment, because they are at high risk for the development of ascending UTI. Asymptomatic bacteriuria is many times as frequent in diabetic as in nondiabetic women, for unknown reasons. It is not clear if these patients should be treated.

Urethritis

Most of the infections that cause purulent urethritis without cystitis are sexually transmitted. Urethritis may be gonococcal or nongonococcal. Most cases of nongonococcal urethritis are thought to be caused by strains of *Chlamydia trachomatis*, certain mycoplasmas (e.g., *Ureaplasma urealyticum*), or combinations of these species, but disagreement exists on this subject. Furthermore, in some cases the causative agent of urethritis is simply not known. For details, see Chapter 14, "Neisseriae" and Chapter 27, "Chlamydiae."

Pyelonephritis

■ CASE 2: BACTERIAL PYELONEPHRITIS IN AN INFANT

D., a 3-month-old boy, was gaining weight very slowly. On examination, the only clinical or laboratory abnormality was the finding of 3×10^5 *E. coli* per ml of urine. D. was treated with intravenous ampicillin for 1 week and began to gain weight more rapidly. However, after 6 weeks, he again stopped gaining weight and was found to have *E. coli* bacteriuria. Over the next 2 months, the laboratory reported comparable bacterial counts with the same organism on two more occasions. Radiological studies showed reflux of urine from the bladder into the ureter and scarring of the pelvis of the left kidney. No obstruction was seen. A tentative diagnosis of **bacterial pyelonephritis** was made. D. was treated with intravenous ampicillin followed by oral ampicillin for 6 weeks in an attempt to eradicate the infection. This regimen was successful, and D. had no further problems with UTI.

⊙ CASE 3: PYELONEPHRITIS AND BACTEREMIA

Mr. P., a 65-year-old man, was admitted to the hospital with acute urinary tract obstruction due to prostatic hypertrophy. He was confused, had a temperature of 40.1°C, and his blood pressure was lower than normal. Cultures of his urine and blood yielded *Proteus vulgaris*. A urinary catheter was placed to relieve the obstruction. He was diagnosed with bacterial pyelonephritis with secondary bacteremia. After treatment with antibiotics, he underwent cystoscopy and resection of his hypertrophied prostate gland without further significant problems.

Pathobiology

In contrast to cystitis, pyelonephritis is an invasive infection that leads to fever, flank pain, and tenderness; peripheral leukocytosis is present usually. These signs are seen in the case of Mr. P. The urine of patients with pyelonephritis often contains microscopic **white blood cell casts**, elongated structures composed of cells that were tightly packed in the tubules and excreted in a proteinaceous matrix. Their presence indicates involvement of the renal tubules. Some patients with pyelonephritis, like Mr. P, develop bacteremia, which may lead to shock and death. Renal abscesses are also occasional complications of bacterial pyelonephritis.

Treatment of pyelonephritis

These patients should be treated for longer periods of time than those with simple cystitis, i.e., 2 weeks or more. Longer treatment than for cystitis makes sense because these infections involve deeper tissues, from which it may be difficult to eradicate the bacteria. For uncomplicated pyelonephritis, 2 weeks of treatment is as effective as 6 weeks. Physicians tend to prefer bactericidal over bacteriostatic drugs for the treatment of pyelonephritis, but this preference is not based on the results of controlled clinical studies. Patients with pyelonephritis are usually treated in the hospital, often with drugs given intravenously. Empiric therapy that is reliably effective against Gram-negative bacteria should be used initially (e.g., a broad-spectrum β-lactam, an aminoglycoside, or a quinolone). Upon availability of antimicro-

bial susceptibility tests for the recovered etiologic agent, therapy may be changed to a more narrow-spectrum, less expensive, less toxic drug, such as trimethoprim–sulfamethoxazole. Once the patient's condition improves, oral antibiotic therapy may be used. In men with suspected prostatitis, prolonged treatment with an appropriate drug likely to penetrate the prostate is advisable, e.g., trimethoprim–sulfamethoxazole, doxycycline, or a quinolone. Most renal abscesses can be cured by antibiotic treatment alone, but some require a drainage procedure. Pyogenic perinephric abscesses usually require drainage.

"Complicated" UTI and Nosocomial Infections
Pathobiology

UTI occurring in patients with a structurally normal urinary tract are called uncomplicated UTI. Infections in patients with anatomic abnormalities, stones, or indwelling catheters are called complicated UTI. The latter have a tendency to relapse unless the predisposing factors can be removed. In the case of Mr. P., resection of the prostate and removal of the catheter contributed to his cure. Nosocomial UTI—i.e., UTI acquired in the hospital—are usually the consequence of instrumentation, mainly catheterization of the bladder. The selective action of antibiotics commonly used in hospitalized patients tends to favor infection by species of bacteria that are relatively resistant to antibiotics.

Treatment of complicated UTI

UTIs acquired in the hospital are often caused by bacteria that are resistant to orally administered antibiotics and require treatment with a broad-spectrum β-lactam or an aminoglycoside. Prophylactic administration of antibiotics in the catheterized patient is not recommended, because the result is usually simply to postpone the infection by a day or so and to select resistant bacteria. The usual indication to start treatment is the development of fever. Treatment in such patients will usually keep the infection under control but will not eradicate it. Eradication usually requires removal of the foreign body (e.g., the catheter).

Recurrent Infections: Relapse versus Reinfection
Pathobiology

Among the most significant problems in the management of patients with UTI is the tendency of the infection to recur. Ms. C. exemplifies the situation. Recurrence may be either a **relapse**, i.e., the reappearance of the original infection, or more commonly, **reinfection**, the occurrence of a new infection. Relapse is caused by the same strain of organism that caused the original infection and often occurs shortly after cessation of treatment. This timeframe suggests that the causative agent has persisted in the urinary tract or nearby, possibly because of an anatomic problem such as an obstruction or a stone. In contrast, reinfection may be caused by the original organism or a different one, and can occur at any time after treatment is stopped. It does not suggest an anatomic abnormality. Ms. C. experienced reinfections, as the offending organism was different in each attack.

Treatment of recurrent UTI

The greatest challenge in treating patients with UTI is not usually the management of the initial infection but the problem of recurrence. We have already emphasized the importance of distinguishing between relapse and reinfection, because the management of these two types of recurrences is different.

In patients with frequent reinfections, the major goal is to interrupt the cycle of colonization of the introitus and infection of the bladder. Success is achieved with drugs such as trimethoprim–sulfamethoxazole or some quinolones, which reach high concentrations not only in the urine but also in vaginal secretions. Special studies to search for anatomic abnormalities, by x-rays or ultrasound, for example, are not usually called for because the likelihood of finding abnormalities is very low. However, such studies may be indicated in very young patients or in those with unusual frequency of recurrence.

Relapse of infection, by contrast, signals either a structural abnormality (stone, obstruction, bladder dysfunction) or invasion of deep tissues (pyelonephritis, renal abscess, bacterial prostatitis) and merits not only long-term treatment with antibiotics but also urological studies and radiographic studies (e.g., intravenous pyelogram) to detect the abnormality.

CONCLUSION

The lining of the urinary tract is open to the exterior of the body, and, not surprisingly, often becomes colonized by fecal bacteria. Organisms successful at colonizing tend to be those capable of adhering to the epithelial cells and not readily washed away by the urine.

The defense mechanisms of this system of the body are different from those that operate at many other sites. Here, neither white cells nor antibodies occupy center stage. Rather, the major role is played by mechanical factors, especially the normal flow of urine. Accordingly, interruptions in these defenses predispose persons to colonization and infection. A particularly important feature of these infections is that they recur unless the underlying predisposing factor is found and the condition corrected. An optimal approach to treatment and prevention must take these facts into account.

SUGGESTED READINGS

Bacheller CD, Bernstein JM. Urinary tract infections. Med Clin of N Amer 1997;81:719–730.

Johnson JR, WE Stamm. Urinary tract infections in women: diagnosis and treatment. Ann Intern Med 1989;111: 906–917.

Mobley HTL, Warren JW, eds. Urinary tract infections: molecular pathogenesis and clinical management. Washington, DC: American Society for Microbiology, 1995.

Scheinfeld J, Schaeffer AJ, Cordon-Cardo C, Rogatko A, Fair WR. Association of the Lewis blood-group phenotype with recurrent urinary tract infections in women. N Engl J Med 1989;320:773–777.

Schoolnik GK. How *Escherichia coli* infects the urinary tract. N Engl J Med 1989;320:804–805.

Stamm WE, Hooton TM. Management of urinary tract infections in adults. New Engl J Med 1993;329:1328–1334.

Stark RP, DG Maki. Bacteriuria in the catheterized patient. What quantitative level is relevant? N Engl J Med 1984;311: 560–564.

Zhanel GC, GKM Harding, DRP Guay. Asymptomatic bacteriuria. Which patients should be treated? Arch Intern Med 1990;150:1389–1396.

CHAPTER 61

Skin and Soft Tissue

FRANCIS P. TALLY

Inflamed hangnails, infected cuts, and athlete's foot occur so frequently that we scarcely notice. These mild and usually inconsequential conditions represent the less serious extreme of the infections of the skin. The other extreme includes less frequent but potentially serious diseases, such as herpes zoster, candidiasis, or bacterial cellulitis. Infections of the skin may be caused by viruses, fungi, or bacteria. In addition, many diseases that affect other organs have cutaneous manifestations. Visible skin lesions may indicate systemic infections by viruses (e.g., smallpox, measles, chickenpox), fungi (e.g., cryptococcosis, blastomycosis), or bacteria (e.g., syphilis, tuberculosis, scarlet fever, meningococcemia).

Primary infections of the skin and systemic infections with cutaneous manifestations are discussed throughout this book in the context of specific agents (see Chapter 11, "*Staphylococcus*"; Chapter 12, "The Streptococci"; Chapter 18, "*Pseudomonas*"; Chapter 40, "Warts"; Chapter 34, "Paramyxoviruses: Measles"; and Chapter 48, "Subcutaneous Mycoses"). This chapter is limited to bacterial skin infections and emphasizes those with important pathobiological implications. Because these infections frequently involve the "soft tissues" underlying the skin, subcutaneous fat, and superficial fasciae, they are also included in this discussion.

An understanding of the pathogenesis of skin and soft tissue infections requires knowledge of its anatomy and physiology. The skin is divided into three distinct layers: the epidermis, dermis, and fat layer. The **epidermis** is a thin, self-renewing epidermal sheet that covers the body. Over most of the body, it is about the thickness of two of the sheets of this book (0.1 mm) and is devoid of vessels and nerves. The basal cells of the epidermis, the **keratinocytes**, divide, differentiate, and are eventually sloughed from the skin surface. As they rise from the basal layer to the skin surface, they become more stratified and produce a cornified layer of dead cells, the **stratum corneum**. This outermost epidermal layer consists of dead keratinocytes rich in the tough fibrous protein **keratin** and held together by intercellular neutral lipids. The stratum corneum is the major physical barrier that prevents environmental chemicals and microorganisms from entering the body. In addition to the keratinocytes, the epidermis contains other cell types, the **Langerhans cells** and the pigment-containing **melanocytes**. Langerhans cells are fixed tissue macrophages. They represent a distal outpost of the immune system and process antigens that breach the stratum corneum.

Skin appendages, including hairs, oil (sebaceous) glands, and sweat glands, originate from the basal layer of the epidermis. They invaginate into the dermis and exit at the surface through the epidermis. Bacteria may bypass the stratum corneum by traversing these conduits.

The **dermis** is several millimeters thick and is separated from the epidermis by a basement membrane. The fibrous proteins **collagen** and **elastin** are embedded in a glycoprotein matrix and constitute the strong supportive dermal structure. Through the dermis courses a rich plexus of blood vessels and lymphatics. Interruption of dermal blood flow predisposes to infection by restricting access of humoral and cellular defenses against invaders and by compromising the nutrition of the epidermal barrier.

Subcutaneous fat, the third layer of the skin, consists predominantly of lipid cells. These cells serve as heat insulators, shock absorbers, and depots of caloric reserves. Below this layer is a **superficial fascia** that separates the skin from muscles. As described below, any or all of these layers of "soft tissue" may be involved in a given infectious process.

Encounter

The skin is sterile only at birth. It is soon colonized by a flora that includes both anaerobic and aerobic bacteria that ranges from 10^2 to 10^4 CFU (colony forming units)/square centimeter of surface. Many factors affect the distribution, composition, and density of this flora, few of which are understood. These factors include not only the environmental climate, which differs throughout the world, but also the microclimates of the body. The "tropical swamps" of the axilla and the groin are markedly different from the "deserts" of the back.

The two properties that make the skin hostile to bacterial growth are **exfoliation** and **dryness**. The constant sloughing of the stratum corneum dislodges many of the bacteria that adhere to its surface. The importance of dryness can be seen when occlusive dressings are applied: within 2 or 3 days bacterial counts may increase from 10^2 to over 10^7 CFU per cm^2. Accordingly, bacterial counts are much higher in the moister areas of the skin than in drier regions. Other factors that help limit bacterial growth are low pH, low temperature, and chemical composition. The skin has a pH of approximately 5.5, the result of hydrolysis of sebum lipids by the skin bacteria themselves. Growth of some microorganisms is further hindered by the skin's low temperature, which averages about 33°C. Parts of the skin are also salty owing to the evaporation of sweat. This saltiness may encourage the growth of salt-resistant species, such as *Staphylococcus epidermidis*. Some organisms are also inhibited by the lipid content of the skin surface.

The bacterial flora of the skin, like that of mucous membranes, also helps protect the host from invasion by pathogens, and skin infections are more likely to occur when this flora is wiped out. The mechanisms that account for the protection of the skin by normal flora are not known but may include saturation of binding sites, competition for nutrients, and production of bacteriocins and other inhibitory chemicals.

Members of the resident flora of the skin are of low virulence and rarely cause significant infections. Included in the flora are **resident bacteria,** which multiply on the skin and are regularly present, and **transient bacteria,** which survive on the skin for only a short period of time. Members of the transient flora are deposited on the skin either from mucous membrane "fallout" or from the environment. Evidence suggests that specific adhesins are required for some bacteria to adhere to the skin before they are able to colonize it.

The dry and exposed areas of the skin are normally colonized with Gram-positive bacteria (including *S. epidermidis*, micrococci, anaerobic Gram-positive cocci, and both anaerobic and aerobic diphtheroids). *Propionibacterium acnes*, a Gram-positive rod, thrives in the sebaceous areas. Facultative and anaerobic Gram-negative rods more often colonize the axilla and groin regions and other moist areas, such as the web of the toes. For unknown reasons, the skin of bedridden patients with serious medical illnesses often has increased colonization of Gram-negative bacilli.

The most important organisms of the transient flora are the common pathogens of cutaneous infections, *S.*

Table 61.1. Members of the Skin Flora and the Infections They Cause

Resident Flora
  Propionibacterium acnes
  Staphylococcus epidermidis—infection around foreign bodies (prosthetic devices, etc.)
  Micrococci
  Anaerobic Gram-positive cocci
  Aerobic Gram-negative bacilli (low numbers)
  Pityrosporum ovale (a yeast)

Transient Flora
  Bacteria
    Frequent:
    Staphylococcus aureus—abscesses, toxic shock, and bacteremia
    Streptococcus pyogenes—cellulitis, lymphangitis
    Infrequent:
    Haemophilus influenzae—cellulitis
    Clostridia—gangrene
    Francisella tularensis—tularemia
    Bacillus anthracis—anthrax
    Pseudomonas aeruginosa—hot-tub infection
    Pseudomonas cepacia—foot infection ("foot rot")
    Mycobacterium marinum—"fish tank cellulitis"
  Fungi
    Candida albicans—diaper rash, chronic paronychia
    Dermatophytes—tinea infections (ringworm)
  Viruses
    Frequent:
    Herpes simplex virus 1 and 2—perioral ("cold sore") and genital infection
    Papilloma—warts
    Infrequent:
    Molluscum contagiosum—wartlike lesions

---

aureus and *Streptococcus pyogenes*. These organisms are found more often on exposed skin than on areas normally protected by clothing. *S. aureus* is found commonly on the face and upper body rather than on the trunk and legs, probably because the reservoir for this organism is the upper respiratory tract. Table 61.1 lists some of the important pathogens that transiently colonize the skin and the infections they cause.

Entry, Spread, and Multiplication

Infectious agents enter the skin and its underlying soft tissues by two routes:

- **From the outside,** via cuts, wounds, insect bites, skin disease, or other breaks in the integrity of the stratum corneum.
- **From within,** from underlying tissue or carried by blood or lymph.

Once microorganisms have penetrated the skin, they may spread locally and invade the lymphatics or the bloodstream. As a result, infections that are originally confined to the skin and soft tissues may ultimately cause complications in other areas of the body. An example of staphylococcal osteomyelitis following a skin abscess is discussed in Chapter 11, "*Staphylococcus*".

The spread of some bacteria is associated with specific virulence factors; an example is **hyaluronidase** (also called **spreading factor**), an extracellular enzyme made both by *S. pyogenes* and *S. aureus* (see Chapter 11, "*Staphylococcus*"). Other enzymes, such as hemolysins, lipases, collagenase, and elastases are elaborated by cutaneous pathogens and probably play a role in pathogenesis (see Chapter 9, "Damage by Microbial Agents"). **In general, *S. aureus* infections tend to localize, e.g., form abscesses, whereas *S. pyogenes* infections spread more extensively through tissues.**

What is the role of cellular and humoral immunity in the skin? Neutrophils are attracted to the infected area by chemoattractants elaborated by the bacteria, tissue macrophages, and activation of complement via the alternative pathway. A local antimicrobial effort is mounted by the epidermal macrophages, the Langerhans cells, through the elaboration of cytokines. Patients with acquired and congenital immunodeficiences have an increased frequency of certain skin infections, e.g., *Candida*, which suggests that cellular immunity is important in skin defenses. When microorganisms breach the stratum corneum and begin to multiply, the host's defenses are mobilized to the skin as elsewhere. When the defenses are defective, infections of the skin become frequent events.

Damage

Cellular damage to the skin and soft tissues may be mediated by toxins, degradative enzymes, and the induction of the host cellular responses that destroy tissues. The kind of infection caused by the invasion of microorganisms in the skin depends on the level of penetration and on the host response. Infections of skin and soft tissue may be divided into three classes:

- Exogenous infections that result from direct invasion from the external environment
- Endogenous infections due to invasion from an internal source, such as the blood or an infected organ
- Toxin-induced skin diseases, caused by toxins produced at a distant site

EXOGENOUS INFECTIONS

Controversy exists about whether potent pathogens are able to directly penetrate the normal skin when present in high concentrations, or whether they enter via imperceptible microscopic lesions. Without a noticeable break in the skin, high numbers of potent pathogens are required to produce exogenous skin and soft tissue in-

fection. Experimental studies have shown that colonization of the skin by more than 10^6 S. aureus per square centimeter of skin is required to cause skin lesions. Normally, bacteria grow to these high densities only under special circumstances, such as when the skin is very dirty or is kept moist for prolonged periods of time. Once the skin barrier is broken from trauma or surgery, infection may be caused by as few as 10 to 100 *S. aureus* per cm². A number of conditions predispose to skin invasion, including excessive moisture, trauma, introduction of a foreign body, pressure, and compromised blood supply.

Excessive moisture may result from the use of occlusive dressings or from wet diapers in babies. Obese people accumulate moisture in their intertriginous folds. **Immersion infection** is seen in people who spend long periods of time in wet or swampy areas and who cannot allow their footwear to dry out, such as troops during training or combat. Moisture induces skin maceration and a breakdown of the stratum corneum. It is estimated that among United States foot soldiers in Vietnam, disability was more often associated with skin infections than with combat-associated wounds. Staphylococci and streptococci are frequently responsible for these infections, but water-borne Gram-negative bacteria may also be involved. The modern era has heralded a new type of immersion infection, that acquired by bathing in hot tubs containing high numbers of *Pseudomonas aeruginosa* (see Chapter 18, "*Pseudomonas*").

Trauma is the most common factor leading to skin and soft tissue infection. Trauma may be mild, as in a torn hangnail or cracks in the skin caused by athlete's foot. Major forms of trauma that place the patient at risk include surgery ("organized trauma"), gunshot wounds, crush injuries (automobile accidents), or burns, in which large areas of skin are denuded and left open. Infections in surgical wounds are a major cause of morbidity in postoperative patients. Infections are also the primary cause of mortality in burn victims.

Many procedures used in the hospital breach the skin. The most common of these procedures is the use of **percutaneous** ("through the skin") **catheters**. The list of such devices has grown enormously and includes central venous lines, peritoneal dialysis catheters, tubes to drain body cavities, temporary pacemaker lines, chemotherapy infusion lines, and parenteral nutrition lines. Indeed, the most common reason for premature removal of these catheters is bacterial infection. Another type of skin infection in hospitalized patients are the cutaneous lesions that develop secondary to pressure injury, the so-called bed sores. Constant pressure leads to skin necrosis and frequently to secondary infection.

Any condition that compromises the blood supply predisposes the skin to invasion by causing barrier breakdown and limiting defenses. Blood supply compromise may occur following peripheral vascular disease, as in diabetics, elderly patients, or patients with

Table 61.2. Some Frequent Exogenous Infections of the Skin and Soft Tissues

Disease	Organisms
Folliculitis	Staphylococci, *Pseudomonas*
Abscesses	Staphylococci
Impetigo	Streptococci, staphylococci
Erysipelas	Streptococci
Lymphangitis	Streptococci
Cellulitis	Streptococci, staphylococci, *Haemophilus influenzae* (in children)
Synergistic cellulitis	Streptococci, enteric bacteria, anaerobes
Fasciitis	Streptococci, enteric bacteria, anaerobes

vasculitis. In the diabetic patient, compromise of the vascular supply is often accompanied by peripheral sensory neuropathy; these patients are sometimes not aware of traumatic damage to their skin. Secondary infections may also follow certain noninfectious skin diseases known as atopic dermatitis or pemphigus vulgaris.

The skin responds to invading microorganisms in a limited number of ways, which fall into three general categories:

- **Spreading infections**, called **impetigo** when confined to the epidermis, **erysipelas** when involving the dermal lymphatics, and **cellulitis** when the major focus is the subcutaneous fat layer.
- **Abscess formation**, known as folliculitis, boils (furuncles), and carbuncles.
- **Necrotizing infections**, including fasciitis and gas gangrene (myonecrosis).

The organisms commonly implicated are listed in Table 61.2. Cellulitis is illustrated in the following case.

Streptococcal Cellulitis

▊ CASE 1

A 27-year-old emergency medical technician was seen for a slight infection around the nail of his left index finger (medically called **paronychia**). The lesion was drained and a culture of the pus grew a group A β-hemolytic streptococcus (*S. pyogenes*). The patient was not given antimicrobial agents because the physician believed that drainage was sufficient. Five days later, the patient complained of fever and severe pain in the forearm, which had become swollen and red (erythematous). His temperature was 40.2°C, and he was sweaty and hot. A patchy rash extended from the left upper arm to the shoulder. Lymph nodes in the axilla were enlarged and tender. The patient was admitted to the hospital with a diagnosis of **streptococcal cellulitis**. He was

treated successfully with high doses of penicillin. Blood cultures drawn before starting chemotherapy also yielded group A *S. pyogenes*.

Cellulitis refers to an acute inflammatory process that involves subcutaneous tissue, characterized by areas of redness, induration, heat, and tenderness. The borders of these areas usually blend with the surrounding tissues, which distinguishes it from erysipelas in which the lesions are frequently sharply demarcated. Cellulitis may spread rapidly and is often accompanied by lymphangitis and inflammation of the draining lymph nodes. Over 90% of cases are caused by *S. aureus* and group A streptococci, while the rest are attributed to a variety of bacteria. In children, infection with *Haemophilus influenzae* type b is an important cause of cellulitis, and it may be characterized by a blue tint of the overlying erythema (see the case described in Chapter 65, "Head and Neck"). Cellulitis associated with cat or dog bites or scratches is often due to *Pasteurella multocida* (see Chapter 70, "Zoonoses"). This organism is a normal inhabitant of the oral flora of many domestic and wild animals. When injected into human skin through a bite or scratches, it spreads rapidly and causes painful cellulitis.

The pathological processes in cellulitis develop rapidly and may progress within 24–48 hours from a minor injury to severe septicemia. Characteristically, the tissues contain few organisms but undergo a marked inflammatory response, probably caused by the toxins and inflammation-provoking compounds elaborated by the invading bacteria. The ability of group A streptococci to spread through the tissues is aided by hyaluronidase and other spreading factors mentioned above.

Impetigo is a characteristic infection of the epidermis, manifested by intraepidermal vesicles filled with exudate, which eventually result in a weeping and crusting lesion (Fig. 61.1). It is caused either by group A strepto-

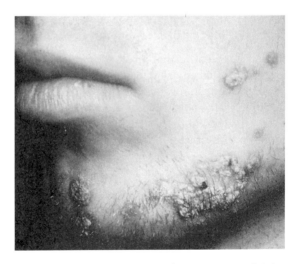

Figure 61.1. A case of impetigo, showing a superficial crusting infection of the face.

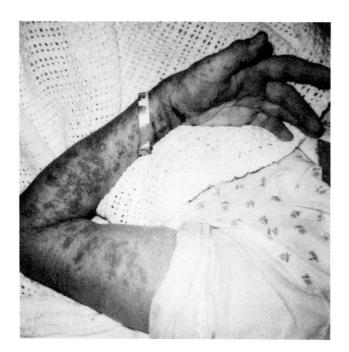

Figure 61.2. A case of erysipelas due to *S. pyogenes* in a patient with a preexisting skin disease (psoriasis).

cocci or staphylococci. It is a common disease of children, and is seen mainly in exposed areas of the body during warm and moist weather. It is not usually associated with systemic signs or symptoms.

Erysipelas is a more serious disease, characterized by tender, superficial erythematous and edematous lesions. The infection spreads primarily in the superficial lymphatics of the dermis (Fig. 61.2). The rash is usually confluent but is sharply demarcated from the surrounding normal skin, and it extends rapidly. It is seen most frequently in adults with edema of the extremities and often occurs on the face. The most common organisms that cause erysipelas are group A streptococci. Infection of the deep lymphatics, or **lymphangitis**, is also caused by group A streptococci. Erysipelas used to be one of the most serious complications of surgery and puerperal sepsis (postpartum infection, see Chapter 12, "The Streptococci"), and it carried a high mortality rate. Its severity and incidence have markedly decreased over the last few decades. The decline can be explained only partially by the widespread use of penicillin to treat streptococcal infections.

Skin Abscesses

CASE 2

A 37-year-old roofer came to the emergency room with a painful swelling on the left side of his neck and fever (Fig. 61.3). He had previously been healthy except for occasional boils. Three days before, he noted a minor irritation around

some whiskers. The lesion progressed to the size of a walnut, which prevented him from buttoning his shirt. Physical examination revealed a febrile (temperature 38.8°C) healthy man in mild distress. A 2 × 3 cm mass with a soft center was noted on his left anterior cervical area at the beard line, surrounded by a rash. Needle aspiration of the mass yielded about 1 ml of pus which, under the microscope, showed large Gram-positive cocci in clusters and many neutrophils. A culture grew *S. aureus*. The abscess was incised and drained, and he was successfully treated with antibiotics.

Cutaneous abscesses usually begin as superficial infections in and around hair follicles, called **folliculitis**. Folliculitis is a pustular eruption usually associated with *S. aureus*. In the follicle, bacteria are somewhat sequestered from defense mechanisms and are capable of forming microabscesses. If not controlled, these abscesses enlarge to become **furuncles**, better known as **common boils**. If a number of boils cluster together to form a large multifocal infection, the lesion is called a **carbuncle**. Furuncles may be a recurring and frustrating problem in patients, especially young ones, who are chronic nasal carriers of virulent *S. aureus*. Although these lesions are confined to the skin, they may be a source of bacteremia and complications, as in the case of osteomyelitis described in Chapter 11, "*Staphylococcus*".

The pathological processes that lead to abscess formation involve a massive influx of neutrophils and walling-off of the infected site. The walling-off of the infected site is caused by deposition of fibrin (fostered by staphylococcal coagulase), and by stimulation of fibroblasts to produce a fibrous capsule. The result is a well-organized infection, containing necrotic white blood cells and huge numbers of bacteria, i.e., pus. The pathological steps that lead to abscess formation include tissue destruction by the invading organisms and by the massive release of lysosomal enzymes from lysing neutrophils, as well as deposition of fibrin (see Chapter 11). The unique physicochemical characteristics of abscesses are discussed in Chapter 30, "Strategies to Combat Bacterial Infections." Therapy of an abscess is usually two-pronged: removal of pus by incision and drainage, and when warranted, treatment with antimicrobial agents.

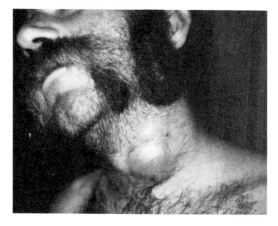

Figure 61.3. Skin abscess in the neck developing from an infected hair follicle of the beard.

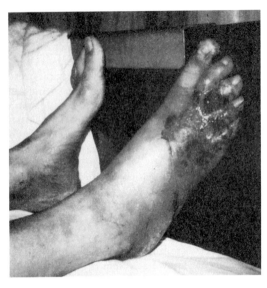

Figure 61.4. Necrotizing cellulitis of the foot due to a mixed anaerobic–aerobic infection. The patient was diabetic and the infection arose from an ulcer on the sole of the foot.

Necrotizing Infections

CASE 3

A slightly feverish 57-year-old diabetic woman came to the emergency room after 2 days of pain in her right forefoot. When her pain started, she had noticed tenderness and serious (watery) discharge between her third and fourth toes. She had been bothered recently by an ulcer on the sole of her foot, apparently caused by constant scraping against her shoe. On physical examination she appeared ill and had a temperature of 39.8°C. Her right foot was swollen with patchy erythema, cyanosis, and signs of necrosis. There was crusting and oozing around her third and fourth toe (Fig. 61.4).

Cultures of the exudate and the blood were taken and the patient was started on antibiotics. After 24 hours she showed no clinical improvement and the infection continued to move up her leg. She was taken to the operating room, and multiple incisions revealed necrotic fasciitis extending to the upper thigh. As much necrotic tissue as possible was removed. Cultures from the wound grew the anaerobic Gram-negative rod *Bacteroides fragilis* and an enteric bacterium, *Enterobacter*. Her blood cultures were negative. She slowly recovered and underwent a second operation for closure of her wound.

This case illustrates **synergistic necrotizing fasciitis**, probably started by the entry of bacteria through the ulcer on the sole of the patient's foot. Diabetics frequently suffer from poor skin circulation and lack of local sensation, which may have been the reason for the development of the ulcer. The infection spread rapidly along the superficial fascia that separates subcutaneous fat and muscle. The vessels and nerves that supply the skin course this fascia, and their destruction leads to the patchy necrosis and cutaneous anesthesia that characterize such a rapidly spreading and dangerous infection.

Although tissue necrosis occurs to some extent in most infections, the term **necrotizing infection** (or **gangrenous infection**) is reserved for those in which extensive necrosis is the outstanding characteristic. Gas from bacterial metabolism is sometimes found in these lesions (see Chapter 20, "The Clostridia"). Necrotizing infections of the skin are often caused by *S. pyogenes*, or as in this case, by the synergistic combination of enteric Gram-negative rods and strict anaerobes, such as *Bacteroides* or clostridia (see Chapter 15, "*Bacteroides* and Abscesses"). If a necrotizing infection is suspected, the diagnosis should be confirmed by inspection of the fascia on surgical exploration. This disease must be distinguished from the more severe clostridial gas gangrene or myonecrosis, which involves the muscle (see Chapter 20). Antibiotic treatment of necrotizing fasciitis is rarely successful, probably because of the compromised blood supply; extensive surgical debridement is mandatory.

INVASION FROM WITHIN

The skin may become infected by microorganisms that spread from another infected site, either by direct extension from an underlying focus or via the bloodstream. Such secondary infections occur in both immunocompetent and immunosuppressed hosts but with different degrees of incidence and severity. Some of the types of skin infections that occur from within are listed in Table 61.3. Systemic infections are manifested in a variety of ways:

- **Abscesses.** These may result from intravascular infections such as endocarditis, particularly when due to *S. aureus*.
- **Necrosis.** This manifestation is seen in chronic meningococcemia or in overwhelming meningococcal septicemia, in which large areas of confluent necrosis of the skin may be present. This condition, called **purpura fulminans**, is the skin manifestation of disseminated intravascular coagulation (Fig. 61.5). Milder forms of necrosis are also seen, for example, in disseminated gonorrhea. Immunocompromised hosts are susceptible to a unique skin lesion called **ecthyma gangrenosum**, usually seen with *P. aeruginosa* septicemia. A case of this disease is presented below.
- Many infections are accompanied by **rashes** or exanthems. These conditions are seen in a large variety of infections caused by rickettsiae, other bacteria, and viruses. They are subdivided into hemorrhagic rashes, often accompanied by necrosis (as in meningococcemia, see Fig. 61.5) and macular (spotted) rashes (as in typhoid fever or Rocky Mountain spotted fever). Rashes are prominent in several viral infections, such as measles and rubella, and are

known as the **viral exanthems** (see Chapter 34, "Paramyxoviruses" and Table 61.4).

- A large number of cutaneous lesions are themselves **noninfectious** but are secondary to septicemia or other systemic infections. They include hemorrhages, petechiae, and special manifestations of subacute bacterial endocarditis called Osler nodes and Janeway spots (see Chapter 64, "Intravascular Infection"). They are caused by vasculitis, probably as a result of deposition of immune complexes.

Table 61.3. Examples of Sources of Endogenous Skin Infections

A. Direct Extension
 1. Osteomyelitis—draining sinus
 2. Septic arthritis—draining sinus
 3. Lymphadenitis
  a. Tuberculosis
  b. Atypical mycobacteriosis
  c. Streptococcal or staphylococcal infection
 4. Oral infection—dental sepsis
  a. Actinomycosis (lumpy jaw)
  b. Mixed cellulitis
 5. Intra-abdominal—necrotizing infection
 6. Herpes simplex
 7. Zoster varicella

B. Hematogenous Spread
 1. Bacteremia
   Meningococcus
   Staphylococcus
   Pseudomonas
 2. Endocarditis
 3. Fungemia—*Candida*
 4. Viremia—varicella, measles
 5. Recurrent viral infections
   Herpes simplex
   Zoster
 6. Rickettsioses
   Rocky Mountain spotted fever
   Epidemic or endemic typhus

CASE 4

A 52-year-old man underwent chemotherapy with cytotoxic agents for an aggressive lymphoma. As the result of the chemotherapy, his white blood cell count fell to fewer than 100 cells per microliter of blood. The patient suddenly developed shaking chills and fever and complained of pain over his left shoulder. Examination of the area showed an erythematous round area with a central vesicle (Fig. 61.6). Because of the suspicion of Gram-negative bacteremia, the

---

Table 61.4. Some Viral Diseases with Cutaneous Manifestations

Disease	Etiological agent	Principal cutaneous manifestation
Herpes simplex	Herpes simplex virus	"Cold sore" on lip Vesicles in genital area
Herpes zoster	Varicella virus	Shingles—vesicles over specific dermotome(s)
Chickenpox (varicella)	Varicella virus	Vesicles, becoming purulent, then dry, crusted lesions
Measles	Measles virus	Maculopapular rash
German measles	Rubella virus	Maculopapular rash
Smallpox (eradicated)	Smallpox virus	Uniform pustular vesicles

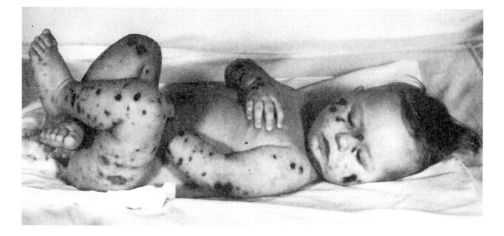

Figure 61.5. Hemorrhagic purpura due to disseminated intravascular coagulation in a child with meningococcal septicemia.

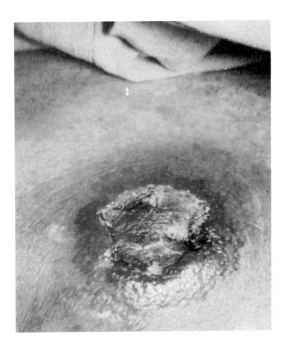

Figure 61.6. Ecthyma gangrenosum, a necrotic skin lesion due to *P. aeruginosa*.

patient was started on broad-spectrum antimicrobial agents. Within a few hours, the area on the left shoulder developed a necrotic center with surrounding erythema, a lesion known as **ecthyma gangrenosum**. A biopsy of the lesion showed that it contained an infarcted blood vessel teeming with bacteria. Cultures of the biopsy material and the blood grew *P. aeruginosa*. The patient responded to the antimicrobial chemotherapy with resolution of fever and clearing of the skin lesions.

This case exemplifies a specific skin lesion resulting from seeding of the skin with *P. aeruginosa*. One of the characteristics of endogenous infection with this organism is arteritis resulting in infarction of the skin from vascular insufficiency. *P. aeruginosa* grows in the infarcted area and causes necrosis by the production of exotoxin A and other toxins (see Chapter 18, "*Pseudomonas aeruginosa*"). In this case, biopsy of the necrotic area revealed no neutrophil infiltrate because of the patient's granulocytopenia. Instead, infarction of blood vessels by bacterial emboli occurred, with destruction of the arterial wall and bacterial invasion of the surrounding tissues.

This characteristic lesion is usually diagnostic of Gram-negative bacteremia, with *P. aeruginosa* the most common organism encountered. Other Gram-negative rods may also be involved, e.g., *Klebsiella* and *Serratia*; occasionally, *S. aureus* also causes these manifestations. Disseminated fungal infections, including those due to *Aspergillus* and *Cryptococcus*, can cause the same characteristic lesions. It is imperative that the physician treat early—before bacteriological confirmation—because the mortality rate in untreated granulocytopenic patients with Gram-negative bacteremia is 50% within 24 hours.

CUTANEOUS RESPONSES TO BACTERIAL TOXINS

The skin responds to toxins elaborated during infections that take place at a distant site. An example is scarlet fever, a pharyngitis caused by certain strains of group A streptococci that elaborate an exotoxin called **erythrogenic factor**. This toxin spreads through the bloodstream and is responsible for the red rash, "strawberry tongue" and desquamation of the skin of the extremities. Scarlet fever used to be a serious disease of childhood; the marked decrease in its severity over the last century has defied explanation.

Staphylococci cause two specific toxin-induced skin diseases: **scalded skin syndrome** and **toxic shock syndrome**. Staphylococcal scalded skin syndrome, a disease of infants, results from the action of a toxin, **exfoliatin**, that separates the epidermis by destroying the intracellular connections (desmosomes). The result resembles skin scalded with hot water. The other staphylococcal toxin skin disease, toxic shock syndrome, is presented below.

CASE 5

A 24-year-old man had an operation to repair an inguinal hernia. Five days later, he developed shaking chills and a rash started on his trunk and rapidly spread to the head and extremities. He became progressively sicker over the next 48 hours, developing a sore throat, headache, myalgias (muscle pains), vomiting, diarrhea, and postural dizziness (dizzy when upright, suggesting low blood pressure). On physical examination he had a diffuse rash with some blanching on pressure. His eyes were inflamed with conjunctivitis, and he had an erythematous pharynx and a "strawberry" tongue. His inguinal wound was draining a brown odorless material.

Laboratory examination revealed a high white blood cell count and elevated high serum creatinine (5.7 mg/dl), indicating acute renal failure. A Gram stain of the material from the wound showed Gram-positive cocci in clusters and grew *S. aureus*. The organism tested positive for the toxic shock syndrome toxin. The patient ultimately showed desquamation of his hands and trunk (Fig. 61.7). He was placed on antibiotics and eventually recovered.

This case is a typical clinical presentation of toxic shock syndrome (TSS). The disease is caused by an exotoxin produced by *S. aureus* strains that cause minor infections, such as small surgical wounds. This syndrome was first described in children in the early 1970s. It be-

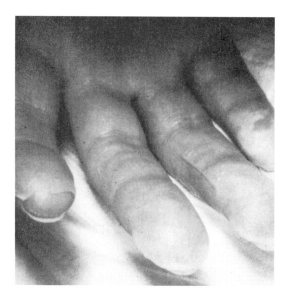

Figure 61.7. Desquamation of the skin of the hand in a patient with staphylococcal toxic shock.

came widely known in the early 1980s when young menstruating women using "super tampons" developed this impressive syndrome: if untreated, TSS can be fatal. The tampons used facilitated the colonization of the vagina with *S. aureus*; the toxin was then absorbed to act systemically. Today tampon-associated TSS is rare; more commonly it occurs after an infection, as illustrated in this case. A similar syndrome can also occur in patients with severe and disseminated *S. pyogenes* infection.

CONCLUSION

The skin and its underlying soft tissues protect the body from hostile influences in the environment. To penetrate these barriers, infectious agents are most often helped by traumatic breaks, the bite of insects, or other skin diseases. Microorganisms may also lodge in the skin and soft tissues as the result of hematogenous or lymphatic dissemination. The resulting diseases are extraordinarily varied and are caused by a wide variety of mechanisms. Thus, the hallmark of infectious diseases of the skin and soft tissues is variety in the clinical presentation.

The skin also acts as a diagnostic window for a multitude of diseases. The clinician can acquire a wealth of critical information by careful examination of the skin.

SUGGESTED READINGS

Feingold DS, Hirschmann JV. Approach to the patient with skin or soft tissue infection. In: Infectious Diseases, 2nd ed. Gorbach SL, Bartlett JG, Blacklow NR, eds. 1998; 1261–1262.

Noble WC. Microbial skin disease: its epidemiology. London: Edward Arnold, 1981.

Swartz M. Skin and soft tissue infections. In: Mandel GL, Douglas RG, Bennett JE, eds. Principles and practice of infectious diseases. 4th ed. New York: John Wiley, 1995; 909–944.

CHAPTER 62

Bone, Joints, and Infections of Muscles

GERALD MEDOFF

BONE INFECTIONS

Infections of bone, or **osteomyelitis**, may result from bloodborne infections (hematogenous) or from the direct introduction of microorganisms from external (environmental) or contiguous sources (soft tissues or joints). A special type of infection from contiguous sources occurs in the bones of the feet of individuals with diabetes. The pathophysiology of the diseases, the types of infecting agents, and the kinds of treatments and prognoses are frequently different. For this reason, they will be discussed separately.

Hematogenous Osteomyelitis

■ CASE

O., a 15-year-old boy, received an injury to the lower part of his right thigh in a high school football game. The pain was so intense he had to leave the game. The pain then subsided for several hours but returned that night, and he developed chills followed by a fever to 103°F. A physician who saw him the next day noted that the lower right thigh was hot, swollen, and tender. The knee joint was normal with full range of motion. The patient had a temperature of 101°F. The physician noted several small boils on the neck and chest of the patient. Some were scarred and crusted and the patient admitted squeezing them in the past 2 days. X-rays of the right femur showed soft tissue swelling without any abnormalities of the bone.

O. was diagnosed with acute hematogenous osteomyelitis. The most likely infecting organism was *Staphylococcus aureus*. This diagnosis becomes even more plausible when the pathophysiology of the infection is understood. Several features of the history and physical examination of the patient point to this diagnosis.

- The trauma to the leg suffered in the football game damaged the distal femur and probably resulted in

rupture of small blood vessels and formation of hematoma or blood clot in the bone. The disruption in the normal anatomical barriers made the bone more susceptible to infection.

- Manipulation of the boils by the patient probably resulted in bacteremia, with *S. aureus* a likely infecting organism. Bloodborne *S. aureus* could have then seeded the traumatized bone and caused the infection.

- The history of chills and fever, as well as pain and inflammation over the area of trauma, indicate that an infection is in progress. The normal x-ray does not rule out osteomyelitis because it may take several weeks for the characteristic changes in the bone to appear (periosteal proliferation or elevation, loss of bone cortex, bone lysis, etc.). These changes often appear later in the course of an infection because about 50% of bone must be destroyed before bone lysis can be detected on x-ray. A radionuclide bone scan is more likely to be positive early in the disease because it measures inflammation, although not infallibly.

Pathophysiology

Bone has a high rate of synthesis and resorption, two processes that depend on a rich vascular supply. Many bloodborne infections therefore involve actively growing sites; hematogenous osteomyelitis thus occurs mostly in children and adolescents, at a time of life when long bones are growing rapidly. The most frequent sites are the growing ends (metaphysis, Fig. 62.1) of long bones, where growth and rapid turnover occur. Osteomyelitis most often occurs at these sites when the bone has suffered severe trauma with disruption of blood vessels and hematoma formation.

The anatomy of the vascular supply of the metaphysis also predisposes this area to infection. The capillaries from the nutrient arteries of bone make sharp loops close to the growth plate. They then expand to large si-

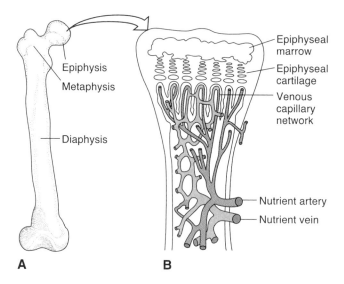

Figure 62.1. A. Femur showing epiphysis, metaphysis, and diaphysis. B. Schematic representation of the vascular supply of a long bone.

nusoidal vessels which connect with the venous network of the medullary cavity. The sudden increase in diameter of these vessels slows blood flow and results in sludging of red blood cells (Fig. 62.1). Areas where sludging of blood cells occurs are ideal for the growth of bacteria, because microclots form spontaneously in areas of slow blood flow. Clots retain bacteria and shield them from neutrophils, thus allowing the bacteria to proliferate. The result is inflammation, small areas of bones necrosis, and an acid pH, all of which cause more tissue destruction and more bacterial growth. The endothelial cells in the capillary loop and sinusoids in the bone lack phagocytic properties, which also predisposes these areas to infection.

Diagnosis and treatment

In the case presented, O.'s local pain and the systemic signs of infection (chills and fever) indicated a serious disease, acute osteomyelitis, which calls for admission to the hospital. Blood cultures should be obtained and the patient started on antibiotics. Since about 90% of the patients with this clinical presentation are infected with *S. aureus*, a β-lactamase-resistant penicillin or a cephalosporin is usually used empirically. If the patient has specific predisposing conditions, other bacterial etiologies are more likely (e.g. *Salmonella* infection in patients with sickle cell disease, *Pseudomonas aeruginosa* in drug users). In the case, aspiration or biopsy of bones for culture would be indicated to make identification of the organism more certain.

Treatment of osteomyelitis requires a high daily dose of antibiotic that is continued for 4 to 6 weeks. High doses are necessary to penetrate bone tissue, but it is not clear why osteomyelitis requires long-term treatment. The areas of bone necrosis that result from

the infection are likely to shield the bacteria from body defenses. These areas have to be resorbed, which is a slow process. Meanwhile, antibiotics may help keep the bacteria in check and prevent them from spreading to adjacent areas.

If appropriate treatment is started early in the course of the infection, before much bone necrosis occurs, patients respond quickly and cure can be achieved in greater than 90% of cases. If fever and pain continue for 24–48 hours after treatment is started, surgical drainage may be indicated. Blood cultures will be positive in about one-third of cases, which may obviate the need for surgery to determine the infectious agent.

Although *S. aureus* is the most frequent infecting organism in hematogenous osteomyelitis, other organisms can also cause the disease. Often the clinical setting in which these infections occur gives a clue about the organisms involved in the infection. Table 62.1 lists other infecting organisms and the clinical situations that suggest them.

The course of the untreated disease

Unfortunately, the diagnosis was missed in the case presented. O. was given an oral antibiotic by his physician and sent home. He was not seen again by a physician for another 2 weeks, when he returned to the emergency room because of continued fever and pain in his leg. A repeat x-ray of O.'s leg showed definite osteomyelitis (Fig. 62.2) and he was admitted to the hospital and started on intravenous treatment with a cephalosporin. Unfortunately, his disease had progressed to the subacute and chronic phase of osteomyelitis. By now the compromised blood supply resulted in small avascular pieces of bone or **sequestra**. The blood supply was disrupted by the pressure caused by inflammation. The chance of medical cure had significantly lessened because of the delay in diagnosis. Over the next few years, the patient had a slowly progressive

Table 62.1. Some Predisposing Causes and Etiologic Organisms Leading to Osteomyelitis

Predisposing causes	Etiologic organisms
Infancy	Group B streptococci
Childhood	*Haemophilus influenzae*
Sickle cell disease	*Salmonella* spp.
Immunosuppression	Opportunistic fungi, *Nocardia, Pseudomonas*
Residing in an endemic area	*Coccidioides immitis, Histoplasma capsulatum*
Trauma to the jaw	*Actinomyces israelii*
Animal exposure	*Brucella* spp.
Pulmonary tuberculosis	*Mycobacterium tuberculosis*

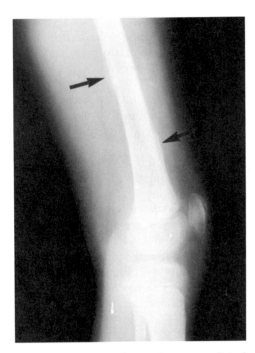

Figure 62.2. X-ray showing changes in osteomyelitis showing sclerosis and periosteal changes.

infection with several acute flares each year. Over the next 10 years, he spent many days in the hospital and had multiple surgical procedures to drain pus and cut away infected dead bone (Fig. 62.3). He suffered several fractures because of the weakened bone and finally, at the age of 25, had to have his leg amputated because it was feared that the infection would spread into his hip joint and pelvis. Thus an infection that should have been easily treated with antibiotics was converted into a more complex disease (chronic osteomyelitis) which required vigorous medical and surgical intervention, culminating in amputation of the leg to preserve the patient's life.

Hematogenous osteomyelitis at different ages

Infants. The clinical presentation of hematogenous osteomyelitis depends a great deal on the age of the patient. the various clinical presentations are due to the changing characteristics of the bone in different age groups. In the infant, the bone is soft and the periosteum is loosely attached to the cortex. Infection can therefore spread and rupture through the thin cortical bone into the subperiosteal space. Subperiosteal abscesses are common in this age group and lead to a stimulation of periosteal bone formation at this inappropriate site, as periosteal cells transform into osteoblasts. This new bone formation is disorganized and produces a weakened bone called an *involucrum* (Fig. 62.4) Osteomyelitis in the infant can be a devastating disease because early in life the capillaries of the metaphysis extend into the epiphyseal growth plate. the infection can then

spread by this route into the epiphysis and seriously affect growth of the bone. In addition, the infection can also rupture into the joint space and cause infectious arthritis. Consequently, osteomyelitis in the infant can result in a severe destructive process with significant deformity of bone and abnormalities of growth which can affect the patient for the rest of his or her life (Fig. 62.5).

Children. Between the age of one and puberty, infection is generally contained in the metaphysis because the bone is more calcified and there are no vessels connecting the metaphysis and the epiphysis. Also, the periosteum is more tightly adhered to the cortex in this age group, so that rupture of infection into the subperiosteal space and formation of involucrum is less likely. Thus, the purulent infectious process will probably be contained in bone, but it has other consequences. Within the bone, pressure builds and results in occlusion of arterioles and clot formation in the capillaries.

Necrosis of bone is the end result in the formation of the necrotic sequestrum (see Fig. 62.3). This area is no longer in contact with the vasculature and acts as a foreign body on which organisms can proliferate out of reach of host defenses and antibiotics. Ultimately, the sequestrum must be resorbed (by the body) or removed surgically if the infection is to be cured. With increasing

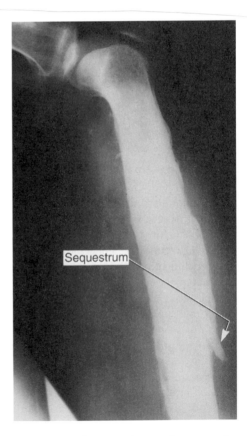

Figure 62.3. X-ray showing changes in more advanced osteomyelitis with extensive bone lesions. Sequestrum, an area of bone necrosis, is indicated by the arrow.

age, this complication is even more likely because the bone is more calcified and the periosteum even more attached to bone. This is what happened to O.

Adults. Hematogenous osteomyelitis also occurs in adults, in whom the most commonly involved bones are the vertebrae of the spine. The reason for the preferential involvement is unknown; it may relate to the degenerative changes and vascular proliferation in the disc space between the vertebrae that normally occur with age. The infection almost always begins in the disc space and then spreads to the two contiguous vertebrae. Abnormalities of the disc space with erosion of the vertebral plates on x-ray is always infectious and not a malignancy. This rule is one of the most reliable in radiology (see Fig. 11.2).

S. aureus is still the most frequent infecting organism, but vertebral osteomyelitis is also frequently caused by Gram-negative bacteria. Several reasons probably exist for this etiology. First, Gram-negative bacteremia resulting from sources in the bowel, gallbladder, and urinary tract is more frequent in the population over the age of 60. Second, the pelvic veins flow into the paravertebral plexus (Batson's plexus), and infection of bone may occur from drainage of infected pelvic organs (such as the bladder and kidneys) which empty their blood into the complex ramifications and anastomoses of this venous system. Because of the variety of possible causes of vertebral osteomyelitis, cultures and a determination of antibiotic sensitivity are imperative. If blood cultures are negative, tissue biopsies must be obtained. Aspiration or needle biopsy of the disc space can be done with guidance from x-rays or a CAT scan. Most of these infections respond to medical therapy, but the neurologic status of the patient must be carefully followed because the infection may spread from the vertebral body into the subdural or subarachnoid space through the rich venous and arterial plexus of the paravertebral circulation (Fig. 62.6). Sensory or motor changes imply spread of the infection into the epidural space and may necessitate surgical drainage to prevent permanent damage to the

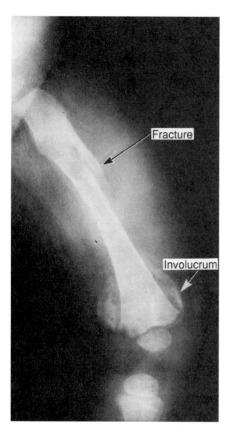

Figure 62.4. Involucrum secondary to extensive periosteal reaction and fracture due to weakened infected bone.

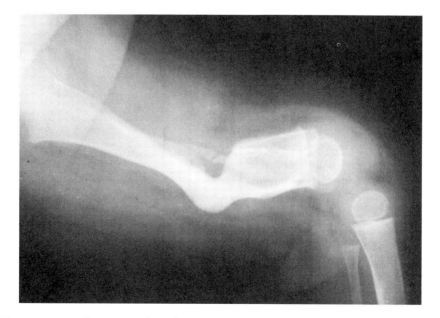

Figure 62.5. Deformity resulting from pathological fracture secondary to osteomyelitis.

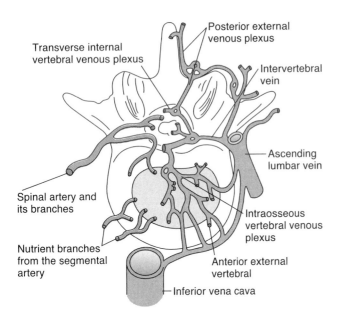

Figure 62.6. Vascular supply of a vertebral body showing the connections of the rich venous and arterial plexus of the paravertebral circulation.

nerves of the spinal cord. Thus, proper management of these cases requires a good understanding of anatomy, neurology, and pathophysiology.

Osteomyelitis Secondary to External or Contiguous Foci of Infection

Bone infection may also result from the direct introduction of microorganisms from an external or contiguous source. Penetrating trauma is an obvious example of this type of infection. Another type is postoperative infection, particularly when surgery involves placement of a prosthesis or fixation device, which is done, for example, to stabilize a hip fracture (Fig. 62.7). These infections are often difficult to treat both because the bone has been traumatized and the foreign body can act as an avascular sanctuary for the persistence of bacteria. The problem of whether or not to remove the fixation device or prosthesis is a particularly complex one. On the one hand, the device is necessary for appropriate fixation of the bone (it has been put there for a good reason, i.e., to stabilize a fracture); on the other hand, its presence may prevent the elimination of bacteria. These decisions require close interactions between surgeons and internists to determine if and when removal is appropriate.

Although *S. aureus* is still the most common infecting organism in this type of osteomyelitis, others are also common. Frequently, the type of pathogen reflects the circumstances of the trauma and the area of the body involved. Contamination of the wound with soil often leads to infection by Gram-negative bacteria. Postoperative infections are frequently due to *S. aureus*. A wound may become contaminated with bacteria that are part of

the fecal flora, particularly in an incontinent patient with a hip fracture. *Staphylococcus epidermidis* infection is more likely to occur in the presence of a prosthesis.

Osteomyelitis in Diabetic Patients

A special category of osteomyelitis occurs in diabetics because of the vascular insufficiency and nerve damage characteristic of diabetes. Skin and soft tissue ulcerations on the feet of such patients may penetrate into the bone (see Fig. 61.4). These infections are usually caused by a mixed bacterial flora, with the actual species reflecting the area of involvement. *S. aureus*, *Streptococcus* species, Gram-negative bacteria, and anaerobic bacteria are all commonly involved. These infections are particularly difficult to treat because the organisms grow in necrotic bone with poor vascular supply. Therapy involves the use of antibiotics effective against the specific organisms, plus careful surgical debridement. Because of the poor vascular supply to the bone in diabetics, phagocytic cells and antibiotics penetrate poorly into the infected area, and therapy is often unsuccessful. Unfortunately, amputation is frequently the end result of a trivial soft tissue infection of the foot. Good foot care is therefore essential to the survival of a patient with diabetes.

INFECTION OF JOINTS

Pathobiology

A swollen, red hot, painful joint in a patient with fever raises questions similar to those in a patient with

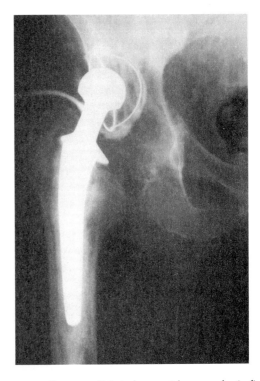

Figure 62.7. Osteomyelitis in bone with a prosthetic fixation device.

osteomyelitis. First, is an infection present? Noninfectious inflammatory joint disease secondary to trauma, gout, pseudogout, or rheumatoid arthritis can also present in this manner. Second, if an infection is present, how did it get there? As in osteomyelitis, infection can be seeded from a bacteremic focus, introduced directly into the joint by trauma, or a medical or surgical procedure, or can extend into the joint space from the bone. Third, what is the infecting organism? All three of these questions can usually be answered by obtaining a complete history, doing a careful physical examination, and analyzing fluid obtained by aspiration of the joint. The diagnosis of infection is confirmed by inflammatory white cells and other abnormalities that indicate infection in the joint fluid.

Synovial fluid consists of water, electrolytes, and other low-molecular-weight substances filtered from plasma, as well as components synthesized and secreted by synovial cells. Serum proteins are present in normal synovial fluid but in lower concentrations than in plasma. Because fibrinogen is absent, normal synovial fluid does not clot. The inflammatory reaction in synovial fluid is caused by the interaction of serum proteins, phagocytic host cells, and microorganisms.

It is important to recognize that diagnosis of one joint disease does not preclude a second. Therefore, a joint deformed by arthritis can become infected with bacteria, particularly if that joint has recently been operated on or if steroids have been injected into it. The key to understanding the disease process is to obtain joint fluid for analysis and culture.

Infections of the joints can be caused by bacteria, viruses, and fungi. These possibilities can be differentiated by the clinical presentation of the patient and by the results of laboratory tests on the joint fluid. In general, bacterial infections are more common than the other types of infections and produce a higher number of white blood cells in the joint fluid, with a predominance of neutrophils. The frequency with which specific bacterial agents cause septic arthritis varies with age. Again, *S. aureus* is the most common overall cause and affects all age groups. *Haemophilus influenzae* type b is most frequent in infants between the ages of 6 months and 3 years. The gonococcus is the leading cause in sexually active adults and accounts for 30% to 50% of hospital admissions for suppurative arthritis in adults under 30 years of age.

The etiologic organism causing septic arthritis can be identified by Gram stain and culture of joint fluid. Even if the Gram stain is negative, antibiotic treatment should be started immediately after joint fluid and blood are obtained for culture to prevent continued infection and destruction of the structures in the joint. Table 62.2 lists the relative frequency of infecting organisms and the clinical situations in which they are most likely to occur. Certain organisms like the gonococcus, *S. aureus*, and several spirochetes have an unusual tropism for the joints. The reason for this predilection is unknown.

Treatment

In addition to appropriate high-dose antibiotic therapy given parenterally the infected synovial fluid should be drained. Drainage can be performed by repeated aspirations or by open surgical drainage. Usually, aspiration is attempted first, and surgery is used only when aspiration fails. Open drainage is always performed in septic arthritis of the hip joint. Open drainage is required to prevent necrosis of the head of the femur which results because the blood supply to this part of the bone is too tenuous. Once again, a review of anatomy helps understand infectious process.

Table 62.2. Most Frequent Causes of Bacterial Arthritis by Age

Organism	Children			Adults
	Neonates	2 months–2 years	3–10 years	
Staphylococcus aureus	10–25%	1–10%	10–25%	25–75%
Streptococcus species (group A, viridans, microaerophilic, anaerobic *S. pneumoniae*	1–10%	10–25%	10–25%	10–25%
Group B streptococci	10–25%	Rare	Rare	1–10%
Haemophilus influenzae, type b	Rare	25–75%	1–10%	Rare
Neisseria	Rare	1–10%	10–25%	10–25%*
Gram-negative bacilli	10–25%	1–10%	1–10%	1–10%
Anaerobes	Rare	Rare	Rare	Rare
Other	1–10%	Rare	1–10%	Rare

* Generally adults less than 30 years of age.

Table 62.3. Pathogenesis of Muscle Infections

Pathogenesis	Clinical presentations	Principal specific etiologies
Localized and spread from a contiguous site	Gas gangrene	*Clostridium perfringens,* occasionally other clostridial species
	Synergistic myositis or gangrene	Mixed infections; anaerobic bacteria and enteric bacteria
	Muscle abscesses Gram-negative bacteria	*Staphylococcus aureus,* Group A streptococci
	Miscellaneous	Mycobacterium, *Nocardia Actinomyces,* fungi
Hematogenous spread	Bacterial	Group A, B streptococci *Staphylococcus aureus,* Gram-negative bacteria
	Fungal	*Candida, Aspergillus, Histoplasma capsulatum, Coccidioides immitis*
	Mycobacterial	Typical and atypical mycobacteria
	Parasitic malaria, filariasis, etc.	*Trichinella spiralis, Dracunculus medinensis*
	Viral	Echovirus, coxsackievirus, Epstein-Barr virus

INFECTIONS OF MUSCLE (MYOSITIS)

Pathobiology

All of us have experienced the muscle aches and stiffness (myalgia) that commonly occur when we have a viral illness ("the flu"). In fact, these myalgias are prominent features of a variety of infections including viral illness, rickettsial infection, and even osteomyelitis and bacterial endocarditis. Fever is often accompanied by muscle pains or myalgias. Infecting organisms are rarely directly involved in myalgias. More often, muscle involvement is indirect, probably because of the accelerated catabolism of skeletal muscle, part of the so-called acute phase response that accompanies sepsis and trauma. This catabolism is probably mediated by several products of macrophages (monokines) including interleukin-1 and tumor necrosis factor. The systemic symptoms resulting from these macrophage products are mediated by the increased synthesis of prostaglandin E2, which in turn activates muscle proteases. The same substances lead to the production of fever in the hypothalamus. These events explain why inhibitors of prostaglandin synthesis, like aspirin, help resolve both fever and muscle aches.

Specific Muscle Infections

Specific infections of skeletal muscle are uncommon. When they occur, they may be caused by a wide range of organisms including bacteria, fungi, viruses, and parasitic agents. Muscles may be invaded either from contiguous sites of infection or by hematogenous spread from a distant focus. The kinds of infection and their frequency depend on the host, geographic area, or eating habits of the patient.

Several of the clinical presentations are so distinctive that they readily suggest the etiologic agent. For example, the presence of gas in muscle suggests gas gangrene secondary to *Clostridium perfringens.* Generalized muscle pain and peripheral eosinophilia in a patient who has eaten undercooked pork should raise the possibility of trichinosis.

CONCLUSION

Table 62.3 lists several of the more common causes of infectious myositis and their specific clinical presentations. Therapy of nonspecific myalgia is usually symptomatic. When a specific etiologic agent is identified, therapy should be directed at this agent. Prompt drainage of abscesses and extensive surgical debridement may be necessary if necrotic tissue is present.

SUGGESTED READINGS

Norden C, Gillespie WJ, Nade S. Infections in bones and joints. Blackwell Scientific Publications, 1994.

Smith JW, Piercy EA. Infectious arthritis. In: Mandell G, Bennett JE, Dolion R. Principles and practice of infectious diseases. 4th ed. New York: Churchill Livingstone, 1995: 1032–1038.

Swartz MN. Myositis. In: Mandell G, Bennett JE, Dolion R. Principles and practice of infectious diseases. 4th ed. New York: Churchill Livingstone, 1995:929–935.

Waldvogel FA, Medoff G, Swartz MN. Osteomyelitis: a review of clinical features, therapeutic considerations and unusual aspects (parts 1, 2, and 3). N Engl J Med 1970;282:198, 260, 316.

Waldvogel FA, Vesey H. Osteomyelitis: the past decade. N Engl J Med 1980;303:360.

ELLEN WHITNACK

S epsis is somewhat inaccurately referred to as "blood poisoning." Before describing sepsis in detail, consider the following two cases illustrating "sepsis, old and new."

CASE 1

George L., a 48-year-old farmer, cut his thumb one day while installing the spreaders on his combine. The next morning, the thumb was sore and the skin surrounding the cut was red. Mr. L., who needed to get his soybeans in before the rain started, resumed combining until well after dark. By the time he got back to the house, the thumb was swollen and throbbing, and some yellowish–white pus was oozing out. Mr. L. noticed two red streaks going up the inside of his forearm. As he thought that he'd better get his thumb looked at, he suddenly had a shaking chill and felt queasy. His wife drove him 17 miles to the county hospital. By the time they arrived, Mr. L.'s temperature had reached 39.7°C. He was flushed and ill-appearing, with a pulse of 125 and a blood pressure of 100/60, compared to his usual of 145/85. Blood cultures were drawn, and Mr. L. was started on intravenous fluids and an antibiotic active against staphylococci and streptococci. By morning he was somewhat better and by the following day his symptoms had disappeared. His subsequent recovery and wound healing were uneventful. The blood cultures were found to be positive for *Staphylococcus aureus* on the second day of his illness.

CASE 2

Laura J., a 59-year-old woman with cervical carcinoma, underwent extensive pelvic surgery to remove the tumor, including removal of all pelvic organs, removal of a segment of ileum to construct a new bladder, and a colostomy. At first she seemed to be recovering well. During the evening of the third postoperative day, the nurse on the evening shift noticed that Mrs. J.'s respiratory rate, which had been 16–18 per minute, was 26. Mrs. J. said she did feel sick. She was not short of breath or in much pain, and her temperature was actually subnormal—36.2°C. The next morning, Mrs. J. had some fever, 38.3°C, but she continued to feel fairly well. Her wound showed no sign of infection, and her abdomen was no more tender than expected. That afternoon, however, Mrs. J. was clearly in trouble. She was flushed, anxious, and restless; her blood pressure was down from 135/75 to 105/58, and her temperature was 39.2°. Blood cultures were drawn, antibiotics were started, and intravenous fluids were infused rapidly, which brought her blood pressure up. Thereafter, Mrs. J.'s condition worsened. By morning, she was short of breath and had excess fluid throughout her lungs. Intravenous fluids were cut back; and a vasopressor was now required to maintain her blood pressure. She was moved to the intensive care unit for monitoring. To better assess her hemodynamic status, the superior vena cava and one pulmonary artery were catheterized (the latter via the jugular vein, right atrium, and right ventricle). Mrs. J. was found to have a cardiac output nearly double the normal for a resting adult of her size, but her systemic vascular resistance was extremely low. This finding accounted for her low blood pressure despite the high cardiac output. Over the next 24 hours, Mrs. J. continued to do poorly; her urine output dropped nearly to zero, and she required mechanical ventilation to maintain oxygenation. The surgeon decided that reexploration was warranted because of persistent sepsis in the presence of broad-spectrum antimicrobial therapy. At surgery, the suture line attaching the ileum to the colon was found to be partially disrupted, with leakage of bowel contents, intense inflammation of the mesentery, and early abscess formation. Appropriate repairs were made and drains were inserted. Thereafter, Mrs. J. recovered slowly but completely. The blood cultures remained sterile.

SEPSIS

What Is Sepsis?

Sepsis is an ancient Greek word meaning, roughly, "putrefaction." Throughout earlier medical history, the term *septic* has been used to describe an inflammatory

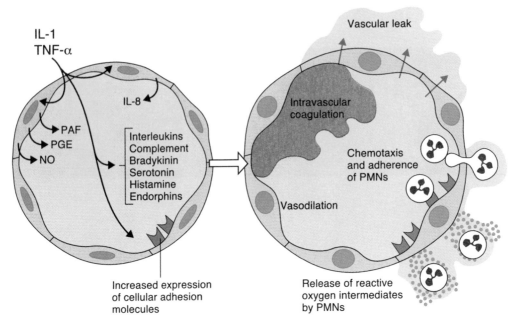

Figure 63.1. Vasculature effects in sepsis. The release of IL-1 and TNF-α causes the outpouring of a number of cytokines and other effectors. In turn, this leads to intravascular coagulation, vasodilation, increased neutrophil adherence to vessel walls, and vascular leakage.

process yielding foul-smelling pus, such as a septic wound or a septic abortion. In the past, the pus was considered to be pathologic only if it was malodorous; the white, odorless pus commonly encountered in wounds was considered essential for proper healing ("laudable pus"). This thinking changed with the microbiologic discoveries of Pasteur and Lister. Although the term *septic* for a local infection is still used, the requirement for a foul odor has long since been dropped with the recognition that any pus usually represents infection. If a wound must be infected, it is indeed better that leukocytes are drawn to the wound site and pus is produced. However, it is even better if the wound does not become infected in the first place.

Microbiologic discoveries in the last century also provided an explanation of why patients with septic wounds sometimes get so sick: the microbes spread, first to the lymphatics (hence the red streaks on Mr. L.'s arm) and then to the bloodstream, producing "septic blood"—**septicemia**—and "pyemia"—pus in the blood, or as we now call it, **leukocytosis**. A matter of considerable debate was whether the patient became sick because of the effects of the microbes, whether the illness was caused by microbial toxins in the blood itself, or carried throughout the body by the circulation? What was clear was that a local process had become systemic.

Early on it was recognized that viable bacteria could be present in the blood—a condition called **bacteremia**—without the presence of illness. On the other hand, if a severe systemic illness was present, bacteremia could often be found; thus septicemic patients were bacteremic by definition. What, then, is **sepsis**? Until quite recently, sepsis and septicemia were essentially synonyms, and still are in many texts. However, in the past 20 years or so, ideas about the nature of septicemia/sepsis have evolved in two ways.

First, sepsis has become as much a **physiologic** as it is a clinical or microbiologic term. ("Clinical" means determined at the bedside by signs and symptoms, as opposed to laboratory tests and invasive procedures). The widespread use of hemodynamic monitoring in intensive care units has shown that patients with clinical sepsis—fever or hypothermia, tachycardia, subnormal blood pressure, and subnormal urine output—characteristically have an increased **cardiac output** and a greatly decreased **peripheral vascular resistance**, as in Mrs. J.'s case. Patients with these "septic hemodynamics" are not necessarily bacteremic; indeed, they need not have a bacterial infection at all. In these cases, sepsis may result from infections with fungi (especially *Candida*), parasites (falciparum malaria), tuberculosis (sepsis tuberculosis gravissima), and even viruses (adenovirus). In bacterial sepsis, which is by far the most common type, half or more of the patients do not have bacteremia.

Second, we now realize that the sepsis syndrome results from the release of **cytokines** from host cells (macrophages) stimulated by microbial substances (Table 63.1 and Fig. 63.1). It is the host's own molecules, not the microbe's, that are the proximate cause of sepsis, although in certain special cases (e.g., clostridial α-toxin) bacterial toxins may contribute to the pathogenesis of the illness by a direct toxicity. Sepsis is therefore the final common path of host response to a variety of microbial molecules.

For these reasons, the term *septicemia* in the old sense of bacteremia plus severe systemic illness is becoming outdated; the preferred term is now *sepsis*. Sepsis is now defined according to various degrees of severity. For our purposes, we will define sepsis as a severe systemic illness marked by characteristic hemodynamic derangements and organ malfunction, brought about by the interaction of certain microbial products with host reticuloendothelial cells.

Sepsis leaves no organ or system untouched. In protracted cases of sepsis, such as those complicating abdominal surgery, one organ after another may fail. This condition is called the **multi-organ dysfunction syndrome (MODS)**. The following organs are affected:

Brain: Septic patients commonly are confused, delirious, stuporous, or comatose.

Heart: Myocardial contractility is depressed in sepsis. The heart compensates by dilating and beating faster, so that cardiac output is actually increased. In some patients, compensatory mechanisms fail, and cardiac output drops to low levels shortly before death.

Vasculature: Despite the high cardiac output, blood pressure falls because of massive peripheral vasodilation. The combination of very low blood pressure (in adults, defined as < 90 mm Hg systolic or > 40 mm below baseline) and high cardiac output has been termed "warm shock," because the patient has warm or even flushed skin, in contrast to other common forms of shock. It may seem paradoxical to call this condition "shock," because the low blood pressure could be counteracted by the high cardiac output. The justification for the term "shock" is that despite the high cardiac output, inadequate perfusion of selected vascular beds occurs, particularly in the kidney, liver, and gut. This lack of perfusion in selected vascular beds is called **distributive shock**. Sometimes, late in the course of sepsis, cardiac output falls and peripheral vasodilation is replaced by vasoconstriction. The skin becomes pale and cold, the hands and feet are bluish–purple, and the patient expires in

Table 63.1. Putative Mediators of Sepsis

Mediator	Physiologic effects
Tumor necrosis factor	Mimics sepsis syndrome; margination of neutrophils is particularly striking after TNF administration
Interleukin-1	Fever, increased adhesiveness of endothelial cells and leukocytes, endothelial procoagulant activity
Interleukins-2, -4, -6, -8	Hypotension, capillary leak, decreased myocardial contractility, synthesis of "acute phase" proteins (e.g., fibrinogen) by the liver, leukocyte chemotaxis
Hageman factor (factor XII), tissue factor, factor X	Coagulation, fibrinolysis
Complement cascade	Neutrophil chemotaxis, neutrophil aggregation, capillary leak
Endorphins	Hypotension
Leukotrienes and thromboxane	Platelet aggregation, neutrophil adhesion, capillary leak, decreased myocardial contractility
Prostaglandins (especially E_2 and I_2)	Hypotension, neutrophil adhesion to endothelium, fever, muscle aches, muscle proteolysis
Bradykinin (via factor XII and kallikrein)	Hypotension, capillary leak
Serotonin	Pulmonary hypertension, capillary leak
Histamine	Hypotension, capillary leak
Platelet-activating factor (PAF) (currently a hot research topic)	Hypotension, capillary leak, platelet aggregation, leukocyte activation, decreased myocardial contractility
Phagocyte products—lysosomal proteins, oxygen free radicals	Endothelial cell damage, capillary leak
Myocardial depressant factor (can be passively transferred)	Decreased myocardial contractility
Endothelin 1	Vasocontriction, especially in the kidney
Endothelial relaxing factor (? nitric oxide)—another hot research topic	Hypotension

"cold shock," similar to that seen after a massive heart attack or hemorrhage. However, it is possible to die of sepsis without ever reaching this phase.

Clotting system: Endothelial damage can lead to extensive microvascular thrombosis, or **disseminated intravascular coagulation (DIC).** DIC consumes platelets and clotting factors, which increases the tendency of bleeding. As a result, thrombosis and bleeding may be present at the same time. Activation of the fibrinolytic system counteracts the thrombosis, but adds to the coagulopathy because some fibrin degradation products inhibit clotting.

Lung: In sepsis, the **capillaries** are generally leaky; in the lung, capillary endothelial damage may be enhanced by activated neutrophils which adhere to the pulmonary endothelium in large numbers, spewing oxygen radicals. Fluid exudes into the interstitium and alveolar spaces, the lung becomes soggy and stiff, and adequate gas exchange is impossible. This condition is called the **adult respiratory distress syndrome (ARDS).** Oxygen must be pumped into the patient's lungs under pressure using a ventilator.

Kidney: Acute renal failure due to **acute tubular necrosis** occurs. As Dr. Myron Greengold succinctly put it (*JAMA*, 1995), "the lungs leak, the kidneys don't."

Liver: Stasis of bile, focal necrosis, and jaundice are common.

Gastrointestinal tract: Hemorrhagic necrosis of the mucosa occurs, probably at least in part because of ischemia. Loss of mucosal integrity can lead to **hemorrhage.**

Endocrine and metabolic effects: Sepsis is a **catabolic state,** with massive proteolysis, lipolysis, and glycogenolysis. Stress hormones (cortisol, catecholamines, glucagon) circulate in high levels. Oxygen metabolism is deranged: an abnormally high fraction of the oxygen sent to the tissues is returned to the heart unused, either because some vascular beds are not perfused or because some cells are too metabolically impaired to use the oxygen delivered to them. Either way, in the absence of a functioning Krebs cycle, glycolysis proceeds at a high rate and the pyruvic acid formed is reduced to lactic acid, resulting in **lactic acidosis.**

ENCOUNTER

Most cases of sepsis result from infections with endogenous bacterial flora. Before mid-century, the group A streptococcus (see Chapter 12, "Streptococci") was the leading cause of sepsis, with *Staphylococcus aureus* (see Chapter 11, "Staphylococcus") second. Most cases caused by these Gram-positive cocci resulted from wounds, puerperal fever, and abortions. Other infections leading to sepsis included pyelonephritis (**urosepsis**), generally caused by enteric Gram-negative bacilli

such as *Escherichia coli,* and intra-abdominal infections such as appendicitis with rupture, generally caused by mixtures of enterics and anaerobes such as *Bacteroides fragilis. Neisseria meningitidis* occasionally caused fulminant sepsis in healthy people with no more predisposition than, perhaps, a viral upper respiratory tract infection (see Chapter 59, "Respiratory System").

All of these infections still exist, particularly staphylococcal sepsis and urosepsis. Streptococcal sepsis, rare in recent years, may be making a comeback (see Chapter 12, "Streptococci"). However, since World War II, the population of chronically ill, debilitated, immunocompromised, and therefore hospitalized people has expanded, to the point that the majority of cases of sepsis now arise in hospitalized patients (nosocomial sepsis). Hospitalized patients—and the various lines and tubes that penetrate their skin and body orifices—tend to become colonized with a special population of hospital microbes brought to them on the inadequately washed hands of personnel. In the 1950s, the leading cause of nosocomial sepsis was "hospital staph." In the 1960s and 1970s, probably because of the use of antibiotics, the major cause of sepsis was an ever more antibiotic-resistant population of enteric Gram-negative bacilli and nonfermenters such as *Pseudomonas aeruginosa* (see Chapter 18). The 1980s saw a resurgence of staph and other Gram-positives. Currently, **"Gram-negative sepsis"** and **"staph sepsis"** are running about even. Between them, they cause perhaps 300,000 cases of sepsis a year, of which about a third are fatal.

ENTRY, SPREAD, AND MULTIPLICATION

Most cases of sepsis start with a localized infection, including not only tissue infections but infected foreign bodies such as intravenous catheters (**"line sepsis"**). Sepsis can also occur following damage to an epithelial surface that is normally heavily colonized, e.g., the colonic mucosa. Damage permits the passage of bacteria or bacterial products into the circulation, and defects in clearance mechanisms allow otherwise insignificant bacterial growth to get out of hand. For sepsis to occur, three things seem to be necessary:

- A large population of infecting or colonizing microorganisms. Defects in the host's containment and clearance mechanisms and strong microbial resistance to host defenses must also be present.
- The presence of bacterial products capable of stimulating the release of host cytokines. Many microbes can cause sepsis, but some rarely do; for example, enterococci (see Chapter 12, "Streptococci") seem to be nontoxic organisms that cause febrile bacteremia frequently, but full-blown sepsis rarely.
- The widespread dissemination of these microbial products to the host's reticuloendothelial system. Bacteremia is one way to achieve requirement, but

microbial products can also be disseminated from a localized source, particularly from the gastrointestinal tract or the peritoneal cavity, as happened in Mrs. J.'s case.

As noted above, defects in host defenses predispose to sepsis. Although *Neisseria meningitidis* causes sepsis in healthy people, and some cases of staphylococcal sepsis arise for no apparent reason, the vast majority of sepsis occur in patients with defects in host defenses. These defects include:

- **Disruption or penetration of anatomical barriers.** Wounds, intravascular catheters, and contaminated intravenous drugs and medications are obvious examples. Others include ischemic necrosis (as in the gut) and tumors. Cytotoxic chemotherapy damages rapidly dividing cells including intestinal epithelium.
- **Devitalized tissue.** Necrotic tissue has no blood supply and therefore no phagocytes, complement, or antibody to protect it. It is also a rich culture medium.
- **Granulocytopenia and defective granulocyte function.** Neutrophils are the first line of defense against many bacteria as well as fungal hyphae and pseudohyphae. Granulocytopenia, as occurs, for instance, during chemotherapy with agents toxic to the bone marrow, predisposes to infections from bacteria and such fungi as *Candida*. Patients with diabetes are notoriously susceptible to bacterial infections of all kinds, including sepsis. In diabetes, the number of granulocytes is normal, but adherence, chemotaxis, ingestion, oxidative burst, and killing are all impaired. These defects are more pronounced if the diabetes is poorly controlled.
- **Complement defects.** Homozygous deficiencies in classical pathway components and in C3 are associated with bacteremia and sepsis in some affected patients. A rare defect in the alternate pathway, properdin deficiency, predisposes to fulminant sepsis with *N. meningitidis*. Deficiencies in late components (C5–C9) create a susceptibility to neisserial infections also, but these infections are apt to be milder (less bacteriolysis, less release of toxic bacterial components). Cirrhosis and severe burn injury are complement-deficient states because of decreased syntheses and increased complement; the result is impaired neutrophil chemotaxis. Premature infants too, are short of complement. All of these patient groups have an increased incidence of sepsis.
- **Immune defects.** Loss of opsonic and bactericidal antibody (humoral defects) and loss of the ability to activate macrophages in response to specific antigenic stimuli (cellular defects) predispose to sepsis. Humoral immune defects, such as occur in B-cell malignancies, protein-losing states such as burns, and AIDS are particularly associated with bacterial infections, including sepsis.
- **Splenic malfunction or absence.** Loss of the spleen creates a humoral immunodeficiency, particularly in primary antibody responses. Additionally, without the spleen, clearance of encapsulated bacteria from the blood is impaired. Persons who lack a functioning spleen (for example, sickle-cell patients) are susceptible to fulminant sepsis due to bacteria such as *Streptococcus pneumoniae, Haemophilus influenzae,* and *N. meningitidis*. Such persons are immunized against these bacteria to the extent possible (see Chapter 67, "Infections of the Compromised Patient") and warned not to take flulike illnesses lightly. Some take antibiotics on a long-term basis for prophylaxis.

DAMAGE

Mediators of the sepsis syndrome

We have alluded to "microbial molecules" that interact with host macrophages to initiate the chain of events leading to the sepsis syndrome. In Gram-positive bacteria, these include such cell-wall components as peptidoglycan and teichoic or lipoteichoic acids. In Gram-negative bacteria, the molecule that incites the sepsis syndrome is **endotoxin** or **lipopolysaccharide (LPS)**, specifically its **lipid A** moiety, which is the main component of the outer leaflet of the outer membrane (see Chapter 3, "Biology of Infectious Agents"). Endotoxin is one of the most extensively studied of all bacterial molecules. In animals its administration elicits many features of experimental sepsis; in humans, LPS (in small doses) causes fever, chills, rapid breathing, and a mild version of the cardiovascular alterations seen in sepsis: decreased myocardial contractility, increased cardiac output, decreased systemic vascular resistance, and hypotension.

Although the mechanism by which LPS produces its many effects has not been determined in all cases, it appears that LPS may not be *directly* responsible for any of them. LPS is nontoxic (except at unrealistically high doses) in a strain of mice called C3H/HeJ unless the mice first receive a transplant of normal marrow. These mice have a mutant gene encoding a defective protein (perhaps a component of the signal transduction pathway) required for the response of macrophages to stimulation by LPS. The transplanted marrow supplies normal, responsive macrophages. Thus it appears that the macrophage, not the microbe, actually causes the sepsis syndrome.

How does the macrophage cause the sepsis syndrome? LPS binds to the CD14 protein on the macrophage surface, triggering production of a cytokine called **tumor necrosis factor-α (TNF)** or **cachectin** (Fig. 63.1). (The former name comes from the ability of TNF to cause necrosis of transplantable tumors in mice, the latter from its ability to produce wasting in animal models of certain chronic parasitic infections.) TNF, like LPS, can induce a sepsis-like state in experimental animals and is the only host mediator known to do this when administered alone. TNF stimulates the macrophages to produce interleukin-1β (IL-1). TNF and IL-1 have the largest number of target genes of any known natural substances. They act synergistically on macrophages (in a sort of positive feedback loop) and on other cells, particularly neutrophils and endothelial cells, to alter their surfaces by expressing certain membrane proteins and to produce a variety of additional mediators. In fact, once sepsis is underway, the endothelial cell may be the key cell, both as target and effector. Elucidating the secondary effects of TNF and IL-1 is complex as the list of mediators gets ever longer. It is not always clear whether a given mediator produces its effects directly or through additional mediators. Some of the mediators of sepsis, shown in Table 63.1, include interleukins, the complement cascade, the clotting cascade, bradykinin, serotonin, histamine, endorphins, phagocytic products (oxygen radicals, lysosomal enzymes), arachidonic acid metabolites (prostaglandins and leukotrienes). Other substances synthesized by endothelial cells, particularly platelet-activating factor and nitric oxide, may also be mediators. Both of these substances are candidates for the final common pathway of capillary leak and hypotension.

Why does the body self-destruct? Can the process be stopped?

We normally think of the body as self-protective, and expect that its response to insult will be in the direction of damage control and repair. In sepsis, however, the host seems bent on self-destruction. Why is this? Is sepsis a "maladaptive" or "excessive" response—a defense system evolved to deal with cuts and earaches and gonorrhea that becomes deleterious when it must scale up to meet massive microbial challenges for which it was never designed? Or is the sepsis syndrome, however deadly, a protective mechanism, such that the host would die even faster without it? What good are TNF, IL-1, and all the mediators in the acute response to an infecting organism?

Recall the CH3/HeJ mouse, which does not respond to LPS. These mice are killed by a much lower inoculum of Gram-negative bacilli than are normal mice, and are protected by pretreatment with TNF and IL-1. Or consider a mouse model of infection with *Listeria monocytogenes*, in which anti-TNF antibody exacerbates the disease; or a model of granuloma formation in mycobacterial infection, in which anti-TNF prevents killing of the mycobacteria by the granulomas. These observations suggest that TNF is part of a legitimate system of host defense. Many of the mediators of sepsis have, in fact, been shown to protect the host in various animal models of infection. Furthermore, sepsis is not simply an

inflammatory response run riot. Along with all the mediators, anti-inflammatory cytokines (such as IL-4 and IL-10) and mediator-blocking agents can be found, suggesting that sepsis is a regulated, orchestrated host response.

These issues are not simply academic. For the question arises: if sepsis is brought about by host mediators, might treatment designed to counteract these mediators be beneficial? And even if the mediators are important in host defense, could that function not be entrusted to antibiotics? In the past 10 years, several human trials have tested antibodies to endotoxin, antibodies to TNF, soluble receptors for TNF, blocking agents for IL-1 receptors, and blocking agents for platelet-activating factor receptors. The results of these trials may be simply summarized: the animal experiments and preliminary human trials have been promising, while the randomized controlled trials disappointing. It now appears that much more information needs to be learned about the sepsis syndrome—in particular, the nature of the defect in oxygen utilization, and the minute-to-minute, cytokine-by-cytokine evolution of the syndrome in the individual patient—before this approach will be fruitful.

DIAGNOSIS AND TREATMENT

The signs of sepsis may be obvious, as in Mr. L.'s case, or subtle, as in Mrs. J.'s. Delay in diagnosis is particularly likely when there is no fever. Easily overlooked or misinterpreted signs of early sepsis include decreased (rather than increased) temperature, increased respiratory rate, increased heart rate, nausea, and mental confusion. Blood pressure may not fall much at first. Early changes in the results of routine laboratory studies are likewise nonspecific. They may include either leukocytosis or leukopenia and perhaps a fall in the level of serum bicarbonate, reflecting the development of lactic acidosis.

In about half of patients with sepsis, the blood cultures will be positive, although the bacteria may take a few days to grow. In some critically ill patients, the diagnosis of sepsis becomes apparent when the central catheters are placed, revealing the characteristic hemodynamic changes. Very few acute illnesses other than sepsis produce a rise in cardiac output and a fall in systemic vascular resistance.

The mainstays of therapy of sepsis are optimization of oxygen delivery to the tissues, drainage of pus, debridement of devitalized tissue and, of course, antibiotics. Sepsis is, as mentioned, a state of oxygen starvation. An abnormally low fraction of oxygen is extracted from the arterial blood, but if more oxygen is supplied, more will be extracted. Measures to promote oxygen delivery include high oxygen content of the air supplied to the patient; use of a ventilator to keep the airways under pressure throughout the respiratory cycle; intravenous fluids to maintain the blood volume; transfusions, if needed, to increase the hemoglobin content of the blood (but not too much—red cells increase the viscosity of the blood, with deleterious effects on microcirculatory flow); and adrenergic drugs to maintain tissue perfusion pressure, increase myocardial contractility, and correct some of the maldistribution of the circulation. Debridement of devitalized tissue and drainage of pus are essential, as illustrated by Mrs. J., who did not get better, despite antibiotics, until her abscess was drained.

An interesting issue is whether antibiotics might actually be temporarily deleterious even as they control the infection. After all, if antibiotics kill bacteria, they will cause the release of toxic bacterial components such as endotoxin. A transient deleterious effect of antibiotic therapy has, in fact, been demonstrated in two clinical situations: bacterial meningitis, which is essentially sepsis within the central nervous system (see Chapter 58, "Central Nervous System"), and massive bacteremia in immunocompromised, granulocytopenic patients. In ordinary cases of sepsis, a deleterious effect of antibiotics is not so obvious, although it is common to see patients get worse before they get better. However, antibiotics must be prescribed: the infection must be controlled, or the patient will die. Even with the best treatment, the mortality of sepsis that has reached the shock stage is ≥ 50%.

In the future patients with sepsis may be given a "cocktail" of anticytokine antibodies, soluble receptors to act as decoys for mediators, receptor-blocking agents, and inhibitors of mediator synthesis to tide them over while the antibiotics do their work. The trick will be to reduce the deleterious effects of host mediators without neutralizing their ability to perform essential defensive functions.

SUGGESTED READINGS

Lynn WA, Cohen J. Adjunctive therapy for septic shock: a review of experimental approaches. Clin Infect Dis 1995;20: 143–158.

Majno G. The ancient riddle of σγψισ (sepsis). J Infect Dis 1991;163:937–945.

Young LS. Sepsis syndrome. In: Mandell G, Bennett JE, Dolion R. Principles and practice of infectious diseases. 4th ed. New York: Churchill Livingstone, 1995:690–704.

CHAPTER 64

Intravascular Infection

A. W. KARCHMER

A variety of microorganisms gain entry to the intravascular space and are passively carried throughout the circulatory system, either suspended in the plasma or within various cellular components of blood. Usually, entry of microorganisms into the circulatory tree represents a brief phase of an infection that is centered primarily in another organ system. However, for some bacteria and protozoa, the primary site of infection is within the vascular system, i.e., the cellular components of blood or the structural elements of the circulatory system. For example, *Plasmodium* species (the cause of malaria), *Babesia microti* (the cause of babesiosis), and *Bartonella bacilliformis* (the agent of Oroya fever) produce disease by invading or adhering to erythrocytes. Occasionally, microorganisms infect the endothelial surface of a specific component of the cardiovascular system. These intravascular infections are called **endarteritis** when involving an artery, **endocarditis** when affecting an endothelial site in the heart, and **phlebitis** if localized in the lumen of a vein.

Infective phlebitis occurs mainly by direct spread from an adjacent focus of infection or when intravascular foreign bodies (such as catheters) that have been implanted in veins become infected. **Infective endarteritis** arises in an analogous manner and, on rare occasions, when congenital arterial anomalies (patent ductus arteriosus, coarctation of the aorta) or diseased arterial endothelium (atherosclerotic plaques) become infected during transient bacteremia. **Infective endocarditis**, with the exception of episodes that arise as a consequence of cardiac surgery or intracardiac instrumentation, results from seeding of endothelial sites by microorganisms that are transiently present in the circulatory tree. Most vascular endothelial infections are caused by bacteria and, rarely, by fungi. Infective endocarditis is the prototype of spontaneously occurring intravascular endothelial infections and is the focus of this chapter. The term *endocarditis* will refer here to *infectious endocarditis*.

CASE

Mrs. A.D., a 75-year-old woman with a history of a systolic ejection heart murmur and mild aortic stenosis, hypertension, and diabetes, was admitted to the hospital because of 6 weeks of intermittent fevers, malaise, weakness, and loss of appetite. The day prior to admission she noted her temperature was 41.2°C and discovered that she was 14 lb below her usual weight.

On examination, Mrs. D. was pale, her temperature was 38.1°C, heart rate 100, and blood pressure 150/90 mm Hg. Three small hemorrhages were noted on the right palpebral conjunctiva. The fundi were normal. She was edentulous. On cardiac examination, a grade III/VI systolic ejection heart murmur was heard at the base of the heart suggesting aortic stenosis and a grade I/VI, brief, high-pitched decrescendo diastolic murmur was heard at the left sternal border, indicating aortic insufficiency. The spleen could not be palpated.

Laboratory tests revealed a hematocrit of 27% (normal is greater than 36%), a normal leukocyte count, a sedimentation rate of 92 mm/hr (normal is less than 15 mm/hr), a creatinine level of 1.9 mg/dl (normal is less than 1.3 mg/dl), and a urine analysis which showed 25–30 red blood cells/high-power field, but no white blood cells or casts. Six blood cultures obtained over 48 hours were all positive for *Streptococcus bovis*.

Treatment for subacute bacterial endocarditis was started with 3 million units of penicillin intravenously every 4 hours. On the sixth hospital day, the patient was found unresponsive with a dilated left pupil. An emergency cranial CAT scan revealed a large left parietal hematoma. The patient died on the eighth hospital day.

Autopsy confirmed vegetations on the aortic valve at the closure line. The valve was bicuspid and thickened. A Gram stain of the vegetation confirmed the presence of Gram-positive cocci. Small embolic infarcts were noted in the myocardium and in the slightly enlarged spleen. There were changes of focal glomerulonephritis and several small infarcts in both kidneys. A massive subarachnoid and left parietal intracerebral hemorrhage from an apparent leaking aneurysm (a mycotic aneurysm or sac-like dilatation, which results from growth of bacteria in the vessel wall) was also noted.

DEFINITION AND CLASSIFICATION OF ENDOCARDITIS

Infective endocarditis is usually localized on one of the cardiac valves, but it may also occur on one of the cordae tendineae or on areas of the atrial or ventricular wall. Endocarditis can be classified according to the tempo of the clinical illness, the microbiological cause, or the clinical setting or site of infection. Patients presenting with a markedly febrile, toxic course lasting only days to several weeks have acute endocarditis, whereas those with lower fevers, an illness marked by anorexia, weakness, and weight loss, and who have been symptomatic for several weeks, have **subacute endocarditis.** Subacute endocarditis, which is typically caused by less virulent nonpyogenic bacteria, occurs on structurally abnormal valves. **Acute endocarditis,** which is caused by more invasive pyogenic bacteria, may involve either structurally abnormal or normal valves. The tendency nowadays is to avoid such classifications in favor of brief descriptions that include the microbiological cause, the type and site of the infected valve, and predisposing event. Thus, "α-hemolytic streptococcal native valve endocarditis," "*Staphylococcus aureus* tricuspid valve endocarditis in an intravenous drug abuser," or "*Staphylococcus epidermidis* prosthetic aortic valve endocarditis" provide more precise diagnoses and give specific indications regarding therapy and prognosis.

EPIDEMIOLOGY

Over the past two decades, the incidence of endocarditis in the developed countries has ranged from 1.7 to 4.2 cases/100,000 person-years. Endocarditis accounts for approximately 1 in 1000 admissions to large general hospitals. The median age of patients with endocarditis has increased steadily since the preantibiotic era; in the 1920s, the median age was less than 30 years, whereas currently more than 50% of cases occur in persons over 50 years of age.

The type of structural heart disease that serves as the predisposing factor for endocarditis has also changed. Thus, **acute rheumatic fever** has declined in developed countries as a predisposing factor for endocarditis. The common predisposing causes for endocarditis are now **congenital cardiac defects** (especially bicuspid aortic valves, ventricular septal defects, tetralogy of Fallot, and patent ductus arteriosus), **degenerative valvular disease** (calcific valvular disease), and **mitral valve prolapse** with mitral regurgitation. In recent reports, about 20% of en-

docarditis patients were found to have infection on a prolapsing regurgitant mitral valve. **Prosthetic heart valves** have also become an important site for the establishment of endocarditis. Between 15% to 30% of patients with endocarditis are not known to have had a prior valvular abnormality.

Endocarditis may affect older people for the following reasons:

- People with congenital heart disease now live longer.
- Prosthetic valves to correct valve dysfunction are implanted more frequently in this age group.
- The age of the general population and therefore that of patients with degenerative valve disease has increased.
- The prevalence of rheumatic heart disease (a disease with onset at a younger age) has decreased.
- The precipitating circumstances for transient bacteremia resulting in endocarditis, such as genitourinary tract infections and manipulations, colonic pathology (benign polyps and malignancy), and nosocomial bacteremias are more common in the elderly.

However, the current epidemic of intravenous drug abuse has raised the incidence of endocarditis among younger persons. In these patients, the structures affected are different. Typically, endocarditis in persons who do not abuse drugs involves a previously abnormal **aortic** or **mitral valve.** In intravenous drug abusers, it affects not only previously abnormal left heart valves, but in half the cases, it involves a normal **tricuspid valve.**

ENCOUNTER

Endocarditis is caused by many different microorganisms, but the most prevalent are streptococci, enterococci, and staphylococci (Table 64.1). Specific organisms show a preference for the type of valve that is infected (native vs. prosthetic) and the event or site causing the endocarditis-inciting bacteremia (e.g., dental source, intravenou s drug abuse, nosocomial infection).

The organisms that cause native valve endocarditis tend to differ in acute and subacute infections. In acute endocarditis, *S. aureus* accounts for 60% of cases, the rest being caused by pneumococci, streptococci, and aerobic Gram-negative bacilli. In contrast, in subacute endocarditis, α-hemolytic and nonhemolytic streptococci cause 60% of infection, with enterococci, coagulase-negative staphylococci, and fastidious Gram-negative rods causing the rest. Among the streptococci causing the subacute illness, *Streptococcus mitior, S. bovis, S. sanguis,* and *S. mutans* predominate and account for 70% of the isolates.

The organisms that cause infection among intravenous drug users vary depending upon whether infection involves the tricuspid valve (or occasionally the pulmonic

Table 64.1. Microbiology of Infective Endocarditis

Organism	Native valve endocarditis	Intravenous drug abuse	Prosthetic valve endocarditis	
			Onset in first year following surgery	Onset more than a year following surgery
Streptococci				
α-hemolytic, nonhemolytic	30	8	5	30
S. bovis	10	<5	<5	<5
Other	<5	<1	<1	<1
Enterococci	10	8	<5	10
Staphylococci				
S. aureus	30	55	10	15
Coagulase-negative	5	<5	55	15
Gram-negative aerobic rods	<5	8	5	<5
Fastidious Gram-negative rods[a]	5	<1	<1	8
Fungi	<5	5	5	<1
Miscellaneous	<5	<5	10[b]	<5
Polymicrobial	<1	5	<5	<1
Culture-negative	5	8	10	

[a] Includes *Haemophilus* sp., *Actinobacillus actinomycetemcomitans*, *Cardiobacterium hominis*, *Eikenella*, and *Kingella*.
[b] Includes *Corynebacterium* sp.

valve) or the valves of the left heart. In these patients, *S. aureus* causes 75% of right-sided endocarditis, whereas a broader range of organisms cause left-sided infection (*S. aureus,* 25%; streptococci, 15%; enterococci, 25%; Gram-negative bacilli, 8%; and fungi, 10%.) *S. aureus* isolated from drug users with endocarditis are often resistant to methicillin. With increasingl y effective blood culture technology a rickettsia, *Coxiella burnetii* (especially in western Europe), and *Bartonella* species have been identified as infrequent but important causes of subacute endocarditis. Previously, endocarditis caused by these organisms was often classified as culture-negative.

The microbiology of prosthetic valve endocarditis depends on the time after surgery when infection becomes symptomatic. During the initial year after valve placement, many infections are nosocomial and often the result of perioperative wound contamination. Paralleling other nosocomial infections, staphylococci cause 65% of cases during this first year, with Gram-negative rods, corynebacteria, and fungi each accounting for 5%. Prosthetic valve endocarditis with symptoms beginning more than a year after valve surgery is community-acquired and the consequence of transient bacteremias similar to those which give rise to native valve endocarditis. Accordingly, these infections are caused by streptococci, *S. aureus*, enterococci, and fastidious Gram-negative coccobacilli. Coagulase-negative staphylococci remain an important cause of these infections. In the first-year patients, 80% of these coagulase-negative staphylococci are β-lactam antibiotic resistant *S. epidermidis*, whereas in patients who become infected later, other, often β-lactam sensitive, staphylococcal species are more common. This pattern suggests that late-onset staphylococcal prosthetic endocarditis, is probably acquired as a consequence of transient bacteremia.

ENTRY AND COLONIZATION

Transient bacteremia is a common event (Chapter 63, "Sepsis"). It occurs when heavily colonized mucosal surfaces are traumatized and even spontaneously when mucosal surfaces are diseased (Table 64.2). For example, spontaneous bacteremia was documented in 10% of patients with severe gingival disease who were studied prior to a dental procedure. Despite the frequency of bacteremia and the broad spectrum of organisms that gain entry into the circulatory system, endocarditis remains a relatively rare occurrence. A small group of bacteria, the majority of which are not notably virulent, cause the majority of cases. Also puzzling is that these infections are confined primarily to the aortic and mitral valves and are not seen in the vast expanse of the remaining vascular endothelial surface. What factors operate to produce this uniform pattern?

The role of nonbacterial thrombotic vegetations

Normal vascular endothelium is resistant to bacterial infection, as can be inferred from the relative infrequency of endocarditis involving normal heart valves as well as from the difficulty of inducing endocarditis in laboratory animals. Microscopic examination of the traumatized valve in experimental animal models reveals that intravenously injected bacteria initially adhere to aggregates of platelets and fibrin, the so-called **nonbacterial thrombotic vegetations.**

Several lines of evidence suggest that nonbacterial thrombotic vegetations play a prominent permissive role in the development of endocarditis in humans. First, this type of vegetations occurring in patients with chronic disease and malignancy (so-called marantic endocarditis) is seen at the exact valve sites most commonly involved in infective endocarditis. Second, the cardiac abnormalities associated with endocarditis promote the formation of platelet–fibrin aggregates in these same sites. Cardiac abnormalities that allow blood to flow from a very high-pressure area through a narrowing into a low-pressure reservoir (ventricular septal defects, mitral and aortic valve regurgitation) are commonly associated with endocarditis. This flow pattern results in a **Venturi effect,** in which a low-pressure area is formed immediately downstream and to the sides of the narrowed orifice. This effect, combined with turbulent flow, allows platelet–fibrin aggregates to form on the endothelium at the low-pressure side of regurgitant aortic or mitral valves and ventricular septal defects. Additionally, high-velocity jet streams of blood flowing through these regurgitant valves and septal defects injure the endothelium on the wall of the left atrium, the right ventricle, or the chordae tendineae–anterior mitral valve leaflet. In turn, platelet–fibrin thrombi form at the sites of endothelial injury and serve as a niche for infective endocarditis (Fig. 64.1). Interestingly, cardiac lesions that

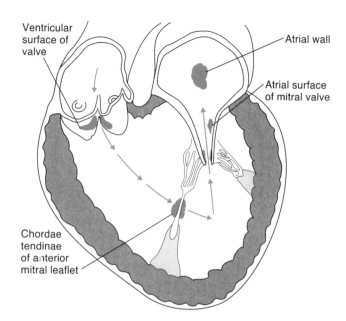

Figure 64.1. The location of endocarditic vegetations resulting from high-velocity regurgitant blood flow. The *arrows* indicate the high-velocity stream of blood. Regurgitant flow through the orifice of an incompetent aortic valve results in vegetations on the ventricular surface of the valve or on the chordae tendineae of the anterior mitral leaflet. Regurgitant flow across the incompetent mitral valve into the low-pressure left atrium allows vegetations to form on the atrial surface of the mitral valve (or at the site of jet stream impact on the atrial wall).

Table 64.2. Frequency of Transient Bacteremia in Selected Settings

Type of Event	Percentage of patients with bacteremia	Common organisms recovered
Oral cavity		
Dental extractions	30–80	Streptococci, diphtheroids, *S. epidermidis*
Tooth rocking	85	
Chewing paraffin	50	
Gingival surgery	30–85	
Airway		
Tonsillectomy	38	Streptococci, *Haemophilus* spp., diphtheroids
Bronchoscopy (rigid scope)	15	Streptococci, *S. epidermidis,* aerobic Gram-negative rods
Gastrointestinal tract		
Upper gastrointestinal endoscopy	8–12	Streptococci, *S. epidermidis,* diphtheroids, *Neisseria*
Colonoscopy	2–10	Aerobic Gram-negative rods, streptococci, *Bacteroides*
Urinary tract		
Urethral dilation	20–36	Aerobic Gram-negative rods, diphtheroids, streptococci
Cystoscopy	17	
Transurethral prostatic resection	10–45	
Genital tract		
Parturition	0–5	Aerobic Gram-negative rods, streptococci
Intrauterine device insertion/removal	0	

result in low-pressure gradients (ostium secundum atrial septal defect) or low flow and reduced turbulence (chronic congestive heart failure) are rarely associated with infective endocarditis.

Microbial Virulence Factors

Although a broad array of bacteria gain entry to the circulation, only a limited number are common causes of endocarditis. To cause endocarditis, organisms must not only enter the circulation but also survive host defenses, adhere to the thrombotic vegetation or valve endothelium, replicate on the valve surface, and promote further vegetation formation. For this sequence to culminate in endocarditis requires a complex interaction between infective agent, host defenses, endothelium, plasma components of the coagulation system, platelets, and host proteins. The precise molecular and quantitative interactions vary among specific agents and remain incompletely understood. Some elements of these interactions have been inferred by study of organisms causing endocarditis and their ability to do so in animal models.

To cause endocarditis, organisms that reach the cardiac valve must be resistant to the complement-mediated bactericidal activity of serum, as well as escape phagocytosis and killing by neutrophils. Such organisms must also be able to adhere to the thrombotic vegetation or the valve epithelium. Structures in the bacterial cell wall or extracellular polysaccharides have been implicated in ligand–receptor interactions resulting in the adherence of selected organisms. *S. mutans, S. sanguis,* and *S. bovis,* which are common causes of endocarditis, produce extracellular dextran which mediates vigorous adherence of these organisms to platelet–fibrin aggregates on the aortic valve. Also, the ability to produce dextran by streptococci isolated from blood cultures is strongly associated with endocarditis. Adherence of streptococci to fibrin is also facilitated by a cell envelope protein previously identified as an oral cavity adhesin; this protein is associated with virulence of streptococcal strains in an animal model of endocarditis. It has been suggested that cell wall lipoteichoic acid and a protein with major homology to the streptococcal oral adhesins promote adherence of enterococci to platelet–fibrin aggregates.

Endocarditis-producing organisms, including *S. aureus, Enterococcus faecalis,* and *S. sanguis,* bind more vigorously to fibronectin than do organisms rarely implicated in the disease, suggesting a role for this host protein in mediating microbial adherence to cardiac valves. Binding of *S. aureus* and coagulase-negative staphylococci to fibronectin-coated foreign devices correlates with device infection and has been suggested as a possible important step in initiating prosthetic valve infection as a consequence of bacteremia. Fibronectin is present on the surface of nonbacterial thrombotic vegetations and is exposed as subendothelial matrix when the endothelium is injured. However, this protein is not present on intact normal endothelium. Fibrinogen, on the other hand, binds to normal endothelial cells and may mediate adherence of *S. aureus* to normal valve endothelium in the absence of platelet–fibrin thrombi. This effect occurs through the fibrinogen binding protein of the *S. aureus* cell surface (clumping factor) and may account for acute endocarditis without prior valvular disease. Interestingly, coagulase, which is used to identify *S. aureus* (versus coagulase-negative species), does not promote adherence to thrombotic vegetations and is not a virulence factor associated with endocarditis. The reason may be that coagulase is secreted into the medium rather than being bound to the bacterial surface.

After adherence to the valve, bacteria must survive and replicate if endocarditis is to occur. The virulence factors that initially favor bacterial survival are not well known. Platelets activated with thrombin release low-molecular-weight, cationic, microbicidal proteins which kill some *S. aureus* and α-hemolytic streptococci. Resistance to these platelet microbicidal proteins by adherent organisms may be an important factor in progression from valvular adherence to endocarditis. A capsular polysaccharide on coagulase-negative staphylococci may enhance their resistance to clearance by host defenses and thus facilitate development of prosthetic valve endocarditis by strains that contaminate the valve intraoperatively.

Vegetation formation and bacterial growth feed upon one another. When a vegetation is colonized by bacteria, it tends to grow by continued deposition of platelets and fibrin. α-hemolytic streptococci promote platelet aggregation and stimulate valve endothelial and stromal cells to express a tissue factor (tissue thromboplastin) that prompts continued fibrin deposition and thus growth of the vegetation. Coagulase-positive staphylococci stimulate the formation of vegetation both by the release of tissue thromboplastin and by the local activation of coagulation. In turn, the vegetation allows increased bacterial proliferation, leading to dense populations of organisms (10^8 to 10^9 bacteria/gram of tissue). The relative absence of phagocytic cells in vegetations permits bacterial growth to proceed unimpeded by host defenses. On the other hand, experimental data suggest that phagocytic cells limit infection at extracardiac, intravascular sites and on the tricuspid valve (perhaps a reason why bacteremic infection of these sites is infrequent). When animals with experimental endocarditis are treated with anticoagulation or fibrinolytic therapy, the size of the vegetations is reduced.

SPREAD AND DAMAGE

A vegetation is the cardinal pathologic feature of infective endocarditis (Fig. 64.2). Classically, vegetations occur along the line of valve closure on the low-pressure surface of the regurgitant valve or septal defect, or at the

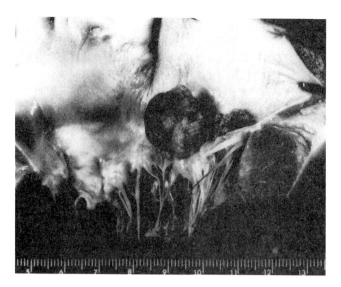

Figure 64.2. Vegetation on a heart valve from a patient with bacterial endocarditis.

site of a jet stream lesion. Vegetations vary in size from a few millimeters to a centimeter or larger and may be single or multiple. Microscopically, vegetations are a mass of fibrin, platelets, and clumps of bacteria; neutrophils are rare. Microorganisms deep in vegetations are often metabolically inactive, whereas the more superficial one are actively proliferating. The broad array of symptoms and signs associated with endocarditis (Table 64.3) are due to:

- Persistent bacteremia
- Release of cytokines, resulting in constitutional symptoms
- Tissue destruction by infecting organisms
- Fragmentation of vegetations into the circulation, causing peripheral emboli
- Stimulation of antibodies, which combine with bacterial antigens to form circulating immune complexes.

Organisms proliferating near the surface of the vegetation are continuously shed into the blood. Although the number of organisms in the blood varies over time, infective endocarditis is characterized by continuous bacteremia. Bacteremia undoubtedly mediates the release of cytokines, resulting in the constitutional symptoms associated with endocarditis, e.g., fever, sweats, fatigue, anorexia, and weight loss.

Damage of tissues in endocarditis may occur at the intracardiac site of infection or at a remote site that has been infected during bacteremia. **Intracardiac damage** most commonly involves distortion and destruction of valve leaflets, rupture of a chordae tendineae, or in the case of infected prosthetic valves, destruction of a valve leaflet, impaired mobility of the valve mechanism, and paravalvular flow due to dehiscence from the annulus. The resulting valvular dysfunction may precipitate congestive

heart failure. Infection may also extend beyond the valve leaflet into the annulus to cause a perivalvular abscess.

Clinical clues to invasive infection, especially following aortic valve endocarditis, include fever that persists despite appropriate antimicrobial therapy, new electrocardiographic conduction changes (a consequence of the anatomic proximity of the atrioventricular conduction system, the bundle of His, and the bundle branches to the mitral and aortic annulus), and pericarditis (a consequence of extension of infection into the pericardial space). Vegetations, valve function, hemodynamic status, and perivalvular–myocardial abscess are now demonstrable by transthoracic or transesophageal echocardiography. Although intracardiac complications can occur with all microbial causes of endocarditis, they are more common when the cause is a virulent pyogenic bacterium and when infection involves prosthetic valves (particularly within the initial year after valve surgery). These complications are a major cause of endocarditis-related mortality. Nevertheless, they are often amenable to surgical correction.

Infection of remote sites often complicates endocarditis caused by pyogenic bacteria. Included among such infections are septic arthritis, osteomyelitis, splenic or kidney abscess, and meningeal or parenchymal brain abscesses. Infection in the vasa vasorum of larger arteries and arteritis beginning at the site of arterial occlusion from septic emboli in patients with *S. aureus* endocarditis give rise to **mycotic aneurysms**. These lesions, which can occur in any artery, are usually asymptomatic until they rupture (see case).

Emboli are recognized clinically in 25% to 35% of

Table 64.3. Symptoms and Signs Associated with Infective Endocarditis

Symptom	Frequency (%)	Sign	Frequency (%)
Fever	90	Fever	90
Weakness	50	Murmur	85
Sweats	30	Embolic event	35
Anorexia	50	Peripheral manifestations	
Weight loss	60		
Malaise	60	Osler's nodes	10
Myalgia-arthralgia	15	Petechiae	25
		Janeway lesion	5–10
		Retinal lesion	<5
Back pain	10	Stroke	20
Confusion	10	Splenomegaly	25–50
		Septic complications	20

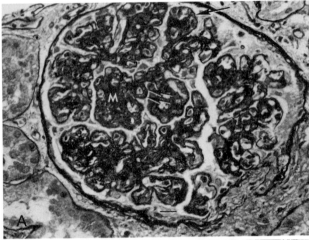

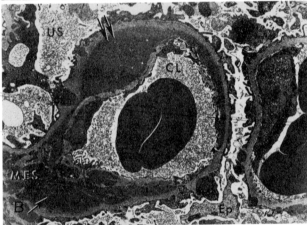

Figure 64.3. Immune complex glomerulonephritis. A. Glomerulus stained with PAS (×450). A membranoproliferative pattern is present with expansion of the mesangium, hypercellularity, cells in the capillary lumen (*single arrow*), and a double-contoured basement membrane characteristic of subendothelial immune complex deposition (*double arrow*). **B.** Electron micrograph of a glomerular tuft revealing electron-dense immune complex deposits in the mesangium (*single arrow*) and subendothelial capillary space (*double arrow*). The basement membrane splits to surround the subendothelial deposits, giving rise to the double-contoured appearance noted in **A.** These deposits will be stained by fluorescent tagged antihuman IgG in a lumpy-bumpy distribution. *Mes* = mesangium; *Ep* = epithelial cell; *US* = urinary (Bowman's) space.

patients and are found at autopsy in 45% to 65% of patients with this disease. They may cause arterial occlusion, infarction, and other secondary complications in virtually any organ. Clinically, they are most notable as the cause of embolic stroke, acute myocardial infarction, and abdominal, flank, and back pain resulting from intestinal, splenic, and renal infarction, respectively. In tricuspid valve endocarditis caused by *S. aureus*, septic pulmonary artery emboli with secondary pneumonia, lung abscess or pyo-pneumothorax are prominent components of the clinical picture.

Circulating **immune complexes** that contain antigen from the causative organisms are detectable in the majority of patients; the concentration of these complexes has been correlated with prolonged duration of the disease, occurrence of extracardiac manifestation, and reduced serum complement concentrations. Tissue injury mediated by deposition of circulating immune complexes has been described in the skin, choroid plexus, spleen, and synovium. Clinical findings such as Osler's nodes, petechiae, vasculitic purpura, and arthralgia have been attributed to the deposition of immune complexes in skin, arterial wall, and synovium.

Glomerulonephritis is the best documented immune-mediated complication of endocarditis (see Chapter 12, "Streptococci"). Endocarditis is associated with a continuum of immune renal injury, from focal embolic glomerulonephritis (a lesion with few clinical consequences), to diffuse proliferative glomerulonephritis that results in an active urine sediment and is commonly associated with decreased creatinine clearance. In patients with prolonged episodes of subacute streptococcal endocarditis, circulating immune complexes, which form intravascularly under conditions of antibody excess, deposit in a subendothelial location in the glomerulus. Immunofluorescent studies reveal IgG and early complement components on the glomerular basement membrane in a lumpy-bumpy distribution (Fig. 64.3). Among patients with subacute endocarditis, glomerulonephritis is probably frequent, generally mild (primarily focal) and remits with effective therapy of the infection. Acute staphylococcal endocarditis causes an immune-mediated glomerulonephritis as a consequence of antigen deposition at the glomerular basement membrane and activation of the alternate complement pathway. This lesion may be found in more than 25% of patients with *S. aureus* endocarditis of less than 2 weeks' duration.

DIAGNOSIS

The diagnosis of endocarditis is suggested by the clinical picture and is confirmed by documenting persistent bacteremia, i.e., multiple positive blood cultures for the same organisms over 24 to 48 hours. Likewise, blood cultures positive for the organisms that commonly cause endocarditis should raise suspicion of this diagnosis, even in the absence of other clinical findings. Without prior antibiotic therapy, at least 95% of patients with endocarditis have positive blood cultures. In almost all of these patients, one of the initial two cultures will be positive. Depending upon the susceptibility of the organism, administration of antibiotics during the preceding 2 weeks may significantly reduce the frequency of positive blood cultures. Therefore, to avoid false-negative blood cultures, cultures should be obtained before antibiotics are given. Transthoracic echocardiography, followed by transesophageal echocardiography if necessary, is a highly sensitive and specific approach to the identification of vegetations on valves and intracardiac complications. Although this approach is not suitable for screening patients with little clinical evidence of endocarditis, it can aid in identifying typical vegetations in patients in whom the disease is highly suspected. Other laboratory tests that are frequently abnormal in patients with endocarditis, e.g., hematocrit, sedimentation rate, urine analysis, circulating immune complex concentration, and rheumatoid factor, are not helpful in making a specific diagnosis.

TREATMENT

Effective treatment for endocarditis requires that the causative agent be identified and its antimicrobial susceptibility be determined. This information allows the design of an effective antimicrobial regimen. Because host defenses are not very effective at inhibiting bacteria within vegetations, bactericidal antibiotics or combinations of antibiotics are required for optimal therapy. Antibiotics are administered parenterally to achieve high serum concentrations, necessary to penetrate into the depths of relatively avascular vegetations. The reduced metabolic state of organisms deep in vegetations may render these cells difficult to eradicate and supports the prolonged antibiotic courses advocated for most patients with infective endocarditis. The increasing prevalence of enterococci that are resistant to penicillins, vancomycin, and the aminoglycosides (high-level resistance to streptomycin and gentamicin)—and staphylococci that are resistant to methicillin (also resistant to all semisynthetic penicillinase-resistant penicillins, cephalosporins, and carbapenems)—may result in endocarditis that is difficult to treat with antibiotics. Fungi and antibiotic-resistant Gram-negative rods may also cause endocarditis that is difficult to treat with antibiotics. Surgery to excise valves infected by antibiotic-resistant organisms may allow eradication of these infections. Additionally, the survival of patients with intracardiac complications, such as valve dysfunction that leads to congestive heart failure or perivalvular abscess, has been greatly enhanced by surgery to debride sites of infection, restore anatomic defects, and replace a dysfunctional valve with a prosthesis.

PREVENTION

The value of prophylactic antibiotics to prevent endocarditis in patients at risk is uncertain because no carefully controlled studies have been performed. Nevertheless, animal studies support the use of antibiotic prophylaxis. Patients at risk typically include those with heart valve lesions who undergo procedures that may lead to bacteremia with organisms that are the most common causes of endocarditis. Therefore, it is recommended that patients with known rheumatic heart disease or heart valve malformations from other causes be given penicillin just prior to, and for a short time after, such procedures as cleaning and extraction of teeth. To cover the enterococcus, an aminoglycoside should be added to the penicillin prior to invasive maneuvers in the gastrointestinal or genitourinary tracts. Prophylactic use of antibiotics is particularly important in patients who have a prosthetic heart valve. Bacterial endocarditis in such patients has such a poor prognosis that attempts to prevent it are mandatory.

SUGGESTED READINGS

Baddour LM. Virulence factors among gram-positive bacteria in experimental endocarditis. Infect Immun 1994;62: 2143–2148.

Karchmer AW. Infective endocarditis. In: Braunwald E, ed. Heart disease. 5th ed. Philadelphia: W.B. Saunders, 1996.

Livornese LL, Jr., Korzeniowski OM. Pathogenesis of infective endocarditis. In: Kaye D, ed. Infective endocarditis. 2nd ed. New York: Raven Press, 1992:19–35.

Scheld WM, Sande MA. Endocarditis and intravascular infections. In: Mandell GL, Bennett JE, Dolin R, eds. Mandel, Douglas and Bennett's Principles and practice of infectious diseases. 4th ed. New York: Churchill Livingstone, 1995: 740–783.

Head and Neck Infections

ARNOLD L. SMITH

Infections of the head and neck occur most commonly when organisms from contiguous mucosal surfaces extend into the soft tissue and interstitial spaces of this area by extension. Less commonly, organisms may be seeded from the bloodstream. Regardless of the route by which the infectious agents reach the tissue, manifestations of head and neck infections that come to medical attention are due to **inflammation**. Infections of these parts of the body result in cellulitis, lymphadenitis, or abscesses of soft tissues. The resulting swelling may be readily recognized, for example, when it causes facial cellulitis, or when it affects a physiological function (such as swallowing).

INTRODUCTION

The **air-filled cavities** of the head (sinuses, mastoids, middle ear) are lined with respiratory epithelium (Fig. 65.1). Infections of these spaces result when their normal drainage route becomes blocked. With **blockage**, the ciliated respiratory epithelium, which normally functions to remove bacteria by entrapping them in mucus and propelling the mucus out, can no longer function. Once aerobic bacteria have reached their maximum growth, oxygen in the blocked cavity is depleted and anaerobes can grow. High densities of bacteria release fragments of cell envelopes (such as lipopolysaccharide or murein subunits), which elicit an inflammatory response, leading to swelling and more blockage. The inflammation produces the symptoms of such infections.

ENCOUNTER AND ENTRY

Frequently, infection of the soft tissue or lymph nodes of the head and neck is due to a previous infection with viruses or group A streptococci, which served to disrupt the integrity of the epithelial surface. Histological examination of respiratory mucosa during acute viral infec-

tions shows loss of ciliated epithelial cells and thinning of the mucosal layer. Extension of this process results in physical loss of continuity of the epithelium and allows bacteria to enter the underlying soft tissue and produce cellulitis or overwhelm the defenses in the lymph nodes, causing lymphadenitis.

In **sinusitis**, the ostia may become blocked because of a viral upper respiratory infection, or more commonly, by allergy, both of which produce edema. In the **middle ear**, eustachian tube dysfunction may occur congenitally (as in infants with cleft palate who lack the muscle to open the medial orifice of the eustachian tube), or as a result of a viral upper respiratory tract infection, or can be caused by allergies. Because the cavity of the middle ear is contiguous with the mastoid air cells, individuals with acute otitis media also have mastoiditis, which is an acute inflammatory reaction in the mastoid ear cells.

The most common bacterial infections of the head and neck and their etiologies are listed in Table 65.1. The bacteria that cause infections of the head and neck are those commonly isolated from the surface of the upper respiratory tract, i.e., *Streptococcus pneumoniae, Haemophilus influenzae, Staphylococcus aureus, Streptococcus pyogenes,* and anaerobic bacteria. Four clinical cases are discussed below.

■ CASE 1. OTITIS MEDIA

E., a 14-month-old girl, came down with the same "cold" that her sister had had for the past 3 days. She then stopped taking her bottle, became irritable, and developed a temperature of 39.8°C. She continued to feed poorly and had a low-grade fever and irritability, which prompted her mother to take her to a physician. In the doctor's office, the nurse used a tympanometer to measure the mobility of E.'s ear drum, and told the mother that E. had an ear infection. On further otoscopic examination, the physician agreed, and prescribed the antibiotic amoxicillin.

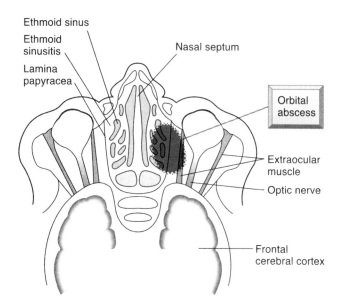

Figure 65.1. Superior view of the face sectioned through the level of the ethmoid sinus.

E.'s mother had many questions:

1. Should E.'s sister be brought in and checked for an ear infection?
2. Is an ear infection contagious?
3. How does a machine (the tympanometer) diagnose an ear infection?
4. Should a culture be obtained before antibiotics are prescribed?
5. How can the doctor be sure that amoxicillin is the right antibiotic for E.?
6. Are there complications of ear infections?

Otitis media is one of the most common infections seen by family physicians and pediatricians. The majority of cases occur in children between 6 and 36 months of age, the average child having two episodes per year during the first 3 years of life. Why are children especially sensitive to this type of infection? A likely predisposing cause is that the medial orifice of the eustachian tube is patulent in infancy. Supine feeding (giving a bottle at bedtime) permits reflux of pharyngeal contents into the lumen of the eustachian tubes, producing chemical irritation which results in inflammation and occlusion. Dysfunction of the eustachian tubes is also facilitated by upper respiratory infections of the abundant lymphoid tissue around the medial orifice, such as those caused by respiratory syncytial virus, influenza A or B, or adenovirus. Members of the normal upper respiratory flora (pneumococci, *H. influenzae,* and, occasionally, *S. aureus, Branhamella catarrhalis,* and group A streptococci) become entrapped in the middle ear and proliferate. A previous viral infection may also predispose to bacterial replication in the middle ear by direct damage to the respiratory epithelium lining that cavity.

The signs and symptoms of inflammation of the middle ear reflect the anatomy of this region. Early in the course of the infection, submucosal edema and hemorrhage lead to the outpouring of exudate into the lumen. As the middle ear cavity fills with fluid, the tympanic membrane becomes relatively immobile, which impairs hearing. Mobility can be measured by pneumatic otoscopy (changing the air pressure on the ear drum while looking at it), or by tympanometry (a technique that measures the ability of the ear drum to reflect sound at various air pressures). In the normal ventilated ear, tension on the tympanic membrane varies with the pressure exerted on it. When fluid is present in the middle ear, the tympanic membrane cannot stretch with changes in pressure, and the acoustic impedance (or compliance) does not change. This is how the nurse diagnosed the infection.

In **chronic otitis media**, the epithelium of the middle ear undergoes marked histological changes: mucus-secreting cells increase in number and may even form glands. Mucin is secreted into the middle ear, possibly in order to entrap and "wash out" bacteria and inflammatory debris. These changes are elicited by bacterial cell wall material and secreted toxins. The usual exit route for fluids, the eustachian tube, continues to be occluded. Drainage of the fluid either by using drugs that restore eustachian tube function or by direct drainage through a tube inserted through the ear drum, returns the metaplastic epithelium and ventilates the middle ear.

Table 65.1. Infections of the Head and Neck

Infections of air-filled cavities
    Otitis media
    Sinusitis
    Mastoiditis
Infections of structures contiguous to air-filled cavities
    Orbital cellulitis or abscess
    Cavernous sinus thrombosis or thrombophlebitis
    Lateral sinus thrombosis or thrombophlebitis
    Cervical adenitis
Infections of soft tissues
    Conjunctivitis
    Fascial cellulitis
    Abscess of canine fossa
    Lymphadenitis
    Parapharyngeal abscess
        Paratonsillar
        Pteromaxillary
        Lateral neck
    Thyroiditis
Infections of embryonic remnants
    Branchial cleft cellulitis or abscess
        Thyroglossal duct cellulitis or abscess

The middle ear may become infected with any of the bacteria present in the upper respiratory tract. As with upper respiratory tract infections (e.g., sinusitis), the primary pathogens are pneumococci and *H. influenzae* (together these bacteria cause 80% of the total). Antibiotics active against these two species have proven effective in the treatment of otitis media, alone or in combination. Thus, empirical antibiotic administration directed against the most common pathogens is justifiable in this disease. However, in several studies it is clear that acute otitis media can resolve without antibiotic administration. It is not necessary to aspirate the middle ear fluid (a painful procedure) for culture and susceptibility testing.

Although most ear infections treated with antibiotics resolve without complication, chronic and recurrent episodes of otitis media may lead to sequelae such as brain abscess or meningeal epidural abscess. Usually the patient has had a perforated ear drum. In such cases, the pathogens include not only members of the upper respiratory flora, but occasionally enteric Gram-negative bacilli that gain access to the middle ear through the perforated ear drum.

CASE 2. CELLULITIS IN THE ORBIT OF THE EYE

B., a 14-year-old girl, has had intermittent problems with allergies, which manifest primarily as a runny nose, watery eyes, and episodes of fullness in the front part of her face and nose. One morning, she developed fever, headache, cough, and had a foul taste in her mouth. She interpreted this as another one of her allergies and took an antihistamine pill and some antipyretics. However, the next morning, she awoke with a severe headache, felt terribly ill, and could not open her left eye. Her pediatrician noted marked redness and swelling around her eye and a slight exudate from the eyelids. When she retracted her left eyelids she found that B.'s left eye was slightly deviated down and laterally. She recommended that B. should immediately see an ear, nose, and throat (ENT) physician as she probably had a serious illness, orbital cellulitis.

B. and her family wondered what was going on.

1. What is orbital cellulitis?
2. Why should B. see an ENT physician if the problem is with her eye?
3. How are B's allergies related to her cellulitis?
4. Are antibiotics necessary?

Orbital cellulitis is acute inflammation of the connective tissue of the eye socket and is a complication of acute sinusitis. The anterior and lateral border of the ethmoid sinuses form the medial and superior border of the orbit. The orbit is then separated from the ethmoid sinus by the **lamina papyracea**, which is literally a paper-thin piece of bone. Infection in the ethmoid sinus may break through this thin piece of bone and enter the orbit. If the cellulitis becomes localized, an intraorbital but extraocular abscess may develop (see Fig. 65.1).

B's physician quickly recognized the disease, because of the region of the orbit affected (superior and medial) and the displacement of the eye down and out. Had she measured it, the physician would have found that the eyeball was exophthalmic, i.e., it protruded out of the orbit. It is difficult to appreciate this protrusion without a measuring device. **Exophthalmus** is caused by the edema and inflammatory exudate in the orbit, literally making the cavity smaller and forcing the eye out. As might be expected, other signs of orbital cellulitis include limitation of the movement of the eye as the muscles become edematous and stretched. In addition, stretching of the optic nerve may decrease visual acuity, a very serious complication, and lead to blindness.

Because the source of orbital cellulitis is the sinus, the treatment of choice is surgical drainage of the involved ethmoid. Drainage decompresses the orbit and allows the eyeball to return to its normal place. Treatment of this infection should also include the administration of antibiotics. As with other infections of the head and neck, bacteria isolated from the infected sites are from the oral pharyngeal flora. In the more virulent infections, such as the one experienced by B., there is a higher probability that *S. aureus will* be isolated. Here, antibiotics should be active against *S. aureus* as well as members of the upper respiratory tract flora.

CASE 3. FACIAL CELLULITIS

R., a 14-month-old baby boy, was not sleeping through the night and seemed hungry all of the time. His mother started supplementing his food with a bottle of milk containing cereal. One afternoon, when he awoke from his nap, his mother noted that he was fussy, had a low-grade temperature, and had a slight swelling of his right cheek. She thought he might have bumped it with the bottle as he frequently did when feeding himself in the crib. That evening when she put him to bed, he seemed a little improved but still irritable and his right cheek was somewhat swollen and had a slightly purplish hue. His temperature seemed increased, but other than that, he seemed well. The next morning, his mother thought that he was worse. She took his temperature and found that it was 41.6°C. She took him to the family doctor who told her that R. would need hospitalization for antibiotic treatment of **facial cellulitis**.

His mother had many questions:

1. Was this cellulitis different from the kind that she had on her hand after working in the garden?
2. Why did R. need to be hospitalized to receive antibiotics for cellulitis?

3. How did the bacteria get into R.'s cheek?
4. Will the antibiotics cure R.?

Facial cellulitis in infants is almost exclusively caused by *H. influenzae* type b. If R. had been immunized with the vaccine containing the capsular carbohydrate of *H. influenzae,* the disease would not have occurred. The pathogenesis is not entirely clear, but it is likely that minor facial trauma allows blood to seep into the soft tissues. When transient *H. influenzae* bacteremia occurs, the organisms seed and grow in the traumatized subcutaneous tissue using the extravasated red blood cells as a source of nutrition (the name "haemo-philus" [blood-loving] is apt: it requires, among other cofactors, heme for growth). Because the soft tissue was seeded via the bloodstream, R. is at risk for other infectious complications of *H. influenzae* bacteremia, such as meningitis, septic arthritis, and osteomyelitis, and R. requires hospitalization for vigorous treatment and careful observation.

Because *H. influenzae* does not make cell-damaging exotoxins, the inflammation in tissues is often minimal. Often, as in R.'s case, the distinction between a slight bruise on the face and cellulitis is difficult to make. The telling clues are the swelling that is out of proportion to the magnitude of the facial trauma, and that the infant has a high fever. One of the reasons R.'s physician suspected that the etiological agent was *H. influenzae* was the typical purplish (not reddish) hue of the inflamed region and his knowledge that the family refused *H. influenzae* b vaccine for religious reasons. The reason for this special coloration is not known, but it is characteristic.

H. influenzae cellulitis resolves with the administration of appropriate antibiotics. Because secondary diseases due to *H. influenzae* are serious, the usual treatment is to administer antibiotics intravenously until the cellulitis has resolved.

▌ CASE 4. PARAPHARYNGEAL ABSCESS

Before going to bed one evening, Ms. J., a 19-year-old college student, noticed "a scratchy throat" with slight pain. Over the next 4 days, she had an increasingly sore throat and her right ear began to ache. She thought she had a fever and took aspirin. On the morning of the sixth day of her illness, Ms. J. found that she could barely open her mouth to eat breakfast. When she did get food in, it was difficult for her to swallow. Her roommate noted that her voice was of lower pitch and decreased in volume, as though she had something hot in her mouth. She went to the infirmary, where the physician, after looking in her mouth, told her that hospitalization was necessary for additional tests and possibly surgery.

Ms. J. had several questions:

1. How could surgery help a sore throat?

2. Don't sore throats go away by themselves?
3. Does her roommate have to worry about catching this illness?

Ms. J. had symptoms that are typical of a parapharyngeal abscess. In her case, the most likely diagnosis was that of a **peritonsillar abscess**. This diagnosis was evident by examination of the mouth. Tonsils lie between the two palatal pillars, with their superior poles overlying a portion of the superior pharyngeal constrictor muscle and their medial portion, the medial pterygoid muscle. These are two of the four muscles that function to open the mouth. Inflammation behind the tonsil adjacent to these muscles causes their dysfunction. **Trismus,** the inability to open one's mouth, is caused by dysfunction of the medial pterygoid, while the inability to initiate swallowing is due to dysfunction of the superior pharyngeal constrictor. Failure to elevate the palate results from edema in that area; this leads to a muffled, "hot potato" voice, even though the tongue is unaffected. Ms. J. could swallow, as there was no mechanical obstruction to a bolus of food entering her esophagus, but inflammation of the superior constrictor made it difficult to initiate the process (Fig. 65.2). In the mouth of patients with peritonsillar abscess, the tonsil appears medially and downward displaced and, on palpation, may feel as though it is floating. This is caused by the pus pushing it from behind.

Bacteria that cause this illness are, as in most head and neck infections, those commonly found in the oral pharynx. Most of these organisms are commensals, but group A streptococci are responsible for approximately half of the cases of peritonsillar abscess. The infection seems first to cause a cellulitis of the peritonsillar tissues, followed by local necrosis. The aerobic and anaerobic flora of the oral pharyngeal epithelium then gain access to the necrotic tissue in the interstitial space.

The primary therapy is surgical drainage. Antibiotic therapy of choice for this disease should include a drug (such as penicillin G) active against common mouth anaerobes and aerobes but also against *S. aureus*. In most cases, the choice is a semisynthetic penicillin that is resistant to staphylococcal β-lactamase.

▌ CASE 5. CONJUNCTIVITIS

J. was an active 9-year-old boy who returned from summer camp in good health. The next day he awoke with swelling of his right eye and the sensation that he had "something stuck" in this eye. His left eye felt fine. His mother took him to a physician when she noted that the inside of both his upper and lower eyelid looked "bloody" and tears from that eye were blood-tinged. The examining physician noted a tender, palpable lymph node just in front of the right ear and a mild runny nose. In spite of J. now having blurred vision in the right eye, the physician placed a patch over the eye and told the mother that J. had a "virus" and all would be well in 5 days.

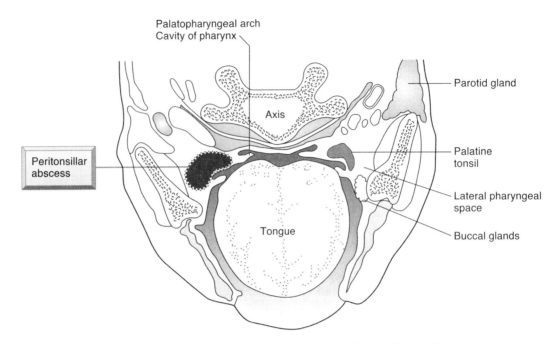

Figure 65.2. Cross-section of the oropharynx through the tonsils.

The mother questioned the physician's wisdom and asked several questions:

1. Why is the other eye not involved if it is a virus?
2. Didn't the bloody tears indicate something in the eye?
3. Could she and J.'s father develop the eye infection?
4. Shouldn't antibiotics be prescribed for an eye infection?

Conjunctivitis is an extremely common infection in children and young adults. Conjunctivitis can be caused by viruses, bacteria, or obligate intracellular organisms such as the chlamydiae. Conjunctivitis should be distinguished from more serious conditions such as **keratitis** or **iritis**. A distinguishing feature of keratitis is impaired vision, eye pain, and photophobia, in addition to diffuse inflammation of the eye, gritty irritation, and excessive lacrimation. When conjunctivitis occurs alone, it is caused by *H. influenzae* (42%), adenovirus (22%), and the pneumococcus (12%); *B. catarrhalis* and staphylococci together comprise approximately 5%.

The only clinically distinguishing features between adenoviral disease and bacterial conjunctivitis is that the former is usually accompanied by upper respiratory symptoms (up to one-half in some studies), hyperplasia of lymphoid follicles beneath the conjunctiva, and hyperemia of the palpebral conjunctiva as well as conjunctival hemorrhages on the globe. In addition, "hemorrhagic" conjunctivitis is almost exclusively adenovirus disease. In 75% of patients, adenoviral conjunctivitis is also accompanied by a diffuse superficial keratitis in which subepithelial corneal infiltrates are present. This causes transient blurring of the vision. Adenoviral keratoconjunctivitis is more commonly associated with preauricular lymphadenopathy. In this case, history and physical examination alone enabled the physician to make the correct diagnosis.

Organisms are introduced into the eye probably by direct contact with hands of carriers. Rarely, the agent is introduced into the eye by respiratory droplets. Serious infections of the anterior portion of the eye are due to herpes simplex virus (HSV), *Pseudomonas aeruginosa* in individuals who wear contact lenses, and, in undeveloped nations, *Chlamydia trachomatis*. HSV (and varicella zoster virus) cause vesicular lesions on the eyelid in addition to the usual symptoms of conjunctivitis. No other distinguishing feature exists between HSV conjunctivitis and adenoviral conjunctivitis. The significance of **herpes simplex conjunctivitis** is that severe keratitis develops in 50% of all ocular herpes infections; it is the most common cause of severe corneal ulceration in children in the U.S. Moreover, herpes simplex keratitis is second only to trauma in causing acquired blindness in children. Because of the serious nature of herpetic keratoconjunctivitis and the high risk of recurrence, these patients should be cared for by an ophthalmologist. **Varicella zoster conjunctivitis** occurs in approximately 4% of all the children with chickenpox. Because the virus is delivered to the skin via the vascular compartment, vesicles present on the lateral aspect of the tip of the nose invariably predict involvement of the eye; vesicles at this location reflect the involvement of the nasociliary branch of the first division of the trigeminal nerve. Thus, subsequent involvement of the anterior structures of the eye is inevitable.

Symptomatic treatment of adenoviral conjunctivitis consists of removing exudate, if it is matted, with a saline-moist cotton and patching to relieve pain. Chemotherapeutic agents active against adenovirus are not available. In patients with suspected bacterial conjunctivitis, the administration of an **antibiotic ointment** (polymyxin and bacitracin) four times a day increases the rate of resolution over that seen with placebo alone. Other acceptable ophthalmic preparations contain tetracycline, gentamicin, or erythromycin.

Herpetic infections of the eye are treated with idoxuridine, trifluorothymidine, vidarabine, and acyclovir. Available data suggest that the overwhelming majority of herpetic corneal ulcers treated with trifluorothymidine resolve within 2 weeks. Ideal administration of topical antiviral agents to the eye is every 1–2 hours.

Within 3 days, J.'s signs and symptoms were gone. The physician removed his eye patch and no further treatment was administered. If the physician's initial diagnosis had been incorrect, a reasonable approach would be to reexamine the eye, seeking evidence of herpes simplex, and to have administered antibiotic ointment if there was no herpes, but if exudate was still present.

CASE 6. CERVICAL LYMPHADENITIS

M. is an 18-year-old Caucasian woman who had lived in Minneapolis all of her life. She and her family were in good health and proud of the fact that no family members had ever been hospitalized. Six weeks after arriving at the University of Wisconsin, she experienced a mild sore throat and a low-grade temperature (100°F orally). On going to bed that night, she noted a small, slightly tender lump beneath the angle of her jaw. Upon awakening in the morning, the lump was the size of a walnut, more tender, and she felt feverish although her temperature was not higher. At the Student Health Service, a physician told M. that she would need a throat culture and some blood tests before she could prescribe treatment.

The physician told M. that she had cervical adenitis and that a throat culture was needed to determine if group A streptococci were the likely etiological agents. The blood test was a complete blood count with differential and a screening for heterophile antibody.

Upon hearing this report, M.'s parents had many questions:

1. Is this a life-threatening illness?
2. Is this cancer?

3. Why did she need blood tests?
4. Should the physician prescribe antibiotics?

Cervical adenitis, inflammation of the lymph nodes in the neck, may be caused by many infectious agents. Because these lymph nodes receive drainage from the mouth, gums, posterior pharynx, as well as the face, cheek, and nose, it is conceivable that many infectious agents can produce swelling and tenderness of lymph nodes. Depending on the nature of the infectious agent in the lymph node, the influx of cells causing the swelling consists of neutrophils or histiocytes and lymphocytes. Table 65.2 lists the agents that can cause cervical adenitis. Some generalizations can be drawn about these agents. In general, bacterial infections cause disease that is isolated to one cervical lymph node and make the center lymph node necrose (i.e., cause suppuration). In contrast, viral infections of the cervical lymph nodes are rarely localized exclusively to one region, such as the neck; lymph nodes that can be readily detected by palpation in other parts of the body are also swollen. In addition, only bacterial infections of the lymph nodes produce suppuration.

The physician's approach to the patient with cervical adenitis relies heavily on epidemiological considerations. From inspection of Table 65.2, it is clear that numerous agents might be the cause of the disease. Infections of certain agents only occur in certain parts of the world (i.e., trypanosomiasis in tropical countries and *Pseudomonas pseudomallei* in southeast Asia). Other important information consists of recent contact with animals (important for the diagnosis of tularemia, plague, and cat scratch disease) and immunization status, which is important in determining if the patient has measles, rubella, or mumps.

In this individual, a common cause of cervical adenitis, tuberculosis, can be excluded. Tuberculosis of the cervical lymph glands occurs in individuals with pulmonary tuberculosis who inoculate the mouth through coughing. Rarely, it is acquired through the ingestion of milk contaminated with *Mycobacterium tuberculosis*. In the continental U.S., the overwhelming majority of *M. tuberculosis* infections (other than those in HIV-infected individuals) occurs in individuals recently emigrated to this country and in native Americans. Thus, *M. tuberculosis* is unlikely on epidemiological grounds. Moreover, the rapidity of onset of the swelling is also evidence against this being a tuberculous infection.

The major etiological agents that need to be considered in M.'s case are *S. pyogenes* (group A streptococcus), *S. aureus*, and Epstein-Barr virus (EBV) infection. In individuals with Epstein-Barr virus infection, there is usually sore throat, fever, and swelling in the neck. In addition, approximately one-half of the EBV-infected patients have headache, severe loss of appetite, malaise, and muscle aches, and one-fifth have muscle aches and

Table 65.2. Agents of Lymphadenitis

Agent	Generalized lymphadenopathy	Isolated cervical disease	Suppuration
Bacterial			
Streptococcus pyogenes, group A	+	+	+
Staphylococcus aureus	0	+	+
Atypical mycobacteria	0	+	+
Corynebacterium diphtheriae	0	+	0
Mycobacterium tuberculosis	+	+	+
Brucella spp.	+	0	0
Francisella tularensis	0	+	+
Strict anaerobes	0	+	0
Yersinia pestis	0	+	+
Cat-scratch agent	0	+	+
Pseudomonas pseudomallei	0	+	+
Viral			
Measles	+	0	0
Rubella	+	0	0
EBV	+	0	0
Adenovirus (groups 3 and 7)	0	+	0
Herpes simplex	0	+	0
Cytomegalovirus	+	0	0
Mumps	0	0	0
HIV	+	0	0
Fungal			
Histoplasma capsulatum	+	0	0
Coccidioides immitis	+	+	0
Aspergillus spp.	0	+	0
Parasitic			
Toxoplasma gondii	+	0	0
Trypanosoma brucei	+	0	0

chills. As might be expected, the virus does not localize only on one side of the pharynx; thus, most cervical adenitis due to EBV infection is bilateral.

The test ordered by the physician was a **heterophile antibody titer.** This antibody is present in 90% of the cases. Because it may not be present at the time of initial symptoms, the physician should repeat these tests 2 weeks later if the antibody is initially absent. Most bacterial cervical adenitis presents with symptoms much like M.'s with unilateral swelling of a single lymph node and minimal upper respiratory or constitutional complaints. The most common bacterial etiology is group A streptococcus or *S. aureus*. Finding the group A streptococcus in the pharynx would strengthen the diagnosis. Needle aspiration of the lymph node (with or without suppuration) is the only definitive means of assuring the diagnosis. Thus, the prudent physician should administer an antibiotic active against both bacteria. The importance of finding group A streptococci in the throat is

that treatment should be continued for at least 10 days to assure eradication of the *Streptococcus* and to prevent sequelae.

SUGGESTED READINGS

Brook I. Microbiology of retropharyngeal abscesses in children. Am J Dis Child 1987;141:202.

Henderson FW, Collier AM, Sanyal MA, Watkins JM, Fairlough DL, Clyde WL, Denny FW. A longitudinal study of respiratory viruses and bacteria in the etiology of acute otitis media with effusion. N Engl J Med 1982;306:1377.

Johnson JT, Yu VL. Infectious diseases and antimicrobial therapy of the ears, nose and throat. Philadelphia: W.B. Saunders, 1997.

Meyerhoff WL, Giebink GS. Pathology and microbiology of otitis media. Laryngoscope 1982;92:273.

Schlossberg D. Infections of the head and neck. New York: Springer Verlag, 1987.

Siegel JD. Eye infections encountered by the pediatrician. Pediatr Infect Dis 1986;5:741.

Sexually Transmitted Diseases

PENELOPE J. HITCHCOCK

For review of the individual agents of sexually transmitted diseases, see Chapters 14, "*Neisseria*"; 24, "Syphilis"; 27, "Chlamydiae"; 38, "Human Retroviruses"; 40, "Warts"; 41, "Herpesviruses"; 51, "Intestinal and Vaginal Protozoa."

Sexually transmitted diseases (**STDs**) are a broad but relatively well-defined group of infectious diseases, generally with acute manifestations that often progress to a chronic clinical picture. STDs rank among the most important of all infectious diseases with regard to the physical, psychological, and economic damage they cause to humans.

The agents of STDs are highly varied (Table 66.1); they include representatives of such different groups as the pyogenic cocci (gonococci), spirochetes (*Treponema pallidum* of syphilis), fastidious Gram-negative rods (*Haemophilus ducreyi* of chancroid), strict intracellular bacteria (*Chlamydia trachomatis*), viruses (herpes simplex viruses 1 and 2, human papillomaviruses, and HIV), protozoa (*Trichomonas vaginalis*), and arthropods (scabies, pubic lice). There are other agents of STDs but these are encountered less frequently in developed countries.

THE MAGNITUDE OF THE PROBLEM

During the last half of this century, the incidence of STDs has dramatically increased worldwide. In the last 25 years, several new STDs have been recognized worldwide and dramatic increases have been documented in most STDs in the U.S. Adolescent and minority populations have been disproportionately affected. In 1996, more than 14 million cases of STDs, including HIV, occurred; 63% of them were in people less than 24 years old.

Annually, approximately 750,000 new cases of gonorrhea occur in the U. S., at an enormous physical, emotional, and social cost (Table 66.2). Gonorrhea alone costs an estimated $1 billion each year. Twenty-five percent of gonorrhea cases are in teenagers. In addition, gonococcal antibiotic resistance has been on the rise in the last decade. The public is becoming aware of the large increase in chlamydial infections, with an annual incidence in the U.S. of about 4 million cases.

STDs that cause genital ulcer disease, such as syphilis and chancroid, have declined between 1992 and 1997, but these infections remain an important problem in certain geographic areas, such as the rural Southern U.S. and in inner cities, particularly among African-Americans. In these settings, the cycle of infection reflects failure to diagnose and treat these diseases, a pattern that is driven by poverty and lack of access to health care. Genital herpes, on the other hand, does not appear to be decreasing in any segment of the population or region. An estimated 47 million North Americans are afflicted with genital herpes (HSV), 80% of whom are unaware of being infected.

Recently, certain types of human papillomavirus (HPV) infection have been recognized as the cause of cervical cancer. An estimated 28 million North Americans are infected with genital HPV; the majority of these infections involve low-risk types associated with genital warts. Some, however, involve cervical dysplasias and cervical cancer. For reasons that are not understood but are likely to be linked to a functional immune system, only a small number of infected women progress to cervical cancer (15,000/year) and only one in three die of this surgically treatable condition.

POPULATION DYNAMICS

Efforts at prevention and control of STDs require an understanding of the factors that contribute to their

Table 66.1. Sexually Transmitted Diseases and Their Agents

Disease	Agent
Chlamydial infection	*Chlamydia trachomatis* (all biovars but L)
Gonorrhea	*Neisseria gonorrhoeae*
Genital herpes	Herpes simplex virus type II and type I
Warts, anogenital cancer	Human papillomavirus
Trichomoniasis	*Trichomonas vaginalis*
AIDS	HIV
Chancroid	*Haemophilus ducreyi*
Syphilis	*Treponema pallidum*
Lymphogranuloma venereum (LGV)	*Chlamydia trachomatis* (L biovars)
Granuloma inguinale	*Donovania granulomatis*
Candidiasis	*Candida albicans*
Bacterial vaginosis	*Gardnerella vaginalis*

spread and progression. Although STDs share a common mode of transmission, each of them presents unique challenges to diagnosis, therapy, and prevention. A large number of biological and social forces are also involved in the dynamics of STD transmission. To make sense of this multitude of variables, it is convenient to separate them according to a model proposed by May and Anderson, which states that the rate of movement of an STD throughout the population depends on: (1) the **transmissibility** of the infectious agent; (2) the **rate of new partner acquisition** as well as the partners' sexual history, and (3) the **duration of infectiousness**. Each of the variables in this model is affected by biological, behavioral, and social risk factors.

The Transmissibility of the Agent (or Infectivity Rate)

The infectivity rate is defined as the risk of acquiring infection during a single contact with an infected partner. For each STD, the rate varies not only with behavioral factors but also with the biological properties of the host and the agents (Table 66.3). Each pathogen has unique pathophysiological parameters that affect the infectivity rate. For example, the number of organisms necessary to establish infection, the **infectious dose**, varies both with the agent and with individual host factors. In each case, gender, genetic susceptibility, age of exposure, coinfection with other infectious organisms, and immunological status must be considered.

Behavioral factors, including drug and alcohol use, contraceptive practices, circumcision, douching, and specific sexual practices, also affect the infectivity rate. Consider HIV, which possesses specific surface molecules for attachment to host cell receptors found primarily on rectal epithelial cells as well as lymphocytes. Sexual behavior is an important factor here since anal intercourse facilitates the spread of the virus. Several studies on risk-taking behavior among teenagers showed that risk-taking may be a characteristic of a subset of this population. Thus, smoking, alcohol and other substance abuse, a high number of sexual partners, and excessive automobile speeding are coassociated high-risk behaviors.

The Rate of New Partner Acquisition

The rate of new partner acquisition is defined as the number of new partners an individual has over a specified period of time. This parameter depends on the probability that any given partner may be infected. The greater the number of partners, the greater the chance that one of them is infected. Surveys indicate that most people have only a few sexual partners over their lifetime and that propagation of STD epidemics is actually attributable to a small number of individuals with a large number of sexual partners, referred to as the **core**. Thus, the number of sexual partners an individual has, determines membership in the core. Sexual activity among core members sustains the disease, sexual activity outside the core spreads the disease.

Common characteristics of STD core members include living in an urban environment, low socioeconomic status, age range between 15 and 30 years old, often minority ethnicity, and illicit drug use and prostitution. The size of the core may differ with each pathogen and is influenced both by the infectivity rate and the duration of the infection. It is important to note that asymptomatic infections, such as those caused by chlamydiae or HIV, are usually not confined to a core.

In considering the degree of risk involved in a sexual encounter, each person must take into account the probability that the partner is a core member; this, of course, requires being able to identify a core member. This is often difficult to determine because identification depends on such variables as the length of the relationship prior to sexual activity, the circumstances under which the partners meet, and the ability to obtain accurate risk-related information from the partner prior to sexual activity.

Duration of Infectivity

The duration of infectivity is the length of time that an individual is capable of transmitting the infection. Included in this factor are biological characteristics of both the pathogen and the host. Some pathogens (e.g., chlamydiae) commonly cause asymptomatic disease; carriers of chlamydiae do not know they are infected and do not seek treatment. Thus they remain able to

---

Table 66.2. Dimensions of the STD Problem

- In the last 25 years, several new STDs have been recognized worldwide, and dramatic increases have been documented in most STDs in the U.S.; adolescents and minority populations have been disproportionately affected; this year over 9 million cases of STDs, including HIV infection, will occur—63% of which will be in people less than 24 years of age.

Gonorrhea—*Neisseria gonorrhoeae*
- Approximately half to three quarters of a million new cases annually
- Overall slight decrease in incidence, but increases in African-American teenage boys; 25% of cases occur in teenagers
- Rates more than 40 times higher in African-Americans than in Caucasians
- Four new types of antibiotic resistance emerged in the last decade. Between 1991 and 1995, the percentage of isolates with plasmid-mediated penicillin resistance declined from 13.1% to 6.8%, whereas isolates with chromosomally mediated penicillin resistance increased slightly (from 6.4% to 7.0%). The number of plasmid-mediated isolates resistant to ciprofloxacin, one of the currently recommended drugs for gonorrhea, is increasing.
- Estimated annual cost almost $1 billion

Chlamydial infection—*Chlamydia trachomatis*
- Most common bacterial STD with an estimated 4 million cases annually
- Incidence increasing
- The apparent rise in incidence may reflect the effectiveness of screening and case-finding techniques, e.g., sensitive and specific diagnostic tests
- Control complicated by frequency of asymptomatic disease, cost and technical difficulty of diagnostic tests, lack of single-dose therapy.
- Comprehensive annual cost estimated at more than $2.8 billion

Pelvic inflammatory disease (PID)
- An estimated 1 million cases each year, due to untreated or inadequately treated gonococcal and chlamydial infections. This figure is probably an underestimate.
- Responsible for 15–30% of infertility and 50% of tubal pregnancies (both of which are increasing)
- Comprehensive annual costs estimated to exceed $7.0 billion

Syphilis—*Treponema pallidum*
- In 1995, over 16,500 primary and secondary cases were reported
- Infectious syphilis at highest level in over 40 years
- Increases concentrated in African-American men and women; rates over 60 times higher than in Caucasians
- Decrease in women in most states, echoed by a decrease in congenital cases since 1983

Genital herpes—Herpes Simplex Virus (HSV) I and II
- Approximately 47 million North Americans infected; 500,000 new cases annually
- First visits to physicians for genital HSV increased 7-fold between 1966 and 1989
- Annual costs roughly $100 million

Chancroid—*Haemophilus ducreyi*
- In 1995, fewer than 1000 cases were reported
- Increased more than 500% during 1980s; a sharp decline that started in 1990 continues

Genital warts—Human papillomavirus (HPV)
- Estimated 24–40 million people infected
- Approximately 500,000 to 1 million new cases annually
- First visits to physicians for genital warts increased by 33% in 1995

AIDS—Human Immunodeficiency Virus (HIV)
- Approximately 180,000 AIDS cases in first 10 years of epidemic; 1–1.5 million person believed to be HIV-infected. Almost 400,000 North Americans have died from AIDS. One in five living with AIDS was infected as a teenager.
- 56,000–71,000 new AIDS cases expected annually.
- Increase in AIDS cases now greater in women than men.
- AIDS projected to be among top five causes of death in women 15–44 years of age.

---

transmit the disease. If the carrier state involves partial immunity, the number of infectious organisms may be so low that the person is asymptomatic but still infectious. Antimicrobial sensitivity is also an important factor in duration of infectivity; if an agent is drug-resistant, treatment will fail and the infective period will be increased.

Factors that affect the duration of infectivity include access to and use of health care as well as attitudes and behaviors of health care providers. Access to health care

Table 66.3. Factors Involved in the Transmission of STDs

Transmission or complica-tion rate	Rate and nature of partner exchange	Duration of infectiousness or active infections	Sociocultural context
Sexual practices[a]	Number of partners/time[a]	Infecting organism	Socioeconomic status[a]
Age of coital debut[a]	Type of partner[a] (e.g., membership in core)	Host response	Residence[a]
Age		Health care behavior[a]	Educational status[a]
Genetic susceptibility	Age	routine STD screening	Religion[a]
Gender	Age of coital debut[a]	early diagnosis and therapy of symptoms	Race
Contraceptive method[a]	Gender	compliance with therapy	Ethnicity[d]
Alcohol use[a,b]		compliance with partner notification	Marital status[a]
Drug use (intravenous and other)[a,b]		Vaccine use	Sexual preference[a]
Smoking[a,b]		Douching and other intravaginal preparations	
Prior/coexisting STDs			
Intravaginal and intra-anal preparations (including douching)[a]			
Circumcision status[a,c]			

[a] Behavioral factor.
[b] A number of studies have focused on risk-taking behavior among adolescents. The data suggest that aggregate risk taking may be a characteristic of a subset of adolescents. For example, smoking, alcohol and other substance abuse, having high numbers of sexual partners, and excessive automobile speeding are high-risk behaviors that are highly coassociated.
[c] Geographical analysis of HIV seroprevalence and the presence of tribal-based taboos against the practice of circumcision has revealed high positive correlation in Africa. Additional studies are in progress to determine the cause–effect relationship between intact foreskin and increased transmission of HIV. Such transmission could be facilitated by the poor hygiene often associated with the lack of circumcision, the associated increased prevalence of genital ulcer diseases (e.g., chancroid, syphilis, herpes), or both.
[d] An example of how race and ethnicity are different with respect to risk markers is as follows: Among different ethnic groups of African-Americans, anthropological data suggest that gender–power relationships, which significantly influence STD rates, vary systematically by region of residence. This variability appears to reflect the country of origin and the patrilineal or matrilineal social heritage for distinct African-American groups. For example, preliminary data suggest that black women descendent from patrilineal societies have higher rates of STDs than those descendent from matrilineal societies.

is affected by the location of the clinic, the speed with which care can be obtained, and the cost of the services. The likelihood that an individual will seek care is influenced by such factors as the stigma associated with using an STD facility, knowledge of the existence of the facility, and the perception of the quality of services provided.

Other factors that influence the duration of infectivity include the existence of effective screening programs (dependent on accurate, sensitive, easy-to-use and inexpensive diagnostic tests), **partner notification** (which is essential in preventing "ping-pong" transmission even if one partner is treated), and effective treatment protocols (the fewer the doses, the more likely compliance will occur; the ideal is a single effective dose given at the time of diagnosis). Duration of infectivity also depends on access to programs designed to influence behavior (such as the use of condoms) and the availability of vaccines (as well as their effectiveness, distribution, acceptance, and administration).

Finally, all variables that influence the spread of infection are affected by the **sociocultural context** in which the infection occurs. This context is time-dependent, and influenced by historical and current political, economic, and biotechnological forces. Each society defines what is considered normal and acceptable sexual behavior. Ultimately, all the factors that dictate individual and institutional beliefs, values, intentions, and behaviors affect the transmissibility of STDs (Table 66.3).

GROUPS AT RISK

The multiple, long-term, devastating consequences of STDs disproportionately affect women and infants (Table 66.4). STDs are especially prevalent among the young. In the United States 63% of all STD cases occur in persons less than 25 years old. The problems of STDs among the young are likely to worsen because sexual activity among teenagers is increasing and adolescents often reject precautions, in part because of a perception of invulnerability. Biological factors also compound these behavioral risk factors. Thus, features of the cervical anatomy of adolescents (primarily cervical ectopy) increase the likelihood of chlamydial or gonococcal infection. Hormone changes in puberty alter the vaginal flora and natural mucus barriers to infection, and immunological naiveté facilitates the acquisition and progression of STDs.

The current STD epidemic in the United States also disproportionately affects minority groups. Both the incidence of STDs and long-term sequelae are consistently higher among non-Caucasians. During the second half of the 1980s, syphilis increased enormously among low-income, inner-city heterosexuals and their children. In the 1980s, the incidence of gonorrhea decreased in Caucasians of both sexes and increased in African-Americans. A recent survey showed that African-American males were approximately three times more likely than Caucasians to be seropositive to herpes simplex virus type 2 (HSV-2). The difference between females was sixfold.

Although non-Caucasian women comprise 17% of the total female population of the United States, they represent a disproportionate share (33%) of consultations for pelvic inflammatory disease (PID). In addition, ectopic pregnancy was 1.5 times as common among minority females as among whites. Furthermore, minority teenagers with ectopic pregnancies were almost 6 times more likely to die as their white counterparts.

ENCOUNTER AND ENTRY

Most of the STD-causing agents enter the body at local sites, through the mucosal or squamous epithelial layers of the vagina, cervix, urethra, rectum, or oral

---

Table 66.4. STD Complications in Women and Infants

STDs have frequent, severe, and irreversible complications, particularly for women and children

10–40% of women with untreated chlamydial and/or gonococcal cervicitis develop PID

Approximately 17–25% of women with PID become infertile

Risk of potentially fatal tubal pregnancy increases 6–10 fold after PID; tubal pregnancy is the leading cause of maternal death in African-American women

Several biotypes of HPV are associated with cervical cancer, which kills almost 5000 North American women yearly and is the second most common cause of cancer deaths in women worldwide

STDs cause spontaneous abortion, stillbirth, premature delivery, low birth weight, and permanently disabling infant infections

---

pharynx. An exception is HIV. Although HIV is transmitted primarily by sexual contact, contaminated blood products or hypodermic needles are also a source of infection.

It is possible to make a few other generalizations regarding the STDs and their agents. Nearly all the agents of STDs are relatively sensitive to chemical and physical factors and are practically never found free in the environment. Animal reservoirs are also unknown for most of these agents, thus the asymptomatic human carrier is the most frequent reservoir. The limited distribution of these agents makes these diseases theoretical candidates for eradication, but formidable medical, social, and political obstacles lie in the way of achieving it.

SPREAD AND MULTIPLICATION

All the agents that cause STDs are able to resist the host's nonspecific defense mechanisms and are infectious, i.e., are able to attach to and enter tissue with relative ease. The fact that chronic manifestations of STDs are relatively frequent indicates that the agents often cause asymptomatic disease and are not easily eliminated by specific immune responses. The strategies employed to withstand antimicrobial defenses are varied and should be reviewed by reading the chapters on specific agents

DAMAGE

The acute manifestations of the most frequent STDs fall into three groups: (1) **mucopurulent cervicitis and urethritis**, as in gonorrhea and chlamydial infection; (2) **genital ulcer disease**, as in syphilis, chancroid, and genital herpes; and (3) **dysplasia and cancer**, as in genital warts or cervical cancer.

With the exception of HIV, the STD-causing agents tend to cause primary lesions at or near the site of entry. It is not uncommon for these lesions to be so indolent as to go unnoticed or to be located at an anatomical site as to be invisible. As a consequence, diagnosis and treatment are often delayed, enabling the transmission and progression of the disease to continue.

The most serious consequences of STDs relate to their progression to chronic infections. These include:

- **Pelvic inflammatory disease (PID)**, an ascending infection of the uterus and fallopian tubes caused by gonococci and chlamydia
- **Anogenital cancer,** including **cervical cancer,** caused by some human papillomavirus types
- Secondary and tertiary **syphilis**
- **Recurrent herpes** infection

Many of these chronic infections cause additional adverse sequelae, including:

- **Fallopian tube scarring and adhesions** of surrounding tissues, resulting in **ectopic pregnancy, infertility,** and **chronic pelvic pain.**
- **Congenital diseases** such as in syphilis, herpes, papillomatosis, and chlamydial infection.
- **Increased risk of acquiring HIV,** due to genital ulcers (found in syphilis, chancroid, and herpes) or altered genital mucosa (found in gonorrhea and chlamydial infection).
- **Adverse outcomes of pregnancy** including premature termination, fetal wastage, low birth weight, and premature rupture of membranes.

SELECTED SEXUALLY TRANSMITTED DISEASES

Pelvic Inflammatory Disease

Pelvic inflammatory disease (**PID**), or **female upper reproductive tract infection,** is an ascending infection of the uterus, fallopian tubes, ovaries, and adjacent peritoneal linings. PID frequently results in severe, irreversible sequelae such as infertility, ectopic pregnancy, and chronic pelvic pain. A case of post-chlamydial PID is described in Chapter 14 ("*Neisseria*").

PID is the most serious and most costly common consequence of STD affecting women. It is estimated that in the United States, 10 to 15% of women of reproductive age have had at least one episode of PID, and that annually between 750,000 and 1,000,000 new cases are added to this figure. The highest annual incidence occurs in sexually active females who have approximately a 1 in 8 chance of developing PID.

Pathobiology

The events that lead to PID are not well understood. It is likely that almost all cases involve the ascending spread of infection from the lower to the upper genital tract. A proportion of cases progresses to develop chronic sequelae.

Most cases of PID are caused by the sexually transmitted organisms *Neisseria gonorrhoeae* or *Chlamydia trachomatis,* and follow cervicitis and urethritis. Other organisms implicated in the etiology of PID include *Mycoplasma hominis, Mycoplasma genitalium, Ureaplasma urealyticum,* and numerous aerobic and anaerobic bacteria. These bacteria are referred to as **endogenous** because they are often isolated from the lower tract in the absence of any disease. Little is known about the pathogenesis of these infections. Usually, a primary episode of gonococcal and chlamydial PID is followed by subsequent episodes of PID caused by the endogenous organisms. The pathogenesis of gonococcal and chlamydial PID, as well as their clinical manifestations, probably represent nonspecific inflammatory responses to bacterial invasion that result in tissue damage, as well as the specific immune responses to gonococci or chlamydiae.

Several anatomical factors appear to be important in the pathogenesis of gonococcal or chlamydial PID:

- Gonococcal or chlamydial cervical infection may damage the endocervical canal, break down the mucus plug in the endocervix, and allow these pathogens, as well as endogenous vaginal organisms to ascend into the upper genital tract.
- Increase in the size of the **zone of ectopy** (extension of the columnar epithelium onto the ectocervix) may result in increased susceptibility to infection by these organisms because these cells are preferential sites of microbial attachment and invasion. Age-related changes in the zone of ectopy, cervical mucus, or host defense mechanisms may play a role in determining whether lower genital tract infections linger, spread to the endometrium and fallopian tubes, or are resolved.

Other host defenses are probably useful in preventing centripetal spread of organisms. These include: tubal ciliary movement (unidirectional towards the uterus); flow of mucus in the tubal lumen (towards the uterus); and myometrial contractions during menses (resulting in sloughing of the endometrium).

Several hormonal factors appear to be important in the pathogenesis of PID. **Oral contraceptives** may increase risk of cervical chlamydial infection. Experimentally, both estrogen and progesterone are reported to facilitate the growth and survival of chlamydial infection; however, oral contraceptives decrease the penetrability of the cervical mucus, thus interfering with ascent of infection. Oral contraceptives also increase the size of the zone of cervical ectopy where chlamydiae and gonococci attach. Most cases of gonococcal PID occur within 7 days of the onset of menses; hormonal changes during the menstrual cycle may lead to changes in the cervical mucus plug, permitting passage of organisms, particularly when estrogen levels are high and progesterone levels are relatively low. The reflux of infected blood during menstrual uterine contractions may also provide a route of entry into the fallopian tubes.

Types of PID

Gonococcal PID. The ability to cause PID is not equally distributed among all strains of gonococci. Strains with a major outer membrane protein called IB are much more likely to cause PID. The pathophysiological changes that occur have been studied in fallopian tube explants exposed to gonococci (Chapter 14, "*Neisseria*"). In the presence of these organisms, motility of ciliated epithelial cells slows and ultimately ceases. Ciliated cells are selectively sloughed from the epithelial surface, apparently due to the toxic action of lipopolysaccharide (LPS) or murein fragments. Gonococci attach to nonciliated epithelial cells via pili and outer membrane protein II and induce phagocytosis. The organisms replicate within phagosomal vesicles and move to the basal portion of the cells and exit into the subepithelium to cause inflammation.

The inflammatory response to gonococcal infection is mediated by a number of soluble factors. Damage to ciliated cells may be caused in part by **tumor necrosis factor (TNF)**, which is released from fallopian tube explants after incubation with viable gonococci or purified LPS. PID causing strains of gonococci elicit the formation of **complement component C5a**, a chemoattractant for neutrophils. Experimental evidence suggests gonococci in the upper tract may be protected by a coating of antibodies and complement.

Chlamydial PID

The steps in infection of chlamydial PID include attachment of the organisms to cells, probably via specific receptor–ligand interactions, but these steps have not been confirmed. The chlamydial major outer membrane protein appears to be involved in these interactions. The organisms actively induce uptake by stimulating endocytosis. Phagolysosomal fusion does not occur probably owing to the function of ill-defined surface components of the **elementary bodies** (the infectious form of the organism). The chlamydia-containing phagosomes, referred to as **inclusions**, are visible in histologic preparations. Within the phagosomes, elementary bodies differentiate into **reticulate bodies** (the metabolic form of the organism). The life cycle of these organisms is described in detail in Chapter 27 ("Chlamydiae").

Not all elementary bodies within an inclusion differentiate, a point of possible clinical significance for the following reason. It is not known if the remaining elementary bodies are infective, but it is likely that they are resistant to bacteriostatic antibiotics such as tetracycline; thus, they may represent a dormant form that could be responsible for treatment failure and recurrence. Ultimately, the reticulate bodies reorganize into new elementary bodies and, in time, are released from the host cell to infect adjacent cells.

Chlamydial infections incite a greater mononuclear immune response that those caused by gonococci, but neutrophils are also seen, mainly in the early phases of the inflammatory response. The chronic sequelae of chlamydial disease may be due to cell-mediated immunity. A surface protein of the organisms, known as the 57 kDal heat shock protein, may be the target antigen of a delayed hypersensitivity reaction. In epidemiological studies, high titers of antibodies against this protein have been shown to be prognosticators of tubal scarring, a long-term sequelae of PID.

Coinfections by gonococci and chlamydiae

The high prevalence of gonococcal and chlamydial coinfection has prompted recommendations that patients with either infection be treated for both (see "Treatment"). Experimentally, simultaneous gonococcal infection facilitates chlamydial replication in cervical epithelia by about 100-fold. It has been proposed that stimulation of endocytosis in nonciliated epithelial cells by the first parasite leads to alterations in the surface structure of these cells which allow ready uptake of the second parasite. Thus, one pathogen may facilitate the engulfment of the second one.

Bacterial vaginosis and PID

Bacterial vaginosis (BV) is an asymptomatic or mildly symptomatic disruption of the normal vaginal flora. Lactobacilli (especially species that produce hydrogen peroxide) are suppressed, while a variety of species including *Gardnerella vaginalis*, anaerobic streptococci, *Bacteroides* species, and genital mycoplasmas increase in numbers. Whether BV predisposes women to polymicrobial PID remains speculative. To date, no host factor has been identified that increases susceptibility to PID, with the possible exception of the use of intrauterine devices (IUDS). IUDs may increase the risk of BV by hindering the mechanisms that eliminate bacteria from the upper female genital tract. Recently, BV has been shown to increase the risk for premature rupture of membranes and premature delivery in pregnant women.

Risk Factors for PID

The role of sexual behavior in the development of PID and its sequelae is not well understood. However, multiple sexual partners, young age at first sexual intercourse, high frequency of sexual intercourse, douching, and high rate of acquiring new sexual partners within the 30 days prior to developing PID appear to be risk factors. Both high-risk sexual behaviors and prevalence of STDs are more frequent in adolescents and young adults, thus, these groups have a higher incidence of PID. Several biological risk factors also change with age, namely lower titers of protective antibody, larger zones of cervical ectopy that may facilitate attachment of pathogens, and easier penetrability of the cervical mucus plug, which facilitates pathogen ascent. The difference in the incidence of PID among ethnic groups is smaller than that of lower genital tract infections. This observation contradicts the assumption that race is a marker for poor health-care behaviors. Low socioeconomic status is probably a better marker for high-risk sexual and poor health behaviors that result in the greater prevalence of STDs and PID in the population.

Contraceptive practices also influence the occurrence of PID. The use of an IUD increases the risk of this complication, primarily in the first several months after insertion. In contrast to IUDs, combined estrogen/progesterone oral contraceptive pills and barrier methods are slightly protective against PID. Barrier contraceptive methods should, therefore, be recommended over IUDs, particularly to young, nulliparous women who are sexually active with more than one partner. It has been repeatedly shown that vaginal douching is also associated with PID.

PID results in infertility and ectopic pregnancy, but its exact frequency is unknown. Estimates have ranged from 15 to 30% of all active PID cases. In addition, an estimated 50% of ectopic pregnancies are caused by previous PID. Ectopic pregnancy is the principal cause of pregnancy-related mortality among African-American women in the U.S.

HIV and STDs

The AIDS pandemic has focused attention on STDs for several reasons (Table 66.5). The relationships between HIV infection and other STDs are unique, complex, and intriguing. They explain, in part, the global spread of the HIV epidemic and may provide insights into the pathogenesis of all sexually transmitted infections. Furthermore, these relationships have compelling implications in efforts to control HIV.

Aside from sexual behavior, the two obvious relationships between HIV infection and other STDs are: (1) increased transmission of HIV due to other STDs; (2) alteration in the history, diagnosis, or response to therapy of other STDs due to HIV infection.

The Bidirectional Interplay Between HIV and STDs

The risk of HIV transmission is increased 3- to 5-fold in the presence of both the genital ulcer diseases (e.g., syphilis) and nonulcerative STDs (e.g., gonorrhea and chlamydial infection). Human papillomavirus infection and anogenital warts do not appear to facilitate HIV transmission, perhaps because they do not usually cause breaks in the skin or mucous membranes.

As with other infections, the compromised immune system of AIDS patients results in particularly serious manifestations of other STDs. The available information is not conclusive, but data suggest that HIV prolongs the duration of genital ulcer disease, resulting in more persistent lesions, more frequent recurrences, and more common treatment failures. In addition, these patients often have atypical presentations that result in misdiagnosis. Although not definitive, the infectiousness and prevalence of genital ulcer disease may be increased by HIV infection.

Table 66.5. Interrelationship Between STDs and AIDS

Most STDs increase the risk of HIV transmission at least 3–5 fold

HIV infection makes it more difficult to treat several other STDs (e.g., syphilis and chancroid)

STDs and HIV infection can greatly amplify each other, so STD control is critical to HIV prevention

HIV infection probably potentiates the progression of HPV infection to anogenital (primarily cervical) cancer

---

HIV infection also appears to affect systemic manifestations of STDs. Systemic complications, such as PID or disseminated gonococcal infection, seem to be accelerated in AIDS patients. HIV infection possibly increases progression of human papillomavirus-associated neoplasia. The diagnosis, treatment, and progression of syphilis are altered in AIDS patients.

In the past, the potential significance of the bidirectional interplay between HIV infection and other STDs has not been fully appreciated. If HIV coinfection prolongs infectivity of certain STDs, and if the same STDs facilitate transmission of HIV, the two infections should greatly amplify one another. The increases in HIV and STD incidence may well contribute to the rapid spread of HIV in some heterosexual populations and may represent "epidemiological synergy" between diseases that are linked by a common mode of transmission.

A 1955 study conducted in Tanzania showed that increased treatment of symptomatic STDs correlated with a 42% reduction in HIV seroconversion. To determine a causal relationship between STD treatment and the spread of HIV, the National Institutes of Allergy and Infectious Diseases is sponsoring a detailed, large-scale study in Uganda. When such data become available, it will be possible to recommend and implement comprehensive STD prevention and control treatments.

How is the Transmission of HIV Enhanced by Other STDs?

It is likely that the inflammatory changes that accompany STDs facilitate HIV entry by altering the barrier function of the genital mucosal epithelium. In fact, HIV has been isolated directly from genital ulcers in both men and women. It is recognized that intercourse during menses increases risk of HIV transmission, therefore it is likely that mucosal irritation, friability, and bleeding may shorten the route to target cells and impair the function of natural defenses. These defenses normally include an intact mucus layer and tight junctions between epithelial cells.

Other factors may play a role in facilitating the transmission of HIV (Table 66.5). It is well known that HIV enters lymphocytes and macrophages. STD-induced inflammation increases the number of these cells, thereby increasing the number of target cells for HIV invasion. The result may reduce the HIV infectious dose.

The interrelationship between AIDS and other STDs may also involve an interplay at the systemic level of the immune response. Several STD pathogens activate T lymphocytes, which may lead to increased susceptibility to HIV infection and possibly to HIV replication.

Molecular interactions may also contribute to the pathogenesis of HIV infection and other STDs. For example, herpes simplex virus may potentiate HIV infection by stimulating the expression of surface receptors needed for HIV attachment. Conversely, HIV gene products have been shown to be potent intracellular trans-activating factors. These factors may enhance the growth of herpesvirus and human papillomavirus.

PREVENTION AND CONTROL

Prevention and control of sexually transmitted diseases is a multifaceted problem. Depending upon the circumstances, the objective may be prevention of infection, transmission, disease, or disease progression. These objectives can be achieved through a number of approaches: effective vaccines, interruption of transmission and progression through behavioral interventions, and curative medical interventions. The tools necessary to achieve these objectives include information about the prevalence of known high-risk behaviors and corresponding effective behavioral interventions, safe, efficacious vaccines, diagnostic tests, effective therapeutics, an efficient network of health care facilities, and trained, effective health care professionals.

In an ideal world, we would have safe, efficacious **vaccines** that were universally implemented, and an acceptable, infallible **barrier method** for STD prophylaxis would be available. This method could be used without partner cooperation or knowledge, i.e., controlled by either a male or a female. Furthermore, we would have fail-safe diagnostic tests as well as screening tests that were given regularly to all sexually active people. STDs and sexual behavior would be completely de-stigmatized and dealt with in a value-neutral fashion. Partner notification would be conducted in this socially acceptable atmosphere and therefore would be more effective. In addition, we would have reliable prognostic indicators for disease resolution or progression, not to mention the availability of single-dose curative therapies effective in both acute and chronic stages for each bacterial, viral, and parasitic STD. The health care system would be efficient, adequately funded, oriented towards disease prevention, pleasant, and accessible. Health care providers would be expertly trained medically, psychologically and socially to prevent as well as to treat STDs. In addition, all of these tools would be inexpensive, i.e., less than $1 cost to patient.

In reality, almost all of these tools are still in the realm of fantasy. We have no vaccines for STDs except for hepatitis B, and that vaccine is underused. For some STDs, medical therapy is either unavailable (e.g., viral diseases) or problematic (e.g., antimicrobial resistance). Given that we are interested in preferentially facilitating practical goals, how would we order our priorities for technological advances?

Development and use of inexpensive, simple, rapid diagnostic tests that are appropriate for resource-limited settings, such as inner cities (where the majority of STDs occur), is a fundamental component of STD prevention and control. Such tests are particularly important for diagnosis of STDs in women. In resource-limited settings, clinical algorithms based on recognition of symptoms and signs of STDs have been useful for diagnosis and treatment of urethritis and genital ulcer disease in men, but are far less useful for diagnosis of STDs in women. The special requirements of resource-limited settings force us to conclude that useful diagnostics tests should be: (1) inexpensive: provider cost less than $1.00 (U.S.) per patient; (2) simple: no equipment and minimal training required; (3) rapid: results available before the patient leaves the clinic; (4) performed on convenient specimens: simple to collect, socioculturally acceptable, no separation or preparation needed; (5) able to utilize stable reagents: long shelf life, no refrigeration required; (6) packaged simply: functional, low cost; and (7) appropriately sensitive and specific: dependent, in part, on the potential morbidity and cost for undetected infection and the cost of the resulting treatment. Examples of diagnostic tests with the appropriate format are the occult fecal blood card and the urine glucose dipstick. No such STD test presently exists. In the future, public health conscious physicians will need to emphasize this medical need so that rapid, simple, inexpensive tests are preferentially developed over those that are fancier, but also prohibitively expensive for this population.

The second order on the wish list is for safe and effective, single-dose therapies. Noncompliance is a formidable problem when treatment regimens involve multiple-dose therapy for prolonged periods, especially when treatment exceeds the duration of symptoms. Again, therapies should be inexpensive, have a long shelf life, have minimal side effects and be safe for use during pregnancy. Theoretically, this approach should decrease the likelihood of antibiotic resistance. An example of such an advance is the recent development of azithromycin (an erythromycin-like macrolide antibiotic), a single-dose treatment for chlamydial infection.

There is general consensus that prevention of sexually transmitted STDs, including HIV infection, will be facilitated by the development of safe and effective female-controlled **chemical barriers** called topical **microbicides.** A microbicide effective not only against the most common agents of STDs but also those of genital ulcers would have a substantial impact on HIV transmission. The male condom, which is very effective if used consistently and correctly, requires male cooperation, which can run into personal, social, or cultural barriers. Specifically, the need for a method implemented by women is grounded on the high prevalence of consensual sex, sex without the use of condoms, and risky behaviors that occur without the partner's knowledge. Just as hormonal contraceptives and intrauterine devices have dramatically enhanced women's ability to avoid unwanted pregnancy, effective female-controlled microbicides are urgently needed to enhance a woman's ability to avoid STDs. In addition, effective chemical barriers may reduce female-to-male as well as male-to-female transmission.

The ideal microbicide should be colorless, odorless, tasteless, stable, easy to store, fast acting, effective pre- and postcoitus, inexpensive, available without prescription, and safe for repeated use. Such microbicides could ideally be formulated with or without spermicidal activity. Noncontraceptive microbicides would be very useful for women who wish to become pregnant. Indeed, a person's contraceptive choice may change over a lifetime, but, as long as they remain sexually active, individuals may either desire or require protection from STDs.

The role of the health care provider is an integral part of an STD prevention and control program. Currently many medical school curricula lack focused STD training. Ideally, an integrated approach, including basic biomedical, clinical, epidemiological, and behavioral training, would be most effective.

The good news is that although each STD presents unique diagnostic, therapeutic, and prevention challenges, all STDs (by definition) share a common mode of transmission. Interruption of transmission and progression may be accomplished most effectively through behavioral approaches. Important areas for intervention include sexual and contraceptive practices, patterns of partner selection and change, substance use, health care utilization, and health care provider attitudes.

Although much research is needed to identify both target behaviors and effective interventions for heterogeneous populations, our current understanding has allowed us to move forward while awaiting results from ongoing and future studies. Behavioral interventions based on decreasing partner numbers, use of barrier methods and, in some populations, delay of onset of sexual activity are being implemented. Interestingly, the role of the health care provider is critical, as in the case of vaccines where the single most important determinant of vaccine use is physician recommendation. Early studies indicate health care providers appear to be a critical component of an effective information delivery system, especially for adolescents.

As mentioned earlier, target populations include adolescents and all groups comprised of individuals who have multiple partners (i.e., greater than 10 per lifetime). Use of commercial television for social-marketing campaigns (e.g., condom advertisements) may be effective. However, given the limited impact of public service announcements, positive treatment of STD risk issues in sexually explicit television programs and movies may be the most effective and cost-effective way to influence and sustain behavior change, as evidenced somewhat by campaigns to increase seat belt usage and decrease cigarette smoking.

CONCLUSION

In summary, the STD epidemic is a complex, multifaceted problem that mandates multifaceted approaches for prevention and control. Vaccines, diagnostics, therapeutics, health care delivery systems, and behavioral interventions will each play an important part in achieving these interrelated goals.

SUGGESTED READINGS

Hitchcock PJ. Adolescents and sexually transmitted diseases. AIDS Patient Care STDs. 1966;10:79–85.

Hitchcock PJ. Screening and treatment of sexually transmitted diseases: an important strategy for reducing the risk of HIV transmission. AIDS Patient Care STDs. 1966;10:710–715.

Hitchcock PJ, Wasserheit JN, Harris JR, Holmes KK. Sexually transmitted diseases in the AIDS era: development of STD diagnostics for resource-limited settings in a global priority. Sex Transmit Dis 1991;18:133–135.

Holmes KK, Mardh P-A, Sparling PF, et al, eds. Sexually transmitted diseases. New York: McGraw-Hill, 1990.

NIAID Expert Committee on Pelvic Inflammatory Disease. Pelvic inflammatory disease: research directions in the 1990s. Sex Transmit Dis 1991;18:46–64.

Stone A, Hitchcock PJ. Vaginal manifestations. *AIDS* 1994; 8(Suppl 1):S285–S293.

Wasserheit JN. Epidemiological synergy: inter-relationships between HIV infection and other STDs. In: Chen L, Segal S, Sepulveda J, eds. AIDS and reproductive health. New York: Plenum, 1992.

Infections of the Compromised Patient

WILLIAM G. POWDERLY

A person is considered to be compromised when suffering either from the disruption of specific defenses of a particular organ or system, or from systemic abnormalities of humoral or cellular immunity. Usually, it is possible to predict the general type of infection such a patient is likely to acquire, depending on the component of the defense mechanisms that is disturbed. However, when the immune deficiency is general and profound, the patient may acquire any of a number of different infections, several of which may even occur at the same time.

Researchers have learned a great deal about the body's normal defense mechanisms by studying what happens when they become impaired. In fact, our knowledge of the relative importance of humoral and cellular immunity is derived from observing patients with immunodeficiencies. Thus, we note that persons with agammaglobulinemia are especially susceptible to extracellular bacteria that cause acute inflammation, whereas those with defects in cell-mediated immunity fall prey more readily to viruses, fungi, mycobacteria, and other intracellular agents of chronic diseases. Opportunistic infections have assumed immense importance in modern medicine, primarily because many of the major technological advances in therapeutics have been accompanied by iatrogenic disruption of body defense mechanisms. The practical need to understand the risk factors associated with defects in defenses against invading microorganisms cannot be overestimated.

In most cases, infections of immunocompromised patients are caused by commonly known pathogens. However, severe forms of immunocompromise open the door to infections by organisms not typically considered to be virulent, including many that are common in the normal flora and the environment. Unexpected extremes have been reached in scattered cases of infections of heart valves and other vital tissues by mushrooms (in their mycelial form) and colorless algae! This underscores how the definition of virulence must include not only the obvious pathogenic properties of microorganisms, but also the range of susceptibility of the patient.

This chapter recapitulates the consequences of risk factors mentioned throughout this book, presenting them according to the type of abnormality or defect in specific defense mechanisms.

CASE

A 17-year-old female, who came to the hospital with fever and bruising, was diagnosed with acute myelogenous leukemia. Remission of the leukemia was achieved with chemotherapy, and allogeneic (nontwin) bone marrow transplantation was attempted in the hope of curing her leukemia. Five days after transplantation, she had no detectable circulating white blood cells and 2 days thereafter she became febrile. Blood cultures taken at this time were positive for *Escherichia coli*. She responded well to antibiotics, and defervesced rapidly.

Eight days later, the patient again became febrile, and blood cultures were positive for *Candida albicans*. Although she was placed on antifungals, she remained febrile for 4 days but her temperature rapidly dropped to normal after removal of a venous catheter that had been implanted in her subclavian vein for intravenous drug administration. At this time (19 days post-transplantation), white blood cells started to appear in her circulation, indicating that the transplanted marrow had successfully engrafted and was beginning to function.

Thirty-one days after transplantation, the patient became short of breath, and chest x-ray showed a diffuse pneumonia. A lung biopsy revealed the presence of *Pneumocystis carinii*. Treatment with trimethoprim/sulfamethoxazole was started and she slowly responded to therapy. She was discharged from the hospital 2 months after her transplantation, but 10 days later, the patient developed a painful cutaneous herpes zoster infection. She remained well for the next 3 months, although she had developed mild chronic graft-versus-host disease. She returned again to the hospital 5 months after her transplantation, complaining of fever and shortness of breath. Physical examination and chest x-ray revealed a lobar pneumonia, and both blood and sputum cultures grew *Streptococcus pneumoniae*. She responded well to penicillin therapy and remained healthy thereafter.

Patients who have undergone bone marrow transplantation provide an extreme example of the profound disturbances of normal body defenses that can predispose to infection. For example, disruption of anatomic barriers by radiation and chemotherapy, which cause skin and mucosal ulcerations, provides entry sites for invasive organisms. Severe neutropenia is characteristic of the immediate post-transplant period, and although granulocyte recovery begins in the third week after transplantation, qualitative defects remain for some time. Cellular immune function, which now depends on donor macrophages and T cells, remains abnormal for several months. It is also compromised by the use of immunosuppressive therapy to treat graft-versus-host disease. Although IgG and IgM levels may return to normal after 45 months, B-cell function remains disturbed and antibody levels to specific organisms, such as pneumococci, may remain depressed for years.

In the following sections, we review the disturbances in various body defense mechanisms and their consequences in affected individuals.

ABNORMALITIES OF LOCAL HOST DEFENSE

The body is protected from microbial invasion by the mechanical and biochemical barrier provided by skin and mucous membranes and by the presence of a normal commensal flora. Disruption of these local mechanical barriers may occur as a result of instrumentation (e.g., intravenous or urinary catheterization), surgery, drugs, or burns. Under these circumstances, the infecting organisms are usually members of the commensal flora resident at the site. For example, breaching the skin with intravenous catheters may introduce *Staphylococcus epidermidis* into the bloodstream, with subsequent septicemia (Chapter 63, "Sepsis").

The consequences of immunological or biochemical impairment at the level of the integuments are less well understood. For example, we do not know with certainty if secreted IgA immunoglobulins or lysozyme contributes to resistance to infection. We suspect, however, that people with IgA deficiency are more prone to sinusitis, pneumonia, and gastrointestinal infections (e.g.,

giardiasis). Persons with genetic defects in lysozyme have not been found.

Burns are an extreme example of the critical role of the intact integument on resistance to infection. Necrotic skin tissue is an excellent culture medium for bacteria, thus increasing the size of the inoculum. In addition, the thermal injury itself leads to a poorly understood suppression of white blood cell function. It is not surprising that skin and subcutaneous tissue infections and septicemias with *Staphylococcus aureus* or *Pseudomonas aeruginosa* are major challenges in the management of patients with severe burns.

The normal bacterial flora may be disrupted as the result of antibiotic treatment, which may in turn lead to superinfection by organisms resistant to the drug. This happens particularly often in the intestine, sometimes as the result of antibiotic "prepping" of patients for abdominal surgery. Pseudomembranous colitis due to *Clostridium difficile* is a complication of such therapy (Chapter 20, "Clostridia").

Some tissues possess additional local defense mechanisms. In the lungs, for example, the combination of mucous production by goblet cells and ciliary activity of the respiratory epithelial cells serves to trap microbes and carry them out of the lungs. Disruption of this disposal system predisposes to pneumonia (Chapter 59, "Respiratory System"). An extreme example of this occurs in cystic fibrosis, a chronic hereditary condition characterized by the production of abnormally thick mucus. These patients experience recurrent pneumonia, and their lungs are often colonized by the opportunistic bacterium *P. aeruginosa*. Most patients are unable to clear this organism from the respiratory tract and may die from respiratory failure after repeated episodes of pneumonia.

DISTURBANCE IN PHAGOCYTIC NUMBERS AND FUNCTION

Once the first line of defense is breached, **neutrophils** assume a critical role in checking the spread of invasive disease. Defects in neutrophil activity, either qualitative or quantitative, predispose patients to infection with certain bacteria and fungi (Table 67.1). Examples of such defects include: (1) a decreased number of phagocytic cells; (2) impairment of their chemotactic response; and (3) lowering of their ability to kill microorganisms.

Granulocytopenia, which is a decrease in the number of circulating neutrophils, clearly predisposes to infection. Myelosuppressive cancer chemotherapy is the most common cause of granulocytopenia in hospitals. Neutropenia also occurs in bone marrow failure due to aplasia, autoimmune disease, hematological malignancy, or invasion of the bone marrow by a tumor. Serious infections, usually accompanied by bacteremia, are a frequent and often life-threatening problem in these hosts.

Table 67.1. Common Causes of Compromise and Their Consequences

Impaired function	Common infecting organisms	Sites commonly affected
Barrier		
Integument	Pyogenic cocci, enteric bacteria	Skin, subcutaneous connective tissue
Normal microbial flora	Pyogenic cocci, enteric bacteria, *Clostridium difficile*, *Candida albicans*	Skin, intestine
Phagocyte functions		
Chemotaxis	*Staphylococcus aureus*, enteric bacteria	Skin, respiratory tract
Neutropenia	*S. aureus*, enteric bacteria	Skin, respiratory tract
Microbial killing	*S. aureus, Aspergillus*	Skin, visceral abscesses
Humoral functions		
Hypogammaglobulinemia	Pyogenic bacteria	Any site
IgA deficiency	Pyogenic bacteria	Respiratory tract
Lack of spleen	Pneumococcus, *H. influenzae*	Septicemia
Complement deficiency		
C1q, C2, or C3	Pyogenic bacteria	Bacteremia, meningitis
C5, C6, C7, C8, or C9	*Neisseria*	Meningitis, arthritis
Cell-mediated immunity	Viruses, fungi, protozoa, intracellular bacteria	Any site

The most important correlation is between the number of circulating neutrophils and the risk of infection. The rate of infection clearly increases as the number of neutrophils decreases (Fig. 67.1). Disruptions in the integrity of the skin and gastrointestinal tract, which are often the result of chemotherapy or radiation therapy, are also important in the pathogenesis of these infections. The organisms responsible are usually derived from the patient's own flora, particularly that of the bowel. Gram-negative enteric bacilli and staphylococci are the most common bacterial pathogens. Prolonged antibacterial therapy also predisposes to colonization by fungi. *Candida* and *Aspergillus* are the most important causes of fungal sepsis and mortality in this population.

Chemotactic dysfunction of phagocytes is uncommon and usually congenital in origin. Defective neutrophil chemotaxis may result from inadequate signaling of the neutrophil, abnormalities of neutrophil receptors for chemoattractants, or disorders in cell locomotion. *S. aureus* is the most important pathogen in these patients, who are usually seen with recurrent cutaneous or deep abscesses.

Abnormalities in microbial killing power are usually inherited. Of the many disorders that have been described, the most common is chronic **granulomatous disease,** a condition in which neutrophils fail to mount a respiratory burst during phagocytosis. The cause of this deficiency is a defect in the enzyme NADPH oxidase, and hydrogen peroxide is not formed. Patients with this disorder are at risk of infection with catalase-positive organisms, especially *S. aureus*. A Gram-negative rod, *Serratia marcescens*, also causes infections in these patients, as do fungi (especially *Aspergillus*). These organisms are relatively resistant to the nonoxidative killing mechanisms of neutrophils. On the other hand, bacteria such as pneumococci and other streptococci that make their own hydrogen peroxide but have no catalase, are likely to be killed by the defective neutrophils. These defective neutrophils are still effective against these bacteria because they still contain the enzyme myeloperoxidase. This enzyme uses the hydrogen peroxide made by bacterial metabolism to produce lethal radicals (Chapter 6,

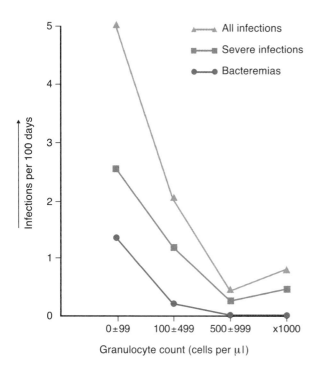

Figure 67.1. Relationship between the incidence of infection and the absolute neutrophil count in patients with acute nonlymphocyte leukemia. The incidence of infection rises as the neutrophil count decreases.

"Constitutive Defenses"). In effect, these bacteria commit suicide.

ABNORMALITIES IN HUMORAL IMMUNITY

Immunoglobulin deficiency may be congenital (e.g., Bruton's X-linked agammaglobulinemia) or acquired (e.g., common variable immunodeficiency). Acquired hypogammaglobulinemia may also arise as a result of conditions that lead to protein loss (nephrotic syndrome, intestinal lymphangiectasia), cancers of cells that make immunoglobulins (multiple myeloma, chronic lymphocytic leukemia), or burns. Defective B-lymphocyte function also occurs following bone marrow transplantation, as noted in the case above. The predominant infectious disease problem in these patients is recurrent upper and lower respiratory tract infection due to encapsulated bacteria, reflecting the important role of antibodies in opsonization of encapsulated bacteria.

Complement deficiencies are rare and are also characterized by predisposition to infection with encapsulated bacteria (see Table 6.4). *Neisseria* are a special problem for patients with deficiencies of any of the late complement components (C6, C7, C8, or C9), because complement-mediated lysis is required to kill these organisms. Many bacteria infect patients with defects earlier in the complement cascade. Most clinically significant complement deficiencies are congenitally acquired.

The **spleen** plays an important role in humoral immunity, both as a source of complement- and antibody-producing B cells, and as the organ primarily responsible for the removal of opsonized microbes from the bloodstream. Defects in spleen function may result from splenectomy or diseases such as sickle cell anemia. In these situations, patients are at risk of infection with encapsulated bacteria, e.g., pneumococci and *Haemophilus*. These bacterial infections may be fulminant in patients with splenic deficiency. Bacteremia and septic shock often result, and mortality is high unless appropriate therapy is given rapidly.

DISORDERS OF CELL-MEDIATED IMMUNITY

Defects in the function or number of macrophages and T lymphocytes lead to an increased risk of infection with bacteria that survive intracellularly, as well as with viruses, fungi, and protozoa (Table 67.1).

Patients with defective cell-mediated immunity are divided into two groups, depending on whether their defect is congenital or acquired. Primary disorders of cell-mediated immunity are usually diagnosed in childhood and are lethal. These patients usually die from opportunistic infections before adulthood.

Acquired defects in cell-mediated immunity are seen in an increasingly large population of patients treated in

hospitals. The enormous success of transplant surgery is a consequence of the development of drugs (such as cyclosporin) that suppress the graft-versus-host response and prevent rejection of the transplant. However, these **immunosuppressive drugs** also interfere with normal cell-mediated immunity, and all of these patients are at increased risk of opportunistic infection. Some immunosuppressive drugs, especially corticosteroids, are also used to treat a variety of inflammatory diseases. Cell-mediated immunity is also disturbed in patients with lymphoma.

The most profound example of defective cell-mediated immunity occurs in acquired immunodeficiency syndrome (Chapter 67, "AIDS"). Here, depletion of CD4$^+$-helper T cells due to HIV infection leads almost inevitably to death from uncontrolled opportunistic infection or malignancy. Patients have profound disturbances of cell-mediated immunity, especially that mediated by cytotoxic lymphocytes and macrophages, and develop infections with eukaryotic agents (e.g., *Pneumocystis carinii)*, viruses (e.g., cytomegalovirus), and intracellular bacteria (e.g., mycobacteria).

MANAGEMENT OF INFECTION IN COMPROMISED HOSTS: GENERAL CONSIDERATIONS

As with all infections, treatment in the immunocompromised host should be directed against the specific infecting organism. However, defective host response heightens the risk of severe infection, and there may be an urgent need to begin treatment presumptively, based on the most likely etiological possibilities. Knowing the type of immune defect, the likely resident microbial flora, the site and clinical features of the infection, and some epidemiological features often makes it possible to predict the likely infecting organism. For example, in granulocytopenic patients, broad-spectrum antibiotics with activity against both Gram-positive bacteria and Enterobacteriaceae and other Gram-negative bacteria should be given at the first sign of infection, such as fever. Patients with decreased spleen function should be treated with drugs active against pneumococci and *H. influenzae*. A diffuse pneumonia involving most of the lung in a patient with AIDS is most likely due to *P. carinii*. However, this is not always the case, and it is often necessary to specifically identify the causative organism so that appropriate treatment may be started or toxic therapy avoided. Therefore, whenever possible, specimens should be obtained before starting therapy. The clinician and the microbiology laboratory should coordinate to assure the recovery and identification of opportunistic pathogens. Unless warned, the microbiological laboratory may consider *S. epidermidis* a contaminant from the skin and not report it.

It is particularly important to attempt to reverse the

immune defect; whenever practical, iatrogenic causes should be eliminated. Catheters should be removed, or at least changed; immunosuppressive drugs should be discontinued whenever possible. In some transplant recipients, it may even be necessary to allow the transplant to be rejected by suspending immunosuppressive therapy in order to permit an adequate host response to infection. In other cases, replacement therapy is beneficial. Passive administration of immunoglobulins decreases the incidence of infection in patients with hypogammaglobulinemia. Granulocyte transfusions may benefit some granulocytopenic patients with refractory Gram-negative bacterial infections.

Preventive measure are also important in the care of these patients. Simple procedures such as care with use and insertion of catheters, careful hand washing, and appropriate isolation techniques may reduce the incidence of opportunistic infection acquired in hospitals. Some vaccines (e.g., against influenza virus or pneumococci) may be beneficial. It is essential to remember that live vaccines should be given with caution to immunocompromised hosts because even attenuated viruses may cause severe disease in these patients. Prophylactic antibiotics are rarely beneficial; major exceptions are the use of penicillin to prevent pneumococcal infections in children with sickle cell disease, and the use of trimethoprim/sulfamethoxazole or pentamidine to prevent *Pneumocystis* pneumonia in patients with severe defects in cell-mediated immunity (see Chapter 68, "AIDS").

SUGGESTED READINGS

Holland SM, Gallin JI. Evaluation of the patient with suspected immunodeficiency. In: Mandell GL, Bennett JE, Dolin R, eds. Principles and practice of infectious diseases. 4th ed. New York: Churchill Livingstone; 1995:149–157.

Mazur H. Management of opportunistic infections associated with HIV infection. In: Mandell GL, Bennett JE, Dolin R, eds. Principles and practice of infectious diseases. 4th ed. New York: Churchill Livingstone, 1995:1280–1293.

Piot P, Merson M. Global perspectives on HIV infection and AIDS. In: Mandell GL, Bennett JE, Dolin R, eds. Principles and practice of infectious diseases. 4th ed. New York: Churchill Livingstone, 1995;1164–1173.

Rubin RH, Young LS. Clinical approach to infection in the compromised host. 2nd ed. New York: Plenum Publishing, 1988.

Acquired Immunodeficiency Syndrome

WILLIAM G. POWDERLY

As of 1995, it is estimated that between 1.5 and 2.5 million persons in the U.S. have been infected with human immunodeficiency virus (HIV), the causative agent of acquired immunodeficiency syndrome (AIDS). The World Health Organization estimates that approximately 25 million persons are infected worldwide. By 1995, over 250,000 people have died of AIDS in the U.S. alone. Unless curative therapy is developed, most infected individuals will develop AIDS and eventually die from its consequences. In the interim, infected individuals may infect others.

The impact of this disease cannot be overemphasized. In 1995, AIDS was the leading cause of death in the U.S. among men 20–45 years of age, and was rapidly rising among women. In some parts of Africa, AIDS is the leading cause of death among young adults.

AIDS is a constellation of clinical illnesses, primarily opportunistic infections and malignancies (Table 68.1), that are the consequence of the destruction of the immune system by HIV. AIDS is the final manifestation of HIV infection that occurred many years previously (on average 10 years). HIV infection is continuous and relentless in its progression. The progressive nature of the infection has been well characterized, and several methods are used to classify its stages (see tables 38.3 and 38.4). This chapter describes the course of a typical HIV infection in terms of these progressive stages. The virology of HIV is discussed in detail in Chapter 38, "Retroviruses."

■ CASE

Early Acute HIV Infection

J.P., a 26-year-old married bisexual man who worked as a hospital phlebotomist, was seen in his physician's office complaining of a 1-week history of fever, swollen lymph nodes, and headache. He stated that he had unprotected sexual contact with a new male partner 3 weeks previously. On examination, he had a red, inflamed pharynx; enlarged cervical lymph nodes; and a red splotchy rash all over his body.

J.'s complaints and manifestations are nonspecific and common. His presentation is typical of many viral infections, including those caused by HIV and the Epstein-Barr virus (see Chapter 40, "Warts"). The clinician should consider the possibility of HIV infection, if the patient has risk factors for HIV, homosexual or bisexual men, intravenous drug users, or their sexual partners. J. has a number of risk factors for HIV infection; he is bisexual, has had multiple sex partners who could have been infected, and he is a hospital phlebotomist.

Could J. have been infected with HIV? Acute illness occurs in 50–90% of persons 24 weeks after infection by HIV. In the majority of such cases, the only symptoms are mild fever and sore throat. A small subgroup may have fever, myalgias, lethargy, pharyngitis, arthralgias, lymphadenopathy, and a maculopapular rash of the trunk. Some patients have aseptic meningitis, and the headache that J. complains of may have been caused by mild meningeal irritation. The illness typically lasts 3–14 days and complete recovery is the rule, even in patients with neurological complications.

Can HIV be diagnosed at this stage? Antibodies against HIV are usually not detectable initially. However, various methods of detecting viral RNA in the blood have been developed. Although patients with acute HIV infection usually have high levels of viral RNA, follow-up serological testing is needed to confirm a diagnosis. No specific therapy is available for acute HIV disease. Although HIV test results of patients at this stage will probably be negative, the result can be used to establish a baseline for future testing.

Table 68.1. AIDS-Defining Illnesses[a]

1. Multiple or recurrent bacterial infections (two in a 2-year period), affecting a child less than 13 years of age; these include septicemia, pneumonia, meningitis, bone or joint infection, or internal abscess caused by *Haemophilus influenzae*, streptococci, or other pyogenic bacteria

2. Candidiasis of the esophagus, trachea, bronchi, or lungs

3. Disseminated coccidioidomycosis

4. Extrapulmonary cryptococcosis

5. Chronic cryptosporidiosis, with diarrhea for more than 1 month

6. Cytomegalovirus infection

7. Mucocutaneous herpes simplex virus infection persisting for more than 1 month

8. HIV encephalopathy

9. Disseminated histoplasmosis

10. Isosporiasis, with diarrhea for over 1 month

11. Kaposi's sarcoma

12. Primary lymphoma of the brain

13. Non-Hodgkin's lymphoma of B cell or unknown phenotype, including Burkitt's lymphoma

14. Lymphoid interstitial pneumonia affecting a child under 13 years

15. Disseminated mycobacterial infection (not *M. tuberculosis*)

16. Extrapulmonary tuberculosis

17. *Pneumocystis carinii* infection

18. Progressive multifocal leucoencephalopathy

19. Recurrent *Salmonella* infection

20. Toxoplasmosis of the brain

[a] Any of these diseases indicates a diagnosis of AIDS, in the presence of laboratory evidence of HIV infection.

Diagnostic Tests for HIV

After counseling about the implications and possible outcome of HIV testing, J. had an HIV test, which was negative. He returned for follow-up 6 weeks later. His symptoms had resolved completely and he felt well. Serological testing at this time revealed a positive enzyme-linked immunosorbent assay (ELISA for HIV) signifying antibodies specific to HIV. A Western blot confirmed this result.

How accurate are the tests for HIV? Can we be sure J. is infected? A definitive diagnosis of infection could be achieved by culturing the virus, but culturing HIV is difficult in early infection. As noted above, measurement of viral RNA by various polymerase chain reaction (PCR) methodologies can detect HIV early in infection, but these tests are rarely used as screening tests for infection because of their expense. HIV infection is generally diagnosed by detecting circulating antibodies to the virus. Unlike most antibody tests, in which the presence of specific antibodies signifies past infection with the agent in question, a positive HIV antibody test signifies current infection. Any individual who has HIV antibodies must be assumed to have active infection that can be transmitted to others. It is important, therefore, that such individuals receive counseling about the issues involved in transmission so that spread can be minimized.

Specific anti-HIV antibodies generally appear 6–12 weeks after infection. However, studies using PCR (Chapter 55, "Diagnostic Principles") to test for specific HIV RNA have shown that, rarely, some infected individuals do not develop antibodies for several months or years after exposure. These unusual individuals have a false-negative serological test for HIV. In addition, some patients in the terminal phases of AIDS have negative serological tests (presumably because of severe B-cell dysfunction). However, patients with advanced disease can usually be identified by other than serological means.

The most common method for testing for HIV antibodies is the ELISA. This test is performed by adding a sample of the patient's serum to small wells to which HIV antigens are bound. If antibodies are present, they will complex with the antigen. Anti-immunoglobulin antibody linked to an identifier enzyme is then added to bind to the complex. Although this test is highly sensitive (more than 99%), it is not completely specific, and false-positive results occur. When screening a large population (such as the adults in the U.S.), even a false-positive rate of less than 0.01% means that many individuals who are not infected will be misidentified. Such persons could face potential discrimination in insurance, employment, and housing. The incidence of false-positives, no matter how low, is a strong argument against indiscriminate testing without obtaining the permission of the patient.

For these reasons, ELISA-positive results should be verified with a more specific test. In most laboratories, this test is a Western blot (see Fig. 55.5). This test detects antibodies to specific viral polypeptides. The Western blot is a sensitive and specific way to test for HIV antibodies; however, it is too time-consuming and expensive to be used for primary screening purposes.

Rarely, some people exhibit nonspecific cross-reactivity in serological HIV tests and may be difficult to distinguish from patients with early HIV infection. The true pattern can usually be determined by repeating the Western blot after 34 months. By then, a person with true infection will usually have developed new antibodies to different epitopes (which show up in the Western blot), whereas those with nonspecific reactivity will have the same pattern as before. Waiting for repeat HIV tests can be a difficult time for patients, who will need counseling and support to help them understand the limitations of technology.

Other assays to determine the presence of HIV infection are available, but are not always useful. The p24 antigen is the viral core protein, produced by the *gag* gene, and its presence denotes active viral replication. However, this antigen is not detectable in the serum of all patients and thus not useful diagnostically. HIV can be cultured from lymphocytes of most infected individuals, but this test is technically difficult and is rarely used outside of research settings. Direct testing of viral load by PCR-based methods is also available, and is increasingly used to assess the need for and effectiveness of antiretroviral therapy.

ENCOUNTER AND ENTRY

J. has clearly seroconverted (from negative to positive) and is infected with HIV. How did he get his infection? HIV is transmitted primarily by direct inoculation of infected blood or body fluids into the host. Thus, the epidemiology of HIV mirrors that of viruses spread by such means, e.g., hepatitis B and C. Most cases of HIV infection are acquired sexually and sexual practices that are associated with trauma, such as receptive anal intercourse, facilitate the spread of the virus. Other sexually transmitted diseases, especially chancroid, are associated with an increased risk of HIV transmission, possibly because the epithelial barrier is breached by the genital ulcers. In the U.S. and other Western countries, HIV initially infected mainly homosexual men and was wrongly perceived as an exclusive disease of that community. However, in other parts of the world, sexual transmission of HIV is predominantly heterosexual. In the U.S., the number of cases of HIV infection acquired by heterosexual contact has risen steadily. Some evidence shows that women may be more easily infected than men, but transmission clearly occurs in both directions.

Contact with infected blood or blood products is another important form of transmission of HIV. Initially, this mode of transmission was recognized because of the occurrence of AIDS in people with hemophilia who had been given infected factor VIII and factor IX, or who had received HIV-infected blood transfusions. Transmission through infected blood and blood products has considerably diminished since blood donor testing and treatment of plasma to inactivate the virus was instituted. However, this mode of transmission has not been eliminated completely. Because of the "window period" in early infection, blood donors with early HIV infection may not have developed HIV antibodies.

Bloodborne spread of HIV remains a considerable problem among intravenous drug users who share needles and syringes. Individuals who exchange sex for drugs may then infect their sexual partners. Infected women may infect their children in utero (**vertical transmission**). Between 15% and 30% of these infants will be infected with the virus, although antiretroviral therapy of pregnant women substantially lowers the risk of transmission to their babies. The reason why all such children are not infected is unknown, although it may be related, in part, to maternal immune responses to HIV and to the level of HIV circulating in the mother's blood. Transmission may also occur during birth process and via breast milk.

HIV is also a worrisome occupational problem for health care workers. Exposure to HIV-infected blood, predominantly through needlestick injuries, is now a significant hazard for health care workers. The risk of infection after such exposure is low; it is estimated that 1 in 300 such exposures leads to infection. Very few cases of AIDS resulting from needlestick injuries have been documented. Transmission in the opposite direction (i.e., from infected health care worker to patient) has also been documented on at least one occasion, in the case of an infected dentist. Universal precautions (assuming all blood or other fluids are potentially infected) are important to prevent this kind of transmission.

We can see, therefore, that J. could have been infected in a number of ways. He is a bisexual man with a recent new sexual partner, and he is also a phlebotomist who may have had exposure to infected blood. Statistically, it is most likely that he acquired HIV from sexual contact.

When should people be tested for HIV infection? Persons with HIV disease seek medical attention at different stages of the disease. Many patients with early HIV infection do not seek medical attention and do not know they are infected until they develop AIDS. However, most patients are seen by a physician before they develop AIDS. Many seek to be tested for HIV, because they perceive that some aspect of their lifestyle may put them at risk. Others consult a physician with complaints that are not obviously due to HIV disease, and the diagnosis is made when their physician counsels them to be tested for HIV.

Consequences of Being HIV-Positive

J. returned to his physician's office 2 weeks later to get the results of his antibody tests. When told he is HIV-positive, he became anxious and asked, "Does this mean I have AIDS?"

The period following a definitive diagnosis of HIV infection is a difficult time for a patient. Patients are anxious about the possibility of AIDS and worried about transmission of the virus to close family members. Counseling patients is, therefore, important at this point. Patients should be taught how the virus is spread and educated fully of their duty to protect other people, especially their sexual contacts. Infected persons should be informed that abstinence from sexual intercourse is the only sure way of avoiding transmission. Sexual practices that do not involve contact with semen or vaginal secretions are considered safe. Condom use is essential if patients are going to continue to have sexual intercourse. Patients should be reassured that casual contact with others does not pose a risk of transmission.

In addition to informing his male and female sexual partners that he is HIV-positive and taking precautions not to infect them, J. needs to consider his occupation. If his hospital duties include the performance of invasive procedures, he should think about transferring to another position.

Will J. get AIDS? Probably yes. The probability of progression to AIDS can be estimated by determining the degree of immunodeficiency. The most helpful measurement is the level of **T-lymphocyte** subsets. Because the **CD4** (**T4** or **helper-inducer**) **T-lymphocytes** are a specific target of HIV, measurement of the number of these cells in the circulation indicates the degree of immune impairment and thus the risk of developing AIDS. The normal CD T-cell count in adults ranges from 800–2000 cells/mm^3. Progressive loss of these cells over time is the usual pattern of progressive HIV infection (Fig. 68.1). However, by itself, the CD T-cell count is not an absolute indicator of the probability of developing AIDS. Many asymptomatic HIV-infected persons have CD T-cell counts of less than 200 cells/mm^3; but in general, the lower the CD T-cell count, the greater the risk of impending AIDS. The rate of decline of CD T cells over time may also give important prognostic clues. In addition, the viral load, as reflected by measurements of the HIV plasma RNA, also provides important prognostic information—perhaps even more important than the CD4 T-cell count. The higher the viral load in the plasma, the more rapid the progression of a patient to clinical AIDS or death.

Once HIV enters the body, it rapidly disseminates to many organs, especially the lymphoreticular system and the brain. Initial infection may, in fact, be associated with a profound, albeit temporary, loss of CD4+ T cells (and even opportunistic infections in occasional patients). With the appearance of an immune response, the levels of viral RNA in the plasma decrease dramatically and the virus is sequestered within lymph nodes. Unlike other chronic virus infections (such as the herpesviruses), HIV is never truly latent and active viral replication occurs at a high rate within lymph nodes. Recent information suggests that a high turnover of virus and of CD4+ T cells occurs on a daily basis until the body's reserve of lymphocytes is depleted. Pathologically the lymph nodes are progressively destroyed at the same time, and ultimately the virus escapes this partial surveillance and high plasma levels of virus are seen again as the disease progresses.

Symptoms or clinical illnesses that suggest immunodeficiency also help identify patients who are likely to progress more rapidly to AIDS. Consequently, a careful history should be taken regarding fever, night sweats, unintentional weight loss, or unexplained diarrhea. The presence of *Candida* infection in the mouth (thrush) also indicates a poor prognosis. Despite these prognostic markers, we cannot tell precisely how quickly any particular patient will progress to AIDS. The mechanisms controlling the rate of progression are not well understood, and factors such as genetic variability (i.e., the

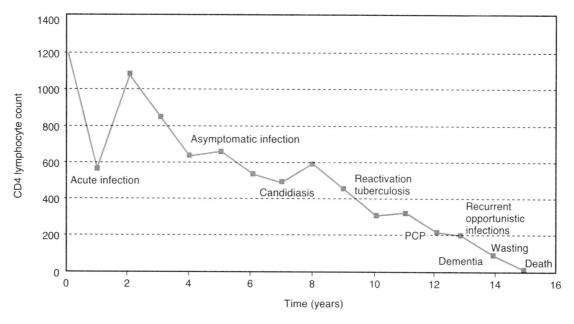

Figure 68.1. The natural history of HIV disease.

host), viral phenotype, and viral load are potentially important.

Because most HIV-infected individuals develop progressive immunodeficiency, they should be assessed for occult infections that may become problematic later. Tuberculin skin testing and chest x-ray should be performed, because reactivation tuberculosis is extremely common in HIV-infected persons. Patients who test positive should be treated prophylactically with isoniazid. Patients with positive serology for syphilis require intensive antitreponemal therapy, particularly if neurosyphilis is suspected. Baseline **cytomegalovirus (CMV)** and *Toxoplasma gondi* antibody testing identifies persons at risk for reactivation disease by these agents. HIV-positive individuals are also candidates for vaccination against pneumococcal disease and annual immunization against influenza. Because patients are also at risk for hepatitis B, they should be tested for antibodies against this virus, and those who are negative should be offered vaccination against it.

Progression to AIDS

J.'s CD4 T-cell count was measured and found to be 750 cells /mm³. He was otherwise completely well.

At this point, J. was advised that he had no evidence of significant immune impairment. He was told to return to his physician every 6 months, for CD4 T-count measurement evaluation.

Unfortunately, J. did not keep his scheduled appointments. Four years later, he returned to his physician's office complaining of a blistering rash on his left shoulder and upper torso. He also complained of sore throat and white spots in his mouth. Examination showed oral thrush; enlarged, nontender cervical, axillary, and inguinal lymph nodes; and a vesicular (blistering) rash in a dermatomal distribution consistent with shingles. At this time, his CD4 T-cell count was 280 cells/mm³.

Acute HIV infection is followed by a latent period during which infected individuals are asymptomatic and appear healthy. The duration of this period is variable and ranges from 18 months to over 15 years. The median time is approximately 10 years. Although we refer to this period as asymptomatic, many patients, in fact, have complaints that are not obviously linked to HIV infection or to the associated immunodeficiency. For example, HIV-infected persons are particularly prone to skin complaints. The reason is unknown, but infection of the epidermal Langerhans cells may be a contributory factor. Many patients complain of excessively dry skin and pruritus; seborrheic dermatitis with eczema; folliculitis; and psoriasis. Onset of severe psoriasis, eczema, or folliculitis in a previously healthy adult should raise the possibility of HIV infection. Furthermore, reactivation of **herpes zoster** (**shingles**), as occurred with J., may also be a sentinel of HIV infection. Patients are also prone to recurrent **herpes simplex** infection, **molluscum contagiosum**, and drug eruptions. In addition, a type of skin cancer, cutaneous **Kaposi's sarcoma**, may be the first manifestation of AIDS. It is characterized by blue–violet palpable, nonpruritic, painless lesions.

Patients in this stage may also present with localized or generalized lymphatic enlargement, as J. did. Painless generalized lymphadenopathy is a common manifestation of HIV disease, but has no prognostic significance. On the other hand, localized adenopathy or changes in already enlarged nodes may be early signs of infection or malignancy and should be investigated.

Recurrent mucocutaneous candidiasis (vaginal or oral in women, oral in men) and extensive oral aphthous ulcerations (canker sores) are common early manifestations of HIV infection and identify patients at greater risk of soon developing AIDS. **Hairy leukoplakia** (plaques of thickened mucosa on the tongue and elsewhere in the mouth) is caused by Epstein-Barr virus and also occurs early in HIV disease.

Abnormal laboratory findings may also be found early in HIV disease. Many infected individuals have isolated hematologic cytopenias, usually anemia, lymphopenia, or thrombocytopenia. Abnormalities in liver function tests, which are also common, are usually due to previous or concurrent viral hepatitis.

AIDS-Related Complex and Early AIDS

The progressive loss of CD4 T cells and the oral *Candida* infection suggest that J.'s cell-mediated immunity has significantly diminished since his physician last saw him. J. does not yet have AIDS. However, he can be classified as having AIDS-related complex (ARC). Although patients with ARC may not develop AIDS for several years, ARC is a poor prognostic sign and is an indication for starting specific antiretroviral treatment. J. should start prophylactic therapy to prevent *Pneumocystis carinii* infection.

Table 68.2. AIDS-Related Complex (ARC)

Unexplained weight loss (10% of body weight in 6 months)

Fevers +/− night sweats persisting for 1 month

Unexplained diarrhea persisting for 30 days

Recurrent oral candidiasis

Multidermatomal herpes zoster

Oral hairy leukoplakia

Chronic debilitating fatigue

The status of patients in the natural progression of HIV infection is routinely assessed in three ways: by ongoing clinical evaluation for HIV- and AIDS-related conditions, by a CD4 T lymphocyte count, and by quantification of HIV viral burden. HIV viral burden is typically measured in blood using a nucleic acid-based test, such as a DNA probe or polymerase chain reaction assay. Such tests have been shown to have significant prognostic power in predicting progression to AIDS and long-term survival. The decision to initiate antiretroviral therapy is usually based one or more of these three assessments. Although there remains some controversy about when antiretroviral therapy should begin in early HIV infection, the presence of an AIDS-defining illness, a CD4 count < 500 cells/mm^3, or a viral burden of >5,000 viral genomes/mm^3 of blood have been used as criteria for initiating therapy.

Treatment with zidovudine (AZT) as a single agent showed that the progression to AIDS could be modestly delayed, but other indicators of HIV progression, such as CD4 T cell counts and viral burden progress in spite of therapy after a few months. The progression of therapy in spite of antiviral treatment results from the emergence of resistant HIV viruses during therapy. Resistant mutants arise promptly because the viral reverse transcriptase is prone to errors. In the case of AZT and other reverse transcriptase inhibitors, the mutations occur in the viral gene encoding this enzyme. The emergence of resistance can be prevented by combining antiretroviral agents that act at different steps of viral replication or that require distinct mutations to confer resistance. Today, most patients are treated initially with three or more active drugs (e.g., two reverse transcriptase inhibitors and a protease inhibitor). Combination antiretroviral regimens typically induce long-lasting reductions in viral burden and rises in CD4 T cell counts, and these regimens have contributed to a recent and significant reduction in AIDS-related deaths in the United States (Figure 38.6).

Pneumocystis pneumonia is a preventable disease. Prospective studies of HIV-positive patients have shown that at least one-third of patients with CD4 T-cell counts less than 200 cells/mm^3 develop *Pneumocystis* pneumonia within 3 years. The risk is considerably greater if the patients are also symptomatic (i.e., have fever, night sweats, weight loss, or oral candidiasis). The risk of this infection may be substantially reduced with prophylactic therapy using trimethoprim–sulfamethoxazole or aerosolized pentamidine. *Pneumocystis* pneumonia is less clearly correlated with CD4 T-cell counts in children. HIV-infected infants with CD4 T-cell counts less than 1500 cells/mm^3 should be considered candidates for prophylaxis.

Clinical Manifestations of AIDS

J.'s physician prescribed zidovudine and trimethoprim–sulfamethoxazole tablets. Ten days later, J. stopped the trimethoprim–sulfamethoxazole because of an itchy rash but did not inform his doctor. Six months later, he turned up at a local emergency room complaining of a 6-day history of gradually worsening dry cough and shortness of breath. His temperature was 40°C and his chest x-ray showed a diffuse bilateral interstitial pneumonia. Examination of fluid from bronchoalveolar lavage revealed *P. carinii*.

J. now has AIDS. The signs and symptoms of *Pneumocystis* pneumonia place him in that category, but any of a number of other opportunistic infections, singly or in groups, would lead to the same diagnosis. Table 68.1 indicates the major infections associated with AIDS, most of which are due to intracellular agents usually controlled by cell-mediated immunity. These infections are often the result of endogenous reactivation of previously acquired organisms, rather than newly acquired infection.

Most AIDS-related infections do not occur until the CD4 count falls below 200 cells/mm^3. Kaposi's sarcoma is the major exception to this rule because its occurrence seems to be independent of the underlying T-cell depletion, although it is more frequent at lower CD4 counts. Infections in AIDS patients are characterized by a high density of organisms and disseminated disease, as well as infections with multiple organisms. These infections are rarely cured. Control of disease consequently requires prolonged acute therapy as well as long-term use of antimicrobial agents to prevent relapses.

Lung Infections

Pneumonia caused by *Pneumocystis* is the most frequent opportunistic infection associated with AIDS and occurs in between 25% and 60% of all patients. The typical symptoms are fever, cough, and shortness of breath. Although this infection typically affects the lung, it may involve other sites, especially the liver, lymph nodes, and choroid. Although treatable, *Pneumocystis* pneumonia is associated with a mortality of 10–20% from irreversible respiratory failure.

An opportunistic infection such as *Pneumocystis* pneumonia does not mean that patients will automatically develop multiple medical problems and soon die. The use of specific antiretroviral therapy, such as zidovudine, and anti-*Pneumocystis* drugs has led to an improvement in the quality and length of life for AIDS patients. Many people are able to live and work normally for some time. Nevertheless, no specific curative therapy is available, and the progressive decline in immunity continues. Progressive deterioration with repeated episodes of infection is the normal pattern for patients with advanced HIV disease.

Gastrointestinal Infections

After the episode of pneumonia, J. made a complete recovery and was able to return to work. He took zidovudine and aerosolized pentamidine for *Pneumocystis* prophylaxis. J. had no problems for about a year, when he saw his physician and complained of difficulty in swallowing and diarrhea. His diarrhea was intermittent, but could be as severe as 20 bouts of loose watery stools per day. On examining his mouth, multiple white plaques on his palate and tongue were seen.

Gastrointestinal problems are common in patients with AIDS. Infection of the mouth and pharynx with *Candida* is almost universal in patients with profound immunodeficiency, but is usually manageable. A substantial number of patients go on to develop esophageal candidiasis, which may cause pain and difficulty on swallowing, leading to considerable weight loss. Esophageal infection may also be caused by the herpes viruses, herpes simplex and cytomegalovirus (CMV), although they more typically involve other sites. Herpes simplex causes recurrent skin infections, especially perirectally, that can become resistant to therapy. CMV typically causes disseminated disease with viremia. Involvement of the colon may lead to severe abdominal pain and diarrhea. CMV infection of the eye presents as blurred vision and may lead to blindness.

Diarrhea is a common problem in patients with advanced AIDS and may be severe and difficult to diagnose and treat. It may be caused by a large number of agents, including:

- CMV and other viruses;
- Enteric Gram-negative bacteria such as *Salmonella* and *Shigella* (with accompanying bacteremia);
- Mycobacterial infection (especially the *Mycobacterium-avium* complex [MAC]) that affects the small bowel and colon and causes malabsorption and diarrhea;
- Intestinal parasites such as *Giardia, Isospora, Cryptosporidium,* and microsporidia.

Malignancies such as Kaposi's sarcoma or lymphoma involving the stomach or colon may also cause gastrointestinal symptoms. Furthermore, HIV itself may infect the cells of the gastrointestinal tract and cause an enteropathy leading to diarrhea.

To investigate J.'s intestinal distress, it will be necessary to culture his stool for bacteria and to examine it microscopically for parasites. If this examination does not give an answer, it may be necessary to perform invasive tests.

Mycobacterial and Fungal Infections

J., was found to have esophageal candidiasis and *Salmonella* infection. Following treatment, his symptoms resolved. Two months later, he was admitted to the hospital with a high fever, cough, and shortness of breath. His x-ray showed a lobar pneumonia and sputum cultures grew *Streptococcus pneumoniae.* He responded rapidly to penicillin treatment.

Although *Pneumocystis* is a frequent cause of pneumonia in AIDS patients, other causes must be considered, such as pneumococci, *Haemophilus influenzae,* and enteric Gram-negative rods. Tuberculosis is another important cause of pneumonia in AIDS, and it may disseminate widely to cause lymphadenitis, hepatitis, or meningitis.

Although most opportunistic infections occur during severe immunodeficiency, tuberculosis is an exception and may occur earlier, when the immune function of AIDS patients is only mildly impaired (i.e., in the "asymptomatic" phase). Consequently, HIV infection should be considered in the event of pulmonary tuberculosis in previously healthy young adults or adolescents. Infected patients can easily spread tuberculosis to household and other close contacts. Indeed, the rise in incidence of tuberculosis in the U.S. that began in the late 1980s can be attributed to a large extent to the spread of tuberculosis among HIV-infected persons and their close contacts.

Disseminated infection with the *Mycobacterium-avium* complex is also common in AIDS. Although this organism may cause pneumonia, it more typically causes disseminated disease, particularly in the lymph–reticular organs and the gastrointestinal tract. Typically, patients develop fever, night sweats, weight loss, and enlarged livers and spleens. Some also develop diarrhea. Similar symptoms are seen in patients with disseminated fungal infection, such as **histoplasmosis**, which is common in patients from the midwestern U.S. and Latin America. Disseminated **coccidioidomycosis** is found in patients from the southwestern U.S.

Infections of the Nervous System

After the episode of pneumonia, J. returned to work. Four months later, he developed high fever and a new headache. He went to his doctor's office and although his examination was normal, his doctor recommended a spinal tap. The cell count and glucose and protein levels were normal, but an India ink smear of cerebrospinal fluid showed it to be packed with *Cryptococcus neoformans.* J. responded well to antifungal treatment.

Opportunistic infections may also cause neurological problems in AIDS patients. Fever and headache are the most common presentations of infection with the fungus *C. neoformans,* which typically causes meningitis. J.'s case illustrates one of the major problems of treating such infections in a patient with AIDS. His spinal fluid is teeming with fungi, yet because of his immune defect, he is unable to mount an effective inflammatory response (thus his normal cell count and glucose and protein levels).

Other opportunistic infections can affect the brain. Reactivation of infection with the parasite *Toxoplasma gondii* typically causes a brain abscess. Such patients may present with headache, confusion, or seizures. Infection with another virus, the **JC papovavirus**, causes a progressive and fatal encephalopathy. CMV causes retinitis and occasionally encephalitis.

Infections by HIV Itself

J. became increasingly concerned about his weight loss. In fact, when his records were reviewed, his weight loss over the previous year was 90 lb, although he felt he was eating fairly well. He also noted fevers, night sweats, and intermittent bouts of severe diarrhea.

J. has progressive AIDS. HIV itself can directly affect many organs of the body, such as the intestine and the kidney. **HIV nephropathy** is manifested by proteinuria, the nephrotic syndrome, and kidney failure, and may respond to antiretroviral therapy. Myopathy and myositis both occur and may be related to HIV infection or the effects of drug therapy. Cardiomyopathy also occurs. One of the most distressing features of late AIDS is a wasting syndrome that is characterized by profound weight loss with concomitant loss of muscle mass. The pathogenesis of wasting syndrome in AIDS is unclear; however, it carries a grave prognosis and usually portends an early demise.

Oncological Manifestations in Advanced AIDS

Later, J. returned to his physician with several purple–red skin lesions on his legs and trunk. These lesions are biopsied, and Kaposi's sarcoma is diagnosed.

It is important to realize that the illnesses we associate with AIDS are changing in frequency and importance. As physicians become more adept in treating and preventing infections such as *Pneumocystis* pneumonia, other infections (e.g., those due to mycobacteria and CMV) assume greater importance. Neurological manifestations of HIV (see below) and malignancies have also assumed more importance. As patients live longer with profound immunodeficiency, malignancies are seen more frequently. The two most common malignancies are Kaposi's sarcoma and lymphoma.

Recent evidence suggests that Kaposi's sarcoma may be associated with a newly recognized human herpes virus. It is most commonly seen in male homosexuals with HIV disease. Its occurrence is independent of underlying immunocompromise, although it behaves more aggressively and is more difficult to treat as the CD4 T-cell count falls. In its mildest form, it may merely cause localized skin disease without significant morbidity. In

severe cases of Kaposi's sarcoma, lesions are widely disseminated and involve the lymph nodes, gastrointestinal tract, and lungs. Severe cases may be fatal.

Both Hodgkin's disease and non-Hodgkin's lymphoma occur more frequently in HIV-infected patients. The latter is an increasingly important problem. Involvement of the central nervous system is common and usually associated with poor prognosis. Epstein-Barr virus has been associated with most cases of central nervous system lymphoma, suggesting a probable role for this virus in the pathogenesis of this tumor.

Neurological Manifestations in Advanced AIDS

J. missed his next two doctor's appointments, and the next time he came to the office he was accompanied by his parents who noticed that he had become more forgetful and withdrawn. They informed the physician that J. was fired

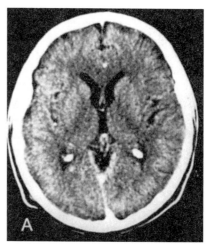

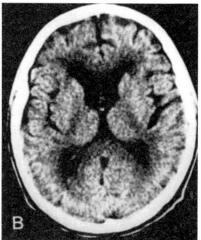

Figure 68.2. Computed tomography of the brain in a patient with AIDS. A. Normal CT scan. **B.** Scan from the same patient 4 months later when he presented with mental slowing and confusion. Note the profound loss of brain substance and consequent enlargement of the fluid-filled ventricles.

from his job because he was constantly late and could not concentrate on tasks. When his physician examined him, J. appeared inattentive and, although he knew who and where he was, he had problems remembering simple commands. The physician ordered a computed tomographic (CT) scan of his head, which showed profound brain atrophy.

Although opportunistic infections and lymphomas can involve the nervous system in AIDS, by far the most common neurological problems are caused by HIV itself. HIV is a lentivirus and, like many others in this group, is neurotropic. Infection of the nervous system occurs early in the disease, probably soon after exposure. The presence of HIV in the nervous system has been documented by viral culture of brain tissue, in situ hybridization demonstrating viral DNA sequences, and electron micrographic identification of retroviral particles. Within the central nervous system, the virus resides predominantly in macrophages and cells derived from macrophages, although the pathogenesis of HIV-associated neuronal damage is unclear.

Manifestations of nervous system involvement may occur at any stage of HIV disease. Acute primary infection may be complicated by aseptic meningitis, encephalitis, myelitis, or inflammatory neuropathies such as Guillain-Barré syndrome. Later in HIV disease, patients may have peripheral neuropathies, both motor and sensory, or spinal cord syndromes, resembling subacute combined degeneration of the cord. The most common form of neurological disease, however, is HIV-associated encephalopathy, which leads to progressive dementia, as in the case of J. In its earliest form, HIV dementia may consist of generalized mental slowing, difficulty concentrating, and forgetfulness, all of which must be differentiated from the depression that often accompanies HIV infection. In the later stages of HIV dementia, patients have profound deficits in cognitive, motor, and sensory functions, and may be totally unable to care for themselves. CT scans of the brain often show considerable atrophy (Fig. 68.2). Severe dementia is almost inevitably fatal.

Outcome

Two weeks later, J.'s parents called the physician to tell him that J. died at home that day.

J.'s outcome is typical of the usual course of HIV infection and it appears that most, if not all, HIV-infected individuals die of AIDS. Although HIV disease is, as yet, incurable and fatal, its progression varies. With improved antiretroviral therapy and use of prophylactic antimicrobial therapy, HIV infection may be a chronic disease in some patients.

GENETIC AND DEVELOPMENTAL PREDISPOSITION TO AIDS

Would the course of J.'s illness have been different if he had been a female? Probably not, although some of the indicator diseases may have been different. As mentioned earlier, recurrent vaginal candidiasis may be a common and troublesome complaint in HIV-infected women. In addition, increasing evidence shows that human papilloma virus infection may behave more aggressively in persons with HIV infection. Consequently, cancer of the uterine cervix may emerge as an important complication.

We do not know if AIDS behaves differently in various ethnic groups. Because most drug therapeutic studies have been performed mainly in Caucasian males, we are not certain that treatment is as effective in women or in other ethnic groups. It should be noted that there are no indications that drug treatment is ineffective or harmful; thus, no person should go untreated because he or she belongs to a particular racial group or gender.

HIV infection in children follows a similar course, with progressive immunodeficiency, recurrent opportunistic infections, and neurological involvement. However, the pace of the disease is much more rapid in infants. Transmission is usually vertical (i.e., acquired from the mother) and between 13% and 40% of babies born to HIV-infected mothers acquire HIV infection. Zidovudine therapy of the mother during the last two trimesters and labor may reduce this transmission rate by over 60%. The median time to progression to AIDS for these children is only 2 years and, consequently, their life expectancy is short. In addition to their opportunistic infections, most infants fail to thrive (i.e., have an abnormal growth rate) and many have developmental delays secondary to HIV brain infection. Recurrent bacterial infections (otitis, pneumonia) are common and are related to B-cell dysfunction. However, as with adults, antiretroviral treatment and prophylactic therapy for infection improve the quality and quantity of life. Most children with vertically acquired HIV infection have an indolent course with slow progression (8 or more years) to clinical disease; however, 15–20% of such children rapidly progress to symptomatic disease and death within 2–4 years after birth.

MANAGEMENT OF HIV-INFECTED PATIENTS

Management of the HIV-infected patient involves a long-term commitment from physicians and other members of the health team not only to medical care but also to support and to educate the patient and the family. Patients need to be alerted about symptoms that require prompt medical attention, such as changes in fever patterns or new onsets of cough or headache. Physicians must be prepared to deal with the many complaints that develop and distinguish those that herald important complications. Patients must be educated about the modes of transmission so that new cases can be prevented. In addition, the members of the health care team need to help the patient cope with the changing social dimensions of the disease. Confidentiality and maintenance of employment and insurance benefits are prime concerns. Most patients with AIDS wish to be treated as much as possible at home. Family and friends also need support and education.

Starting antiretroviral therapy early in the disease has been shown to delay the progression of HIV infection. Later in disease, these therapies can prolong survival. Nucleoside analogs, such as zidovudine, didanosine, zalcitabine, stavudine, and lamivudine, act by inhibition of reverse transcriptase, the retroviral-specific DNA polymerase (see Chapter 38, "Retroviruses"). Nevirapine and delavirdine are non-nucleoside inhibitors of reverse transcriptase. Several inhibitors of HIV protease have been developed and have been shown to prevent viral replication and to prolong survival (given alone or in combination with nucleoside analog) in patients with advanced infection. Other steps in viral replication, such as viral adherence to target cells and release from infected cells, are also potential target cells for antiviral agents. Immunomodulatory therapy, designed to boost the host's response to HIV infection, is also being studied. This kind of therapy may be particularly important since the appearance of an immune response appears to be associated with substantial reduction in viral load. Genetic therapy approaches attempting to induce resistance, interfere with viral replication or induce antiviral immunity are also under study. In a manner analogous to the therapy of tuberculosis, chemotherapy for HIV involves combinations of agents acting at different sites to achieve synergism and delay the emergence of resistant viruses.

PREVENTION

By far, the best approach to AIDS is prevention. Development of an effective vaccine would eliminate the future threat of this disease. However, the development of an HIV vaccine has been hampered by many problems. One is our incomplete understanding of the host immune response to the virus; although many individuals develop neutralizing antibodies to HIV, their role in vivo is unclear. Thus, circulating antibodies effectively clear the bloodstream of infectious virus yet fail to prevent the progression of HIV infection. In addition, HIV shows great variability in its major antigens (Chapter 38, "Retroviruses"). Finally, the testing of HIV vaccines for protective efficacy requires putting people at risk for infection and, thus, raises ethical concerns. Even after vaccines are developed and applied, it may be decades before AIDS ceases to be a major problem.

Until vaccines are developed, education to reduce transmission of HIV remains the only effective way of tackling its spread. Controversial though they may be, the most effective approach to AIDS prevention is education and the use of measures to reduce sexual spread (such as condoms) and intravenous drug use.

CONCLUSION

AIDS is a devastating disease that will continue to have a profound effect on society. Scientifically, it has enhanced our understanding of the human immune system. The practice of medicine has been irrevocably changed with the recognition of this new incurable disease. In Western societies, the crisis has forced us to face issues such as the economics and inequity of health care delivery and discrimination in employment and insurance. Despite our recognition of these problems, the sobering truth is that mortality will continue to increase and the devastation caused by this virus will continue for the foreseeable future. AIDS will decimate communities in the developing world that lack the resources to treat infected individuals or to prevent further transmission. Little relief is in sight.

SUGGESTED READINGS

Broder S, Merigan T, Bolognesi D, eds. Textbook of AIDS medicine. Baltimore: Williams and Wilkins, 1994.

Chaisson RE, Volberding PA. Clinical manifestations of HIV infection. In: Mandell G, Bennett JE, Dolin R, eds. Principles and practice of infectious diseases. 4th ed. New York: Churchill Livingstone, 1995;1217–1252.

Sande MA, Volberding PA, eds. The medical management of AIDS. 4th ed. Orlando: WB Saunders, 1995.

Spooner KM, Lane HC, Masur H. Guide to major clinical trials of antiretroviral therapy administered to patients infected with human immunodeficiency virus. Clin Infect Dis 1996;23:15–27.

Congenital and Neonatal Infections

JANET R. GILSDORF

ROGER G. FAIX

etuses and babies up to 4 weeks old are susceptible to a variety of infections that are unique to this period of life. Congenital (also called intrauterine or prenatal) infections are those that occur during fetal life and result from maternal infection that has been transmitted to the fetus. Neonatal infections (those occurring during the first 4 weeks after birth) are generally acquired by the baby from microbial agents present in the maternal birth canal or the environment. Both congenital and neonatal infections are characterized by microorganisms and clinical presentations that are uncommon in older children or adults. Agents such as *Toxoplasma gondii*, cytomegalovirus (CMV), and rubella virus may cause devastating infections in the developing fetus, but are relatively minor or asymptomatic in neonates or older infants. Conversely, agents such as *Escherichia coli* and herpes simplex virus cause overwhelming and often fatal infections in neonates, but do not usually infect fetuses, probably because these organisms do not cross the placental barrier easily.

SPECIAL IMMUNOLOGICAL PROBLEMS OF THE FETUS AND THE PREGNANT MOTHER

The development of the mammalian fetus poses an immunological paradox; the immune systems of the mother and her developing fetus must be modulated to avoid mutual rejection. The fetus is antigenically distinct from its mother, but suppression of certain aspects of the maternal immune system during pregnancy, the limited number of transplant antigens expressed by the fetal unit (fetus and placenta), and a variety of other factors act in harmony to prevent maternal rejection of the fetus. In addition, the fetal immune system is not fully mature,

thus preventing **"graft versus host"** type of rejection of maternal tissues by the fetus.

The humoral immune responses of the fetus are detectable as early as 2 months of gestation but do not "ripen" until about 2 years of age. This "fetal immunodeficiency" is caused by many factors, including the inability of fetal and neonatal mononuclear cells to produce macrophage-activating factors. In the absence of cytokines (such as α-interferon), neither a cytotoxic proliferative response nor an immune response can be mounted effectively. In the mother, although cytokines are present in the placental circulation, they are not transported to the fetus, where they might activate the immune response of her "graft," i.e., the baby. In addition to the lack of cytokines, the fetal cellular antimicrobial machinery is also defective. Placental or neonatal macrophages permit the intracellular replication of certain microorganisms (such as *T. gondii*), whereas macrophages from adults kill them.

The fetus is protected from infection by several special defense mechanisms including the **fetal membranes**, which shelter it from external microorganisms, and the **placenta**, which protects the fetus from many maternal microorganisms. The mother further protects her fetus by endowing it with considerable quantities of immunoglobulins, largely of the IgG class. At term, the fetal concentration of IgG antibodies may be greater than that of the mother, as the placenta actively transports these molecules into the fetal circulation by a mechanism of receptor-mediated endocytosis. Conversely, a baby born several months prematurely may not have received a full complement of maternal antibodies, which contributes to the increased risk of infection of such babies. IgM does not cross the intact placenta but may be synthesized by an infant in response to an infection. Maternal IgG is slowly metabolized by the newborn infant; some maternal antibodies, such as those against bacterial polysaccharides, are undetectable in the infant's serum 2–4 months after birth whereas other antibodies, such as those against measles and HIV, may persist for as long as 12–15 months. In addition, breast milk contains secretory IgA antibodies that appear to protect nursing infants against certain gastrointestinal pathogens.

PRENATALLY ACQUIRED INFECTIONS

■ CASE

Baby L. was born at 37 weeks' gestation, following an uneventful pregnancy to a 28-year-old healthy mother. His two siblings had been born with no difficulties and are healthy at ages 2 and 4 years. On physical examination about 30 minutes postdelivery, the baby was found to weigh 2 kg (well below the 3rd percentile for a term baby) and to have a head circumference of 28 cm (well below the 3rd percentile for a term baby). He was pale and had numerous nonblanching purplish spots on his trunk, back, face, and all four extremities. His vital signs were stable and his cardiopulmonary examination was unremarkable. He had an enlarged liver and spleen. The urine grew CMV on viral culture, thus establishing the diagnosis of congenital CMV infection.

The parents had many questions about their son and his illness. The physician reassured them that they had not done anything to contribute to the child's illness. On the other hand, the parents were troubled by the fact that this child was sick even though their two previous children were normal. The answer to the parent's question: "How could our baby get an infection before he was even born?" requires an understanding of the establishment of intrauterine infections.

Comment

This baby presents clinical signs and symptoms typical of prenatal infections, including signs of poor intrauterine growth and evidence of multisystem disease (including microcephaly, a rash compatible with thrombocytopenia, and hepatosplenomegaly). Notably, the symptoms of this infection were present at the time of birth. Also characteristic of many intrauterine infections is the fact that the mother was asymptomatic during her pregnancy.

Microbial Agents

A variety of microbial agents can infect the human fetus, including bacteria, viruses, and parasites (Table 69.1). Among the bacterial agents that actively infect fetuses are the spirochete of syphilis, *Treponema pallidum*, and *Mycobacterium tuberculosis*. A number of viruses may infect human fetuses, and those with the highest morbidity and mortality to the fetus include rubella virus and CMV. Varicella virus, parvovirus, enterovirus, hepatitis B, and human immunodeficiency virus (HIV) also occasionally infect the fetus but result in different clinical pictures from the classical intrauterine infection as described in the case. One animal parasite, *T. gondii*, is also an important intrauterine pathogen.

Although many other infectious agents do not directly infect the fetus, maternal illness may indirectly affect the outcome of pregnancy. For example, maternal Gram-negative bacterial infections (typhoid fever, septicemia, or urinary tract infection), malaria, or measles may result in abortion, stillbirth, or premature delivery due to hypoxia, high fever, or other metabolic abnormalities in the mother.

ENCOUNTER AND ENTRY

During pregnancy, mothers may become infected with agents that invade the blood and, thus, possibly in-

---

Table 69.1. Infectious Agents Causing Congenital Intrauterine Disease

	Persistent postnatal infection	Teratogenic	Trimester of greatest impact on fetus		
			1st	2nd	3rd
Bacteria					
Treponema pallidum	+	−	−	+	+
Mycobacterium tuberculosis	−	−	−	+	
Viruses					
Cytomegalovirus	+	+		?	
Rubella	+	+	+ +	+	−
Varicella zoster	+	+	+	−	+
Parvovirus B19	−	−	+	+	−
Herpes simplex	+	−	+	+	+
?HIV	+	?		?	
Protozoa					
Toxoplasma gondii	+	−	+	+	−

fect the fetus. For example, pregnant women may acquire *T. pallidum*, herpes simplex virus, or CMV through sexual contact. Mothers may also be infected by person-to-person or airborne transmission of *M. tuberculosis*, varicella, rubella, and CMV. Fomites in the environment may harbor microbial agents that may infect a pregnant mother; e.g., *Toxoplasma* cysts are present in the feces of cats and in raw or undercooked meat.

Microorganisms enter into a fetus in one of two ways: (1) through amniotic leaks that allow direct access of organisms from the vaginal tract (such leaks develop rarely and only late in pregnancy), and (2) from the mother's blood (organisms using this route encounter a variety of host defense factors in the placenta, including the villous trophoblasts, tissue macrophages, and locally produced immune factors such as antibodies or lymphokines). When infection of the placenta occurs, it may or may not progress to fetal infection (Fig. 69.1), depending on the infecting agent and the integrity of the placental defenses.

Timing of the maternal infection is an important determinant of fetal infection and outcome. For unknown reasons, *M. tuberculosis* appears incapable of crossing the placental barrier before approximately 26 weeks of pregnancy. The placenta can be breached by *T. pallidum* before then, but induction of pathologic changes in fetal tissue does not result before the fifth month of gestation. On the other hand, *T. gondii*, CMV, rubella virus, and parvovirus can infect the fetus during the first trimester, when the impact on fetal development is greatest. Infection late in pregnancy with these organisms usually has no adverse effects on the fetus. Varicella zoster infection

may, on rare occasions, have teratogenic effects, but only if the mother is infected during the first or early second trimester. However, when maternal varicella infections occur within 5 days of delivery, the baby is at high risk of serious, overwhelming infection because the virus will readily cross the placenta and the baby will be born before protective maternal antibodies are made. In this circumstance, the newborn should be treated with varicella zoster immune globulin to try to prevent severe infection.

DAMAGE

Three types of effects on the growing and developing fetus may result from intrauterine infection.

- One is the interference with normal organogenesis, which may result in structural abnormalities in tissues and organs. Thus, congenital rubella may result in cataracts and defects of the retina, patent ductus arteriosus, pulmonary artery stenosis, pulmonary valvular stenosis, or sensorineural deafness. The types and extent of teratogenic effects on the fetus are highly dependent on the time when maternal infection occurs during gestation. Specific fetal tissues, such as the eyes and heart, are most susceptible to viral damage during discrete periods of organogenesis in the first half of pregnancy.
- The second effect on the developing fetus results from the inflammatory reaction in response to tissue infection. For example, congenital CMV or toxoplasmosis infections may result in cerebritis, which may lead to cerebral atrophy and intracranial calcifications.
- The third effect relates to **placental insufficiency** due to placental infection. Inflammation, edema, and fibrosis associated with placental infection may compromise normal growth and development of the fetus, leading to low birth weight, premature birth, or fetal death.

Although the damage to fetal cells and organs occurs prenatally at the time of the infection, the effects of the damage may not become clinically apparent until several months after birth. For example, deafness or mental retardation as a result of congenital rubella or CMV infection may not manifest clinically until children have reached an age in which language and other cognitive skills can be evaluated. In addition, certain tissue damage continues after birth in some congenital infections (such as rubella, CMV, and untreated syphilis) as the microbes continue to replicate after delivery.

DIAGNOSIS

Significant exposure of a mother to a potentially damaging infectious agent during pregnancy warrants

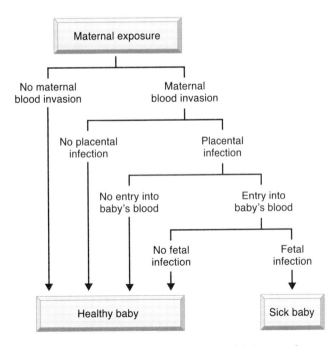

Figure 69.1. Sequence of events in the establishment of congenital infections.

attempts to document the presence of a resultant infection, because this information may be important in making decisions regarding gestational therapy or termination of the pregnancy. During pregnancy, detection of either IgM antibodies specific for the microbial agent or a rising titer of specific IgG antibodies in the mother's serum may be helpful in assessing the risk of congenital toxoplasmosis, CMV, rubella, or syphilis. Other maternal organism-specific tests, such as darkfield microscopy, antigen detection, or polymerase chain reaction (PCR), may be warranted in suggestive clinical settings. If gestational maternal infection with an agent of congenital infection is strongly suspected, antenatal specific testing of amniotic fluid or fetal blood may be useful to better determine if fetal infection has occurred. Such information may be useful for parental counseling and for making decisions regarding transplacental fetal therapy and continuation of the pregnancy. Unfortunately, many agents that cause congenital infection frequently produce minimal or no symptoms in the mother and consequently arouse no suspicion until after the infant is born.

In an ill neonate, such as the one presented in the case history, an attempt should be made to identify the presence of an infecting agent in appropriate tissue specimens or body fluids. Urine, saliva, buffy coat, or cerebrospinal fluid specimens should be cultured for CMV, and nasopharyngeal specimens, urine, buffy coat, and cerebrospinal fluid should be cultured for the presence of rubella virus. Techniques for culturing *Toxoplasma* and *T. pallidum* are not available in routine diagnostic laboratories. Darkfield examination of material from the base of an oral or skin lesion may reveal the presence of *T. pallidum*, and an immunoassay may identify CMV or *T. pallidum* antigens in tissue specimens. Careful inspection for placental trophozoites by a skilled pathologist may facilitate prompt detection of congenital infection with *Toxoplasma*. PCR techniques that amplify organism-specific DNA in appropriate specimens may greatly enhance the ability to detect even small numbers of pathogens.

Culture, antigen-detection, and PCR techniques may be unavailable or require a number of days before an agent is detected, thus the diagnosis of congenital infection may rely on evidence of the immune response in the baby. Because IgG antibodies readily pass through and sometimes are concentrated by the placenta, the presence of such antibodies in the baby is not, by itself, diagnostic of intrauterine infection unless the concentration of antibody in the infant is substantially greater than that in the mother (e.g., fourfold higher titer in specimens processed at the same time in the same lab). Maternal IgG antibodies cannot be distinguished easily from those produced by a congenitally infected newborn. Maternal IgM antibodies, on the other hand, do not readily cross the placenta; thus, the presence of CMV, rubella virus, or *Toxoplasma* specific IgM antibodies in a baby strongly suggests that the baby has been infected and is generating an immune response. Unfortunately, not all infants with culture-proven congenital infection have organism-specific IgM at the time of diagnostic evaluation, so the absence of IgM does not necessarily exclude congenital infection.

The interpretation of serological data in newborns may be complicated by maternal–fetal blood transfusion or by suppression of fetal production of antibodies by the infectious process itself. A useful way to retrospectively diagnose congenital infections using serology is to monitor the antibody titer in the baby over several months. Because the half-life of maternal IgG is approximately 20 days, most of the maternal IgG will have been degraded after several months, and any IgG detectable in the baby is most likely to be of infant origin. Thus, in the congenitally infected baby, IgG antibody will stay the same or increase over time, whereas in an uninfected baby, specific antibodies of maternal origin will eventually disappear.

TREATMENT

The availability and success of treatment for congenitally acquired infections varies with the infectious agent. Penicillin G is highly effective in treating congenital syphilis if given more than 1 month before delivery. If syphilis is detected during pregnancy, penicillin given to the mother is readily delivered through the placenta to the fetus and the infection will be adequately treated most of the time. Infants infected with *Toxoplasma* have been successfully treated with a combination of pyrimethamine and sulfadiazine, although the optimal dosage and duration of therapy remain uncertain. Therapy of fetal *Toxoplasma* infection with maternal spiramycin followed by pyrimethamine and sulfonamide has been reported to decrease mortality and improve long-term outcome. Presently, no widely accepted, proven treatment is available for congenital rubella or CMV. The development of new antiviral agents with apparent improved efficacy against CMV in immunocompromised individuals suggests that, in the future, effective antimicrobial agents against CMV with acceptable toxicity may be available.

PREVENTION

Prevention of congenital infections depends on assuring excellent health of the mother. Appropriate immunization during childhood (or postpartum in nonimmune mothers) protects a mother and her baby against rubella. Similarly, immunization of individuals living in endemic areas against *M. tuberculosis* with BCG vaccine may protect some mothers and babies against tuberculosis. Routine prenatal examination will reveal syphilis or tuberculosis in infected mothers, and adequate treatment of the mother will prevent ongoing infection in her baby. Good hygiene practices including appropriate handwashing may protect susceptible pregnant mothers from primary toxoplasmosis infection after exposure to cat feces containing *T. gondii* cysts or from primary CMV infection after exposure to secretions and body fluids of young children (who frequently excrete CMV). Adequate cooking of meat will prevent ingestion of infectious *Toxoplasma* cysts.

PERINATALLY ACQUIRED INFECTION

▌CASE

C.C. is a 14-day-old baby brought to the emergency room with a 24-hour history of fever to 38.9°C, poor feeding, lethargy, and irritability. The baby was born at term to a 22-year-old mother following an uneventful pregnancy. C.C. was discharged home with his mother 24 hours after delivery and had reportedly been doing well at home until the previous day, when the mother had to wake the baby for feeding. The baby then nursed only weakly and only for a short period of time.

Workup in the emergency room revealed a high peripheral white blood cell count (24,000/mm^3 with 68% segmented, 20% bands, and 12% lymphocytes). Examination of the cerebrospinal fluid revealed the presence of 230 white blood cells, 90% of which were neutrophils, which suggests an acute bacterial infection. The cerebrospinal fluid had an elevated protein content (830 mg/dl), and a low glucose concentration (20 mg/dl with a concomitant serum glucose of 80 mg/dl; see Chapter 58, "Central Nervous System" for a detailed explanation of these findings), also in keeping with a bacterial infection. A Gram stain of the cerebrospinal fluid showed Gram-positive cocci in chains, and the culture grew group β-hemolytic streptococci (*Streptococcus agalactiae*). The baby was given penicillin G and gentamicin as initial therapy. After a rocky hospital course characterized by apneic spells, seizures, and later, poor feeding, the baby was sent home following a 21-day course of antibiotic therapy. At age 8 months, he was delayed in achieving appropriate developmental milestones.

This baby was apparently healthy and normal at birth and developed acute symptoms suggestive of infection at 2 weeks of age. Thus, the infection was most likely acquired after birth rather than before it. The presence of an inflammatory reaction and the recovery of pathogenic bacteria from the cerebrospinal fluid confirms that this baby is suffering from bacterial meningitis, common kinds of severe perinatally acquired infection.

Unlike many other animal species, human infants at birth are incomplete in many aspects of their development and possess an immature immune system. The newborn is supplied by the mother with antibodies from the circulation and protective factors in breast milk. Breast milk contains IgA type antibodies, white blood cells, and lysozyme. The growth of Gram-negative enteric bacteria in the intestinal tract is suppressed in breast-fed babies, possibly by the growth of Gram-positive lactobacilli and bifidobacterial species and by the presence of iron-sequestering protein, lactoferrin. Epidemiological studies in India and England, for example, have shown that low-birth-weight babies fed breast milk developed fewer infections than those who were formula-fed.

Although neonates have maternal antibodies, they are obviously not protected against organisms to which their mothers have not generated an immune response. In addition, they are unable to generate antibodies against certain types of antigens, particularly polysaccharides. Terminal components of the complement cascade, especially important for defense against Gram-negative enteric bacteria, are present at a concentration less than 20% of that found in older children and adults. Also, the neonatal cellular immune system is suppressed as evidenced by decreased natural killer (NK) cytotoxicity and antibody-dependent cell-mediated cytotoxicity (ADCC). Phagocytic defenses are compromised by a smaller neutrophil storage pool, reduced ability to adhere to endothelium and migrate to infectious foci, and variable deficiencies in ingestion and killing of microbes. Secretory IgA and other elements of mucosal immunity are not adequately developed until several weeks or more after birth. Thus, otherwise normal healthy neonates are, to some extent, immunocompromised (Table 69.2). The risk of life-threatening infection is even greater in premature babies because their immune systems are more immature, their mucoepithelial surfaces are often colonized by multiply-resistant flora selected by frequent broad-spectrum empiric antibiotic therapy, and their care sometimes requires procedures that invade the skin and mucous membrane barriers, such as intravenous lines, chest tubes, or endotracheal tubes.

The risks to the neonate are great indeed. Without proper attention to sanitary measures such as good handwashing, bathing with clean water, and pasteurized milk (if fresh maternal breast milk is not used), the rate

---

Table 69.2. Factors That Place Newborn Infants at Increased Risk of Infection

Primary (inherent)
  1. Immature host defenses
  2. Naive, inexperienced immune system

Secondary (environmental)
  1. Hospital environment exposes them to drug-resistant pathogenic organisms
  2. Medical intervention invades protective barriers of skin and mucous membranes

of infant mortality can be prodigious. Survival of the first few years of life is only of recent origin even in developed countries, and has yet to be realized in many developing ones.

Microbial Agents

The most common types of bacteria that cause perinatally acquired infections are present in the maternal vaginal tract and include *E. coli*, group B β-hemolytic streptococci, *Listeria monocytogenes*, and *Haemophilus influenzae*. Other bacteria that are present in the baby's postnatal environment may also cause neonatal infection, and include other Gram-negative enteric bacilli, *S. aureus*, *M. tuberculosis*, and coagulase-negative staphylococci.

Several viruses are unique in their predilection for neonates. Herpes simplex virus, most commonly type 2, can cause serious multiorgan system infection that may clinically resemble acute bacterial sepsis. Perinatal transmission of varicella zoster virus or enteroviruses may also result in overwhelming infection with multiorgan failure. Human immunodeficiency virus (HIV) may be transmitted perinatally, although infected babies are usually asymptomatic during the neonatal period. Hepatitis B virus is frequently transmitted perinatally from a carrier mother to her baby. However, neonates infected with hepatitis B virus are generally asymptomatic and when symptoms do develop, they occur following the usual 2- to 3-month incubation period. Respiratory syncytial virus may induce apnea and particularly virulent forms of pneumonia and bronchiolitis.

Fungal infections with *Candida albicans* as well as with other *Candida* species play an increasingly important role in infections of sick, hospitalized neonates, especially those born prematurely. Animal parasites are not an important cause of neonatally acquired infections in the U.S., as neonates are seldom exposed to the environmental conditions required for transmission. *Chlamydia trachomatis* and *Neisseria gonorrhoeae* may infect the ocular and respiratory mucous membranes during birth and may cause neonatal conjunctivitis.

Although the baby described in the case was infected with group B streptococci, his clinical presentation was identical to that of babies with meningitis caused by other bacterial pathogens.

ENCOUNTER AND ENTRY

Babies are exposed to the agents causing perinatal infections in various ways. The bacterial agents causing neonatal sepsis, such as *E. coli*, group B streptococci, *Listeria monocytogenes*, and *Haemophilus influenzae* all normally colonize the maternal vaginal tract. During vaginal delivery, the skin and mucous membranes of the infant are exposed to these bacteria. Within the first 24–48 hours after birth, babies become colonized with

these organisms, particularly on their nasopharynx, skin, and around the umbilical stump. Colonization of the neonatal gastrointestinal tract occurs more slowly. Babies may also be exposed at the time of delivery to bloodborne agents that do not readily cross the placenta. This seems to be the most common mechanism of perinatal acquisition of hepatitis B virus and HIV.

A variety of environmental hazards also promotes the invasion of the human neonates by bacteria and fungi (Table 69.2). During labor, many infants are monitored for evidence of fetal distress by the application of monitoring devices to the fetal scalp as it presents in the vaginal tract. This procedure may allow access of skin organisms to the baby's blood. In addition, after the umbilical cord is severed, the healing stump provides a potential route for bacterial invasion. Many prematurely born newborns require intensive medical support such as intratracheal intubation with artificial ventilation, alimentation, antibiotic therapy through intravenous lines, and a variety of other therapeutic or diagnostic procedures that are invasive or potentially injurious to the otherwise protective barriers of the skin and mucous membranes. The increasing use of glucocorticoids and other potentially immunomodulating agents for a variety of indications may further compromise marginal host defenses and facilitate pathogenic invasion.

DAMAGE

The effect of perinatally acquired infections on the neonate is extremely variable and depends on the type of organism, the organ or organ systems infected, and the degree of relative immunosuppression of the baby. The early clinical manifestations of infections in neonates are often nonspecific, and include poor feeding, lethargy, or irritability. The outcome may depend on the speed with which antimicrobial and supportive therapy are initiated. Bacterial sepsis or meningitis can progress rapidly to severe neonatal illness or death within 12–24 hours. Even with timely, appropriate antibiotic therapy, the mortality of neonatal sepsis is between 10% and 40%, and significant neurological sequelae are seen in 20–50% of survivors of neonatal meningitis.

The extent of involvement and the morbidity of perinatally acquired infections varies greatly from baby to baby. Herpes simplex infection may involve a single organ such as the skin, with cutaneous vesicles being the only sign of infection, or it may be a serious multiorgan systemic infection involving the liver, central nervous system, lungs, and skin, ultimately resulting in severe brain damage or death. In contrast, hepatitis B is generally asymptomatic in the neonates but neonates infected with hepatitis B virus are at extremely high risk (more than 90%) of becoming chronic carriers of hepatitis B and, as young adults, are at risk for hepatic cirrhosis or hepatocellular carcinoma.

DIAGNOSIS

Diagnosis of a perinatally acquired infection depends on the recognition of suggestive signs and symptoms. Temperature instability, poor feeding, lethargy, or irritability may be the only presenting sign and symptom of neonatal septicemia and/or meningitis, and may be very subtle. Thus, the possibility of perinatal infection should be considered in neonates exhibiting even these nonspecific symptoms. Other, more specific symptoms, such as conjunctivitis or skin rash, may suggest a more focal infectious process.

Diagnosis is firmly established by the detection of an etiological agent in potentially infected body sites. However, the causative agents may not always be recovered by culture, sometimes because of antimicrobial therapy given before collection of specimens or because specimens likely to reveal the organism cannot easily be obtained (such as lung, liver, or brain biopsy specimens). Detection of viral or bacterial antigens or nucleic acids in serum, urine, cerebrospinal fluid, or other appropriate body fluids in these situations may reveal the causative agent. Antigen detection is routinely available for group B streptococci, E. coli K1 (which cross-reacts with the group B capsule of Neisseria meningitidis), HIV, and hepatitis B virus. In situations such as neonatal herpes simplex infections, for which culture is often difficult or nonrewarding and antigen detection probes are not readily available, the diagnosis may be supported by detection of an immune response in the baby, either by evidence of antigen-specific IgM antibodies, a rise in antigen-specific IgG antibody, or a concentration of antigen-specific IgG from the acute phase serum that is significantly higher than that of the mother.

TREATMENT

Successful treatment of perinatally infected babies is greatly influenced by the type of microbial agent, the availability of specific antimicrobial therapy, the rapidity with which appropriate therapy is instituted, the severity of the infection, and the underlying state of health. A variety of effective and relatively safe antimicrobial agents are available for the treatment of neonatal septicemia due to E. coli, H. influenzae, group B streptococci, and L. monocytogenes. In addition, antifungal agents are effective in treating fungal infections. The antiviral agent acyclovir has been shown to be effective in treating neonates with herpes simplex virus infections. In general, the efficacy of treatment and the outcome improve with early initiation of treatment. Selection of antimicrobial therapy must usually be made empirically, based on the likely pathogens for the clinical setting, since recovery and/or identification of the invading microbe is not immediate. The dosing levels and dosing intervals of drugs differ in neonates from those in older children or adults because neonates have decreased renal and hepatic elimination of most drugs and increased volumes of distribution of many drugs. Provision of appropriate life support therapy may also be necessary to support such vital functions as respiration and perfusion that are often deranged during the acute phase of infection. Careful surveillance during therapy is necessary to assure successful eradication of the infection, minimize potential antimicrobial toxicity, and institute appropriate rehabilitative therapy as needed.

PREVENTION

Because prematurely born infants are at greater risk of perinatal infection than full-term neonates, prevention of premature delivery prevents a significant number of neonatal infections. Prematurely born babies often require prolonged hospital care and invasive medical interventions; therefore, strict attention to infection control practices in the care of ill neonates (e.g., handwashing and equipment decontamination) also decreases the risk of neonatal infection.

Other preventive strategies involve the mother. Immunization of the mother against tetanus, for example, provides protective transplacental antibodies to infants greater than 28 weeks gestation and greatly reduces the potential for neonatal tetanus. Gestational screening for maternal hepatitis B infection permits effective immunoprophylaxis for the infant at birth. Intrapartum maternal administration of penicillin reduces the risk of early-onset group B streptococcal disease in newborn infants. Policies to maximize the benefits and minimize the costs and risks of this chemoprophylactic approach continue to evolve. The development of maternal vaccines, antimicrobial prophylaxis, and other preventive strategies against important perinatal pathogens is ongoing.

SUGGESTED READINGS

Feigin RD, Adcock LM, Miller DJ. Postnatal bacterial infections. In: Fanaroff AA, Martin RJ, eds. Neonatal–perinatal medicine: diseases of the fetus and infant. St. Louis: Mosby-Yearbook, 1992.

Greenough A, Osborne J, Sutherland S, eds. Congenital, perinatal and neonatal infections. Edinburgh: Churchill Livingstone, 1992.

McCracken GH Jr, Freij BJ. Infectious diseases of the fetus and newborn. In: Feigin RD, Cherry JD, eds. Textbook of pediatric infectious diseases. Philadelphia: WB Saunders, 1992.

Remington JS, Klein JO, eds. Infectious diseases of the fetus and newborn infant. Philadelphia: WB Saunders, 1995.

Zoonoses

VICTOR L. YU

Diseases that are transmitted from animals to humans are called **zoonoses** or **zoonotic diseases.** The existence of an animal reservoir makes zoonoses difficult to control. Consider, for example, the problems involved in controlling rodents that are infected with the plague or Hantavirus in the deserts of the southwestern United States or controlling large herds of wildebeests that carry sleeping sickness in Central Africa. Animal-related diseases have caused untold damage to people in the past, and continue to be of enormous concern, especially in tropical areas of the world.

Zoonoses are defined as infectious diseases that are naturally transmitted between vertebrate animals and humans. The word is derived from the Greek *zoon* meaning animal, and *nosos*, meaning disease. Persons at greatest risk of acquiring zoonoses are those who work in close proximity to animals, such as farmers, veterinarians, slaughterhouse workers, and animal researchers. The most common sources of zoonotic diseases are domestic animals, such as pets and farm animals. Over 100 million cats and dogs are kept as pets in the United States, and over 30 human diseases can be acquired from them, although each is rare.

With the international movement of animals, importation of zoonotic diseases from one geographic locale to another takes place with increasing frequency. A scary incident took place in 1989, when an Ebola-like virus caused a fatal epidemic among monkeys from Asia in a Reston, Virginia quarantine facility. Five American animal workers contracted the infection from the monkeys but did not show symptoms. Hundreds of other persons had potentially been exposed to this virus.

Adaptation to a host is basic to the survival of many microorganisms. Prolonged interaction between the host and individual microbial species results in a balanced relationship that allows both to survive. In some zoonoses, the pathogenic organism is part of the commensal flora of the animal (for example, organisms associated with animal bites). Usually, animals involved show no apparent disease despite carriage of a zoonotic organism (for example, histoplasmosis in birds). Arthropod vectors of zoonoses do not often demonstrate abnormal physiology or behavior despite carriage of an infecting organism. On the other hand, if the infecting agent invades previously unexposed animal or human populations, infections may be extraordinarily destructive, as evolutionary host defenses have not had sufficient time to develop. Explosive epidemics may occur if the microorganism is not quickly identified and contained. Outbreaks of plague and histoplasmosis are examples of such epidemics.

Many organisms have adapted to specific hosts. For example, individual species of *Brucella*, the etiologic agent of brucellosis, prefer different mammalian hosts: *Brucella melitensis* infects sheep and goats, *B. abortus* cattle, *B. suis* pigs, *B. canis* dogs, and *B. rangiferii tarandi* reindeer.

ENCOUNTER

Transmission of zoonotic agents from animals to humans has two scenarios: 1. **People are "dead-end-hosts,"** accidental intruders in an animal-to-animal chain and cannot transmit the agent further. 2. **People may transmit** an agent acquired from animals to other people and/or animals.

In the second scenario, the organisms travel from animals to humans; from humans, they are transmitted to other humans or even other animals. The route of transmission may change in the process. For instance, plague bacilli enter the human body via flea bites, multiply, and may then go from person to person by inhalation of droplets produced by the cough of patients. (Fig. 70.1) Similarly, the virus of Korean hemorrhagic fever may be acquired by eating food contaminated with the excreta of rodents, but can then spread by the respiratory route. In salmonellosis the organisms are acquired by eating contaminated animal products and can then spread via the fecal–oral route to other people.

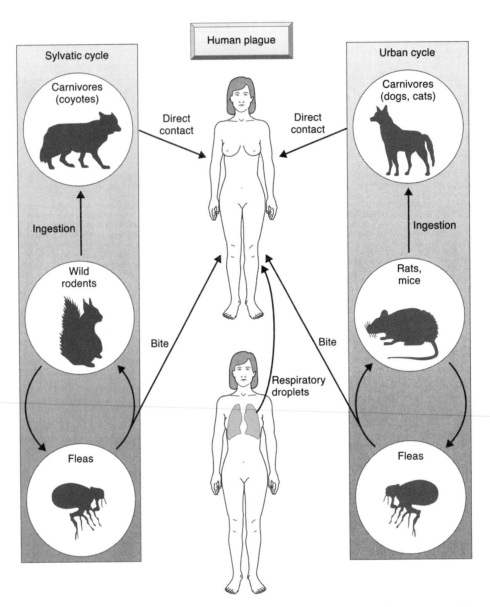

Figure 70.1. Plague is perpetuated in rodent reservoirs and spread to humans via three cycles. 1 (left). Sylvatic cycle among wild rodents via transmission by fleas. Other mammals including skunks and coyotes may also acquire the organism by ingestion of infected animals. **2 (right).** Urban cycle which is transmitted by the rat flea among urban rat populations. **3 (center).** Human plague can be transmitted by contact with infected animal tissue, bite of the fleas, or by infected aerosols from other humans.

The **pathogenesis** of zoonotic diseases in the animal reservoir often gives clues about their transmission to humans. The most successful organisms are those that cause an indolent, low-grade disease in the animal but which are easily spread. Control of these zoonotic diseases is extremely difficult. For example, leptospirosis is a chronic, often asymptomatic infection of rats and domestic animals, especially dogs. The organisms multiply in the kidney tubules and are excreted in the urine. The disease can then be acquired by people who come in contact with contaminated urine, e.g., by swimming in an irrigation ditch. Similarly, cows infected with tuberculosis can shed the tubercle bacilli in their milk without undue signs of disease. In all these cases, the animals become shedders, because the agents are able to persist for long periods of time. Persistence is sometimes caused by the localization of the organisms in sheltered sites, such as the kidney tubules (*Leptospira*) or the mammary glands (*Brucella*).

ENTRY

The agents of zoonoses gain access to the human host in customary ways: penetration of the skin, inhalation, and ingestion. Few microorganisms can directly penetrate the skin or mucous membranes of humans, and few can traverse the distance between hosts. But evolutionary innovations have allowed some organisms to overcome these physical and biological barriers. Many organisms use an intermediary **vector** that can serve both the delivery and entry functions. For example, a tsetse fly that carries the trypanosomes of sleeping sickness bridges the distance between infected cattle and people, introducing the organisms when it bites.

In zoonoses transmitted by arthropod vectors, the microorganisms may undergo developmental changes within the vectors. Particularly elaborate examples are seen in the protozoa of malaria or sleeping sickness. In other zoonoses, developmental changes take place within a vertebrate host, as in the case of tapeworms and other metazoan parasites. Finally, organisms involved in yet other zoonoses undergo developmental changes in the external environment, such as soil, bodies of water, food, or plants. For example, hookworm eggs hatch in soil and the larvae simply wait for a mammalian host.

The diversity of modes of transmission is well illustrated by a group of related diseases, the viral hemorrhagic fevers. These illnesses are found in tropical climates and have similar clinical manifestations; they include Hantavirus infection, Lassa fever, Marburg virus disease, Crimean–Congo hemorrhagic fever, and Ebola hemorrhagic fever. All these infections can be transmitted from person to person by direct contact. The intriguing aspect of transmission of these viruses is how they reach the human host from their animal reservoir. The Lassa virus is frequently present in mice and is transmitted to humans by ingestion of foodstuff contaminated with mouse urine. The Marburg virus is transmitted from monkeys to humans by direct contact. The Crimean–Congo hemorrhagic fever virus is transmitted from domestic animals to humans via tick bites, and it is thought that the Ebola virus is transmitted by aerosols and direct contact with blood. The Hantaviruses are probably transmitted by infected aerosols of urine or feces of rodents.

Direct Penetration

The epidermis of the skin may be breached in a number of ways to permit entry of microorganisms. One obvious mechanism is direct entry through minute **abrasions** or open **wounds** (Table 70.1). The organisms themselves may directly penetrate the skin. For instance, the fungi that cause athlete's foot produce an enzyme that hydrolyzes the keratin of the stratum corneum, whereas hookworms have "teeth" that allow them to chew their way through the epidermis. Microorganisms may also gain entry via arthropod vectors by stings or bites (Table 70.2); animals themselves may neatly solve the problem of entry by biting the host (Table 70.3)

The anatomic sites that are usually penetrated by infectious agents include those that come in contact with the organisms as well as those that are more likely to experience abrasions or wounds. Thus, exposed extremities tend to be sites of infection in erysipeloid, anthrax, and cat scratch fever.

Arthropod vectors

This fascinating mode of transmission is the most complex because it requires living intermediaries. Some arthropod vectors function as "flying syringes" (mosquitoes or biting flies), whereas others jump (fleas), or crawl (ticks or mites) (Table 70.2). Transmission by arthropod vectors can be either mechanical or biological. In mechanical transmission the vector simply transports the pathogen. Biting flies, for instance, often serve as mechanical vectors. After feeding on an infected animal, the insect digests the blood meal and contaminates its mouth and feces. When it moves to a human, microorganisms are transmitted with the next bite. In an even more passive mode of transmission, insects may transmit diseases without biting, just by contaminating foodstuff with organisms they carry on their legs. *Salmonella* may be transported by house flies that pick up the organisms from the feces of diseased animals.

In biological transmission, part of the developmental cycle of the microorganism must take place within an arthropod vector. This type of transmission is most often seen in protozoa. For instance, in American trypanosomiasis (Chagas disease), the organisms multiply and pass through various developmental stages within reduviid bugs. Ingested trypanosomes multiply in the bug's gut and transform into flagellar forms. The insect feces are infective. They enter the human host when the insect's feces are deposited at the site of the bite during feeding; the trypanosomes gain access when the host rubs them into the skin while scratching the insect bite.

Animal bites

Animal bites introduce floras from two sources into deep tissue: the flora from the skin of the recipient, and, more often, the flora found in the mouth and teeth of the biting animal. Table 70.3 lists the common pathogens that are transmitted by bites.

The most common pathogen associated with animal bites, especially by cats, is a bacterium, *Pasteurella multocida*, which cause skin and soft tissue infections at the site of inoculation and can also cause disseminated infections following invasion of the bloodstream. A condition known as rat-bite fever can be caused by one of two organisms, a Gram-negative called *Streptobacillus moniliformis* or a spirochete, *Spirillum minor*. Both organisms are members of the oropharyngeal flora of rats.

Viral diseases that can be transmitted through animal bites include rabies and a herpes virus of monkeys. The latter is usually transmitted by the bites of monkeys in a zoo or a laboratory. Both viruses are present in the saliva

Table 70.1. Direct Skin Penetration

Disease	Organism name	Group	Animal
Bacteria			
Anthrax[a,b]	*Bacillus anthracis*	Gram-positive aerobic spore former	Domestic mammals (herbivores)
Brucellosis[a,b]	*Brucella melitensis*	Gram-negative rods	Goats, sheep
	B. abortus		Cattle
	B. suis		Swine
	B. canis		Dogs
Erysipeloid	*Erysipelothrix rhusiopathiae*	Gram-positive rods	Swine, poultry, fish
Leptospirosis[b]	*Leptospira interrogans*	Spirochete	Rodents, foxes, domestic animals
Melioidosis[b]	*Pseudomonas pseudomallei*	Gram-negative rods	Rodents
Glanders[a]	*Pseudomonas mallei*	Gram-negative rods	Equines, domestic mammals
Tularemia[a,b,c]	*Francisella tularensis*	Gram-negative rods	Rabbits, rodents
Viruses			
Foot and mouth disease	Aphthovirus	Picornavirus family	Cattle
Orf (contagious ecthyma)	Parapox virus	Poxvirus family	Sheep, goats
Vesicular stomatitis	Vesicular stomatitis virus	Rhabdovirus family	Cattle, horses virus
Parasite			
Cutaneous larva migrans (creeping eruption)	*Ancylostoma caninum* (dog hookworm)	Nematode	Dogs, cats, carnivores
	Ancylostoma braziliense (dog and cat hookworm)	Nematode	
Fungi			
Dermatophytes	Zoophilic trichophytons, microsporums	Fungi	Dogs, cats, cattle
Miscellaneous			
Cat scratch fever[d]	Unknown	Gram-negative rods	Cats, dogs suspected

Alternative portals:
[a] Inhalation.
[b] Ingestion.
[c] Arthropod vector.
[d] Animal bite.

of the biting animal, and both are neurotropic. They migrate to the central nervous system and cause paralysis, encephalitis, and even respiratory arrest.

Inhalation

Zoonotic microorganisms may be inhaled in two ways: 1) from infected droplets aerosolized from the respiratory tract of animals, as in the case of bovine tuberculosis; or 2) from an inanimate reservoir, generally soil, that is contaminated with excreta or carcasses of infected animals. Examples are anthrax and Q fever, which are caused by spore-forming organisms that are resistant in the environment. As can logically be expected, the primary clinical manifestation of zoonoses acquired by inhalation is pneumonia (Table 70.4). Disseminated infections occur after invasion of the bloodstream.

Ingestion

Most zoonoses that are acquired by ingestion are caused by bacteria or animal parasites (Table 70.5). The bacterial diseases are acquired by the direct ingestion of the organisms, usually in contaminated foodstuffs. Salmonellosis has emerged as one of the most prevalent zoonotic diseases in the U.S. The reservoir for *Salmonella* includes poultry, eggs, and dairy products. It has been suggested that the addition of antibiotics to animal feed has increased the infectivity of this organism in humans. Animal parasites are usually ingested as ova or cysts. In some cases, the ova or cysts must be activated in the human host as part of the developmental cycle of the parasite. In others a cyst may contain viable organisms.

DAMAGE

The clinical manifestations of zoonotic infections generally depend on the **portal of entry**. If the route is in-

Table 70.2. Arthropod Vectors

Disease	Vector	Organism	Microbial Group	Animal Reservoir
Bacteria				
Lyme Disease	Tick	*Borrelia burgdorferi*	Spirochete	Rodents, deer
Plague—bubonic[c]	Flea	*Yersinia pestis*	Gram-negative rods	Urban rats, rodents
Relapsing fever	Tick	*Borrelia species*	Spirochete	Rodent, wild mammals
Tularemia[a,b,c]	Tick, biting flies	*Francisella tularensis*	Gram-negative rods	Rodents, wild mammals, birds
Rocky Mountain spotted fever	Tick	*Rickettsia rickettsii*	Rickettsia	Wild rodents, dogs
Scrub typhus	Mite (chigger)	*Rickettsia tsutsugamushi*	Rickettsia	Wild rodents, rats
Murine typhus	Flea	*Rickettsia typhi*	Rickettsia	Rats
Rickettsialpox	Mite	*Rickettsia akari*	Rickettsia	Mice
Ehrlichiosis	Ticks	*Ehrlichia canis*	Ehrlichia	Canines, especially dogs
Viruses				
Yellow Fever	Mosquito	Flavivirus	Togavirus family	Primates
Encephalitis	Mosquito	Alphavirus	Togavirus family	Birds, horses
Eastern Equine				
Western Equine				
Venezuelan Equine				
St. Louis	Mosquito	Flavivirus	Togavirus family	Birds
California	Mosquito	Bunyavirus	Bunyavirus family	Mammals, wild rodents
Rift Valley fever	Mosquito	Bunyavirus	Bunyavirus family	Sheep, goats, cattle
Crimean-Congo Hemorrhagic fever	Tick	Bunyavirus	Bunyavirus family	Domestic mammals, rodents
Colorado tick fever	Tick	Orbivirus	Reovirus family	Rodents
Protozoa				
Babesiosis	Tick	*Babesia species*		Domestic and wild animals
Leishmaniasis (Kala-azar, cutaneous Leishmaniasis)	Sandfly	*Leishmania species*		Dogs, foxes, rodents, wild mammals
American trypanosomiasis	Reduviid bug (kissing bug)	*Trypanosoma cruzi*		Dogs, cats, opossums, armadillos, wild mammals
African sleeping sickness	Tsetse fly	*Trypanosoma species*		Reptiles, cattle, wild animals

Alternative portals:
[a] Inhalation.
[b] Ingestion.
[c] Skin penetration.

halation, the primary disease is usually pneumonia. If the organisms penetrate the skin, the primary manifestations are cellulitis near the site of entry, often followed by regional lymphadenitis (plague, tularemia, anthrax). The organisms may then disseminate to other tissues via the bloodstream. Ingestion of the organisms leads to early gastrointestinal symptoms and later systemic symptoms following dissemination through the bloodstream. In parasitic zoonoses, the clinical manifestations depend on the target organ favored by the released organism. In cysticercosis, for example, central nervous system dysfunction results from encystment of the larvae

in the brain; in trichinosis, myalgias result from the encystment of the larvae in skeletal muscles; in echinococcosis, abdominal pains result from enlarging cysts in the liver; in giardiasis, diarrhea and malabsorbtion result from invasion of the small intestine by trophozoites; in Lyme disease, neurologic, cardiac, and arthritic symptoms arise from spirochetal invasion of the central nervous system, heart, and joints.

All of these clinical manifestations are seen in tularemia, since the causative bacillus, *Francisella tularensis,* may enter humans via **multiple portals.** When it penetrates the skin via minute abrasions, a papule develops

Table 70.3. Animal Bite

Disease	Organism name	Group	Animal
Bacteria			
Pasteurellosis[a]	*Pasteurella multocida*	Gram-negative rods	Dogs, cats, birds, and wild mammals
Rat bite fever[a,b]	*Spirillum minor*	Spirochete	Rats, mice, cats
	Streptobacillus moniliformis	Gram-negative rods	Rats, rodents, turkeys
"DF-2"	*Capnocytophaga canimorsus*	Gram-negative rods	Dogs
Viruses			
Rabies	Rabies virus	Rhabdovirus	Domestic mammals skunks, foxes, opossums, bats, cattle
Herpes B encephalomyelitis	*Herpesvirus simiae* (Monkey pox virus)	Herpes virus	Monkeys
Fungi			
Blastomycosis	*Blastomyces dermatitidis*		Dogs

Alternative portal:
[a] Skin penetration.
[b] Ingestion.

Table 70.4. Inhalation

Disease	Organism name	Group	Animal reservoir	Inhalant
Bacteria				
Anthrax (Woolsorter's disease)	*Bacillus anthracis*	Gram-positive anaerobic spore-forming rod	Goats, sheep	Spores from wool, animal hides
Tuberculosis	*Mycobacterium tuberculosis*	Acid-fast bacillus	Domestic mammals	Contaminated respiratory secretions
Q fever	*Coxiella burnetii*	*Rickettsia*	Domestic animals	Soil and fomites contaminated with animal excretions
Ornithoses (psittacosis)	*Chlamydia psittaci*	*Chlamydia*	Parrots, turkeys, birds	Dried excreta from infected birds
Fungi				
Histoplasmosis	*Histoplasma capsulatum*		Birds, bats	Microconidia from contaminated soil
Viruses				
Lymphocytic[a,b] choriomeningitis	Lymphocytic choriomeningitis virus	Arenavirus family	Mice, hamsters rodents	Infected aerosols

Alternative portals:
[a] Skin penetration.
[b] Animal bite.

at the site of entry and later ulcerates. Regional lymphadenopathy and fever (ulceroglandular form) soon follows. The organisms can accidentally be inoculated into the skin or the conjunctiva during the skinning of an infected carcass, resulting in symptoms of conjunctivitis and cervical lymphadenopathy (oculoglandular form). The bacteria can also be inhaled as a result of a laboratory accident or via dust contaminated with excretions from infected rodents. The disease is then characterized by pharyngitis, pneumonia, fever, and muscle aches (pneumonic form). In addition, the organisms may be transmitted by bites of ticks or flies, resulting in systemic manifestations at various sites. If the portal of entry into the human host differs from that of the animal, the clinical manifestations differ correspondingly. For example, ornithosis in birds results in diarrhea and systemic signs because the chlamydiae enter via the gastrointestinal tract. In humans, the same organisms cause pneumonia

Table 70.5. Ingestion

Disease	Organism name	Group	Animal	Ingestant (contaminated foodstuff)
Bacteria				
Brucellosis[a]	*Brucella melitensis* *B. abortus*	Gram-negative rods	Goats, cattle	Dairy products
Campylobacter infection	*Campylobacter jejuni*	Gram-negative rods	Domestic mammals, fowl	Milk, water, meat, poultry
Listeriosis[a]	*Listeria monocytogenes*	Gram-positive rods	Domestic mammals, rodents, birds	Vegetables, water, cheese
Salmonellosis	*Salmonella* species (not *S. typhi*)	Gram-negative rods	Fowl, domestic mammals, turtles	Milk, eggs, meat, poultry, shellfish
Tuberculosis[b]	*Mycobacterium bovis*	Acid-fast bacillus	Cattle	Milk
Virus				
Lassa fever[2]	Arenavirus family		Mouse	Contaminated food
Protozoa				
Giardiasis	*Giardia lamblia*		Wild animals	Cyst in water
Cryptosporidiosis	*Cryptosporidium*		Calves	Oocysts
Toxoplasmosis	*Toxoplasma gondii*		Cat	Oocysts from cat feces; tissue cyst from uncooked meat
Helminths				
Tapeworms	*Taenia saginata*	Cestode	Cattle	Larva (cysticercus) in undercooked beef
	Taenia solium	Cestode	Pigs	Larva (cysticercus) in undercooked pork; ova in soil
	Diphyllobothrium latum	Cestode	Fish	Larvae in raw fish
	Echinococcus	Cestode	Dogs, sheep, reindeer, caribou, wolves	Ova
Anisakiasis	*Anisakis*	Nematode	Marine fish	Larva in undercooked fish
Trichinosis	*Trichinella spiralis*	Nematode	Pigs, domestic mammals, wild mammals, rodents	Larval cysts
Visceral larva migrans	*Toxocara canis* (roundworm of dogs)	Nematode	Dog	Ova in soil

Alternative portals:
[a] Skin penetration.
[b] Inhalation.

and cough because they usually enter via the respiratory route.

Finally, it should be noted that when an organism has remained in close contact with the host for many generations, clinical symptoms tend to be latent or subacute. For example, lassitude is a cardinal symptom in many parasitic infections.

CONTROL

The control of zoonoses must be multidisciplinary because of the various animal reservoirs and modes of transmission of the agents. Control measures often depend on such varied disciplines as human and veterinary medicine, sanitary engineering, and in some instances, entomology, and wildlife zoology. Some appropriate interventions include: eradication of the infected animal reservoir (slaughter of infected domestic or wild animals), protection of the animals before they can become infected (improved sanitary practices, vaccination, antibiotics), killing the organisms before they can come in contact with humans (pasteurization of milk, cooking of food), or for zoonoses that depend on arthropod vectors, the eradication of flies, mosquitoes, etc. (insecticide application, sanitation). Experience has taught us that single approaches do not work as well as an integrated attack on several sanitary and medical fronts.

SUGGESTED READINGS

Acha PN, Szyfres B. Zoonoses and communicable diseases common to man and animals. 2nd ed. Washington, DC: Pan American Health Organization, WHO, 1989.

Butler T. Plague and other *Yersinia* infections. New York: Plenum Press, 1983.

Last JM, ed. Maxcy-Rosenau public health and preventive medicine. 11th ed. New York: Appleton-Century-Crofts, 1980.

Steele JH, ed. CRC handbook series in zoonoses. Boca Raton, FL: CRC Press, 1979–1982.

Weinberg AN. Zoonoses. In: Mandell G, Douglas R, Bennet J, eds. Principles and practice of infectious diseases. 4th ed. New York: Churchill Livingstone, 1995: 2790–2795.

CHAPTER 71

Fever: A Clinical Sign of Infection

SUZANNE F. BRADLEY

WHAT IS NORMAL BODY TEMPERATURE?

Rigors (shivering), sweats, chills, flushing, tachycardia, lethargy, and increased warmth of skin have been recognized as signs and symptoms of disease since ancient times. Although crude mercury thermometers had been available for more than a century, the significance of increased body temperature and its association with the signs and symptoms of disease (fever) was not fully appreciated until 1871, when Carl Wunderlich reported his detailed studies of body temperature.

Generally, **normal body temperature** ranges from 97.3–99.5°F or 36.3–37.5°C in healthy humans. Body temperature normally fluctuates 0.5–0.9°F, with the lowest measurements noted between 2–8 am and the highest between 4–9 pm (diurnal variation). Temperature measurements vary when measured at different body sites. Rectal temperature measurements are generally 1°F higher than oral temperature measurements. Normal temperatures may be higher in females and lower in newborns and the debilitated elderly. Therefore, the accepted "normal temperature" of 98.6°F or 37°C, an average value, may have little clinical meaning. Within these limitations, temperatures above 99.4°F orally and 100.4°F rectally are generally accepted as abnormal in immuncompetent adults. Abnormal temperatures in newborns and the elderly may be lower.

Every elevated temperature does not necessarily require evaluation for underlying disease. Normal elevations of body temperatures of 1–1.5°F may be observed transiently in healthy persons after vigorous exercise or eating. A brief local increase in oral temperature measurements can occur after smoking, gum chewing, or drinking warm liquids. Following a self-limited febrile infection, some patients continue to take their temperature even though the illness has resolved. A diary that details early morning and evening temperatures, measurements when the patient feels warm, and associated activities may be a helpful tool to determine whether a temperature is abnormal or merely reflects daily activities or normal diurnal variation.

ABNORMAL REGULATION OF THERMOREGULATION (HYPERTHERMIA)

Humans regulate their body temperature by voluntary and involuntary means. A person who feels too cool will move to a warmer environment or put on warmer clothing. To minimize loss of body heat, **peripheral vasoconstriction** occurs via α-adrenergic receptors of the sympathetic nervous system. Heat may be generated through the involuntary contraction of skeletal muscle (shivering) and increased catabolism. Conversely, cooling is accomplished through movement to a cooler environment, removal of excess clothing, vasodilatation mediated via β-adrenergic receptors, and sweating (via cholinergic receptors). Dysregulation of normal thermoregulatory mechanisms leading to increased body temperature is termed **hyperthermia**.

Patients with mild hyperthermia (heat exhaustion) may feel lethargic, thirsty, and with clammy skin and signs of mild dehydration. In patients with **severe hyperthermia** (heat stroke), high temperatures, delirium, coma, warm dry skin, signs of severe dehydration, organ failure, cardiac arrythmias, and death may ensue. Treatment includes rehydration and immersion in cooling baths. Because hyperthermia is not mediated by endogenous pyrogens, antipyretics are not effective in lowering body temperature.

Persons with impairment of any aspect of thermoregulation may be at increased risk of hyperthermia. The elderly, demented individuals, and patients with cerebrovascular accidents and other neuropsychiatric disorders may have impaired thermal perception. Conditions that impair mobility may prevent an individual from removing themselves from a warm environment. Drugs with α-adrenergic activity may prevent vasodilatation, and those that increase fluid loss (diuretics) or have anticholinergic side effects (antipsychotics, antiemetics) may impair sweating. Patients with skin disorders that impair sweating may be at risk, as are those with cervical spinal cord injuries that impair the sympathetic nervous system leading to dysregulated thermoregulatory responses. Endocrine disorders such as hyperthyroidism and pheochromocytoma or increased skeletal muscle activity as seen in generalized seizures may also lead to hyperthermia.

THE PATHOPHYSIOLOGY OF FEVER

Fever is a normal physiologic phenomenon regulated by the central nervous system. Thus, fever differs in its pathophysiology from the dysregulated phenomenon of hyperthermia. Fever is caused by the release of **inflammatory mediators (endogenous pyrogens)**, stimulated by invading pathogens, e.g., bacteria, viruses, fungi, and parasites. (See Chapter 6, "Constitutive Defenses"). The microbial products that elicit this response are surface components (e.g., endotoxin, lipoteichoic acids, muramyl dipeptide, mannan), and exotoxins (staphylococcal TSST-1). Antigen–antibody complexes can also stimulate endogenous pyrogen production. Endogenous pyrogen activity has been attributed to several **cytokines**, interleukin-1 (IL-1), tumor necrosis factor (TNF), IL-6, macrophage inflammatory protein-1 (MIP-1), and α- and β-interferon (IFN). In addition, IL-2, gamma-interferon (γ-IFN), and others may indirectly cause fever by stimulating the production of these cytokines. The relative contributions of each of these cytokines to the febrile response are not clear. Many different cells contribute to the production of these mediators, but most are probably produced by monocytes and macrophages. Endogenous pyrogens presumably travel to the brain via the circulation, although TNF and IL-1 are frequently not detected by assays of the blood in patients with overwhelming infection.

Circulating endogenous pyrogens probably act at those portions of the brain that have fenestrated capillaries and thus lack a complete blood–brain barrier. These areas, the **circumventricular organs**, are close to the preoptic/anterior hypothalamus and brainstem, which are important regulatory centers for autonomic and endocrine functions. One circumventricular organ, the organum vasculosum of the lamina terminalis (OVLT), appears to be important in the development of fever and recognition of cytokines in certain animals. It is not known which specific cells within the circumventricular organ respond to endogenous pyrogens.

The result of the action of endogenous pyrogens is an increase in **prostaglandin E₂** (PGE₂) levels. It is thought that local PGE₂ production in the OVLT stimulates neu-

ronal pathways to the hypothalamus and brainstem, which in turn results in the development of fever. Areas within the preoptic hypothalamus are important in thermoregulation (preoptic area), the secretion of hormones such as vasopressin and corticotropin-releasing hormone, regulation of blood flow (paraventricular nucleus), and the control of appetite (lateral hypothalamus). In addition to the sleep–wake centers located in the hypothalamus and brainstem, these centers account not only for the generation of fever, but also for its associated symptoms of chilling, rigors, cool clammy skin, anorexia, and lethargy.

Fever does not increase unimpeded while an infection persists. The preoptic hypothalamus contains multiple cell populations whose firing rate is temperature-dependent. It has been suggested that such warmth-sensitive neurons have an inhibitory effect on other neurons responsible for the generation of heat. Endogenous pyrogens may work by inhibiting these "warm" neurons, leading to an increase in the normal thermoregulatory set point in the hypothalamus.

The new elevated thermoregulatory set point is maintained by a complex negative feedback loop. Endogenous pyrogen production leads to increased corticotropin-releasing, factor-mediated stimulation of the hypopituitary–adrenal axis. The **adrenal glucocorticoids** so produced then inhibit cytokine production. Other factors with antiendogenous pyrogen activity, such as melanocyte-stimulating hormone and arginine vasopressin, may be produced by the central nervous system. Increased levels of the endogenous pyrogens themselves may downregulate their own production. In addition, target end organ cells, stimulated by cytokines, decrease their responsiveness to a specific mediator by downregulating the expression of the surface receptors for that cytokine, and in some instances, shed them.

As a result, patients who have reached the hypothetical thermoregulatory set point will begin to sweat and their vessels dilate to dissipate excess heat. If the patient's temperature falls below the thermoregulatory set point, the cycle begins again with rigors, chills, and vasoconstriction ensuing. External means of cooling a patient with fever, such as using ice packs and cooling blankets, will only further stimulate the body to reach its higher thermoregulatory set point. Frequent bouts of rigors and chills may be more uncomfortable to the patient than the fever itself. To prevent recurrence of fever, the disease that causes the fever must be treated and the thermoregulatory set point lowered through the use of **antipyretic agents** (aspirin, nonsteroidal anti-inflammatory drugs, acetaminophen) that inhibit endogenous pyrogen and PGE₂ production.

FEVER AS A BENEFICIAL HOST RESPONSE

In the last two centuries, fever has been perceived as a dangerous affliction to be eliminated by physician and layperson alike. However, until the 1800s and the advent of antipyretics, fever was seen as a potent ally purging patients of the bad humors that caused disease. The evolution of fever in unrelated species, plus the presence of multiple cytokines with redundant endogenous pyrogen activity, suggest that fever confers some survival advantage to the host.

In infected reptiles and fish, inhibiting fever results in increased mortality. Patients with bacteremia or peritonitis who are unable to mount a febrile response are more likely to die than those who develop fever. Inhibition of the febrile response with antipyretics has been associated with prolonged shedding of rhinovirus and delayed healing of varicella lesions.

In addition, endogenous pyrogens not only cause fever, but influence the recruitment and function of many types of cells. Not unexpectedly, some of these cells function optimally at higher body temperatures. Thus, phagocytosis and killing by neutrophils and macrophages is enhanced at elevated temperatures. Antigen presentation by macrophages, helper T-cell–dependent antibody production, lymphocyte proliferation, cytotoxic T-cell function, and production of IFN-γ, IL-1, and IL-2 all increase at higher temperatures.

Endogenous pyrogens decrease levels of trace metals (iron and zinc) which many bacteria require for growth. In addition, temperatures of 39–41°C directly inhibit the growth of some bacteria (pneumococci, gonococci, *Treponema pallidum, Mycobacterium leprae)*, fungi *(Sporotrichum schenkii)*, and some parasites in vitro. Motility, capsule formation, and cell wall formation may be inhibited and antimicrobial susceptibility may increase at increased temperatures. Because many of these microorganisms prefer to grow at cooler temperatures, they infect distal appendages. Local heating has been reported to be effective in the treatment of infection caused by chromomycosis, sporotrichosis, chancroid, and leishmaniasis.

In the past, physicians used artificial fever therapy, probably induced by infection with malaria, to treat leprosy, tumors, and other diseases. Recently, the artificial induction of fever in mammals has been shown to increase resistance to bacterial, fungal, and viral infections. In 1927, malarial therapy for neurosyphilis was sufficiently successful to earn its discoverer the Nobel Prize.

In animal studies, injection of recombinant endogenous pyrogens prior to or within a few hours of infection has been shown to reduce mortality, and sometimes the microbial load. Conversely, increased mortality has been seen when antibodies to endogenous pyrogens were given prior to some infections. Thus, evidence exists that fever may have a beneficial role in the host response to infection.

FEVER AS AN ADVERSE HOST RESPONSE

Unfortunately, the story of fever versus microbes is not clearly that of hero versus villain. Excessive production of endogenous pyrogens, the sepsis syndrome, may result in necrosis of tissues, end organ failure, shock, and even death. Monoclonal antibodies against TNF, an antagonist of the IL-1 receptor, and other cytokine inhibitors appear to confer protection in animals, but subsequent studies in humans have shown less promise for their therapeutic use. Future therapies must aim to control excessive endogenous pyrogen production without loss of the beneficial effects of these cytokines.

Moderate fever alone is not dangerous and generally does not require medical intervention except for patient comfort. Although one could argue that inhibiting fever may be detrimental, it should be recognized that an increase in temperature of 1°C or more over 37°C leads to a 13% rise in oxygen consumption. Very high fevers (106°F or 41°C) considerably increase host metabolic demands and place considerable stress on the cardiovascular system. Congestive heart failure and ischemia may result; thus, decreasing body temperature is essential in some patients. In the setting of very high fever, external cooling to rapidly reduce body temperature is appropriate when used in conjunction with antipyretics. Organ damage and death can theoretically occur when temperatures exceed 107°F.

Temperatures higher than 103°F or 40°C have been associated with generalized seizures in children. Children with prior seizures are likely to have further episodes, and there is little evidence that the early use of antipyretics and anticonvulsants is helpful in preventing further seizures. Fortunately, neurologic sequelae and resulting learning disabilities are very rare. Congenital malformations in the newborns of women who had high fevers while pregnant have also been reported.

EVALUATION OF ELEVATED TEMPERATURE

Elevated body temperature is a sign of possible disease. The temperature amplitude itself does not predict whether a patient has serious disease. Classic fever patterns, when present, may suggest specific diseases: Hodgkin's disease (Pel-Ebstein fever), malaria (tertian and quartan fever), yellow fever, dengue (saddle back or biphasic fever), or spirochetal diseases post-treatment (Jarisch-Herxheimer reaction).

A careful clinical history, including present illness, past medical history, prescription and nonprescription medications, travel history, pets, family history, and review of systems is essential in order to narrow the diagnostic possibilities. A thorough physical examination looking for signs involving specific organ systems may further confirm or exclude clinical suspicions. How fast this evaluation is performed and treatment is initiated depends on the clinical status of the patient. A patient who appears clinically well can be evaluated and treated at a more leisurely pace than the patient who appears to be severely ill.

Infections are the most common causes of fever. Fortunately, the majority of infections encountered in routine practice get better with time, regardless of whether treatment is initiated. Malignancies, granulomatous diseases, vasculitis, autoimmune diseases, drug reactions, and others may also present as febrile illnesses. Sometimes the etiology of fever defies easy diagnosis. This uncommon clinical syndrome, termed **fever of unknown** or **undetermined origin** (FUO), remains one of the greatest clinical challenges in medicine.

FEVERS OF UNKNOWN ORIGIN (FUO)

■ CASE

Mr. J. is an 82-year-old man who felt well until 1 year ago, when he noted a significant decline in his vision, intermittent jaw pain, and headaches associated with night sweats, anorexia, weight loss of 20 lb, and occasional temperatures greater than 101.5°F. Prior examination revealed a decline in vision, mild anemia, and an erythrocyte sedimentation rate (ESR) of 129 mm/hr (normal 0–20). The change in vision, anemia, anorexia, and elevated ESR was ascribed to "old age," and the jaw pain to poor dentition. He was treated with multiple antibiotics for "sinusitis" and "bronchitis," although he denied productive cough or pain over his sinuses.

Mr. J. has no allergies and takes no medications. He is a retired insurance salesman who has traveled throughout the United States. He lives with his wife, a dog, and a cat. His medical and family history are unremarkable. He looks relatively well, but his clothes fit loosely. Physical examination is unremarkable except for a temperature of 102°F, a resting pulse of 105 beats/min, and tenderness over the right temple. No sinus tenderness is elicited by palpation and the chest examination is normal.

The following questions arise:

- Given the duration and severity of his symptoms, what are the most likely diagnoses that would explain Mr. J.'s fever?
- Does Mr. J. require an extensive inpatient evaluation?
- How might you begin to evaluate the potential causes for Mr. J.'s symptoms?

Mr J. has a fever of unknown origin (FUO) of longstanding duration. He looks relatively well, so that it is not likely that he has an occult abscess, tuberculosis, or malignancy. His workup does not necessarily require hospitalization. Dismissing patient symptoms as normal consequences of aging is unwise. Declining vision, jaw pain, and ESR greater than 100 mm/hr in an elderly man strongly suggests temporal arteritis. An outpatient temporal artery biopsy revealed granulomas consistent with this diagnosis. With corticosteroid therapy, the patient's fever and jaw pain resolved, he regained weight, and his vision and anemia rapidly improved.

What is FUO?

FUO is usually defined as the presence of temperatures higher than 101°F or 38.3°C noted on multiple occasions over a 3-week period. A possible etiology of that fever must not be evident following reasonable intensive diagnostic evaluation over a period of approximately 1 week. This definition excludes most self-limited causes of fever that usually resolve spontaneously or prolonged fevers that are diagnosed promptly.

The diseases that cause FUO usually are not rare or unusual, but are often the atypical presentation of common diseases. Diagnosis is frequently delayed not because too few tests were ordered but because the physician overlooked significant clues to the diagnosis or misinterpreted their significance. Diagnosis may be particularly difficult in the very young or very old who are unable to adequately perceive, interpret, and communicate their symptoms. Repeated clarification of the history and reexamination of the patient can be extremely valuable. Each symptom, physical finding, and laboratory abnormality should be thoroughly evaluated and used to guide the judicious ordering of invasive or expensive diagnostic tests.

The spectrum of diseases responsible for FUOs changes with time as technological advances lead to improvements in diagnosis. The advent of computerized tomography, magnetic resonance, and radionucleotide imaging has removed from the FUO category many patients with **abscesses**, **bacterial endocarditis**, and **collagen vascular diseases** (autoimmune/immune complex-mediated diseases).

While we have become more successful in determining many causes of FUO, changes in the population result in new challenges. The spectrum of diseases causing FUO may vary in patients who are immunocompromised, e.g., HIV-infected patients, transplant recipients, the elderly, and those who develop FUO in the hospital. In general, infection remains the most common cause of FUO, followed by neoplasms, collagen vascular diseases, and granulomatous diseases (Table 71.1). Very rarely, patients will cause fever by injecting themselves with pyrogenic substances (fraudulent fever) or manipulate the temperature-measuring device so that they appear to have fever (factitious fever).

Treatment

Even with improvements in diagnostic technology, 10% of FUO patients still defy diagnosis. Fortunately, most patients with undiagnosed FUO do well. Greater than 95% of patients under the age of 35 spontaneously recover without therapy. In persons over the age of 65, spontaneous resolution is rare, and a serious disease is usually ultimately found. Empiric trials of antitubercular therapy, corticosteroids, and anti-inflammatory agents may be tried in patients with persistent FUO, but only if the patient's clinical

Table 71.1. Differential Diagnosis of Fevers of Unknown Origin (FUO)

Category	Cases (%)
Infections	30–40
Abscesses (intra-abdominal)	
Hepatic, biliary	
Tuberculosis	
Endocarditis	
Cytomegalovirus infection	
HIV infection	
Malignancies	20–30
Hematologic	
Leukemias (monocyte-derived)	
Lymphomas (Hodgkin's disease, non-Hodgkin's)	
Myeloma	
Solid tumors	
Hypernephroma (renal)	
Hepatoma (liver)	
Collagen vascular diseases	10–15
Rheumatoid arthritis (Still's disease)	
Systemic lupus erythematosus	
Rheumatic fever	
Arteritis (temporal arteritis, polyarteritis nodosa)	
Granulomatous diseases	5–10
Sarcoidosis	
Inflammatory bowel disease (Crohn's disease)	
Granulomatous hepatitis	
Miscellaneous	10–20
Pulmonary embolus	
Drug fever	
Hematoma	
Occupational (metal fume fever)	
Periodic (Familial Mediterranean fever)	
Thermoregulatory disorders[a]	
Cervical spinal cord injuries	
Endocrine diseases (hyperthyroidism, Addison's disease)	
Congenital skin disorders	
Factitious[b]/Fraudulent fever	
No diagnosis	10–15

[a] Although included as FUO, the elevated body temperatures in these disorders are not fever, but hyperthermia.

[b] Although included as FUO, patients manipulate temperature-measuring devices, giving the illusion that they are febrile.

condition is deteriorating rapidly and only after exhaustive attempts to make the diagnosis have failed.

CONCLUSION

It is important to interpret elevated body temperature measurements only after careful assessment of the patient. Not all elevated body temperatures are fever. Fever may be a beneficial host response. Some elevations of body temperature require treatment, others only careful observation. Treat the underlying cause, not just the elevated body temperature! The treatment of hyperthermia is different from that of fever. Some etiologies of fever may be difficult to discern. A careful approach is essential for diagnosis, and empirical therapy should be used only as a last resort.

SUGGESTED READINGS

Kazanjian PH. Fever of unknown origin: review of 86 patients treated in community hospitals. Clin Infect Dis 1992;15: 968.

Knockaert DC, Vanneste LJ, Vanneste SB, Bobbaers HJ. Fever of unknown origin in the 1980's: an update of the diagnostic spectrum. Arch Intern Med 1992;152:51.

Larson EB, Featherstone HJ, Petersdorf RG. Fever of undetermined origin: diagnosis and follow-up of 105 cases, 1970–1980. Medicine 1982;61:269.

Mackowiak PA, ed. Fever: basic mechanisms and management. New York: Raven Press, 1991.

Mackowiak PA, Worden G. Carl Reinhold August Wunderlich and the evolution of clinical thermometry. Clin Infect Dis 1994;18:458.

Miralles P, Moreno S, Perez-Tascon M, Cosin J, Diaz MD, Bouza E. Fever of uncertain origin in patients infected with the human immunodeficiency virus. Clin Infect Dis 1995; 20:872.

Saper CB, Breder CD. The neurologic basis of fever. N Engl J Med 1994;330:1880.

CHAPTER 72

Nosocomial and Latrogenic Infections

DAVID R. SNYDMAN

OVERVIEW

Approximately 5% of all patients develop an infection during their stay in the hospital. These hospital-acquired conditions are known as **nosocomial infections.** An infection that is the result of intervention by a physician, in or out of a hospital, is known as **iatrogenic.** Nosocomial infections often result in a prolonged hospital stay and are extraordinarily costly in terms of morbidity and even mortality. It is estimated that about 5 billion dollars are spent each year for the management of hospital-acquired infections in the U. S.

A number of factors related to hospitalization predispose patients to the risk of a hospital-acquired infection. The most important factors are those that violate the host's own defenses. Invasive procedures produce **new portals of entry** for microorganisms from the patient's own flora or from the environment. Examples of invasion are the use of devices such as endotracheal tubes, mechanical ventilators, intravenous or intra-arterial catheters, and surgical procedures in general.

Broadly speaking, the incidence of nosocomial infections is related to the severity of the underlying disease, i.e., patients who have a high likelihood of dying during their hospitalization also run a higher risk of developing nosocomial infections. In contrast, patients who are admitted with less severe disease are at lesser risk of acquiring infections in the hospital. This underscores the need for improved management of the severely compromised patient. Unfortunately, it is estimated that only about one-third to one-half of all nosocomial infections are preventable even under the most favorable conditions.

AGENTS OF NOSOCOMIAL AND IATROGENIC INFECTIONS

Generally speaking, the organisms that cause nosocomial and iatrogenic infections are similar to those found elsewhere in the community. The most common causative agents may not be especially pathogenic; in fact, sometimes they are even less pathogenic than those that cause disease outside of the hospital.

A salient example is the emergence of *Serratia marcescens* as a hospital-acquired pathogen. This bacterium was thought to be so benign that it was used in the 1950s to trace the movement of air in a subway system, and to determine the movement of bacteria into the urethra through the catheter–meatal interface. This "nonpathogen" has become the source of significant nosocomial infections, although it rarely causes disease outside the hospital.

Like many pathogens associated with nosocomial infections, *S. marcescens* has acquired significant antibiotic resistance. Gram-negative bacterial strains that possess plasmid-mediated, multiple antibiotic resistance are commonly encountered in nosocomial infections. Plasmid transfer occurs among different strains of the same species and even among different genera. **Transfer of antibiotic resistance** has been demonstrated in the urine of patients with Foley catheters and on patient's skin. Presumably, transfer of antibiotic resistance takes place in the gastrointestinal tract as well. Antibiotic-resistant pathogens have become so common that we regularly encounter methicillin-resistant *Staphylococcus aureus*, and aminoglycoside-resistant Gram-negative bacteria in nosocomial infections. Examples of nosocomial pathogens are listed in Table 72.1. The list of pathogens that can cause nosocomial infections encompasses the agents of practically all infections.

ENCOUNTER

A hospital is a microenvironment in which organisms can be transferred in a variety of ways from one individ-

Table 72.1. Common Hospital-acquired Infections and Frequently Associated Organisms

Type of infection	Most common organism
Surgical wounds	*Staphylococcus aureus* *Escherichia coli* *Streptococcus faecalis*
Pneumonia	*Klebsiella pneumoniae* *Pseudomonas aeruginosa* *Staphylococcus aureus* *Enterobacter* spp. *Escherichia coli*
Intravenous catheter	*Staphylococcus epidermidis* *Staphylococcus aureus* *Streptococcus faecalis* *Candida* spp.
Urinary catheter	*Escherichia coli* *Streptococcus faecalis* *Pseudomonas aeruginosa* *Klebsiella* spp.

ual to another, or from the hospital staff to the patients (Fig. 72.1). Transmission between individuals may be direct, by hand contact, or indirect, by inhalation, ingestion, or puncture through the integument. For example, methicillin-resistant staphylococci spread directly between patients or via hospital personnel. Tubercle bacilli are transmitted through aerosolization and inhalation. Viral agents, such as those of varicella or influenza, may be spread through the air to susceptible immunocompromised individuals. Blood used for transfusions may be contaminated with hepatitis A, B, and C viruses, or HIV. Food handlers may contaminate food eaten by patients, and physicians and nurses may introduce microorganisms into deeper tissues during operations or while dressing surgical or other wounds. Unusual epidemics can sometimes be traced to **specific carriers** among members of the hospital staff. For example, well-documented epidemics caused by group A streptococci have been attributed to carriers who had contact with patients in the operating room. In one epidemic, the organisms were located in the carrier's vagina, from where they were presumably aerosolized through normal body movements.

Microorganisms that spread to patients may be **endemic** to the hospital environment. Notable examples include the fungi that cause aspergillosis, which may be present as more or less visible mildew on moist room walls or construction panels. Infections by exogenous organisms may also be acquired from improperly sterilized surgical instruments and even contaminated disinfectant solutions. Fortunately, these events are rare in a proper hospital setting.

Patients acquire nosocomial infections as the result of breaks in their own defenses and from their inability to combat infection. These breaks usually occur as the result of **invasive diagnostic or therapeutic interventions** that physicians perform on patients. For these reasons, the most common nosocomial infections affect the urinary tract, because catheterization of the bladder is frequently used with bedridden patients. The commonly used Foley catheter bypasses the normal mucosal barriers and facilitates the entry of organisms that colonize the skin or the urinary introitus. The next most frequent type of infection is that of surgical wounds, followed by respiratory tract infections; both involve invasive procedures.

ENTRY

Skin Penetration

The skin barrier is breached by intravenous catheters or devices used to measure intravascular pressure. The longer these devices stay in place, the higher the risk of both local infection and bacteremia. This underscores the need for vigilance in the care of patients with indwelling devices. In national surveys in the U.S., the rate of nosocomial bacteremia has almost doubled in the decade of the 1980s, and that due to *Staphylococcus epi-*

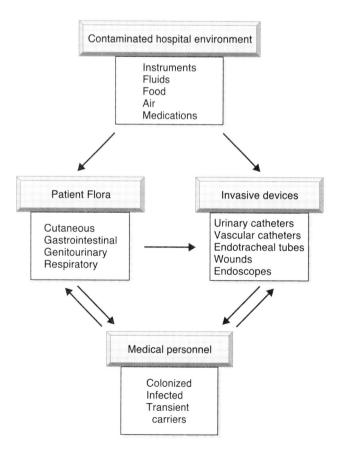

Figure 72.1. Sources of hospital-acquired infections.

dermidis, tripled. In the writer's institution, 1 in 100 patients develops hospital-acquired bacteremia; half of these cases are due to the implantation of intravascular devices.

Another example that illustrates the role of the normal skin in protecting from microbial invasion is that of burn victims. Frequently, patients who have extensive second or third degree burns will become colonized with bacteria, especially *Pseudomonas aeruginosa*. Necrotizing lesions at the site of skin damage are accompanied by sepsis, the major cause of death in burn victims.

Inhalation

The most common cause of nosocomial pneumonia is the use of an **endotracheal tube**. This bypasses the normal epithelial defenses and allows the entry of organisms via aerosols. In the early 1960s, when mechanical ventilation of the lungs was being developed, it was recognized that epidemics of Gram-negative pneumonia occurred because nebulized mists contained bacteria-laden aerosols. An understanding of the problem prompted in ventilator design, which have virtually eliminated the ventilator as a source of hospital-acquired pneumonia. Patients with endotracheal tubes still develop pneumonia, but now the offending organisms tend to come from the patient's stomach or intestine, which then colonize the nasopharynx. From here, the bacteria may be aspirated into the lungs. Other examples of nosocomial infections acquired by inhalation can be seen in hospital epidemics of influenza and varicella, which are particularly dangerous for immunocompromised patients.

Ingestion

Epidemics of nosocomial infection sometimes result from the ingestion of pathogenic bacteria. The organisms are often those associated with community-acquired infections, such as *Salmonella*, hepatitis A virus, and rotavirus, the latter being most frequent among neonates or infants. Epidemics of salmonellosis in hospitals usually result from eating foods contaminated during preparation. They have also resulted from the use of contaminated animal products used for diagnostic purposes, such as carmine dye.

Inanimate Environment

The complexity of a hospital environment provides innumerable opportunities for the encounter of patients with microorganisms. Some of these encounters are specific to the hospital environments and do not usually occur elsewhere. An example is the use of **contaminated intravenous solutions**, which have caused many epidemics. Contamination rarely takes place at the point of manufacture; more commonly, it occurs during the **handling of bottles and infusion lines.**

Instruments and dressings improperly sterilized before surgery also provide a possible source of infection.

A separate technology has developed to solve the problem of determining if autoclaves and sterilizing ovens perform their expected task. Thus, it is customary to insert a vial containing bacterial spores with the material to be autoclaved, and to determine spore viability afterward. Deviance from established procedures may result in improper sterilization and in contamination of surgical or other wounds.

MODEL INFECTIONS

▮ CASE 1: URINARY TRACT INFECTION

Mr. H., a 67-year-old man, underwent a transurethral prostatectomy for cancer of the prostate. Because of concern about postoperative bleeding from straining during urination, he had a Foley catheter placed into the bladder. Three days later, Mr. H. developed a urinary tract infection with low-grade fever, some pain, and pyuria. Quantitative urine counts yielded 3×10^5 colonies of *Escherichia coli* per ml of urine. The organisms were resistant to all tested antibiotics except for the aminoglycosides. Within 2 days, Mr. H. developed bacteremia with hypotension and shock. Physicians were eventually able to control the bacteremia with gentamicin therapy. Fortunately, Mr. H. recovered completely and was discharged.

How did Mr. H. acquire this infection? This case is a classic example of a nosocomial infection of the urinary tract. The use of Foley catheters for more than 1 or 2 days often results in contamination of the bladder, especially by fecal coliforms. Currently, catheters are usually provided with an expandable collection bag for urine, thus making a closed system. Nonetheless, the risk of bacteriuria is cumulative and still occurs at a rate between 5% and 8%/day. The risk of bacteriuria is related to the skill of the person inserting the catheter, the sex and age of the patient, and the duration of catheterization.

▮ CASE 2: NOSOCOMIAL WOUND INFECTION

Ms. Z., an 82-year-old woman with rheumatic heart disease, underwent a mitral valve replacement along with surgery for a coronary artery bypass graft. Her postoperative course was complicated by bleeding in the mediastinum, which required more surgery. She did well after these operations and was discharged after 12 days. Three weeks later, Ms. Z. noticed some purulent drainage along the wound site on her chest. She continued to have pain but did not tell her family, assuming that the pain was related to her healing process. When she returned to see the surgeon 1 month later, she reported her pain and low-grade fever. The surgeon noted that there was considerable drainage at the wound site. Probing the wound, he noticed a lot of pus.

Ms. Z. was hospitalized again for radical debridement (cleaning) of her chest wound. Cultures of the pus yielded *S. epidermidis*. She was treated intravenously with vancomycin for 6 weeks and her wound was debrided with the wires in her sternum removed. At the end of this period, she required a plastic surgical procedure and a muscle flap to close the wound. After 2 more months of hospitalization, she was discharged and continued her convalescence at home.

This case illustrates the problem of surgical wound infections and the serious impact they can have on the patient's recovery. Wound infections of the mediastinum complicate between 1% and 5% of open heart surgeries. If the infection reaches deep portions of the chest, its effect can be extremely serious. Patients frequently require multiple surgical interventions with removal of devitalized bone, cartilage, and other tissue.

Surgical wound infections are the most costly of all nosocomial infections. Some are clearly preventable. They are frequently due to *S. aureus*, but the example used here illustrates that *S. epidermidis*, a normal skin commensal, may also be a significant pathogen. In the case of Ms. Z., the source of the infection was probably her own skin flora. As with other infections, the establishment depends on the size of the inoculum, the pathogenic potential of the invading organisms, and the state of host defenses. All of these factors should be taken into account before planning surgical treatment. In cases where infection would be devastating, as in artificial hip implants, surgeons may go to great lengths to prevent wound infections, such as using laminar air flow systems and prophylactic antibiotics.

▉ CASE 3: PRIMARY BACTEREMIA

Fifty-nine-year-old Mr. S. was hospitalized with acute myocardial infarction. His disease was so severe that he required a catheter to measure his cardiac pressure and output. Unfortunately, the catheter was left in place for several more days than was probably necessary. Six days after his infarction, Mr. S. developed fever, leukocytosis, and inflammation at the site of insertion of the catheter. Four blood cultures all revealed the presence of *S. aureus*. He was treated with intravenous antibiotics; however, a new cardiac murmur was noted 7 days into therapy. An echocardiogram revealed the development of a tricuspid valve vegetation. Mr. S. required 4 weeks of antibiotic therapy for his hospital-acquired, catheter-related endocarditis.

This case illustrates an example of primary bacteremia, which is defined as bacteremia that cannot be ascribed to another focus of infection. Primary bacteremia is frequently either the result of a contaminated intravenous line or associated with granulocytopenia in the immunosuppressed leukemic patient.

From the bottle to the intravenous catheter, intravenous therapy provides many potential sources of contamination. The risk of intravenous catheter-related infection is generally influenced by the type of catheter and the duration of catheterization. Patients who have large-bore catheters that require surgical insertion have the highest risk. If the catheter is left in place for 48 hours or longer, the patient has a 23% risk of bacteremia. In the example cited, the patient developed endocarditis, a rare but recognized complication. The usual pathogens tend to be *S. aureus*, *S. epidermidis*, a variety of Gram-negative rods, or *Candida* (Table 72.1).

Another example of primary bacteremia is generally seen in leukemia or lymphoma patients who are granulocytopenic as a result of cancer chemotherapy. These patients frequently become bacteremic, primarily from an intestinal focus. The usual pathogens in this setting are Gram-negative rods, which may originate from the patient's endogenous flora or may be exogenously acquired in the hospital.

▉ CASE 4: NOSOCOMIAL PNEUMONIA

Ms. J. was hospitalized for therapy of acute leukemia. Over a 3-week period, her blood cell count remained low as a result of her chemotherapy. At the end of this period, she developed a pulmonary infiltrate and sinusitis. She was treated with broad-spectrum antibiotics but failed to respond. Her lung involvement progressed and an open lung biopsy was performed. A species of *Aspergillus* (*A. fumigatus*) was cultured from this material. She was started on amphotericin B but became progressively more ill and died within a week.

Nosocomial aspergillosis, while not common, has recently been seen more often among immunosuppressed patients. A number of reported epidemics have been linked to hospital construction and contamination of air conditioning systems. Large numbers of fungal spores in the air lead to nasal or bronchial colonization. Immunosuppression and the resultant granulocytopenia, along with broad-spectrum antibacterial antibiotics, help the organism become established in the airways.

This case illustrates a relatively uncommon mode of acquisition of organisms that cause nosocomial pneumonia. More often, patients aspirate stomach or nasopharyngeal contents as a result of their debilitation. Infections acquired in this manner are frequently caused by a mixed aerobic–anaerobic bacterial flora. Unfortunately, nosocomial pneumonia is the least preventable of all hospital-acquired infections and is associated with the highest mortality rate.

CASE 5. NOSOCOMIAL BLOODBORNE DISEASE

Dr. T. developed a needlestick injury while recapping a needle from a patient who abused intravenous drugs. About 2 months later, Dr. T. developed arthralgias, fatigue, malaise, and jaundice. He slowly recovered but lost 3 months of work. He was diagnosed as having hepatitis B.

For decades, hepatitis B has been recognized as a nosocomial hazard for both health workers and patients. Needlestick transmission is a recognized hazard, with rates of transmission approaching 25%. Blood transfusions constituted a major threat to patients before the early 1970s. Fortunately, the risk of transmission of hepatitis B virus has been recognized, and using hepatitis B surface antigen (HBsAg) screening has significantly reduced the bloodborne transmission of this virus.

The incidence of needlestick injuries has been significantly reduced by the practice of recapping needles, which accounts for 30% of these injuries. Hepatitis B can be prevented by vaccination, which should be given to all health workers. However, needlestick transmission of hepatitis C and HIV can still occur, and, for the unaware, hepatitis B still poses a problem.

CONTROL

Control of nosocomial infections requires awareness by all health care professionals. Hand washing between patient contacts is a simple but much neglected procedure. It can decrease transmission of microorganisms between hospital staff and patients. The use of aseptic techniques during surgical and other invasive procedures, as stressed in surgical training, significantly prevents these infections.

Hospitals have **infection control committees**, whose responsibility is to oversee all aspects of infection control within the institution. They supervise surveillance of hospital-acquired infections, establish policies and procedures to prevent such infections, and have the power to intervene when necessary in investigations of epidemics or other problems. Most hospitals have specific personnel, called **infection control practitioners**, who are assigned these tasks and function as the "eyes and ears" of the committee. These individuals are responsible for tracing epidemics, monitoring infection rates, and determining the level of isolation of patients. However, there is still a good deal to be learned. Intense efforts are directed at preventing infections in the increasing number of immunocompromised hosts and in devising effective means to prevent nosocomial pneumonias.

SUGGESTED READINGS

Bennett JV, Brachman PS, eds. Hospital infections. 6th ed. Boston: Little, Brown, 1997.

Martone WJ, Garner JS. Proceedings of the third decennial international conference on nosocomial infections. Am J Med 1991;91(Suppl 3B).

Wenzel RP, ed. Prevention and control of nosocomial infections, 3rd ed Baltimore: Williams and Wilkins, 1997.

Food-borne Diseases

DAVID R. SNYDMAN

Food-borne infections are a significant public health problem. In the U.S., these infections are a major cause of morbidity, although an infrequent cause of mortality. Between 1983 and 1987, 909 outbreaks were reported to the Centers for Disease Control from virtually all 50 states. The number of ill people reported to the health authorities in these outbreaks totaled more than 50,000, with 134 deaths. Studies suggest that the true incidence of infection related to food probably is 10–100 times more frequent.

A food-borne disease outbreak is defined by two criteria: (a) two or more persons must experience a similar illness, usually gastrointestinal, after ingestion of the same food; and (b) epidemiological analysis must implicate the food as the source of the illness. However, exceptions exist in this definition. For example, one case of botulism constitutes an outbreak for the purposes of epidemiological investigation and control because of the possibility that others may be involved.

The most common diseases in the U.S. acquired by **ingestion of contaminated food** are those usually called **food poisoning**. These diseases are caused by the consumption of food contaminated with bacteria, bacterial toxins, parasites, viruses, and chemicals. Bacteria cause approximately two-thirds of the food-borne outbreaks in the U.S. for which an etiology can be determined (Table 73.1). However, it should be noted that only in 44% of food-borne disease outbreaks is the etiology confirmed.

This chapter discusses major food poisoning illnesses that occur in the United States. The chapter is organized according to the three main types of food-borne illnesses:

- **Intoxications due to a toxin preformed in the food;** in these cases, the organism does not have to be alive to cause disease. Examples of causative bacteria are *Staphylococcus aureus, Clostridium botulinum,* and *Bacillus cereus.*

- **Intoxications due to toxins manufactured in the body** after live organisms such as *Vibrio cholerae* or *Clostridium perfringens* are ingested.
- **Intestinal invasive diseases,** such as gastroenteritis due to invasive organisms, e.g., *Salmonella* and *Campylobacter.*

The distinction between food-borne illnesses caused by toxin-producing organisms and those caused by invasive pathogens is important clinically and epidemiologically. In general, **diseases due to toxin-forming organisms** such as *S. aureus* have a short incubation period and are characterized by upper gastrointestinal complaints, such as nausea and vomiting. Diarrhea is less frequent, and constitutional symptoms, e.g., fever and chills, are uncommon. In contrast, **food poisonings caused by invasive organisms,** such as *Salmonella,* usually have a longer incubation period and are characterized by fever, chills, and lower gastrointestinal complaints. Diarrhea, often bloody or containing pus or mucus, is more prominent in these diseases than nausea or vomiting. Therefore, food poisoning is generally characterized by whether the symptoms of intoxication or invasion are more prominent. Some overlap exists in this classification scheme, because organisms such as *Shigella* and *Salmonella* may have invasive properties as well as the ability to produce toxin.

In the U.S., the most frequently recognized agents of bacterial food poisoning are generally limited to a dozen organisms (see Table 73.1). *Salmonella* outbreaks dominate the confirmed outbreaks and constitute over half of the reported cases of food-borne illness. This noted dominance is due, in part, to the ease with which the disease is recognized and to the awareness of physicians and the public. Shigellae are the next most frequent cause of food-borne outbreaks and are associated with 20% of reported cases. *S. aureus* and *C. perfringens* are the next most frequent and are associated with 56% of reported cases. *Campylobacter,* hepatitis A and Norwalk viruses,

Table 73.1. Recent Major Food-borne Outbreaks in the United States[a]

Year	Etiologic agent	Circumstances
1997	Hepatitis A	153 cases associated with eating frozen strawberries imported from Mexico and served in Michigan public schools
1996	*Cyclospora cayetanensis*	> 40 individual outbreaks and > 850 persons ill due to contaminated raspberries imported from Guatemala and distributed nationwide
1996	Enterohemorrhagic *E. coli*	Juice and cider made with "dropped" apples harvested from the ground. Sixty-six illnesses and one death in Western U.S. and Canada
1995	Norwalk virus	34 clusters of viral gastroenteritis cases associated with oysters harvested from Florida baywaters
1994	*Salmonella enteritidis*	Multistate outbreak due to contamination of a national brand of ice cream contaminated at the factory; an estimated 224,000 persons became ill
1993	Enterohemorrhagic *E. coli*	> 500 cases of hemorrhagic colitis associated with undercooked hamburgers served at 93 fast food restaurants in several states (four children died)
1991	*Vibrio cholerae*	Four cases in nontravelers associated with tainted coconut milk imported from Thailand
1990	*Clostridium perfringens*	700 cases of food poisoning in a Missouri prison associated with beef and chicken tacos
1988	*Campylobacter jejuni*	120 cases traced to raw milk served at a vacation Bible school in Kansas
1988	*Shigella sonnei*	3175 illnesses among people who ate raw tofu salad at an outdoor music festival in Michigan (117 hospitalized)

[a] Selected from among approximately 500 outbreaks each year reported to the Centers for Disease Control.

and other pathogens cause illness less frequently. Parasites and chemical agents acquired from food are the least frequent causes of food-borne disease. Features of the principal food-borne diseases are shown in Table 73.2.

It is important to note that **etiological patterns vary throughout the world.** Etiology depends on many factors, such as food preferences, awareness by physicians and the public, and laboratory capabilities. For example, in the U.S., food poisoning by *Salmonella* and *Shigella* represents about 70% of the outbreaks. In contrast, *C. perfringens* is implicated in over 90% of the recognized food-borne illness in England and Wales. Japan has yet different etiological patterns, with *Vibrio parahaemolyticus* gastroenteritis representing over 50% of reported outbreaks. For travelers from the U.S. to countries such as Mexico, the most common cause of diarrhea ("turista") is an enterotoxigenic strain of *Escherichia coli*.

INTOXICATIONS

CASE 1

Staphylococcus aureus

As the aircraft cruised at 35,000 feet, the cabin attendants passed out a lunch meal that included ham sandwiches. Two hours later, two-thirds of the passengers aboard the 747 jet plane developed nausea and vomiting. Diarrhea occurred in about one-third of those affected. The waiting lines for the facilities trailed down the aisle. As a result of such epidemics, rules for serving the cockpit crew different meals went into effect.

The following questions arise:
1. What was the cause of the outbreak?
2. How could one kind of meal have affected such a large number of individuals?

In the epidemic described, about two-thirds of the passengers were served ham sliced by a chef who had a pustular lesion on his hand. *S. aureus* was isolated from the lesion and an identical strain was isolated from the ham. The passengers had ingested food contaminated with one of the many *S. aureus* toxins. (For details, see Chapter 11, "*Staphylococcus*.")

Encounter

Staphylococcal food-borne outbreaks are characterized by explosive onset 1–6 hours after consuming contaminated food. Attack rates are usually quite high because very small quantities of staphylococcal enterotoxin can cause illness. In outbreaks involving single families and uniform doses of enterotoxin, virtually 100% of individuals are affected. The **staphylococcal enterotoxin is resistant to heat** and can remain in food after cooking, even though the causative organism has been killed.

Outbreaks from staphylococci may occur at any time of the year, but most are reported during the warm weather months. Staphylococci are carried by so many people that food preparation in almost any setting may be involved. Most outbreaks are reported from large gatherings, e.g., schools, group picnics, clubs, and restaurants. Many different foods have been implicated, including ham, canned beef, pork, or any salted meat, and cream-filled cakes or pastries such as cream puffs. Potato and macaroni salads are occasionally involved. Foods that have a high content of salt (ham) or sugar (custard) selectively favor the growth of staphylococci.

Foods that are involved in outbreaks have usually been cut, sliced, grated, mixed, or ground by workers who are carriers of enterotoxin-producing strains of staphylococci. Although animal carcasses may be contaminated before processing, competitive growth from other members of the normal flora usually limits the staphylococci. Therefore, transmission is from the food handler to the food product. Most commonly, the contaminated food has been allowed to sit at room temperature for some time before preparation or cooking, thus allowing the toxin to be produced in significant quantities.

Diagnosis

The signs and symptoms of staphylococcal food poisoning are primarily profuse vomiting, nausea, and abdominal cramps, often followed by diarrhea. In severe cases, blood may be observed in the vomitus or stool. Rarely, hypotension and marked prostration may occur, but recovery is usually complete within 24 to 48 hours.

Staphylococcal food poisoning should be considered in anyone with severe vomiting, nausea, cramps, and some diarrhea. A history of ingesting meats of high salt or sugar content may be helpful. The best epidemiological clue, especially if a number of individuals are ill, is the short incubation period (1 to 6 hours). Of the bacterial food-borne diseases, only *B. cereus* has similar symptoms, with a short incubation period and a marked

vomiting syndrome. However, because the *B. cereus* vomiting syndrome is closely associated with rice consumption, the epidemiological distinction can usually be easily made.

Diagnosis can be confirmed by culturing the suspected food, the skin or nose of the food handler, or occasionally, the vomitus or stools of affected individuals. The recovered *S. aureus* may be phage-typed to prove that the isolated strains are identical (see Chapter 11, "*Staphylococcus*"). Detection of staphylococcal enterotoxin will be the ultimate means of making the diagnosis when an appropriate test becomes generally available.

■ CASE 2

Clostridium perfringens

A group of college dormitory residents sat down for a turkey feast at a nearby restaurant at 6 PM. They consumed turkey, giblets, gravy, and "all the fixins." At approximately 2 AM, the first of many of the group awoke with severe intestinal cramps and watery diarrhea. Most of the students in the group became ill with similar symptoms at approximately 6 AM. Several required hospitalization in the college infirmary. Fortunately, the wave of diarrhea resolved within 24 hours.

The following questions arise:

1. What is the likely agent of this disease?
2. What is the pathophysiology of this type of diarrhea?
3. How could such an outbreak be prevented?

Encounter

The lengthy time between ingestion of suspected food and onset of symptoms, the clinical manifestations, and

---

Table 73.2. Some Characteristics of Bacterial Food Poisoning

Organism	Mechanism	Incubation period (hr)	Vehicles	Features
S. aureus	Heat-stable toxin	1–6	Ham, pastry, baked goods	Vomiting
B. cereus	Heat-stable toxin	1–6	Fried rice	Vomiting
	Heat-labile toxin	8–24	Cream sauce	Diarrhea
Salmonella	Invasion	16–48	Chicken, beef, eggs, milk	Fever, diarrhea
Campylobacter	Invasion	16–48	Chicken, beef, milk	Fever, diarrhea
V. parahemolyticus	Invasion (toxin?)	16–72	Shellfish	Fever, diarrhea
Y. enterocolitica	Invasion (toxin?)	16–72	Milk, tofu	Diarrhea
E. coli	Toxin	16–72	Salads	Diarrhea
	0157:H7 (vero toxin)	16–48	Beef	Fever, diarrhea
C. perfringen	Toxin	8–12	Beef, poultry, gravy	Diarrhea

the fact that most of the persons present at the meal got sick point to *Clostridium perfringens* as the likely cause of the outbreak. *C. perfringens* food poisoning is the fourth most common cause of food-borne disease in the U.S. Because the diagnosis is often difficult to establish, reported cases probably represent a small fraction of the actual cases that occur.

Epidemics of *C. perfringens* are usually characterized by high attack rates. The incubation period in most outbreaks varies between 8 and 14 hours (median of 12 hours), but can be as long as 74 hours. For reasons that are not clear, more cases of *C. perfringens* food poisoning are reported in the fall and winter months. The nadir of reported cases occurs in the summer, in marked contrast to outbreaks of *Salmonella* and staphylococcal food poisoning. It may be that the kinds of food usually implicated in *C. perfringens* outbreaks, such as stews, are eaten less frequently in the summer.

Outbreaks caused by this organism are most frequently reported from institutions or large gatherings. The latter is probably a reporting artifact, because only such groups recognize the illness as food poisoning. In the late 1940s, it was discovered that *C. perfringens* caused outbreaks of a severe and often lethal intestinal disease labeled **enteritis necroticans** that affected people in Germany and New Guinea (where it is termed "pig-bel," see below).

Pathophysiology

This form of food poisoning often occurs when poultry, meat, or fish is precooked and then reheated before serving. Spores of the organisms resist the first heating and then germinate in the food. The second heating must be inadequate to kill them; therefore, they are ingested either as spores or as vegetative cells. In the intestine, the organisms sporulate, forming the toxin.

Diarrhea is caused by a heat-labile protein enterotoxin with a molecular weight of approximately 34,000 daltons. The clostridial toxin differs from cholera toxin in several respects. Its activity is maximal in the ileum and minimal in the duodenum, which is opposite to that of cholera toxin. Clostridial enterotoxin inhibits glucose transport, damages the intestinal epithelium, and causes protein loss into the intestinal lumen; no such effects are observed with cholera toxin. Recently, *C. perfringens* enterotoxin has been detected in the stools of affected individuals. Enterotoxin activity disappears quickly from the stool but can be measured in serum.

Immunity in this disease is not well understood. One study has found that 65% of Americans and 84% of Brazilians have antienterotoxin activity in serum. The significance of this finding is unknown at present; in none of the outbreaks studied to date has blood drawn before an outbreak been available. Such examples would permit the study of a possible correlation between antienterotoxin immunity and the disease. In animal studies, enterotoxin antiserum blocks the action of the toxin on ligated rabbit loops. It is not known, however, if the presence of antibody in serum has any effect on toxin activity in the intestine.

Another disease rarely seen in the U.S. but caused by *C. perfringens* is enteritis necroticans ("pig-bel"), which is characterized by high attack rates in children in New Guinea, coupled with a high mortality. Although both enteritis necroticans and *C. perfringens* food poisoning that occurs in the U.S. are caused by the same organisms, the two diseases are quite different. Outbreaks of "pig-bel" have been clearly associated with the consumption of pork in large native feasts. At these feasts, improperly cooked pork is consumed in large quantities over 34 days.

As its name suggests, enteritis necroticans is a severe necrotizing disease of the small intestine. After a 24-hour incubation period, illness ensues with intense abdominal pain, bloody diarrhea, vomiting, and shock. The mortality rate is about 40%, usually due to intestinal perforation. The disease is caused by a toxin known as β-toxin, a 35-kilodalton protein that is unusually sensitive to proteases and is thus rapidly inactivated by the intestinal enzyme trypsin. The disease usually affects people who eat large, high-protein meals that overwhelm the ability of the intestinal trypsin to neutralize the toxin.

Clinical Features

C. perfringens food poisoning is generally characterized by watery diarrhea and severe cramping abdominal pain, usually without vomiting, beginning 8 to 24 hours after the suspected meal. Fever, chills, headache, or other signs of infection are usually not present.

The illness lasts 24 hours or less. Rare fatalities have been recorded in debilitated or hospitalized patients who are victims of clostridial food poisoning.

Diagnosis

The diagnosis of *C. perfringens* food poisoning should be considered in any diarrheal illness characterized by abdominal pain and moderate to severe diarrhea, unaccompanied by fever and chills. Many individuals usually are involved in the outbreak; the suspected food is beef or chicken that has been stewed, roasted, or boiled and then allowed to stand without proper refrigeration. The incubation period is 8 to 14 hours; occasional outbreaks have incubation periods as short as 5 to 6 or as long as 22 hours.

A form of food poisoning caused by *Bacillus cereus* may have similar symptoms and can only be ruled out by bacteriological study. Enterotoxigenic *E. coli* may also produce these symptoms, although low-grade fever is often present. *Vibrio cholerae* produces more profuse diarrhea, which helps differentiate it from clostridial intoxication. *Salmonella* or *Campylobacter* infections are usually accompanied by fever, a longer incubation period, and more marked systemic signs.

Because *C. perfringens* may be isolated from normal stools, it is helpful to use an established serotyping schema to distinguish between the approximately 20 different serotypes. In an outbreak, the same serotype of *C. perfringens* should be recovered from all affected individuals and from the food they ate. If food specimens are not available, the diagnosis may be made by isolating organisms of the same serotype from the stool of most ill individuals but not from that of suitable controls. In the absence of either of these findings, culturing 10^5 or more organisms per gram of the suspected food is highly suggestive of the diagnosis.

■ CASE 3

Bacillus cereus

Six medical students returned to class after a lunch break in Chinatown. Lunch consisted of hot and sour soup, spring rolls, fried rice, and three other Chinese entrées. Two hours later, while listening to Prof. S. expound on the hazards of mushroom poisoning, four of the six felt the urge to vomit and had to excuse themselves from class.

The following questions arise:
1. Which food is most likely to have contributed to this early-onset form of food poisoning?
2. How could the food have become contaminated?

Encounter

B. cereus has been increasingly recognized as a significant cause of food poisoning since about 1970. One percent or less of all food poisoning outbreaks in the U.S. are caused by this organism. Data from other countries are still generally sparse.

The incubation period for the outbreaks of emetic illness is usually 2–3 hours, whereas that for the diarrheal outbreaks is 6 to 14 hours. The clear-cut association between the vomiting syndrome and fried rice deserves emphasis. Most outbreaks of *B. cereus* vomiting syndrome in the U.S. and in Great Britain implicate this dish as the vehicle. The diarrheal illness, however, has been caused by a variety of vehicles including boiled beef, sausage, chicken soup, vanilla sauce, and puddings.

B. cereus is found in about 25% of foodstuffs sampled, including cream, pudding, meat, spices, dry potatoes, dry milk, spaghetti sauces, and rice. Contamination of food products generally occurs before they are cooked. The organisms grow if the food is maintained at 30 to 50°C during preparation. Spores survive extreme temperatures and, when allowed to cool relatively slowly, germinate and multiply. No evidence exists that human carriage of the organism or other means of contamination play a role in transmission.

Contamination of rice by *B. cereus* is attributed to the practice common in Oriental restaurants of allowing large portions of boiled rice to drain unrefrigerated to avoid clumping. The flash frying in the final preparation of certain rice dishes (e.g., fried rice) does not raise the temperature sufficiently to destroy the preformed heat-stable toxin.

Pathophysiology

Several **extracellular toxins** produced by strains of *B. cereus* may contribute to their virulence, including an enterotoxin that causes fluid accumulation in the rabbit intestine and stimulates the adenyl cyclase–cyclic AMP system in intestinal epithelial cells (see Chapter 9, "Damage").

A second presumptive toxin has been isolated from a strain of *B. cereus* implicated in an outbreak of vomiting-type illness. Cell-free culture filtrates from this strain do not produce fluid accumulation in rabbit intestine, do not stimulate the adenyl cyclase–cyclic AMP system, and only produce vomiting when fed to rhesus monkeys. This "vomiting toxin" is heat-stable.

Clinical Features

Food poisoning due to *B. cereus* has two main clinical manifestations, diarrheal and emetic. The diarrheal, long incubation form of the illness is characterized by a long incubation period, diarrhea (96%), abdominal cramps (75%), and vomiting (23%). Fever is uncommon. The duration of disease ranges from 20 to 36 hours, with a median of 24 hours.

The emetic form of the illness has as its predominant symptoms vomiting (100%) and abdominal cramps (100%). Diarrhea is only present in one-third of affected individuals. The duration of this illness ranges from 8 to 10 hours with a median of 9 hours. In both types of illness, the disease is usually mild and self-limited.

The vomiting syndrome must be differentiated from *S. aureus* food poisoning. As stated above, the association with fried rice is epidemiologically useful in differentiating the two organisms.

FOOD POISONING DUE TO INVASIVE ORGANISMS

■ CASE 4

Salmonella Gastroenteritis

Forty-eight hours after eating poorly cooked chicken, Mr. T. developed fever, shaking chills, abdominal cramps, and blood-tinged diarrhea. The illness lasted several days, and fever and diarrhea gradually abated. Mr. T. is a 65-year-old individual with a silent abdominal arterial aneurysm. Unbeknownst to him or his physician, the organisms causing his febrile diarrheic episode seeded the bloodstream and invaded the aneurysm. Ten days after the initial episode, Mr. T. developed more fever and chills, and his aneurysm expanded. Blood cultures were positive for *Salmonella* serovar *typhimurium*. Surgery and antibiotics were required. Fortunately, Mr. T. survived.

This case underscores the invasive potential of several bacteria associated with food poisoning. A number of organisms are associated with invasiveness; particularly common agents are *Salmonella* and *Campylobacter*. More uncommon bacterial causes are *Vibrio parahaemolyticus, Yersinia enterocolitica,* and a specific strain of *E. coli.* Invasiveness is generally associated with the presence of neutrophils in the stool and systemic signs such as fever, chills, myalgias, and headache. These organisms are discussed in Chapter 16, "Enteric Bacteria: Secretory Diarrhea," and Chapter 17, "Invasive and Tissue-damaging Enteric Bacteria").

Other Invasive Agents of Food Poisoning

Vibrio parahaemolyticus

The organism, like *Vibrio cholera,* is often associated with contaminated shellfish. The organism tends to behave as one of the "invasive" pathogens, rather than as a toxin-producing pathogen, such as *V. cholera.*

Yersinia enterocolitica

Y. enterocolitica is a Gram-negative rod that has recently been implicated as a cause of food poisoning. Contaminated milk has been one well-documented source. The type of infection due to this organism is generally invasive, although a heat-stable enterotoxin has been described. Tissue invasion, frequently mimicking acute appendicitis, is common in this infection. At surgery, the appendix of such patients may be normal but the mesenteric lymph nodes surrounding the appendix will be markedly inflamed.

Escherichia coli

Although *E. coli* is part of the host's normal flora, some toxigenic and enteropathogenic strains are associated with food poisoning. Toxigenic *E. coli* occurs in about 50% of travelers' diarrhea (Chapter 16). These organisms are ingested by travelers through contaminated salads, raw fruits, and vegetables. This syndrome is usually associated with watery diarrhea. Fever is less common. The organisms make both a heat-labile and heat-stable enterotoxin.

Another toxigenic strain of *E. coli* causes a syndrome of bloody diarrhea, generally without fever. The causative agent is a "vero toxin"-producing strain of *E. coli* (serotype O157:H7). The mechanism of action of this toxin appears to be identical to that of *Shigella,* the agent of bacillary dysentery. A rare consequence of this illness in children is hemolytic uremia syndrome (see Chapter 17), which can lead to severe kidney damage and hemolytic anemia. The agent has been epidemiologically connected to poorly cooked hamburger.

"Arizona"

The organism called "Arizona" is a motile Gram-negative rod closely related to *Salmonella.* It has been implicated in outbreaks of gastroenteritis and enteric fever. Foods that have been implicated have included eggs or poultry. Because "Arizona" is similar to *Salmonella,* contaminated animal products should be considered the usual vehicles of "Arizona"-related food poisoning.

The syndromes of "Arizona" infection are also very similar to salmonellosis. Gastroenteritis, enteric fever, bacteremia, or localized infection have been described. In addition, the incubation period is similar to *Salmonella.* Usually, symptoms develop 24 to 48 hours after ingestion of contaminated food. Fever, headache, nausea, vomiting, abdominal pain, and watery diarrhea may occur, as well as marked prostration. Symptoms may persist for several days. Therapy and prevention are also similar to those employed for salmonellosis.

Listeria monocytogenes

This organism has become increasingly recognized as a food-borne pathogen. *Listeria monocytogenes* is a Gram-positive, motile rod that is relatively heat-resistant; it withstands pasteurization of milk. *Listeria* is widely distributed in nature and is found in the intestinal tract of various animals and humans, as well as in sewage, soil, and water.

The syndromes usually associated with listeriosis include meningitis, bacteremia, or focal metastatic disease. Frequently, gastrointestinal symptoms such as diarrhea precede the bacteremic disease. The organism has a propensity to affect adults who are either immunosuppressed or pregnant. The evidence that listeriosis is food-borne is accumulating from investigations of several recent epidemics. Contaminated cole slaw and raw and pasteurized milk have been implicated as vehicles for epidemic listeriosis. The source of sporadic *Listeria* infection is less well understood.

CONTROL AND PREVENTION

The common theme that characterizes all food-borne illnesses is the improper handling of food before its consumption. In a study of factors responsible for food-borne outbreaks in the U.S. over a 15-year period, it was shown that inadequate refrigeration was the single most frequent factor (Table 73.3). Usually, other factors are also associated with a specific outbreak, such as advance preparation of food without adequate storage or improper reheating. To a lesser degree, contaminated equipment, cross-contamination, and poor personal hy-

Table 73.3. Factors that Contributed to Food-borne Disease Outbreaks in the United States

Factor	Percentage implicated[a]
Inadequate refrigeration	47
Food prepared too far in advance of service	21
Infected person with poor personal hygiene	21
Inadequate cooking	16
Inadequate holding temperature	16
Inadequate reheating	12
Contaminated raw ingredient	1
Cross-contamination	7
Dirty equipment	7

[a] Percentage values total more than 100% because more than one factor may contribute to food-borne outbreak.

giene of food preparation personnel may contribute to outbreaks.

The ubiquity of *Salmonella, Campylobacter, B. cereus,* and *C. perfringens* makes it mandatory that food be cooked properly and stored at low temperatures. Control of food-borne illnesses is based on the inhibition of bacterial growth, prevention of contamination after preparation, and destruction of potential pathogens with cooking. In general, foods should be heated to internal temperatures of 165°F, but lower temperatures for longer periods of time are also effective. (Perhaps you should think twice before ordering steak tartare, sushi, or other uncooked or undercooked meat or fish.) Once cooked or processed, foods must be held at temperatures of 40°F or below.

Although these control measures are standard, many places where food preparation takes place do not abide by them. It is through diligent efforts of public health officials that reported outbreaks are investigated and food preparation techniques corrected. Therefore, recognition and reporting of food-borne illness becomes essential in the control of the problem. Education of the public, nurses, physicians, and eating establishment personnel is crucial to the control of food-borne illness. Carriage of most of the organisms considered in this chapter is not a problem, with the exception of staphylococci. Because staphylococcal carriage is necessary for the development of this illness, food handlers must be educated to watch for boils and pustules.

TREATMENT

Because these illnesses are generally self-limited and, for the most part, toxin-mediated, **antibiotics play no major role** either in therapy or prophylaxis. **Fluid replacement** is a major consideration in all of these illnesses. Occasionally, individuals with diseases caused by the more invasive pathogens such as *Salmonella, Shigella, Listeria,* or *Campylobacter* may require antibiotic therapy.

SUGGESTED READINGS

Boyce TG, Swadlow DL, Griffin PM. *Escherichia coli* 0157:H7 and the hemolytic uremic syndrome. N Engl J Med 1995;333:364–368.

Centers for Disease Control. Foodborne disease outbreaks. Annual summary.

Cliver DO. Foodborne diseases. San Diego: Academic Press, 1990.

Doyle MP, ed. Foodborne bacterial pathogens. New York: Dekker, 1989.

Hedberg CW, MacDonald KL, Osterholm MT. Changing epidemiology of food-borne disease: a Minnesota perspective. Clin Inf Dis 1994;18:671–682.

Answers to Self-assessment Questions

PART I. Principles
Chapter 2/Normal Microbial Flora

1. Aspiration pneumonia due to the entry of diverse members of the oral flora into lungs, facilitated by defective ciliary action or factors that increase aspiration (e.g., sedation, drugs, etc.). Peritonitis by entry of members of the fecal flora into the peritoneal cavity via a ruptured appendix or a traumatic break in the intestinal wall. Cystitis caused by fecal *Escherichia coli* due to stasis in the urine flow (e.g., catheterization). Subacute bacterial endocarditis caused by oral α-hemolytic streptococci due to their introduction into the circulation of a patient with heart valve disease. *Pneumocystis carinii* pneumonia in AIDS patients due to impaired immune responses. Many other examples could be cited.

2. Normal flora, especially of the gut, is a constant source of low-level antigenic stimulation. The resulting antibodies and cell-mediated immunity are probably involved in defense against certain infections. Some of the antibodies may cross-react with heterologous cell constituents, such as red blood cells of a different ABO type. It is conceivable that some of these antibodies may be involved in autoimmune reactions.

3. The resident flora wards off external pathogens by prior colonization of available sites and by forming metabolites (such as acids, H_2S) that are inimical to invaders. The immune response against members of the normal flora may have cross-reactivity against possible pathogens.

4. The most colonized parts of the body are the mouth and the large intestine, followed by the vagina and the skin. Transiently, microorganisms may be found in the rest of the digestive and respiratory systems. More rarely, the lower urinary tract may be colo-

nized by small numbers of microorganisms. The deep tissues are normally sterile.

5. The main groups are Gram-positive cocci and Gram-negative rods, mainly strict anaerobes.

6. The effects of the normal flora may be observed by comparing germ-free and conventional animals as well as humans whose flora has been disturbed by antimicrobial therapy or surgical interventions.

Chapter 3/Biology of Infectious Agents

1. Prokaryotes lack internal membrane-bound organelles; they do not have a distinct mitotic apparatus and are not capable of endocytosis. With some exceptions, prokaryotes have a murein cell wall. Prokaryotic ribosomes are smaller than those of eukaryotes and differ in sensitivity to antibiotics. Lacking a nuclear membrane, transcription and translation may be directly coupled in prokaryotes.

2. Smallness makes for faster diffusion of substrates and metabolites. The distance between structural parts makes it possible to connect them directly, as with the transcriptional and translational machineries.

3. Gram-positives have a thick murein layer lacking lipopolysaccharide (endotoxin); Gram-negatives have a thin one with a distinct outer membrane containing lipopolysaccharide. Gram-negatives have pili (fimbriae); Gram-positives generally do not.

4. The outer membrane of Gram-negatives serves to protect the inner membrane from hydrophobic toxic compounds by virtue of its lipopolysaccharide outer leaflet. To make passage of substrates possible, this membrane has pores formed by proteins called porins. These pores have a molecular size exclusion of 600–700 daltons. Transport mechanisms for specific larger compounds such as iron chelates also exist. Lipopolysaccharide functions as endotoxin, which causes fever, and in large doses, shock.

5. Penicillin works by covalently binding to penicillin-binding proteins involved in the synthesis of cell wall murein. Other biosynthetic processes are not inhibited; thus, the cells "outgrow their coats" and, via the activity of autolysins, burst in hypotonic media.

6. Facilitated diffusion, group translocations, and active transport (via permeases) are the principal mechanisms.

7. DNA replication starts at the replicative origin and proceeds bidirectionally until the replication machinery reaches the terminus. In growing bacteria, the rate of replication is nearly independent of the growth rate. To accommodate for growth that is faster than the rate of replication, bacteria initiate new rounds of replication before the previous ones have finished.

8. Inhibition of protein synthesis does not necessarily cause death because ribosomes may just be released prematurely from mRNA but remain available for future use. Bactericidal protein-inhibiting antibiotics bind to ribosomes and render them inactive even after removal of the drug.

9. Bacterial flagella are organs of propulsion and serve in chemotaxis toward attractants such as nutrients and away from toxic repellents. Pili (fimbriae) participate in the adherence of bacteria to surfaces such as those of animal cells, thus facilitating colonization.

10. Bacteria obtain energy by fermentation, using an organic electron receptor, or respiration, using an inorganic electron receptor, usually oxygen. Fermentation is usually carried out in the absence of oxygen; thus, fermentative bacteria may be obligate or facultative anaerobes. Facultative anaerobes and obligate aerobes require oxygen (or other inorganic electron acceptors such as nitrate or sulfate) to respire. Oxygen is generally toxic to obligate anaerobes.

11. The law of bacterial growth states that the number of cells is a direct function of the number of cells present and an exponential function of a rate constant. In the real world, this condition obtains only for short periods of time, when neither nutrients nor toxic metabolites are limiting.

12. Feedback inhibition results in diminution of enzyme activity but not in the amount of enzyme. Control of gene expression results in reduction in the synthesis of gene products, e.g., enzymes, but not in the activity of the formed enzyme.

13. Repression of enzyme synthesis via a repressor, attenuation via early termination of mRNA synthesis are two examples.

14. Bacteria respond to lethal challenges by exhibiting global responses that involve activation and inhibition of selected genes. In some cases, the genes involved are transcribed by special σ factors of RNA polymerase.

Chapter 5/Biological Basis for Antibacterial Action

1. Mention the sudden availability of such substances after World War II, the concept of selective toxicity, examples of specific metabolic targets. Give examples of diseases that can be effectively treated. Discuss the general concept of drug resistance, its importance in medicine, and why antibiotics should be used prudently (e.g., not against insensitive agents and with a view toward resistance).

2. Sulfonamides compete with para-aminobenzoic acid for the synthesis of folic acid, needed for the synthesis of purines, thymine, thiamine, and other metabolites. Bacteria must make their own folic acid and cannot take it up from the medium. Animal cells can take up preformed folic acid, therefore, and are not affected by these drugs.

3. Bactericidal drugs kill bacteria; bacteriostatic ones inhibit their growth. Bactericidal drugs are needed to rid the body of persistent bacteria that cannot be readily cleared by body defenses. This is especially true in bacterial endocarditis and meningitis, or in any infection when the leukocyte count is very low (as after cancer chemotherapy). On the other hand, some bactericidal drugs may take longer to act than bacteriostatic ones, allowing for the accumulation of toxins.

4. Acquired resistance occurs with: (*a*) inactivation of the drug by hydrolysis (e.g., β-lactamases) or chemical modification (e.g., acetylases); (*b*) replacement of a sensitive enzyme by a resistant one (e.g., sulfonamide-resistant enzymes in folic acid synthesis); (*c*) decreased binding affinity for ribosomes (e.g., aminoglycosides); (*d*) decrease transport into cells (e.g., aminoglycosides); and (*e*) increased exit from cell (e.g., tetracyclines). Natural resistance occurs from: (*a*) low accessibility to the target (e.g., Gram-negative bacteria and penicillin), and (*b*) absence of a target (e.g., mycoplasmata, which lack murein, and penicillin).

5. Association with bacteria, penetration into periplasm in Gram-negatives, interaction with penicillin-binding proteins, and activation of an autolysin are the steps involved in β-lactam antibiotics. The most common resistance mechanism affects the first step by hydrolysis of the drugs by β-lactamases.

6. Tetracycline binds to bacteria and is transported into cytoplasm where it inhibits the formation of initiation complex in protein synthesis; resistance is by an increased exit from the cells. Chloramphenicol and macrolides (lincomycin, erythromycin) inhibit the chain elongation step; resistance to chloramphenicol is by acetylation of the drug, to

macrolides by modification of ribosome or mRNA. Aminoglycosides cause translational misreading and inhibit elongation of protein chains; resistance is by enzymatic modification of drugs.

7. Antifungal agents generally work by inhibiting the synthesis of fungal cell sterols (ergosterol), which are different from animal cell sterols (cholesterol).

8. Two drugs decrease the chance of a mutant resistant to both arising. (This is particularly important with infections characterized by a large number of infecting bacteria, such as tuberculosis). A separate advantage of two drugs is that, together, they may cover a wider spectrum of sensitive bacteria. (This is particularly useful in life-threatening infections). Use of multiple antibiotics may be undesirable because of possible antagonism, additive (or synergistic) toxicity, and the emergence of drug resistance among the bacteria and drug sensitization among the patients.

Chapter 9/Damage by Microbial Agents

1. Toxins lyse host cells by destroying membranes via the hydrolysis of compounds such as lecithin (e.g., clostridial lecithinases) or by inserting into membranes to make pores (e.g., staphylococcal α-toxin–a homogeneous pore former, and streptococcal streptolysin O–a heterogeneous pore former).

2. The B portion binds to receptors on the surface of target cells, allowing the A portion (active) to enter and cause damage. In some toxins, the A and B portion are part of the same molecule (e.g., diphtheria toxin), in others they are two separate entities (e.g., cholera toxin).

3. Toxins that work as extracellular hydrolases need not penetrate cells to act (e.g., hyaluronidase, streptokinase). Also, any cytolytic toxins that need not enter cells to cause damage need not possess a B portion.

4. Antitoxins to purified toxin protect against the disease in humans and experimental animals. Nontoxigenic mutants do not cause disease in experimental animals. All isolates from patients with the disease are toxigenic.

5. Cholera toxin acts by ADP-ribosylating G protein, which, in this form, cannot hydrolyze GTP. This modified G protein is locked in a conformation that keeps stimulating adenylate cyclase to make cAMP.

6. Tetanus toxin works on the central nervous system to inhibit the release of inhibitory neurotransmitters, causing neuromuscular excitation. Botulinum toxin works on peripheral nerves causing a presynaptic block in the release of acetylcholine, which results in muscle relaxation.

7. A toxoid should be highly immunogenic and minimally toxic. It should lead to the formation of effective antitoxins. Other practical features include

stability, reasonable solubility, and ease of preparation.

8. Exotoxins are secreted proteins; endotoxins are cell membrane lipopolysaccharides. Exotoxins have a limited repertoire of individual activities; endotoxins act on a variety of cells and the complement system. Exotoxins are usually more potent.

9. In low amounts, endotoxins cause local inflammation via activation of macrophages and complement. Systemically, endotoxin in low amounts causes fever.

10. In high amounts, endotoxins cause shock via the increase in interleukin-1 and tumor necrosis factor, plus disseminated intravascular coagulation by activating the clotting mechanisms.

PART II. Infectious Agents: Bacteria
Chapter 11–Staphylococci: Abscesses and Other Diseases

1. Abscesses and other pyogenic infections of almost any tissue or organ, staphylococcal food poisoning, toxic shock syndrome, and scalded skin syndrome are the most frequent staphylococcal diseases.

2. Staphylococci are Gram-positive cocci that make sizable colonies on regular agar media, form grape cluster–like cellular arrangements, and secrete extracellular proteins, some of which are virulence factors. Many staphylococci are salt-resistant, one reason why they can (and do) reside on the skin. The main types are the coagulase-positive *S. aureus* (the most common pathogenic staph), *S. epidermidis* (an opportunistic pathogen that colonizes surfaces, such as those of prosthetic devices and plastic catheters), *S. saprophyticus*, and other opportunistic pathogens.

3. Staphylococci that cause abscesses and other pyogenic infections, scalded skin syndrome, and toxic shock may be acquired either from the environment or may be members of the flora of the patient. Staphylococci that cause food poisoning are ingested with contaminated food.

4. Staphylococci generally enter deep tissues through trauma-induced openings but subtler ways of penetration cannot be discounted. Once inside, they ward off the action of phagocytes by producing a cytotoxin (α-toxin), a catalase that impedes oxidative killing by neutrophils, and coagulase that renders the organisms less accessible. The presence of protein A hinders the opsonic activity of antibodies. The pathogenesis of staphylococcal pyogenic infections is extraordinarily multifactorial and it becomes difficult to dissect the role of the major virulence factors. Other staphylococcal diseases (toxic shock syndrome, scalded skin syndrome, food poisoning) can be attributed to the action of a single toxin.

5. Pyogenic infections elicit inflammatory responses. Toxic shock toxin induces the formation of a number of cytokines. The body responds to staphylococcal enterotoxin in the gastrointestinal tract by trying to eliminate the organism via diarrhea. Not much is known about scalded skin syndrome.

6. Pyogenic infections require drainage and the administration of antibiotics. The abscesses formed impede the penetration and activity of many antibiotics, as well as the normal host defenses. Penicillin resistance became a hallmark of staphylococci only after the widespread use of antibiotics became established. Scalded skin and toxic shock syndromes require systemic physiological support.

Chapter 12/Streptococci

1. Streptococci make chains by always dividing along the same plane and remaining attached after cell division. They carry out fermentative metabolism only. Some are strict anaerobes, others indifferent to oxygen. They are divided by the type of hemolysis (α, β, γ). β-Hemolytic streptococci can be further divided into groups (A, B, etc.) according to the serology of their C carbohydrate.

2. Streptococci are helped in their spread by making extracellular hydrolases such as hyaluronidase, streptokinase (a fibrinolysin), and DNAase.

3. M proteins (of which there are some 80 serological types) are strongly antiphagocytic. In some individuals, a cross-reactive autoimmune response may be elicited by the M protein.

4. The main diseases are pyogenic infections and postsuppurative glomerulonephritis and rheumatic fever (due to group A, β-hemolytic streptococci) and subacute bacterial endocarditis (by α-hemolytic streptococci).

5. Postsuppurative rheumatic fever is thought to result either from cross-reactivity between myocardial and streptococcal components (i.e., M protein) or from the production of a streptococcal cardiotoxin. Postsuppurative glomerulonephritis has several theories, including cross-reactivity, deposition of streptococcal antigens in the glomeruli followed by an in situ reaction with circulating antibodies, deposition of circulating immune complexes, and nephrotoxic action of streptococcal toxins.

6. Diagnostic problems include differentiating potential pathogens from harmless commensals in the throat. Material from postsuppurative sequelae does not usually carry the organisms and the diagnosis is usually not made on a bacteriological basis.

Chapter 13/Pneumococcus and Bacterial Pneumonia

1. Pneumococcal pneumonia is usually community-acquired. The reservoir is human beings, with the organism typically colonizing the nasopharynx of a small proportion of normal individuals who stay healthy. Illness rarely occurs without predisposing factors, including aspiration (due to poor cough reflex or lowered consciousness), debilitation, sickle cell anemia, various tumors, lack of spleen. The disease is seen most often in the winter and spring. Cases are usually sporadic but outbreaks may occur under crowded conditions.

2. The capsule of the pneumococcus is thought to be its main virulence factor as it impedes phagocytosis. A comparison of encapsulated and unencapsulated isogenic strains (identical except in the capsule) has shed light on this issue. A comparison of other traits between isogenic capsulated strains may uncover other virulence factors.

3. (a) Inflammation begins with an outpouring of clear fluid into the alveoli. (b) Early consolidation brings in neutrophils and red blood cells. (c) Late consolidation leads to the solidification of the tissue ("hepatization") with a greater number of neutrophils. (d) In resolution, neutrophils are replaced by macrophages.

4. The disease may progress very rapidly in elderly patients; thus, early and vigorous intervention is called for. Individuals without spleens are predisposed to a severe septicemic form of the disease, which occurs because of the inadequate ability to clear the organism from the bloodstream. These individuals are often treated prophylactically with monthly injections of long-acting penicillin (or daily oral erythromycin in those with allergy to penicillin).

5. Sputum from the respiratory tree may contain Gram-positive cocci that resemble pneumococci under the microscope. Positive sputum cultures may be due to contamination of the material with commensal pneumococci from the oropharynx. Positive blood or cerebrospinal fluid cultures (because they are obtained from normally sterile regions) are generally diagnostic.

Chapter 14/Neisseriae: Gonococcus and Meningococcus

1. Gonococci are Gram-negative, oxidase-positive diplococci. Meningococci look the same but are usually more heavily encapsulated. Meningococci are more likely to cause serious systemic disease.

2. When a male partner infects the female, the organisms cause urethritis by adherence to epithelial cells via pili, extracellular multiplication, spread up the genital tract, penetration into nonciliated cells, passage to the base of these cells, and extrusion into the submucosal tissue causing an inflammatory response. If the infection reaches the fallopian tubes, the resulting inflammation will cause scarring and

impair ciliary function of the epithelial cells. This allows other organisms from the vagina to reach the peritoneal cavity and cause inflammation in the abdominal pelvis.

3. Early diagnosis and treatment, partner notification, behavioral interventions (use of condom, decreasing number of sexual partners), and vaccination with a vaccine, when an effective one becomes available.

4. The main problem is the antigenic variation in one of the main antigenic components, the pilin protein of pili. In addition, to be effective, a vaccine must elicit secretory immunity.

5. Gonorrhea may lead to salpingitis and ectopic pregnancy, pelvic inflammatory response, scarring of the urethra in males, arthritis, and other systemic infections. It is a major cause of female infertility.

Chapter 15/*Bacteroides* and Abscesses

1. *B. fragilis* causes abscesses in the peritoneal cavity, the lungs, and other sites. Untreated, such conditions may be life-threatening. Infections by anaerobes were often not recognized because anaerobic cultures were not generally carried out.

2. *Bacteroides* are Gram-negative, strictly anaerobic rods found in large amounts in the vertebrate gut and mouth. These organisms are fermentative and resist oxygen although they cannot grow in its presence.

3. *B. fragilis* is among the most oxygen-tolerant of the human strict anaerobes, probably because it makes both superoxide dismutase and catalase. It makes a capsule that protects it from phagocytosis and may be involved in attachment to cell surfaces. Neuraminidase and other hydrolytic enzymes may play a role in pathogenesis.

4. Abscesses caused by anaerobes and mixed flora organisms are often not accessible to drugs and require drainage. Many anaerobes are resistant to common antibiotics and treatment requires special drugs. Bacteriological diagnosis requires specialized anaerobic techniques.

Chapter 16/Enteric Bacteria: "Secretory" (Watery) Diarrhea

1. Through the digestive system there is flow of liquids that may propel microorganisms along, unless these stick to surfaces or reside in crevices. IgA antibodies are secreted throughout most of the digestive tract. In the mouth, lysozyme of saliva is active against certain bacteria. The stomach has low pH and pepsin, the small intestine has the pancreatic enzymes plus bile salts, the large intestine has a metabolically active resident flora.

2. *Salmonella, Shigella,* certain strains of *E. coli, Campylobacter, Yersinia,* and *Vibrio cholerae* cause intestinal infections. They can be distinguished on the basis of biochemical reactions and their serological differences.

3. Most enteropathogenic bacteria have adhesins that permit them to bind to the surface of gut cells. All of the Gram-negative ones have endotoxins. Enterotoxins are produced by certain strains of *E. coli, S. aureus, C. perfringens,* and *V. cholerae.* Invasiveness properties of *Shigella* are associated with the production of cytocidal toxins. *Yersinia* has recently been found to possess a protein, invasin, that allows it to enter epithelial cells.

4. Different strains of *E. coli* cause the following diseases: in the intestine, enterotoxigenic or watery diarrhea from the colon, enteropathogenic or watery diarrhea from the ileum, enteroinvasive or dysentery disease, enterohemorrhagic or hemorrhagic colitis. In the urinary tract, *E. coli* causes cystitis, pyelonephritis, prostatitis. In young infants, *E. coli* strains may cause septicemia and meningitis.

5. Treatment of watery bacterial diarrhea should be aimed at fluid replacement and physiological support and, if necessary, at eliminating the causative agents. Treatment of dysentery should be aimed at eliminating the causative agent.

6. Immunization is not likely to work unless secretory IgA antibodies are formed. Vigorous prophylactic antimicrobial therapy might eliminate the normal flora and give opportunistic organisms the chance to colonize.

Chapter 17/Invasive and Tissue-damaging Enteric Bacterial Pathogens: Bloody Diarrhea and Dysentery

1. The steps are: ingestion; spread from small intestine to mesenteric lymph nodes; primary bacteremia; multiplication in macrophages, especially in liver; septicemia (fever); spread to gallbladder; reinfection of small intestine (inflammation, ulceration of Peyer's patches leading to diarrhea, hemorrhage, perforation).

2. EHEC strains can cause a characteristic nonfebrile bloody diarrhea known as hemorrhagic colitis. Deaths are caused by the hemolytic-uremic syndrome (HUS), a complication of hemorrhagic colitis consisting of hemolytic anemia, thrombocytopenia, and renal failure. These deaths are most commonly in young children, and are now the most frequent cause of acute renal failure in children in the U.S.

3. Typhoid bacilli, at a minimum, must be able to resist the acid in the stomach, invade the small intestine, survive within macrophages, withstand the action of bile, cause local inflammation.

4. Within the body, the organisms' resistance to bile contributes to the carrier state. Ability to reside in macrophages may also be involved. Outside of the body, the ability to survive in water and food is present.

5. Avoidance of contaminated foods and prevention to fecal contamination. In addition, in the case of Shigella, sanitation after direct contact with patients (especially infants)

6. Invasive salmonellosis

Chapter 18/*Pseudomonas aeruginosa:* Ubiquitous Pathogen

1. Pseudomonads are Gram-negative aerobic rods with polar flagella. They can utilize a wide variety of substrates, which is why certain specialized strains are being tried for the cleanup of oil spills and toxic wastes. Their hardiness makes them ubiquitous inhabitants of sinks, faucets, and other water supplies.

2. *P. aeruginosa* causes infections of the lung in cystic fibrosis and in intubated patients on respirators; infections on the skin in burn victims; septicemia in immunodeficient patients, sometimes with necrotic lesions in the skin; endocarditis in intravenous drug addicts; local or system infections after surgery or trauma; urinary tract infections in persons with urine stasis due to kidney stones or catheterization.

3. See Answer 2.

4. Some virulence factors are: exotoxin A, cell necrosis by ADP-ribosylation of elongation factor 2 of protein synthesis; elastase, by breakdown of elastin; phospholipase C by breakdown of cell membranes; endotoxin.

5. Patients with *Pseudomonas* infections are often immunodeficient and require vigorous antimicrobial therapy. However, the organisms are relatively drug-resistant. Problems may be encountered with access of drugs, as in cystic fibrosis and burn patients.

Chapter 19/*Bordetella pertussis* and Whooping Cough

1. Local effects are inflammation due to pertussis toxin, which inactivates phagocytic action, and to tracheal cytotoxin; cough due to accumulation of mucus; hypoxia due to bronchial obstruction and secondary bacterial pneumonia. Systemic manifestations are low-grade fever, possibly due to endotoxin; heightened sensitivity to histamine and serotonin, due to increase in cAMP by the bacterial adenylate cyclase; encephalopathy, probably due to pertussis toxin.

2. Systemic manifestations are due to the formation of exotoxins, such as exotoxin A and adenylate cyclase, that may act at a distance. Hypoxia may result in systemic manifestations.

3. Pertussis toxin ADP-ribosylates adenylate cyclase to increase its activity and increase the production of cAMP. Bacterial adenylate cyclase itself raises the cAMP concentration. Tracheal cytotoxin kills ciliated respiratory epithelial cells by an unknown mechanism. Endotoxin works primarily by increasing the production of interleukin-1 and tissue necrosis factor.

4. The pro is that the vaccine is highly effective in preventing whooping cough. The cons are that the vaccine may cause fever and local pain in about 1 of 5 children, convulsions in a small number (about 1 in 2000 children), serious brain complication in very few (fewer than 1 in 100,000 children). The incidence of serious complications is probably less than that of whooping cough, which is a serious and potentially life-threatening disease, although the precise odds are not known.

Chapter 20/Clostridia

1. Spore formation explains the ability of clostridia to survive at high temperature, e.g., in certain prepared foods. These organisms make powerful hydrolytic enzymes (some of which are exotoxins) that help explain why they are often involved in the decomposition of dead animals and plants, which, by itself, may account for the common finding of clostridia in soils. The fact that these organisms are strict anaerobes does not help explain their location because they are often found in well-oxygenated substrates such as top layers of soils.

2. Pseudomembranous colitis is caused by the overgrowth of *Clostridium difficile* as the result of vigorous therapy with antibiotics that affect most members of the normal bacterial flora. Patients at risk are obviously those who receive this class of antibiotics for whatever reason.

3. Botulinum toxin is resistant to acid in the stomach, whereas tetanus toxin is not. In fact, botulinum toxin is activated in the stomach. In addition, tetanus toxin is not absorbed by the small intestine, while botulinum toxin is. The reason that infant botulism is usually a mild disease is probably because, in that condition, the organisms are found in the large intestine where the toxin is absorbed more poorly than from the small intestine.

4. Tetanus toxin works on the CNS to inhibit the release of inhibitory neurotransmitters, causing neuromuscular excitation. Botulinum toxin works on peripheral nerves causing a presynaptic block in the release of acetylcholine, which results in muscle relaxation.

5. Immunization against *C. difficile* is unlikely to work because the organism resides in the large intestine, where antibodies are not apt to be effective. In addition to this reason, immunization against botulism and clostridial gas gangrene is an effective

measure because these diseases are not widespread and the toxins belong to an inconveniently large number of antigenic types.

Chapter 21/*Legionella*: Parasite of Cells

1. *Legionella* survive in bodies of water and grow in association with protozoa found in such habitats. This aquatic habitat leads to the presence of the organisms in water supplies. In addition, the organisms are relatively resistant to high temperatures and are sometimes found in hot water tanks. From such locations, the organisms may be acquired by inhalation of aerosols of contaminated water.

2. Outbreaks of legionellosis are probably due to the contamination of water supplies used by many people, such as guests of hotels.

3. *Legionella* pneumonia is an interstitial infection of the submucosal tissue of the alveoli of the lung, and the organisms replicate within alveolar macrophages. Pneumococcal pneumonia is more of a superficial infection of the alveolar lumen; the organisms do not replicate intracellularly.

4. The inoculum of *Legionella pneumophila* normally encountered can be handled adequately by most healthy individuals. The establishment of the disease often requires some degree of immune compromise, thereby allowing intracellular replication of the microorganisms. Activation of macrophages leads to inhibition of intracellular replication.

5. The main ones are the pseudomonads, which may be acquired by inhalation or by penetration through the skin.

Chapter 22/*Helicobacter pylori*: Pathogenesis of a "Slow" Bacterial Infection

1. Biopsies showed chronic active gastritis with many neutrophils and mononuclear leukocytes in the lamina propria and the glandular epithelium. Curved, rod-shaped bacteria were seen on the mucosal surfaces of all biopsies. Cultures grew *H. pylori*.

2. These organisms produce urease, which splits urea into carbon dioxide and highly basic ammonia. In the stomach, microbial proliferation causes hypochlorhydria due to gastric inflammation.

3. *H. pylori* positive for CagA induce high degrees of inflammation and damage in the gastric mucosa. Mucosal levels of interleukin-8 (IL-8) are significantly higher in persons with harboring cagA+, which may explain the link between these cagA+ strains and peptic ulcer disease.

4. Cell proliferation in chronic *H. pylori* infection may increase the likelihood of DNA damage by such mutagens as N-nitrosamines or inflammation-related free radicals. These mutagens are associated with reduced concentrations of ascorbic acid in gastric juice, an important defense mechanism against oxidative DNA damage. The risk of gastric cancer may also be related to certain strain characteristics of *H. pylori*. Infection with a cagA+ strain is associated with a twofold increase in risk of gastric adenocarcinoma, perhaps because of the heightened inflammatory response that develops after infection with such strains.

5. In chronic *H. pylori* infection, the host mounts an apparently ineffective immune response, thus a vaccine would have to elicit a different, as yet unknown, kind of response.

6. Endoscopic gastric tissue specimens can be studied by histologic examination, microbiological culture, and rapid urease testing. Biochemical confirmation of *H. pylori* includes positive tests for urease, catalase, and oxidase. Noninvasive tests include serology to detect specific circulating antibodies and the urea breath tests.

Chapter 23/Mycobacteria: Tuberculosis and Leprosy

1. Resistance to drying and to chemicals such as dilute acids.

2. Stain with a red dye (fuchsin) solution containing detergents to permeabilize the waxy coat. Rinse. Treat briefly with dilute hydrochloric acid. Rinse. Counterstain with methylene blue.

3. By causing pulmonary infections and, eventually, the coughing up of the bacteria-laden content of caseous lesions, mycobacteria become abundant in the human environment. The bacteria are spread by aerosolization. Resistance to drying allows them to remain in the environment, e.g., dust, for long periods of time.

4. The ability of the organisms to withstand life inside macrophages and, thus, to cause cell-mediated immunity. Tissue damage is attributable to granuloma formation, delayed type hypersensitivity, and formation of interleukin-1 and tumor necrosis factor.

5. In those who develop disease, tissue damage is due to the cell-mediated immunity, which, if progressive, may be responsible for death in chronic tuberculosis. However, the majority of infected individuals, as determined by a positive response to tuberculin, never get ill with tuberculosis. Presumably, cell-mediated immunity is walling off the infection locally with minimal collateral damage to the host. Moreover, in the absence of the cell-mediated immunity response (as in some patients with AIDS), tubercle bacilli may grow rapidly and cause progressive systemic disease and rapid death.

6. AIDS patients with tuberculosis are likely to develop extrapulmonary disease, involving the lymph nodes, the bone marrow, the genitourinary tract, and the central nervous system. Patients with AIDS

react like the small group of people who develop rapidly advancing or miliary tuberculosis soon after primary infection. The reason for these manifestations is the depletion of CD4$^+$ T cells which, with the associated loss of macrophage function, leads to the impairment of cell-mediated immunity.

7. These patients respond to treatment as do other tuberculosis patients. With effective therapy, the disease progress is arrested. On the other hand, the unfortunate patient with AIDS who acquires multidrug-resistant tuberculosis is likely to develop disease that is persistent and usually fatal.

8. The hallmark of both diseases is cell-mediated immunity. In its presence, tuberculoid leprosy resembles secondary tuberculosis in fundamental ways, although different organs and tissues are usually affected. The absence of cell-mediated immunity leads to lepromatous leprosy, which resembles systemic progressive tuberculosis but is a proportionately more frequent outcome.

9. The first step is usually the microscopic examination of smears of clinical material stained by the acid-fast method or immunofluorescent dyes. This technique may fail because of inexperience by the operator or because the concentration of bacteria is too low. Culturing clinical material requires long incubations (sometimes 3 weeks or more) because the organisms grow slowly. Serological techniques may reveal the presence of antibodies or cell-mediated immunity, neither of which indicates active disease. Newer genetically based techniques (e.g., the polymerase chain reaction or other DNA amplification methods), if commercially developed, may allow rapid diagnosis.

Chapter 24/Syphilis: Disease with a History

1. In primary syphilis, antibodies are not likely to be formed in sufficient titer until nearly the end of this phase. Antibodies may contribute to resolution of secondary syphilitic lesions. In tertiary syphilis, antibodies are unlikely to play a large role because the organisms are not found in many of the lesions. However, antibodies may prevent the multiplication and further spread of the organisms.

2. There are no simple answers to this phenomenon. Healing of local lesions is probably due to local reactions that contain the organisms at the site but do not prevent their systemic spread.

3. Suggestions for autoimmunity in tertiary syphilis are the absence of organisms from many of the lesions and the Wasserman-type serological test, which is based on the presence of antibodies against a normal tissue component, cardiolipin. Positive

Wasserman serology is seen in other diseases, such as lupus erythematosus, which are strongly suspected of being autoimmune diseases.

4. It depends on the nature of the contact. A patient with primary syphilis is highly contagious because of open sores in genital areas. However, the skin and mucosal lesions of secondary syphilis are teeming with organisms and contact with these lesions may lead to spread of the disease.

5. The organisms are apparently only found in humans. They are still sensitive to drugs such as penicillin. The simultaneous injection of repeated doses of penicillin to every human may well lower the human load of treponemes. However, in some of the lesions of tertiary syphilis (gummas), the organisms are still present and may not be accessible by drugs. Thus, a public health surveillance of all known patients with syphilis and their contacts would be required.

6. There are many answers, such as: try to grow the organisms in culture, clone their genes, and study possible virulence factors and antigens; try to set up an animal model that allows the detailed analysis of immunological events during the three stages of the disease.

Chapter 25/Lyme Disease

1. B. *burgdorferi* is a thin, helical-shaped rod with bundles of flagella contained within its outer membrane. Unlike *T. pallidum*, it can be cultivated in artificial media and is arthropod-borne.

2. Emphasize the reservoirs (small rodents, deer), the need for vigilance and protection from various forms of ticks, the geographic distribution (both coasts of U.S., some midwestern states), early symptoms (skin, joints), the seriousness of systemic and neurological manifestations, and available chemotherapy. You may want to mention the history of the disease and how the mothers of infected children helped in its elucidation (Chapter 56).

3. Both have analogous three stages, neurological manifestations late in disease, respond to antibiotics.

4. Primary—erythema migrans. Secondary—neuritic pain of skin, arthralgias. Tertiary—impairment in certain cortical functions (forgetfulness, lethargy, fatigue, hearing impairment).

5. The majority of the patients have the HLA-DR4 or HLA-DR2 specificities. The arthritis in these patients typically does not respond to antibiotic therapy. Such reactions may continue for some time after the organisms have been killed, possibly because of cross-reactive antigens.

Chapter 26/*Bartonella*

1. Cat scratch disease (in immunocompetent persons) and bacillary angiomatosis (in immunocompro-

mised persons), due to *Bartonella henselae*; trench fever and bacteria and blood vessel tumorlike proliferations, due to *Bartonella quintana*; and Oroya fever and Verruca Peruana, due to *Bartonella bacilliformis*.

2. Tumorlike proliferations of blood vessels in the skin and visceral organs

3. Patients with cat scratch fever usually have normal defenses, which may limit the proliferation of the organisms. Patients with bacillary angiomatosis are usually immune-compromised, which allows greater bacterial multiplication.

4. *Bartonella henselae* is introduced into human skin by a scratch or bite from a cat, thus it causes a disease in scattered individuals only. Classical *B. quintana* infections, as during World War I, are transmitted by the human body louse, allowing person-to-person transmission and epidemic spread of the disease. In the present day, *B. quintana* is spread among individuals who do not have lice. However, it is possible that *B. quintana* is spread between individuals by contaminated intravenous needles or perhaps other arthropods.

Chapter 27/Chlamydiae: Genital and Respiratory Pathogens

1. Replicating chlamydiae (reticulate bodies) are larger than transit forms (elementary bodies), are metabolically active, and are much more sensitive to manipulation and environmental influences. The likely biochemical basis for the change between the two forms is that elementary bodies are surrounded by structural proteins rich in disulfide bridges. Under reducing conditions, as obtained when inside phagosomes, these bridges are broken, unraveling the surface proteins and allowing the reticulate bodies to metabolize, to grow, and to divide.

2. Mainly, by causing acute inflammation, elicited by cell lysis. The immune response plays an important role, for example, in the process of scarring. Tissue scarring may be due to a delay-type hypersensitivity response to specific chlamydial antigens, such as hsp60.

3. Genital infections by chlamydiae are a public health problem mainly by virtue of their ability to cause secondary infections, such as those that lead to salpingitis, and to subsequent ectopic pregnancy and pelvic inflammatory disease.

4. Polymerase chain reaction (PCR), the other a ligase chain reaction (LCR), have greatly improved the sensitivity and specificity of chlamydial detection. Other methods (1) fluorescent antibody staining of patient specimens with microscopic evaluation (and

(2) an enzyme-linked immunoassy (EIA). The "gold standard" has been to isolate the organisms in cell cultures but, false-negative results arise. Also, it seems possible that chlamydiae that persist in the body may be noninfectious for in vitro cell cultures.

5. Especial attention must be paid to potential carriers, because carriers of chlamydiae do not know they are infected and do not seek treatment. The high prevalence of gonococcal and chlamydial coinfection has prompted recommendations that patients with either infection be treated for both. The risk of HIV transmission is increased 3- to 5-fold in the presence of both the genital ulcer diseases (e.g., syphilis) and nonulcerative STDs (e.g., gonorrhea and chlamydial infection).

Chapter 28/Rocky Mountain Spotted Fever and Other Rickettsiae

1. Most rickettsioses are arthropod-borne; Q fever may be acquired by inhalation.

2. On the one hand, rickettsiae are capable of at least some energy metabolism, which sets them aside from the chlamydiae. On the other hand, with the exception of the organism of trench fever, they are strict intracellular parasites and are not known to grow outside cells.

3. Rocky Mountain spotted fever is a vasculitis due to the localization of the organisms in endothelia of small vessels. Cell damage, possibly caused by the growth of the organisms or by cell-mediated immunity, leads to localized hemorrhages. These are seen as the skin rashes characteristic of the disease.

4. One way to study rickettsiae is to grow them in animal cells in culture. Rickettsiae may be isolated from cell constituents and some of their in vitro properties studied. In addition, rickettsial genes may be cloned into suitable host bacteria or other cells.

Chapter 29/*Mycoplasma*: Curiosity and Pathogen

1. *Mycoplasma* do not have a rigid cell wall; therefore, they are sensitive to altered osmolarity of their environment. Some, but not all of them, require sterols for growth. They have the smallest known genomes of free-living cellular organisms.

2. Humans are the only known reservoir of *Mycoplasma pneumoniae*. The organism is acquired by inhalation and causes disease without prolonged colonization. *M. pneumoniae* bind to epithelial cells of the lower respiratory tree but not of the alveoli. The organisms impair ciliary function by the formation of toxic compounds, possibly hydrogen peroxide. The immune response appears to contribute to symptoms in this infection.

3. *Mycoplasma* pneumonia is an infection of the mucosa

of the airways, not of the alveoli. It is a bronchopneumonia, not a lobar pneumonia, as with pneumococci, not an interstitial pneumonia, as in legionellosis.

4. *Mycoplasma* are not detected on regular bacteriological media and require specialized techniques for growth in the laboratory.

PART II. Infectious Agents: Viruses
Chapter 31/Biology of Viruses

1. They do not maintain their physical integrity during replication but their nucleic acid is separated from the capsid.

2. The nucleic acid and capsid proteins of icosahedral viruses are loosely connected, whereas those of helical viruses are tightly connected and must "fit" properly in order to assemble correctly.

3. See Figure 31.2.

4. The nucleic acid of host cells does not have enzymes that can replicate negative-strand (−) RNA.

5. It is subject to splicing, contains a 5′ methylguanosine cap, and a 3′ polyadenylate chain.

6. Poxviruses replicate in the cytoplasm, where the DNA-synthesizing enzymes are not found.

7. Frame-shift of the same region of nucleic acid, giving different coding sequences and coding for overlapping genes.

8. Lytic infections lead to cell death. Latent infection occurs when the virus replicates alongside the host cell. Persistent infections occur when the virus continues to replicate faster than the host cell but does not cause appreciable clinical manifestations.

9. Viruses spread via the nerves (neural), the blood (hematogenous), and by the olfactory route (through the cribriform plate).

10. In the blood, viruses spread free, associated with monocytes and lymphocytes, or with red blood cells.

11. Antibodies contribute by forming immune complexes and by stimulating the host to make antibodies against some of its own component (molecular mimicry).

12. Attentuated live vaccines may induce both local and systemic immunity. The virus may persist in the body and cause renewed antigenic stimulation. The virus may spread within the population, thus "vaccinating" nonvaccinated individuals.

13. NK cells appear before CTLs and are not virus-specific.

14. Interferons are not made by antibody-producing cells, but by fibroblasts, lymphocytes, and macrophages. They are not specific but may affect a large number of virus infections. They inhibit viral replication by promoting degradation of viral mRNA and thus the synthesis of viral proteins.

15. Viruses are detected by viral cultivation in cell culture or in animals, immunofluorescence, morphological detection of viral particles or inclusion bodies, detection of virus-specific nucleic acid sequences, detection of specific antibodies.

Chapter 32/Picornaviruses: Polio, Enteroviruses, and the Rhinoviruses

1. Polio used to be a nearly endemic disease in the very young, in whom CNS manifestations were not as severe or frequent as in adolescents. With sanitation, early contact was less frequent, the disease more often caused paralytic manifestations.

2. See Table 32.1—all of these viruses may cause asymptomatic infection and meningitis.

3. Poliovirus is a positive-strand virus and its genomic RNA acts as mRNA. The first step in the replication cycle is uncoating. Replication and assembly take place in the cytoplasm. A viral protein called VPg is attached to the 5′ end. A single polyprotein is synthesized in the cytoplasm using the host protein synthesizing apparatus. Post-translational cleavage reactions cut the polyprotein into structural and nonstructural proteins. Nonstructural proteins are proteases involved in polyprotein cleavage and one is an RNA-dependent RNA polymerase. The structural proteins assemble to make the capsid.

4. See Table 32.2.

5. It suggests that a disease that is not known to be transmitted except between humans could be eradicated. The experience with smallpox vaccination and follow-up of known cases suggests strategies that may be successful with polio as well.

6. Rhinoviruses bind to specific receptors on respiratory epithelial cells. Most of the serotypes bind to the same receptor, others to a second receptor. The major group receptor is the intracellular adhesion molecule-1 (ICAM-1), a member of the immunoglobulin supergene family known to play a role in cell adhesion in the immune response.

7. There is a correlation between the severity of the cold and the amount of rhinovirus that can be recovered. Large amounts of virus are found without tissue destruction. Nasal secretions of persons with a cold contain large amounts of the vasoactive substance bradykinin. Direct stimulation of nerve endings in the nasal mucosa produces some of the manifestations of the cold.

Chapter 33/Arthropod-borne Viruses

1. Arboviruses cause viral encephalitides, hemorrhagic fevers, yellow fever, and dengue fever.

2. Because they are arthropod-borne, transmission depends on the presence of vectors in a region and how these are affected by the weather.

3. Positive-strand virus RNA functions as the m-RNA for the production of virus-encoded proteins. Negative-strand virus RNA must first be transcribed, but

animal cells do not have enzymes with such an activity; thus, a virion-associated enzyme must enter infected cells.

4. The natural life cycle for the viruses that cause encephalitides is from bird to bird, via the bite of mosquitoes. Horses acquire the virus, but they seldom play a role in human infection. The equine viremic phase is so short that it is unlikely a horse would be bitten by a mosquito during that time. Mosquitoes do not become sick with the virus and, once infected, can spread it for the rest of their lives (one season). The normal hosts of the virus (birds) are also relatively unaffected, thus permitting a stable life cycle. The frequency of encounter is dictated by the proximity of humans to the animal reservoir and the insect vector.

5. Horses are important sentinel animals, alerting that the virus has escaped its normal biological boundaries and is a threat to humans.

Chapter 34/Paramyxoviruses: Measles, Mumps, Slow Viruses, and the Respiratory Syncytial Virus

1. They cause extensive fusion of infected host cells (syncytia formation).

2. The single-stranded, nonsegmented RNA genome with negative sense is transcribed into individual mRNAs, which are translated into measles proteins. This virus replicates in the nucleus—which is unusual for RNA viruses.

3. Both the humoral and the cellular immune responses modulate the outcome of measles. Measles-specific globulin given shortly after exposure to the virus ameliorates the infection, but cellular immunity is probably the major determinant of protection. Agammaglobulinemic patients tolerate measles well, but those with congenital or acquired cellular immune deficits get severe or fatal infection. Measles infection itself decreases cellular immunity and measles patients are at an increased risk of reactivating herpes simplex infections and tuberculosis. They transiently lose delayed hypersensitivity to tuberculin and other antigens.

4. The current recommendation is that the live attenuated virus vaccine be given at 15 months of age because nearly all maternal antibody to measles is gone by that age. However, delaying vaccination leaves infants at risk for measles between the time that the maternally derived protection has waned until they are vaccinated.

5. By vaccination with the attenuated virus vaccine of all children after 15 months of age and surveillance for new cases that would require intensive vaccination in that region. For the vaccine to "take" effectively, widespread immunodeficiency among children in certain developing countries should be addressed, partly by improving nutrition.

Chapter 35/Rabies

1. In developed countries, the disease in dogs has been controlled with canine vaccines, and human rabies cases have become very rare. Surveillance in these countries is still important, because the rabies virus is still commonly found in wild animals. In many developing countries, canine rabies persists and thousands of people are vaccinated for exposure to potentially rabid animals.

2. Did a bite or break of the skin really occur? Has rabies been reported in the region where the bite occurred? Was the biting animal rabid – is it available for laboratory diagnosis or did it escape? Is the species known commonly to carry the virus? Can the biting animal be observed?

3. Members of the Rhabdoviridae family of RNA viruses, known to infect many mammals, including humans. Virions are shaped like a bullet, contain an external glycoprotein coat located outside a peripheral matrix protein, have a helical ribonucleoprotein core, and an unsegmented single-stranded RNA. The genome is of negative polarity; thus, the virion contains an RNA-dependent viral RNA transcriptase. The replication cycle of this virus takes place entirely in the cytoplasm of infected cells and results in the formation of numerous viral particles. Masses of nucleocapsids accumulate in the cytoplasm to form Negri bodies.

4. Human treatment consists of three steps: local wound treatment, passive administration of antibody (antiserum or immunoglobulin), and vaccination.

Chapter 36/Influenza and Its Virus

1. See Figure 36.1. Replication steps, after attachment and penetration: Uncoating, nucleocapsid to nucleus. Viral replicas make mRNA from viral (−) strand. "Stealing" 5′ cap and 3′ polyA chains. M-RNA ← cytoplasm to make viral proteins. Viral (−) strands made in nucleus from (+) strands (segments). Viral segments assemble on cytoplasm; membrane at sites of insertion of envelope proteins; bud out of infected cell; a peculiarity is the segmented genome.

2. Antigenic variation (shifts and drifts) in animal reservoirs causes epidemics. Pandemics are caused by antigenic shifts.

3. They are involved in attachment of virions to host cells, antigenic variation. *HA* is involved in phagolysosomal fusion, *NA* in virion release from the cell.

4. They all use a "cassette" mechanism, whereby silent genes are rearranged on the genome to be placed under the control of an active promoter.

5. This drug blocks influenza virus replication by interfering with the ion channel of the viral M2 protein through which the inner core of the virion is acidified.

Chapter 37/Rotaviruses and Other Viral Agents of Gastroenteritis

1. Most rotavirus infection in the U.S. affects children 6 months to 2 years of age. Most individuals have experienced infection and are immune to severe disease due to rotavirus by age 4. Malnourished children are at increased risk for complications of dehydration. Some children develop rotavirus from an encounter with an individual who is asymptomatically shedding virus.

2. Rotavirus-induced disease peaks in the winter and wanes in the warmer months. The rotaviruses cause an annual epidemic that moves from west to east, peaking first in October and November in Mexico and the Southwestern states, progressing across the country during winter months and peaking in Northeastern North America in March and April.

3. Yes, immunity to rotaviruses is long lasting.

4. Antigen detection assays, such as ELISA, are widely available for rotavirus detection.

Chapter 38/Human Retroviruses: AIDS and Other Diseases

1. Small spherical virion surrounded by a lipid envelope; genome contains two identical RNA molecules resembling eukaryotic mRNA with a 5′ cap structure and a 3′ poly A sequence. The replication cycle includes binding to the CD_4 receptor molecule via the envelope glycoprotein; fusion of the envelope with the cell membrane. Genomic RNA is released into the cytoplasm, including reverse transcriptase. Synthesis of DNA by reverse transcriptase, generating a double-stranded DNA molecule. Integration into host cell chromosomes via integrase, by joining the ends of each LTR to cut cellular DNA. Synthesis of progeny virus by transcribing viral DNA into messenger RNA by host cell RNA polymerase. Assembly at the cell surface and release without cell lysis.

2. See Table 38.1.

3. There are many ways to approach this question and you should choose the one that you are most comfortable with.

4. There are many points that could be considered. Examples are that we do not understand how helper lymphocytes are killed or impaired, or why the infection of a small proportion of them has such devastating effects.

5. The antigenic variation of HIV is a problem. Are antibodies against any viral antigen likely to protect? How about for cell-mediated immunity? Vaccine testing faces difficult ethical and practical issues.

6 and 7. See the answer for question 3.

Chapter 39/Adenoviruses

1. See Figure 39.1.

2. Adenoviral gene expression takes place in three phases termed pre-early, early, and late; each phase is characterized by the synthesis of a specific set of viral proteins. The proteins required for viral DNA replication are synthesized before the proteins that make up the virus particle. This assures the accumulation of a large pool of viral DNA before the packaging of viral DNA into capsids begins.

3. A single DNA strand is copied at each viral replication fork, while in host cell replication, both strands are copied concurrently. The synthesis of all new viral DNA is continuous, whereas in host cells one strand is produced continuously, but the other is synthesized discontinuously, as short pieces that must be joined to produce the finished strand. Host chromosome replication occurs once in a division cycle; viral replication is uncoordinated and takes place continuously over a period of time.

4. First, the accumulation of cellular mRNAs in the cytoplasm is prevented, probably by inhibiting the transport of host messages from the nucleus to the cytoplasm. Second, a virally encoded protein appears to inhibit the utilization of existing host mRNAs in the cytoplasm.

5. Adenoviruses prevent the inhibition of protein synthesis via two small RNA molecules (VA RNAs) encoded by viral genes. One of the host proteins (DAI) critical in the inhibition of protein synthesis by interferon is converted to its active form by double-stranded RNA (dsRNA). dsRNA is produced in the course of infection by adenoviruses. The VA RNAs fold into partially double-stranded structures and bind to DAI, preventing its activation by authentic dsRNA.

6. Respiratory infections, pharyngoconjunctivitis, acute respiratory disease, gastrointestinal infection, conjunctivitis, epidemic keratoconjunctivitis are caused by adenoviruses.

Chapter 40/Warts

1. Nonenveloped DNA viruses; circular, double-stranded genomes; transmission by direct inoculation; replication in skin and mucous membranes; long-term latent carriage in epithelial cells; transformation and cancer formation.

2. In warts, the viruses complete their full growth cycle. Progeny are shed from the lesion surface. In associated cancers, replication is restricted. Only a couple of genes are expressed, which lead to cell transformation.

3. Warts are painful, unsightly, chronic, transmissible, can damage the larynx and airways, and can slowly lead to skin or genitourinary malignancies.

4. There are no antiviral drugs that specifically inter-

fere with wart virus replication, largely because these viruses are completely dependent on host cell machinery. The virus persists in a latent form for years and can "wait out" any treatment interval.

5. Only a small percentage of infected people have recognizable symptoms; they spread infection unwittingly. Major wart proteins have not yet been cloned or tested as vaccine candidates.

Chapter 41/Herpes Simplex and Its Relatives

1. Herpesviruses include neurotropic herpes viruses: HSV-1, HSV-2, VZV; and lymphotropic herpes viruses: EBV, HHV-6, HHV-7, CMV.
2. Binding and uncoating cascade of gene expression—immediate, early, late; DNA replication; assembly in nucleus; maturation and spread by budding from nuclear and cytoplasmic membranes; destruction of cell; latency in proper host cell occurs with expression of 1 (HSV-1 or 2) to 10 (EBV) of the many viral genes.
3. Antibodies are effective at preventing primary infection; otherwise cellular immunity is important. Impaired cellular immunity leads to severe or frequent primary or recurrent infections.
4. Initiating treatment quickly enough to completely abort the infection is impossible. Drugs have no effect on the latent state of viruses. The virus may reactivate at a later date, regardless of the nature or duration of treatment.
5. Define risk groups. Identify behaviors that lead to spread of infection and educate with respect to these. Characterize immunogenic proteins. Develop animal models of infections and test vaccines.
6. Counsel with compassion. Educate patients regarding true (rather than mythical) risks and means of preventing spread. Employ acyclovir when appropriate.

Chapter 42/Viral Hepatitis

1. These viruses use either a "hit and run" infectious strategy (hepatitis A and hepatitis E viruses) that results in acute infection that is cleared by the immune system, or a "hide and infiltrate" strategy (hepatitis B, hepatitis C, hepatitis delta, and hepatitis G viruses) that can lead to chronic infection.
2. The HBV replication cycle involves the attachment of the large surface antigen to an unidentified receptor, uptake, and uncoating. In the nucleus, the par-

tially double-stranded nicked viral DNA is converted into a double-stranded, molecule (cccDNA). The RNA on the plus strand and the pol protein on the minus strand are removed, the gapped single-stranded region is filled in, and the resulting termini are ligated. cccDNA serves as the template for transcription of viral RNA, which is synthesized by a host RNA polymerase. Viral RNA is used as a template for reverse transcription, resulting in the formation of viral DNA. HDV is a subviral agent incapable of replicating alone. HDV requires the presence of hepatitis B virus as a helper to provide the envelope proteins needed for HDV assembly.
3. HBV encodes two enhancer elements that have binding sites for host transcription factors uniquely enriched in liver cells. Also, hepadnaviruses only infect cells that express an appropriate receptor(s) on their surface
4. See Table 42.2
5. An effective vaccine against HBV is available. It consists of HBsAg particles obtained from yeast that harbor recombinant DNA. This vaccine is also effective against HDV. No vaccine is available to prevent HCV infection. An inactivated HAV vaccine has proven to be both safe and effective; however, boosters are required for long-term protection. Efforts to develop an HEV vaccine are currently underway.

Chapter 54/Addressing Emerging Infectious Diseases

1. See Table 54.1
2. Weather anomalies leading to an increase in the rodent population in certain regions. Increased contact of humans with rodents
3. See Table 54.1
4. *Staphylococcus aureus*, especially MRSA strains, vancomycin-resistant enterococci. Prudent use of available drugs, development of new antibiotics, especially novel classes that may result in lesser microbial resistance.
5. Strengthening surveillance and response capability domestically and internationally. Addressing research priorities. Improving prevention and control strategies. Strengthening the public health infrastructure at the local, state, and federal levels. Assistance to other countries to strengthen their national infectious disease surveillance systems.

Review of the Main Pathogenic Bacteria

Organism	Gram Reaction, Morphology, Other Distinguishing Traits	Common Habitat and Mode of Encounter	Main Pathogenic Mechanism(s)	Typical Disease(s)	Relevant Chapters
Staphylococcus aureus	Positive, cocci in grapelike arrays	Nose, skin (carriers), breaks through skin and mucous membranes, ingestion of toxin-containing food	Acute inflammation and abscess formation involving many extracellular toxins (coagulase, leukocidin, catalase, toxic shock toxin, enterotoxins) and cell surface components (capsule, murein, teichoic acid, protein A)	Pyogenic infections and abscesses of many organs (e.g., subcutaneous tissue, bone marrow, endocardium), septicemia, toxic shock, food poisoning	11, 61, 62, 73
Staphylococcus epidermidis	Positive, cocci in grapelike arrays	Skin, intestine (normal flora), breaks in skin and mucous membranes	Adherence and colonization of prostheses, intravenous devices via a slime layer	Infections of implanted devices, compromised patients	11, 67
Group A streptococci	Positive cocci in chains, β-hemolytic	Throat (carriers), breaks through skin and mucous membranes	Inflammation due to surface components (M protein, lipoteichoic acids, hyaluronic acid, C5a peptidase, murein), extracellular enzymes (hemolysin, streptokinase, pyrogenic exotoxins); postsuppurative sequelae due to as yet uncertain factors	Skin diseases (e.g., erysipelas, impetigo), tonsillitis, scarlet fever, septicemia, rheumatic fever, glomerulonephritis	12, 61, 64
Other β-hemolytic streptococci	Positive (some normal flora), cocci in chains	Large intestine, vagina	Inflammation involving capsular polysaccharides	Neonatal septicemia and meningitis	12, 69
α-Hemolytic streptococci	Positive (some normal flora), cocci in chains	Throat, intestine, G.U. tract	Colonization of damaged heart valves due to adhesion of organisms transiently in blood	Bacterial endocarditis, rarely others	12, 64
Pneumococcus (*S. pneumoniae*)	Positive, diplococci, α-hemolytic	Throat (carriers), inhalation, hand contact	Inflammation facilitated by resistance to phagocytosis (capsule)	Pneumonia, empyema, meningitis, endocarditis, etc.	13, 59
Meningococcus (*Neisseria meningitidis*)	Gram-negative diplococci	Throat (carriers), inhalation, hand contact	Inflammation facilitated by resistance to phagocytosis (capsule), endotoxin	Septicemia, meningitis	14, 58
Gonococcus (*N. gonorrhoeae*)	Gram-negative diplococci	Genital tract (carriers, some asymptomatic), contact with secretions	Inflammation due to endotoxin, pili and surface protein adhesins, IgA1 protease	Urethritis, salpingitis, pelvic inflammatory disease	14, 66
Haemophilus influenzae	Gram-negative, small rods, nutritionally fastidious	Throat (carriers), inhalation, hand contact	Inflammation facilitated by resistance to phagocytosis (capsule), endotoxin, IgA1 protease, pili, outer membrane protein	Meningitis (infants, 3 months to 2 years) with sequelae, respiratory infections, cellulitis	58, 65

Organism	Gram Reaction, Morphology, Other Distinguishing Traits	Common Habitat and Mode of Encounter	Main Pathogenic Mechanism(s)	Typical Disease(s)	Relevant Chapters
Bacteroides spp.	Gram-negative, rods, anaerobes	Intestine, vagina (normal flora)	Inflammation of sensitive sites after entry of organisms from intestinal, oral flora	Abscesses (e.g., in peritoneum, lungs) often as part of mixed flora	15, 61
Escherichia coli	Gram-negative, rods, many strains differing in pathogenic mechanisms (ETEC, EPEC, EHEC, etc.)	Fecally contaminated bodies of water, foods, personal contact, ingestion	Various forms of diarrhea, dysentery, due to enterotoxins, endotoxin, Shiga-like toxins, adhesins; some of these factors are also involved in deep tissue infections	Secretory diarrhea (tourist disease), cystitis, septicemia, meningitis	16, 57, 60, 69, 73
Shigella spp.	Gram-negative, rods, several species differing in pathogenicity	Fecally contaminated bodies of water, foods, personal contact, ingestion (small inoculum suffices)	Inflammation due to invasion of small intestine mucosa helped by Shiga toxin, adhesins	Dysentery (inflammatory disease)	17, 57
Klebsiella pneumoniae	Gram-negative, rods, heavily encapsulated	Usually, inhalation of oral contents	Inflammation facilitated by resistance to phagocytosis (capsule), perhaps endotoxin	Pneumonia, other inflammations in compromised patients	16, 59, 67
Proteus spp.	Gram-negative, rods, urea splitters (grow at high pH)	Probably fecal contamination from same individual	Inflammation, usually of urinary tract	Urinary tract inflammatory disease; associated with urinary calculi formation	16, 60
Vibrio cholerae	Gram-negative, curved rods	Bodies of water, ingestion	Massive watery diarrhea due to cholera toxin (ADP-ribosylating) adhesins	Cholera (intense watery diarrhea)	16, 57
Salmonella spp.	Gram-negative, rods, species differing in pathogenicity (incl. S. typhi)	Fecally contaminated foods, personal contact, some strains zoonotic, ingestion	Able to multiply in macrophages due to largely unknown factors, diarrhea probably due to toxins	Typhoid and related fevers, gastroenteritis, septicemia	17, 57
Pseudomonas aeruginosa	Gram-negative, rods, oxidative metabolism only	Water, soils, foods, inhalation, ingestion, penetration through breaks in epithelia	Toxins (toxin A [ADP-ribosylating] elastase, exotoxin S, endoxotin), adhesins, alginate in cystic fibrosis	Pyogenic infection in burn patients, diabetics; lung infection in cystic fibrosis	18, 63, 67
Bordetella pertussis	Gram-negative, small rods, nutritionally fastidious	Throat (carriers), inhalation, hand contact	Pertussis toxin (ADP-ribosylating), adenylate cyclase, tracheal cytotoxin, adhesins	Whooping cough	19, 59

Organism	Gram Reaction, Morphology, Other Distinguishing Traits	Common Habitat and Mode of Encounter	Main Pathogenic Mechanism(s)	Typical Disease(s)	Relevant Chapters
Other enterics (*Enterobacter, Citrobacter, Serratia, Campylobacter, Yersinia*)	Gram-negative, rods	Usually fecal contamination, some derived from rodents	Virulence factors not well known, but probably include endotoxins	Various forms of diarrheas, dysenteries; some cause systemic disease and local inflammations	16, 57
Helicobacter pylori	Gram-negative, rods	Frequently found in stomach	Inflammation due to uncharacterized factors	Gastritis, perhaps gastric ulcers	22, 57
Clostridium difficile	Gram-positive, spore-forming rods, anaerobes	Intestine (normal flora?)	Toxins	Pseudo-membranous colitis	20
C. botulinum	Gram-positive, spore-forming rods, anaerobes	Soil, contaminated food, intestine; ingestion of preformed toxin (adult botulism)	Botulinum toxin	Botulism (flaccid paralysis), infant and wound botulism	20
C. tetani	Gram-positive, spore-forming rods, anaerobes	Soil, contaminated food, intestine; punctures of skin, wounds	Tetanus toxin	Tetanus (spastic paralysis)	20
C. perfringens and others	Gram-positive, spore-forming rods, anaerobes	Soil, contaminated food, intestine: wound contamination, ingestion	Lecithinase, other hydrolytic enzymes	Myonecrosis, gas gangrene, food poisoning	20, 73
Legionella pneumophila	Gram-negative, small rods, nutritionally fastidious	Water (air conditioning cooling systems, building water supply); inhalation, ingestion	Induces cellular response by as yet uncertain mechanisms	Pneumonia, system infections	21
Mycobacterium tuberculosis and others	Acid-fast (non-Gram-stainable), thin rods, slow growing	Human environment and secretions (*M. tuberculosis*), soil, waters (*M. avium-intracellulare* et al.)	Chronic inflammation due to bacterial persistence in macrophages, release of cytokines, adjuvant effect	Primary and secondary tuberculosis, *M. avium-intracellulare* etc., typically infect AIDS patients	23, 59, 68

Organism	Gram Reaction, Morphology, Other Distinguishing Traits	Common Habitat and Mode of Encounter	Main Pathogenic Mechanism(s)	Typical Disease(s)	Relevant Chapters
M. leprae	Acid-fast (non-Gram-stainable), thin rods, slow growing	Human environment and secretions	Chronic inflammation due to bacterial persistence in macrophages, release of cytokines	Tuberculoid and lepromatous leprosy	23
Treponema pallidum	Non-Gram-stainable, thin, helical rods, motile, not cultivable	Infected persons, acquired by intimate contact with human secretions	Chancre in first stage, acute inflammation in second, chronic inflammation and perhaps autoimmune-like sequelae in third; virulence factors not know	Syphilis	24, 66
Borrelia burgdorferi	Non-Gram-stainable, thin, helical rods	Wild animal reservoir, transmitted to humans via tick bite	Three stages of infection, vaguely reminiscent of syphilis; virulence factors not known, but some preference for attachment to brain gangliosides	Lyme disease	26
Bartonella henselae	small, gram-negative rods, nutritionally fastidious	Cat scratch or bite, lice, iv pataphernalia	Elicot granulomatous and suppurative response	Cat scratch fever, bacillary angiomatosis	26
Chlamydia trachomatis	Non-Gram-stainable, small organism in two forms (elementary [EB] and reticulate bodies [RBI]), strict intracellular parasite, not culturable extracellularly	Humans, direct contacts with genital and other secretions containing EB	Inflammation due to host cell destruction caused by intracellular growth of RB	Genital infection with possible PID, lymphogranuloma, pneumonia, neonatal conjunctivitis	27, 66
Rickettsia spp.	Non-Gram-stainable, small intracellular rods, strict intracellular parasite, not culturable extracellularly	Animal reservoirs, insect vectors, possibly human carriers in epidemic typhus	Damage to vascular endothelia due to multiplication of the organisms; leakage of fluid, leading to damage of vital organ function	Rocky Mt. spotted fever, various types of typhus, Q fever	28
Ehrichip sp.	Small, gram-negative rods, strict intracellular parasites	Ticks	Grow in white blood cells	Human mouocytic ehrlichiosis, human granulocytic ehrichiosis	28
Mycoplasma spp.	Small, non-Gram-stainable, lacking cell wall, some needing sterols for growth	Human carriers, animals, environment	Damage to respiratory epithelium, loss of ciliary function; perhaps due to organism's metabolites, including hydrogen peroxide	Bronchopneumonia, especially in young adults; genital and intrauterine infections	29, 59

The following charts refer to pathogenic characteristics of bacteria. Complete these charts as a method of reviewing this subject matter.

Capsulated Bacteria of Medical Importance

	Genus and Species		
1.	Pneumococcus	6.	Staphylococcus aureus (some strains)
2.	Meningococcus	7.	Escherichia coli (some strains)
3.	Haemophilus influenza	8.	Gonococcus (some strains)
4.	Klebsiella pneumoniae	9.	Bacteroides fragilis (some strains)
5.	Streptococcus pyogenes (some strains)		

Medically Important Strict Anaerobes

	Gensus and Species		
1.	Clostridium difficile	6.	Bacteroides fragilis
2.	C. botulinum	7.	Several other Bacteroides
3.	C. tetani	8.	Actinomyces bovis
4.	C. perfringens	9.	Some streptococci
5.	Several other clostridia	10.	Other members of the normal flora

Typically Pyogenic (pus-producing) Bacteria

	Genus and Species		
1.	Staphylococcus aureus	4.	Gonococcus
2.	S. epidermidis	5.	Pseudomonas aeruginosa
3.	Streptococcus pyogenes	6.	Pneumococcus

Major Bacterial Toxins (see Table 9.1, p. 117)

Review of the Main Pathogenic Viruses

Virus	Group or Family	Nucleic Acid, Cellular Site of Replication, State if Enveloped	Other Important Attributes	Disease(s) and Systems Involved	Relevant Chapters
Poliovirus	Picornaviruses	RNA (+ strand), cytoplasm	Makes polyprotein; lyses host cells; travels from intestine to anterior horn of spinal cord, medulla	Poliomyelitis; CNS, GI	32
Coxsackie and other enteroviruses	Picornaviruses	RNA (+ strand), cytoplasm	Infants are at particular risk	Meningitis herpangina, exanthems	32
Rhinoviruses	Picornaviruses	RNA (+ strand), cytoplasm	Many serotypes	Common cold	32
Arbovirus encephalitis	Togaviruses, Flaviviruses, Bunyaviruses	RNA (+ strand), (Bunyavirus (−) strand), cytoplasm, enveloped	Many kinds, arthropod-borne, often animal reservoirs, vascular damage in CNS	Eastern, Western equine, St. Louis, Japanese B, other encephalitis	33
Rubella	Togaviruses	RNA (+ strand), cytoplasm enveloped	Causes exanthems	Rubella	33
Measles	Paramyxoviruses	RNA (+ strand), nucleus, enveloped	Damage due to host response; causes cell fusion; depresses cellular immunity	Measles and its complications; subacute sclerosing panencephalitis by related viruses	34
Respiratory syncytial virus	Paramyxoviruses	RNA (+ strand), cytoplasm, enveloped	Syncytia formation due to cell fusion	Bronchiolitis in children	34
Rabies	Rhabdoviruses	RNA (− strand), cytoplasm, enveloped	Spreads by neural path, first up, then down axons	Rabies	35
Influenza	Orthomyxo-viruses	RNA (− strand), segmented genome, nucleus, enveloped	Antigenic variation (shifts and drifts) in hemagglutinin and neuroaminidase; human and animal reservoirs	Influenza and its complications	36
Rotavirus	Reoviruses	RNA, double-stranded, segments, cytoplasm, enveloped	Seasonal occurrence of disease	Most common agent of gastroenteritis, especially in children	37
HIV	Retroviruses	RNA (+ strand), two identical copies, nucleus, enveloped	Must integrate into host genome via reserve transcriptase for replication, antigenic	AIDS	38

Virus	Group or Family	Nucleic Acid, Cellular Site of Replication, State if Enveloped	Other Important Attributes	Disease(s) and Systems Involved	Relevant Chapters
Adenovirus	Adenoviruses	DNA, double-stranded (terminally redundant), nucleus	Many antigenic types, oncogenic; gene expression during replication is temporally regulated	Gastroenteritis, acute respiratory disease, conjunctivitis	39
Papillomavirus	Papovaviruses	DNA, double-stranded, circular, nucleus	Many antigenic types, some more oncogenic; some are sexually transmitted	Warts, cervical carcinoma	40
Herpes simplex	Herpesviruses	DNA, double-stranded, nucleus, enveloped	Persistent infections; capable of latency; not often extracellular	Fever blisters (genital and nongenital), ocular, CNS infection	41
Epstein-Barr virus (EBV) cytomegalovirus (CMV), varicella-zoster	Herpesviruses	DNA, double-stranded, nucleus, enveloped	Similar replication cycle as in herpes simplex; capable of cell transformation (especially EBV)	Infectious mononucleosis, CMV infection and chickenpox	41
Hepatitis A	Picornaviruses	RNA (+) strand, cytoplasm, enveloped	Usually food- or waterborne	Hepatitis	32, 42
Hepatitis B	Hepadnaviruses	DNA, double-stranded with single-stranded portions, nucleus, enveloped	Replicates via an RNA intermediate, transmitted sexually, congenitally, or parenterally	Hepatitis	32
Smallpox	Poxviruses	DNA, double-stranded, nucleus, enveloped	Disease has been eradicated via vaccination; viruses of this type may be useful for recombinant vaccines	Smallpox	

Review of the Medically Important Fungi (see Tables 46.2, p. 429; 47.1, p. 433; 48.1, p. 436)

Review of the Main Pathogenic Animal Parasites (see Tables 50.1, p. 449; 51.1, p. 464; 52.2, p. 477; 53.1, p. 481)

Figure and Table Credits

FIGURES

Figure 3.1. Redrawn from Kobayashi GS, et al. In: Szaniszlo PJ, ed. Fungal dysmorphism. New York: Plenum Publications, 1985.

Figure 3.2. Modified from DiRienzo JM, et al. The outer membrane proteins of Gram-negative bacteria: biosynthesis, assembly, and function. Ann Rev Biochem 1978;47:481.

Figure 3.8. Redrawn from Blumberg P, Strominger JL. Interaction of penicillin with the bacterial cell wall: penicillin-binding proteins and penicillin-sensitive enzymes. Bacteriol Rev 1974;38:291–335.

Figure 3.9. From Spratt B. Distinct penicillin binding proteins involved in the division, elongation and shape of *Escherichia coli* K12. Proc Natl Acad Sci USA 1975;72:2999.

Figure 3.10. Redrawn from Kaback HR. Ion gradient coupled transport. From Andreoli TE, Hoffman JS, Sanastil DD, et al. Physiology of membrane disorders. New York: Plenum Publications, 1986:387–407.

Figure 3.13. Courtesy of Drs. C.C. Brinton and J. Carnham.

Figure 3.15. Adapted from Boyd RF, Hoerl BG. Basic medical microbiology. Boston: Little, Brown, 1986.

Figure 4.6. Redrawn from Wilson G, Dick HM. In: Topley and Wilson's Principles of bacteriology, virology, and immunity. 7th ed. Baltimore: Williams & Wilkins, 1983.

Figure 4.8. Redrawn from Neihardt, et al. Physiology of the bacterial cell. Sunderland, MA: Sinauer Associates, Inc., 1990.

Figure 4.10. Redrawn from Neihardt FC, et al. Physiology of the bacterial cell.

Sunderland, MA: Sinauer Associates, Inc. 1990.

Figure 5.1. Adapted from Strehler BL. Implications of aging research for society. Fed Proc 1975;34:6.

Figure 5.2. Adapted from Gale EF, et al. The molecular basis of antibiotic action. 2nd ed. New York: John Wiley & Sons, 1981.

Figure 5.6. Redrawn from Medoff G, et al. Potentiation of rifampicin and 5-fluorocytosine and antifungal antibiotics by amphotericin B. Proc Natl Acad Sci USA 1972;69:196.

Figure 6.4. From Knobel HR, Villinger W, Isliker H. Chemical analysis and electron microscopy studies of human C1q prepared by different methods. Eur J Immunol 1975;5:78–82.

Figure 6.5. From Bhakdi S, Tranum-Jensen J. Mechanism of complement cytolysis and the concept of channel-forming proteins. Phil Trans Roy Soc London B 1984;306:311.

Figure 6.6. From MacRae EK, Pzyzwansky KB, Cooney MH, Spitzagel IK. Scanning electron microscopic observations of early stages of phagocytosis of *E. coli* by human neutrophils. Cell Tiss Res 1980;209:65–70.

Figure 7.6. Courtesy of K. Ziegler, R. Cotran, and E. Unanue.

Figure 13.1 Courtesy of Dr. Stuart S. Sagel.

Figure 13.2 From Schering Slide Library, Schering Corp., Kenilworth, NJ, copyright owner. All rights reserved.

Figure 13.3 From Wood WB, Jr. Studies on the cellular immunology of acute bacterial infections. Harvey Lectures 1951–1952;47:72–98.

Figure 14.1 From Schering Slide Library, Schering Corp., Kenilworth, NJ, copyright owner. All rights reserved.

Figure 14.6 From McGee Z, et al. Pathogenic mechanisms of *Neisseria gonorrheae*: observation on damage to human fallopian tubes in organ culture by gonococci of colony type 1 or type 4. J Infect Dis 1981;143:413–422.

Figure 15.1 Courtesy of Coy Laboratories, Ann Arbor, MI.

Figure 17.2 Redrawn from Taussig MJ. Processes in pathology and microbiology. 2nd ed. Oxford, UK: Blackwell Scientific Publications, 1984.

Figure 17.3 Courtesy of Dr. Stanley Falkow. Panel B is reproduced with permission from Jones BD, Ghori N, Falkow S.J. Exptl Med 1994;180:15–23.

Figure 19.2 From Muse KE, et al. Scanning electron microscopic study of hamster tracheal organ cultures infected with *Bordetella pertussis*. J Infect Dis 1977;136:771–777.

Figure 19.4 Redrawn from a figure provided courtesy of Dr. W.E. Goldman.

Figure 20.1 From Schering Slide Library, Schering Corp., Kenilworth, NJ, copyright owner. All rights reserved.

Figure 21.1 From Elliot JA, Winn WC, Jr. Treatment of alveolar macrophages with cytochalasin D inhibits uptake and subsequent growth of *Legionella pneumophila*. Infect Immunol 1986;51:33.

Figure 22.2 From the Journal of Clinical Investigation 1994;94:4–8.

Figure 22.3 Redrawn from the Journal of Clinical Investigation 1994;94:4–8.

Figure 23.2 Data from Huebner RE and Castro KG. The changing face of tuberculosis. Annu Rev Med 1995;46:47–55.

Figure 23.3 Data from 1989 Tuberculosis Statistics in the United States, Centers for Disease Control, Atlanta, GA.

Figure 23.4 Adapted from Myers JA. The natural history of tuberculosis in the human body. JAMA 1965;194:1086.

Figure 24.2 Courtesy of Dr. E.M. Walker, Department of Microbiology and Immunology, UCLA School of Medicine, Los Angeles, CA.

Figure 24.3 Redrawn from Taussig MJ. Processes in pathology and microbiology. 2nd ed. Oxford, UK: Blackwell Scientific Publications, 1984.

Figure 24.4 From Kutty K, Sebastion JL, Berg DD, Mewis BA, and Kochar MS. Kochar's concise textbook of medicine. 3rd ed. Baltimore: Williams & Wilkins, 1998.

Figure 27.2C Courtesy of Drs. L. Hodinka and P.R. Wyrick.

Figure 28.1 Courtesy of Dr. D.J. Silverman, School of Medicine, University of Maryland, Baltimore, MD.

Figure 28.4 Courtesy of Dr. Gustav Dammin, Harvard Medical School, Cambridge, MA.

Figure 29.1 Courtesy of Dr. Gary Shackleford.

Figure 29.2 Courtesy of W.A. Clyde, Jr.

Figure 29.3 From Hu PC, et al. Surface parasitism by *Mycoplasma pneumoniae* of respiratory epithelium. J Exp Med 1977;145:1328.

Figure 30.1 Courtesy of Dr. D.J. Krogstad.

Figure 31.1 Redrawn from White DO, Fenner F. Medical virology. 3rd ed. New York: Academic Press, 1986.

Figure 31.2 Redrawn from Taussig MJ. Processes in pathology and microbiology. 2nd ed. Oxford, UK: Blackwell Scientific Publications, 1984.

Figure 31.3 Redrawn from Taussig MJ. Processes in pathology and microbiology. 2nd ed. Oxford, UK: Blackwell Scientific Publications, 1984.

Figure 31.7 Modified from Wold S, et al. In: Nayak DP, ed. Molecular biology of animal viruses. Vol. 2. New York: Marcel Dekker, Inc., 1978.

Figure 32.1 From Lyons AS, Petracelli RJ. Medicine: an illustrated history. New York: Harry N. Abrams, 1978.

Figure 32.7 From Dick EC, Jennings LC, Mink KA, Wartgow CD, Inhorn SL. Aerosol transmission of rhinovirus colds. J Infect Dis 1987;156:442–448.

Figure 32.8 From Jennison. Aerobiology 1947;17:106.

Figure 34.1 Modified from Morgan EM, Rapp F. Measles virus and its associated diseases. Bacteriol Rev 1977;41:636–666.

Figure 34.3 From Morgan EM, Rapp F. Measles virus and its associated diseases. Bacteriol Rev 1977;41:636–666.

Figure 34.4 Redrawn from Krugman S, Katz S. Infectious diseases of children. St. Louis: CV Mosby, 1981:145.

Figure 34.5 From Emond RTD. Color atlas of infectious diseases. London: Wolfe Medical Publications, 1987.

Figure 35.1 Courtesy of Dr. Makonnen Fekadu, Centers for Disease Control, Atlanta, GA.

Figure 35.2 Courtesy of Dr. Makonnen Fekadu, Centers for Disease Control, Atlanta, GA.

Figure 37.1 Modified from LeBaron CW, Lew J, Glass RI, et al. Annual retrovirus epidemic patterns in North America: results of a 5-year retrospective survey of 88 centers in Canada, Mexico, and the United States. JAMA 1990;264:984.

Figure 37.2 Courtesy of A. Kapikian.

Figure 37.3 Modified from Fields BN, et al, eds. Virology. New York: Raven Press, 1990.

Figure 38.5 Courtesy of Dr. M. Gonda.

Figure 39.1 *A* from Burnett RM. Cell 1991;67:145–154. *B* redrawn from Philipson and Pettersson. Advances in tumor virus research. Vol. 18. New York: Academic Press.

Figure 39.3 *A* from Kelly TJ, Jr. Adenovirus DNA replication. In: Ginsberg HS, ed. The adenoviruses. New York: Plenum Publishing, 1984:278, 298. *B* and *C* redrawn from Kelly TJ, Jr. Adenovirus DNA replication. In: Ginsberg HS, ed. The adenoviruses. New York: Plenum Publishing, 1984:278, 298.

Figure 40.1 Courtesy of Dr. K.V. Shah.

Figure 41.6 From Hsiung GD, Mayo DR, Lucia HL, Landry ML. Genital herpes: pathogenesis and chemotherapy in a guinea pig model. Rev Infect Dis 1984;6:33–50.

Figure 42.1 Adapted from Ganew D. Hepadnaviruses. In: Fields BN, Knipe DM, Howley PM eds. Fundameutal Virology. 3rd ed. Philadelphia: Lippincott-Raven, 1996

Figure 42.2 Courtesy of Dr. John Jerin.

Figure 42.3 Adapted from Ganew D. Hepadnaviruses. In: Fields BN, Knipe DM, Howley Mieds. Fundameutal Virology. 3rd ed. Philadelphia: Lippincott-Raven, 1996

Figure 43.4 Modified from Corey L, et al. Intravenous acyclovir for the treatment of primary genital herpes. Ann Intern Med 1983;98:914–921.

Figure 43.5 Redrawn from Straus S, et al. Suppression of recurrent genital herpes with oral acyclovir. Trans Assoc Am Phys 1984;97:278–283.

Figure 45.4 From Cole GT, Nozawa Y. Dimorphism. In: Cole GT, Kendrick B, eds. Biology of conidial fungi. New York: Academic Press, 1981.

Figure 45.5 Courtesy of Laurel Krewson.

Figure 45.6 Courtesy of Dr. R.D. Diamond.

Figure 45.8 Courtesy of Dr. B.H. Cooper.

Figure 50.2 Redrawn from Friedman MJ. Erythrocytic mechanism of sickle cell resistance to malaria. Proc Natl Acad Sci USA 1978;75:1994.

Figure 50.7 Courtesy of Drs. M.S. Bartlett and J.W. Smith, Indiana University School of Medicine.

Figure 50.11 Redrawn from Ross R, Thompson D. Proc Roy Soc London, series B 1910;82:411–415.

Figure 51.3 Courtesy of Dr. Stanley L. Erlandsen, Washington University School of Medicine, St. Louis, MO.

Figure 57.3 Modified from Cawley JR. Infectious diarrhea. Am J Med 1985;78 (Suppl 6B) 65–71.

Figure 58.2 Redrawn from Menkes JH. Viral neurological infections in children. Hosp Pract 1977;12:100–109.

Figure 58.4 Courtesy of Dr. E.J. Bottone, Mount Sinai Hospital, New York.

Figure 59.2 Data from Monto AS, Ullman BM. JAMA 1974;227:164–169.

Figure 59.3 Data from Glezen WP, et al. N Engl J Med 1973;288:498–505. Redrawn from Virology. The Upjohn Co., 1983.

Figure 59.4 From Jennison. Aerobiology 1947;17:106.

Figure 59.5 Courtesy of Dr. G. Shackleford.

Figure 59.6 Courtesy of Dr. G. Shackleford.

Figure 59.7 Courtesy of Dr. S.S. Sagel.

Figure 59.10 Courtesy of Dr. C. Kuhn.

Figure 59.11 Courtesy of Dr. C. Kuhn.

Figure 59.12 Courtesy of Dr. C. Kuhn.

Figure 60.1 Redrawn from Fass RJ, et al. Urinary tract infection. Practical aspects of diagnosis and treatment. JAMA 1973;225:1509–1513.

Figure 60.3 Redrawn from Fass RJ, et al. Urinary tract infection. Practical aspects of diagnosis and treatment. JAMA 1973;225:1509–1513.

Figure 62.6 Adapted from Medoff G. Osteomyelitis: a review of clinical features, therapeutic considerations, and unusual aspects. N Engl J Med 1970;282:260–266.

Figure 64.1 Adapted from Rodbard S. Blood velocity and endocarditis. Circulation 1963;27:18–28.

Figure 67.1 Redrawn from Joshi J. Schimpff S. Infections in the compromised host. In: Mandell G, Douglas G, Bennett JE, eds. Principles and practice of infectious diseases. New York: John Wiley & Sons, 1985:697.

TABLES

Table 6.4. Adapted from Klein J. Immunology. Oxford, UK: Blackwell Scientific, 1990, Table 8.6; and Abbas AK, Lichtman AH, Pober JS. Cell and molecular immunology. Philadelphia: WB Saunders, 1991, Table 13.5.

Table 6.5. Adapted from Abbas AK, Lichtman AH, Pober JS. Cell and molecular immunology. Philadelphia: WB Saunders, 1991, Table 13.2.

Table 8.3. Modified from a table by Mark Klempner.

Table 13.1 Adapted from Hendley JO, Sande MA, Stewart PM, et al. Spread of *Streptococcus pneumoniae* in families. I. Carriage rates and distribution of types. J Infect Dis 1975;13:55–61.

Table 31.1 From Murphy FA. In: Fields BN, Knipe DM, eds. Fundamental virology. New York: Raven Press, 1991; Tyler KL, Fields BN. In: Lannette EH, et al, eds. Laboratory diagnosis of infectious diseases. Vol. 2. New York: Springer-Verlag, 1988.

Table 34.2 From Hall CB, Douglas RW. Modes of transmission of respiratory syncytial virus. J Pediatr 1981;99:100.

Table 36.1 Adapted from unpublished material of B. Murphy.

Table 36.4 Adapted from unpublished material of B. Murphy.

Table 38.2 From Centers for Disease Control and Prevention, HIV-AIDS Surveillance Report 1997; 9:8

Table 38.3 Adapted from Centers for Disease Control. 1993 Revised classification system for HIV infection and expanded surveillance case definition for AIDS among adolescents and adults. MMWR 1992;41[No. RR-17].

Table 54.1 From World Health Report, 1995.

Table 54.2 From McGinnis JM, Foege W. JAMA 1993;270:2207.

Table 54.3 Pinner RW, Teutsch SM, Simonsen L, et al. Trends in infectious diseases mortality in the United States. JAMA 1996;272:189–193.

Table 54.4 Adapted from Morse SS. Emerg Infect Dis 1995;1:7–15.

Table 54.5 Adapted from Satcher D. Emerging infections: getting ahead of the curve. Emerg Infect Dis 1995;1:1–6.

Table 54.8 From U.S. News and World Report, July 1993.

Table 56.4 Data from Hall CB, Douglas RW. J Pediatr 1981;99:100.

Table 57.1 From Keusch GT, Gorbach SL. Ecology of the gastrointestinal tract. In: Berks SE, et al, eds. Gastroenterology. 4th ed. Philadelphia: WB Saunders, 1985.

Table 57.3 Adapted from Gorbach SL. Infectious diarrhea. In: Sleisenger WH, Fordtran SS, eds. Gastrointestinal disease. Pathophysiology, diagnosis, and management. Philadelphia: WB Saunders, 1983:956.

Table 64.2 Adapted from Everett ED, Hirschmann JV. Transient bacteremia and endocarditis prophylaxis. A review. Medicine 1977;56:61–77.

Table 67.1 Adapted from Johnston RB. Recurrent bacterial infections in children. N Engl J Med 1984;310:1237–1243.

Index

Page numbers in *italics* refer to figures; those followed by the letter "t" refer to tables.

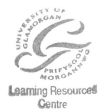